Clinical Pharmacology

D R Laurence MD FRCP

Professor Emeritus of Pharmacology and Therapeutics,
School of Medicine, University College London, London, UK

P N Bennett MD FRCP

Reader in Clinical Pharmacology, University of Bath, and
Consultant Physician, Royal United Hospital, Bath, UK

M J Brown MA MSc MD FRCP

Professor of Clinical Pharmacology, University of Cambridge; Consultant
Physician, Addenbrooke's Hospital, Cambridge and Director of Studies
Gonville and Caius College, Cambridge, UK

EIGHTH EDITION

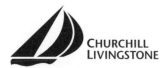 **CHURCHILL
LIVINGSTONE**

EDINBURGH LONDON NEW YORK PHILADELPHIA SYDNEY TORONTO 1997

CHURCHILL LIVINGSTONE
A Medical Division of Harcourt Brace and Company
Limited

First edition 1960
Second edition 1962
Third edition 1966
Fourth edition 1973
Fifth edition 1980
Sixth edition 1987
Seventh edition 1992
Eighth edition 1997
   Reprinted 1998

TRANSLATIONS
Previous editions translated into
Italian, Chinese, Spanish,
Serbo-Croat, Russian

Standard edition ISBN 0 443 04990 4

International Student Edition first published 1996
International Student Edition of 8th edition published 1997

International Student Edition ISBN 0 443 05114 3

British Library Cataloguing in Publication Data
A catalogue record for this book is available from the British
Library

Library of Congress Cataloging in Publication Data
A catalog record for this book is available from the
Library of Congress

Produced by Addison Wesley Longman China Limited,
Hong Kong
NPCC/02

The
publisher's
policy is to use
**paper manufactured
from sustainable forests**

Contents

Preface

For your own satisfaction and for mine, please read this preface![1]

> This book is about the scientific basis and practice of drug therapy. It is particularly intended for medical students and doctors and indeed for anyone concerned with evidence-based drug therapy.

The scope and rate of drug innovation increases.

Doctors are now faced with a professional lifetime handling drugs that are new to themselves — drugs that do new things as well as drugs that do old things better; drugs that become familiar during training will be superseded.

We do not write only for readers who, like us, have a special interest in pharmacology. We try to make pharmacology easy for those whose primary interests lie elsewhere but who recognise that they need some knowledge of pharmacology if they are to meet their moral and legal 'duty of care' to their patients. We try to tell them what they need to know wthout burdening them with irrelevant information and we try to make the subject interesting.[2] We are very serious, but seriousness does not always demand wearying solemnity.

All who prescribe drugs would be wise to keep in mind that the expectations of patients and of society in general are becoming ever more exacting and that doctors who prescribe casually or ignorantly now face not only increasing criticism but also civil (or even criminal) legal charges.

The ability to handle new developments depends, now more than ever, on comprehension of the principles of pharmacology. These principles are not difficult to grasp and are not so many as to defeat even the busiest doctors who take on themselves the responsibility of introducing manufactured medicines into the bodies of their patients.

The principles of pharmacology and drug therapy will be found in chapters 1–8 and they are applied in the subsequent specialist chapters which are offered as a reasonably brief solution to the problem of combining practical clinical utility with some account of the principles on which clinical practice rests.

How much practical technical detail to include has been difficult to decide. In general, more such detail is provided for therapeutic practices that are complex or potentially dangerous *and* urgent, where there may be no time for consultation with colleagues or search in libraries, e.g. anaphylactic shock; less, or even no detail is given on therapy

---

[1] St Francis of Sales: Preface to Introduction to the devout life (1609).

[2] An author, poet and critic (Philip Larkin: 1922–85) has said that he judged fiction thus: 'Could I read it? If I could read it, did I believe it? If I believed it, did I care about it? and if I cared about it, what was the quality of my caring, and did it last?' It would be presumptuous (as well as dangerous) for the authors of a textbook to aspire to satisfy the criteria for fiction, so we will say only that we have been mindful of them in writing this book.

that is generally conducted only by specialists or that can wait on such consultation, e.g. anticancer drugs and i.v. oxytocin. But always, especially with modern drugs with which the prescriber may not be familiar, the manufacturer's current literature should be consulted.

Use of the book. Students are, or should be, concerned to understand, to develop a rational, critical attitude to drug therapy and they should therefore chiefly concern themselves with how drugs act and interact in disease and with how evidence of therapeutic effect is obtained and evaluated. To this end they should read selectively and should not impede themselves by attempts to memorise lists of alternative drugs and minor differences between them, or arbitrary practical details, such as dosage or solution strength, which should never be required of them in examinations; the only way reliably to fix these in the mind is by actual prescribing.

The role and status of a textbook. If a book is to be a useful guide to drug use it must offer clear conclusions and advice. If it is to be of reasonable size, alternative acceptable courses of action will often have to be omitted. What is recommended should be based on sound evidence where this exists, and on an assessment of the opinions of the experienced where it does not. Exceptions to all advice will occur,[3] and part of the clinician's professionalism lies in knowing when to depart from an accepted source. Nor can a textbook take account of all possible modifying factors, e.g. personality, intercurrent disease, metabolic differences, in any individual case.

The status of a textbook as a practical guide has been expressed in a legal judgement where an accusation of negligent treatment made against a doctor was supported by showing that he had not followed the orthodox treatment as stated in various textbooks. The judge said that textbook writers were writing of a subject in general and not of a particular patient. A doctor was entitled to use common sense, experience, and judgement as far as they fitted into a particular case. 'It would be a sorry day for the medical profession if it were to be said that no doctor ought to depart one tittle from that which he saw written in a textbook.'[4] Statements in textbooks were no substitute for the judgement of the physician in charge of the case. 'His Lordship could not follow slavishly the views expressed in textbooks . . . .'[4]

The guide to further reading at the end of each chapter is comprised of a few references to original papers, to referenced editorials and review articles from a small range of English language journals that are likely to be available in even the most modest hospital library in order to enable anyone, anywhere, to gain access to the original literature and to informed opinion, and also to provide interest and sometimes amusement. We urge students to select a title that looks interesting and to read the article. We do not attempt to document all the statements we make, which would be impossible in a book of this size.

Formulary. It is assumed that the reader will possess a formulary, local or national, and so the text has not been encumbered with exhaustive lists of preparations, although it is hoped that enough have been mentioned to cover much routine prescribing, and many drugs have been included solely for identification.

London, Bath, Cambridge   D.R.L.
1997   P.N.B.
       M.J.B.

---

[3] Control of manufacturers' therapeutic claims is properly exercised by government regulatory authority, but limitation of doctors' freedom to prescribe what they have reason to believe best for the patients should be resisted on principle (although cost is increasingly regarded as overriding principle). The solution to bad doctoring is education, not the imposition of limitations on conscientious and informed doctors. But if doctors *will* prescribe carelessly then society will take away their freedom. See isotretinoin, clozapine.

[4] Lancet (1960) 1: 593.

Acknowledgements

It is not possible for three individuals to cover the whole field of drug therapy from their own knowledge and experience, and we are deeply grateful to all those who have, with such good grace, given us their time and energy to supply valuable facts and opinions for this and previous editions; they principally include:

Dr E S K Assem, Dr Stella Barnass, Dr N B Bennett, Dr D C Brown, Dr M Davis, Dr E D Gilby, Dr Sheila Gore, Professor J Guillebaud, Professor D H Jenkinson, Dr C J Lovell, Dr H Ludlam, Professor P J Maddison, Dr P T Magee, the late Professor Sir William Paton, Professor B N C Prichard, Dr J P D Reckless, Dr Gillian Robinson, Dr C J R Singer, Dr J A Vale, Dr C Ward, Professor P L Weissberg, Dr T G Wreghitt.

Other acknowledgements are made in the appropriate places.

Much of any merit this book may have is due to the generosity of those named above as well as others too numerous to mention who have put their knowledge and practical experience of the use of drugs at our disposal. We hope that this collective acknowledgement will be acceptable. Errors are our own.

In addition, permission to quote directly from the writings of some authorities has been generously granted and we thank the authors and their publishers who have given it. If we have omitted any acknowledgement that ought to have been made we will make such amends as we can as soon as we can.

Particular thanks are due to Janice Urquhart (Project Editor) and Kathleen Orr (Copy Editor).

D.R.L.
P.N.B.
M.J.B.

For Churchill Livingstone:

Publisher: Timothy Horne
Project Editor: Janice Urquhart
Copy Editor: Kathleen Orr
Project Controller: Kay Hunston
Design Direction: Erik Bigland

Note from the authors and publishers

Medical knowledge is rapidly increasing and constantly changing. This is particularly true of medicinal therapeutics. The authors and publishers have, as far as it is possible, taken care to ensure that the text of this book is accurate and up-to-date at the time of publication. Readers are, however, strongly advised to ensure that they have access to current standards of practice, and, in the case of drugs, to current manufacturers' Data Sheets (Summaries of Product Characteristics), and to current national formularies.

1

Topics in drug therapy

The therapeutic situation

> Poisons in small doses are the best medicines; and useful medicines in too large doses are poisonous (William Withering, 'discoverer' of digitalis, 1789).

The use of drugs[1] to increase human happiness by elimination or suppression of diseases and symptoms and to improve the quality of life in other ways is a serious matter and involves not only technical, but also psychosocial considerations.

Overall, the major benefits of modern drugs are on **quality** of life (measured with difficulty), and exceed those on **quantity** of life (measured with ease).[2]

---

[1] A World Health Organization Scientific Group has defined a drug as 'any substance or product that is used or intended to be used to modify or explore physiological systems or pathological states for the benefit of the recipient'. WHO 1966 Technical Report Series no. 341: 7. A less restrictive definition is 'a substance that changes a biological system by interacting with it'.

A *drug* is a single chemical substance that forms the active ingredient of a *medicine* (a substance or mixture of substances used in restoring or preserving health). A medicine may contain many other substances to deliver the drug in a stable form, acceptable and convenient to the patient. The terms will be used more or less interchangeably in this book. To use the word 'drug' intending only a harmful, dangerous or addictive substance is to abuse a respectable and useful word.

We therefore begin this book with a series of essays on what we think are important topics.

Medicines are part of our way of life from birth, when we enter the world with the aid of drugs, to death where drugs assist (most of) us to depart with minimal distress and perhaps even with a remnant of dignity. In between these events we regulate our fertility, often, with drugs. We tend to take such usages for granted.

But during the intervals remaining, an average family experiences illness on one day in four and between the ages of 20 and 45 years a lower-middle-class man experiences approximately one life-endangering illness, 20 disabling (temporarily) illnesses, 200 nondisabling illnesses and 1000 symptomatic episodes: the average person in the USA can expect to have about 12 years of bad health in an average lifespan.[3] And medicines play a major role in these. 'At any time, 40–50% of adults [UK] are taking a prescribed medicine.'[4]

Before treating any patient with drugs, doctors should have made up their minds on 8 points:

1. Whether they should interfere with the patient at all and if so —
2. What alteration in the patient's condition they hope to achieve.
3. That the drug they intend to use is best capable of bringing this about.
4. How they will know when it has been brought about.
5. That they can administer the drug in such a way that the right concentration will be attained in the right place at the right time and for the right duration.

6. What other effects the drug may have and whether these may be harmful.
7. How they will decide to stop the drug.
8. Whether the likelihood of benefit, and its importance, outweighs the likelihood of damage, and its importance, i.e. to consider benefit versus risk, or efficacy in relation to safety.

> **Drug therapy** involves a great deal more than matching the name of the drug to the name of a disease; it requires knowledge, judgement, skill and wisdom, but above all a sense of responsibility.

A book can provide knowledge and can contribute to the formation of judgement, but it can do little to impart skill and wisdom, which are the products of example of teachers and colleagues, of experience and of innate and acquired capacities.

'It is evident that patients are not treated in a vacuum and that they respond to a variety of subtle forces around them in addition to the specific therapeutic agent.'[5] *When a patient is given a drug the responses are the resultant of numerous factors:*

- The pharmacodynamic effect of the drug and interactions with any other drugs the patient may be taking
- The pharmacokinetics of the drug and its modification in the individual due to genetic influences, disease, other drugs
- The physiological state of the end-organ — whether, for instance, it is over- or underactive
- The act of medication, including the route of administration and the presence or absence of the doctor
- The doctor's mood, personality, attitudes and beliefs
- The patient's mood, personality, attitudes and beliefs
- What the doctor has told the patient
- The patient's past experience of doctors
- The patient's estimate of what has been received and of what ought to happen as a result
- The social environment, e.g. whether supportive or dispiriting.

---

[2] Consider, for example, the worldwide total of suffering relieved and prevented *each day* by anaesthetics (local and general) and by analgesics, not forgetting dentistry which, because of these drugs, no longer strikes terror into even the most stoical as it has done for centuries.

[3] Quoted in: Anderson J A D (ed) 1979 Self medication. MTP Press, Lancaster; USA Public Health Service 1995.

[4] George C F 1994 Prescribers' Journal 34: 7. A moment's reflection will bring home to us that this is an astounding statistic which goes a long way to account for the aggressive promotional activities of the highly competitive international pharmaceutical industry; the markets for medicines are colossal.

[5] Sherman L J 1959 American Journal of Psychiatry 116: 208.

The relative importance of these factors varies according to circumstances. An unconscious patient with meningococcal meningitis does not have a personal relationship with the doctor, but patients sleepless with anxiety because they cannot cope with their family responsibilities may be affected as much by the interaction of their own personalities with that of the doctor as by the benzodiazepine prescribed by the latter; and the same applies to appetite suppressants in food addicts.

The physician may consciously use all of the factors listed above in therapeutic practice. But it is still not enough that patients get better, it is essential to know **why** they do so. This is because potent drugs should only be given if their pharmacodynamic effects are needed; many adverse reactions have been shown to be due to drugs that are not needed, including some severe enough to cause hospital admission.

Drugs can do good

Medically this good may sometimes seem trivial, as in the avoidance of a sleepless night in a noisy hotel or of social embarrassment from a profusely running nose due to seasonal pollen allergy (hay-fever). Such benefits, however, are not necessarily trivial to recipients, concerned to be at their best in important matters, whether of business, of pleasure or of passion, i.e. with quality of life.

Or the good may be literally life-saving, as in serious acute infections (pneumonia, septicaemia) or in the prevention of life-devastating disability from severe asthma, from epilepsy or from blindness due to glaucoma.

Drugs can do harm

This harm may be relatively trivial, as in hangover from a hypnotic or sleepiness from an H_1-receptor antihistamine used for hay-fever (though these effects may be a cause of serious road traffic accidents).

The harm may be life-destroying, as in the rare sudden death following an injection of penicillin, rightly regarded as one of the safest of antibiotics, or the destruction of the quality of life that occasionally attends the use of drugs that are effective in asthma and rheumatoid arthritis (adrenocortical steroids, penicillamine).

There are risks in taking medicines just as there are risks in food and transport. There are also risks in not taking medicines when they are needed, just as there are risks in not taking food or in not using transport when they are needed.

Efficacy and safety do not lie solely in the molecular structure of the drug. Doctors must choose which drugs to use and must apply them correctly in relation not only to their properties, but also to those of the patients and their disease. Then patients must use the prescribed medicine correctly (see Compliance).

Uses of drugs/medicines

> **Drugs are used in three principal ways:**
> - to cure disease: primary and auxiliary
> - to suppress disease
> - to prevent disease: (prophylaxis): primary and secondary.

Cure implies primary therapy (e.g. in bacterial and parasitic infections) when the disease is eliminated and the drug is withdrawn; or auxiliary therapy (as with anaesthetics and with ergometrine and oxytocin in obstetrics).

Suppression of diseases or symptoms is used continuously or intermittently to maintain health without attaining cure (as in hypertension, diabetes mellitus, epilepsy, asthma) or to control symptoms (such as pain and cough) whilst awaiting recovery from the causative disease.

Prevention (prophylaxis). In *primary prevention*, the person does not have the condition and is to be prevented from getting it. In malaria, vaccinations and contraception the decision to treat healthy people is generally easy. But in breast cancer, the use of tamoxifen, which can itself rarely cause endometrial cancer (which is detectable and treatable) raises complex scientific and psychosocial issues.

In *secondary prevention* the patient has the disease and the objective is to reduce risk factors and to retard progression (e.g. aspirin and lipid-lowering drugs in atherosclerosis and post-myocardial infarction).

PHYSICIAN-INDUCED (IATROGENIC) DISEASE

The most shameful act in therapeutics, apart from actually killing a patient, is to injure a patient who is but little disabled or who is suffering from a self-limiting disorder. Such iatrogenic disease,[6] induced by misguided treatment, is far from rare.

Doctors who are temperamentally extremist will do less harm by therapeutic nihilism than by optimistically overwhelming patients with well-intentioned polypharmacy. If in doubt whether or not to give a drug to a person who will soon get better without it, don't.

In 1917 the famous pharmacologist, Sollmann, felt able to write:

> Pharmacology comprises some broad conceptions and generalisations, and some detailed conclusions, of such great and practical importance that every student and practitioner should be absolutely familiar with them. It comprises also a large mass of minute details, which would constitute too great a tax on human memory, but which cannot safely be neglected.[7]

The doctor's aim must be not merely to give the patient what will do good, but to give **only** what will do good, or at least more good than harm.

BENEFITS AND RISKS

Benefits of drugs are manifest to doctor and patient

and also, it might be thought, obvious to even the most unimaginative healthy people who find themselves dismayed by some aspects of modern technology.

Modern technological medicine has been criticised, justly, for following the tradition of centuries by waiting for disease to occur and then trying to cure it rather than seeking to prevent it from occurring in the first place.

Although many diseases are partly or wholly preventable by economic, social and behavioural means, these are too seldom adopted and also are slow to take effect. In the meantime people continue to fall sick and to need and to deserve treatment.

In any case we all have eventually to die of something and, even after excessive practising of all the advice on how to live a healthy life, the likelihood that the mode of death for most of us will be free from pain, anxiety, cough, diarrhoea, paralysis (the list is endless) seems so small that it can be disregarded. Drugs already provide immeasurable solace in these situations, but better drugs are needed and their development should be encouraged.

Doctors know the sick are thankful for drugs just as even the most dedicated pedestrians and environmentalists struck down by a passing car are thankful for a motor ambulance to take them to hospital.

Benefits of drugs in individual diseases are discussed throughout this book and will not be further expanded here. But a general discussion of risk is appropriate.

Unavoidable risks

A risk-free drug would be one for which:

- The physician knew exactly what action was required and used the drug correctly
- The drug did that and nothing else, either by true biological selectivity or by selective targeted delivery
- Exactly the right amount of action, not too little, not too much, was easily achieved.

These criteria may be **completely** fulfilled, e.g. in a streptococcal infection sensitive to penicillin in patients whose genetic constitution does not render them liable to an allergic reaction to penicillin.

---

[6] *Iatrogenic* means 'physician-caused', i.e. disease consequent on following medical advice or intervention.

[7] Sollman T A 1917 Manual of pharmacology. Saunders, Philadelphia.
The information explosion of recent decades will one day be brought under better control when prescribers can, from their desktop computer terminals, enter the facts about their patient (e.g. age, sex, weight, principal and secondary diagnoses) and receive suggestions for which drugs should be considered, with proposed doses and precautions. The limitations on such a service are financial and logistic; the technology exists now. In the meantime, prescribers *must* ensure that they are aware of the basic information contained in manufacturers' data sheets and standard formularies.

These criteria are **partially** fulfilled in insulin-deficient diabetes. But the natural modulation of insulin secretion in response to need (food, exercise) does not operate with injected insulin and even sophisticated technology cannot yet exactly mimic the normal physiological responses. The criteria are still further from realisation in, for example, hyperlipidaemias and schizophrenia.

The reasons why criteria for a risk-free drug are not met are as follows:

- *Drugs may be insufficiently selective*. As the concentration rises, a drug that is highly selective at low concentrations will begin to affect other target sites (receptors, enzymes); a disease process (cancer) is so close to normal cellular mechanisms that perfectly selective cell kill is impossible.
- *Drugs may be highly selective*, but the mechanism affected has widespread functions and interference with it cannot be limited to one site only, e.g. propranolol, aspirin.
- *Prolonged modification of cellular mechanisms* can lead to permanent change in structure and function, e.g. carcinogenicity.
- *Insufficient knowledge of disease processes* (atherosclerosis) and of drug action can lead to interventions that, though undertaken with the best intentions, are harmful.
- *Patients are genetically heterogeneous* to an enormous degree and may have an unpredictable immunological response to drugs.
- *Dosage adjustment* according to need is often unavoidably imprecise, e.g. in depression.
- *Ignorant and casual prescribing*.

Reduction of drug risk

This can be achieved by:

- *Better knowledge of disease* (research); as much as 40% of useful medical advances derive from basic research that was not funded with a practical outcome in view.
- *Site-specific delivery*: drug targeting
  — by topical (local) application
  — by target-selective carriers.
- *Site-specific effect*: by molecular manipulation.
- *Informed*, careful and responsible prescribing.

Three major grades of risk

These are: unacceptable, acceptable and negligible. In the presence of life-threatening disease and with sufficient information on both the disease and the drug, then decisions, though they may be painful, present relatively obvious problems. But where the disease risk is remote, e.g. mild hypertension, or where drugs are to be used to increase comfort or to suppress symptoms that are, in fact, bearable, or for convenience rather than for need, then the issues of risk acceptance are less obvious.

Risks should not be considered without reference to benefits any more than benefits should be considered without reference to risks.

> Risks are among the facts of life. In whatever we do and in whatever we refrain from doing, we are accepting risk. Some risks are obvious, some are unsuspected and some we conceal from ourselves. But risks are universally accepted, whether willingly or unwillingly, whether consciously or not.[8]

Two broad categories of risk

First are those that we accept by *deliberate choice*, even if we do not exactly know their magnitude, or we know but wish they were smaller, or, especially where the likelihood of harm is sufficiently remote though the consequences may be grave, we do not even think about the matter. Such risks include transport and sports, both of which are inescapably subject to potent physical laws such as gravity and momentum, and surgery to rectify disorders that could either be tolerated or treated in other ways, e.g. hernia, much cosmetic surgery.

Second are those risks that are imposed on us in the sense that they cannot be significantly altered by individual action. Risks such as those of food additives, e.g. preservatives, colouring, air pollution and some environmental radioactivity are imposed by man. But there are also risks imposed by nature, such as skin cancer due to excess ultraviolet radiation in sunny climes, as well as some radioactivity.

It seems an obvious truth that unnecessary risks

---

[8] Pochin E E 1975 British Medical Bulletin 31: 184.

should be avoided, but there is disagreement on what risks are truly unnecessary and, on looking closely at the matter, it is plain that many people habitually take risks in their daily and recreational life that it would be a misuse of words to describe as necessary.

It is also the case that some risks, though known to exist, are, in practice, ignored other than by conforming to ordinary prudent conduct. These risks are negligible in the sense that they do not influence behaviour, i.e. they are neglected.[9]

In general it has been suggested that, in medical cases, concern ceases when risks fall below about 1 in 100 000 so that the procedure then becomes regarded as 'safe'. In such cases, when disaster occurs, it can be difficult indeed for individuals to accept that they 'deliberately' accepted a risk; they feel 'it should not have happened to me' and in their distress they may seek to lay blame on others where there is no fault or negligence, only misfortune (see Warnings).

The benefits of chemicals used to colour food verge on or even attain negligibility, although some are known to cause allergy in man. Yet our society permits their use.

There is general agreement that drugs prescribed for disease are themselves the cause of a significant amount of disease (adverse reactions), of death, of permanent disability, of recoverable illness and of minor inconvenience, e.g. in one study (USA) 3% of hospital emergency room visits were attributable to adverse drug reactions.

Risk has two elements
● The likelihood or probability of an adverse event
● Its severity.

Whenever a drug is given a risk is taken

The risk is made up of the properties of the drug, of the prescriber, of the patient and of the environment; it is often so small that second thoughts are hardly necessary, but sometimes it is substantial.

---

[9] Sometimes the term *minimal risk* is used to mean risk about equal to going about our ordinary daily lives; it includes travel on public transport, but not motor bicycling on a motorway.

The doctor must weigh the likelihood of gain for the patient against the likelihood of loss. There are often insufficient data for a rational decision to be reached, but a decision must yet be made, and this is one of the greatest difficulties of clinical practice. Its effect on the attitudes of doctors is often not appreciated by those who have never been in this situation. The patients' protection lies in the doctors' knowledge of the drug and of the disease, and experience of both, together with knowledge of the patient.

Drugs that are capable of killing or disabling patients at doses within the therapeutic range continue to be used where the overall balance of benefit and risk is judged favourable. This can be very difficult for the patient who has suffered a rare severe adverse reaction to understand and to accept (see below).

In some chronic diseases in which suppressive drugs will ultimately be needed they may not benefit the patient in the early stages. For example, victims of early parkinsonism or hypertension may be little inconvenienced or hazarded by the disease, as yet, and the premature use of drugs can exact such a price in side-effects (including fatigue, which may be unrecognised as a side-effect and which is common with, for example, β-adrenoceptor blockers) that patients prefer the untreated state; what patients will tolerate depends on their personality, their attitude to disease, their occupation, mode of life and relationship with their doctor (see Compliance).

PUBLIC VIEW OF DRUGS AND PRESCRIBERS

The current public view of modern medicines, ably fuelled by the mass media, is a compound of vague expectation of 'miracle' cures with outrage when anything goes wrong. It is also unreasonable to expect the public to trust the medical profession (in collaboration with the pharmaceutical industry) to the extent of leaving to them all drug matters.

The public wants benefits without risks and without having to alter its unhealthy ways of living; a deeply irrational position. But it is easy to understand that a person who has taken into his body a chemical with intent to relieve suffering, whether or not it is self-induced, can feel profound anger when harm ensues.

Expectations have been raised and now, at the end of the 20th century with the manifest achievement of technology all around us, the naive expectation that happiness can be a part of the technological package is increasingly seen to be unrealisable.

Patients are aware that there is justifiable criticism of the standards of medical prescribing, indeed doctors are in the forefront of this; as well as justifiable criticism of promotional practices of the profitably rich, aggressive, international pharmaceutical industry.

There are obvious areas where some remedial action is possible:

- *Improvement of prescribing* by doctors, including better communication with patients, i.e. doctors must learn to feel that introduction of foreign chemicals into their patients' bodies is a serious matter, which the majority do not seem to feel at present.[10]
- Introduction of *no-fault compensation schemes* for serious drug injury (some countries already have these; see p. 10).
- *Free public discussion* of the issues between the medical profession, industrial drug developers, politicians and other 'opinion-formers' in society, and patients (the public).
- *Restraint* in promotion *by the pharmaceutical industry* including self-control by both industry and doctors in their necessarily close relationship, which the public is inclined to regard as a conspiracy, especially when the gifts and payments made to doctors get into the news.

If restraint by both parties is not forthcoming, and it may not be, then both doctor and industry can expect more control to be exercised over them by politicians responding to public demand. If doctors

do not want their prescribing to be restricted, they should prescribe better.

CRITICISMS OF MODERN DRUGS

Extremist critics have attracted public attention for their view that modern drug therapy, indeed modern medicine in general, does more harm than good; others, whilst admitting some benefits from drugs, insist that this is medically marginal. These opinions rest on the undisputed fact that favourable trends in many diseases preceded the introduction of modern drugs and were due to economic and environmental changes, sanitation, nutrition, housing. They also rest on the claim that drugs have not changed *expectation of life* or *mortality* (as measured by national mortality statistics) and that drugs can cause illness (adverse reactions).

If something is to be measured then the correct criteria must be chosen. Overall mortality figures are an extremely crude and often an irrelevant measure of the effects of drugs whose major benefits are so often on quality of life rather than on its quantity.

Two examples of inappropriate measurements will suffice:

1. In the case of many infections it is not disputed that environmental changes have had a greater beneficial effect on health than the subsequently introduced antimicrobials. But this does not mean that environmental improvements alone are sufficient in the fight against infections. When comparisons of illnesses in the pre- and post-antimicrobial eras are made, like is not compared with like. Environmental changes achieved their results when mortality from infections was high and antimicrobials were not available; antimicrobials were introduced later against a background of low mortality as well as of environmental change; decades separate the two parts of the comparison, and observers, diagnostic criteria and data recording changed during this long period.[11] It is evident that determining the value of antimicrobials is not simply a matter of looking at mortality rates.

2. About 1% of the UK population has *diabetes mellitus* and about 1% of death certificates mention dia-

---

[10] Doctors who seek to exculpate themselves from serious, even fatal, prescribing errors by appealing to the undoubted difficulties presented by the information explosion of modern times are increasingly less likely to get sympathy (except perhaps from some colleagues), and increasingly more likely to be told, 'If you can't stand the heat, get out of the kitchen' (a dictum attributed to Harry S Truman, US President 1945–52: though he assigns it to US Army General, Harry Vaughan). Pharmacists stand ready and willing to relieve doctors of the burden of prescribing.

[11] Lever A F 1977 Lancet 1: 352.

betes. This is no surprise because all must die and insulin is no cure[12] for this lifelong disease. A standard medical textbook of 1907 stated that juvenile-onset 'diabetes is in all cases a grave disease, and the subjects are regarded by all assurance companies as uninsurable lives: life seems to hang by a thread, a thread often cut by a very trifling accident'. The modern young diabetic is accepted by most, if not all, life insurance companies with no or only modest financial penalty, the premium of a person 5–10 years older. Before insulin replacement therapy was available few survived beyond 3 years[13] after diagnosis; they died for lack of insulin. It is unjustified to assert that a treatment is worthless just because its mention on death certificates (whether as a prime or as a contributory cause) has not declined. The relevant criteria for juvenile-onset diabetes are *change in the age* at which the subjects die and the *quality of life* between diagnosis and death, and both of these have changed enormously.

DRUG-INDUCED INJURY[14] (also Ch 8)

Responsibility for drug-induced injury raises important issues affecting medical practice and development of needed new drugs, as well as of law and of social justice.

Negligence and strict and no-fault liability

All civilised legal systems provide for compensation to be paid to a person injured as a result of using a product of any kind that is defective due to negligence (fault: failure to exercise reasonable care).[15] But there is a growing opinion that special compensation for serious personal injury, beyond the modest sums that general social security systems provide, should be automatic and not dependent on fault and proof of fault of the producer, i.e. there should be 'liability irrespective of fault', 'no-fault liability' or 'strict liability'.[16] After all, victims need assistance (compensation) regardless of the cause of injury and whether or not the producer and, in the case of drugs, the prescriber deserves censure. The question why a person who has suffered injury due to the biological accident of disease should have to depend on social security payments whilst an identical injury due to a drug (in the absence of fault) should attract special added compensation receives no persuasive answer except that this is what society seems to want.

Many countries are now revising their laws on liability for personal injury due to manufactured products and are legislating Consumer Protection Acts (Statutes) which include medicines, for 'drugs represent the class of product in respect of which there has been the greatest pressure for surer compensation in cases of injury'.[17]

Issues that are central to the debate include:

- *Capacity to cause harm* is inherent in drugs in a way that sets them apart from other

---

[12] A cure *eliminates* a disease and may be withdrawn when this is achieved.

[13] Even if given the best treatment. 'Opium alone stands the test of experience as a remedy capable of limiting the progress of the disease', wrote the great Sir William Osler, successively Professor of Medicine in Pennsylvania, McGill, Johns Hopkins and Oxford Universities, in 1918, only three years before the discovery of insulin.

[14] This discussion is about drugs that have been properly manufactured and meet proper standards, e.g. of purity, stability, as laid down by regulatory bodies or pharmacopoeias. A *manufacturing defect* would be dealt with in a way no different from manufacturing errors in other products.

[15] A plaintiff (person who believes he/she has been injured) seeking to obtain compensation from a defendant (via the law of negligence) must prove three things: 1, that the defendant owed a duty of care to the plaintiff; 2, that the defendant failed to exercise reasonable care; and 3, that the plaintiff has suffered actual injury as a result.

[16] The following distinction is made in some discussions of product liability:
   strict liability: compensation is provided by the producer/manufacturer.
   no-fault liability or scheme: compensation is provided by a central fund.

[17] Royal Commission on Civil Liability and Compensation for Personal Injury 1978 HMSO, London: Cmnd. 7054. Although the Commission considered compensation for death and personal injury suffered by any person through manufacture, supply or use of products, i.e. all goods whether natural or manufactured, and included drugs and even human blood and organs, it made no mention of tobacco and alcohol.

manufactured products; and harm often occurs in the absence of fault.

- *Safety*, i.e. the degree of safety that a person is entitled to expect, and adverse effects that should be accepted without complaint, must often be a matter of opinion and will vary with the disease being treated, e.g. cancer or insomnia.
- *Causation*, i.e. proof that the drug in fact caused the injury, is often impossible, particularly where it increases the incidence of a disease that occurs naturally.
- *Contributory negligence*. Should compensation be reduced in smokers and drinkers where there is evidence that these pleasure-drugs increase liability to adverse reactions to therapeutic drugs?

Principles of a workable compensation scheme for injury due to drugs

- *New unlicensed drugs undergoing early trial in small numbers of subjects* (healthy or patient volunteers): the developer should be strictly liable for all adverse effects.
- *New unlicensed drugs undergoing extensive trials* in patients who may reasonably expect benefit: the producer should be strictly liable for any serious effect.
- *New drugs after licensing by an official regulatory body*: liability for serious injury should now be shared with the community, which is expecting to benefit from new drugs.
- *Standard drugs in day-to-day therapeutics*:
  1. there should be a no-fault scheme, operated by or with the assent of government, that has authority, through tribunals, to decide cases *quickly* and to make awards. This body would have authority to reimburse itself from others — manufacturer, supplier, prescriber — wherever that was appropriate. (The basic funding of the scheme would be via a levy on all manufacturers of medicinal products.) An award must not have to wait on the determination of prolonged, vexatious, adversarial, expensive court proceedings.
  2. Patients would be compensated where:
     - causation is proved on 'balance of probability'[18]
     - the injury was serious
     - the event was rare and remote and not reasonably taken into account in making the decision to treat.

- *The concept of defect*, i.e. whether the drug or the prescriber or indeed the patient can be said to be 'defective' so as to attract liability, is a highly complex matter and indeed is a curious concept as applied to medicine.

Nowhere has a scheme that meets all the major difficulties yet been implemented. This is not because there has been too little thought, it is because the subject is so difficult.

COMPLEMENTARY AND TRADITIONAL MEDICINE

Because practitioners of complementary[19] and traditional medicine are severely critical of modern drugs, because they use drugs according to their own special beliefs, and because they are currently attracting more attention than previously (in so-called developed societies), it is appropriate to discuss drug use in complementary medical systems here.

Public disappointment that scientific medicine can neither guarantee happiness nor wholly eliminate the disabilities of degenerative diseases in long-lived populations, as well as the fact that drugs used in modern medicine can cause serious harm, naturally lead to a revival of interest in alternatives that alluringly promise efficacy with complete safety. These range from revival of traditional medicine to adoption of the more modern cults,[20] e.g. homoeopathy (see overleaf).

A proposition belongs to science if we can say what kind of event we would accept as refutation (and this is easy in therapeutics). A proposition (or theory) that cannot clash with any possible or even conceivable event (evidence) is outside science, and this in general applies to cults: everything is interpreted in terms of the theory of the cult; the possibility that the basis of the cult is false is not entertained. This appears to be the case with medical cults, which join Freudianism, and indeed religions, as outside science (after Karl Popper). Willingness to follow where the evidence leads is a

---

[18] This is the criterion for (UK) civil law, rather than 'beyond reasonable doubt', which is the criterion of criminal law.

[19] The term *complementary* seems to make a less ambitious claim than *alternative* medicine, and is preferred.

distinctive feature of conventional scientific medicine.

> A scientific approach does not mean a patient must be treated as a mere biochemical machine. It does not mean the exclusion of spiritual, psychological and social dimensions of human beings. But it does mean treating these in a rational manner.

Traditional or indigenous medicinal therapeutics has developed since before history in all societies. It

comprises a mass of practices varying from the worthless to highly effective remedies, e.g. digitalis (England), quinine (South America), reserpine (India), atropine (various countries). It is the task of science to find the gems and to discard the dross,[21] and at the same time to leave intact socially valuable supportive aspects of traditional medicine.

Complementary medicine caters, in general, for people whom scientific medicine cannot or does not help: it does not compete with the successful mainstream of scientific medicine, but offers comfort especially to two classes of person:

- those with a bad prognosis or severe organic functional disability
- those whose disorder has a major psychological component and/or who are deeply unhappy.

Features common to complementary medicine cults are absence of scientific thinking, naive acceptance of hypotheses, uncritical acceptance of causation, e.g. reliance on anecdote, and assumption that if recovery follows treatment it is due to the treatment (the *post hoc ergo propter hoc*[22] fallacy), and close attention to the patient's personal feelings. Lack of understanding of how therapeutic effects may be measured is also a prominent feature. Exponents often state that comparative controlled trials of their medicines versus conventional medicines are impracticable because the classic double-blind randomised controlled designs are inappropriate and in particular do not allow for the individual approach characteristic of complementary medicine. But modern therapeutic trial designs can cope with this. A number of scientifically unsatisfactory trials comparing homoeopathic with con-

---

[20] A *cult* is a practice that follows a dogma, tenet or principle based on theories or beliefs of its promulgator to the exclusion of demonstrable scientific experience (definition of the American Medical Association).

The profusion of medical cults tells its own story. Scientific medicine changes in accord with evidence obtained by scientific enquiry applied with such intellectual rigour as is humanly possible. But this is not the case with cults, the claims for which are characterised by absence of rigorous intellectual evaluation and unchangeability of beliefs. Medical cults and practices listed in a publication of the World Health Organization (Bannerman R H et al (eds) 1983 Traditional medicine and health care coverage. WHO, Geneva) include: homoeopathy, anthroposophical medicine, applied kinesiology, kirlian photography, reflexology, osteopathy, chiropractic, rolfing, breathing, radiesthesia, radionics, orgone therapy, pyramid therapy, naturopathy, dianetics, interferential therapy, aromatherapy, biochemics, orthomolecular medicine, bioenergetics, enlightenment intensive. The list speaks for itself, and leaves the question why, if each cult has the efficacy claimed by its exponents, conventional medicine and indeed the other cults are not swept away. Some practitioners use conventional medicine and, where it fails, turn to cult practices. Where such complementary practices give comfort they are not to be despised, but their role and validity should be clearly defined. No community can afford to take these cults at their own valuation; they must be tested, and tested with at least the rigour required to justify a therapeutic claim for a new drug. It is sometimes urged in extenuation that traditional and cult practices do no harm to patients, unlike synthetic drugs. But even if that were true (which it is not), investment of scarce resources in delivering what may be ineffective, though sometimes pleasing, experiences, e.g. dance therapy, exaltation of flowers, and the admittedly inexpensive urine therapy, means that resources are not available for other desirable social objectives, e.g. housing, art subsidies, medicine. We do not apologise for this diversion to consider medical cults and practices, for the world cannot afford unreason, and the antidote to unreason is reason and the rigorous pursuit of knowledge, i.e. evidence-based medicine.

---

[21] Traditional medicine is being fostered particularly in countries where scientific medicine is not accessible to large populations for economic reasons, and destruction of traditional medicine would leave unhappy and sick people with nothing. For this reason governments are supporting traditional medicine and at the same time initiating scientific clinical evaluations of the numerous plants and other items employed, many of which contain biologically active substances. The World Health Organization is supportive to these programmes.

[22] Latin: after this, therefore on account of this.

ventional medicines have been done (some with an outcome favourable to homoeopathy), but a lot more study is needed if either advocates or critics are to change their attitudes or their beliefs.

But there remain extremists who contend that they understand scientific method, and reject it as invalid for what they do and believe, i.e. their beliefs are not, in principle, refutable. This is the position taken up by magic and religion where subordination of reason to faith is considered a virtue.

This book is not an appropriate place to attempt a broad discussion of complementary medicine. But it is useful to list some common beliefs of its practitioners and then to consider homoeopathy, a cult that particularly relies on drugs used in an unconventional or unscientific way.

False beliefs

- *That synthetic modern drugs are toxic, but products obtained in nature are not.[23]*
- *That traditional (prescientific) medicines have special virtue.*
- *That scientific medicine will accept evidence that remedies are effective only where the mechanism is also understood.*
- *That scientific medicine recognises no form of evaluation other than the strict randomised controlled trial.*
- *That collection and formal analysis of data on*

[23] Herbal teas containing pyrrolidizine alkaloids (*Senecio, Crotalaria, Heliotropium*) cause serious hepatic veno-occlusive disease. *Comfrey* (*Symphitum*) is similar but also causes hepatocellular tumours and haemangiomas. *Sassafras* (carminative, antirheumatic) is hepatotoxic. *Mistletoe* (*Viscum*) contains cytotoxic alkaloids. *Ginseng* contains oestrogenic substances which have caused gynaecomastia: longterm users may show 'ginseng abuse syndrome' comprising CNS excitation; arterial hypotension can occur. *Liquorice* (*Glycyrrhiza*) has mineralocorticoid action. An amateur 'health food enthusiast' made himself a tea from 'an unfamiliar [to him] plant' in his garden: unfortunately this was the familiar foxglove (*Digitalis purpurea*): he became very ill but happily he recovered. Other toxic natural remedies include lily of the valley (*Convallaria*) and horse chestnut (*Aesculus*). 'The medical herbalist is at fault for clinging to outworn historical authority and for not assessing his drugs in terms of today's knowledge, and the orthodox physician is at fault for a cynical scepticism with regard to any healing discipline other than his own' (Penn R G 1983 Adverse Drug Reaction Bulletin: no 102).

therapeutic outcomes, failures as well as successes, is inessential.
- *That scientific medicine rests on acceptance of rigid and unalterable dogmas.*
- *That, if a patient gets better when treated in accordance with certain beliefs, this provides evidence for the truth of these beliefs.*

The whole patient

Complementary medicine particularly charges that conventional medicine seriously neglects patients as whole integrated human beings (body, mind, spirit) and treats them too much as machines. Conventional practitioners may well feel uneasily that there has been and still is truth in this, that some doctors have been seduced by the enormous successes of medical science and technology and have become liable to look too narrowly at their patients and too easily to rely on a prescription where a much broader (holistic) approach is required. It is evident that such an approach is likely to give particular satisfaction in psychological and psychosomatic conditions for which conventional doctors in a hurry have been all too ready to think that a prescription meets all the patients' needs.[24]

Homoeopathy

The following will suffice to give the flavour of the principal complementary medicine cult involving medicines and the kind of criticism that it has to contend with.

Homoeopathy[25] is a system of medicine founded by Samuel Hahnemann (German physician: 1755–1843) and expounded by him in the *Organon of the rational art of healing.*[26] Hahnemann described his position:

[24] A randomised controlled trial in irritable bowel syndrome of routine medical treatment versus the same management plus individual psychotherapy has shown that the psychotherapy was beneficial in both short- and longterm progress. Svendlund J et al 1983 Lancet 2: 589.

[25] Greek: *homos*: same; *patheia*: suffering.

[26] 1810: trans. Wheeler C E 1913: Dent, London.

After I had discovered the weakness and errors of my teachers and books I sank into a state of sorrowful indignation, which had nearly disgusted me with the study of medicine. I was on the point of concluding that the whole art was vain and incapable of improvement. I gave myself up to solitary reflection, and resolved not to terminate my train of thought until I had arrived at a definite conclusion on the subject.[27]

By understandable revulsion at the medicine of his time, by experimentation on himself (a large dose of quinine made him feel as though he had a malarial attack) and by search of records he 'discovered' a 'law' that is central to homoeopathy (and from which the name is derived):[28]

Similar symptoms in the remedy remove similar symptoms in the disease. The eternal, universal law of Nature, that every disease is destroyed and cured through the similar artificial disease which the appropriate remedy has the tendency to excite, rests on the following proposition: that only one disease can exist in the body at any one time.

In addition to the above, he 'discovered' that the effect of drugs but not of trace impurities is potentiated by dilution (provided the dilution is shaken correctly, i.e. by 'succussion', even to the extent that an effective dose may not contain a single molecule of the drug. It has been pointed out[28] that the 'thirtieth potency' (1 in 10^{60}), recommended by Hahnemann, provided a solution in which there would be one molecule of drug in a volume of a sphere of literally astronomical circumference. That a dose in which no drug is present (including sodium chloride prepared in this way) can be therapeutically effective is explained by the belief that there is a spiritual energy diffused throughout the medicine by the particular way in which the dilutions are shaken (succussion) during preparation, or that the active molecules leave behind some sort of 'imprint' on solvent or excipient.[29] The absence of potentiation of the inevitable contaminating impurities is attributed to the fact that they are not incor-

porated by serial dilution. It also seems that solid formulations may be inactivated during dispensing, by machine or hand counting carried out incorrectly.

Thus, writes a critic, 'We are asked to put aside the whole edifice of evidence concerning the physical nature of materials and the normal concentration-response relationships of biologically active substances in order to accommodate homoeopathic potency'.[30] But no hard evidence that tests the hypothesis is supplied to justify this, and we are invited, for instance, to accept that sodium chloride merely diluted is no remedy, but that 'it raises itself to the most wonderful power through a well-prepared dynamisation process' and stimulates the defensive powers of the body against the disease.

Pharmacologists generally feel that in the absence of conclusive evidence from empirical studies that homoeopathic medicines can *reproducibly* be shown to differ from placebo in clinical studies conducted according to modern scientific standards, there is no point in discussing the hypotheses of homoeopathy. Such evidence as has appeared has proved vulnerable to methodological criticism.[31] But empirical studies can be made without accepting any particular theory of causation; nor should the results of good studies be disregarded because the proposed theory of action seems incredible or is unknown.

Conclusion. There is a single fundamental issue between conventional scientific medicine and traditional and complementary medicine (though it is often obscured by detailed debates on individual practices); the issue is: *What constitutes acceptable evidence*, i.e. what is the nature, quality and interpretation of evidence that can justify general adoption of modes of treatment and acceptance of hypotheses?

---

[27] Hahnemann S 1805 Aesculapius in the balance. Leipsic.

[28] Clark A J 1937 General pharmacology, Heffter's Handbuch. Springer, Berlin.

[29] Homoeopathic practitioners repeatedly express their irritation that critics give so much attention to dilution. They should not be surprised considering the enormous implications of their claim.

[30] Cuthbert A W 1982 Pharmaceutical Journal 15 May: 547.

[31] See Reilly D et al 1994 Is evidence for homoeopathy reproducible? Lancet 344: 1601-1606 and subsequent correspondence Lancet (1995) 345: 251–253.

Prescribing, consumption and economics

The reasons for taking a drug history from patients are:

- Drugs are a cause of disease. Withdrawal of drugs can cause disease, e.g. adrenal steroid, antiepileptic.
- Drugs can conceal disease, e.g. adrenal steroid.
- Drugs can interact causing positive adverse effect, or negative adverse effect, i.e. therapeutic failure.
- Drugs can give diagnostic clues, e.g. ampicillin and amoxycillin causing urticaria in infectious mononucleosis — a diagnostic adverse effect, not a diagnostic test.
- Drugs can cause false results in clinical chemistry tests, e.g. plasma cortisol, urinary catecholamine, urinary glucose.
- Drug history can assist choice of drugs in the future.
- Drugs can leave residual effects after administration has ceased, e.g. chloroquine, digoxin, adrenal steroid.
- Drugs available for independent patient self-medication are increasing in range and importance.

(See also Appendix 2, The prescription.)

Prescribing should be **appropriate**.[32]

Appropriate [prescribing is that] which bases the choice of a drug on its effectiveness, safety and convenience relative to other drugs or treatments (e.g. surgery or psychotherapy), and takes cost into account only when those criteria for choice have been satisfied. In some circumstances appropriateness will require the use of more costly drugs. Only by giving appropriateness high priority will [health payers] be able to achieve their aim of ensuring that patients' clinical needs will be met (Report).

Prescribing that is **inappropriate** is the result of several factors:

- Giving in to patient pressure to write unnecessary prescriptions. The extra time spent in careful explanation will, in the long run, be rewarded.
- 'There is a tendency to continue patients, especially the elderly, on courses of medicinal treatment over many months or even years without proper review of their medication.'
- Doctors 'frequently prescribe brand-name drugs rather than cheaper generic equivalents, even where there is no conceivable therapeutic advantage in so doing. The fact that the brand-name products often have shorter and more memorable names than their generic counterparts' contributes to this. (Report) (see also Ch. 6).
- 'Insufficient training in clinical pharmacology. Many of the drugs on the market may not have been available when a general practitioner was at medical school.[33] The sheer quantity of new products may lead to a practitioner becoming over-reliant on drugs companies' promotional material, or sticking to 'tried and tested' products out of caution based on ignorance' (Report).
- Failure of doctors to keep up-to-date (see Doctor compliance).

Cost-containment

Cost-containment in prescription drug therapy attracts increasing attention. It may involve two particularly contentious activities:

1. *Generic substitution*, where a generic formulation (p. 72) is substituted (by a pharmacist) for the

---

[32] The text on *appropriate prescribing* and some quotations (designated *Report*) are based on a UK Parliamentary Report (The National Health Service Drugs Budget 1994 HMSO London). Twelve Members of Parliament took evidence from up to 100 organisations and individuals orally and/or in writing. It is both a surprise and a pleasure to be able to quote with approval from such a source. DRL, PNB, MJB.

[33] This statement illustrates a common and serious misunderstanding of the role of medical schools. Their role is to teach the scientific basis of clinical pharmacology and drug therapy so that doctors can handle existing and future drugs intelligently, using current data sheets, formularies, etc. It is not to attempt to teach enormous numbers of impossible-to-remember facts, the deadening effect of which on a thinking approach would be disastrous.

proprietary formulation prescribed by the doctor.

2. *Therapeutic substitution*, where a drug of different chemical structure is substituted for the drug prescribed by the doctor. The substitute is of the same chemical class and is deemed to have similar pharmacological properties and to give similar therapeutic benefit. Therapeutic substitution is a particularly controversial matter where it is done without consulting the prescriber, and legal issues may be raised in the event of adverse therapeutic outcome.

The following facts and opinions are worth thinking about:

— The UK National Health Service (NHS) spending on drugs has been 9–11% per year (of the total cost) over nearly 50 years.

— 80% of the total cost of drugs is spent by general practitioners, i.e. in primary care.

— The total number of prescription items rose by 34% between 1980 and 1992.

— People over the age of 65 years receive on average 13 prescriptions per year — twice as many as the population in general.

— 'The average cost per head of medicines supplied to people aged over 75 is nearly five times that of medicines supplied to those below pensionable age (currently in UK women 60 years: men 65)' (Report).

— '*Underprescribing* can be just as harmful to the health of patients as overprescribing.'

It is crucially important that incentives and sanctions address quality of prescribing as well as quantity: 'it would be wrong if too great a preoccupation with the cost issue in isolation were to encourage underprescribing or have an adverse effect on patient care' (Report).

Reasons for underprescribing include: lack of information or lack of the will to use available information (in economically privileged countries there is, if anything, a surplus of information); fear of being blamed for adverse reactions (affecting doctors who lack the confidence that a knowledge of pharmacological principles confers); fear of sanctions against over-costly prescribing.

— Prescription frequency and cost per prescription is lower for older than for younger doctors. There is no reason to think that the patients of older doctors are worse off as a result.

Repeat prescriptions

Long-repeat prescriptions (above 6 months) can be classified[34] thus:

● For the specific pharmacodynamic (therapeutic) effect of the drug

● As a way of maintaining a relationship (by both doctor and patient); the prescription provides contact that can be kept impersonal, e.g. unhappiness manifesting itself as unpleasant bodily symptoms, but without identifiable disease

● As a gift — a symbol of a wish to do something when the prescriber cannot think of anything better

● To fulfil socially motivated patient demands, e.g. weight reduction

● As a way of terminating the consultation.

About two-thirds of general (family) practice prescriptions are for repeat medication (half issued by the doctor at a consultation and half via the receptionist without patient contact with the doctor): 95% of patients' requests are acceded to without further discussion; 25% of patients who receive repeat prescriptions have had 40 or more repeats; 55% of patients aged over 75 years are on repeat medication.

Many patients taking the same drug for years are doing so for the best reason, i.e. firm diagnosis for which effective therapy is available, such as epilepsy, diabetes, hypertension, but many are not.

WARNINGS AND CONSENT

Doctors have a professional duty to inform and to warn, so that patients, who are increasingly informed and educated, may make meaningful personal choices which it is their right to do (unless they opt to leave the choice to the doctor, which it is also their right to do).

---

[34] Harris C M 1980 British Medical Journal 281: 57.

> **Warnings to patients are of two kinds:**
> - Warnings that will affect the patient's choice to accept or reject the treatment
> - Warnings that will affect the safety of the treatment once it has begun, e.g. risk of stopping treatment, occurrence of drug toxicity.

Just as engineers say that the only safe aeroplane is the one that stays on the ground in still air on a disused airfield or in a locked hangar, so the only safe drug is one that stays in its original package. If drugs are not safe then plainly patients are entitled to be warned of their hazards, which should be **explained** to them, i.e. probability, nature and severity.

There is no formal legal or ethical obligation on doctors to warn all patients of all possible adverse consequences of treatment. It is their duty to adapt the information they give (not too little, and not so much as to cause confusion) so that the best interest of each patient is served. If there is a 'real' (say 1–2%) risk inherent in a procedure of some misfortune occurring, then doctors should warn patients of the possibility that the injury may occur, however well the treatment is performed. Doctors should take into account the personality of the patient, the likelihood of any misfortune arising and what warning was necessary for each particular patient's welfare.[35] Doctors should consider what their particular individual patients would wish to know (i.e. would be likely to attach significance to) and not only what they think (paternalistically) that the patients ought to know.

It is part of the professionalism of doctors to tell what is appropriate to the individual patient's interest. If things go wrong doctors must be prepared to defend what they did or, more important in the case of warnings, what they did not do, as being in their patient's best interest; and courts of law will look critically at doctors who seek to justify under-information by saying that they feared to confuse or frighten the patient (or that they left it to the patient to ask, as one doctor did). The increasing availability of patient information leaflets (PILs) prepared by the manufacturer indicates the increasing trend to give more information. Doctors should know what their patients have read (or not read, as is so often the case) when patients express dissatisfaction.

Evidence that extensive information on risks causes 'unnecessary' anxiety or frightens patients suggests that this is only a marginal issue and it does not justify a general policy of withholding of information.

Legal hazards for prescribers

Doctors would be less than human if, as well as trying to help their patients, they were not also concerned to protect themselves from allegations of malpractice (negligence) (see Regret avoidance). The legal position regarding a doctor's duty has been pungently put by a lawyer specialising in the field:

> The provision of information to patients is treated by (English) law as but one part of the way a doctor discharges the obligation he owes to a patient to take reasonable care in all aspects of his treatment of that patient. The provision of information is a corollary of the patient's right to self-determination which is a right recognised by law. Failure to provide appropriate information will usually be a breach of duty and if that breach leads to the patient suffering injury then the basis for a claim for compensation exists.[36]

The keeping of appropriate medical records, written at the time of consultation (and which is so frequently neglected) is not only good medical practice, it is the best way of ensuring that there is an answer to unjustified allegations, made later, when memory has faded;[37] for example, allegations by patients that they would have declined a treatment that has done harm if the doctor had given a proper warning.

---

[35] Legal correspondent 1980 British Medical Journal 280: 575.

[36] Ian Dodds-Smith.

[37] A Professor of Clinical Pharmacology who has made special studies of prescribing and patient information writes: **'What should a prescriber record in the notes?'** Given the existing format of general practitioner notes and the limited time available for each consultation, it seems unlikely that detailed information will be recorded in the notes. A compromise is therefore inevitable. My suggestion

FORMULARIES AND 'ESSENTIAL' DRUGS

Increasingly, doctors recognise that they need guidance through the bountiful menu (thousands of medicines) so seductively served to them by the pharmaceutical industry. Principal sources of guidance are the pharmaceutical industry ('prescribe my drug') and governments ('spend less'); also the developing (profit-making) managed care/insurance bodies ('spend less'); and the proliferating drug bulletins offering independent, and supposedly unbiased advice ('prescribe appropriately').

Even the pharmaceutical industry, in its more sober moments, recognises that their ideal world in which doctors, advised and informed by industry alone, were free to prescribe whatever they pleased,[38] to whomsoever they pleased, for as long as they pleased with someone other than the patient paying, is an unrealisable dream of a 'never-never land'.

The industry knows that it has to learn to live with restrictions of some kinds and one of the means of restriction is the **formulary**, a list of formulations of medicines with varying amounts of added information. A formulary may list all nationally licensed medicines prescribable by health professionals, or list only preferred drugs.

It may be restricted to what a third party payer will reimburse, or to the range of formulations stocked in a hospital (and chosen by a local drugs and therapeutics committee, which all hospitals or groups of hospitals should have), or the range agreed by a partnership of general practitioners or primary care health centre.

All restricted formularies are heavily motivated to keep costs down without impairing appropriate prescribing (p. 15). They should make provision for prescribing outside their range in cases of special need with an 'escape clause'.

Despite enormous individual variation it seems that most doctors do about 75% of their prescribing from about 100 formulations (not 100 different drugs), but the maximum number of preparations used by an individual doctor can be as high as 500.

'Essential' drugs. Economically disadvantaged countries may need help to construct formularies.

Technical help has been forthcoming since 1977 from the World Health Organization (WHO) with its *Model List of Essential Drugs*, i.e. drugs (or representatives of classes of drugs) 'that satisfy the health care needs of the majority of the population; they should therefore be available at all times in adequate amounts and in the appropriate dosage forms'. Countries needing such advice can use the list as a basis for their own choices (WHO also publishes model prescribing information).[39]

The list is updated every few years and contains about 300 items. The current list is provided as Appendix 1 to this chapter.

The pharmaceutical industry dislikes the concept that some drugs may be classed as *essential* and therefore others, by implication, are deemed *inessential*. But the WHO programme has attracted much interest and approval (see WHO Technical Report Series: The use of essential drugs: current edition).

---

is that doctors should make a point of recording the fact that they have warned patients about treatments which are potentially hazardous. Specific examples include the description of dietary precautions to be taken if a monoamine oxidase inhibitor has been prescribed and the issue of steroid treatment cards to patients given prednisolone. Similarly, it would be wise to record that a young woman given a retinoid for acne is taking adequate contraceptive precautions, or that a patient taking carbimazole for thyrotoxicosis had been warned to report to the surgery in the event of a severe sore throat.
'Despite all of these uncertainties, the good news is that patients who receive leaflets are more satisfied than those who do not. Satisfied patients are less likely to complain, and are therefore presumably less likely to take legal action against prescribers' (George C F 1994 Prescribers' Journal 34: 7–11).

[38] It is difficult for us now to appreciate the naive fervour and trust in doctors that allowed them almost unlimited rights to prescribe (in the early years of the UK National Health Service: founded in 1948). Beer was a prescription item in hospitals until, decades later, an audit revealed that only 1 in 10 bottles reached a patient. More recently (1992):
'There could be fewer Christmas puddings consumed this year. The puddings were recently struck off a bizarre list of items that doctors were able to prescribe for their patients. They were removed by Health Department officials without complaint from the medics, on the grounds they had "no therapeutic or clinical value".' (Lancet (1992) 340: 1531).

---

[39] There is an agency for WHO publications in all UN countries.

Compliance

Successful therapy, especially if it is longterm, comprises a great deal more than choosing a standard medicine. It involves patient and doctor compliance.[40] The latter is liable to be overlooked (by doctors), for doctors prefer to dwell on the deficiencies of their patients rather than of themselves.

PATIENT COMPLIANCE

Patient compliance is the extent to which the actual behaviour of the patient coincides with medical advice and instructions: it may be complete, partial, erratic, nil, or there may be overcompliance. To make a diagnosis and to prescribe evidence-based effective treatment is a satisfying experience for doctors, but too many assume that patients will gratefully or accurately do what they are told, i.e. obtain the medicine and consume it as instructed. This assumption is wrong.

The rate of **nonpresentation** (or redemption) of prescriptions[41] (UK) is around 5% but up to 20% or even more in the elderly (who pay no prescription charge). Where lack of money to pay for the medicine is not the cause, this is due to lack of motivation. Incredibly (to doctors) it has been found that the patients feel that what the doctor has to offer has no worth, a fact on which doctors should meditate.

Having obtained the medicine, some 25–50% (sometimes even more) of patients either fail to follow the instruction to a significant extent (taking 50–90% of the prescribed dose), or they do not take it at all.

Patient noncompliance is identified as a major factor in therapeutic failure in both routine practice and in scientific therapeutic trials; but, sad to say, doctors are too often noncompliant about remedying this. All patients are potential noncompliers;[42] good compliance cannot be reliably predicted on clinical criteria, but noncompliance often can be.

In addition to therapeutic failure, undetected noncompliance may lead to the best drug being deemed ineffective when it is not, leading to substitution by second-rank drugs.

Noncompliance may occur because

- the patient has not understood the instructions, so cannot comply,[43] or
- understands the instructions, but fails to carry them out.

Prime factors for poor patient compliance

- Patient dissatisfaction with the doctor, poor patient–doctor relationship
- Lack of motivation
- Forgetfulness (unintentional noncompliance)
- Deliberate intention (see below)
- Lack of information
- Frequency and complexity of drug regimen.

---

[40] The term *compliance* has been objected to as having overtones of obsolete, authoritarian attitudes, implying 'obedience' to doctors' 'orders'. But this seems oversensitive and an abuse of language and the suggested alternatives, adherence and cooperation, do not have quite the right meaning. We retain **compliance**, pointing out that it applies equally to those doctors who neither keep up-to-date, nor follow prescribing instructions, e.g. in official Data Sheets.

[41] Many factors are associated with prescription nonredemption. Perhaps the cameo of a person least likely to redeem a prescription is a middle-aged woman, not exempt from prescription charges (in UK National Health Service) who has a symptomatic condition requiring an 'acute' prescription that is issued by a trainee general practitioner on a Sunday (Beardon P H G et al 1994 British Medical Journal 307: 846).

[42] Even where the grave consequences of noncompliance are understood (glaucoma: blindness) (renal transplant: organ rejection), significant noncompliance has been reported in as many as 20% of patients; psychologists will be able to suggest explanations for this.

[43] **Cautionary tales:**
— A 62-year-old man requiring a metered-dose inhaler (for the first time) was told to 'spray the medicine to the throat'. He was found to have been conscientiously aiming and firing the aerosol to his anterior neck around the thyroid cartilage, four times a day for two weeks (Chiang A A, Lee J C 1994 New England Journal of Medicine 330: 1690).
— A patient thought that 'sublingual' meant able to speak two languages; another that tablets cleared obstructed blood vessels by exploding inside them (E A Kay) — reference, no doubt, to colloquial use of the term 'clot-busting drugs' (for thrombolytics).
— These are extreme examples, most are more subtle and less detectable. Doctors may smile at the ignorant naivety of patients, but the smile should be replaced by a blush of shame at their own deficiencies as communicators.

Poor patient–doctor relationship and **lack of motivation** to take medicines as instructed offer a major challenge to the prescriber whose diagnosis and prescription may be perfect, but yet loses efficacy by patient noncompliance.

Unpleasant disease symptoms, particularly where these are recurrent and known by previous experience to be quickly relieved, provide the highest motivation, i.e. self-motivation, to comply. But particularly where the patient does not feel ill, side-effects are immediate, and benefits are perceived to be remote, e.g. in hypertension, where they may be many years away in the future, then doctors must consciously address themselves to motivating compliance.

The best way to motivate patient compliance is to cultivate the patient–doctor relationship. Doctors cannot be expected actually to like all their patients, but it is a great help (where liking does not come naturally) if they make a positive effort to understand how individual patients must be feeling about their illnesses and their treatments, i.e. to empathise with their patients. This is not always easy, but its achievement is the action of the true professional, and indeed is part of their professional duty of care.

A casual or, worse, an authoritarian, approach impairs this all-important relationship and is liable to cause the patient to evade questions about compliance or even to lie in order to avoid the unpleasantness of censure by the doctor authority-figure. The nature of the relationship is principally in the hands of the doctor.

Unintentional noncompliance, or forgetfulness,[44] may be addressed by associating drug-taking with cues in daily life (breakfast, bedtime), by special packaging (e.g. calendar packs) and by enlisting the aid of others (e.g. carers, teachers).

'Intelligent' or wilful noncompliance.[45] Patients decide they do not need the drug or they do not like the drug, or take 2–3-day drug holidays.

Lack of information. Oral instructions alone are not enough; one-third of patients have been found unable to recount instructions immediately on leaving the consulting room. Lucid and legible labelling of containers is essential, as well as patient-friendly information leaflets, which are increasingly available via doctors and pharmacists and as package inserts. (In hospitals, pharmacists have been known to throw away patient package inserts because they present problems for their administrative routine.)

Frequency and complexity of drug regimen. Many studies attest to compliance being inhibited by:

- *Polypharmacy*: more than three drugs to be taken concurrently
- *More than three drug-taking occasions* in the day (the ideal of one occasion only is often unattainable).

Other substantial factors for poor compliance

- Adverse drug reactions (these may cause 'intelligent' noncompliance)[45]
- Anxiety
- Psychiatric conditions
- Inappropriate health beliefs
- Family instability
- Poverty, homelessness, drug abuse.

Suggestions to doctors *to enhance patient compliance* are:

- Form a nonjudgemental alliance or partnership with the patient

---

[44] Where noncompliance, whether intentional or unintentional, is medically serious it becomes necessary to bypass self-administration (unsupervised) and to resort to directly observed (i.e. supervised) oral administration or to injection (e.g. in schizophrenia).

[45] Of the many causes of failure of patient compliance the following case must be unique:
On a transatlantic flight the father of an asthmatic boy was seated in the row behind two doctors. He overheard one of the doctors expressing doubt about the longterm safety in children of inhaled corticosteroids. He interrupted the conversation, explaining that his son took this treatment; he had a lengthy conversation with one of the doctors, who gave his name. As a consequence, on arrival, he faxed his wife at home to stop the treatment of their son immediately. She did so, and two days later the well-controlled patient had a brisk relapse that responded to urgent treatment by the family doctor (who had been conscientiously following guidelines recently published in an authoritative journal). The family doctor later ascertained that the doctor in the plane was a member of the editorial team of the journal that had so recently published the guidelines that were favourable to inhaled corticosteroid (Cox S 1994 Is eavesdropping bad for your health? British Medical Journal 309: 718).

- Provide oral and written information adapted to the patient's understanding and medical and cultural needs
- Give the patient an opportunity to ask questions
- Plan administration to fit the patient's lifestyle
- Use patient-friendly packaging, e.g. calendar packs, where appropriate; or monitored-dose systems, e.g. boxes compartmented and labelled
- Use fixed-dose combinations or sustained-release (or injectable depot) formulations to simplify drug taking, as appropriate; arrange direct observation of each dose in exceptional cases
- See the patient regularly and not so infrequently that the patient feels the doctor has lost interest
- Use computer-generated reminders for repeat prescriptions.

Directly observed therapy (DOT) (a reliable person supervises *each* dose). In addition to the areas where it is obviously in the interest of patients that they be supervised, e.g. children, DOT is employed (even imposed) where free-living uncooperative patients may be a menace to the community, e.g. multiple-drug-resistant tuberculosis.

What every patient needs to know[46]

- An account of the disease and the reason for prescribing
- The **name** of the medicine
- The **objective**
  - to treat the **disease** and/or
  - to relieve **symptoms**, i.e. how important the medicine is, whether the patient can judge its efficacy and when benefit can be expected to occur
- How and when to take the medicine
- Whether it matters if a dose is missed and what, if anything, to do about it (see p. 23)
- How long the medicine is likely to be needed
- How to recognise adverse effects and any action that should be taken, including effects on car driving
- Any interaction with alcohol or other medicines.

A remarkable instance of noncompliance, with hoarding, was that of a 71-year-old man who attempted suicide and was found to have in his home 46 bottles containing 10 685 tablets. Analysis of his prescriptions showed that over a period of 17 months he had been expected to take 27 tablets of several different kinds daily.[47]

From time to time there are campaigns to collect all unwanted drugs from homes in an area. Usually the public are asked to deliver the drugs to their local pharmacies. In one UK city (600 000 population) 500 000 'solid dose units' (tablets, capsules, etc.) were handed in (see Opportunity cost); such quantities have even caused local problems for safe waste disposal.

Factors that are *insignificant* for compliance are: age[48] (except at extremes), gender, intelligence (except at extreme deficiency) and education level (probably).

Overcompliance. Patients (up to 20%) may take more drug than is prescribed, even increasing the dose by 50%. In diseases where precise compliance with frequent or complex regimens is important, e.g. in glaucoma where sight is at risk, there have been instances of obsessional patients responding to their doctors' overemphatic instructions by clock-watching in a state of anxiety to avoid the slightest deviance from timed administration of the correct dose, to the extent that their daily (and nightly) life becomes dominated by this single purpose.

---

[46] After Drug and Therapeutics Bulletin (1981) 19: 73. *Patient information leaflets.* In economically privileged countries original or patient-pack dispensing is becoming the norm, i.e. patients receive an unopened pack just as it left the manufacturer. The pack contains a Patient Information Leaflet (PIL) (which is therefore supplied with each repeat prescription). Its content is increasingly determined by regulatory authority. The requirements to be comprehensive and, in this litigous age, to protect both manufacturer and regulatory authority, to some extent impair the patient-friendliness of PILs. But studies have shown that patients who receive leaflets are more satisfied than those who do not. Doctors need to have copies of these leaflets so that they can discuss with their patients what they are (or are not) reading.

[47] Smith S E et al 1974 Lancet 1: 937.

[48] But the elderly are commonly taking several drugs — a major factor in noncompliance — and monitoring compliance in this age group becomes particularly important. The over-60s (UK) are, on average, each receiving two or three medications.

Evaluation of patient compliance. Merely asking patients whether they have taken the drug as directed is not likely to provide reliable evidence;[49] and it can be assumed that anything that can happen to impair compliance, will happen sometimes. Estimations of compliance are based on studies using a variety of measures.

Requiring patients to produce containers when they attend the doctor, who counts the tablets, seems to do little more than show the patient that the doctor cares about the matter (which is useful); and a tablet absent from a container has not necessarily entered the patient's body. On the other hand, although patients are known to practise deliberate deception, to maintain effective deception successfully over long periods requires more effort than most patients are likely to make. The same applies to the use of monitored-dosage systems (e.g. compartmented boxes) as memory aids and to electronic containers that record times of opening.

Measuring the drug or a marker substance (e.g. riboflavine, phenol red, or even digoxin in tiny doses) in blood, urine or saliva, at least demonstrates that the drug has entered the body, but patients have been found who take the drug only on the day of a clinic visit; and routine random testing is plainly impracticable.

Some pharmacodynamic effects, e.g. heart rate with beta-adrenoceptor blocker, provide a physiological marker as an indication of the presence of drug in the body.

Compliance in new drug development

Noncompliance, discovered or undiscovered, can invalidate therapeutic trials (in which it should always be monitored). In new drug development trials the diluting effect of undetected noncompliance (prescribed doses are increased) can result in unduly high doses being initially recommended (licensed) (with toxicity in good compliers after

marketing), so that the standard dose has soon to be urgently reduced (this has probably occurred with some new nonsteroidal anti-inflammatory drugs).

DOCTOR COMPLIANCE

Doctor compliance is the extent to which the behaviour of doctors fulfils their professional duty:

- not to be ignorant
- to adopt new advances when they are sufficiently proved (which doctors are often slow to do)[50]
- to prescribe accurately[51]
- to refrain from inappropriate prescribing
- to tell patients what they need to know
- to warn, i.e. to recognise the importance of the act of prescribing.

Anyone who has had the opportunity to inspect medical prescriptions in hospitals and in a primary care setting will surely conclude that if doctors wrote personal bank cheques as badly as they write prescriptions they would soon be in financial trouble, and would change their ways.

In one study in a university hospital, where standards might be expected to be high, there was an error of drug use (dose, frequency, route) in 3% of prescriptions and an error of prescription writing (in relation to standard hospital instructions) in 30%. Many errors were trivial, but many could have resulted in overdose, serious interaction or undertreatment.

In other hospital studies error rates in drug administration of 15–25% have been found, rates rising rapidly where 4 or more drugs are being given concurrently, as is often the case; studies on hospital in-patients show that each receives about 6 drugs, and up to 20 during a stay is not rare.

It has been found that merely providing information (on antimicrobials) did not influence prescribing, but gently asking physicians to justify their

---

[49] Hippocrates (5th cent. BC) noted that patients are liars regarding compliance. The way the patient is questioned may be all-important, e.g. 'Were you able to take the tablets?' may get a truthful reply where, 'Did you take the tablets?' may not, because the latter question may be understood by the patient as implying personal criticism (Pearson R M 1982 British Medical Journal 285: 757).

[50] See Bobbio M et al 1994 Completeness of reporting trial results: effect on physicians' willingness to prescribe. Lancet 343: 1209.

[51] Accuracy includes legibility: a doctor wrote Intal (sodium cromoglycate) for an asthmatic patient: the pharmacist read it as Inderal (propranolol): the patient died. See also, Names of drugs.

prescriptions caused a marked fall in inappropriate prescribing.

On a harsher note, of recent years, doctors who have given drugs, of the use of which they have later admitted ignorance (e.g. route of administration and/or dose), have been charged with manslaughter[52] and have been convicted. Shocked by this, fellow doctors have written to the medical press offering understanding sympathy to these, sometimes junior, colleagues; 'There, but for the grace of God, go I'.[53] But the public response is not sympathetic. Doctors put themselves forward as trained professionals who offer a service of responsible, competent provision of drugs which they alone have the legal right to prescribe. The public is increasingly inclined to hold them to that claim, and, where they seriously fail, to exact retribution.

> If you don't know about a drug, find out before you act, or take the personal consequences, which, increasingly, may be very serious indeed.

Underdosing

Use of suboptimal doses of drugs in serious disease, sacrificing efficacy for avoidance of serious adverse effects, has been documented. It particularly affects drugs of low therapeutic index (see Index), i.e. where the effective and toxic dose ranges are close, or even overlap, e.g. heparin, anticancer drugs, aminoglycoside antimicrobials. In these cases dose adjustment to obtain maximum benefit with minimum risk requires both knowledge and attentiveness — qualities that are not always in abundant supply.

It has been reported that when data from therapeutic drug monitoring (of plasma concentration) show underdose, and are presented to clinicians, they have sometimes even then failed to increase the dose of, e.g. heparin, aminoglycosides (see Regret avoidance).

The clinical importance of missed dose(s)

Even the most conscientious of patients will miss a dose or doses occasionally. Patients should therefore be told whether this matters and what they should do about it, if anything.

> **Missed dose(s) may lead to:**
> - loss of efficacy (acute disease)
> - resurgence (chronic disease)
> - rebound or withdrawal syndrome.

Loss of efficacy relates to the **pharmacokinetic properties** of the drugs. With some short $t^{1}/2$ drugs there is a simple issue of a transient drop in plasma concentration below a defined therapeutic level. But with others there may be complex issues such as recovery of negative feedback homoeostatic mechanisms (e.g. adrenocortical steroids). Therapeutic effect may not decline in parallel with plasma concentration. With some drugs a single missed dose may be important (e.g. oral contraceptives), with others (long $t^{1}/2$) several doses may be omitted before there is any serious decline in efficacy (e.g. thyroxine).

These pharmacokinetic considerations are complex and important, and are, or should be, taken into account by drug manufacturers in devising dosage schedules and informative Data Sheets. Manufacturers should aim at one or two doses per day (not more), and this is generally best achieved with drugs having relatively long biological effect $t^{1}/2$, or where the biological effect $t^{1}/2$ is short, by using sustained-release formulations.

Discontinuation syndrome (recurrence of disease, rebound, or withdrawal syndrome) may occur due to a variety of mechanisms (see Index).

Placebo medicines

> A **placebo**[54] is any component of therapy that is without specific biological activity for the condition being treated.

---

[52] Unlawful killing in circumstances that do not amount to murder (which requires an intention to kill), e.g. causing death by negligence that is much more serious than mere carelessness; reckless breach of the legal duty of care.

[53] Attributed to John Bradford, an English preacher and martyr (16th cent), on seeing a convicted criminal pass by.

[54] Latin: *placebo*, I shall be pleasing or acceptable.

Placebo medicines are used for two purposes:

- As a control in scientific evaluation of drugs (see Therapeutic trials) (see p. 57)
- To benefit or please a patient, not by any pharmacological actions, but by psychological means.

All treatments have a psychological component, whether to please (placebo effect) or, occasionally, to vex (negative placebo or nocebo[55] effect).

A placebo medicine is a vehicle for 'cure' by suggestion, and is surprisingly often successful, if only temporarily. All treatments carry placebo effect: physiotherapy, psychotherapy, surgery, entering a patient into a therapeutic trial; even the personality and style of the doctor; but the effect is most easily investigated with drugs, for the active and the inert can often be made to appear identical so that comparisons can be made.

The deliberate use of drugs as placebos is a confession of failure by the doctor. Failures however are sometimes inevitable and an absolute condemnation of the use of placebos on all occasions would be unrealistic.

> A **placebo-reactor** is an individual who reports changes of physical or mental state after taking a pharmacologically inert substance.

Placebo-reactors are suggestible people and likely to respond favourably to any treatment. They have misled doctors into making false therapeutic claims. **Negative reactors**, who develop adverse effects when given a placebo, exist but, fortunately, are fewer.

Some 35% of the physically ill and 40% or more of the mentally ill respond to placebos. Placebo reaction is an inconstant attribute; a person may respond at one time in one situation and not at another time under different conditions. However, there is some consistency in the type of person who tends to react to any therapeutic intervention. In one study on medical students, psychological tests revealed that those who reacted to a placebo tended to be extraverted, sociable, less dominant, less self-confident, more appreciative of their teaching, more aware of their autonomic functions and more neurotic than their colleagues who did not react to a placebo under the particular conditions of the experiment.

The use of placebo medicines may be considered:

- for mild psychological disorders
- to sustain a patient with chronic incurable disease
- to sustain a patient when the diagnosis is in doubt
- where to attempt to disabuse patients of their beliefs would be without benefit and even cruel.

Do not use placebos alone. Conditioning theory leads us to expect that placebo effects would be greatest when used along with treatments having strong specific effect. Continued use of inert remedies alone leads to 'placebo sag';[56] placebo benefits are unlikely to last more than a few weeks, but patients may become dependent on a prescription and demand that it be continued indefinitely.

There is a cogent reason for avoiding deliberate placebo (drug) therapy: it is that the patient, reasonably, interprets the advice to take medicine as meaning that the doctor admits a physical basis for the symptoms; so that when later, the placebo effect having declined, an attempt is made to attribute a psychological cause, this will not be accepted.

Placebos should be prescribed only after a serious attempt to avoid using them has failed, and then only briefly; the placebo should consist of an innocuous and cheap substance (vitamin mineral supplements can be used), unless patients pay for it themselves, when high cost greatly potentiates its effect.

In addition to the psychological suggestion inherent in any act of medication, deliberate confident oral suggestion has been shown to raise the threshold for pain and indeed to reverse pharmacodynamic effects at least temporarily. Such psychological effects are operative in any enthusiastically pursued therapeutic regimen.

It is of great importance that all who administer drugs should be aware that their attitudes to the

---

[55] Latin: *nocebo*, I shall injure; the term is little used.

[56] Chaput de Saintonge D M, Herxheimer A 1994 Lancet 344: 995–8.

treatment may greatly influence the result. Undue scepticism may prevent a drug from achieving its effect and enthusiasm or confidence may potentiate the actions of drugs.

Tonics are placebos. They may be defined as substances with which it is hoped to strengthen and increase the appetite of those so weakened by disease, misery, overindulgence in play or work, or by physical or mental inadequacy, that they cannot face the stresses of life. The essential feature of this weakness is the absence of any definite recognisable defect for which there is a known remedy.

Since tonics are placebos, they **must** be harmless.[57]

Pharmacoeconomics

Even the richest societies cannot satisfy the appetite of their citizens for health care based on their real needs, on their wants and on their (often unrealistic) expectations.

Health care resources are rationed[58] in one way or another, whether according to national social policies or to individual wealth. The debate on supply is not about whether there should be rationing, but about what form rationing should take; whether it should be explicit or concealed (from the public).

Doctors prescribe, patients consume and, increasingly throughout the world, third (purchasing) parties (government, insurance companies) pay the bill with money they have obtained from increasingly reluctant healthy members of the public.

The purchasers of health care are now engaged in serious exercises to contain drug costs in the short term without, it is hoped, impairing the quality of medical care, or damaging the development of useful new drugs (which is an enormously expensive and longterm process). This can be achieved successfully only if **reliable** data are available on costs and benefits, both absolute and relative. The difficulties of generating such data, not only during development, but later under actual-use conditions, are enormous and a new breed of professional has arisen to meet the need: the health economist.

> **Economics** is the science of the distribution of wealth and resources. Prescribing doctors, who have a duty to the community as well as to individual patients, cannot escape involvement with economics.

The economists' objective

The objective is to enable needs to be defined so that available resources may be deployed according to priorities set by society, which has an interest in fairness between its members. The question is whether resources are to be distributed in accordance with an unregulated power struggle between professionals and associations of patients and public pressure groups — all, no doubt, warm-hearted towards deserving cases of one kind or another, but none able to view the whole scene; or whether there is to be a planned evaluation that allows division of the resources on the basis of some visible attempt at fairness.

A health economist[59] writes:

> The economist's approach to evaluating drug therapies is to look at a group of patients with a particular disorder and the various drugs that could be used to treat them. The costs of the various treatments and some costs associated with their use (together with the costs of giving no treatment) are then considered in terms of impact on health status (survival and quality of life) and impact on other health care costs (e.g. admissions to hospital, need for other drugs, use of other procedures).

> 'Economists are often portrayed as people who want to focus on cost, whereas in reality they see everything in terms of a balance between costs and benefits.'[59]

---

[57] Tonics (licensed) available in the UK include: Gentian Mixture, acid (or alkaline) (gentian, a natural plant bitter substance, and dilute HCl or sodium bicarbonate): Labiton (thiamine, caffeine, alcohol, all in low dose).

[58] The term rationing is used here to embrace the allocation of priorities as well as the actual withholding of resources (in this case, drugs).

[59] Prof Michael Drummond.

Three economic concepts have particular importance to the thinking of every doctor who takes up a pen to prescribe, i.e. to distribute resources.

- *Opportunity cost* means that which has to be sacrificed in order to carry out a certain course of action, i.e. costs are benefits foregone elsewhere. If money is spent on prescribing, that money is not available for another purpose; wasteful prescribing can be seen as an affront to those who are in serious need, e.g. institutionalised mentally handicapped citizens who everywhere would benefit from increased resources.
- *Cost-effectiveness analysis* is concerned with how to attain a given objective at minimum financial cost, e.g. prevention of postsurgical venous thromboembolism by heparin, warfarin, aspirin, external pneumatic compression. Analysis includes cost of: materials, adverse effects, any tests, nursing and doctor time, duration of stay in hospital (which may greatly exceed the cost of the drug).
- *Cost-benefit analysis* is concerned with issues of whether (and to what extent) to pursue objectives and policies; it is thus a broader activity than cost-effectiveness analysis and puts monetary values on the quality as well as on the quantity (duration) of life.

Allied measures include cost-minimisation analysis and cost-utility analysis. Economic analysis requires that both quantity and quality of life be measured. The former is easy, the latter is hard.

Quality of life

Everyone is familiar with the measurement of the benefit of treatment in saving or extending life, i.e. life expectancy: the measure is the quantity of life (in years). But it is evident that life may be extended and yet have a low quality, even to the point that it is not worth having at all. It is therefore useful to have a unit of health measurement that combines the quantity of life with its quality to allow individual and social decisions to be made on a sounder basis than mere intuition.

To meet this need economists have developed the *quality-adjusted-life-year* (QALY); estimations of years of life expectancy are modified according to

estimations of quality of life. **Quality of life has four principal dimensions:**[60]

1. physical mobility
2. freedom from pain and distress
3. capacity for self-care
4. ability to engage in normal work and social interactions.

The approach to measure quality of life has been developed into a questionnaire to measure what the subject perceives as personal health. The assessments are being refined to provide improved assessment of the benefits and risks of medicines to the individual and to society. Plainly quality of life is a major aspect of what is now called *outcomes research*.

But, we emphasise, there have been serious criticisms of QALYs, not only for being based on poor data (which should be remediable), but more importantly on ethical grounds. They may lead to unfair decisions when used to make resource allocation decisions between, for example: the rich and the poor, the educated and the uneducated, the old and the young, as well as between groups of patients having very different diseases.

Self-medication

To feel unwell is common, though the frequency varies with social and cultural circumstances.

People commonly experience symptoms or complaints and commonly want to take remedial action. In one study of adults randomly selected from a large population, 9 out of 10 had one or more complaints in the 2 weeks before interview; in another of premenopausal women a symptom occurred as often as 1 day in 3; in both studies a medicine was taken for more than half these occurrences.

Modern consumers (patients) wish to take a greater role in the maintenance of their own health and are often competent to manage (uncomplicated) chronic and recurrent illnesses (not merely short-term symptoms) after proper medical diagno-

---

[60] Williams A 1983. In: Smith G T (ed) Measuring the social benefits of medicine. Office of Health Economics, London.

sis and with only occasional professional advice, e.g. use of histamine H_2-receptor blocker, topical corticosteroid and antifungal, and oral contraceptive. They are understandably unwilling to submit to the inconvenience of visiting a doctor for what they rightly feel they can manage for themselves, given adequate information.

Increased consumer autonomy leads to satisfied:

- consumers (above)
- governments (lower drug bill)
- industry (profits)
- doctors (reduced work load).

The pharmaceutical industry enthusiastically estimates that extending self-medication to all potentially self-treatable illnesses could save 100–150 million general practitioner consultations per year (in the UK: population 57 million). But there will also be added costs as pharmacists extend their responsibilities for supply and information.

Regulatory authorities are increasingly receptive to switching hitherto prescription-only medicines (POM) for self-medication (over-the-counter, OTC, sale) via pharmacies (P) or via any retail outlet (general sale). The operation is known as POM-OTC or POM-P 'switch'. It requires particularly exacting standards of safety.

Self-medication is appropriate for:

- short-term relief of symptoms where accurate diagnosis is unnecessary
- uncomplicated cases of some chronic and recurrent disease (a medical diagnosis having been made and advice given).

Safety in self-medication (an overriding requirement) depends on four items:

- *The drug* — its inherent properties, dose and duration of use, including its power to induce dependence
- *The formulation* — devised with unsupervised use in mind, e.g. low dose
- *Information* — available with all purchases (printed) and rigorously reviewed (by panels of potential users) for user-friendliness and adequacy for a wide range of education and intellectual capacity
- *Patient compliance.*

Doctors must recognise the increasing importance of questioning about self-medication when taking a drug history.

GUIDE TO FURTHER READING

Beardon P H G et al 1993 Primary non-compliance with prescribed medication in primary care. British Medical Journal 307: 846

Branch R A et al 1992 The formulary: An educational tool for clinical pharmacology. Clinical Pharmacology and Therapeutics 51: 481

Chaput de Saintonge, Herxheimer A 1994 Harnessing placebo effects in care. Lancet 344: 995

Cohen E P 1988 Direct-to-the-public advertisements of prescription drugs. New England Journal of Medicine 318: 373

Controversies in treatment 1994 How can hospitals ration drugs? British Medical Journal 308: 901 (a debate)

Drummond M F, Jefferson T O (BMJ Economic Evaluation Working Party) 1996 Guidelines for authors and peer reviewers of economic submissions to the BMJ. British Medical Journal 313: 275 (an excellent review of pharmacoeconomic evaluation)

Editorial 1988 When to believe the unbelievable. Nature 333: 787 (A report of an investigation into experiments with antibodies in solutions that contained no antibody molecules (as in some homoeopathic medicines). The editor of Nature took a three-person team (one of whom was a professional magician, included to detect any trickery) on a week-long visit to the laboratory that claimed positive results. Despite the scientific seriousness of the operation it developed comical aspects (codes of the contents of test tubes were taped to the laboratory ceiling); the Nature team, having reached an unfavourable view of the experiments 'sped past the [laboratory] common-room filled with champagne bottles destined now not to be opened'). Full reports in this issue of Nature (28 July 1988), including an acrimonious response by the original scientist, are highly recommended reading, both for scientific logic and for entertainment. See also Nature 1994 370: 322

Editorial 1994 Over-the-counter drugs. Lancet 343: 1374

Feely J et al 1990 Hospital formularies: need for continuous intervention. British Medical Journal 300: 28

Kessler D A et al 1994 Therapeutic-class wars. Drug promotion in a competitive market place. New England Journal of Medicine 331: 1350

Kleijnen J et al 1994 Placebo effect in double-blind clinical trials. Lancet 344: 1347

Laporte J-R et al 1983 Drug utilisation studies: a tool for determining the effectiveness of drug use. British Journal of Clinical Pharmacology 16: 301

Lenert L A, Markowitz D R, Blaschke T F 1993 *Primum non nocere?* Valuing the risk of drug toxicity in therapeutic decision making. Clinical Pharmacology and Therapeutics 53: 285

Levy G 1993 A pharmacokinetic perspective on medicament non-compliance. Clinical Pharmacology and Therapeutics 54: 242

MacLennan A H, Wilson D H, Taylor A W 1996 Prevalence and cost of alternative medicine in Australia. Lancet 347: 569

Melmon K L et al 1983 The undereducated physician's therapeutic decisions. New England Journal of Medicine 308: 1473

Michel J-M 1985 Why do people like medicines? A perspective from Africa. Lancet 1: 210

Morse D I 1996 Directly observed therapy for tuberculosis: spend now or pay later. British Medical Journal 312: 719

Mullan K 1988 Writing a wrong [a legal action against a doctor and a pharmacist for negligence in prescribing and dispensing]. British Medical Journal 297: 470

Pullar T 1991 Compliance with drug therapy. British Journal of Clinical Pharmacology 32: 535

Robinson R 1993 Economic evaluation and health care. What does it mean? British Medical Journal 307: 670

Rosenzweig P, Brohier S, Zipfel A 1993 The placebo effect in healthy volunteers. Clinical Pharmacology and Therapeutics 54: 578

Schaffner W et al 1983 Improving antibiotic prescribing in office practice. A controlled trial of three educational methods. Journal of the American Medical Association 250: 1728

Slevin M L 1992 Quality of life: philosophical question or clinical reality? British Medical Journal 305: 466

Steel K et al 1981 Iatrogenic illness on a general medical service at a university hospital. New England Journal of Medicine 304: 638

Thomas K B 1994 The placebo in general practice. Lancet 344: 1066

Walley T, Davey P 1995 Pharmacoeconomics: a challenge for clinical pharmacologists. British Journal of Clinical Pharmacology 40: 199

Wright E C 1993 Non-compliance — or how many aunts has Matilda? Lancet 342: 909

Wyatt J, Walton R 1995 Computer based prescribing: improves decision making and reduces cost. British Medical Journal 311: 1181

Appendix 1: The World Health Organization model list of essential drugs

We reprint the current list[1] (by permission). Whilst the WHO programme was instituted particularly to help developing countries, the list has interest and lessons for all societies facing, as they now are, the problems of delivering economically affordable health care to all. We commend a study of the list to all our readers (see also p. 18).

Any national or local group of health workers wishing to produce a formulary to provide for the needs of their own community would be well advised to study the current version in addition to other sources.

Explanatory notes

We print the list in full. *Antiviral drugs* are not included because of limited efficacy.

Drugs marked * represent an example of a therapeutic group, i.e. various other drugs could serve as an alternative, e.g. on cost grounds.

Complementary drugs are for use where, for any reason, drugs in the main list are unavailable, or there are exceptional medical circumstances, e.g. bacterial resistance, rare disorders.

Spelling of drug names. The World Health Organization devises recommended International Nonproprietary Names (rINN): These are becoming universal; most do not give rise to any confusion, but occasionally we insert an alternative name or spelling.

Not every entry in the list is discussed in this book.

1. Anaesthetics

1.1 General anaesthetics and oxygen
ether, anaesthetic
halothane
ketamine
nitrous oxide
oxygen
* thiopental

1.2 Local anaesthetics
* bupivacaine
* lidocaine (lignocaine)

1.3 Preoperative medication
atropine
chloral hydrate
* diazepam
* morphine
* promethazine

2. Analgesics, antipyretics, non-steroidal anti-inflammatory drugs and drugs used to treat gout

2.1 Non-opioids
acetylsalicylic acid (aspirin)
allopurinol
colchicine
* ibuprofen
* indometacin
paracetamol

2.2 Opioid analgesics
* codeine
* morphine
COMPLEMENTARY DRUG
* pethidine

3. Antiallergics and drugs used in anaphylaxis
* chlorphenamine
* dexamethasone
epinephrine (adrenaline)
hydrocortisone
* prednisolone

4. Antidotes and other substances used in poisonings

4.1 General
* charcoal, activated
ipecacuanha

4.2 Specific
atropine
deferoxamine (desferrioxamine)
dimercaprol
* DL-methionine.
methylthioninium chloride (methylene blue)
naloxone
penicillamine
potassium ferric hexacyanoferrate(ll)·2H$_2$O (Prussian blue)
sodium calcium edetate
sodium nitrite
sodium thiosulfate

5. Antiepileptics
carbamazepine
* diazepam
ethosuximide
phenobarbital
phenytoin
valproic acid

6. Anti-infective drugs

6.1 Anthelminthics

---

[1] The use of essential drugs. WHO Technical Report Series 850: Geneva 1995.

6.1.1 *Intestinal anthelminthics*
albendazole
levamisole
* mebendazole
niclosamide
piperazine
praziquantel
pyrantel

6.1.2 *Antifilarials*
diethylcarbamazine
ivermectin
COMPLEMENTARY DRUG
suramin sodium

6.1.3 *Antischistosomals*
metrifonate
oxamniquine
praziquantel

6.2 Antibacterials

6.2.1 *Penicillins*
* amoxicillin
ampicillin
benzathine benzylpenicillin
benzylpenicillin
* cloxacillin
phenoxymethylpenicillin
* piperacillin
procaine benzylpenicillin

6.2.2 *Other antibacterials*
* chloramphenicol
doxycycline
* erythromycin
* gentamicin
* metronidazole
spectinomycin
* sulfadimidine
* sulfamethoxazole +
trimethoprim
* tetracycline
COMPLEMENTARY DRUGS
chloramphenicol
ciprofloxacin
clindamycin
nalidixic acid
nitrofurantoin
trimethoprim
Additional reserve drugs may be
needed

6.2.3 *Antileprosy drugs*
clofazimine
dapsone
rifampicin

6.2.4 *Antituberculosis drugs*
ethambutol
isoniazid
pyrazinamide

rifampicin
rifampicin + isoniazid
streptomycin
COMPLEMENTARY DRUG
thioacetazone + isoniazid

6.3 Antifungal drugs
amphotericin B
griseofulvin
* ketoconazole
nystatin
COMPLEMENTARY DRUG
flucytosine

6.4 Antiprotozoal drugs

6.4.1 *Antiamoebic and antigiardiasis
drugs*
* diloxanide
* metronidazole
COMPLEMENTARY DRUG
chloroquine

6.4.2 *Antileishmaniasis drugs*
* meglumine antimoniate
pentamidine

6.4.3 *Antimalarial drugs*
(a) For curative treatment
* chloroquine
primaquine
* quinine
COMPLEMENTARY DRUGS
mefloquine
* sulfadoxine + pyrimethamine
* tetracycline
(b) For prophylaxis
chloroquine
mefloquine
proguanil

6.4.4 *Antitrypanosomal drugs*
(a) African trypanosomiasis
melarsoprol
pentamidine
suramin sodium
COMPLEMENTARY DRUG
eflornithine
(b) American trypanosomiasis
benznidazole
nifurtimox

6.5 Insect repellents
diethyltoluamide

7. Antimigraine drugs

7.1 For treatment of acute attack
acetylsalicylic acid (aspirin)
ergotamine
paracetamol

7.2 For prophylaxis
propranolol

**8. Antineoplastic and
immunosuppressant drugs
and drugs used in palliative
care**

8.1 Immunosuppressant drugs
* azathioprine
ciclosporin (cyclosporin/e)

8.2 Cytotoxic drugs
asparaginase
bleomycin
calcium folinate
chlormethine
cisplatin
cyclophosphamide
cytarabine
dacarbazine
dactinomycin
* doxorubicin
etoposide
fluorouracil
levamisole
mercaptopurine
methotrexate
procarbazine
vinblastine
vincristine

8.3 Hormones and antihormones
* prednisolone
tamoxifen

8.4 Drugs used in palliative care
The drugs are included in the
relevant sections of the model
list, according to their
therapeutic use, e.g. analgesics

9. Antiparkinsonism drugs
* biperiden
levodopa + * carbidopa

10. Drugs affecting the blood

10.1 Antianaemia drugs
ferrous salt
ferrous salt + folic acid
folic acid
hydroxocobalamin
COMPLEMENTARY DRUG
* iron dextran

10.2 Drugs affecting coagulation
desmopressin
heparin

phytomenadione
protamine sulfate
warfarin

11. Blood products and plasma substitutes

11.1 Plasma substitutes
* dextran 70
* polygeline

11.2 Plasma fractions for specific uses
albumin, human
COMPLEMENTARY DRUGS
* factor VIII concentrate
* factor IX complex (coagulation factors II, VII, IX, X) concentrate

12. Cardiovascular drugs

12.1 Antianginal drugs
glyceryl trinitrate
* isosorbide dinitrate
* propranolol
verapamil
COMPLEMENTARY DRUG
atenolol

12.2 Antidysrhythmic drugs
lidocaine (lignocaine)
* propranolol
verapamil
COMPLEMENTARY DRUGS
atenolol
isoprenaline
* procainamide
* quinidine

12.3 Antihypertensive drugs
* hydralazine
* hydrochlorothiazide
* nifedipine
* propranolol
COMPLEMENTARY DRUGS
atenolol
* captopril
methyldopa
* reserpine
* sodium nitroprusside

12.4 Cardiac glycosides
digoxin

12.5 Drugs used in vascular shock
dopamine

12.6 Antithrombotic drugs
acetylsalicylic acid (aspirin)

COMPLEMENTARY DRUG
streptokinase

13. Dermatological drugs

13.1 Antifungal drugs (topical)
benzoic acid + salicylic acid
* miconazole
sodium thiosulfate
COMPLEMENTARY DRUG
selenium sulfide

13.2 Anti-infective drugs
* methylrosanilinium chloride (gentian violet)
* neomycin + * bacitracin
silver sulfadiazine

13.3 Anti-inflammatory and antipruritic drugs
* betamethasone
* calamine lotion
* hydrocortisone

13.4 Astringent drugs
aluminium diacetate

13.5 Keratoplastic and keratolytic agents
benzoyl peroxide
coal tar
dithranol
fluorouracil
* podophyllum resin
salicylic acid

13.6 Scabicides and pediculicides
benzyl benzoate
permethrin

13.7 Ultraviolet-blocking agents
COMPLEMENTARY DRUGS
p-aminobenzoic acid, sun protection factor 15
* benzophenones, sun protection factor 15
* zinc oxide

14. Diagnostic agents

14.1 Ophthalmic drugs
fluorescein
* tropicamide

14.2 Radiocontrast media
* amidotrizoate
barium sulfate
* iopanoic acid
* propyliodone
COMPLEMENTARY DRUG
* meglumine iotroxate

15. Disinfectants and antiseptics

15.1 Antiseptics
* chlorhexidine
hydrogen peroxide
* polyvidone iodine

15.2 Disinfectants
* calcium hypochlorite
glutaral

16. Diuretics
* amiloride
* furosemide (frusemide)
* hydrochlorothiazide
COMPLEMENTARY DRUGS
* mannitol
spironolactone

17. Gastrointestinal drugs

17.1 Antacids and other antiulcer drugs
aluminium hydroxide
* cimetidine
magnesium hydroxide

17.2 Antiemetic drugs
metoclopramide
* promethazine

17.3 Antihaemorrhoidal drugs
* local anaesthetic, astringent and anti-inflammatory drug

17.4 Anti-inflammatory drugs
hydrocortisone
sulfasalazine

17.5 Antispasmodic drugs
* atropine

17.6 Cathartic drugs
* senna

17.7 Drugs used in diarrhoea

17.7.1 Oral rehydration
oral rehydration salts (glucose-electrolyte solution)

17.7.2 Antidiarrhoeal (symptomatic) drugs
* codeine

18. Hormones, other endocrine drugs and contraceptives

18.1 Adrenal hormones and synthetic substitutes
* dexamethasone
hydrocortisone
* prednisolone

COMPLEMENTARY DRUG
fludrocortisone

18.2 Androgens
COMPLEMENTARY DRUG
testosterone

18.3 Contraceptives

18.3.1 Hormonal contraceptives
* ethinylestradiol +
    * levonorgestrel
* ethinylestradiol +
    * norethisterone
COMPLEMENTARY DRUGS
medroxyprogesterone acetate
    (depot)
* norethisterone
norethisterone enantate

18.3.2 Intrauterine devices
copper-containing device

18.3.3 Barrier methods
condoms with or without
    spermicide (nonoxinol)
diaphragms with spermicide
    (nonoxinol)

18.4 Estrogens
* ethinylestradiol

18.5 Insulins and other antidiabetic agents
insulin injection (soluble)
intermediate-acting insulin
* tolbutamide

18.6 Ovulation inducers
COMPLEMENTARY DRUG
* clomifene

18.7 Progestogens
norethisterone
COMPLEMENTARY DRUG
medroxyprogesterone acetate

18.8 Thyroid hormones and antithyroid drugs
levothyroxine
potassium iodide
* propylthiouracil

19. Immunologicals

19.1 Diagnostic agents
tuberculin, purified protein
    derivative (PPD)

19.2 Sera and immunoglobulins
anti-D immunoglobulin (human)
antiscorpion sera
* antitetanus immunoglobulin
    (human)

antivenom serum
diphtheria antitoxin
immunoglobulin, human normal
* rabies immunoglobulin

19.3 Vaccines

19.3.1 For universal immunisation
BCG vaccine (dried)
diphtheria-pertussis-tetanus
    vaccine
diphtheria-tetanus vaccine
hepatitis B vaccine
measles-mumps-rubella vaccine
measles vaccine
poliomyelitis vaccine
    (inactivated)
poliomyelitis vaccine (live
    attenuated)
tetanus vaccine

19.3.2 For specific groups of individuals
influenza vaccine
meningococcal vaccine
rabies vaccine
rubella vaccine
typhoid vaccine
yellow fever vaccine

20. Muscle relaxants (peripherally acting) and cholinesterase inhibitors
* alcuronium
* neostigmine
pyridostigmine
suxamethonium
COMPLEMENTARY DRUG
vecuronium bromide

21. Ophthalmological preparations

21.1 Anti-infective agents
* gentamicin
* idoxuridine
silver nitrate
* tetracycline

21.2 Anti-inflammatory agents
* prednisolone

21.3 Local anaesthetics
* tetracaine (amethocaine)

21.4 Miotics and antiglaucoma drugs
acetazolamide
* pilocarpine
* timolol

21.5 Mydriatics
atropine

COMPLEMENTARY DRUG
epinephrine (adrenaline)

22. Oxytocics and antioxytocics

22.1 Oxytocics
* ergometrine
oxytocin

22.2 Antioxytocics
* salbutamol

23. Peritoneal dialysis solution
intraperitoneal dialysis solution
(of appropriate composition)

24. Psychotherapeutic drugs

24.1 Drugs used in psychotic disorders
* chlorpromazine
* fluphenazine
* haloperidol

24.2 Drugs used in mood disorders
* amitryptiline
lithium carbonate

24.3 Drugs used for sedation and in generalised anxiety disorders
* diazepam

24.4 Drugs used in obsessive-compulsive disorders and panic attacks
clomipramine

25. Drugs acting on the respiratory tract

25.1 Antiasthmatic drugs
* aminophylline
beclometasone
epinephrine (adrenaline)
* salbutamol
COMPLEMENTARY DRUG
* cromoglicic acid (sodium cromoglycate)

25.2 Antitussives
* codeine

26. Solutions correcting water, electrolyte and acid-base disturbances

26.1 Oral rehydration
oral rehydration salts (glucose-electrolyte solution)
potassium chloride

26.2   Parenteral
glucose
glucose with sodium chloride
potassium chloride
sodium chloride
sodium hydrogen carbonate
* compound solution of sodium
    lactate

26.3   Miscellaneous
water for injection

27.   Vitamins and minerals
ascorbic acid
* ergocalciferol
iodine
* nicotinamide

pyridoxine
* retinol
riboflavin
* sodium fluoride
thiamine
COMPLEMENTARY DRUG
calcium gluconate

The list of essential drugs may be considered against the background of the available marketed medicines worldwide.

A major standard reference work (Martindale 1996 The extra pharmacopoeia. 31st edn., Pharmaceutical Press, London), describes 62 500 preparations or groups of preparations from 17 different countries.

Appendix 2: The prescription

The prescription is the means by which medicines that are not considered safe for sale directly to the public are delivered to patients. Its format is officially regulated to ensure precision in the interests of safety and efficacy and to prevent fraudulent misuse; full details will be found in national formularies and prescribers have a responsibility to comply with these.

Prescriptions of pure drugs or of formulations from the British National Formulary (BNF)[1] are satisfactory for almost all purposes. The composition of many of the preparations in the BNF is laid down in official pharmacopoeias, e.g. British Pharmacopoeia (BP). There are also many national and international pharmacopoeias.

Traditional extemporaneous prescription-writing art, defining drug, base, adjuvant, corrective, flavouring and vehicle is obsolete, as is the use of the Latin language. [However certain convenient Latin abbreviations survive for lack of convenient English substitutes (chiefly in hospitals where instructions are given to nurses and not to patients). They are listed below, without approval or disapproval.]

The elementary requirements of a prescription are that it should state what is to be given to whom and by whom prescribed, and give instructions on how much should be taken how often, by what route and for how long or total quantity to be supplied, as below.

---

1. **Date.**

2. **Address of doctor.**

3. **Name and address of patient: age** is also desirable for safety reasons; in the UK it is a legal requirement for children under age 12 years.

4. ℞

   This is a traditional esoteric symbol[2] for the word 'Recipe' — 'take thou', which is addressed to the pharmacist. It is pointless; but since many doctors gain a harmless pleasure from writing ℞ with a flourish before the name of a proprietary preparation of whose exact nature they are ignorant, it is likely to survive as a sentimental link with the past.

5. **The name and dose of the medicine.**
   Abbreviations. Only abbreviate where there is an official abbreviation. Never use unofficial abbreviations or invent your own; **it is not safe to do so**.

   Quantities (after BNF)
   — 1 gram or more: write 1 g etc.
   — Less than 1 g: write as milligrams: 500 mg, not 0.5 g.
   — Less than 1 mg: write as micrograms, e.g. 100 micrograms, not 0.1 mg.
   — For decimals a zero should precede the decimal point where there is no other figure, e.g. 0.5 mL, not .5 mL, or for a range, 0.5 to 1 g.
   — Do not abbreviate microgram, nanogram or unit.
   — Use millilitre, ml or mL, not cubic centimetre, cc.
   — Home/domestic measures, see below.

   State dose and dose frequency; for 'as required', specify minimum dose interval or maximum dose per day.

6. **Directions to the pharmacist**, if any: 'mix', 'make a solution'. Write the total quantity to be dispensed (if this is not stated in 5 above); or duration of supply.

---

[1] Supplied free to all doctors practising in the UK National Health Service and to medical students.

[2] Derived from the eye of Horus, ancient Egyptian sun god.

7. **Instruction for the patient**, to be written on container by the pharmacist. Here brevity, clarity and accuracy are especially important. It is dangerous to rely on the patient remembering oral instructions. The BNF provides a list of recommended 'cautionary and advisory labels for dispensed medicines' representing a balance between 'the unintelligibly short and the inconveniently long', e.g. 'Do not stop taking this medicine except on your doctor's advice'.

Pharmacists nowadays use their own initiative in giving advice to patients.

8. **Signature of doctor.**

Example of a prescription for a patient with an annoying unproductive cough.

1,2,3, as above
4. ℞
5. Codeine Linctus, BNF, 5 ml
6. Send 60 ml
7. Label: Codeine Linctus [or NP]. Take 5 ml twice a day and on retiring.
8. Signature of doctor.

Computer-issued prescriptions must conform to recommendations of local professional bodies. If altered by hand (undesirable), the alteration must be signed.

Medicine containers. Reclosable child-resistant containers and blister packs are increasingly used, as is dispensing in manufacturers' original sealed packs containing a patient information leaflet. These add to immediate cost but may save money in the end (increased efficiency of use, and safety).

Unwanted medicines. Patients should be encouraged to return these to the original supplier for disposal.

Drugs liable to cause dependence or be the subject of misuse. Doctors have a particular responsibility to ensure, (1) they do not create dependence, (2) the patient does not increase the dose and create dependence, (3) they are not used as an unwitting source of supply to addicts. To many such drugs special prescribing regulations apply (see BNF).

Abbreviations (see also Weights and measures, below)

ac: ante cibum	before food
bd: bis in die	twice a day (bid is also used)
BNF	British National Formulary
BP	British Pharmacopoeia
BPC	British Pharmaceutical Codex
i.m.: intramuscular	by intramuscular injection
IU	International Unit
i.v.: intravenous	by intravenous injection
NP: nomen proprium	proper name
od: omni die	every day
om: omni mane	every morning
on: omni nocte	every night
pc: post cibum	after food
po: per os	by mouth
PR: per rectum	by the anal/rectal route
prn: pro re nata	as required. It is best to add the maximum frequency of repetition, e.g. Aspirin and Codeine Tablets, 1 or 2 prn, 4-hourly
PV: per vaginam	by the vaginal route
qds: quater die sumendus	4 times a day (qid is also used)
q or qq: quaque	every, e.g. qq6 h = every 6 h
qqh: quarta quaque hora	every 4 hours
qs: quantum sufficiat	a sufficiency, enough
rep: repetatur	let it be repeated, as in rep. mist(ura), repeat the mixture
sc: subcutaneous	by subcutaneous injection
sos: si opus sit	if necessary. It is useful to confine sos to prescriptions to be repeated once only and to use prn where many repetitions are intended
stat: statim	immediately
tds: ter (in) die sumendus	3 times a day (tid is also used).

Weights and measures

In this book doses are given in the metric system, or in international units (IU) when metric doses are impracticable.

Equivalents:
1 litre (l or L) = 1.76 pints
1 kilogram (kg) = 2.2 pounds (lb)

Abbreviations:
1 gram (g)
1 milligram (mg) (1×10^{-3} g)

1 microgram^3 $(1 \times 10^{-6}\,\text{g})$
1 nanogram^3 $(1 \times 10^{-9}\,\text{g})$
1 decilitre (dL) $(1 \times 10^{-1}\,\text{l})$
1 millilitre (mL) $(1 \times 10^{-3}\,\text{l})$

Home/domestic measures. A standard 5 ml spoon and a graduated oral syringe are available. Otherwise the following approximations will serve:

> 1 tablespoonful = 14 ml (or mL)
> 1 dessertspoonful = 7 ml (or mL)
> 1 teaspoonful = 5 ml (or mL)

Percentages, proportions, weight in volume

Some solutions of drugs (e.g. local anaesthetics, adrenaline) for parenteral use are labelled in a variety of ways: percentage, proportion, or weight in volume (e.g. 0.1%, 1:1000, 1 mg per mL). Also, dilu-

tions may have to be made by doctors at the time of use. Such drugs are commonly dangerous in overdose and great precision is required, especially as any errors are liable to be by a factor of 10 and can be fatal. Doctors who do not feel confident with such calculations (because they do not do them frequently) should feel no embarrassment,[4] but should recognise that they have a responsibility to check their results with a competent colleague or pharmacist before proceeding.

---

[3] Spell out in full in prescribing.

---

[4] Called to an emergency tension pneumothorax on an intercontinental flight, two surgeons, who chanced to be passengers, were provided with lignocaine 100 mg in 10 ml (in the aircraft medical kit). They were accustomed to thinking in percentages for this drug and 'in the heat of the moment' neither was able to make the conversion. Chest surgery was conducted successfully with an adapted wire coat-hanger as a trocar ('sterilised' in brandy), using a urinary catheter. The patient survived the flight and recovered in hospital. Wallace W A 1995 Managing in-flight emergencies: A personal account. British Medical Journal 311: 374.

2

Clinical pharmacology

SYNOPSIS

Clinical pharmacology comprises all aspects of the scientific study of drugs in man. Its objective is to optimise drug therapy and it is justified in so far as it is of practical use.

Over recent years pharmacology has undergone great expansion resulting from technology that allows the understanding of molecular action and the capacity to exploit this. The potential consequences for therapeutics are enormous. All cellular mechanisms (normal and pathological), in their immense complexity are, in principle, identifiable. What seems almost an infinity of substances, transmitters, local hormones, cell growth factors, can be made, modified and tested to provide agonists, partial agonists, inverse agonists and antagonists. And interference with genetic disease processes is now possible. Increasingly large numbers of substances will deserve to be investigated in therapeutics and used for altering physiology to the perceived advantage (real or imagined) of humans.

But, with all these developments and their potential for good, comes capacity for harm, whether inherent in the substances or as a result of human misapplication.[1]

Successful use of the power conferred (by biotechnology in particular) requires understanding of the enormous complexity of the *consequences of interference*. Willingness to learn the principles of pharmacology and how to apply them in individual circumstances of infinite variety is vital to success without harm: to maximise benefit and minimise risk. All these issues are the concern of clinical pharmacologists and are the subject of this book.

The drug and information 'explosion' of the past 55 years combined with medical need has called into being the discipline, clinical pharmacology. The discipline is now recognised as both a health care and an academic specialty; indeed, no medical school can be considered complete without a department or subdepartment of Clinical Pharmacology.

The clinical pharmacologist's role is to provide facts and opinions that are **useful** for optimising the treatment of patients. Therapeutic success with drugs is becoming more and more dependent on the user having at least an outline technical knowledge of both pharmacodynamics and pharmacokinetics. And this outline is quite simple and easy to acquire. However humane and caring doctors may be, they cannot dispense with technical skill.

---

[1]And the mass media, indifferent to the social consequences of their activities and driven to irresponsibility by commerical pressures for audience numbers, promote false expectations to a credulous public. In 1995 a TV programme (UK) was introduced thus, 'The latest contender for the wonder drug of the millennium . . . Howard, 63, has shed his paunch, steadied his palsy and binned his specs . . . Can it rejuvenate the elderly? Give eternal life?' The drug referred to was human growth hormone.

> **Clinical pharmacology** provides the scientific basis for:
>
> - the general aspects of rational, safe and effective drug therapy
> - drug therapy of individual diseases
> - introduction of new medicines.

Pharmacology is commonly practised in concert with other clinical specialties. More detailed aspects comprise:

1. Pharmacology
   - *Pharmacodynamics*: how drugs, alone and in combination, affect the body (young, old, well, sick)
   - *Pharmacokinetics*: absorption, distribution, metabolism, excretion or, how the body, well or sick, affects drugs
2. Therapeutic evaluation
   - Whether a drug is of value
   - How it may best be used
   - Formal therapeutic trials
   - Surveillance studies for both efficacy and adverse effects: pharmacoepidemiology and pharmacovigilance
3. Control
   - Rational prescribing and formularies
   - Official regulation of medicines
   - Social aspects of the use and misuse of medicines, including pharmacoeconomics.

If it is desired to single out a pioneer clinical pharmacologist it would surely be Harry Gold[2] (1899–1972) of Cornell University, USA, whose influential studies in the 1930s showed us how to be clinical pharmacologists. In 1952 he wrote in a seminal article:

> a special kind of investigator is required, one whose training has equipped him not only with the principles and technics of laboratory pharmacology but also with knowledge of clinical medicine . . .

Clinical scientists of all kinds do not differ fundamentally from other biologists; they are set apart only to the extent that there are special difficulties and limitations, ethical and practical, in seeking knowledge from man.[3]

Pharmacology is the same science whether animal or man is investigated. The need for it grows rapidly as not only scientists, but now the whole community, can see its promise of release from distress and premature death over yet wider fields. The concomitant dangers of drugs (fetal deformities, adverse reactions, dependence) only add to the need for the systematic and ethical application of science to drug development, evaluation, and use, i.e. clinical pharmacology.

GUIDE TO FURTHER READING

Alvan G et al 1983 Problem-oriented drug information: a clinical pharmacological service. Lancet 2: 1410

Breckenridge A 1995 Science, medicine and clinical pharmacology. British Journal of Clinical Pharmacology 40: 1

[2]Gold H 1952 'The proper study of mankind is man'. American Journal of Medicine 12: 619. The title is taken from *An Essay on Man* by Alexander Pope (English poet, 1688–1744); the whole passage is relevant to modern clinical pharmacology and drug therapy; it is best read aloud whether the reader be alone or in company.
Know then thyself, presume no God to scan,
The proper study of mankind is man,
Placed on this isthmus of a middle state,
A being darkly wise, and rudely great:
With too much knowledge for the sceptic side,
With too much weakness for the stoic's pride,
 He hangs between; in doubt to act or rest;
In doubt to deem himself a god or beast;
In doubt his mind or body to prefer;
Born but to die, and reas'ning but to err;
Alike in ignorance, his reason such,
Whether he thinks too little or too much;
Chaos of thought and passion, all confused;
Still by himself abused, or disabused;
Created half to rise, and half to fall;
Great lord of all things, yet a prey to all;
Sole judge of truth, in endless error hurled;
The Glory, jest and riddle of the world!

[3]*Self-experimentation* has always been a feature of clinical pharmacology. A survey of 250 members of the Dutch Society of Clinical Pharmacology evoked 102 responders of whom 55 had done experiments on themselves (largely for convenience) (van Everdingen et al 1990 Lancet 336: 1448). A spectacular example occurred at the 1983 meeting of the American Urological Association at Las Vegas, during a lecture on pharmacologically-induced penile erection, when the lecturer stepped out from behind the lectern to demonstrate personally the efficacy of the technique (Zorgniotti A W 1990 Lancet 336: 1200).

Crooks J 1983 Drug epidemiology and clinical pharmacology. Their contribution to patient care. British Journal of Clinical Pharmacology 16: 351

Dollery C T 1996 Clinical pharmocology: future prospects for the discipline. British Journal of Clinical Pharmacology 42: 137

Dukes G 1990 Clinical pharmacology and primary health care in Europe. European Journal of Clinical Pharmacology 38: 315

Grahame-Smith D G 1991 Clinical Pharmacology. Roles and responsibilities in academic research. British Journal of Clinical Pharmacology 32: 151

Laurence D R 1989 Ethics and law in clinical pharmacology. British Journal of Clinical Pharmacology 27: 715

Vane J, O'Grady J 1991 Clinical pharmacology in the pharmaceutical industry. British Journal of Clinical Pharmacology 32: 155

Walley T 1995 Drugs, money and society. British Journal of Clinical Pharmacology 39: 343

The following report, though based on UK experience, has wider relevance:

Walley T, Bligh J, Orme M, Breckenridge A 1994 I. Clinical pharmacology and therapeutics in undergraduate medical education in the UK: current status. British Journal of Clinical Pharmacology 37: 129; II. The future: 137

Discovery and development of drugs

SYNOPSIS

- Preclinical drug development. Discovery of new drugs in the laboratory is an exercise in prediction.
- Techniques of discovery. Sophisticated molecular modelling allows precise design of potential new therapeutic substances and new technologies have increased the rate of development of potential medicines.
- Preclinical studies in animals. A candidate molecule is first studied in vitro and in animals before being tested on humans.
- Prediction. Failures of prediction occur and a drug may be abandoned at any stage, including after marketing. New drug development is a colossally expensive and commercially driven activity.
- Orphan drugs and diseases.

Preclinical drug development

Pharmacology and medicinal chemistry have transformed medicine from an intellectual exercise in diagnosis into a powerful force for the relief of human disease (C T Dollery 1994).[1]

The development of new medicines (drugs) is an exercise in **prediction** from laboratory studies in vitro and in vivo (animals) which forecast what the agent will do to man. Medicinal therapeutics rests on **the two great supporting pillars of pharmacology:**

- **Selectivity**: the desired effect alone is obtained; 'We must learn to aim, learn to aim with chemical substances' (Paul Ehrlich)[2]
- **Dose**: ' ... The dose alone decides that something is no poison' (Paracelsus).[3]

For decades the rational discovery of new medicines has depended on modifications of the molecu-

---

[1] In this chapter we are grateful for permission from Professor Sir Colin Dollery to quote directly and indirectly from his Harveian Oration, 'Medicine and the pharmacological revolution' (1994) Journal of the Royal College of Physicians of London 28: 59–69.

[2] Paul Ehrlich (1845–1915), German scientist who pioneered the scientific approach to drug discovery. The 606th organic arsenical that he tested against spirochaetes (in animals) became a successful medicine (Salvarsan 1910); it and a minor variant were used against syphilis until superseded by penicillin in 1945.

[3] Paracelsus (1493–1541) was a controversial figure who has been portrayed as both ignorant and superstitious. He had no medical degree; he burned the classical medical works (Galen, Avicenna) before his lectures in Basel (Switzerland) and had to leave the city following a dispute about fees with a prominent churchman. He died in Salzburg (Austria) either as a result of a drunken debauch or because he was thrown down a steep incline by 'hitmen' employed by jealous local physicians. *But he was right about the dose.*

lar structures of the increasing numbers of known natural chemical mediators and it had even been predicted that the pace of discovery would decline before the end of the current century as classic pharmacology and pathophysiology reached the limits of application and invention. This prediction has perished before the astonishing evolution of *molecular medicine* (including recombinant DNA technology) of the past 20 years.

The discovery of a truly novel medicine, i.e. one that does something valuable that had previously not been possible (or that does safely what could only previously have been achieved with substantial risk), is most likely when the development programme is founded on precise knowledge, at molecular level, of the biological processes it is desired to change. The commercial rewards of a successful product are potentially enormous and provide a massive incentive to developers to invest and risk huge sums of money.

> Studies of signal transduction, the fundamental process by which cells talk to one another as intracellular proteins transmit signals from the surface of the cell to the nucleus inside, have opened an entirely new approach to the development of therapeutic agents that can target discrete steps in the body's elaborate pathways of chemical reactions. The opportunities are endless.[4]

As a consequence of the exploitation of this technology more potential medicines will be produced and more and more doctors will become involved in clinical testing; it is expedient that they should have some acquaintance with the events and processes that precede their involvement.

New drug development proceeds thus:

- Idea or hypothesis
- Design and synthesis of substances
- Studies on tissues and whole animals (preclinical studies)
- Studies in man (clinical studies)
- Grant of an official licence to make therapeutic claims and to sell
- Post-licensing (marketing) studies of safety and comparisons with other medicines.

It will be obvious from the account that follows that drug development is an extremely arduous, highly technical and enormously expensive operation. Successful developments (1% of compounds that proceed to full test eventually become licensed medicines) must carry the cost of the failures (99%).[5] It is also obvious that such programmes are likely to be carried to completion only when the organisations and the individuals within them are motivated overall by the challenge to succeed and to serve society, as well as to make money.

TECHNIQUES OF DISCOVERY

The newer technologies, the impact of which have yet to be fully felt, include:

Molecular modelling aided by three-dimensional computer graphics (including virtual reality) allows the design of structures based on new and known molecules to enhance their desired, and to eliminate their undesired, properties to create highly selective targeted compounds. In principle all molecular structures capable of binding to a single high-affinity site can be modelled.

Combinatorial chemistry involves the random mixing and matching of large numbers of chemical building blocks (amino acids, nucleotides, simple chemicals) to produce 'libraries' of all possible combinations. This technology can generate billions of

---

[4] Culliton B J 1994 Nature Medicine 1: 1

[5] The cost of development of a new chemical entity (NCE) (a novel molecule not previously tested in humans) from synthesis to market (general clinical use) is estimated at US$ 250 million; the process may take as much as 15 years (including up to 10 years of clinical studies), which is relevant to duration of patent life and so to ultimate profitability; if the developer does not see profit at the end of the process, the investment will not be made. The drug may fail at any stage, including the ultimate, i.e. at the official regulatory body after all the development costs have been incurred. It may also fail (due to adverse effects) within the first year after marketing, which constitutes a catastrophe (in reputation and finance) for the developer as well as for some of the patients.

Pirated copies of full regulatory dossiers have substantial black market value to competitor companies who have used them even to leap-frog the original developer to obtain a licence for their unresearched copied molecule. Dossiers may be enormous, even one million pages or the electronic equivalent, the latter being very convenient as it allows instant searching.

new compounds that are initially evaluated using automated robotic high-throughput screening devices that can handle thousands of compounds a day.[6] These screens utilise radio-labelled ligand displacement on single human receptor subtypes or enzymes on nucleated (eukaryotic) cells. If the screen records a positive response the compound is further investigated using traditional laboratory methods, and the molecule is manipulated to enhance selectivity and / or potency (above).

Proteins as medicines: biotechnology. The targets of most drugs are proteins (cell receptors, enzymes) and it is only lack of technology that has hitherto prevented the exploitation of proteins (and peptides) as medicines. The technology is now available. But yet there are great practical problems of getting the proteins to the target site in the body (they are digested when swallowed and cross cell membranes with difficulty).

Biotechnology involves the use of recombinant DNA technology / genetic engineering to clone and express human genes, for example, in microbial, *Escherichia coli* or yeast, cells so that they manufacture proteins that medicinal chemists have not been able to synthesise; they also produce hormones and autacoids in commercial amounts (such as insulin and growth hormone, erythropoietins, cell growth factors and plasminogen activators, interferons, vaccines and immune antibodies). *Transgenic animals* (that breed true for the gene) are also being developed as models for human disease as well as for production of medicines.

The *polymerase chain reaction* (PCR) is an alternative to bacterial cloning. This is a method of gene amplification that does not require living cells; it takes place in vitro and can produce (in a cost-effective way) commercial quantities of pure potential medicines.

Genetic medicines. Synthetic oligonucleotides are being developed to target defined sites on DNA sequences or genes (double strand DNA: triplex approach) or messenger RNA (antisense approach) so that the production of disease-related proteins is blocked. These oligonucleotides offer prospects of treatment for cancers and viruses without harming healthy tissues.[7]

Gene therapy of human genetic disorders is, 'a strategy in which nucleic acid, usually in the form of DNA, is administered to modify the genetic repertoire for therapeutic purposes' (e.g. cystic fibrosis). 'The era of "the gene as drug" is clearly upon us' (R G Crystal).

Immunopharmacology. Understanding of the molecular basis of immune responses has allowed the definition of mechanisms by which cellular function is altered by a legion of local hormones or autacoids in, for example, infections, cancer, autoimmune diseases, organ transplant rejection. These processes present targets for therapeutic intervention. Hence the rise of immunopharmacology.

PET (positron emission tomography) allows non-invasive pharmacokinetic and pharmacodynamic measurements in previously inaccessible sites, e.g. the brain in intact humans and animals.

Older approaches to discovery of new medicines that continue in use include:

- *Animal models of human disease* or an aspect of it of varying relevance to man
- *Natural products*, the basis for many of today's medicines for pain, inflammation, cancer, cardiovascular problems, etc. Modern technology for screening has revived interest and intensified the search by multinational pharmaceutical companies which scour the world for leads from microorganisms (in soil or

---

[6] 'It is too early to say what success these programmes may have but automation of assays, possibly coupled to similar automation of syntheses, promises to speed up the search for new leads which is the rate-limiting step in the introduction of really novel therapeutic agents. Their value in medicine will depend upon the significance of the control mechanism concerned in the pathogenesis of a disease process. Critics fear that the result may well be large numbers of drugs in search of a disease to treat' (C T Dollery, ibidem). The demand for competent clinical trialists, already great, will increase to meet the demand; the financial rewards to competent (and honest) clinical trialists are great, in the competitive world of drug introduction (see also McNamee D 1995 Lancet 345: 1167).

[7] Cohen J S, Hogan M E 1994 The new genetic medicines. Scientific American (Dec): 50–55.

sewage or even from insects entombed in amber 40 million years ago), from fungi, plants and animals. Developing countries in the tropics (with their luxuriant natural resources) are prominent targets in this search and have justly complained of exploitation ('gene robbery'). Many now require formal profit-sharing agreements to allow such searches

- *Traditional medicine*, which is being studied for possible leads to usefully active compounds
- *Modifications of the structures of known drugs*; these are obviously likely to produce more agents having similar basic properties, but may deliver worthwhile improvements. It is in this area that the much-complained-of *me-too* and *me-again* drugs are developed (sometimes purely for commercial reasons)
- *Random screening* of synthesised and natural products
- New *uses for drugs already in general use* as a result of intelligent observation and serendipity,[8] or advancing knowledge of molecular mechanisms, e.g. aspirin for antithrombosis effect.

Preclinical studies in animals[9]

In general, the following tests are undertaken:

- *Pharmacodynamics*: to explore actions relevant to the proposed therapeutic use, and other effects at that dose
- *Pharmacokinetics*: to discover how the drug is distributed in and disposed of by the body
- *Toxicology*: to see whether and how the drug causes injury (in vitro tests and intact animals) in:
  — single dose studies (acute toxicity)
  — repeated-dose studies (subacute, intermediate and chronic or longterm toxicology)
  — the duration of repeated-dose studies will range as shown below.

INTENDED DURATION OF USE IN MAN	DURATION OF STUDIES ANIMALS
Single dose (or several doses on one day)	14 days
up to 10 days	28 days
up to 30 days	90 days
beyond 30 days	180 days

Special toxicology involves areas in which a particularly horrible drug accident might occur on a substantial scale; all involve interaction with genetic material or its expression in cell division.

— *Mutagenicity* (genotoxicity). A bacterial mutagenicity test which demonstrates the induction of point (gene) mutations is always required. Some mutations result in the development of cancer.

— Definitive *carcinogenicity* (oncogenicity) tests are often not required prior to the early studies in man unless there is serious reason to be suspicious of the drug, e.g. if the mutagenicity test is unsatisfactory; the molecular structure, including likely metabolites in man, gives rise to suspicion; or the histopathology in repeated-dose animal studies raises suspicions.

Full scale (most of the animal's life) carcinogenicity tests will generally only be required if the drug is to be given to man for above one year, or it resembles a known human carcinogen, or it is mutagenic (in circumstances relevant to human use) or it has major organ-specific hormonal agonist action.

It may be asked why any novel compound should be given to man before full-scale formal carcinogenicity studies are completed. The answers are that animal tests are uncertain predictors,[10] that such a requirement would make socially desirable drug development expensive to a seriously detrimental degree, or might even cause potentially valuable novel ventures to cease. For example, tests would have to be done on numerous compounds that are eventually abandoned for other reasons.

---

[8] Serendipity is the faculty of making fortunate discoveries by general sagacity or by accident: the word derives from a fairy tale about three princes of Serendip (Sri Lanka) who had this happy faculty.

[9] Mouse, rat, hamster, guinea pig, rabbit, cat, dog, monkey. Not all are used for any one drug.

[10] A sardonic comment on the relevance for man of carcinogenicity tests in animals was made by investigators who induced cancer in animals using American 'dimes' (10 cent coin) and the plastic of credit cards. They advised the US government to consider banning money as unsafe for humans (Moore G E et al 1977 Journal of the American Medical Association 238: 397).

This may seem right or wrong, but it is how things are at present.

Reproduction studies have to be extensive because of the diversity of physiological processes that may be affected (and because of the potentially horrific consequences of error in this field; see thalidomide): tests include gametes (male and female); fertility; implantation; intrauterine growth into embryo and fetus; parturition; postnatal development (suckling, lactation); later development (growth and behaviour and intellectual function of progeny and their fertility); second generation effects.

It is plain that all the above tests constitute a major laboratory exercise requiring great and diverse scientific skills and big money.

ETHICS[11]

No one will read the above scheme with satisfaction and some people will read it with disgust. Experienced toxicologists point out that:

> The majority of toxicity tests [which particularly are subject to ethical criticism] are firmly based on studies in whole animals, because only in them is it possible to approach the complexity of organization of body systems in humans, to explore any consequences of variable absorption, metabolism and excretion, and to reveal not only direct toxic effects but also those of a secondary or indirect nature due to induced abnormalities in integrative mechanisms, or distant effects of a toxic metabolite produced in one organ that acts on another.[12]

The use of animals would be totally unjustified if results useful to man could not be obtained. In many known respects animals are similar to man, but in many respects they are not. Increasingly, the low-prediction tests are being defined and eliminated. It will be a long time before in vitro tests become sufficiently scientifically robust to eliminate the need for tests in whole animals, but we welcome the progress that is being made towards this end. The incentive to eliminate whole animal tests is not only ethical, it is economic, for whole animals are very expensive to breed and house and keep in health. The European Union instructs researchers to choose non-(whole) animal methods if they are 'scientifically satisfactory [and] reasonably and practically available'.

Prediction

It is frequently pointed out that regulatory guidelines are not rigid requirements to be universally applied. But whatever the intention, they do tend to be treated as minimum requirements if only because research directors fear to risk holding up their expensive coordinated programmes with disagreements that result in their having to go back to the laboratory, with consequent delay and financial loss.

Knowledge of the *mode of action* of a potential new drug obviously greatly enhances prediction from animal studies of what will happen in man. Whenever practicable such knowledge should be obtained; sometimes this is quite easy, but sometimes it is impossible. Many drugs have been introduced safely without such knowledge, the later acquisition of which has not always made an important difference to their use, e.g. antimicrobials. The pharmacological studies are integrated with those of the toxicologist to build up a picture of the undesired as well as the desired drug effects.

In pharmacological testing the investigators know what they are looking for and choose the experiments to gain their objectives.

In toxicological testing the investigators have less clear ideas of what they are looking for; they are screening for risk, unexpected as well as predicted and certain major routines must be done. Toxicity testing is therefore liable to become mindless routine to meet regulatory requirements to a greater extent than are the pharmacological studies. The predictive value of special toxicology (above) is particularly controversial.

---

[11] An admirable discussion of the issues will be found in Paton W 1984 Man and mouse. Oxford, London and in Zbinden G 1990 Alternatives to animal experimentation. Trends in Pharmacological Sciences 11: 104.

[12] Brimblecombe R W, Dayan A D 1993 In: Burley D M, Clarke J M, Lasagna L (eds) Pharmaceutical medicine. Arnold, London.

All drugs are poisons if enough is given and the task of the toxicologist is to find out whether, where and how a compound acts as a poison to animals, and to give an opinion on the significance of the data in relation to risks likely to be run by human beings. This will remain a nearly impossible task until molecular explanations of all effects can be provided. Toxicologists are in an unenviable position. When a useful drug is safely introduced they are considered to have done no more than their duty. When an accident occurs they are invited to explain how this failure of prediction came about. When they predict that a chemical is unsafe in a major way for man, this prediction is never tested.

DRUG QUALITY

It is easy for an investigator or prescriber, interested in pharmacology, toxicology and therapeutics, to forget the fundamental importance of chemical and pharmaceutical aspects. An impure, unstable drug or formulation is useless. Pure drugs that remain pure drugs after 5 years of storage in hot, damp climates are vital to therapeutics. The record of manufacturers in providing this is impressive.

CONCLUSION ON PRECLINICAL TESTING

As drugs are developed and promoted for longterm use in more and relatively trivial conditions, e.g. minor anxiety or mild arterial hypertension, and affluent societies become less and less willing to tolerate small physical or mental discomforts, the demand for and the supply of new medicines will continue to increase. Only profound knowledge of molecular mechanisms will reduce risk in the introduction of new drugs. Occasional failures of prediction are inevitable, with consequent public outcry.

Limited resources of scientific manpower and money will not be used to the best advantage if the public shock over thalidomide (p. 69) and subsequent events is allowed to express itself in governmental regulations requiring a plethora of expensive tests (and toxicity testing is very expensive), many of them of dubious meaning for anything other than the animal concerned. Such a policy would prevent industrial laboratories from devoting resources to investigation of molecular mechanisms of drug action, in the knowledge of which alone lies health with safety.

When the preclinical testing has been completed to the satisfaction of the developer and of the national or international regulatory agency, it is time to administer the drug to man and so to launch the experimental programme that will decide whether the drug is only a drug or whether it is also a medicine. This is the subject of the next chapter.

Orphan drugs and diseases

A free market economy is liable to leave untreated, rare diseases, e.g. some cancers (in all countries), and some common diseases, e.g. parasitic infections (in poor countries).

Where a drug is not developed into a usable medicine because the costs will not be recovered by the developer then it is known as an orphan drug, and the disease is an orphan disease; the sufferer is a health orphan.[13] Drugs for rare diseases inevitably must often be licensed on less than ideal amounts of clinical evidence.

The remedy for these situations lies in government itself undertaking drug development (which is likely to be inefficient) or in government-offered incentives, e.g. tax relief, subsidies, exclusive marketing rights, to pharmaceutical companies and, in the case of poor countries, international aid programmes; such programmes are being implemented.[14]

GUIDE TO FURTHER READING

Black J W 1986 Pharmacology: analysis and exploration. British Medical Journal 293: 252

Bugg C E, Carcon W M, Montgomery J A 1993 Drugs by design. Scientific American (Dec): 60

[13] At the time of writing the cost of treating a patient having the rare genetic Gaucher's liposome storage disease with genetically engineered enzyme is US$ 145 to 400 000 per annum according to severity. Who can and will pay? More such situations will occur.

[14] Official recognition of orphan drug status is accorded in the USA (pop 240M) where the relevant disease affects fewer than 200 000 people; in Japan (pop 121M) for fewer than 50 000 people.

Cohen J S, Hogan M E 1994 The new genetic medicines. Scientific American. (Dec): 50

Crystal R G 1995 The gene as a drug. Nature Medicine 1: 15

DiMasi J A 1995 Success rates for new drugs entering clinical testing in the United States. Clinical Pharmacology and Therapeutics 58: 1

DiMasi J A, Seibring M A, Lasagna L 1994 New drug development in the United States from 1963 to 1992. Clinical Pharmacology and Therapeutics 55: 609

Editorial 1994 Pharmaceuticals from plants: great potential, few funds. Lancet 343: 1513

Hillman A L et al 1991 Avoiding bias in the conduct and reporting of cost-effectiveness: research sponsored by pharmaceutical companies. New England Journal of Medicine 324: 1362

Lachmann P 1992 The use of animals in research. British Medical Journal 305: 1

Lasagna L 1982 Will all new drugs become orphans? Clinical Pharmacology and Therapeutics 31: 285

Lasagna L 1987 On assuring pharmacotherapeutic progress in the 21st century. British Journal of Clinical Pharmacology 23: 659

Meyer B R 1992 Biotechnology and therapeutics: Experimental treatments and limited resources. Clinical Pharmacology and Therapeutics 51: 359

Sykes R 1994 Innovation in the pharmaceutical industry. British Medical Journal 309: 422

Evaluation of drugs in man

SYNOPSIS

This chapter is about evidence-based drug therapy.

New drugs are gradually introduced via clinical pharmacological studies in rising numbers of healthy and/or patient volunteers until enough information has been gained to justify a formal therapeutic study. This is usually a randomised controlled trial where a precisely framed question is posed and answered by treating equivalent groups of patients in different ways.

The key to the ethics of such studies is informed consent by patients, efficient scientific design and review by an independent Research Ethics Committee. The key interpretative factors in the analysis of trial results are calculations of confidence intervals and of statistical significance. Results should be expressed not only as percentage differences but also as the number of patients who have to be treated to obtain one desired outcome.

Finally, surveillance studies detect rare adverse effects and allow accurate comparisons of safety; they also define patterns of drug use in the community. Further trials to compare the new medicine with existing medicines are also necessary.

Topics include

- Experimental therapeutics
- Ethics of research
- Rational introduction of a new drug
- Need for statistics
- Therapeutic trials
  Concepts and terms
  Size and sensitivity of trials
- Meta-analysis
- Research results
- Pharmacoepidemiology.

Experimental therapeutics

As the number of potential medicines produced increases, the problem of who to test them on grows. Clearly there are two main groups: healthy volunteers and volunteer patients (plus, very rarely, non-volunteer patients). It is evident that some drug actions can be demonstrated on healthy people (anticoagulant, anaesthetic) whereas others cannot (antiparkinsonian, antimicrobial) so that to try the latter on healthy volunteers to obtain pharmacokinetic and safety data involves treating man formally as an experimental animal, risking toxicity, however remotely, to obtain information of no benefit to the individual subject; this is increasingly often done and it poses ethical problems (see below).

There are three main reasons why doctors should have a grounding in knowledge of the principles of experimental therapeutics:

1. More and more doctors are personally involved.
2. The results of good research alter clinical practice.
3. The study provides an exercise in ethical and logical thinking (which is always a good thing although it does require a little effort). But plainly doctors cannot read in detail and evaluate for themselves all the published studies (often hundreds) that *might* influence their practice. They therefore turn to specialist review articles and abstracts,[1] including meta-analyses (p. 60) for guidance. But readers must approach these critically.

Ethics of research in man[2]

Modern medicine is accused of callous application of science to human problems and of subordinating the interest of the individual to those of the group (society).[3] Official regulatory bodies rightly require scientific evaluation of drugs. Drug developers need to satisfy the official regulators and they also seek to persuade an increasingly sophisticated medical profession to prescribe their products. For these reasons scientific drug evaluation as described here is likely to increase in volume and the doctors involved will be held responsible for the ethics of what they do even if they played no personal part in the study design.

Therefore we provide a brief discussion of some relevant ethical aspects (and particularly of the randomised controlled trial).

RESEARCH[4] INVOLVING HUMAN SUBJECTS

This may be:

- **Therapeutic:** that which may actually have a therapeutic effect or provide information that can be used to help the participating subjects
- **Nontherapeutic:** that which provides information that cannot be of direct use to them, e.g. healthy volunteers always and patients sometimes.

It may also be *experimental* (involving psychologically intrusive or physically invasive intervention) or solely *observational* (including much epidemiology).

The right to choose

People have the right to choose for themselves whether or not they will participate in research, i.e. they have the right to self-determination or autonomy. They should be given whatever information is necessary for making an informed choice (consent).

---

[1] Many review articles (and there are whole journals devoted to reviews) are of poor quality, merely reporting uncritically the opinions of the original authors. But high-quality critical reviews are to be treasured. A journal titled Evidence-Based Medicine was launched in 1995.

[2] For extensive practical detail, see: *International ethical guidelines for biomedical research involving human subjects;* prepared by the Council for International Organizations of Medical Sciences (CIOMS) in collaboration with the World Health Organization (WHO): Geneva, 1993. (WHO publications are available in all UN member countries.)

[3] *The World Medical Association* declaration of Helsinki (Hong Kong revision 1989) states that 'Concern for the interests of the subject must always prevail over the interests of science and society'. We would qualify this thus: It is not for official bodies totally to forbid public-spirited people who understand what they are doing, from volunteering for research to benefit society. Naturally, Research Ethics Committees will look closely at such proposals. *The General Assembly of the United Nations* adopted in 1966 the International Covenant on Civil and Political Rights, of which Article 7 states, 'In particular, no one shall be subjected without his free consent to medical or scientific experimentation'. (This means that subjects are entitled to know that they are being entered into research even though the research be thought to be 'harmless'.) But yet there are people who cannot give (informed) consent, e.g. mental illness. The need for special procedures for such is now recognised, for there is a consensus that they must not be allowed to become therapeutic 'orphans', and yet they need special protection.

[4] 'The definition of research continues to present difficulties. The distinction between medical research and innovative medical practice derives from the *intent*. In medical *practice* the sole intention is to benefit the *individual patient* consulting the clinician, not to gain knowledge of general benefit, though such knowledge may incidentally emerge from the clinical experience gained. In medical *research* the primary intention is to advance knowledge so that *patients in general* may benefit; the individual patient may or may not benefit directly.' (Royal College of Physicians of London 1996 Guidelines on the practice of ethics committees in medical research involving human subjects).

The issue of (informed) *consent*[5] bulks large in discussions of the ethics of research involving human subjects and is a principal concern of the Research Ethics Committees that are now the norm in medical research.

Some dislike the word 'experiment' in relation to man, thinking that its mere use implies a degree of impropriety in what is done. It is better, however, that all should recognise the true meaning of the word, 'to ascertain or establish by trial',[6] that the benefits of modern medicine derive almost wholly from experimentation and that some risk is inseparable from much medical advance. The duty of all doctors lies in ensuring that in their desire to help patients in general they should never allow themselves to put the individual who has sought their aid at any disadvantage, for 'the scientist or physician has no right to choose martyrs for society',[7] i.e. the ethical principle of *non-maleficence*.

Physicians deal with individuals and have sometimes argued against the statistical therapeutic trial that it does not tell what will happen to any one individual who consults them. This is obviously true, but the knowledge gained from such studies that, with a treatment, $x\%$ recover, $y\%$ improve and $z\%$ are unchanged, with details of unwanted effects, provides a better basis for the choice of therapy for individuals than the often divergent clinical impressions of doctors.

It is, of course, only proper to perform a therapeutic trial when the doctors genuinely do not know which treatment is best, and when they are prepared to withdraw individual patients or to stop the whole trial when at any time they become convinced that it is in the patients' interest to do so.

If it is truly not known whether one treatment is better than another (i.e. there is equipoise)[8] then nothing is lost, at least in theory, by allotting patients at random to those treatments under test, and it is in everybody's interest that good treatments should be adopted and bad treatments abandoned as soon as possible. It is, of course, more difficult to justify testing a new treatment when existing treatments are good than when they are bad, and this difficulty is likely to grow. It involves weighing the needs of future patients who may benefit from the results of a study against those of the patients who are actually taking part, some of whom will receive new (and possibly less effective) treatment, i.e. the principle of *justice*.[9]

The ethics of the randomised controlled trial

Ethical objections have always, often justly, been raised to the *conduct* of individual randomised controlled trials, but of recent years these have been extended to the *principles* on which such trials are based.

It is our view that the critics do not fully understand that history, including recent history, is replete with examples of even the best-intentioned doctors being wrong about the efficacy and safety of (new) treatments and that this situation can and should be remedied by the ethical employment of science.

This has been well summarised in a Report:[10]

> An analysis of the ethical problems of therapeutic trials might begin with a question long familiar to moral philosophy: what is the nature and degree of

---

[5] Consent procedures (e.g. information, especially on risks) bulk larger in research, particularly where it is non-therapeutic, than they do in medical practice.

[6] Oxford English Dictionary.

[7] Kety S. Quoted by Beecher H K 1959 Journal of the American Medical Association 169: 461.

[8] In this situation it has been urged that it need be no concern of patients that they are entered into a research study. Even if it should be the case that there is true equipoise, this (convenient) belief does not allow the requirement for (informed) consent to be bypassed; and doctors often have opinions that would be of interest to patients if they were told of them, which they may not be.

[9] In a disabling disease having no proved treatment, the advent of a potentially effective medicine, unavoidably in *limited supply*, heightens the emotions of all concerned. This was the situation for the first study of interferon-β_{1b} in multiple sclerosis. The manufacturer, seeking to be fair, arranged a lottery for patients (having a certified diagnosis) to enter a randomised placebo-controlled trial. Some patients, when they understood that they might be allocated placebo, became angry (and said so on television). (British Medical Journal (1993) 307: 958: Lancet (1993) 343: 169). It is not obvious how this situation could have been made fairer.

[10] European Journal of Clinical Pharmacology (1980) 18: 129.

certitude required for an ethical decision? More precisely, is there any ethically relevant difference between the use of statistical methods and the use of other ways of knowing, such as experience, common sense, guessing, etc.? When decisions are to be made in uncertainty, is it more or less ethical to choose and abide by statistical methods of defining 'certitude' than to be guided by one's hunch or striking experience? These questions are raised by the assertion that it is ethically imperative to conclude a clinical trial when a 'trend' appears . . . the choice of statistical methods can constitute in many circumstances an acceptable ethical approach to the problem of decision in uncertainty.

As physician-investigators seek knowledge about safety and efficacy of medicines, which is a social good, the dignity of individuals must not be overridden. The therapeutic trial is both ethically required for the social good of more effective medical care and is capable of being designed in ways which respect the wellbeing and rights of individual participants.

Ethical conduct of clinical research

The objective must be that no patients should be worse off than they might have been in the hands of a reasonable and competent physician.

Injury to research subjects

The question of compensation for accidental (physical) injury due to participation in research is a vexed one. Plainly there are substantial differences between the position of healthy volunteers (whether or not they are paid) and that of patients who may benefit and, in some cases, who may be prepared to accept even serious risk for the chance of gain. There is no simple answer. But the topic must always be addressed in any research carrying risk, including the risk of withholding known effective treatment.

The CIOMS/WHO guidelines[2] state:

Research subjects who suffer physical injury as a result of their participation are entitled to such financial or other assistance as would compensate them equitably for any temporary or permanent

impairment or disability. In the case of death, their dependants are entitled to material compensation. The right to compensation may not be waived.

In some societies the right to compensation for accidental injury is not acknowledged. Therefore, when giving their informed consent to participate, research subjects should be told whether there is provision for compensation in case of physical injury, and the circumstances in which they or their dependants would receive it.

There is no consensus on the matter of compensation for psychological injury.

Rational introduction of a new drug

When studies in animals predict that a new molecule may be a useful medicine, i.e. effective and safe in relation to its benefits, then the time has come to put it to the test in man.

We devote substantial space to clinical evaluation of drugs because doctors need to be able to scan reports of therapeutic studies to decide whether they are likely to be reliable and to deserve to influence their prescribing.

When a new chemical entity offers a possibility of doing something that has not been done before or of doing something familiar in a different or better way, it can be seen to be worth testing. But where it is a new member of a familiar class of drug, potential advantage may be harder to detect.

Yet these 'me-too' drugs are often worth testing. Prediction from animal studies of modest but useful clinical advantage is particularly uncertain and therefore if the new drug seems reasonably effective and safe in animals it is also reasonable to test it in man: 'It is possible to waste too much time in animal studies before testing a drug in man'.[11]

Phases of clinical development

Human experiments progress in a commonsense manner that is conventionally divided in four phases.

---

[11] Brodie B B 1962 Clinical Pharmacology and Therapeutics 3: 374.

These phases are divisions of convenience in what is a continuous expanding process beginning with a single subject closely observed in the laboratory and proceeding in tens of subjects (healthy subjects and volunteer patients) through hundreds of patients, to thousands before the drug is agreed to be a medicine by a national or international regulatory authority and is licensed for general prescribing (though this is by no means the end of the evaluation). The process may be abandoned at any stage.

● **Phase 1. Clinical pharmacology (20–50 subjects)**

— Healthy[12] volunteers or volunteer patients, according to the class of drug and its safety

— Pharmacokinetics (absorption, distribution, metabolism, excretion)

— Pharmacodynamics (biological effects) where practicable; tolerance, safety, efficacy.

● **Phase 2. Clinical investigation (50–300)**

— Patients

— Pharmacokinetics and pharmacodynamics in dose-ranging in expanding, carefully controlled studies for efficacy and safety.

● **Phase 3. Formal therapeutic trials (randomised controlled trials; 250–1000+)**

— Efficacy on a substantial scale; safety; comparison with existing drugs.

● **Phase 4. Post-licensing (marketing) studies (2000–10 000+)**

— Surveillance for safety and efficacy: further formal therapeutic trials, especially comparisons with other drugs.

OFFICIAL REGULATORY GUIDELINES AND REQUIREMENTS

For studies in man (see also Ch. 5) these ordinarily include:

● Studies of *pharmacokinetics* and (when other manufacturers have similar products) of *bioequivalence* (equal bioavailability) with alternative products.

● *Therapeutic trials* (reported in detail) that sub-

stantiate the safety and efficacy of the drug under likely conditions of use, e.g. a drug for longterm use in a common condition will require a total of at least 1000 patients (preferably more), of which at least 100 have been treated continuously for about one year. At least three independent trials are likely to be required.

● *Special groups.* If the drug will be used in, e.g. the elderly, then elderly people should be studied if there are reasons for thinking they may react to or handle the drug differently. The same applies to children and to pregnant women (who present a special problem) and who, if they are not studied may be excluded from licensed uses and so become health 'orphans'. Studies in patients having disease that affects drug metabolism and elimination may be needed.

● *Fixed-dose combination* products will require explicit justification for each component.

● *Interaction studies* with other drugs likely to be taken simultaneously. Plainly all possible combinations cannot be evaluated; an intelligent choice, based on knowledge of pharmacodynamics and pharmacokinetics, is made.

● The application for a licence for general use (Product Licence) should include a draft *Data* (information) *Sheet* (or Summary of Product Characteristics)[13] for prescribers and sometimes for patients. This should include information on the form of the product (tablet, capsule, sustained-release, liquid, etc), its uses, dosage (adults, children, elderly where appropriate), contraindications (strong recommendation), warnings and precautions (less strong), side-effects/adverse reactions, overdose and how to treat it.

THERAPEUTIC INVESTIGATIONS

The two classes of endpoint or outcome of therapeutic investigations are:

● The therapeutic effect itself, e.g. sleep, eradication of infection, and/or
● A factor reliably related to the therapeutic effect, a surrogate effect, e.g. blood lipids or glucose, or blood pressure.

---

[12] Moderate to severe adverse events have occurred in about 0.5% of healthy subjects (Orme M et al 1989 British Journal of Clinical Pharmacology 27: 125. Sibille M et al 1992 European Journal of Clinical Pharmacology 42: 393).

[13] Medicines need instruction manuals just as do domestic appliances.

Use of surrogate effects presupposes that the disease process is fully understood. They are employed in diseases for which the true therapeutic effect, i.e. healthy life free from complications, can be measured only by studying large numbers of patients over years. Such longterm (outcome) studies are indeed necessary but are impracticable on organisational, financial and sometimes ethical grounds prior to releasing all new drugs for general prescription. It is in such areas as these that techniques of large-scale surveillance for efficacy, as well as for safety, under conditions of ordinary use (below), are needed to supplement the necessarily smaller and shorter formal therapeutic trials employing surrogate effects.

Therapeutic evaluation

Therapeutic evaluation is conducted in two principal ways:

- *Formal therapeutic trials* (*experimental* cohort studies)
- *Surveillance programmes*, e.g. case-control studies, and *observational* cohort studies (large-scale monitoring for efficacy and/or adverse reactions) (see p. 62).

When a new drug is being developed, the first therapeutic trials are devised to find out the best that the drug can do (and how it works) under conditions ideal for showing efficacy, e.g. uncomplicated disease of mild-to-moderate severity in patients taking no other drugs, with carefully supervised administration by specialist doctors. Interest lies particularly in patients who complete a full course of treatment. If the drug is ineffective in these circumstances there is no point in proceeding with an expensive development programme. Such studies are sometimes called (a little inappropriately) '*explanatory*' or 'fastidious' trials.

If the drug is found useful in these trials, then it becomes desirable next to find out how closely the ideal may be approached in the rough and tumble of routine medical practice: in patients of all ages, at all stages of disease, with complications, taking other drugs and relatively unsupervised. Interest continues in all patients from the moment they are entered into the trial and it is maintained if they fail to complete, or even to start, the treatment; what is

wanted is to know the outcome in all patients deemed suitable for therapy, not only in those who successfully complete therapy.[14] The reasons some drop out may be related to aspects of the treatment. Such trials are therefore analysed according to the clinicians' *initial* intention (*intention-to-treat analysis*), i.e. investigators are not allowed to risk introducing bias by exercising their own judgement as to who should or should not be excluded from the analysis. In these real life, or 'naturalistic', conditions the drug may not perform so well, e.g. minor adverse effects may now cause patient noncompliance which had been avoided by supervision and enthusiasm in the early trials. These naturalistic studies are sometimes called '*pragmatic*' trials.

Formal therapeutic trials are expensive and are hard to administer. Surveillance studies are less precise but compensate for this by their convenience and/or large size and closeness to the realities of ordinary medical practice. **Formal therapeutic trials** are **unlikely** to reveal:

- Adverse effects that are uncommon or occur only after prolonged use, e.g. oral contraceptives and vascular disease; renal damage due to analgesics
- Effects in special subpopulation groups, e.g. pregnancy, intercurrent renal or hepatic disease, since these are generally excluded, reasonably, from at least the early formal therapeutic trials
- Unexpected therapeutic effects, i.e. potential new uses
- Interactions between drugs.

Surveillance studies may remedy these deficiencies.

Conclusions

Drug evaluation comprises formal therapeutic trials followed by surveillance studies.

That considerable progress has been made is unquestionable, but there remains much to be achieved.

There are some who dislike or reject the notion of deliberate experimentation on the sick, feeling that

---

[14] Information on both categories (*use effectiveness* and *method effectiveness*) is valuable. Sheiner L B et al 1995 Intention-to-treat analysis and the goals of clinical trials. Clinical Pharmacology and Therapeutics 57: 1.

a scientific approach implies an unsympathetic or even a malevolent disposition. They forget that in the past positively harmful treatments have been widely used for many years (e.g. bleeding for pneumonia) because of the lack of recognition of the need, as well as lack of knowledge of the techniques, of scientific evaluation of therapy. It has been pointed out that where the worth of a treatment, new or old, is in doubt, there may be a greater obligation to test it critically than to go on prescribing it supported only by habit or wishful thinking.

> The choice before doctors is not whether they should experiment on their patients, but whether they should do so in a planned or in a haphazard fashion.

Modern scientific techniques uncover the most effective treatments whilst exposing the smallest numbers to the less effective or positively harmful; they save lives, time and money. Doctors who think they can assess the value of a treatment by using it on patients in an uncontrolled fashion have the whole history of therapeutics against them.

Though the 'statistical therapeutic comparison' or 'formal therapeutic trial' or 'randomised controlled trial', discussed below, is a powerful tool for advancing therapy, it does not suit every occasion. Sometimes, as in malaria or diabetes, there are clinical or laboratory tests that are accepted surrogate measures that tell whether a treatment is immediately effective, though they may not provide evidence of a marginal difference between effective drugs; in tuberculous meningitis a single recovery was considered adequate evidence of therapeutic efficacy (but carefully planned studies are necessary to define the best regimens).

Need for statistics

In order to decide whether patients treated in one way are benefited more than those treated in another, there is no possibility of avoiding the use of numbers. The mere statement by clinicians that patients do better with this or that treatment is due to their having formed an opinion that more patients are helped by the treatment advocated than by other treatments. The opinion is based on numbers, but having omitted to record exactly how many patients have been treated by different methods and having omitted to ensure that the only variable factor affecting the patient was the treatment in question, researchers can only state a 'clinical impression', instead of facts. This is a pity, for progress is delayed when convinced opinions are offered in place of convincing facts.

> **Statistics** may be defined as 'a body of methods for making wise decisions in the face of uncertainty'.[15] Used properly, they are a tool of great value for promoting efficient therapy.

Over 100 years ago Francis Galton saw this clearly.

> In our general impressions far too great weight is attached to what is marvellous .... Experience warns us against it, and the scientific man takes care to base his conclusions upon actual numbers. The human mind is ... a most imperfect apparatus for the elaboration of general ideas .... General impressions are never to be trusted. Unfortunately when they are of long standing they become fixed rules of life, and assume a prescriptive right not to be questioned. Consequently, those who are not accustomed to original enquiry entertain a hatred and a horror of statistics. They cannot endure the idea of submitting their sacred impressions to cold-blooded verification. But it is the triumph of scientific men to rise superior to such superstitions, to devise tests by which the value of beliefs may be ascertained, and to feel sufficiently masters of themselves to discard contemptuously whatever may be found untrue ... the frequent incorrectness of notions derived from general impressions may be assumed .... [16]

---

[15] Wallis W A et al 1957 Statistics, a new approach. Methuen, London.

[16] Galton F 1879 Generic images. Proceedings of the Royal Institution.

Therapeutic trials

The aims of a therapeutic trial, not all of which can be attempted on any one occasion, are to decide the following:

- Whether a treatment is of value
- How great its value is (compared with other remedies, if such exist)
- In what types of patients it is of value
- What is the best method of applying the treatment; how often, and in what dosage if it is a drug
- What are the disadvantages and dangers of the treatment.

The therapeutic trial is

a carefully, and ethically, designed experiment with the aim of answering some precisely framed question. In its most rigorous form it demands equivalent groups of patients concurrently treated in different ways. These groups are constructed by the random allocation of patients to one or other treatment . . . . In principle the method is applicable with any disease and any treatment. It may also be applied on any scale; it does not necessarily demand large numbers of patients.[17]

This is the classic randomised controlled trial. Three important points in the above definition deserve to be stressed.

- **Equivalent groups of patients by random (chance) allocation.** If the treatment groups differ significantly in age, sex, race, duration of disease, severity of disease or in any other possible hidden or unknown factors, there is confounding, and it will not be possible to attribute differences in outcome to the treatment under investigation, unless there is some way of eliminating the bias that has entered. The best way of forming equivalent groups is by allocating patients to them at random after (not before) the patient has been admitted to the trial.[18]

The function of randomisation is to eliminate sys-tematic biases, and, where they are later found to have occurred (e.g. differences in age or severity of disease), to permit the use of statistical calculations to 'correct' for these.

To allot patients alternately or otherwise system-atically is *not* satisfactory as investigators almost inevitably know into what treatment group a patient will go whilst engaged in deciding whether the patient should enter the trial. They may be con-sciously or unconsciously influenced by this if they have strong feelings about either the patient or the value of the respective treatments. With random allocations in sealed envelopes that are opened only *after* the patient has entered into the trial, allocation bias is eliminated.

But, unsurprisingly, some, even many, patients dislike the idea that the treatment they receive will be determined by chance (they are entitled to be told this), with resulting low recruitment and high drop-out rate. Trial designs are being developed in which patient preferences are taken into account for some or all patients, but they have less discrimina-tion (*statistical power*) than truly randomised stud-ies, for potential biases are uncontrolled, so that they require more subjects.[19]

- **Time and place of treatments.** Treatments must be carried out concurrently (at the same time) and concomitantly (at the same place) for the rea-sons given above and because diseases may vary in severity with both time and place. Thus controls from the past (historical controls) are nearly always unacceptable.

- **Precisely framed question.** Before commenc-ing any therapeutic trial it is essential to formulate exactly the question that is to be answered. For example: 'Is drug X capable of relieving the pain of osteoarthrosis more or less completely, with greater or fewer side-effects and for a shorter or longer time

---

[18] It is not necessary to have equal numbers in each group, especially if the natural history of the disease is well known, when a 2:1 ratio can be used instead of the usual 1:1. Random number series can be adapted to provide unequal groups or allocation may be devised to change during the trial so that more patients are progressively allocated to the most successful treatment — '*play the winner*' allocation.

[19] See Silverman W A 1994 Patients' preferences and randomized trials. Lancet 343: 1586

---

[17] Bradford Hill A 1977 Principles of medical statistics. Hodder and Stoughton, London. If there is a 'father' of the modern scientific therapeutic trial, it is he.

than is drug Y?' The question should be as simple as possible, for to try to discover too much can be a cause of failure, and it should be kept in mind throughout the whole process of designing the trial. Neglect to set down at the start exactly what are the objectives of the study invites failure.

CONCEPTS AND TERMS

Hypothesis of no difference

When it is suspected that treatment A may be superior to treatment B and it is wished to find out the truth, it is convenient to set about it by testing the hypothesis that the treatments are equally effective, or ineffective, as the case may be — the 'no difference' hypothesis (*null hypothesis*). Thus, when two groups of patients have been treated (between-patient comparison) or each patient has had a course of each drug (within-patient comparison) and it has been found that improvement has occurred more often with one treatment than with the other, it is necessary to decide how likely it is that this difference is due to a real superiority of one treatment over the other. To make this decision *we need to understand two major concepts, statistical significance*[20] *and confidence intervals*.

A statistical significance test[21] will tell how often a difference of the observed size would occur due to chance (random influences) if there is, in reality, no difference between the treatments. In clinical practice most agree that where the statistical significance test shows that if the no-difference hypothesis is correct, a difference as large as that observed would only occur five times if the experiment were repeated 100 times, then this is acceptable as sufficient evidence that the null hypothesis is *unlikely* to be true. Therefore the conclusion is that there is (probably) a real difference between the treatments. This level of probability is generally expressed in therapeutic trials as: the difference was 'statistically significant', 'significant at the 5% level' or '$P = 0.05$' (P = percent-

age divided by 100; chance proportion). Statistical significance simply means that the result is unlikely to have occurred if there is *no* genuine treatment difference, i.e. there probably *is* a difference.

If the analysis reveals that, the no-difference hypothesis being true, the observed difference, or greater, would only occur once if the experiment were repeated 100 times, the results are generally said to be 'statistically highly significant', 'significant at the 1% level' or '$P = 0.01$'.

Confidence intervals. If the result of the statistical significance test is that the observed difference is *unlikely* where there is truly *no* difference between treatments, then we need to know the size of the difference, and what degree of assurance, or confidence, we may have in the precision or power of this estimate. To obtain this we need to know the confidence intervals.[22]

Confidence intervals are expressed as a range of values within which we may be 95% (or other chosen %) certain that the true value lies. The range may be broad, indicating uncertainty, or narrow, indicating (relative) certainty.

> **Confidence intervals** reveal the precision of an estimate.

A wide confidence interval points to a lack of information, whether the difference is statistically significant or not, and is a warning (against placing much weight on, or confidence in, the results of small studies). Confidence intervals are extremely helpful in interpretation, particularly of small studies, as they show the degree of uncertainty related to a result — such as the difference between two means — whether or not it was statistically significant. Their use in conjunction with nonsignificant results may be especially enlightening.[23]

A finding of not statistically significant can only be interpreted as meaning there is no clinically useful difference if the confidence intervals of the

---

[20] The main function of that section of statistics that deals with tests of significance is to prevent people making fools of themselves.

[21] Altman D et al 1983 British Medical Journal 286: 1489.

[22] Gardner M J, Altman D G 1986 British Medical Journal 292: 746.

[23] Altman D G et al 1983 British Medical Journal 286: 1489.

result are also stated in the report and are narrow. If the confidence intervals are wide a real difference may have been missed in a trial of the size performed; i.e. absence of evidence that there is a difference is not the same as showing that there is no difference. Small numbers of patients inevitably give low precision or power.

Plainly trials should be devised to have adequate *precision* or *power*, i.e. at least an 80% chance of detecting (at 5% statistical significance, $P = 0.05$) the defined useful target effect (say 15%) within narrow confidence limits. It is not worth starting a trial that has less than a 50% chance of achieving the set objective, because the power of the trial is too low; but such small trials are frequently done and published without any statement of power or confidence interval, which would reveal their inadequacy.

Types of error

Confidence intervals provide us with information on the likelihood of falling into one of the two principal kinds of error of therapeutic experiments:

- Type I error, i.e. finding a difference between treatments when in reality they do not differ.
- Type II error, i.e. finding no difference between treatments when in reality they do differ to an extent doctors would want to know about — the target difference.

It is up to the investigators to decide the target difference[24] and what probability level (for either type of error) they will accept if they are to use the result as a guide to action; this the statistical significance test alone cannot tell them.

The statistical tests do not prove that a difference is due to one treatment being better than another or not better than another, as the case may be; they merely provide probabilities.

> A difference may be statistically significant and have narrow confidence intervals but yet it may be clinically unimportant.

[24] *The target difference.* Differences in trial outcomes fall into three grades: (1) that the doctor will ignore, (2) that will make the doctor wonder what to do (more research needed), and (3) that will make the doctor act, i.e. change prescribing practice.

Double-blind and single-blind techniques

The fact that both doctors and patients are subject to bias due to their beliefs and feelings has led to the invention of the double-blind technique, which is a

control device to prevent bias from influencing results. On the one hand it rules out the effects of hopes and anxieties of the patient by giving both the drug under investigation and a placebo (dummy) of identical appearance in such a way that the subject (the first 'blind' man) does not know which he is receiving. On the other hand, it also rules out the influence of preconceived hopes of, and unconscious communication by, the investigator or observer by keeping him (the second 'blind' man) ignorant of whether he is prescribing a placebo or an active drug. At the same time, the technique provides another control, a means of comparison with the magnitude of placebo effects. The device is both philosophically and practically sound.[25]

A nonblind trial is called an *open trial*.

The double-blind technique should be used if possible whenever evaluation depends on other than strictly objective measurements. There are occasions when it might at first sight seem that criteria of clinical improvement are objective when in fact they are not, e.g. the range of voluntary joint movement in rheumatoid arthritis has been shown to be greatly influenced by psychological factors, and a moment's thought shows why, for the amount of pain patients will put up with is influenced by their mental state.

Sometimes the double-blind technique is not possible because, for example, side-effects of an active drug reveal which patients are taking it or tablets look or taste different; but it never carries a disadvantage, 'only protection against spurious data'. It is not, of course, used with new chemical entities fresh from the animal laboratory, whose dose and effects in man are unknown, although the subject may legitimately be kept in ignorance (single-blind) of the time of administration. Single-blind technique has little use in therapeutics research as it is equally important that the observer also be blind.

[25] Modell W 1958 Journal of the American Medical Association 167: 2190.

Ophthalmologists are understandably disinclined to refer to the double-blind technique; they call it double-masked.

Placebo (dummy) medication as a research tool

Dummy or placebo treatment is used in conjunction with the double-blind technique (see also p. 56).

Its use is not always scientifically necessary nor indeed ethical, for it is not permissible to deprive patients having serious disease of existing effective therapy. In drug trials in, say, epilepsy or tuberculosis, the control groups comprise patients receiving the best available therapy. But the use of placebo does not necessarily require that patients be deprived of effective therapy (where it exists). New drug and placebo may be added against a background of established therapy, e.g. in heart failure.

The pharmacologically inert placebo or dummy is useful to:

● Distinguish the *pharmacodynamic effects* of a drug from the psychological effects of the act of medication and circumstances surrounding it, e.g. increased interest by the doctor, more frequent visits, etc., for these latter may also have placebo efficacy
● Distinguish *drug effects* from fluctuations in disease that occur with time and other external factors, provided active treatment, if any, can be ethically withheld
● Avoid *false negative conclusions*. For example, a therapeutic trial of a new analgesic should consist of comparison of the new drug with a dummy[26] as well as with a proved active analgesic. If all three treatments give the same result, a likely explanation is that the method used (including trial size) is incapable of distinguishing between an active and an inactive drug and so should be modified; whereas if only the new drug and the dummy are used and give identical results, there are two possible explanations, first that the method used is insensitive and second that the new drug has only placebo effect, i.e. is pharmacologically inactive at the dose used.

The use of a placebo or dummy treatment poses

ethical problems but is often preferable to the continued use of treatments of unproven efficacy or safety. It is not inherently unethical. Investigators who propose to use a placebo or otherwise withhold effective treatment should specifically justify their intention. It may be ethically acceptable to seek patient consent to brief withdrawal (for scientific purposes) of effective therapy in minor conditions; but it is unethical even to raise the question in serious disease for which significantly effective therapy already exists.

Consent can be obtained to the use of a placebo without impairing the scientific validity of the procedure if the patient is invited to agree that an inert preparation will (or may) be used (and why it will be used) at some time during the course of treatment, but without specifying exactly when. Generally, patients easily understand the concept of distinguishing between the imagined effects of treatment and those due to a direct action on the body.

In the above circumstances a patient is not the subject of deception in any ethical sense; but a patient given a placebo in the absence of consent is deceived and Research Ethics Committees will, rightly, be slow to agree to this.

Crossover and parallel group studies

Sometimes in chronic stable disease that cannot be cured but can be alleviated it is possible to give each of the treatments and doses under test, including placebo, to each patient, thus conveniently using them as their own controls (a crossover study), e.g. in parkinsonism or hypertension. When this is done it is important to ensure that each drug both precedes and follows each other drug the same number of times,[27] to avoid the risk of systematic bias due to changes with time and 'carry-over' effect, i.e. interaction of the drug given first with that given second. If in an analgesic trial a less effective drug always follows a more effective, the weaker drug may be dismissed as ineffective because the patient's judgement has become influenced by the high

---

[26] Careful ethical design allows a patient unrelieved by a placebo, or by an ineffective new drug, to be quickly given a known active drug.

[27] This kind of programme, done extensively in a single patient has been dignified by the term *n-of-1 trial*; it is intended to optimise drug choice for the individual patient rather than to obtain information that may be applicable to patients in general, so that it is part of medical practice (care) rather than research.

degree of relief provided by the more effective drug. The less effective drug must precede as well as follow both the more effective drug and the dummy (if any). In addition, persistence of a drug or metabolites, and enzyme induction, may influence the response to a subsequent drug.[28] For these reasons between-patient studies are preferred, but they require more subjects.

In acute self-limiting diseases it is plainly impossible to give more than one treatment to one patient and the controls must be other patients, i.e. between-patient or *parallel* groups.

Historical controls

Naturally there is a temptation simply to give a new treatment to all patients and to compare the results with the past, i.e. historical controls. Unfortunately this is almost always[29] unacceptable, even with a disease such as leukaemia, for standards of diagnosis and treatment change with time and severity of disease (infections) fluctuates. The provision stands that controls must be concurrent and concomitant (p. 54).

Some mortal sins of clinical assessment[30]

- *Enthusiasm and scepticism:*
  'A marvellous/useless drug, this.'
- *Change of assessor:*
  'Do the measurements for me Jim/Miss Jones/darling.'
- *Change of time:*
  'Don't worry about the assessment. Go ahead with lunch/X-rays/physiotherapy/your bath.'
- *Squeezing:*
  'You're much better, aren't you, Miss B?' 'Any indigestion yet, Miss B?'
- *Pride:*
  'I'm honest. No need for placebo in my trials.'
- *Impurity:*
  'We're short of cases: she'll have to do.' 'A few aspirins won't make much difference.'
- *Imbalance:*
  'Sex/severity/treatment order, doesn't matter.'
- *Error:*
  'Not quite significant. Let's try sequential analysis.'

SIZE OF TRIALS

Before the start of a therapeutic trial it is necessary to decide when it should stop, for ethical as well as for practical reasons.

The number of patients required for a therapeutic trial depends on what difference the investigator regards as clinically important (the *target difference*) and the number of patients likely to be available. Investigators will turn to statisticians for help. An estimate can be provided only if they will tell the statisticians the target difference and the risks they will tolerate of errors of types I and II, i.e. of accepting a difference where it does not exist and of missing a difference that does exist. The result of this calculation is liable to be a shock to the investigators if they have, a little vaguely, and full of therapeutic enthusiasm, begun by saying that they want to detect 'any' difference, however small, and to be 'quite certain' that it is real.

A trial that offers a better than even chance of detecting a difference of 2:3, i.e. 2 deaths (or other event) in one treatment group against 3 deaths in the other, which can well be a clinically important difference, will require numbers of patients that provide for about 100 deaths (or other event) in the trial. But such a probability (better than even chance) may be thought insufficient, and to become reasonably sure that a difference of this magnitude (2:3) will be detected, a trial involving about 200 deaths will be needed. If the death rate is 20%, then the trial should be planned to include about 1000 patients — a daunting and expensive prospect.

A trial that would detect (with statistical significance at 5% level) a treatment that raised a cure rate from 75% to 85% would require 500 patients for 80% power. Obviously larger differences require fewer patients, and smaller differences require more patients (these figures make it clear why surveillance (observational) techniques of therapeutic

---

[28] 'Carry-over' can be minimised by inserting 'washout' periods between active treatments, but these are not always ethically acceptable.

[29] Criteria for cautiously but usefully employing historical controls are suggested by Bailar J C et al 1984 Studies without internal controls. New England Journal of Medicine 311: 156.

[30] Hart F D et al 1972 Measurement in rheumatoid arthritis. Lancet 2: 28.

evaluation are attracting increasing interest). (See also Sensitivity of trials, below.)

The public demand for speed and early access to potentially important new drugs in, for example, AIDS and myocardial infarction, is leading to the performance of randomised or nonrandomised *heterogeneous megatrials*. In these studies there is some sacrifice of scientific rigour (by using surrogate endpoints and heterogeneous enrolment), which, it is hoped, is compensated by the enormous number of patients in the trial, e.g. 50 000.

Fixed-number trials

It is necessary, after deciding in consultation with a statistician what difference it is realistic to seek and with what precision, having regard to the time, the energy of the investigators and the number of patients available, to agree on the number of patients to be treated, to treat them and then to test the results. This is a fixed-sample trial and at the end there may be disappointment if, when the results are examined, they just miss the agreed acceptable level of statistical significance. Here, having presented their results, clinicians are entitled to express their opinion on their meaning, and the size of the confidence interval will be of great assistance (see above). It is here too that the results of independent workers are helpful; *confirmation by others is an essential process in therapeutic advance* as in all science. It is not legitimate, having just failed (say, $P = 0.06$) to reach the agreed level (say, $P = 0.05$) to take in a few more patients in the hope that they will bring P down to 0.05 or less, for this is deliberately not allowing chance and the treatment to be the sole factors involved in the outcome, as they should be. At least this is the theory, but 'only an investigator with superhuman willpower or completely chaotic records could supervise a clinical trial for months or years without ever looking to see which way the results were drifting'[31] and being influenced by them in deciding when to stop the trial.

Such capricious peeping is statistically unacceptable because it allows the feelings of the investigator to determine when the trial shall stop (and investigators like significant results as do journal editors and drug developers).

---

[31] Peto R et al 1976 British Journal of Cancer 34: 585; 35: 1.

But there is a solution, although it does reduce the power (precision) of the study; it is called *interim analysis* (below).

Variable number trials

Adaptive designs in which the number of subjects is not decided in advance have been developed in response to the evident need for a design that allows continuous or intermittent assessment as the trial proceeds and stops it either as soon as a statistically significant result is reached or when such a result becomes unlikely. The essential feature has to be that the trial is terminated when a predetermined result is attained and not when the investigator, looking at the results to date, thinks it appropriate. (Few investigators would be able to resist picking out the moment when the difference was statistically significant, which inevitably would mean a high rate of false-positive results.) Truly continuous monitoring (*sequential analysis*) imposes severe restrictions and a compromise has been attained; it allows a formal analysis to be conducted at several predetermined intervals and a decision made to stop or to continue. Such **interim analyses** reduce the precision or power of the statistical significance test (see Confidence intervals) but not to a serious degree if they do not exceed four times in a big trial. Such **modified sequential designs** recognise the realities of medical practice and provide a reasonable trade-off between statistical, medical and ethical needs. It is virtually a necessity to have expert statistical advice when undertaking such trials.

If an experiment is ill-designed or ill-conducted it cannot be salvaged by statistics and statisticians are justifiably annoyed if they are invited to attempt such an operation, particularly after the report has been rejected by a journal for poor design and inadequate or wrong statistics. Investigators who get into this situation have only themselves to blame.

SENSITIVITY OF TRIALS

Definitive therapeutic trials are expensive and tedious and may be so prolonged that aspects of treatment have been superseded by the time a result is obtained. Of studies in cancer it is said:

The practical conclusion is that clinical trials can easily monitor death rate ratios between two treatments which are 1:3 or better, but that detection of anything less extreme than 2:3 is very difficult. These summary ratios are very important, and should be written on the shirt-cuffs of all trial organisers, as attempting to study a difference which could not plausibly be as extreme as 2:3 by a clinical trial is a common mistake.[32]

It is plain that a single trial will seldom give a conclusive answer to a therapeutic question. Confirmatory trials by other people in other centres play a major role in reaching reasonable certainty in therapeutics.

A big definitive therapeutic trial is difficult, prolonged (years) and expensive to do;[33] it may give a result that is inconclusive or no longer of great interest, such is the speed of new drug development; furthermore, a single inadvertent serious design fault may render it worthless. Most new drugs are licensed after several small trials which inevitably lack power; a (still controversial) compromise has been reached: meta-analysis (see also Compliance — in new drug development studies).

Meta-analysis

Where numerous trials have been done and the outcomes vary, it is tempting to collect them all together in a *systematic review* and analyse the accumulated results using appropriate statistical methods (it is not acceptable to do a simple addition of groups). This meta[34] (or *overall*) analysis can be enlightening, but the trials selected must meet the criteria of a good scientific study and the final result must be treated with caution. Meta-analyses may involve 100 000 patients or more. But the problems of identifying all suitable trials in the multilingual world literature and of assessing their scientific validity are enormous.[35] There is also *publication bias* to be taken into account, i.e. the preference of both journal editors and authors to publish studies having a positive (interesting) result, and the nonpublication of negative (boring) trials.

Nevertheless meta-analyses are understandably gaining popularity and influence. They are at their best where the measured outcome is unequivocal, e.g. death, stroke.

Results: implementation

The way in which data from therapeutic trials are presented can influence doctors' perceptions of the advisability of adopting a treatment in their routine practice.

Relative and absolute risk

The results of therapeutic trials are commonly expressed as per cent reduction of an unfavourable (or % increase in a favourable) outcome, i.e. as relative risk, and this can be very impressive indeed until the figures are presented as the number of individuals actually affected per 100 people treated, i.e. as absolute risk.

Where a baseline risk is *low*, a statement of relative risk alone is particularly misleading (it implies big benefit where actual benefit is small); e.g., reduction of risk from 2% to 1% is 50% relative risk reduction, but it saves only one patient for every 100 patients treated. But where the baseline is high,

---

[32] Peto M et al 1976 British Journal of Cancer 34: 585.

[33] Cost looms over these huge trials, e.g. US$ 60 million for a myocardial infarction thrombolysis trial (41 000 patients); US$ 25 million for cholesterol-lowering trial (20 000 patients). These intimidating and rising costs stimulate interest in the cheaper observational cohort studies (below) and in heterogeneous megatrials (above).

[34] Meta (Greek) is a prefix loosely applied in various sciences and having a variety of meanings: sharing, action in common, change, and sometimes after, behind.

[35] There is an international body, the Cochrane Collaboration (named after a distinguished epidemiologist and articulate advocate of evidence-based medicine), set up to promote and undertake meta-analyses. It has started an electronic journal, the Cochrane Database of Systematic Reviews. In 1995 it undertook a computer-based international literature search of treatment trials in stroke, supplemented by hand searches. It retrieved about 10 000 articles 'each of which had to be assessed'; and it estimated that at least 300 journals have included stroke trials (Counsell C, Fraser H 1995 British Medical Journal 310: 126).

say 40%, a 50% reduction in relative risk saves 20 patients for every 100 treated.

> To make clinical decisions readers of therapeutic studies need to know: how many patients must be treated[36] (and for how long) to obtain one desired result (*number needed to treat*). This is the inverse (or reciprocal) of absolute risk reduction.

Relative risk reductions can remain high (and thus make treatments seem attractive) even when susceptibility to the events being prevented is low (and the corresponding numbers needed to be treated are large). As a result, restricting the reporting of efficacy to just relative risk reductions can lead to greater — and at times excessive — zeal in decisions about treatment for patients with low susceptibilities.[37]

A real-life example follows:

Antiplatelet drugs reduce the risk of future non-fatal myocardial infarction by 30% [relative risk] in trials of both primary and secondary prevention. But when the results are presented as the number of patients who need to be treated for one non-fatal myocardial infarction to be avoided [absolute risk] they look very different.

In secondary prevention 50 patients need to be treated for two years, while in primary prevention 200 patients need to be treated for five years, for one non-fatal myocardial infarction to be prevented. In other words, it takes 100 patient-years of treatment in primary prevention to produce the same beneficial outcome of one fewer non-fatal myocardial infarction.[37]

In the context of absolute risk, the question whether a low incidence of adverse drug effects is acceptable becomes a serious one.[38]

Absolute risk (and number of patients needed to treat) is frequently unstated in publications. The fact that readers can usually calculate it for them-selves from the published tables is no excuse for not setting it alongside the often over-impressive relative risk. Until journal editors require this of investigators, readers would be wise to DIY (do-it-yourself).

There are other reasons why doctors may be slow to adopt therapeutic advances, as indeed many, particularly nonspecialists, have been shown to be. They include: doubts about how far selected trial patients treated under special supervision represent the 'real world' of general practice; fear of adverse reactions: turgid, unreadable, misleading (above) publications; clinical isolation, and so on. There is also evidence that it is harder to extinguish practices that were once accepted than it is to introduce new practices (no doubt publication bias is a factor in this). Nonspecialist, primary care doctors particularly, need and deserve clear and informative presentation of therapeutic trial results that measure the overall impact of a treatment on the patient's life, i.e. *outcomes research* (morbidity, mortality, quality of life, working capacity, fewer days in hospital, etc.). Without it, they cannot adequately advise patients.

> **Important aspects of therapeutic trial reports**
> - Statistical significance and its clinical importance
> - Confidence intervals
> - Number needed to treat, or absolute risk.

Pharmacoepidemiology

Three important epidemiological approaches (phase 4, p. 51) are used to determine how the results of controlled therapeutic trials are translated

---

[36] See Cooke R J, Sackett D L 1995 The number needed to treat: a clinically useful treatment effect. British Medical Journal 310: 452.

[37] Sackett D L, Cooke R J 1994 Understanding clinical trials: What measures of efficacy should journal articles provide busy clinicians. British Medical Journal 309: 755.

[38] For example, drug therapy for high blood pressure carries risks, but the risks of the disease vary enormously according to severity of disease:
'Depending on the initial absolute risk, the benefits of lowering blood pressure range from preventing one cardiovascular event a year for about every 20 people treated to preventing one event for about every 5000–10 000 people treated. The level of risk at which treatment should be started is debatable' (Jackson R et al 1993 Management of raised blood pressure in New Zealand: a discussion document. British Medical Journal 307: 107).

into performance in the looser conditions of use in the community, and especially to the detection of uncommon adverse reactions. They are not experimental (as is the randomised trial where entry and allocation of treatment are strictly controlled). They are *observational* in that the groups to be compared have been assembled from subjects who are, or who are not (the controls), taking the treatment in the ordinary way of medical care. Observational studies come into their own when sufficiently large randomised trials are logistically and financially impracticable. New statistical approaches enhance the utility of such studies (see also p. 59).

The observational cohort[39] study. Patients receiving the drug are collected and followed up to determine the outcomes (therapeutic and adverse). This is forward-looking (prospective) research. *Prescription event monitoring* (p. 123) is an example, and there is an increasing tendency to recognise that most new drugs should be monitored in this way when prescribing becomes general. Major difficulties include selection of an appropriate control group, the need for large numbers of subjects and for prolonged surveillance. This sort of study is scientifically inferior to the experimental cohort study (randomised controlled trial) and is cumbersome for research on drugs. Happily, clever epidemiologists have devised a partial alternative, the case-control study.

The case-control study. This reverses the direction of scientific logic from forward-looking, 'what happens next' (*prospective*) to a backward-looking, 'what has happened in the past' (*retrospective*)[40] investigation. The investigator assembles a group of patients who have the condition it is desired to investigate, e.g. women who have had an episode of thromboembolism. A control group of women who have not had an episode of thromboembolism is then assembled (e.g. similar age, parity and smoking habits) from hospital admissions for other reasons, or primary care records. A complete drug history is

taken from each group, i.e. the two groups are 'followed up' backwards to determine the proportion in each group that has taken the suspect agent, in this case the oral contraceptive pill.

To solve the question of thromboembolism and the combined oestrogen-progestogen contraceptive pill by means of an observational cohort study required enormous numbers of subjects[41] (the adverse effect is, happily, uncommon) followed over years. An investigation into cancer and the contraceptive pill by an observational cohort would require follow-up for 10–15 years. But a case-control study can be done quickly; it has the advantage that it begins with a much smaller number of cases (hundreds) of disease; though it has the disadvantage that it follows up subjects backwards and there is always suspicion of the intrusion of unknown and so unavoidable biases in selection of both patients and controls. Here again, independent repetition of the studies, if the results are the same, greatly enhances confidence in the outcome.

A major disadvantage of the case-control study is that it requires a definite hypothesis or suspicion of causality. A cohort study on the other hand does not; subjects can be followed 'to see what happens' (event recording). Case-control studies do not prove causation.[42] They reveal associations and it is up to investigators and critical readers to decide what is the most plausible explanation.

Record linkage by computer allows correlation in a population of life and health events with history of drug use. It is being developed as far as resources permit. It includes prescription event monitoring (see above).

---

[39] Used here for a group of people having a common attribute, e.g. they have all taken the same drug.

[40] For this reason Feinstein has named these *trohoc* (*cohort* spelled backwards) studies.

[41] The Royal College of General Practitioners (UK) recruited 23 000 women takers of the pill and 23 000 controls in 1968 and issued a report in 1973. It found an approximate doubled incidence of venous thrombosis in combined-pill takers (the dose of oestrogen has been reduced since this study).

[42] Experimental cohort studies (randomised controlled trials) are on firmer ground with regard to causation. In the experimental cohort study there should be only *one* systematic difference between the groups (i.e. the treatment being studied). In case-control studies the groups may differ systematically in several ways.

IN CONCLUSION

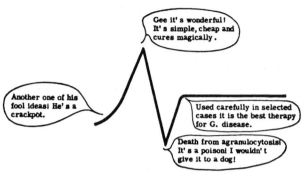

Fig. 4.1 Oscillations in the development of a drug[43]

GUIDE TO FURTHER READING

Ayanian J Z et al 1994 Knowledge and practice of generalist and specialist physicians regarding drug therapy for acute myocardial infarction. New England Journal of Medicine 331: 1136

Carpenter L M 1993 Is the study worth doing? Lancet 342: 221

Chalmers I 1995 What do I want from health research and researchers when I am a patient? British Medical Journal 310: 1315

Chatellier G et al 1996 The numbers needed to treat: a clinically useful nomogram in its proper context. British Medical Journal 312: 426

Cook C H C et al 1988 Another trial that failed. Lancet 1: 524

Editorial 1993 Clinical trials and clinical practice. Lancet 342: 877

---

[43] By courtesy of Dr Robert H Williams and the Editor of The Journal of the American Medical Association.

Egger M, Smith G D 1995 Misleading meta-analysis. Lessons from 'an effective, safe, simple' intervention that wasn't. British Medical Journal 310: 752

Gore S M 1994 The consumer principle of randomization. 343: 58

Grisso J 1993 Making comparisons. Lancet 342: 157

Hellman S et al 1991 Of mice but not men — problems of the randomized clinical trial. New England Journal of Medicine 324: 1585

Levy G 1992 Publication bias: Its implications for clinical pharmacology. Clinical Pharmacology and Therapeutics 52: 115

Mulrow C D 1994 Rationale for systematic reviews (meta-analyses). British Medical Journal 309: 597

Pocock S J 1992 When to stop a clinical trial. British Medical Journal 305: 235 and subsequent correspondence

Rosenberg W, Donald A 1995 Evidence-based medicine: an approach to clinical problem-solving. British Medical Journal 310: 1122

Schmucker D L, Vesell E S 1993 Underrepresentation of women in clinical trials. Clinical Pharmacology and Therapeutics 54: 11

Shapiro S 1989 The role of automated record linkage in the postmarketing surveillance of drug safety: a critique. Clinical Pharmacology and Therapeutics 46: 371; (responses to the article) 387, 391, 478, 479

Silverman W A, Altman D G 1996 Patients' preferences and randomized trials. Lancet 347: 171

Smith G D, Egger M 1994 Who benefits from medical interventions? British Medical Journal 308: 72

Waller P C, Jackson P R, Tucker G T, Ramsay L E 1994 Clinical pharmacology with confidence [intervals]. British Journal of Clinical Pharmacology 37: 309

Official regulation of medicines

SYNOPSIS

- Basis for regulation
- Present-day requirements
- Women as subjects in early tests
- Counterfeit drugs
- Appendix: the thalidomide disaster

Regulation of medicines is concerned with:

- safety
- efficacy
- quality
- supply.

Basis for regulation

Neither patients nor doctors are in a position to decide for themselves across the range of medicines that they use which ones are *pure* and *stable* and *effective* and *safe*. They need assurance that the medicines they are offered fulfil these requirements and are supported by information that permits optimal use. Only governments can provide such assurance, insofar as it can be provided.

The principles of official medicines regulation are of general importance, but the details (with accompanying administrative jargon) of how each country or group of countries administers these principles differ in (biologically) unimportant ways. We therefore restrict ourselves to the principles (below). Efforts are being made (the International Conferences on Harmonization) to minimise the enormous waste of resources caused by the need for drug developers to adapt their research programmes to needlessly diverse national bureaucratic requirements.[1]

Plainly manufacturers and developers are entitled to be told what substances are regulated and what are not[2] and what kinds and amounts of data[3]

---

[1] From the point of view of a multinational pharmaceutical company seeking worldwide marketing the regulatory bodies that its programme *must* satisfy include the Food and Drug Administration (FDA) of the USA, the European Medicines Evaluation Agency (EMEA) of the European Union (EU) (15 countries in 1995; the national regulatory bodies of individual EU members remain but have diminishing importance), and the Japanese Pharmaceutical Affairs Bureau.

[2] However much doctors may mock the bureaucratic 'regulatory mind', regulation provides an important service and it is expedient that doctors should have some insight into its working and some of the very real problems faced by public servants who (generally) are trying to do good without risking losing their jobs.

It is obviously impossible to list substances that will be regulated if anybody should choose one day to synthesise them. Therefore regulation is based on the supply of 'medicinal products', i.e. substances are regulated according to their proposed use; and they must be defined in a way that will resist legal challenge (hence the stilted regulatory language).

The following terms have gained informal acceptance for 'borderline substances' (which may or may not be regulated):
— *nutriceutical*: a food or part of a food that provides medicinal benefits
— *cosmeceutical*: a cosmetic that also has medicinal use.

are likely to persuade a regulatory authority to grant a licence to sell and promote a product (for uses that are defined in the licence). In addition, a good regulatory authority confers protection on a good drug developer.

The principles of official (statutory) medicines regulation are that:

- No medicine shall be supplied without prior licensing by the government.
- A licence shall be granted on the basis of scientific evaluation[4] of:
  - **quality**, i.e. purity, stability (shelf-life)
  - **safety**, in relation to its use: evaluation at the point of marketing is provisional in the sense that it is followed in the community by a pharmacovigilance programme
  - **efficacy** (now often including quality of life and cost-benefit studies)
  - **supply**: i.e. whether the drug is suitable to be unrestrictedly available to the public or whether it should be confined to sales through pharmacies or on doctors' prescriptions; and what printed information should accompany its sale (labelling, leaflets).
- A licence shall specify the clinical indications that may be promoted and shall be for a limited period (5 years) which is renewable on application.
- A regulatory authority may order a drug to be taken off the market at any time for good cause.

---

[3] Manufacturers ignore at their (financial) peril the guidance regulators give on GLP (good laboratory practice), GMP (good manufacturing practice) and GCP (good clinical practice).

[4] Except in the case of traditional herbal medicines (which can be ineffective and/or hazardous), as well as other substances used in the 'legitimate practice' of complementary medicine, for which this requirement cannot be met. Official regulators, finding themselves between 'the rock' of maintaining scientific principles and 'the hard place' of banning complementary medicines that are popular with the public (a political impossibility), have reacted in accordance with the highest traditions of their calling as civil servants. They have produced a compromise mix of reinterpreted regulations with circumspect labelling that will allow these products to continue to be sold without, it is hoped, misleading the public.

Background

The beginning of substantial government intervention in the field of medicines paralleled the proliferation of synthetic drugs in the early 20th century when the traditional and familiar pharmacopoeia[5] expanded slowly and then, in mid-century, with enormous rapidity.

The first comprehensive regulatory law that required premarketing testing was passed in the USA in 1938, following the death of about 107 people due to the use of diethylene glycol (a constituent of antifreezes) as a solvent for a stable liquid formulation of sulphanilamide for treating common infections.[6] It was convenient for children to take; the toxicity (CNS, renal, hepatic) of ethylene glycol was already known. The only premarketing 'tests' were for appearance, fragrance and flavour. The procedure was compatible with the then-existing law in the USA. The head of the company said he was sorry for the deaths but he felt no responsibility.

Other countries did not learn the lesson provided by the USA and it took the thalidomide disaster of 1960–61 (p. 69) to make governments all over the world initiate comprehensive control over all aspects of drug introduction, therapeutic claims and supply. Those governments that already had some control system strengthened it.

Present-day requirements

A modern drug regulatory authority requires the following:

- **Preclinical tests**
  - Tests carried out in animals to allow some

---

[5] *Pharmacopoeia*: a book (often official) listing drugs, their uses, standards of purity, etc.

[6] Report of the Secretary of Agriculture submitted in response to resolutions in the House of Representatives and Senate (USA). 1937 Journal of the American Medical Association 111: 583, 919. Recommended reading. A similar episode occurred as recently as 1990–1992: See Hanif M et al 1995 Fatal renal failure caused by diethylene glycol in paracetamol elixir: the Bangladesh epidemic. British Medical Journal 311: 88. Note: diethylene glycol is cheap.

prediction of potential efficacy and safety in man (see Ch. 3)

— Chemical and pharmaceutical quality checks (purity, stability, formulation, etc.)

● **Clinical (human) tests** (Phases 1,2,3; p. 51) The full process of regulatory review of a truly novel drug (new chemical entity) takes months or, where there are difficulties, several years.

● **Knowledge of the environmental impact of pharmaceuticals**. Regulatory authorities now expect manufacturers to address this concern in their application to market new chemical entities. Aspects include manufacture (chemical pollution), packaging (waste disposal), pollution in immediate use (e.g. antimicrobials) and, more remotely, drugs or metabolites entering the food chain or water where use may be massive, e.g. hormones.

● **Post-licensing (marketing) phase 4 studies**.

REGULATORY REVIEW

An authority normally conducts a review in two stages:

1. To examine preclinical data (sometimes with added tests on healthy volunteers)[7] to determine whether the drug is safe enough to be tested for (predicted) human therapeutic efficacy.
2. To examine the clinical studies to determine whether the drug has been shown to be therapeutically effective with safety appropriate to its use.[8]

If the decision is favourable the drug is granted a Product Licence (for 5 years: renewable) which allows it to be marketed for specified therapeutic uses. The decisions are made by civil servants using independent professional advisers for matters of particular controversy or importance.[9]

---

[7] In the UK tests on healthy volunteers are not subject to official regulation.

[8] Common sense dictates that what, in regulatory terms is 'safe' for leukaemia would not be 'safe' for anxiety.

[9] For example the UK Committee on Safety of Medicines advises the Medicines Control Agency (which represents the Licensing Authority which is, strictly, the Ministry of Health of the UK, thus maintaining ultimate responsibility to parliament).

The authority must satisfy itself of the adequacy of the information to be provided to prescribers in a Summary of Product Characteristics (SPC or Data Sheet) and also, where appropriate, any Patient Information Leaflet (which is particularly important with preparations for longterm use such as oral contraceptives). Where a drug has special advantage, but also has special risk, restrictions on its promotion and use can be imposed, e.g. see isotretinoin and clozapine.

When a novel drug is granted a Product Licence it is recognised as a medicine by independent critics and there is rejoicing amongst those who have spent many years developing it. But the testing is not over, the most stringent test of all is about to begin. It will be used in all sorts of people of all ages and sizes and having all sorts of other conditions. Its use can no longer be so closely supervised as hitherto. Doctors will prescribe it and patients will use it correctly and incorrectly. It will have effects that have not been anticipated. It will be taken in overdose. It has to find its place in therapeutics, a process that may take years.

Post-licensing/marketing surveillance (phase 4) has thus become an essential part of drug evaluation. It is neither easy nor cheap to accomplish efficiently. (Some studies conducted by pharmaceutical companies are thinly disguised promotional exercises.)

The important objective is to obtain information on very large numbers of patients, 10 000–20 000, in *observational* cohort studies, e.g. prescription event monitoring (p. 123) and case-control studies where appropriate; spontaneous reporting of suspected adverse reactions is also encouraged, e.g. by marking the drug with a special symbol ▼ in formularies (in the UK). All new chemical entities become subject to a general *pharmacovigilance* programme.

Further randomised controlled trials (*experimental* cohort studies), especially comparing the new drug with those already available, will continue for a long time in the case of really novel advances.

Discussion

It may be wondered why post-licensing/marketing surveillance and pharmacovigilance should be necessary. Common sense would seem to dictate that safety and efficacy of a drug should be fully defined before it is granted a Product Licence (marketed). Pre-licensing trials with very close supervision are commonly limited to hundreds of patients and this is unavoidable, chiefly because this close supervision is impracticable on a large scale for a very long time.

Post-licensing studies are increasingly regarded as essential to complete the definitive evaluation of drugs under conditions of ordinary use on a large scale, these programmes being preferable to attempts to enlarge and prolong formal therapeutic trials.

It would also seem sensible to require developers to prove that a new drug is not only effective but is actually *needed* in medicine before it is licensed. But a novel drug finds its place only after several, sometimes many, years, and to delay licensing is simply impracticable on financial grounds. This ought not to be so, but it is so. A 'need clause' in licensing is not generally practicable if drug developers are to stay in that business. This is why *comparative* therapeutic studies with existing drugs are not required for licensing in countries having a research-based pharmaceutical industry. A 'need clause' is, however, appropriate for economically deprived countries (see World Health Organization Essential Drugs Programme); indeed such countries have no alternative.

Licensed medicines for unlicensed indications

Doctors may generally prescribe any medicine for any legitimate medical purpose.[10]

But if doctors use a drug for an indication that is not formally included in the Product Licence ('off-label' use) they would be wise to think carefully and to keep particularly good records for, if a patient is dissatisfied, prescribers may find themselves having to justify the use in a court of law. (Written records made at the time of a decision carry substantial weight, but records made later, when trouble is already brewing, lose much of their power to convince, and records that have been altered later, are quite fatal to any defence.)

Manufacturers are not always willing to go to the trouble and expense of the rigorous clinical studies required to extend their licence unless a new use is likely to generate significant profits. They are prohibited by law from promoting an unlicensed use, though this does not stop some of them from doing so.

Unlicensed medicines and accelerated licensing

Regulatory systems sensibly make provision for supply of an unlicensed medicine (e.g. one that has not yet completed its full programme of clinical trials) for patients who, on the judgement of their doctors, have no alternative amongst licensed drugs. The doctor must apply to the manufacturer who may supply the drug for that particular patient and at the doctor's own responsibility. Various terms are used, e.g. supply on a 'named-patient' basis (UK); 'compassionate' drug use (USA). It is illegal to exploit this sensible loophole in supply laws to conduct research. Precise record-keeping of such use is essential.

But there can be desperate needs involving large numbers of patients, e.g. AIDS, and regulatory authorities may respond by licensing a drug before completion of the usual range of studies (making it clear that patients must understand the risks they are taking). Unfortunately such well-intentioned practice discourages patients from entering formal trials and may, in the long run, actually delay the definition of lifesaving therapies.

Decision taking

> It must be remembered always that, though there are risks in taking drugs, there are also risks in not taking drugs, and there are risks in not developing new drugs.

The requirements imposed by regulatory authorities increase as unexpected events occur amidst public outcry against both developers and the authorities.

---

[10] In many countries this excludes supply of drugs such as heroin or cocaine for controlled/supervised maintenance of drug addicts. In the UK such supply is permitted to doctors who hold a special licence.

A perceptive comment on one drug withdrawal was, 'The present system is too slow at detecting risk as well as unduly apt to slam the brakes on hard once it is detected'.[11]

In taking decisions about drug regulation, it has been pointed out,[12] there is uncertainty in three areas:

- Facts
- Public reaction to the facts
- Future consequences of decisions.

Regulators are influenced not only to avoid risk but to avoid regret later (*regret avoidance*) and this consideration has a profound effect whether or not the decision taker is conscious of it; it promotes defensive regulation.

It is self-evident that it is much harder to detect and quantitate a good that is not done, than it is to detect and quantitate a harm that is done. Therefore, although it is part of the decision-taker's job to facilitate the doing of good, the avoidance of harm looms larger. Attempts to convict regulators of failing to do good due to regulatory procrastination, the 'drug lag'[13] do not induce the same feelings of horror in regulators that are induced by the prospect of finding they have approved a drug that has, or may have, caused serious injury and that the victims are about to appear on television.[14] The bitterness of people injured by drugs, whether or not there is fault could be much reduced by the institution of simple, non-adversarial arrangements for compensation (see p. 11).

This is not to ridicule the regulators and their advisers. They are doing their best, and commonly make good and sensible decisions that receive no congratulations.

---

[11] The Times, 24 August 1982.

[12] Lord Ashby 1976 Proceedings of the Royal Society of Medicine 69: 721.

[13] Nevertheless, regulatory authorities have responded by providing a facility for 'fast-tracking' drugs for which clinical need may be urgent, e.g. AIDS (see above).

[14] The very last thing a drug regulator wishes to be able to say is, 'I awoke one morning and found myself famous': Lord Byron (1788–1824) on the publication of his poem, Childe Harold's Pilgrimage.

Women as subjects in early tests

For many years women of 'childbearing potential' have been excluded from early tests (phase 1 and early phase 2) of new drugs because of fears that they might be, or become, pregnant and bear a deformed child. In 1993 the Food and Drug Administration (FDA) (USA) changed this policy:

1. for scientific reasons (early detection of sex differences can be of value in design of later studies)
2. out of respect for women's 'autonomy and decision-making capacity'
3. because it is possible to reduce risk of fetal exposure through protocol design.

The FDA added that,

> Whether removal of the impediments to their participation will increase the number of women in early trials depends partly on drug companies' concerns about [legal] liability.... If we are to achieve broader participation of women in all phases of clinical trials, legitimate issues such as liability will have to be addressed as part of ongoing dialogue among drug developers, scientists, policy makers, health advocates, and women's groups.

Drug developers see the consequences of an allegation that their new drug even may have caused a congenital abnormality as so horrific in its consequences to the company that it seems likely that company-sponsored early studies will continue to be confined to men. However, it is acknowledged that women as subjects of research in general have been under-represented. USA Congress has passed an Act to remedy this in federally funded research.

Counterfeit drugs

Fraudulent medicines make up as much as 6% of pharmaceutical sales worldwide. They present a serious health (and economic) problem in countries with weak regulatory authorities and lacking money to police drug quality. In these countries counterfeit medicines may comprise 20–50% of available products. The trade may involve false labelling of legally manufactured products, in order to play one national market against another; also low-quality manufacture of correct ingredients; wrong ingredients, including added ingredients (e.g. corticosteroids added to herbal medicine for arthritis); no active ingredient; false packaging.

The trail from raw material to appearance on a pharmacy shelf may involve as many as four countries, with the final stages (importer, wholesaler) quite innocent, so well has the process been obscured.

Appendix: A tale to remember: the thalidomide disaster

Thalidomide has provided a terrible lesson to the world in regard to drug development, testing, naming, prescribing and consumption. It deserves to be remembered.

In 1960–61 in [West] Germany an outbreak of phocomelia occurred. Phocomelia means 'seal extremities'; it is a congenital deformity in which the long bones of the limbs are defective and substantially normal or rudimentary hands and feet arise on, or nearly on, the trunk, like the flippers of a seal; other abnormalities may occur simultaneously. Phocomelia is ordinarily exceedingly rare.

Most [West] German clinics had no cases during the 10 years up to 1959. In 1959, in 10 clinics, 17 were seen in 1959, 126 in 1960, 477 in 1961. The European outbreak seemed confined to [West] Germany (though a similar but smaller occurrence was simultaneously noted in Australia), and this, with the steady increase, made a virus infection, such as rubella, seem an unlikely cause. Radioactive fall-out was considered and so were X-ray exposure of the mother, hormones, foods, food preservatives and contraceptives. One doctor, investigating his patients retrospectively with a questionnaire, found that 20% reported taking a proprietary medicine, Contergan, in early pregnancy. He questioned the patients again and 50% then admitted taking it; many said they had thought the drug too obviously innocent to be worth mentioning initially.[15]

In November 1961, the suggestion that a drug, unnamed, was the cause of the outbreak was publicly made by the same doctor at a paediatric meeting, following a report on 34 cases of phocomelia. That night a physician came up to him and said, 'Will you tell me confidentially, is the drug Contergan? I ask because we have such a child and my wife took Contergan'. Several letters followed, asking the same question, and it soon became widely known that thalidomide (Contergan, Distaval, Kevadon, Talimol, Softenon) was probably the cause. It was withdrawn from the [West] German market in November and from the British market in December 1961. By that time reports had also come from other countries. A *case-control study* showed that of 46 cases of phocomelia 41 mothers had taken thalidomide and of 300 mothers with normal babies none had taken thalidomide between the fourth and ninth week of pregnancy.

Prospective *observational cohort studies* were quickly made in antenatal clinics where women had yet to give birth; though few, they provided evidence incriminating thalidomide. The worst had happened, a trivial new drug was the cause of the most grisly disaster in the short history of modern scientific drug therapy. Many thalidomide babies died, but many live on with deformed limbs, eyes, ears, heart and alimentary and urinary tracts.[16]

The [West] German Health Ministry estimated that thalidomide caused about 10 000 birth deformities in babies, 5000 of whom survived and 1600 of whom would eventually need artificial limbs. In Britain there were probably at least 600 live births

---

[15] Illustrating the problems of retrospective research, e.g. case-control studies; enquiries of patients are unreliable.

[16] For pictures of thalidomide deformities, see British Medical Journal (1962) 2: 646, 647; Journal of the American Medical Association (1962) 180: 1106.

of malformed children of whom about 400 survived. The world total of survivors was probably about 10 000.

Thalidomide had been marketed in [West] Germany in 1956 and in Britain in 1958, and in other countries as a sedative and hypnotic and was recommended for use in pregnant women. It had not been tested on pregnant animals. When it was eventually tested it was at first difficult to induce fetal deformity (until it was used on New Zealand White Rabbits).

Thalidomide, skilfully promoted and credulously prescribed and taken by the public—it was also sold without prescription—achieved huge popularity; it 'became [West] Germany's baby-sitter'. It was a routine hypnotic in hospitals and was even recommended to help children adapt themselves to a convalescent home atmosphere and was sold mixed with other drugs for symptomatic relief of pain, cough and fever.

In 1960–61 it had become evident that prolonged use of thalidomide could cause hypothyroidism and peripheral neuritis. The latter effect was the principal reason why approval for marketing in the USA, as Kevadon, had been delayed by the US Food and Drug Administration. Approval had still not been given when the fetal effects were discovered and so general distribution was avoided. Nonetheless some 'thalidomide babies' were born in the USA following indiscriminate premarketing clinical trials.

Thalidomide has anti-inflammatory and immunosuppressant actions and retains a limited specialist use in, for example, lepromatous leprosy,[17] and oral ulceration in AIDS (some cases).

The thalidomide disaster provided the impetus for the introduction of national drug regulatory authorities worldwide.

---

[17] Further cases of congenital malformations were reported in 1994 due to lax control of thalidomide use (Lancet 343, 433: 344, 196). Thalidomide is available in the UK on a 'named-patient' basis only, with a detailed patient information leaflet and with signed patient consent.

GUIDE TO FURTHER READING

Baber N 1994 International conference on harmonization of technical requirements for registration of pharmaceuticals. British Journal of Clinical Pharmacology 37: 401

Bakke O M et al 1995 Drug safety discontinuations in the United Kingdom, the United States and Spain from 1972 through 1993: a regulatory perspective. Clinical Pharmacology and Therapeutics 58: 108

DiMasi J A, Seibring M A, Lasagna L 1994 New drug development in the United States from 1963 to 1992. Clinical Pharmacology and Therapeutics 55: 609

Herxheimer A 1984 Immortality for old drugs. Lancet 2: 1460 and subsequent correspondence

Litvack J I et al 1989 Setting the price for essential drugs: necessity and affordability. Lancet 2: 376

Medicines Control Agency 1994 Guidelines for company-sponsored Safety Assessment of Marketed Medicines (SAMM Guidelines). British Journal of Clinical Pharmacology 38: 95

Merkatz R B et al 1993 Women in clinical trials of new drugs: A change in Food and Drug Administration policy. New England Journal of Medicine 329: 72: also 329: 271, 288, 1815, 1816

Richard B W et al 1987 Drug regulation in the United States and the United Kingdom: the Depo-Provera story. Annals of Internal Medicine 106: 886. An analysis of how drug regulators in the USA and the UK came to opposite conclusions on the same data.

Taylor D 1992 Counterfeiting drugs can kill. British Medical Journal 304: 334

ON THALIDOMIDE

Chamberlain G 1989 The obstetric problems of the [now adult] thalidomide children. British Medical Journal 298: 6

Editorial 1981 Thalidomide: 20 years on. Lancet 2: 510

Mellin G W et al 1962 The saga of thalidomide. New England Journal of Medicine 267: 1184, 1238

6

Classification and naming of drugs

SYNOPSIS

In any science there are two basic requirements: classification and nomenclature (names).

- Classification: drugs cannot be classified and named according to a single rational system because the requirements of pharmacologists, chemists and doctors differ.
- Nomenclature: nor is it practicable always to present each drug under a single name because the formulations in which they are presented as prescribable medicines vary widely and commercial considerations are too often paramount.

  Generic (nonproprietary) names should be used as far as possible except where pharmaceutical bioavailability differences have overriding importance.

Classification

It is evident from the way this book is organised that there is no homogeneous system for classifying drugs that suits all purposes. Drugs are commonly categorised according to the convenience of who is discussing them: clinicians, pharmacologists or medicinal chemists.

Drugs may be classified by:

- *Therapeutic use*, e.g. antimicrobial, antidiabetic, antihypertensive, analgesic
- *Mode* or *site of action*
  - *molecular interaction*, e.g. receptor blockers, enzyme inhibitors
  - *cellular site*, e.g. loop diuretic, catecholamine uptake inhibitor (imipramine)
  - *molecular structure*, e.g. glycoside, alkaloid, steroid.

Nomenclature (names)

The world is moving towards a uniform policy of one drug, one official name. This is a highly desirable objective for ultimate convenience and safety. But in the short term there will be inconvenience as countries (sometimes after a period of use in tandem) adopt the recommended International Nonproprietary Names (see below).

Any drug may have names in all three of the following classes:

1. The *full chemical name*.
2. A *nonproprietary (official, approved, generic) name* used in pharmacopoeias and chosen by official bodies; recommended International Nonproprietary Names (rINN), are chosen by the World Health Organization (WHO), but national and regional differences persist. We have done our best to minimise

some unavoidable differences with, where appropriate, alternative names in the text and index.

3. *A proprietary (brand) name* or names that are the commercial property of a pharmaceutical company/ies.

Example: one drug — three names

1. 3-(10,11-dihydro-5H-dibenz [b,f]-azepin-5-yl) propyl-dimethylamine
2. imipramine
3. Tofranil (UK), Prodepress, Surplix, Deprinol, etc. (various countries)

In this book proprietary names are distinguished by an initial capital letter.

The full chemical name describes the compound for chemists. It is obviously unsuitable for prescribing.

A nonproprietary (generic, approved) name is given by an official (pharmacopoeia) agency, e.g. WHO.

Three principles remain supreme and unchallenged in importance: the need for distinction in sound and spelling, especially when the name is handwritten; the need for freedom from confusion with existing names, both nonproprietary and proprietary, and the desirability of indicating relationships between similar substances.[1]

The generic names **diazepam, nitrazepam, flurazepam** are all of benzodiazepines. Their proprietary names are Valium, Mogadon and Dalmane respectively. Names ending in *-olol* are adrenoceptor blockers: in *-pril* are ACE-inhibitors: in *-olone* are quinolone antimicrobials.

Any industrial company may manufacture a drug that has a well-established use and is no longer under patent restriction, in accordance with official pharmacopoeial quality criteria, and may apply to the regulatory authority for a licence to market. The task of authority is to ensure that these *generic* or *multisource pharmaceuticals* are inter-

changeable, i.e. they are pharmaceutically and biologically equivalent so that a formulation from one source will be absorbed and give the same blood concentrations and have the same therapeutic efficacy as that from another. (Further formal therapeutic trials are not demanded for these well-established drugs.) A prescription for a generic drug formulation may be filled by any officially licensed product that the dispensing pharmacy has chosen (on economic criteria) to purchase (see Generic substitution, p. 15).

The proprietary name is a trade mark applied to particular formulation(s) of a particular substance by a particular manufacturer. Manufacture is confined to the owner of the trade mark or to others licensed by the owner. It is designed to maximise the difference between the names of similar drugs marketed by rivals for obvious commercial reasons. To add confusion, some companies give proprietary names to their generic products in an attempt to capture the prescription market, both proprietary and generic, and some market lower-priced generics of their own proprietaries. When a prescription is written for a proprietary product pharmacists must, under law, dispense that product only, unless they persuade the doctor to alter the prescription or, under law, they have the right to substitute a generic product (this is called *generic substitution*), or a drug of different molecular structure deemed to be pharmacologically and therapeutically equivalent (this is called *therapeutic substitution*). Both these substitutions are designed to reduce cost; they are medically and commercially contentious.[2]

NONPROPRIETARY NAMES

The principal reasons for advocating the habitual use of nonproprietary (generic) names in prescribing are:

Clarity: because it gives information of the class of drug, e.g. nortriptyline and amitriptyline are plainly related, but their proprietary names are Allegron and Lentizol.

---

[1] Trigg R B 1978 Pharmaceutical Journal 220: 181.

[2] In the UK National Health Service hospitals operate generic substitution (but not therapeutic substitution) to allow them to purchase drugs in bulk (cheaply).

There have been cases of prescribers, when one drug had failed, unwittingly changing to another drug of the same group or even to the same drug, thinking that such different proprietary names must mean different drugs. Such occurrences are a criticism of the prescriber, but they are also a criticism of the system that allows such confusion.

Economy: drugs sold under nonproprietary names are usually, but not always, cheaper than those sold under proprietary names.

Convenience: pharmacists may supply whatever version they stock[3] whereas if a proprietary name is used they are normally obliged to supply that preparation alone. They may have to send for the preparation named although they have an equivalent in stock. Mixtures of drugs are sometimes given nonproprietary names, often having the prefix *co-* to indicate more than one active ingredient, e.g. co-amoxiclav for Augmentin, but many are not because they exist for commercial advantage rather than for therapeutic need. No prescriber can be expected to write out the ingredients, so proprietary names are used in many cases, there being no alternative.

International travellers with chronic illnesses will be grateful for international nonproprietary names (INN) (proprietary names often differ from country to country: the reasons are linguistic as well as commercial, see below).

PROPRIETARY NAMES

The principal noncommercial reason for advocating the use of proprietary names in prescribing is consistency of the product, so that problems of quality, especially of bioavailability, are reduced. There is substance in this argument, though it is often exaggerated.

It is reasonable to use proprietary names when dosage, and therefore pharmaceutical bioavailability, are critical so that small variations in the amount of drug available for absorption can have big effects on the patient, e.g. drugs with low therapeutic ratio, digoxin, hormone replacement therapy, adrenocortical steroids (oral), antiepileptics, cardiac antidysrhythmics, warfarin. Also, with the introduction of complex formulations, e.g. sustained-release, it is important clearly to identify these, and use of proprietary names has a role.

The pharmaceutical industry regards freedom to market proprietary names and to advertise or, as it calls the latter, to 'effectively [bring] to the notice of the medical profession', as two of the essentials of the 'process of discovery in a vigorous competitive environment'.[4]

The present situation is that industry spends an enormous amount of money promoting its many names for the same article; and the community, as represented by the UK Department of Health, spends a small sum trying to persuade doctors to forget the brand names and to use nonproprietary names. The ordinary doctor who prescribes for his ordinary patients is the target of both sides.

Whatever the theoretical pros and cons, one thing is plain, that until nonproprietary names approach in brevity and euphony those coined by pharmaceutical companies, the fight for their general use is a losing one. If one of the chief purposes of a drug name is that it should be used by doctors when prescribing, then provision of such nonproprietary names as ceftazidime for Fortum, or zidovudine for Retrovir defeats this purpose.

The search for proprietary names is a 'major problem' for pharmaceutical companies, increasing, as they are, their output of new preparations. A company may average 30 new preparations (not new chemical entities) a year, another warning of the urgent necessity for the doctor to cultivate a sceptical habit of mind.

One firm (in the USA) commissioned a computer to produce a dictionary of forty-two thousand nonsense words of an appropriate scientific look and sound. An official said,

> Thinking up names has been driving us cuckoo around here ... proper chemical names are hopeless for trade purposes, of course .... Doctors are the market we shoot for. A good trade name carries a lot of weight with doctors ... they're more

---

[3] This can result in supply of a formulation of appearance different from that previously used. Patients naturally find this disturbing.

[4] Annual Report, 1963–1964. Association of the British Pharmaceutical Industry.

apt to write a prescription for a drug whose name is short, and easy to spell and pronounce, but has an impressive medical ring . . . . We believe there are enough brand new words in this dictionary to keep us going for years . . . . We don't yet know what proportion of names is unpronounceable . . . how many are obscene, either in English or in other languages, and how many are objectionable on grounds of good taste: 'Godamycin' would be a mild example.[5,6]

The names which 'look and sound medically seductive' are being picked out. 'Words that survive scrutiny will go into a stock-pile and await the inexorable proliferation of new drugs'.[6]

Perhaps the doctors have themselves to blame for this prospect which is made more dismaying by the news that no other officially regulated industry has a faster rate of innovation and product obsolescence.

> In practical terms, most (UK) doctors have a British National Formulary on their desks; it includes a reasonably comprehensive glossary of proprietary drugs with their approved names. The range of drugs prescribed by any individual is remarkably narrow, and once the decision is taken to 'think generic' surely the effort required is small[7]

and, we would add, worthwhile.

Confusing names. The need for both clear thought and clear handwriting is shown by the frequency with which medicines of totally different class have closely similar names, both proprietary and nonproprietary. Serious injury has occurred due to confusion of names and the dispensing of the wrong drug, e.g. Lasix (frusemide) for Losec (omeprazole) [death]; AZT (intending zidovudine) was misinterpreted in the pharmacy and *azathioprine* was dispensed [do not use abbreviations for drug names]; *Daonil* (glibenclamide) for *De-nol* (bismuth chelate) and for *Danol* (danazol). It will be noticed that the generic names are unlikely to be confused with other classes of drugs.

GUIDE TO FURTHER READING

Controversies in therapeutics 1988 The cases for and against prescribing generic drugs. British Medical Journal 297: (Collier J Generic prescribing benefits patients) 1596 (Cruickshank J M Don't take innovative research-based pharmaceutical companies for granted) 1597

George C F 1996 Naming of drugs: pass the epinephrine please. British Medical Journal 312: 1315

Jack D B, Soppitt A J 1991 Give a drug a bad name. British Medical Journal 303: 1606

Taussig H B 1963 The evils of camouflage as illustrated by thalidomide. New England Journal of Medicine 180: 92, Editorial, p. 108

---

[5] Pharmaceutical companies increasingly operate worldwide and are liable to find themselves embarrassed by unanticipated verbal associations. For example, names marketed (in some countries) such as Bumaflex, Kriplex, Nokhel and Snootie conjure up in the minds of native English-speakers associations that may inhibit both doctors and patients from using them (see Jack and Soppitt in Guide to Further Reading).

[6] New Yorker, 14 July 1956.

[7] Editorial 1977 British Medical Journal 4: 980 and subsequent correspondence.

FROM PHARMACOLOGY TO TOXICOLOGY

7

General pharmacology

SYNOPSIS

How drugs act and interact, how they enter the body, what happens to them inside the body, how they are eliminated from it; the effects of genetics, age, and disease on drug action — these topics are important for, although they will generally not be in the front of the conscious mind of the prescriber, an understanding of them will enhance rational decision taking.

Knowledge of the requirements for success and the explanations for failure and for adverse events will enable the doctor to maximise the benefits and minimise the risks of drug therapy.

Pharmacodynamics

- Qualitative aspects: Receptors, Enzymes, Selectivity
- Quantitative aspects: Dose response, Potency, Therapeutic efficacy, Tolerance

Pharmacokinetics

- Time course of drug concentration: Order of reaction; Plasma half-life and steady-state concentration; Therapeutic drug monitoring
- Individual processes: Drug passage across cell membranes, Absorption, Distribution, Metabolism, Elimination
- Drug dosage: Dosing schedules

SYNOPSIS (cont'd)

- Chronic pharmacology: the consequences of prolonged drug administration and drug discontinuation syndromes
- Individual or biological variation: Variability due to inherited influences, environmental and host influences
- Drug interactions: outside the body, at site of absorption, during distribution, directly on receptors, during metabolism, during excretion

Pharmacodynamics is what drugs do to the body: pharmacokinetics is what the body does to drugs.

It is self-evident that knowledge of pharmacodynamics is essential to the choice of drug therapy. But the well-chosen drug may fail to produce benefit or may be poisonous because too little or too much is present at the site of action for too short or too long a time. Drug therapy can fail for pharmacokinetic as well as for pharmacodynamic reasons. The practice of drug therapy entails more than remembering an apparently arbitrary list of actions or indications.

Technical incompetence in the modern doctor is inexcusable and technical competence and a humane approach are not incompatible as is sometimes suggested.

Pharmacodynamics

> Understanding the mechanisms of drug action is not only an objective of the pharmacologist who seeks to develop new and better drugs, it is also the basis of intelligent use of medicines.

Qualitative aspects

It is appropriate to begin by considering what drugs do and how they do it, i.e. the nature of drug action. Body functions are mediated through control systems that involve chemotransmitters or local hormones, receptors, enzymes, carrier molecules and other specialised macromolecules such as DNA. Most drugs act by altering the body's control systems. Some do so unselectively, e.g. general anaesthetic agents and alcohol, and such substances tend to interfere with multiple systems thereby causing unwanted as well as wanted effects. The majority of medicinal drugs act by binding to some specialised constituent of the cell to alter its function selectively and consequently that of the physiological or pathological system to which it contributes. Such drugs are biologically selective and structurally specific in that small modifications to their chemical structure may profoundly alter their effect.

MECHANISMS

An overview of the mechanisms of drug action shows that drugs act on **the cell membrane** by:

● Action on *specific receptors*,[1] e.g. agonists and antagonists on adrenoceptors, histamine receptors, acetylcholine receptors
● Interference with selective *passage of ions across membranes*, e.g. calcium entry (or channel) blockers
● Inhibition of *membrane bound enzymes* and *pumps*, e.g. membrane bound ATPase by cardiac

glycoside; tricyclic antidepressants block the pump by which amines are actively taken up from the exterior to the interior of nerve cells
● Physicochemical interaction, e.g. general and local anaesthetics and alcohol appear to act on the lipid, protein or water constituents of nerve cell membranes.

Drugs act on **metabolic processes within the cell** by:

● *Enzyme inhibition*, e.g. monoamine oxidase by phenelzine, cholinesterase by pyridostigmine, xanthine oxidase by allopurinol
● *Inhibition of transport processes* that carry substances across cells, e.g. blockade of anion transport in the renal tubule cell by probenecid can be used to delay excretion of penicillin, and to enhance elimination of urate
● *Incorporation into larger molecules*, e.g. 5-fluorouracil, an anticancer drug, is incorporated into messenger-RNA in place of uracil
● In the case of successful *antimicrobial* agents, altering metabolic processes unique to microorganisms, e.g. penicillin interferes with formation of the bacterial cell wall, *or by* showing enormous quantitative differences in affecting a process common to both humans and microbes, e.g. inhibition of folic acid synthesis by trimethoprim.

Drugs act **outside the cell** by:

● *Direct chemical interaction*, e.g. chelating agents, antacids
● *Osmosis*, as with purgatives, e.g. magnesium sulphate, and diuretics, e.g. mannitol, which are active because neither they nor the water in which they are dissolved are absorbed by the cells lining the gut and kidney tubules respectively.

RECEPTORS

Most receptors are protein macromolecules. When the agonist binds to the receptor, the proteins undergo an alteration in conformation which induces changes in systems within the cell that in turn bring about the response to the drug. For example, activation of β-adrenoceptors by a cate-

---

[1] A receptor mediates a biological effect, e.g. adrenoceptor; a binding site, e.g. plasma albumin, does not.

cholamine (the *first messenger*) increases the activity of adenylate cyclase which raises the rate of formation of cyclic AMP (the *second messenger*), a modulator of the activity of several enzyme systems that cause the cell to act. Other drug–receptor effects are mediated through control of membrane ion channels closely associated with the receptor, e.g. calcium entry blockers.

Radioligand binding studies[2] have shown that the receptor numbers do not remain constant but change according to circumstances. When tissues are continuously exposed to an agonist, the number of receptors decreases (*down-regulation*) and this may be a cause of tachyphylaxis (loss of efficacy with frequently repeated doses), e.g. in asthmatics who use adrenoceptor agonist bronchodilators excessively. Prolonged contact with an antagonist leads to formation of new receptors (*up-regulation*). Indeed, one explanation for the worsening of angina pectoris or cardiac ventricular dysrhythmia in some patients following abrupt withdrawal of a β-adrenoceptor blocker is that normal concentrations of circulating catecholamines now have access to an increased (up-regulated) population of β-adrenoceptors (see Chronic pharmacology, p. 107).

Agonists. Drugs that activate receptors do so because they resemble the natural transmitter or hormone, but their value in clinical practice often rests on their greater capacity to resist degradation and so to act for longer than the natural substances (endogenous ligands) they mimic; for this reason bronchodilation produced by salbutamol lasts longer than that induced by adrenaline.

Antagonists (blockers) of receptors are sufficiently similar to the natural agonist to be 'recognised' by the receptor and to occupy it without activating a response, thereby preventing (blocking) the natural agonist from exerting its effect. Drugs that have no activating effect whatever on the receptor are termed *pure antagonists*. A receptor occupied by a low efficacy agonist is inaccessible to a subsequent

dose of a high efficacy agonist, so that, in this specific situation, a low efficacy agonist acts as an antagonist. This can happen with opioids.

Partial agonists. Some drugs, in addition to blocking access of the natural agonist to the receptor are capable of a low degree of activation, i.e. they have both antagonist and agonist action. Such substances are said to show *partial agonist activity* (PAA). The β-adrenoceptor antagonists pindolol and oxprenolol have partial agonist activity (in their case it is often called *intrinsic sympathomimetic activity*) (ISA), whilst propranolol is devoid of agonist activity, i.e. it is a pure antagonist. A patient may be as extensively 'β-blocked' by propranolol as by pindolol, i.e. exercise tachycardia is abolished, but the resting heart rate is lower on propranolol; such differences have clinical importance.

Inverse agonists. Some substances produce effects that are specifically opposite to those of the agonist. The agonist action of benzodiazepines on the benzodiazepine receptor in the CNS produces sedation, anxiolysis, muscle relaxation and controls convulsions; substances called β-carbolines which also bind to this receptor cause stimulation, anxiety, increased muscle tone and convulsions; they are inverse agonists. Both types of drug act by modulating the effects of the neurotransmitter gamma-aminobutyric acid (GABA).

Receptor binding (and vice versa). If the forces that bind drug to receptor are weak (hydrogen bonds, van der Waals bonds, electrostatic bonds), the binding will be easily and rapidly reversible; if the forces involved are strong (covalent bonds), then binding will be effectively irreversible. An antagonist that binds reversibly to a receptor can by definition be displaced from the receptor by mass action (see p. 84) of the agonist (and vice versa). If the concentration of agonist increases sufficiently above that of the antagonist the response is restored. This phenomenon is commonly seen in clinical practice — patients who are taking a β-adrenoceptor blocker, and whose low resting heart rate can be increased by exercise, are showing that they can raise their sympathetic drive to release enough noradrenaline (agonist) to diminish the prevailing degree of receptor blockade. Increasing

---

[2] The extraordinary discrimination of this technique is shown by the calculation that the total β-adrenoceptor protein in a large cow amounts to 1 mg (Maguire M E et al 1977 In: Greengard P, Robison G A (eds) Advances in Cyclic Nucleotide Research. Raven Press, New York: 8: 1.

the dose of β-adrenoceptor blocker will limit or abolish exercise-induced tachycardia, showing that the degree of blockade is enhanced as more drug becomes available to compete with the endogenous transmitter. Since agonist and antagonist compete to occupy the receptor according to the law of mass action, this type of drug action is termed *competitive antagonism*. When receptor-mediated responses are studied either in isolated tissues or in intact man, a graph of the logarithm of the dose given (horizontal axis), plotted against the response obtained (vertical axis), commonly gives an S-shaped (sigmoid) curve, the central part of which is a straight line. If the measurements are repeated in the presence of an antagonist, and the curve obtained is parallel to the original but displaced to the **right,** then antagonism is said to be competitive and the agonist to be surmountable.

Drugs that bind *irreversibly* to receptors include phenoxybenzamine (to the α-adrenoceptor). Since such a drug cannot be displaced from the receptor, increasing the concentration of agonist does not fully restore the response and antagonism of this type is said to be insurmountable.

The log-dose-response curves for the agonist in the absence of and in the presence of a *noncompetitive* antagonist are not parallel. Some toxins act in this way, e.g. α-bungarotoxin, a constituent of some snake and spider venoms, binds irreversibly to the acetylcholine receptor and is used as a tool to study it. Restoration of the response after irreversible binding requires elimination of the drug from the body and synthesis of new receptor, and for this reason the effect may persist long after drug administration has ceased. Irreversible agents find little place in clinical practice.

ENZYMES

Interaction between drug and enzyme is in many respects similar to that between drug and receptor. Drugs may alter enzyme activity because they resemble a natural substrate and hence compete with it for the enzyme. For example, enalapril is effective in hypertension because it is structurally similar to that part of angiotensin I which is attacked by angiotensin-converting enzyme (ACE); by occupying the active site of the enzyme and so inhibiting its action enalapril prevents formation of the pressor angiotensin II. Carbidopa competes with levodopa for dopa decarboxylase and the resulting reduction in metabolism of levodopa in the blood (but not in the brain to which carbidopa does not penetrate) is the basis for the use of this combination in Parkinson's disease. Ethanol prevents metabolism of methanol to its toxic metabolite, formic acid, by competing for occupancy of the enzyme alcohol dehydrogenase; this is the rationale for using ethanol in methanol poisoning. The above are examples of competitive (**reversible**) inhibition of enzyme activity.

Irreversible inhibition occurs with organophosphorus insecticides and chemical warfare agents (see p. 148) which combine covalently with the active site of acetylcholinesterase; recovery of cholinesterase activity depends on the formation of new enzyme. Covalent binding of aspirin to prostaglandin G/H synthase inhibits the enzyme in platelets for their entire lifespan because platelets have no system for synthesising new protein and this is why low doses of aspirin are sufficient for antiplatelet action.

Physiological (functional) antagonism

An action on the same receptor is not the only mechanism by which one drug may oppose the effect of another. Extreme bradycardia following overdose of a β-adrenoceptor blocker can be relieved by atropine which accelerates the heart by blockade of the parasympathetic branch of the autonomic nervous system, the cholinergic tone of which (vagal tone) operates continuously to slow it. Bronchoconstriction produced by histamine released from mast cells in anaphylactic shock can be counteracted by adrenaline which relaxes bronchial smooth muscle (β$_2$-adrenoceptor effect) or by theophylline. In both cases, a pharmacological effect is overcome by a second drug which acts via a different physiological mechanism, i.e. there is physiological or functional antagonism.

SELECTIVITY

The pharmacologist who produces a new drug and the doctor who gives it to a patient share the desire that it should possess a selective action so that management of the patient is not complicated by additional and unwanted (adverse) effects.

There are in general two approaches to obtaining selectivity of drug action:

Modification of drug structure

Many drugs are designed to have a structural similarity to some natural constituent of the body, e.g. a neurotransmitter, a hormone, a substrate for an enzyme; they achieve selectivity of action by replacing or competing with that natural constituent. Enormous scientific effort and expertise go into the synthesis and testing of analogues of natural substances in order to create drugs capable of obtaining a specified effect and that alone. The approach is the basis of modern drug design and it has led to the production of adrenoceptor antagonists, histamine-receptor antagonists and many other important medicines. But there are biological constraints to selectivity. Anticancer drugs that act against rapidly dividing cells lack selectivity because they also damage other tissues with a high cell replication rate, such as bone marrow and gut epithelium.

Selective delivery (drug targeting)

The objective of target tissue selectivity can sometimes be achieved by simple topical application, e.g. skin and eye, and by special drug delivery systems, as by intrabronchial administration of β_2-adrenoceptor agonists or corticosteroids (inhaled pressurised metered aerosol for asthma). Selective targeting of drugs to less accessible sites of disease offers considerable scope for therapy as technology develops, e.g. attaching drugs to antibodies selective for cancer cells.

Stereoselectivity. Drug molecules are three-dimensional and many drugs contain one or more *asymmetric* or *chiral* centres in their structures, i.e. a single drug can be in effect a mixture of two non-identical mirror images (like a mixture of left- and right-hand gloves). The two forms which are known as *enantiomorphs* can exhibit very different biological activity, e.g. the S(−) form of warfarin is four times more active than the R(+) form. Many other drugs are available as mixtures of enantiomorphs or racemates. Pharmaceutical develop-

ment of drugs as single enantiomers rather than as racemic mixtures offers the prospect of greater selectivity of action and lessens risk of toxicity.

Quantitative aspects

That a drug has a desired qualitative action is obviously all-important, but it is not by itself enough. There are also quantitative aspects, i.e. the right **amount** of action is required and with some drugs the dose has to be very precisely adjusted to deliver this, neither too little nor too much, to escape both inefficacy and toxicity, e.g. digoxin, lithium, gentamicin. Whilst the general correlation between dose and response may evoke no surprise, certain characteristics of the relation are fundamental to the way drugs are used. These are:

DOSE-RESPONSE CURVES

The extent to which the desired response alters as the dose is changed is defined by the shape of the dose-response curve, which conventionally has dose plotted on the horizontal and response on the vertical axis. A steep-rising and prolonged curve indicates that a small change in dose produces a large change in drug effect, e.g. loop diuretics. By contrast the dose-response curve for the thiazide diuretics soon reaches a plateau; e.g. the clinically useful dose range for bendrofluazide is between 2.5 and 10 mg and increasing the dose beyond this produces no added diuretic effect though it adds to toxicity. The wanted and unwanted effects of drugs have their own dose-response curves (see below). Toxicity is commonest with drugs that have steep dose-response curves for both the wanted and unwanted effects.

POTENCY AND PHARMACOLOGICAL EFFICACY

The terms potency and efficacy are often used imprecisely and so confusingly. It is pertinent to make a clear distinction between them, particularly in relation to claims made for usefulness in therapeutics.

Potency is the amount (weight) of drug in relation to its effect, e.g. if weight-for-weight drug A has a greater effect than drug B, then drug A is more potent than drug B, but the maximum therapeutic effect obtainable may be similar with both drugs. The diuretic effect of bumetanide 1 mg is equivalent to frusemide 50 mg, thus bumetanide is more *potent* than frusemide but both drugs achieve about the same maximum effect. The difference in weight of drug that has to be administered is of no clinical significance unless it is great.

Pharmacological efficacy refers to the strength of response induced by occupancy of a receptor by an agonist (intrinsic activity); it is a specialised pharmacological concept. But clinicians are concerned with *therapeutic efficacy*, as follows.

THERAPEUTIC EFFICACY

Therapeutic efficacy, or effectiveness, is the capacity of a drug to produce an effect and refers to the maximum such effect, e.g. if drug A can produce a therapeutic effect that cannot be obtained with drug B, however much of drug B is given, then drug A has the higher therapeutic efficacy. Differences in therapeutic efficacy are of great clinical importance. Amiloride (low efficacy) can at best cause no more than 5% of the filtered sodium load to be excreted and there is no point in increasing the dose beyond that which achieves this for no greater diuretic effect can be attained; bendrofluazide (moderate efficacy) can cause no more than 10% of the filtered sodium load to be excreted no matter how much drug is administered; frusemide (high efficacy) can cause 25% and more of filtered sodium to be excreted, hence it is called a high efficacy diuretic.

THERAPEUTIC INDEX

When the dose of a drug is increased progressively, the desired response in the patient usually rises to a maximum beyond which further increases in dose elicit no greater benefit but induce only unwanted effects. This is because a drug does not have a single dose-response curve, but a different curve for each action (wanted as well as unwanted), so that new and unwanted actions are recruited if dose is increased after the maximum therapeutic effect has

been achieved. Thus a sympathomimetic bronchodilator might exhibit one dose-response relation for decreasing airways resistance and another for increase in heart rate. Clearly the usefulness of any drug is intimately related to the extent to which such dose-response relations can be separated. Ehrlich (p. 187) introduced the concept of the *therapeutic index* as the maximum tolerated dose divided by the minimum curative dose but, since such single doses cannot be determined accurately, the index is never calculated in this way in man. A dose that has some unwanted effect in 50% of humans, e.g. a specified increase in heart rate, in the case of an adrenoceptor agonist bronchodilator can be related to that which is therapeutic in 50%, e.g. a specified decrease in airways resistance, although in practice such information is not available for many drugs. Nevertheless the therapeutic index does embody a concept that is fundamental in comparing the usefulness of one drug with another, namely, *safety* in relation to efficacy. The concept is expressed diagrammatically in Figure 7.1.

TOLERANCE

Tolerance is said to have developed when it becomes necessary to increase the dose of a drug to

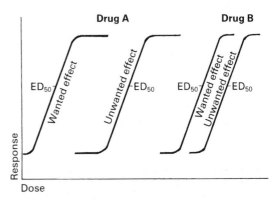

Fig. 7.1 Dose-response curves for two hypothetical drugs
Drug A: the dose that causes maximum wanted effect causes no unwanted effect. The ratio ED_{50} (unwanted effect)/ED_{50} (wanted effect)[3] indicates that it has a large therapeutic ratio: it is thus highly selective in its action
Drug B causes unwanted effects at doses well below that which produces its maximum benefit. The ratio ED_{50} (unwanted effect)/ED_{50} (wanted effect) indicates that it has a small therapeutic ratio: it is thus nonselective

[3] ED_{50} = effective dose in 50% of subjects.

obtain an effect previously obtained with a smaller dose. *Acquired tolerance* is familiar especially with opioids and is due to reduced pharmacological efficacy (p. 82) at receptor sites or to down-regulation of receptors. It can also be due to increased metabolism as a result of enzyme induction. There is commonly cross-tolerance between drugs of similar structure and sometimes between those of dissimilar structure. There is also *natural tolerance* which is not induced by the drug but is due to inherent factors (see Pharmacogenetics, p. 81).

BIOASSAY AND STANDARDISATION

Biological assay (bioassay) is the process by which the activity of a substance (identified or unidentified) is measured on living material: e.g. contraction of bronchial, uterine or vascular muscle. It is used only when chemical or physical methods are not practicable as in the case of a mixture of active substances, or of an incompletely purified preparation, or where no chemical method has been developed. The activity of a preparation is expressed relative to that of a standard preparation of the same substance. The controlled therapeutic trial is a special form of bioassay.

Biological *standardisation* is a specialised form of bioassay. It involves matching of material of unknown potency with an International or National Standard with the objective of providing a preparation for use in therapeutics and research. The results are expressed as *units* of a substance rather than its weight, e.g. insulin, vaccines.

Pharmacokinetics

To initiate a desired drug action is a qualitative choice but, when the qualitative choice is made, considerations of quantity immediately arise; it is possible to have too much or too little of a good thing. To obtain the right effect at the right intensity, at the right time, for the right duration, with minimum risk of unpleasantness or harm, is what pharmacokinetics is about.

Dosage regimens of long-established drugs were devised by trial and error. Doctors learned by experience the dose, the frequency of dosing and the route of administration that was most likely to benefit and least likely to harm. Apart from being laborious and putting patients at risk, this empirical ('suck it and see') approach left some questions unanswered. It did not explain, for example, why digoxin is effective in a once-daily dose, whereas aspirin may need to be given 4 times daily; why a dose of morphine is more effective if it is given intramuscularly than if the same amount is taken by mouth; why insulin is useless unless it is injected. The answers to these questions lie in understanding how drugs cross membranes to enter the body, how they are distributed round it in the blood and other body fluids, how they are bound to plasma proteins and tissues (which act as stores) and how they are eliminated from the body. These processes can now be quantified and allow efficient development of dosing regimens.

Pharmacokinetics[4] is concerned with the rate at which drug molecules cross cell membranes to enter the body, to distribute within it and to leave the body, as well as with the structural changes (metabolism) to which they are subject within it.

The subject will be discussed under the following headings:

- Time course of drug concentration and effect
  First- and zero-order processes
  Plasma half-life and steady-state concentration
  Therapeutic monitoring
- The individual processes
  Drug passage across membranes
  Absorption
  Distribution
  Metabolism (biotransformation)
  Elimination.

Time course of drug concentration and effect

A number of important topics are fundamental to the understanding of this process.

---

[4] Greek: *pharmakon* drug, *kinein* to move.

> - In first-order processes a constant fraction of drug is metabolised/eliminated in unit time.
> - In zero-order processes a constant amount of drug is metabolised/eliminated in unit time.

FIRST-ORDER (EXPONENTIAL) PROCESSES

Drugs taken into the body are subject to processes of absorption, distribution, metabolism and excretion. In the majority of instances the rates at which these processes occur are directly proportional to the concentration of the drug. In other words, transfer of drug across a cell membrane or formation of a metabolite is high at high concentrations and falls in direct proportion to be low at low concentrations (an exponential relationship). This is because the processes follow the Law of Mass Action, which states that the rate of reaction is directly proportional to the active masses of reacting substances. In other words, at high concentrations, there are more opportunities for crowded molecules to interact with each other or to cross cell membranes than at low, uncrowded concentrations. Processes for which rate is proportional to concentration are called first-order.

In doses used clinically, most drugs are subject to first-order processes of absorption, distribution, metabolism and elimination and the knowledge that a drug exhibits first-order kinetics is useful; e.g. it can be predicted that a 50% or 100% increase in dose will lead to an increase in steady-state plasma concentration by the same percentage. The converse will also be true: since rate and concentration are in proportion, when dosing is discontinued, the rate of elimination from plasma falls as the plasma concentration falls and the time for any plasma concentration to fall by 50% ($t^1/2$, the plasma half-life) will always be the same; thus it is possible to quote a single figure for the $t^1/2$ of the drug. Certain simple and valuable calculations are dependent on knowing the $t^1/2$: i.e. estimation of time to eliminate a drug; construction of dosing schedules; prediction of the time to achieve steady-state plasma concentration. In this book $t^1/2$ means *plasma* $t^1/2$ unless otherwise stated.

ZERO-ORDER PROCESSES (SATURATION KINETICS)

Zero-order processes are of particular importance in drug elimination and dosing. As the amount of drug in the body rises, any metabolic processes that have limited capacity become saturated. In other words, the rate of the process reaches a maximum amount at which it stays constant, e.g. due to limited amount of an enzyme, and further increase in rate is impossible despite an increase in the dose of drug. Clearly, these are circumstances in which the rate of reaction is not proportional to dose, and processes that exhibit this type of kinetics are described as rate-limited or dose-dependent or zero-order or as showing *saturation kinetics*. In practice enzyme-mediated metabolic reactions are the most likely to show rate-limitation because the amount of enzyme present is finite and can become saturated. Passive diffusion does not become saturated. There are some important consequences of zero-order kinetics.

Alcohol (ethanol) (see also p. 166) is a drug whose kinetics have considerable implications for society as well as for the individual, as follows.

Alcohol is subject to first-order kinetics with a $t^1/2$ of about one hour at plasma concentrations below 10 mg/dl (attained after drinking about two-thirds of a unit (glass) of wine or beer). Above this concentration the main enzyme (alcohol dehydrogenase) that converts the alcohol into acetaldehyde approaches and then reaches saturation, at which point alcohol metabolism cannot proceed any faster. Thus if the subject continues to drink, the blood alcohol concentration rises disproportionately, for the rate of metabolism remains the same (at about 10 ml or 8 g/h for a 70 kg man), and alcohol shows zero-order kinetics.

Consider a man of average size whose life is unhappy to a degree where he drinks about half (375 ml) a standard bottle of whisky (40% alcohol), i.e. 150 ml of alcohol, over a short period, absorbs it and goes very drunk to bed at midnight with a blood alcohol concentration of about 250 mg/dl.

If alcohol metabolism were subject to first-order kinetics, with a $t^1/2$ of one hour throughout the whole range of social consumption, the subject would halve his blood alcohol concentration each hour and it is easy to calculate that, when he drove his car to work at 08.00 h the next morning, he would have a negligible blood alcohol concentration (less than 1 mg/dl); though, no doubt, a severe hangover might reduce his driving skill.

But at these high concentrations, alcohol is subject to zero-order kinetics and so, metabolising about 10 ml of alcohol per hour, after 8 h the subject will have eliminated 80 ml, leaving 70 ml in his body and giving a blood concentration of about 120 mg/dl. The legal limit for car driving in the UK is a generous 80 mg/dl; at 120 mg/dl his driving skill would be seriously impaired. The subject could have an accident and be convicted of drunk driving on his way to work despite his indignant protests that the blood or breath alcohol determination must be faulty since he has not touched a drop since midnight. He would be banned from the road, and thus have leisure to reflect on the difference between first-order and zero-order kinetics.

This is an example thought up for this occasion, although no doubt something close to it happens in real life often enough, but an example important in therapeutics is provided by **phenytoin**. At low doses the elimination of phenytoin proceeds as a first-order process, i.e. as dose is increased there is a directly proportional increase in the steady-state plasma concentration because elimination increases to match the increase in dose. But gradually, the enzymatic elimination process approaches and reaches saturation, attaining a maximum rate beyond which it cannot increase; the process has become constant and zero-order. Since further increases in dose cannot be matched by increase in the rate of metabolism the plasma concentration rises steeply and disproportionately, with danger of toxicity. No doubt many drugs could exhibit saturation kinetics if a high enough dose were taken. The distinction between first-order and zero-order kinetics becomes a clinically important issue when the change from one to the other occurs within the range of therapeutic dosing. This is the case with alcohol, phenytoin and salicylate (at high therapeutic doses). Clearly saturation kinetics is a significant factor in delay in recovery from drug overdose with, e.g. phenytoin or aspirin.

When a drug is subject to first-order kinetics and by definition the rate of elimination is proportional to plasma concentration, then the $t^1/2$ is a constant characteristic, i.e. a single value can be quoted throughout the plasma concentration range, and this is convenient. If the rate of a process, e.g. removal from the plasma by metabolism, is not directly proportional to plasma concentration, then the $t^1/2$ cannot be constant. Consequently, when a drug exhibits zero-order elimination kinetics no single value for its $t^1/2$ can be quoted for, in fact, $t^1/2$ decreases as plasma concentration falls and the calculations on elimination and dosing that are so easy with first-order elimination become too complicated to be of much practical use. Zero-order absorption processes apply to iron, to depot i.m. formulations and to drug implants, e.g. antipsychotics and sex hormones.

Plasma half-life and steady-state concentration

The manner in which plasma drug concentration rises or falls when dosing is begun, altered or ceased follows certain simple rules which provide a means for rational control of drug effect. Central to understanding these is the concept of half-life. Consider the time course of a drug in the blood after an i.v. bolus injection, i.e. a single dose injected in a period of seconds as distinct from a continuous infusion. Plasma concentration will rise quickly as drug enters the blood to reach a peak; there will then be a sharp drop as the drug distributes round the body (*distribution phase*) which will be followed by a steady decline as drug is removed from the blood by the liver or kidneys (*elimination phase*). If the elimination processes are first-order, the time taken for any concentration point in the elimination phase to fall to half its value is always the same; in other words, the half-life or half-time ($t^1/2$), which is the time taken for the plasma concentration to fall by half, is a constant, as is illustrated in Figure 7.2.

> The $t^1/2$ is the single pharmacokinetic characteristic of a drug that it is most useful to know.

The $t^1/2$ may be used to predict the manner in which plasma concentration alters in response to

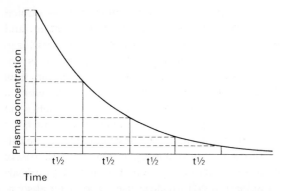

Fig. 7.2 Changes in plasma concentration following an i.v. bolus injection of a drug, in the elimination phase (the distribution phase, see text, is not shown); as elimination is a first-order process, the time taken for any concentration to fall by 50% ($t^1/2$) is the same

starting, altering or ceasing drug administration. These events are illustrated in Figure 7.3 and the subsequent text.

Increases in plasma concentration

When a drug is infused at a constant rate the amount in the body and with it the plasma concentration rise until a state is reached at which the rate of administration of drug to the body is exactly equal to the rate of elimination. This is called the *steady state*, and when it is attained the amount of drug in the body remains constant; the plasma concentration is on a *plateau*. Figure 7.3 depicts the smooth changes in plasma concentration that result from a constant i.v. infusion. Clearly if a drug is given by intermittent oral or intravenous dose, the plasma concentration will fluctuate between peaks and troughs, but in time all the peaks will be of equal height and all the troughs will be of equal depth; this is also called a steady-state concentration, since the mean concentration is constant.[5]

Time to reach steady state

When a drug is administered by constant-rate i.v. infusion it is important to know *when* steady state has been reached, for maintaining the same dosing schedule will then ensure a constant amount of drug in the body and the patient will experience neither acute toxicity nor decline of effect. The $t^1/2$ provides

[5] The peaks and troughs can be of practical importance with drugs of low therapeutic index, e.g. aminoglycoside antibiotics, and it is often necessary to monitor both for safe and effective therapy.

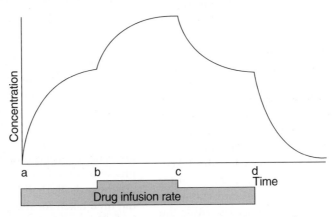

Fig. 7.3 Changes in drug plasma concentration during the course of a constant-rate i.v. infusion
a: The infusion commences and plasma concentration rises to reach a steady state (plateau) in about 5 x $t^1/2$.
b: The infusion rate is increased by 50% and the plasma concentration rises further to reach a new steady state in another 5 x $t^1/2$; this new steady state is 50% greater than the original steady state.
c: The infusion is decreased to the original rate and the plasma concentration returns to the original steady state in 5 x $t^1/2$.
d: The infusion is discontinued and the plasma concentration falls to virtually zero in 5 x $t^1/2$

the answer: with the passage of each $t^1/2$ period of time, the plasma concentration rises by **half** the difference between the current concentration and the ultimate steady-state (100%) concentration.

Thus in $1 \times t^1/2$, the concentration will reach $(100/2)$ 50%,

in $2 \times t^1/2$ $(50 + 50/2)$ 75%,

in $3 \times t^1/2$ $(75 + 25/2)$ 87.5%,

in $4 \times t^1/2$ $(87.5 + 12.5/2)$ 93.75%

in $5 \times t^1/2$ $(93.75 + 6.25/2)$ 96.875% of the ultimate steady state.

When a drug is given at a constant rate (continuous or intermittent) the *time to reach steady state* depends only on the $t^1/2$ and, for all practical purposes, after $5 \times t^1/2$ the amount of drug in the body will be constant and the plasma concentration will be at a plateau.

Changes in plasma concentration

The same principle holds for change from any steady-state plasma concentration to a new steady state brought about by increase or decrease in the rate of drug administration, provided the kinetics remain first-order. Thus when the rate of administration is altered to cause either a rise or a fall in plasma concentration, a new steady-state concentration will eventually be reached and it will take a time equal to $5 \times t^1/2$ to reach the new steady state.

Note that the actual **level** of any steady-state plasma concentration (as opposed to the **time** taken to reach it) is determined only by the difference between the rate of drug administration (input) and the rate of elimination (output). If drug elimination remains constant and administration is increased by 50%, in time a new steady-state concentration will be reached which will be 50% greater than the original.

Decline in plasma concentration

Since $t^1/2$ is the time taken for any plasma concentration to decline by one-half, starting at any steady-state (100%) plasma concentration, in $1 \times t^1/2$ the plasma concentration will fall to 50%, in $2 \times t^1/2$ to 25%, in $3 \times t^1/2$ to 12.5%, in $4 \times t^1/2$ to 6.25% and in $5 \times t^1/2$ to 3.125% of the original steady-state concentration.

Hence the $t^1/2$ can predict the rate and extent of

decline in plasma concentration after dosing is discontinued. The relation between $t^1/2$ and time to reach steady-state plasma concentration applies to all drugs that obey first-order kinetics, as much to dobutamine ($t^1/2$ 2 min) when it is useful to know that an alteration of infusion rate will reach a plateau within 10 min, as to digoxin ($t^1/2$ 36 h) when a constant (repeated) dose will give a steady-state plasma concentration only after 7.5 days.

Plasma $t^1/2$ values are given in the text where they seem particularly relevant. Inevitably, natural variation within the population produces a range in $t^1/2$ values for any drug. For clarity only, single average $t^1/2$ values are given while recognising that the population range may be as much as 50% from the stated figure in either direction.

A few $t^1/2$ values are listed in Table 7.1 so that they can be pondered upon in relation to dosing in clinical practice.

Biological effect. $t^1/2$ is the time in which the biological effect of a drug declines by one half. With drugs that act competitively on receptors (α- and β-adrenoceptor agonists and antagonists) the biological effect $t^1/2$ can be provided with reasonable accuracy. Sometimes the biological effect $t^1/2$ cannot be provided, e.g. with antimicrobials when the number of infecting organisms and their sensitivity determine the outcome.

Therapeutic monitoring

The issues that concern the practising doctor are not

Table 7.1 Plasma $t^1/2$ of some drugs	
Drug	$t^1/2$
dobutamine	2 min
benzylpenicillin	30 min
amoxycillin	1 h
paracetamol	2 h
midazolam	3 h
tolbutamide	6 h
atenolol	7 h
dothiepin	25 h
diazepam	40 h
piroxicam	45 h
ethosuximide	54 h

primarily those of changing drug plasma concentration but relate to drug effect: to the onset, magnitude and duration of action of individual doses. Accurate information about the time course of drug action is less readily obtained than that about plasma concentration. This immediately raises implications about the relation between drug effect and plasma concentration and, particularly, the extent to which useful response may be predicted by measuring the concentration of drug in plasma.

Experience shows that patients differ greatly in the amount of drug required to achieve the same response. The dose of warfarin that maintains a therapeutic concentration may vary as much as 5-fold between individuals, and there are many other examples. This is hardly surprising considering known variation in rates of drug metabolism, in disposition and in tissue responsiveness, and it raises the question of how optimal drug effect can be achieved quickly in each patient, i.e. can drug therapy be individualised? A logical approach is to assume that effect is related to drug concentration at the receptor site in the tissues and that in turn the plasma concentration is likely to be constantly related to, though not necessarily the same as, tissue concentration. Indeed, for many drugs, correlation between plasma concentration and clinical effect is better than that between dose and effect. Yet monitoring therapy by measuring drug in plasma is of practical use only in selected instances. The reasons for this repay some thought.

Plasma concentration may not be worth measuring. This is the case where dose can be titrated against a quickly and easily measured effect such as blood pressure (antihypertensives), body weight (diuretics), prothrombin time (oral anticoagulants) or blood sugar (hypoglycaemics).

Plasma concentration may have no correlation with effect. This is the case with drugs that act irreversibly and these have been named 'hit and run drugs' because their effect persists long after the drug has left the plasma. Such drugs destroy or inactivate target tissue (enzyme, receptor) and restoration of effect occurs only after days or weeks, when resynthesis takes place, e.g. some monoamine oxidase inhibitors, aspirin (on platelets), some anticholinesterases and anticancer drugs.

Plasma concentration may correlate poorly with effect. Inflammatory states may cause misleading results if only total drug concentration is measured. Many basic drugs, e.g. lignocaine, disopyramide, bind to acute phase proteins, e.g. α_1-acid glycoprotein, which are present in greatly elevated concentration in inflammatory states. The consequent rise in total drug concentration is due to increase in bound (inactive) but not in the free (active) concentration and correlation with effect will be poor if only total drug is measured. The best correlation is likely to be achieved by measurement of free (active) drug in plasma water but this is technically more difficult and total drug in plasma is usually monitored in routine clinical practice.

Sometimes the therapeutic effect of a drug declines as dose is increased beyond an optimum point. Nortriptyline is most effective in a range 50–150 µg/l of plasma. The lack of benefit below 50 µg/l is expected, and presumably represents concentrations too low to inhibit the amine pump; loss of effect at concentrations in excess of 150 µg/l is unexpected, and may be due to the α-adrenoceptor blocking effect of nortriptyline which becomes important only at higher concentration. The phenomenon arises because drugs may have more than one action (and so more than one dose response curve) depending on the dose used. An intermediate range in which effective action is obtained is called a *therapeutic window*.

The assay procedure may not measure metabolites of a drug that are pharmacologically active, e.g. some benzodiazepines, or may measure metabolites that are pharmacologically inactive; in either event correlation between plasma concentration and effect is weakened.

Plasma concentration may correlate well with effect. When this is the case, and when the therapeutic effect is inconvenient to measure, dosage may best be monitored according to the plasma concentration (in relation to a previously defined optimum range).

Plasma concentration monitoring has proved useful in the following situations:

● When the desired effect is suppression of infrequent sporadic events such as epileptic seizures or episodes of cardiac dysrhythmia

- When there is no quick and reliable assessment of effect, e.g. mood changes in a depressed patient, and where social environment plays a role as great or even greater than that of the drug
- When lack of therapeutic effect and toxicity may be difficult to distinguish. Digoxin is both a treatment for, and sometimes the cause of, cardiac supraventricular dysrhythmia; a plasma digoxin measurement will help to distinguish whether a dysrhythmia is due to too little or too much digoxin
- To reduce the risk of adverse drug effects, e.g. otic damage with aminoglycoside antibiotics or adverse CNS effects of lithium, when therapeutic doses are close to toxic doses (low therapeutic index)
- To check patient compliance on a drug regimen, e.g. when there is failure of therapeutic effect at a dose that is expected to be effective
- To treat drug overdose.

Interpreting concentration measurements

- A target therapeutic concentration range quoted for a drug should be regarded only as a guide to help to optimise dosing and should be evaluated with other clinical indicators of progress.
- Consider whether a patient has been taking a drug for a sufficient time to reach steady-state conditions, i.e. when 5 $t^1/2$ periods have elapsed since dosing commenced or since the last change in dose. In the case of drugs that alter their own rates of metabolism by enzyme induction, e.g. carbamazepine and phenytoin, it is best to allow 2–4 weeks to elapse between change in dose and plasma concentration measurement. Sampling when plasma concentrations are still rising or falling towards a steady state is likely to be misleading.
- Consider whether *peak* or *trough* concentration should be measured. As a general rule when a drug has a short $t^1/2$ it is desirable to know both; monitoring peak (15 min after an i.v. dose) and trough (just before the next dose) concentrations of gentamicin ($t^1/2$ 2.5 h) helps to provide efficacy without toxicity. For a drug with a long $t^1/2$, it is usually best to sample just before a dose

is due; effective immunosuppression with cyclosporin ($t^1/2$ 27 h) is obtained with trough concentrations of 60–200 $\mu g/l$ when the drug is given by mouth.

Recommended plasma concentrations for drugs appear throughout this book where these are relevant.[6]

Individual pharmacokinetic processes

The following section considers the processes whereby drugs are absorbed into, distributed around, metabolised by and eliminated from the body. Common to all these is the necessity for drugs to pass across cell membranes.

Drug passage across cell membranes

Our bodies are labyrinths of fluid-filled spaces. Some, such as the lumina of the kidney tubules or intestine, are connected to the outside world; the blood, lymph and cerebrospinal fluid are enclosed. These spaces are lined by sheets of cells and the extent to which a drug can cross epithelia or endothelia is fundamental to its clinical use. It is the major factor that determines whether a drug can be taken orally for systemic effect and whether within the glomerular filtrate it will be reabsorbed or excreted in the urine.

Cell membranes are essentially bilayers of lipid molecules with 'islands' of protein and they preserve and regulate the internal environment. Lipid-soluble substances diffuse readily into cells and therefore throughout body tissues. Adjacent epithe-

---

[6] Concentrations of drugs in biological fluids are currently expressed in a dangerously confusing variety of notations, e.g. mg/100 ml, mg/l, micromol/l. Standardisation is desirable and the convention is likely to become molar unit per litre, i.e. SI (Système International) units.

lial or endothelial cells are joined by so-called tight junctions, some of which are traversed by water-filled channels through which water-soluble substances of small molecular size may filter. The jejunum and proximal renal tubule contain many such channels and are called *leaky* epithelia, whereas the tight junctions in the stomach and urinary bladder do not have these channels and water cannot pass; they are termed *tight* epithelia. Special protein molecules within the lipid bilayer allow specific substances to enter or leave the cell preferentially (carrier proteins).

The passage of drugs across membranes is determined by the natural processes of diffusion, filtration and carrier-mediated transport.

PASSIVE DIFFUSION

This is the most important means by which a drug enters the tissues and is distributed through them. It refers simply to the natural tendency of any substance to move passively from an area of high concentration to one of low concentration. In the context of an individual cell, the drug moves at a rate proportional to the concentration difference across the cell membrane, i.e. it shows first-order kinetics; cellular energy is not required, which means that the process does not become saturated and is not inhibited by other substances.

The dominating importance of lipid solubility to drug transfer across membranes is clear. Drugs exhibit greater or lesser degrees of lipid solubility according to environmental pH and the structural properties of the molecule.

The presence of a benzene ring, a hydrocarbon chain, a steroid nucleus or halogen (-Br, -Cl, -F) groups favours lipid solubility. Water solubility is favoured by the possession of alcoholic (-OH), amide (-CO.NH$_2$) or carboxylic (-COOH) groups, and the formation of glucuronide and sulphate conjugates.

It is useful to classify drugs in a physicochemical sense into:

- Those that are variably ionised according to environmental pH (electrolytes) (lipid-soluble or water-soluble)

- Those that are incapable of becoming ionised whatever the environmental pH (un-ionised, non-polar substances) (lipid-soluble)
- Those that are permanently ionised whatever the environmental pH (ionised, polar substances) (water-soluble).

Drugs ionised by environmental pH

Many drugs are weak electrolytes, i.e. their structural groups ionise to a greater or lesser extent, according to environmental pH. Most such molecules are present partly in the ionised and partly in the un-ionised state. The degree of ionisation influences lipid-solubility (and hence diffusibility) and so affects absorption, distribution and elimination.

Ionisable groups in a drug molecule tend either to lose a hydrogen ion (acidic groups) or to add a hydrogen ion (basic groups). The extent to which a molecule has this tendency to ionise is given by the *dissociation* (or ionisation) *constant (Ka)*. This is usually expressed as the pKa, i.e. the negative logarithm of the Ka (just as pH is the negative logarithm of the hydrogen ion concentration). In an acidic environment, i.e. one already containing many free hydrogen ions, an acidic group tends not to lose a hydrogen ion and remains un-ionised; a relative deficit of free hydrogen ions, i.e. a basic environment, favours dissociation of the hydrogen ion from an acidic group which thus becomes ionised. The opposite is the case for a base. The issue may be summarised:

- Acidic groups become less ionised in an acidic environment
- Basic groups become less ionised in a basic (alkaline) environment
- Vice versa.

This in turn influences *diffusibility* since:

- Un-ionised drug is lipid-soluble and diffusible
- Ionised drug is lipid-insoluble and non-diffusible.

The profound effect of environmental pH on the degree of ionisation is best shown when the relation between these is quantified. It is convenient to remember that when the pH of the environment is the same as the pKa of a drug within it, then the ratio of un-ionised to ionised molecules is 1:1. But for every unit by which pH is changed, the un-ionised:ionised ratio changes 10-fold, as Table 7.2 shows.

Table 7.2 pH and ionisation

pH	acid un-ionised:ionised	base un-ionised:ionised
= pKa −2 units	100:1	1:100
= pKa −1 unit	10:1	1:10
= pKa	1:1	1:1
= pKa +1 unit	1:10	10:1
= pKa +2 units	1:100	100:1

pH variation and drug kinetics. Studies of the partitioning of a drug across a lipid membrane according to differences in pH have been developed as the *pH partition hypothesis*. There is a wide range of pH in the gut (pH 1.5 in the stomach; 6.8 in the upper and 7.6 in the lower intestine). But the pH inside the body is maintained within a limited range (pH 7.4 ± 0.04) so that only drugs that are substantially un-ionised at this pH will be lipid-soluble, diffuse across tissue boundaries and so be widely distributed, e.g. into the CNS. Urine pH varies between the extremes of 4.6 and 8.2; thus the amount of drug reabsorbed from the renal tubular lumen by passive diffusion can be very much affected by the prevailing urine pH.

Consider the effect of pH changes on the disposition of aspirin (acetylsalicylic acid, pKa 3.5). In the stomach aspirin is un-ionised and thus lipid-soluble and diffusible. When aspirin enters the gastric epithelial cells (pH 7.4) it will ionise, become less diffusible and so will localise there. This *ion trapping* is one mechanism whereby aspirin is concentrated in, and so harms, the gastric mucosa. In the body aspirin is metabolised to salicylic acid (pKa 3.0) which at pH 7.4 is predominantly ionised and thus remains in the extracellular fluid. Eventually the molecules of salicylic acid in the plasma are filtered by the glomeruli and pass into the tubular fluid which is generally more acidic than plasma and causes a proportion of salicylic acid to become un-ionised and lipid-soluble so that it diffuses back into the tubular cells. Alkalinising the urine with sodium bicarbonate causes more salicylic acid to become ionised and lipid-insoluble so that it remains in the tubular fluid, and is eliminated in the urine. This effect is sufficiently great for alkalinising the urine to be effective treatment for salicylate (aspirin) overdose.

Conversely, acidifying the urine increases the elimination of the base amphetamine (pKa 9.9) (see Acidification of urine, p. 143).

Drugs incapable of becoming ionised

These include digoxin and chloramphenicol. Having no ionisable groups, they are unaffected by environmental pH, are lipid-soluble and so diffuse readily across tissue boundaries. These drugs are also referred to as non-polar.

Permanently ionised drugs

Drugs that are permanently ionised carry groups which dissociate so strongly that they remain ionised over the range of the body pH. Such compounds are termed polar, for their groups are either negatively charged (acidic, e.g. heparin) or positively charged (basic, e.g. ipratropium, tubocurarine, suxamethonium) and all have a very limited capacity to cross cell membranes. This is a disadvantage in the case of heparin which is not absorbed by the gut and must be given parenterally. Conversely, heparin is a useful anticoagulant in pregnancy because it does not cross the placenta (which the orally effective warfarin does and is liable to cause fetal haemorrhage as well as being teratogenic).

The clinical relevance of drug passage across membranes may be illustrated with reference to the following:

Brain and cerebrospinal fluid (CSF). The capillaries of the cerebral circulation differ from those in most other parts of the body in that they lack the filtration channels between endothelial cells through which substances in the blood nominally gain access to the extracellular fluid. There are tight junctions between adjacent capillary endothelial cells which, together with their basement membrane and a thin covering from the processes of astrocytes, separate the blood from the brain tissue. This barrier places constraints on the passage of substances from the blood to the brain and CSF.

Compounds that are lipid-insoluble do not cross it readily, e.g. atenolol, compared with propranolol (lipid-soluble), and CNS side-effects are more prominent with the latter. Therapy with methotrexate (lipid-insoluble) may have no effect on leukaemic deposits in the CNS. Conversely lipid-soluble substances enter brain tissue with ease; thus diazepam (lipid-soluble) given intravenously is effective within one minute for status epilepticus, and effects of alcohol (ethanol) by mouth are noted within minutes; the level of general anaesthesia can be controlled closely by altering the concentration of inhaled anaesthetic gas (lipid-soluble).

Placenta. Chorionic villi, consisting of a layer of trophoblastic cells that enclose fetal capillaries, are bathed in maternal blood. The large surface area and blood flow (500 ml/min) are essential for gas exchange, uptake of nutrients and elimination of waste products. The fetal and maternal bloodstreams are therefore separated by a lipid barrier that allows the passage of lipid-soluble substances but excludes water-soluble compounds, especially those with molecular weight exceeding 600.[7]

This exclusion is of particular importance with short-term use, e.g. tubocurarine (mol. wt 772) (lipid-insoluble) or gallamine (mol. wt 891) used as a muscle relaxant during Caesarian section do not affect the infant; with prolonged use, however, all compounds will eventually enter the fetus to some extent (see Drugs and the embryo and fetus).

FILTRATION

Aqueous channels in the tight junctions between adjacent epithelial cells allow the passage of some water-soluble substances. Neutral or uncharged, i.e. nonpolar, molecules pass most readily since the pores are electrically charged. Within the alimentary tract, channels are largest and most numerous in jejunal epithelium and filtration allows for rapid equilibration of concentrations and consequently of osmotic pressures across the mucosa. Ions such as sodium enter the body through the aqueous channels the size of which probably limits passage to

---

[7] Most drugs have a molecular weight of less than 600 (e.g. diazepam 284, morphine 303) but some have more (erythromycin 733, digoxin 780).

substances of low molecular weight, e.g. ethanol (mol. wt 46). Filtration seems to play at most a minor role in drug transfer within the body except for glomerular filtration, which is an important mechanism of drug excretion.

CARRIER-MEDIATED TRANSPORT

Some drugs move into or out of cells against a concentration gradient, i.e. by active transport. These processes involve endogenous molecules, expend cellular energy and are more rapid than transfer by diffusion. The mechanisms show a high degree of specificity for particular compounds because they have evolved from biological needs for the uptake of essential nutrients or elimination of metabolic products. Thus, drugs that are subject to them bear some structural resemblance to natural constituents of the body. Examples of active transport systems are the absorption of iron by the gut, levodopa across the blood–brain barrier and the secretion of many organic acids and bases by renal tubular and biliary duct cells. Carrier-mediated transport that does not require energy is called *facilitated diffusion*, e.g. vitamin B_{12} absorption; carrier-mediated transport is subject to saturation and can be inhibited.

Absorption

Commonsense considerations of anatomy, physiology, pathology, pharmacology, therapeutics and convenience determine the routes by which drugs are administered. Usually these are:

- Enteral: by mouth (swallowed) or by sublingual or buccal absorption; by rectum
- Parenteral: by intravenous injection or infusion, intramuscular injection, subcutaneous injection or infusion, inhalation, topical application for local (skin, eye, lung) or for systemic (transdermal) effect
- Other routes, e.g. intrathecal, intradermal, intranasal, intratracheal, intrapleural, are used when appropriate.

The features of the various routes, their advantages and disadvantages are now considered.

ABSORPTION FROM THE GASTROINTESTINAL TRACT

The *small intestine* is the principal site for absorption of nutrients and it is also where most orally-administered drugs enter the body. This part of the gut has two important attributes, an enormous surface area (estimated to be 4500 m^2 or about half the size of a football pitch), and an epithelium through which fluid readily filters in response to osmotic differences caused by the presence of food. It follows that drug access to the small intestinal mucosa is important and disturbed alimentary motility can reduce absorption, i.e. if gastric emptying is slowed by food, or intestinal transit is accelerated by gut infection. The colon is capable of absorbing drugs and many sustained-release formulations probably depend on absorption there.

Absorption of ionisable drugs from the *buccal mucosa* is influenced by the prevailing pH which is 6.2–7.2. Lipid-soluble drugs are rapidly effective by this route because blood flow through the mucosa is abundant and entry is directly into the systemic circulation, avoiding the possibility of first-pass (presystemic) inactivation in the liver (see below). The stomach does not play a major role in absorbing drugs, even those that are acidic and thus unionised and lipid-soluble at gastric pH, because its surface area is much smaller than that of the small intestine and gastric emptying is speedy ($t^{1}/_2$ 30 min).

Enterohepatic circulation

This system is exemplified by the bile salts, which are conserved by circulating between liver and intestine about eight times a day. A number of drugs form conjugates with glucuronic acid in the liver and are excreted in the bile. These glucuronides are too polar (ionised) to be reabsorbed; they therefore remain in the gut where they are hydrolysed by enzymes and bacteria to release the parent drug which is then reabsorbed and reconjugated in the liver. Enterohepatic recycling appears to help maintain the effect of sulindac, pentaerythritol tetranitrate and ethinyloestradiol (in many oral contraceptives).

Systemic availability and bioavailability

When a drug is injected intravenously it enters the systemic circulation and thence gains access to the tissues and to receptors, i.e. 100% is available to exert its therapeutic effect. If the same quantity of the drug is swallowed, it does not follow that the entire amount will reach first the portal blood and then the systemic blood, i.e. its availability for therapeutic effect via the systemic circulation may be less than 100%. The anticipated response to a drug may not be achieved unless biological availability is taken into account. In a strict sense, considerations of reduced availability apply whenever any drug intended for systemic effect is given by any route other than the intravenous, but in practice the issue concerns enteral administration. The extent of bioavailability is ordinarily calculated by relating the area under the plasma concentration-time curve (AUC) after a single oral dose to that obtained after i.v. administration of the same amount (by which route a drug is 100% bioavailable). Different pharmaceutical formulations of the same drug can thus be compared. Factors influencing bioavailability may be thought of in three main ways:

Pharmaceutical factors.[8] The amount of drug that is released from a dose form is highly dependent on its formulation. With tablets, for example, particle size (surface area exposed to solution), diluting substances, tablet size and pressure used in the tabletting machine can affect disintegration and dissolution and so the *bioavailability* of the drug. Manufacturers are expected to produce a formulation with an unvarying bioavailability so that the same amount of drug is released with the same speed from whatever manufactured batch or brand

---

[8] Some definitions of enteral dose-forms: *Tablet*: a solid dose form in which the drug is compressed or moulded with pharmacologically inert substances (excipients); variants include sustained-release and coated tablets. *Capsule*: the drug is provided in a gelatin shell or container. *Mixture*: a liquid formulation of a drug for oral administration. *Suppository*: a solid dose-form shaped for insertion into rectum (or vagina, when it may be called a *pessary*); it may be designed to dissolve or it may melt at body temperature (in which case there is a storage problem in countries where the environmental temperature may exceed 37°C); the vehicle in which the drug is carried may be fat, glycerol with gelatin, or macrogols (polycondensation products of ethylene oxide) with gelatin. *Syrup*: the drug is provided in a concentrated sugar (fructose or other) solution. *Linctus*: a viscous liquid formulation, traditional for cough.

the patient may be taking. Substantial differences in bioavailability of digoxin tablets from one manufacturer occurred when only the technique and machinery for making the tablets were changed; also tablets containing the same amount of digoxin but made by different companies, were shown to produce different plasma concentrations and therefore different effects, i.e. there was neither *bioequivalence* nor *therapeutic equivalence*. Physicians tend to ignore pharmaceutical formulation as a factor in variable or unexpected responses because they do not understand it and feel entitled to rely on reputable manufacturers and official regulatory authorities to ensure provision of reliable formulations. Good pharmaceutical companies reasonably point out that, having a reputation to lose, they take much trouble to make their preparations consistently reliable. This is a matter of great importance when dosage requires to be precise (anticoagulants, antidiabetics, adrenal steroids). The following account by Lauder Brunton in 1897 indicates that the phenomenon of variable bioavailability is not recent.

> A very unfortunate case occurred some time ago in a doctor who had prescribed aconitine to a patient and gradually increased the dose. He thought he was quite certain that he knew what he was doing. The druggist's supply of aconitine ran out, and he procured some new aconitine from a different maker. This turned out to be many times stronger than the other, and the patient unfortunately became very ill. *The doctor said, 'It cannot be the medicine',* and to show that this was true, he drank off a dose himself with the result that he died. So you must remember the difference in the different preparations of aconitine,[9]

i.e. they had different bioavailability and so lacked therapeutic equivalence.

Biological factors. Those related to the gut include destruction of drug by gastric acid, e.g. benzylpenicillin, and impaired absorption due to intestinal hurry which is important for all drugs that are slowly absorbed. Drugs may also bind to food con-

stituents — tetracyclines to calcium (e.g. in milk) — and to iron, or to other drugs (e.g. acidic drugs to cholestyramine) and the resulting complex is not absorbed.

Presystemic (first-pass) elimination. Despite the fact that they readily enter gut mucosal cells, some drugs appear in low concentration in the systemic circulation. The reason lies in the considerable extent to which such drugs are metabolised in a single passage through the gut wall and (principally) the liver. This is an important feature of the oral route. As little as 10–20% of the parent drug may reach the systemic circulation unchanged, but the degree of presystemic elimination differs much between drugs and between individuals. Hence the phenomenon of first-pass elimination adds, in some cases significantly, to variation in systemic plasma concentrations, and thus in response to the drugs that are subject to this process. By contrast, if the same dose is given intravenously, 100% becomes systemically available and the patient is exposed to higher concentrations with greater, but more predictable, effect. Once a drug is in the systemic circulation, irrespective of which route is used, about 20% is subject to the hepatic metabolic processes in each circulation because that is the proportion of cardiac output that passes to the liver.

Drugs for which **presystemic elimination** is significant include:

ANALGESICS	ADRENOCEPTOR BLOCKERS	OTHERS
Dextro-propoxyphene	Labetalol	Chlormethiazole
Morphine	Metoprolol	Chlorpromazine
Pentazocine	Oxprenolol	Isosorbide dinitrate
Pethidine	Propranolol	Nortriptyline

If the reader cares to list the *enteral* and *parenteral* doses of the above drugs that achieve comparable effects, the difference introduced by presystemic elimination will be apparent. Note that if a drug produces active metabolites, differences in dose may not be as great as those anticipated on the basis of differences in plasma concentration of the parent drug after intravenous and oral administration.

In severe hepatic cirrhosis with both impaired liver cell function and well developed channels

---

[9] The doctor died of cardiac dysrhythmia and/or cerebral depression. Aconitine is a plant alkaloid and has no place in medicine.

shunting blood into the systemic circulation without passing through the liver, first-pass elimination is reduced and systemic availability is increased. The result of these changes is an increased likelihood of exaggerated response to normal doses of drugs having high hepatic clearance and, on occasion, frank toxicity.

Drugs that exhibit the hepatic first-pass phenomenon do so because of the rapidity with which they are metabolised. The rate at which drug is delivered to the liver, i.e. blood flow, is then the main determinant of its metabolism. Many other drugs are completely metabolised by the liver but at a slower rate and consequently loss in the first pass through the liver is unimportant. The parenteral dose of these drugs does not need to be reduced to account for presystemic elimination. Such drugs include: chloramphenicol, diazepam, phenytoin, theophylline, warfarin.

Advantages and disadvantages of enteral administration

By swallowing

● For systemic effect

Advantages are convenience and acceptability.

Disadvantages are that absorption may be delayed, reduced or even enhanced after food or slow or irregular after drugs that inhibit gut motility (antimuscarinic, opioid). Differences in presystemic elimination are a cause of variation in drug effect between patients. Some drugs are not absorbed (gentamicin) and some drugs are destroyed in the gut (insulin, oxytocin, some penicillins). Tablets taken with too small a quantity of liquid and in the supine position, can lodge in the oesophagus with delayed absorption[10] and may even cause ulceration (sustained-release potassium chloride and doxycycline tablets), especially in the feeble elderly and those with an enlarged left atrium which impinges on the oesophagus.[11]

● For effect in the gut

Advantages are that the drug is placed at the site of action (neomycin, anthelminthics), and with nonabsorbed drugs the local concentration can be higher than would be safe in the blood.

Disadvantages are that drug distribution may be uneven, and in some diseases of the gut the whole thickness of the wall is affected (severe bacillary dysentery, typhoid) and effective blood concentrations (as well as luminal concentrations) may be needed.

Sublingual or buccal sulcus for systemic effect

Advantages are that quick effect is obtained (glyceryl trinitrate, nifedipine and ergotamine are given thus), especially if the tablet is chewed, giving greater surface area for solution. The effect can be terminated by spitting out the tablet.

Disadvantages are the inconvenience if use has to be frequent, irritation of the mucous membrane and excessive salivation which promotes swallowing, so losing the advantages of bypassing presystemic elimination.

Rectal administration

● For systemic effect (suppositories or solutions).
The rectal mucosa has a rich blood and lymph supply and, in general, dose requirements are either the same or slightly greater than those needed for oral use. Drugs chiefly enter the portal system, but those that are subject to hepatic first-pass elimination may escape this if they are absorbed from the lower rectum which drains directly to the systemic circulation. The degree of presystemic elimination thus depends on distribution within the rectum and this is somewhat unpredictable.

Advantages are that a drug that is irritant to the stomach can be given by suppository (aminophylline, indomethacin); the route is suitable in vomiting, motion sickness, migraine or when a patient cannot swallow, and when cooperation is lacking (sedation in children).

---

[10] A woman's failure to respond to antihypertensive medication was explained when she was observed to choke on drinking. Investigation revealed a large pharyngeal pouch that was full of tablets and capsules. Her blood pressure became easy to control when the pouch was removed. Birch D J, Dehn T C B 1993 British Medical Journal 306: 1012.

[11] Ideally solid-dose forms should be taken standing up and washed down with 150 ml (tea cup) of water; even sitting (higher intra-abdominal pressure) impairs passage. At least patients should be told to sit and take 3 or 4 mouthfuls of water (a mouthful = 30 ml) or a cupful. Some patients do not even know they should take water.

Disadvantages are psychological in that the patient may be embarrassed or may like the route too much; rectal inflammation may occur with repeated use and absorption can be unreliable, especially if the rectum is full of faeces.

● **For local effect**, e.g. in proctitis or colitis, an obvious use.

A survey in the UK showed that a substantial proportion of patients did not remove the wrapper before inserting the suppository.

Parenteral administration (for systemic and local effect)

Intravenous (bolus or infusion). An i.v. bolus, i.e. rapid injection, passes round the circulation being progressively diluted each time; it is delivered principally to the organs with high blood flow (brain, liver, heart, lung, kidneys).

Advantages are that the i.v. route gives swift, effective and highly predictable blood concentration and allows rapid modification of dose, i.e. immediate cessation of administration is possible if unwanted effects occur during administration. The route is suitable for administration of drugs that are not absorbed from the gut or are too irritant (anticancer agents) to be given by other routes.

Disadvantages are the hazard if a drug is given too quickly, as plasma concentration may rise at such a rate that normal mechanisms of distribution and elimination are outpaced. (Some drugs will act within one arm-to-tongue (brain) circulation time which is 13 ± 3 seconds; with most drugs an injection given over 4 or 5 circulation times seems sufficient to avoid excessive plasma concentrations.) Local venous thrombosis is liable to occur with prolonged infusion and with bolus doses of irritant formulations, e.g. diazepam, or microparticulate components of infusion fluids, especially if small veins are used. Infection of the intravenous catheter and the small thrombi on its tip are also a risk during prolonged infusions.

Intramuscular injection. Blood flow is greater in the muscles of the upper arm than in the gluteal mass and thigh, and also increases with physical exercise. (Usually these influences are unimportant but one football-playing patient who was given an intramuscular injection of a sustained-release phenothiazine had to be substituted towards the end of the game when he developed an extrapyramidal disorder, presumably due to too rapid absorption of the drug.)

Advantages are that the route is reliable, is suitable for irritant drugs, and depot preparations (penicillins, neuroleptics, medroxyprogesterone) can be used at monthly or longer intervals. Absorption is more rapid than following subcutaneous injection (soluble preparations are absorbed within 10–30 min).

Disadvantages are that the route is not acceptable for self-administration, it may be painful, and if any adverse effects occur to a depot formulation, it cannot be removed.

Subcutaneous injection
Advantages are that the route is reliable and is acceptable for self-administration.

Disadvantages are poor absorption in peripheral circulatory failure. Repeated injections at one site can cause lipoatrophy, resulting in erratic absorption (see Insulin).

Inhalation
● **As a gas**, e.g. volatile anaesthetics.
● **As an aerosol**, e.g. β_2-adrenoceptor agonist bronchodilators. Aerosols are particles dispersed in a gas, the particles being small enough to remain in suspension for a long time instead of sedimenting rapidly under the influence of gravity; the particles may be liquid (fog) or solid (smoke).
● **As a powder**, e.g. sodium cromoglycate. Particle size and air flow velocity are important. Most particles above 5 μm in diameter impact in the upper respiratory areas; particles of about 2 μm reach the terminal bronchioles; a large proportion of particles less than 1 μm will be exhaled. Air flow velocity diminishes considerably as the bronchi progressively divide, promoting drug deposition peripherally.

Advantages are that drugs as gases can be rapidly taken up or eliminated, giving the close control that has marked the use of this route in general anaesthesia from its earliest days. Self-administration is practicable. Aerosols and powders provide high local concentration for action on bronchi, minimising systemic effects; aerosols can also be used for systemic effect, e.g. ergotamine for migraine.

Disadvantages are that special apparatus is needed (some patients find pressurised aerosols difficult to use to best effect) and a drug must be nonirritant if the patient is conscious. Obstructed bronchi (mucus plugs in asthma) may cause therapy to fail.

Topical application

- **For local effect**, e.g. to skin, eye, lung, anal canal, rectum, vagina.

Advantage is the provision of high local concentration without systemic effect (usually[12]).

Disadvantage is that absorption can occur, especially when there is tissue destruction so that systemic effects result, e.g. adrenal steroids and neomycin to the skin, atropine to the eye. Ocular administration of a β-adrenoceptor blocker may cause systemic effects (first-pass elimination is bypassed) and such eye drops are contraindicated for patients with asthma or chronic lung disease.[13] There is extensive literature on this subject characterised by expressions of astonishment that serious effects, even death, can occur.

- **For systemic effect**. Transdermal delivery systems (TDS) release drug through a rate-controlling membrane into the skin and so into the systemic circulation. Fluctuations in plasma concentration associated with other routes of administration are largely avoided, as is first-pass elimination in the liver. Glyceryl trinitrate

and postmenopausal hormone replacement therapy may be given this way, in the form of a sticking plaster attached to the skin[14] or as an ointment (glyceryl trinitrate).

Distribution

If a drug is required to act throughout the body or to reach an organ inaccessible to topical administration, it must be got into the blood and into other body compartments. Most drugs distribute widely, in part dissolved in body water, in part bound to plasma proteins, in part to tissues. Distribution is often uneven, for drugs may bind selectively to plasma or tissue proteins or be localised within particular organs. Clearly, the site of localisation of a drug is likely to influence its action, e.g. whether it crosses the blood–brain barrier to enter the brain; the *extent* (amount) and *strength* (tenacity) of protein or tissue binding (stored drug) will affect the time it spends in the body and thereby its duration of action.

Drug distribution, its quantification and its clinical implications are now discussed.

DISTRIBUTION VOLUME

> The distribution volume of a drug is the volume in which it appears to distribute (or which it would require) if the concentration throughout the body were equal to that in plasma, i.e. as if the body were a single compartment.

---

[12] A cautionary tale. A 70-year-old man reported left breast enlargement and underwent mastectomy; histological examination revealed benign gynaecomastia. Ten months later the right breast enlarged. Tests of endocrine function were normal but the patient himself was struck by the fact that his wife had been using a vaginal cream (containing 0.01% dienestrol) initially for atrophic vaginitis but latterly the cream had been used to facilitate sexual intercourse which took place two to three times a week. On the assumption that penile absorption of oestrogen was responsible for the disorder, exposure to the cream was terminated. The gynaecomastia in the remaining breast then resolved (Di Raimondo C V et al 1980 New England Journal of Medicine 302: 1089).

[13] Two drops of 0.5% timolol solution, one to each eye, can equate to 10 mg by mouth.

[14] But TDS may have an unexpected outcome for, not only may the sticking plaster drop off unnoticed, it may find its way onto another person. A hypertensive father rose one morning and noticed that his clonidine plaster was missing from his upper arm. He could not find it and applied a new plaster. His nine-month-old child, who had been taken into the paternal bed during the night because he needed comforting, spent an irritable and hypoactive day, refused food but drank and passed more urine than usual. The missing clonidine patch was discovered on his back when he was being prepared for his bath. No doubt this was accidental, but children also enjoy stick-on decoration and the possibility of poisoning from misused, discarded or new (e.g. strong opioid, used in palliative care) drug plasters means that these should be kept and disposed of as carefully as oral formulations (Reed M T et al 1986 New England Journal of Medicine 314: 1120).

The pattern of distribution from plasma to other body fluids and tissues is a characteristic of each drug that enters the circulation and it varies between drugs. Precise information on the concentration of drug attained in various tissues and fluids requires biopsy samples and for understandable reasons this is usually not available for humans.[15] What can be sampled readily in humans is *blood plasma*, the drug concentration in which, taking account of the dose, is a measure of whether a drug tends to remain in the circulation or to distribute from the plasma into the tissues. If a drug remains mostly in the plasma, its distribution volume will be small; if it is present mainly in other tissues the distribution volume will be large.

Such information is clinically useful. Consider drug overdose. Removing a drug by haemodialysis is likely to be a beneficial exercise only if a major proportion of the total body load is in the plasma, e.g. with salicylate which has a small distribution volume; but haemodialysis is an inappropriate treatment for overdose with pethidine which has a large distribution volume. These, however, are generalisations and if the knowledge of distribution volume is to be of practical value it must be quantified more precisely.

The **principle** for establishing the distribution volume is essentially that of using a dye to find the volume of a container filled with liquid. The weight of dye that is added divided by the concentration of dye once mixing is complete gives the distribution volume of the dye, which is the volume of the container. Similarly, the distribution volume of a drug in the body may be determined after a single intravenous bolus dose by dividing the dose given by the concentration achieved in plasma.[16]

The result of this calculation, the distribution volume, in fact only rarely corresponds with a physiological body space such as extracellular water or total body water, for it is a measure of the volume a

drug would apparently occupy knowing the dose given and the plasma concentration achieved and assuming the entire volume is at that concentration. For this reason, it is often referred to as the *apparent distribution volume*. Indeed, for some drugs that bind extensively to extravascular tissues, the apparent distribution volume, which is based on the resulting low plasma concentration, is many times total body volume (see list below).

> Distribution volume is the volume of fluid in which the drug appears to distribute with a concentration equal to that in plasma.

The list in Table 7.3 illustrates a range of apparent distribution volumes. The names of those substances that distribute within (and have been used to measure) physiological spaces are in italics.

Table 7.3 Apparent distribution volume of some drugs

(Figures are in litres for a 70 kg person who would displace about 70 l)[17]

Drug	Distribution volume	Drug	Distribution volume
Evans blue	3 (plasma volume)	atenolol	77
heparin	5	diazepam	140
aspirin	11	pethidine	280
inulin	15 (extracellular water)	digoxin	420
gentamicin	18	nortriptyline	1000
frusemide	21	dothiepin	4900
amoxicillin	28	chloroquine	13 000
antipyrine	43 (total body water)		

[15] Positron emission tomography (PET) offers prospect of obtaining similar information. With PET, a positron emitting isotope, e.g. ^{15}O, is substituted for a stable atom without altering the chemical behaviour of the molecule. The radiation dose is very low but can be imaged tomographically. PET can be used to monitor effects of psychoactive drugs on brain metabolism and blood flow, e.g. 'on' and 'off' phases in parkinsonism. Many other applications appear likely.

[16] Clearly a problem arises in that the plasma concentration is not constant but falls after the bolus has been injected. To get round this, use is made of the fact that the relation between the logarithm of plasma concentration and the time after a single intravenous dose is a straight line. The log concentration-time line extended back to zero time gives the theoretical plasma concentration at the time the drug was given. In effect, the assumption is made that drug distributes instantaneously and uniformly through a single compartment, the distribution volume. This mechanism, although seeming artificial, does usefully characterise drugs according to the extent to which they remain in or distribute out from the circulation.

Selective distribution within the body occurs because of special affinity between particular drugs and particular body constituents. Many drugs bind to proteins in the plasma; phenothiazines and chloroquine bind to melanin-containing tissues, including the retina, which may explain the occurrence of retinopathy. Drugs may also concentrate selectively in a particular tissue because of specialised transport mechanisms, e.g. iodine in the thyroid.

PLASMA PROTEIN AND TISSUE BINDING

Many natural substances circulate around the body partly free in plasma water and partly bound to plasma proteins; these include cortisol, thyroxine, iron, copper and, in hepatic or renal failure, by-products of physiological intermediary metabolism. Drugs, too, circulate in the protein-bound and free states, and the significance is that the *free fraction* is pharmacologically active whereas the *protein-bound* component is a reservoir of drug that is inactive because of this binding. Free and bound fractions are in equilibrium and free drug removed from the plasma by metabolism, dialysis or excretion is replaced by drug released from the bound fraction.

Albumin is the main binding protein for many natural substances and drugs. Its complex structure has a net negative charge at blood pH and a high *capacity* but low (weak) *affinity* for many basic drugs, i.e. a lot is bound but it is readily released. Two particular sites on the albumin molecule bind acidic drugs with high affinity (strongly) but these sites have low capacity. Saturation of binding sites on plasma proteins in general is unlikely in the doses in which most drugs are used.

Other binding proteins in the blood include lipoprotein and α_1-acid glycoprotein, both of which carry basic drugs such as quinidine, chlorpromazine and imipramine. Such binding may have implications for therapeutic drug monitoring according to plasma concentration. Thyroxine and sex hormones are bound in the plasma to specific globulins.

---

[17] Litres per kg are commonly used, but give a less vivid image of the implication of the term 'apparent', e.g. chloroquine.

Disease may modify protein binding of drugs to an extent that is clinically relevant as Table 7.4 shows. In *chronic renal failure*, hypoalbuminaemia and retention of (as yet unidentified) products of metabolism that compete for binding sites on protein, are both responsible for the decrease in protein binding of drugs. Most affected are acidic drugs that are highly protein bound, e.g. phenytoin, and special care is needed when initiating and modifying the dose of such drugs for patients with renal failure (see also Drugs and renal disease, p. 494).

Chronic liver disease also leads to hypoalbuminaemia and increase of endogenous substances such as bilirubin that may compete for binding sites on protein. Drugs that are normally extensively protein bound should be used with special caution, for increased free concentration of diazepam, tolbutamide and phenytoin have been demonstrated in patients with this condition (see also Drugs and liver disease, p. 591).

The free, unbound and therefore pharmacologically active percentages of some drugs are listed in Table 7.4 to illustrate the range and, in some cases, the changes caused by disease.

Drugs may *interact* competitively at plasma protein binding sites as is discussed on page 118.

Tissue binding. Some drugs distribute readily to regions of the body other than plasma, as a glance at Table 7.3 will show. These include many lipid-soluble drugs which may enter fat stores, e.g. most

---

Table 7.4 Examples of plasma protein binding of drugs and effects of disease

Drug	% unbound (free)	
warfarin	1	
diazepam	2	(6% in liver disease)
frusemide	2	(6% in nephrotic syndrome)
tolbutamide	2	
clofibrate	4	(11% in nephrotic syndrome)
amitriptyline	5	
phenytoin	9	(19% in renal disease)
triamterene	19	(40% in renal disease)
trimethoprim	30	
theophylline	35	(71% in liver disease)
morphine	65	
digoxin	75	(82% in renal disease)
amoxycillin	82	
ethosuximide	100	

benzodiazepines, verapamil and lignocaine. Less is known about other tissues, e.g. muscle, than about plasma protein binding because solid tissue samples can be obtained only by invasive biopsy, but extensive binding to these tissues delays elimination from the body and accounts for the long $t^1/2$ of chloroquine and amiodarone. Displacement from tissue binding sites may be a mechanism for pharmacokinetic interaction (see p. 119).

Metabolism

Most drugs are treated by the body as foreign substances (xenobiotics) and become subject to its various mechanisms for ridding itself of chemical intruders.

Metabolism is a general term for chemical transformations that occur within the body and its processes change drugs in two major ways:

- by reducing lipid solubility
- by reducing biological activity.

REDUCING LIPID SOLUBILITY

> Metabolic reactions tend to make a drug molecule progressively more water-soluble and so favour its elimination in the urine.

Consider the situation if there were no drug metabolising enzymes.

For simplicity let us assume that a drug is evenly distributed throughout body water. If the compound has a low lipid solubility, about five hours would elapse before half the substance is lost from the body; if the drug is also secreted by the [renal] tubules, this time will be shortened to as little as one hour. However, if the drug is lipid-soluble, the excretion rate will be drastically reduced by back diffusion into the plasma from the tubular segment where the urine is concentrated. About thirty days would elapse before half the drug leaves the body. This extended duration might be an advantage with an antibacterial agent

but would be of doubtful value with an anaesthetic agent. If a drug . . . is also reversibly localised in tissues its half-life would be about 100 years — considerably longer than those of the physician and patient combined![18]

Some environmental chemicals may persist indefinitely in our fat deposits, e.g. dicophane (DDT), with consequences that are as yet unknown.

Drug metabolising enzymes were developed during evolution to enable the body to dispose of lipid-soluble substances such as hydrocarbons, sterols and alkaloids, that are ingested with food.[19]

ALTERED BIOLOGICAL ACTIVITY

The end result of metabolism usually is the abolition of biological activity but various steps in between may have the following consequences:

1. Conversion of a pharmacologically active to an inactive substance: this applies to most drugs
2. Conversion of one pharmacologically active to another active substance: this has the effect of prolonging drug action.

ACTIVE DRUG	ACTIVE METABOLITE
amitriptyline	nortriptyline
codeine	morphine
chloroquine	hydroxychloroquine
diazepam	oxazepam
spironolactone	canrenone

3. Conversion of a pharmacologically inactive to an active substance, i.e. *prodrugs*; the effect may confer advantage or disadvantage. (The process then follows 1, above.)

INACTIVE SUBSTANCE	ACTIVE METABOLITE(S)	COMMENT
benorylate	salicylic acid and paracetamol	possibly reduced gastric toxicity
chloral hydrate	trichloroethanol	gastrointestinal upset is due to chloral hydrate
cholecalciferol	1-α-hydroxy-cholecalciferol	

---

[18] Brodie B B 1964 In: Binns T B (ed) Absorption and distribution of drugs. Livingstone, London.

[19] Fish lose lipid-soluble substances through the gills. They do not need such effective metabolising enzymes and they have not got them.

INACTIVE SUBSTANCE	ACTIVE METABOLITE(S)	COMMENT
cyclophosphamide	4-keto-cyclophosphamide	
enalapril	enalaprilat	less risk of first dose hypotension
levodopa	dopamine	levodopa, but not dopamine, can cross the blood–brain barrier
sulindac	sulindac sulphide	possibly reduced gastric toxicity
sulphasalazine	5-aminosalicylic acid	
talampicillin	ampicillin	less diarrhoea

THE METABOLIC PROCESSES

The liver is by far the most important drug metabolising organ although a number of tissues, including the kidney, gut mucosa, lung and skin also contribute. It is useful to think of drug metabolism in two broad phases:

Phase 1 metabolism brings about a change in the drug molecule by oxidation, reduction or hydrolysis and often introduces a chemically active site into it. The new metabolite may retain biological activity but have different pharmacokinetic properties, e.g. a shorter $t^{1/2}$. The most important single group of reactions is the oxidations, in particular those undertaken by the so-called *mixed-function* (microsomal) *oxidases* which, as the name indicates, are capable of metabolising a variety of compounds. It is because of mixed-function oxidases that we do not need to possess new enzymes for every existing or yet-to-be synthesised drug.

Phase I oxidation of some drugs results in the formation of *epoxides* which are short-lived and highly reactive metabolites. Epoxides are important because they can bind irreversibly through covalent bonds to cell constituents; indeed, this is one of the principal ways in which drugs are toxic to body tissues. Glutathione is a tripeptide that combines with epoxides, rendering them inactive, and its presence in the liver is part of an important defence mechanism against hepatic damage by halothane and paracetamol.

Phase II metabolism involves union of the drug with one of several polar (water-soluble) endoge-

nous molecules that are products of intermediary metabolism, to form a water-soluble conjugate which is readily eliminated by the kidney or, if the molecular weight exceeds 300, in the bile. Morphine, paracetamol and salicylates form conjugates with glucuronic acid (derived from glucose); oral contraceptive steroids form sulphates; isoniazid, phenelzine and dapsone are acetylated. Conjugation with a more polar molecule is also a mechanism by which natural substances are eliminated, e.g. bilirubin as glucuronide, oestrogens as sulphates. Phase II metabolism almost invariably terminates biological activity.

ENZYME INDUCTION

The mechanisms that the body evolved over millions of years to metabolise foreign substances now enable it to meet the modern environmental challenges of tobacco smoke, hydrocarbon pollutants, insecticides, and drugs. At times of high exposure, our enzyme systems respond by increasing in amount and so in activity, i.e. they are *induced*; when exposure falls off, enzyme production lessens. For example, a first alcoholic drink taken after a period of abstinence from alcohol may have quite a significant effect on behaviour but the same drink taken at the end of two weeks' regular imbibing may pass almost unnoticed because the individual's liver enzyme activity is increased so that alcohol is metabolised more rapidly and has less effect, i.e. *tolerance* has been acquired.

Inducing substances in general share some important properties: they tend to be lipid-soluble; they are substrates, though sometimes only minor ones, e.g. DDT, for the enzymes they induce and generally have long $t^{1/2}$. The time for onset and offset of induction depends on the rate of enzyme turnover but significant induction generally occurs within a few days and it passes off over 2 or 3 weeks following withdrawal of the inducer.

It follows that the capacity of the body to metabolise drugs can be altered by certain medicinal drugs themselves and by other substances; clearly this phenomenon has implications for drug therapy. More than 200 substances have been shown to induce enzymes in animals but the list of proven enzyme inducers in man is much more restricted.

Substances that cause enzyme induction in man

barbecued meats	griseofulvin
barbiturates	meprobamate
Brussels sprouts	phenobarbitone
carbamazepine	phenytoin
DDT (dicophane,	primidone
and other	rifampicin
insecticides)	sulphinpyrazone
ethanol (chronic use)	tobacco smoke
glutethimide	

Enzyme induction is relevant to drug therapy for the following reasons:

- Clinically important drug interactions may result, e.g. in failure of oral contraceptives or loss of anticoagulant control.
- Disease may result. Antiepilepsy drugs increase the breakdown of dietary and endogenously formed vitamin D, producing an inactive metabolite — in effect a vitamin D deficiency state, which can result in osteomalacia. The accompanying hypocalcaemia can increase the tendency to fits and a convulsion may lead to fracture of the demineralised bones.
- Tolerance to drug therapy may result in and provide an explanation for suboptimal treatment, e.g. with an antiepilepsy drug.
- Variability in response to drugs is increased. Enzyme induction caused by heavy alcohol drinking or heavy smoking may be an unrecognised cause for failure of an individual to achieve the expected response to a normal dose of a drug.
- Drug toxicity may be more likely. A patient who becomes enzyme-induced by taking rifampicin is more likely to develop liver toxicity after paracetamol overdose by increased production of a hepatotoxic metabolite. (Such a patient will also present with a deceptively low plasma concentration of paracetamol due to accelerated metabolism, see p. 254.)

ENZYME INHIBITION

Consequences of inhibiting drug metabolism can be more profound than those of enzyme induction. Effects of enzyme inhibition by drugs also tend to be more selective than those of enzyme induction. Consequently, enzyme inhibition offers more scope for therapy (see Table 7.5).

Table 7.5 Drugs that act by enzyme inhibition

Drug	Enzyme inhibited	Treatment of
acetazolamide	carbonic anhydrase	glaucoma
allopurinol	xanthine oxidase	gout
benserazide	DOPA decarboxylase	Parkinson's disease
disulfiram	aldehyde dehydrogenase	alcoholism
enalapril	angiotensin converting enzyme	hypertension, cardiac failure
moclobemide	MAO A type	depression
nonsteroidal anti-inflammatory drugs	prostaglandin G/H synthase	pain, inflammation premature labour
selegiline	MAO B type	Parkinson's disease

Enzyme inhibition by drugs is also the basis of a number of clinically important drug interactions (see p. 120).

Elimination

Drugs are eliminated from the body after being partly or wholly converted to water-soluble metabolites or, in some cases, without being metabolised. The physiological processes by which drugs and metabolites leave the body are now considered. To avoid repetition the account refers to **drug** whereas the processes deal with both drug and **its metabolites.**

RENAL ELIMINATION

The following mechanisms are involved.

Glomerular filtration. The rate at which a drug enters the glomerular filtrate depends on the concentration of free drug in plasma water and on its molecular weight. Substances that have a molecular weight in excess of 50 000 are excluded from the glomerular filtrate while those of molecular weight less than 10 000 (which includes almost all drugs)[20]

---

[20] Most drugs have a molecular weight less than 1000.

pass easily through the pores of the glomerular membrane.

Renal tubular excretion. Cells of the proximal renal tubule actively transfer strongly charged molecules from the plasma to the tubular fluid. There are two such systems, one for *acids*, e.g. penicillin, frusemide, and one for *bases*, e.g. amiloride, amphetamine.

Renal tubular reabsorption. The glomerular filtrate contains drug at the same concentration as it is free in the plasma, but the fluid is concentrated progressively as it flows down the nephron so that a gradient develops, drug in the tubular fluid becoming more concentrated than in the blood perfusing the nephron. Since the tubular epithelium has the properties of a lipid membrane, the extent to which a drug diffuses back into the blood will depend on its lipid solubility, i.e. on its pKa and on the pH of tubular fluid. If the fluid becomes more alkaline, an acidic drug ionises, becomes less lipid-soluble and its reabsorption diminishes, but a basic drug becomes un-ionised (and therefore more lipid-soluble) and its reabsorption increases. Manipulation of urine pH is given useful expression when sodium bicarbonate is given to alkalinise the urine to treat overdose with aspirin.

FAECAL ELIMINATION

When a drug intended for systemic effect is taken by mouth, a proportion may remain in the bowel and be excreted in the faeces. Sometimes the objective of therapy is that drug should not be absorbed from the gut, e.g. neomycin. Drug in the blood may also diffuse passively into the gut lumen, depending on its pKa and the pH difference between blood and gut contents. The effectiveness of activated charcoal by mouth for drug overdose depends partly on its adsorption of such diffused drug, which is then eliminated in the faeces (see p. 139).

Biliary excretion. In the liver there is one active transport system for acids and one for bases, similar to those in the proximal renal tubule and, in addition, there is a system that transports un-ionised molecules, e.g. digoxin, into the bile. Small molecules tend to be reabsorbed by the bile canaliculi and in general only compounds that have a molecular weight greater than 300 are excreted in bile.

PULMONARY ELIMINATION

The lungs are the main route of elimination (and of uptake) of volatile anaesthetics. Apart from this, they play only a trivial role in drug elimination. The route however, acquires notable medico-legal significance when ethanol concentration is measured in the air expired by vehicle drivers involved in road traffic accidents (via the breathalyser).

CLEARANCE

Clearance of drug may be calculated for an organ or for the whole body. The term has the same meaning as the familiar *renal creatinine clearance*, which is a measure of removal of endogenous creatinine from the plasma. Clearance values can provide useful information about the biological fate of a drug. Renal clearance of a drug that is eliminated only by filtration by the kidney obviously cannot exceed the glomerular filtration rate (adult male 124 ml/min, female 109 ml/min). If a drug is found to have a renal clearance in excess of this, then it must in addition be actively secreted by the kidney tubules, e.g. benzylpenicillin (renal clearance 480 ml/min).

BREAST MILK

Most drugs that are present in a mother's plasma appear to some extent in her milk though the amounts are so small that loss of drug in milk is of no significance as a mechanism of elimination.[21] Even small amounts, however, may sometimes be of significance for the suckling child whose drug metabolic and eliminating mechanisms are immature.

Whilst most drugs taken by the mother pose no hazard to the child, there are exceptions, as follows:

DRUGS AND BREAST FEEDING[22]

Alimentary tract. Sulphasalazine may cause adverse effects and mesalazine appears preferable.

Anti-asthma. Theophylline and diprophylline are

---

[21] But after mercury poisoning breast milk is a major route of elimination.

[22] Bennett P N (ed) 1996 Drugs and human lactation. Elsevier, Amsterdam.

eliminated slowly by the neonate: observe the infant for irritability or disturbed sleep.

Anticancer. Regard as unsafe because of inherent toxicity.

Antidepressants. Avoid doxepin, a metabolite of which may cause respiratory depression.

Antidysrhythmics (cardiac). Amiodarone is present in high and disopyramide in moderate amounts but effects in the infant have not been reported.

Antiepilepsy. General note of caution: observe the infant for sedation and poor suckling. Primidone, ethosuximide and phenobarbitone are present in milk in high amounts; phenytoin and sodium valproate less so.

Anti-inflammatory. Regard aspirin (salicylates) as unsafe (possible association with Reye's syndrome).

Antimicrobials. Metronidazole is present in milk in moderate amounts; avoid prolonged exposure. Nalidixic acid and nitrofurantoin should be avoided where glucose-6-phosphate dehydrogenase deficiency is prevalent. Avoid clindamycin, dapsone, lincomycin, sulphonamides. Regard chloramphenicol as unsafe.

Antipsychotics. Phenothiazines, butyrophenones and thioxanthenes are best avoided unless the indications are compelling: amounts in milk are small but animal studies suggest adverse effects on the developing nervous system. In particular, moderate amounts of sulpiride enter milk. Lithium is probably best avoided.

Anxiolytics and sedatives. Benzodiazepines are safe if use is brief but prolonged use may cause somnolence or poor suckling.

Beta-adrenoceptor blockers. Neonatal hypoglycaemia is possible. Sotalol and atenolol are present in the highest amounts.

Hormones. Oestrogens, progestogens and androgens suppress lactation in high dose. Oestrogen/progestogen oral contraceptives are present in amounts too small to be harmful but may suppress lactation if it is not well established.

Miscellaneous. Bromocriptine suppresses lactation. Caffeine may cause infant irritability in high doses.

Drug dosage

Drug dosage can be of five main kinds:

- **Fixed dose**. The effect that is desired can be obtained at well below the toxic dose (many mydriatics, diuretics, analgesics, oral contraceptives, antimicrobials) and enough drug can be given to render individual variation clinically insignificant.

- **Variable dose** — with crude adjustments. Here fine adjustments make comparatively insignificant differences and the therapeutic end-point may be hard to measure (depression, anxiety), may change only slowly (thyrotoxicosis), or may vary because of pathophysiological factors (analgesics, adrenal steroids for suppressing disease).

- **Variable dose** — with fine adjustments. Here a vital function (blood pressure, blood sugar), that often changes rapidly in response to dose changes and can easily be measured repeatedly, provides the end-point. Adjustment of dose must be accurate. Adrenocortical replacement therapy falls into this group, whereas adrenocortical pharmacotherapy falls into the group above.

- **Maximum tolerated dose** is used when the ideal therapeutic effect cannot be achieved because of the occurrence of unwanted effects (anticancer drugs; some antimicrobials). The usual way of finding this is to increase the dose until unwanted effects begin to appear and then to reduce it slightly, or to monitor the plasma concentration.

- **Minimum tolerated dose**. This concept is not so common as the one above, but it applies to longterm adrenocortical steroid therapy against inflammatory or immunological conditions, e.g. in asthma and some cases of rheumatoid arthritis, when the dose that provides symptomatic relief may be so high that serious adverse effects are inevitable if it is continued indefinitely. The patient must be persuaded to accept incomplete relief on the grounds of safety. This can be difficult to achieve.

Dosing schedules

Whatever their type, dosing schedules are simply schemes aimed at achieving a desired effect whilst avoiding toxicity. In the discussion that follows it is assumed that drug effect relates closely to plasma concentration, which in turn relates closely to the amount of drug in the body.

The objectives of a dosing regimen where continuing effect is required are:

To specify an initial dose that attains the desired effect rapidly without causing toxicity. Often the dose that is capable of initiating drug effect is the same as that which maintains it. On repeated dosing however, it takes $5 \times t^{1/2}$ periods to reach steady-state concentration in the plasma and this lapse of time may be undesirable. The effect may be achieved earlier by giving an initial dose that is larger than the maintenance dose; the initial dose is then called the *priming or loading dose*, i.e. the priming dose is that dose which will achieve a therapeutic effect in an individual whose body does not already contain the drug.

To specify a maintenance dose: amount and frequency. Intuitively, it might be half the initial / priming dose at intervals equal to its plasma $t^{1/2}$, for this by definition is the time in which the plasma concentration that achieves the desired effect declines by half. Whether or not this approach is satisfactory or practicable, however, depends very much on the $t^{1/2}$ itself, as is illustrated by the following cases:

Case examples

1. *Half-life: 6–12 h*. In this instance, replacing half the initial dose at intervals equal to the $t^{1/2}$ can indeed be a satisfactory solution because dosing every 6–12 h is acceptable.

2. *Half-life: greater than 24 h*. With once-daily dosing (which is desirable for compliance) giving half the priming dose every day means that more drug is entering the body than is leaving it each day, and the drug will accumulate indefinitely. The solution is to replace only that amount of drug that leaves the body in 24 h. This quantity can be calculated once the initial dose and dose interval have been decided and the $t^{1/2}$ is known.

3. *Half-life: less than 3 h*. Dosing at intervals equal to the $t^{1/2}$ would be so frequent as to be unacceptable, and the answer is to use *continuous intravenous infusion* if the $t^{1/2}$ is very short, e.g. dopamine ($t^{1/2}$

2 min; steady-state plasma concentration will be reached in $5 \times t^{1/2} = 10$ min) or, if the $t^{1/2}$ is longer, e.g. lignocaine ($t^{1/2}$ 90 min) to use a priming dose as an intravenous bolus followed by a constant intravenous infusion. Intermittent administration of a drug with short half-life is nevertheless reasonable provided large fluctuations in plasma concentration are acceptable, i.e. that the drug has a large therapeutic index. Benzylpenicillin has a $t^{1/2}$ of 30 min but is effective in a 6-hourly regimen because the drug is so nontoxic that it is possible safely to give a dose that achieves a plasma concentration many times in excess of the minimum inhibitory concentration for sensitive organisms.

PROLONGATION OF DRUG ACTION

- A larger dose is the most obvious way to prolong a drug action. As this is not always feasible, other mechanisms are used.
- Vasoconstriction will reduce local blood flow so that distribution of drug away from an injection site is retarded, e.g. local anaesthetic action is prolonged by combination with adrenaline.
- Slowing of metabolism may usefully extend drug action, as when a dopa decarboxylase inhibitor, e.g. carbidopa, is combined with levodopa (as co-careldopa) for parkinsonism.
- Delayed excretion is seldom practicable, the only important example being the use of probenecid to block renal tubular excretion of penicillin, e.g. when the latter is used in single dose to treat gonorrhoea.
- Molecular structure may be altered to prolong effect, e.g. the various benzodiazepines.
- Pharmaceutical formulation. Manipulating the formulation in which a drug is presented by modified-release[23] systems can achieve the objective of an even as well as a prolonged effect.

Sustained-release (oral) preparations can reduce the frequency of medication to once a day, and com-

---

[23] The term *modified* covers several drug delivery systems. *Delayed-release*: available other than immediately after administration (mesalazine in the colon); *sustained-release*: slow release as governed by the delivery system (iron, potassium); *controlled-release*: at a constant rate to maintain unvarying plasma concentration (nitrate, hormone replacement therapy).

pliance is made easier for the patient. Most long-term medication for the elderly can now be given as a single morning dose. In addition sustained-release preparations may avoid local bowel toxicity due to high local concentrations, e.g ulceration of the small intestine with KCl tablets, and may also avoid the toxic peak plasma concentrations that can occur when dissolution of the formulation and so absorption of the drug are rapid. Some sustained-release formulations also contain an immediate-release component to provide rapid, as well as sustained, effect.

Depot (injectable) preparations are more reliable because the environment in which they are deposited is more constant than can ever be the case in the alimentary tract and medication can be given at longer intervals, even weeks. In general such preparations are pharmaceutical variants, e.g. microcrystals, or the original drug in oil, wax, gelatin or synthetic media. They include phenothiazine neuroleptics, the various insulins and penicillins, preparations of vasopressin, benzathine penicillin and medroxyprogesterone (i.m., s.c.). Tablets of hormones are sometimes implanted subcutaneously. The advantages of infrequent administration and better patient compliance in a variety of situations are obvious.

REDUCTION OF ABSORPTION TIME

This can be achieved by making a soluble salt of the drug which is rapidly absorbed from the site of administration. In the case of s.c. or i.m. injections the same objective may be obtained with *hyaluronidase*, an enzyme which depolymerises hyaluronic acid, a constituent of connective tissue that prevents the spread of foreign substances, e.g. bacteria, drugs. By combining an injection with hyaluronidase, a drug spreads rapidly over a wide area and so is absorbed more quickly. Hyaluronidase can also be used to promote resorption of tissue accumulation of blood and fluid. Ergometrine may be given thus by nurses who are not trained to give i.v. injections.

DOSE, BODY WEIGHT AND SURFACE AREA

When a fixed dose is inappropriate, it is usual to adjust the dose according to body weight.

Adjustment according to body surface area may be more appropriate, for this is directly related to metabolic rate; this is obtained by taking the body weight to the power of 0.7.

FIXED-DOSE DRUG COMBINATIONS

This section refers to combinations of drugs in a single pharmaceutical formulation. It does not refer to concomitant drug therapy, e.g. in infections, hypertension and in cancer, when several drugs are given separately.

Fixed-dose drug combinations are **appropriate** for:

● *Convenience*, with improved patient compliance. This is particularly appropriate when two drugs are used at constant dose, long term, for an asymptomatic condition, e.g. a thiazide plus a β-adrenoceptor blocker in mild or moderate hypertension. The fewer tablets the patients have to take, the more reliably will they use them, especially the elderly who as a group receive more drugs because they have multiple pathology.
● *Enhanced effect*. Single-drug treatment of tuberculosis leads to the emergence of resistant mycobacteria; this effect is prevented or delayed by using two or more drugs simultaneously. Combining isoniazid with rifampicin (Rifinah, Rimactazid) ensures that single drug treatment cannot occur; treatment has to be two drugs or no drug at all. Oral contraception (with an oestrogen and progestogen combination) is used for the same reason.
● *Minimisation of unwanted effects*. Combining levodopa with benserazide (Madopar) or with carbidopa (Sinemet) slows its metabolism outside the central nervous system so that smaller amounts of levodopa can be used; this reduces side-effects.

Fixed-dose drug combinations are **inappropriate**:

● When the dose of one or more of the component drugs may need to be adjusted independently. A drug with a wide dose-range that must be adjusted to suit the patient's response is unsuitable for combination with a drug that has a narrow dose range.

- If the time course of drug action demands different intervals between administration of the components.
- If irregularity of administration, e.g. in response to a symptom such as pain or cough, is desirable for some ingredients but not for others.

CONCLUSIONS

Therapeutic aims should be clear. Combinations should not be prescribed unless there is good reason to consider that the patient needs all the drugs in the formulation and that the doses are appropriate and will not need to be adjusted separately. Rational combinations can provide advantage, just as inappropriate combinations may be dangerous (and identification of a drug causing an adverse effect may be difficult when a combination is used). Thus combinations of iron with folic acid and cyanocobalamin are hazardous if they delay diagnosis of pernicious anaemia. But the fact that iron plus a little folic acid is properly used in pregnancy for routine anaemia prophylaxis simply confirms that combinations can be rationally devised to meet particular needs.

Chronic pharmacology

With many drugs there are differences in pharmacodynamics and pharmacokinetics according to whether their use is in a single dose or over a brief period (acute pharmacology) or longterm (chronic pharmacology). The proportion of the population taking drugs continuously for large portions of their lives increases as tolerable suppressive and prophylactic remedies for chronic or recurrent conditions are developed; e.g. for arterial hypertension, diabetes mellitus, mental diseases, epilepsies, gout, collagen diseases, thrombosis, allergies and various infections. In some cases longterm treatment introduces significant hazard into patients' lives and the cure can be worse than the disease if it is not skilfully managed. In general the dangers of a drug are not markedly increased if therapy lasts years rather than months; exceptions include renal damage due to analgesic mixtures, and carcinogenicity.

INTERFERENCE WITH SELF-REGULATING SYSTEMS

When self-regulating physiological systems (generally controlled by negative feedback systems, e.g. endocrine, cardiovascular) are subject to interference, their control mechanisms respond to minimise the effects of the interference and to restore the previous steady state or rhythm: this is *homeostasis*. The previous state may be a normal function, e.g. ovulation (a rare example of a positive feedback mechanism), or an abnormal function, e.g. high blood pressure. If the body successfully restores the previous steady state or rhythm then the subject has become *tolerant* to the drug, i.e. a higher dose is needed to produce the desired previous effect.

In the case of hormonal contraceptives, persistence of effect on ovulation occurs and is desired, but persistence of other effects, e.g. on blood coagulation and metabolism, is not desired.

In the case of arterial hypertension, tolerance to a single drug commonly occurs, e.g. reduction of peripheral resistance by a vasodilator is compensated by an increase in blood volume that restores the blood pressure; this is why a diuretic is commonly used together with a vasodilator in therapy.

Feedback systems. The endocrine system serves fluctuating body needs. Glands are therefore capable either of increasing or decreasing their output by means of negative (usually) feedback systems. An administered hormone or hormone analogue activates the receptors of the feedback system so that high doses cause suppression of natural production of the hormone. On withdrawal of the administered hormone restoration of the normal control mechanism takes time; e.g. hypothalamic/ pituitary/adrenal cortex system can take months to recover full sensitivity, and sudden withdrawal of administered corticosteroid can result in an acute deficiency state that may be life-endangering.

Regulation of receptors. The number (density) of receptors on cells (for hormones, autacoids or local hormones, and drugs), the number occupied (receptor occupancy) and the capacity of the receptor to respond (affinity, efficacy) can change in response to the concentration of the specific binding molecule or ligand,[24] whether this be agonist or antagonist (blocker). The effects always tend to restore cell function to its normal or usual state. Prolonged high concentrations of agonist (whether administered as a drug or over-produced in the body by a tumour) cause a reduction in the number of receptors available for activation (down-regulation); changes in receptor occupancy and affinity and the prolonged occupation of receptors by inert molecules (antagonists) leads to an increase in the number of receptors (up-regulation). At least some of this may be achieved by receptors moving inside the cell and out again (internalisation and externalisation).

Down-regulation and accompanying receptor changes may explain the tolerant or refractory state seen in severe asthmatics who no longer respond to β-adrenoceptor agonists.

Up-regulation. The occasional exacerbation of ischaemic cardiac disease on sudden withdrawal of a β-adrenoceptor blocker may be explained by up-regulation during its administration, so that on withdrawal an above-normal number of receptors suddenly becomes accessible to the normal chemotransmitter, i.e. noradrenaline (norepinephrine). Up-regulation with rebound sympathomimetic effects may be innocuous to a moderately healthy cardiovascular system, but the increased oxygen demand of these effects can have serious consequences where ischaemic disease is present and increased oxygen need cannot be met (angina pectoris, dysrhythmia, infarction). Unmasking of a disease process that has worsened during prolonged suppressive use of the drug, i.e. resurgence, may also contribute to such exacerbations.

The rebound phenomenon is plainly a potential hazard and the use of a β-adrenoceptor blocker in the presence of ischaemic heart disease would be safer if rebound could be eliminated. β-adrenoceptor blockers that are not pure antagonists but have some agonist (sympathomimetic) activity, i.e. partial agonists may prevent the generation of additional adrenoceptors (up-regulation). Indeed there is evidence that rebound is less or is absent

with pindolol, a partial agonist β-adrenoceptor blocker.

Sometimes a distinction is made between rebound (recurrence at intensified degree of the symptoms for which the drug was given) and withdrawal syndrome (appearance of new additional symptoms). The distinction is quantitative and does not imply different mechanisms.

Rebound and withdrawal phenomena occur erratically. In general, they are more likely with drugs having a short half-life (abrupt drop in plasma concentration) and pure agonist or antagonist action. They are less likely to occur with drugs having a long half-life and (probably) with those having a mixed agonist/antagonist (partial agonist) action on receptors.

ABRUPT WITHDRAWAL

Clinically important consequences are known to occur with the following:

- *Cardiovascular system*: antihypertensives (especially clonidine), β-adrenoceptor blockers.
- *Nervous system:* all depressants (hypnotics, sedatives, alcohol, opioids), antiepileptics, antiparkinsonian agents, tricyclic antidepressants.
- *Endocrine system*: adrenal steroids.
- *Immune inflammation*: adrenal steroids.

Resurgence of chronic disease which has progressed in severity although its consequences have been wholly or partly suppressed, i.e. a catching-up phenomenon, is an obvious possible consequence of withdrawal of effective therapy, e.g. levodopa in Parkinson's disease; in corticosteroid withdrawal in autoimmune disease there may be both resurgence and rebound.

Drug discontinuation syndromes, i.e. rebound, withdrawal and resurgence (defined above) are phenomena that are to be expected. In many cases the exact mechanisms remain obscure but clinicians have no reason to be surprised when they occur, and in the case of rebound they may particularly wish to use gradual withdrawal wherever drugs have been used to modify complex self-adjusting systems, and to suppress (without cure) chronic diseases.

---

[24] Latin: *ligare*, to bind.

OTHER ASPECTS OF CHRONIC DRUG USE

Metabolic changes over a long period may induce disease, e.g. thiazide diuretics (diabetes mellitus), adrenocortical hormones (osteoporosis), phenytoin (osteomalacia). Drugs may also enhance their own metabolism, and that of other drugs (enzyme induction).

Specific cell injury or cell functional disorder occur with individual drugs or drug classes, e.g. tardive dyskinesia (dopamine receptor blockers), retinal damage (chloroquine, phenothiazines), retroperitoneal fibrosis (methysergide), NSAIDs (nephropathy). Cancer may occur, e.g. with oestrogens (endometrium) and with immunosuppressive (anticancer) drugs.

Drug holidays. This term means the deliberate interruption of longterm therapy with the objective of restoring sensitivity (which has been lost) or to reduce the risk of toxicity. Plainly the need for holidays is a substantial disadvantage for any drug. The principal example is methysergide for refractory migraine (see Index). Patients sometimes initiate their own drug holidays (see Patient compliance).

Dangers of intercurrent illness. These are particularly notable with anticoagulants, adrenal steroids and immunosuppressives.

Dangers of interactions with other drugs or food: see index, food, interactions, individual drugs.

Drugs not only induce their known listed primary actions, but they:

- Evoke compensatory responses in the complex inter-related physiological systems that they perturb, and that these systems need time to recover on withdrawal of the drug (gradual withdrawal can give this time; it is sometimes mandatory and never harmful)
- Induce metabolic changes that may be trivial in the short term, but serious if they persist for a long time
- May produce localised effects in specially susceptible tissues and induce serious cell damage or malfunction
- Increase susceptibility to intercurrent illness and to interaction with other drugs that may be taken for new indications.

That such consequences will occur with prolonged drug use is to be expected; with a knowledge of physiology, pathology and pharmacology, combined with an awareness that the unexpected is to be expected ('There are more things in heaven and earth, Horatio, than are dreamt of in your philosophy'[25]) patients requiring longterm therapy may be managed safely, or at least with minimum risk of harm, and enabled to live happy lives.

Individual or biological variation

PRESCRIBING FOR SPECIAL RISK GROUPS

That individuals respond differently to drugs, both from time to time and from other individuals is a matter of everyday experience. Doctors need to accommodate for individual variation, for it may explain both adverse response to a drug and failure of therapy. Sometimes there are obvious physical characteristics such as age, race (genetics) or disease that warn the prescriber to adjust drug dose, but there are no external features that signify, e.g., pseudocholinesterase deficiency, which causes prolonged paralysis after suxamethonium. An understanding of the reasons for individual variation in response to drugs is relevant to all who prescribe. Both pharmacodynamic and pharmacokinetic effects are involved and the issues fall in two general categories: inherited influences and environmental and host influences.

Inherited influences: pharmacogenetics

Consider how individuals in a population might be expected to respond to a fixed dose of a drug; some would show less than the usual response, most would show the usual response and some would show more than the usual response. This type of

---

[25] W Shakespeare (1564–1616) Hamlet: I.V. 166.

variation is described as *continuous* and in a graph the result would appear as a normal or Gaussian (bell-shaped) distribution curve, similar to the type of curve that describes the distribution of height, weight or metabolic rate in a population. The curve is the result of a multitude of factors, some genetic (multiple genes) and some environmental, that contribute collectively to the response of the individual to the drug; they include race, sex, diet, weight, environmental and body temperature, circadian rhythm, absorption, distribution, metabolism, excretion and receptor density, but no single factor has a predominant effect.

Less commonly, variation is *discontinuous* when differences in response reveal a discrete proportion, large or small, who respond differently from the rest, e.g. poor drug oxidisers or fast and slow acetylators of isoniazid. Discontinuous variation most commonly occurs when response to a drug is controlled by a single gene. The term *genetic polymorphism*[26] refers to

> existence in a population of two or more *alleles* (at the same locus), resulting in more than one *phenotype* with respect to the effect of a drug.
>
> Pharmacogenetic polymorphism usually takes the form of different drug metabolising capacities, i.e. genetic differences in a single enzyme.

Pharmacogenetics is concerned with drug responses that are governed by heredity. Inherited factors causing different responses to drugs are commonly biochemical because single genes govern the production of enzymes.

Inherited abnormal responses to drugs mediated by single genes are called **idiosyncrasy** and cause increased, decreased and bizarre responses to drugs.

HERITABLE CONDITIONS CAUSING INCREASED OR TOXIC RESPONSES

Acetylator status

Acetylation is an important route of metabolism for many drugs that possess an $-NH_2$ group.

Population studies have shown that individuals are either rapid or slow acetylators but the proportion of each varies greatly between races as shown in Table 7.6.

Table 7.6 Acetylator status

Ethnic group	Rapid acetylators (%)
Inuit (Canadian Eskimos)	95
Japanese	88
Thais	72
Latin Americans	70
Black Americans	52
White Americans	48
Britons	38
Swedes	32
Egyptians	18

The importance of acetylator status to therapy is illustrated by the following examples:

Isoniazid may cause peripheral neuropathy in slow acetylators on standard doses and pyridoxine is added to the antituberculosis regimen where there is special risk, e.g. in diabetes, alcoholism, renal failure. Acute hepatocellular necrosis with isoniazid is more common in rapid acetylators, perhaps because they more readily form an hepatotoxic metabolite. *Hydralazine* and *procainamide* may cause antinuclear antibodies to develop in the plasma of slow acetylators, and some proceed to systemic lupus erythematosus. *Sulphasalazine* (salicylazosulphapyridine; used for ulcerative colitis) causes adverse effects more frequently in slow acetylators, probably because of the sulphapyridine component which is inactivated by acetylation. *Dapsone* appears to cause more red-cell haemolysis in slow acetylators; rapid acetylators may need higher doses to control dermatitis herpetiformis and leprosy.

Defective carbon oxidation

Variation in response to some drugs can be attributed to genetic polymorphisms of oxidation of their carbon centres. The condition was recognised by abnormal metabolism and response to debrisoquine.[27] Individuals may be classed as extensive or

---

[26] Laurence D, Carpenter J 1994 A dictionary of pharmacology and clinical drug evaluation. University College London Press, London.

[27] The poor oxidiser state was first revealed in the laboratory of R L Smith, Professor of Biochemical Pharmacology, St Mary's Hospital Medical School, London, who was investigating the variable dose requirements of patients

poor oxidisers and the latter are at special risk of adverse effects with standard doses of drugs that include bufuralol, metoprolol, timolol (increased beta-blockade), haloperidol (excessive sedation). There are over 5 million slow oxidisers in the UK population (57m). A similar but distinct condition is characterised by deficiency in metabolism of the antiepileptic mephenytoin: affected individuals may exhibit slow metabolism and increased response to various drugs including propranolol and diazepam.

Glucose-6-phosphate dehydrogenase (G-6-PD) deficiency

G-6-PD activity is important to the integrity of the red blood cell through a chain of reactions:

- It is an important source of reduced nicotinamide-adenine dinucleotide phosphate (NADPH) which maintains erythrocyte glutathione in its reduced form.
- Reduced glutathione is necessary to keep haemoglobin in the reduced (ferrous) rather than in its ferric state (methaemoglobin) which is useless for oxygen carriage.
- Build-up of methaemoglobin in erythrocytes impairs the function of sulphydryl groups, especially those associated with the stability of the cell membrane.

Individuals who are G-6-PD deficient may suffer acute haemolysis if they are exposed to certain *oxidant* substances, including drugs. Characteristically there is an acute haemolytic episode 2–3 days after starting the drug. The haemolysis is self-limiting, only older cells with least enzyme being affected. The condition is common in African, Mediterranean, Middle East and South East Asian races and in their descendants and, throughout the world, affects some 100 million people. As deficiency may result from inheritance of any one of numerous variants of G-6-PD, affected individuals exhibit differing susceptibility to haemolysis, i.e. a substance which affects one G-6-PD deficient subject adversely may be harmless in another. The following guidelines apply:[28]

Drugs that carry a **definite** risk of haemolysis in most G-6-PD deficient subjects include:

Dapsone (and other sulphones), methylene blue, niridazole, nitrofurantoin, pamaquin, primaquine, quinolones, some sulphonamides.

Drugs that carry a **possible** risk of haemolysis in some G-6-PD deficient subjects include:

aspirin, menadione, probenecid, quinidine; chloroquine and quinine (both are acceptable in acute malaria).

Affected individuals are also susceptible to exposure to nitrates, anilines and naphthalenes (found in moth balls). Some individuals experience haemolysis after eating the broad bean, *Vicia faba*, and hence the term 'favism'.

Pseudocholinesterase deficiency

The neuromuscular blocking action of suxamethonium is terminated by plasma pseudocholinesterase. 'True' cholinesterase (acetylcholinesterase) hydrolyses acetylcholine released by nerve endings, whereas various tissues and plasma contain other nonspecific, hence 'pseudo', esterases. Affected individuals form so little plasma pseudocholinesterase that metabolism of suxamethonium is seriously reduced. The deficiency characteristically comes to light when a patient fails to breathe spontaneously after a surgical operation, and assisted ventilation may have to be undertaken for hours. Relatives of an affected individual — for this as for other inherited abnormalities carrying avoidable risk — should be sought out, checked to assess their own risk, and told of the result. The prevalence of pseudocholinesterase deficiency in the UK population is about 1 in 2500.

Malignant hyperthermia (pp 332, 394).

Porphyria (p. 126).

Alcohol (p. 166).

---

receiving the two antihypertensive drugs debrisoquine and bethanidine. He writes: 'I took 40 mg of debrisoquine sulphate; within two hours my blood pressure crashed to 70/50 mmHg and I was unable to stand for four hours due to incapacitating postural hypotension...it was two days until the blood pressure returned to normal. Analysis of my urine revealed that nearly all the dose was excreted as unchanged drug, whereas other subjects who showed little if any cardiovascular response to the same dose of debrisoquine, converted it to the 4-hydroxy metabolite. However, the drama of the clinical response to a single dose of debrisoquine catalysed a search for its explanation and culminated in the uncovering of the first example of a genetic polymorphism of drug oxidation'.

---

[28] Data based on British National Formulary, 1996.

Heritable conditions causing decreased drug responses

- *Resistance to coumarin anticoagulants.* Subjects of this rare inherited abnormality possess a variant of the enzyme that converts vitamin K to its reduced and active form, which enzyme the coumarins normally inhibit; patients require 20 times or more of the usual dose to obtain an adequate clinical response. A similar condition also occurs in rats and has practical importance as warfarin, a coumarin, is used as a rat poison (rats with the gene are dubbed 'super-rats' by the mass media).
- *Resistance to heparin.* Patients with antithrombin III deficiency require large doses of heparin for anticoagulant effect. (The action of heparin is dependent on the presence of antithrombin III in the plasma.)
- *Resistance to suxamethonium.* This rare condition is characterised by increased pseudocholinesterase activity and failure of normal doses of suxamethonium to cause muscular relaxation (cf Cholinesterase deficiency, above).
- *Resistance to vitamin D.* Individuals develop rickets which responds only to huge doses of vitamin D, i.e. × 1000 the standard dose.
- *Bacterial resistance* to drugs is genetically determined and is of great clinical importance.

Conclusion

It is likely that many clinically important single gene differences in response to drugs remain to be discovered. Once a genetic difference, e.g. a metabolic reaction, is understood, it will be possible to predict what will happen when drugs of particular molecular structures are administered. But whether patients should be screened routinely for such differences in drug response is a matter of clinical importance as well as economics and logistics.

Environmental and host influences

A multitude of factors related both to individuals and their environment contribute to differences in drug response. In general, their precise role is less well documented than is the case with genetic factors but their range and complexity are illustrated by the following list of likely candidates: age, sex, pregnancy, lactation, exercise, sunlight, disease, infection, occupational exposures, drugs, circadian and seasonal variations, diet, stress, fever, malnutrition, alcohol intake, tobacco or cannabis smoking and the functioning of the cardiovascular, gastrointestinal, hepatic, immunological and renal systems.[29]

AGE

The neonate, infant and child[30]

Young human beings differ greatly from adults, not merely in size but also in the proportions and constituents of their bodies and the functioning of their physiological systems. These differences are reflected in the way the body handles and responds to drugs and are relevant to prescribing.

- Rectal absorption is efficient with an appropriate formulation and has been used for diazepam and theophyllines; this route may be preferred with an uncooperative infant.
- The intramuscular or subcutaneous routes tend to give unpredictable plasma concentrations, e.g. of digoxin or gentamicin, because of the relatively low proportion of skeletal muscle and fat. Intravenous administration is preferred in the seriously ill newborn.
- Drugs or other substances that come in contact with the skin are readily absorbed as the skin is well hydrated and the stratum corneum is thin; overdose toxicity may result, e.g. with hexachlorophane used in dusting powders and emulsions to prevent infection.

Distribution of drugs is influenced by the fact that total body water in the neonate amounts to 80% as compared to 65% in older children. Consequently:

- Weight-related priming doses of aminoglycosides, aminophylline, digoxin and

---

[29] Vessell E S 1982 Clinical Pharmacology and Therapeutics 31: 1.

[30] A neonate is under 1 month and an infant is 1–12 months of age.

frusemide are larger for neonates than for older children.

- Less extensive binding of drugs to plasma proteins is generally without clinical importance but there is a significant risk of elevation of plasma bilirubin (in the neonate) following its displacement from protein binding sites by vitamin K, X-ray contrast media or indomethacin.

Metabolism. Although the enzyme systems that inactivate drugs are present at birth, they are functionally immature, especially in the preterm baby, and especially for oxidation and for conjugation with glucuronic acid. Inability to conjugate and thus inactivate chloramphenicol causes the fatal 'grey' syndrome in neonates. After the first weeks of life the drug metabolic capacity increases rapidly.

Elimination. Glomerular filtration, tubular secretion and reabsorption are low in the neonate (even lower in preterm babies) only reaching adult values in relation to body surface area at 2–5 months. Therefore drugs that are eliminated by the kidney (e.g. aminoglycosides, penicillins, diuretics) must be given in reduced dose; after about 6 months, body weight- or surface area-related daily doses are the same for all ages.

    Dosage in the young. No single rule or formula suffices for all cases and the dose is established partly by scaling for body-weight and/or surface area (see p. 106) and by making pharmacokinetic and pharmacodynamic measurements when opportunities present. General guidance is available from tables that express the percentage of the adult dose which is suitable for a child according to its age, height and ideal body-weight, e.g. in the British National Formulary.

The elderly

The incidence of adverse drug reactions rises with age in the adult, especially after 65 years because of:

- The increasing number of drugs that they need to take because they tend to have multiple diseases
- Poor compliance with dosing regimens
- Bodily changes of ageing that require modification of dosage regimens.

Absorption of drugs may be slightly slower because gastrointestinal blood flow and motility are reduced but the effect is rarely important.

Distribution is influenced by the following changes:

- There is a significant decrease in lean body mass so that standard adult doses provide a greater amount of drug per kg.
- Total body water is less (and in general the distribution volume of water-soluble drugs is reduced) but body fat is increased, especially in males (and in general lipid-soluble drugs have larger distribution volume). Hence standard doses of drugs ought to be reduced, especially the priming doses of those that are water-soluble.
- Plasma albumin concentration tends to be well maintained in the healthy elderly but may be reduced by chronic disease, giving scope for a greater proportion of unbound (free) drug; this may be important when priming doses are given.

Metabolism is reduced because liver mass and liver blood flow are decreased. Consequently:

- Metabolic inactivation of drugs is slower.
- Drugs that are normally extensively eliminated in first-pass through the liver appear in higher concentration in the systemic circulation and persist in it for longer. There is thus particular cause initially to use lower doses of most neuroleptics, tricyclic antidepressants and cardiac antidysrhythmic agents.
- Capacity for hepatic enzyme induction appears to be lessened.

Elimination. Renal blood flow, glomerular filtration and tubular secretion decrease with age above 55 years, a decline that is not signalled by raised serum creatinine concentration because production of this metabolite is diminished by the age-associated diminution of muscle mass. Indeed, in the elderly, serum creatinine may be within the concentration range for normal young adults even when the creatinine clearance is 50 ml/min (compared to 127 ml/min in adult male). Particular risk of adverse effects arises with drugs that are eliminated mainly by the kidney and that have a small therapeutic ratio, e.g. aminoglycosides, chlorpropamide, digoxin, lithium.

Pharmacodynamic response may alter with age, to produce either a greater or lesser effect than is anticipated in younger adults.

- Drugs that act on the central nervous system appear to produce an exaggerated response in relation to that expected from the plasma concentration, and sedatives and hypnotics may have a pronounced hangover effect. These drugs are also more likely to depress respiration because vital capacity and maximum breathing capacity are lessened in the elderly.
- Response to β-adrenoceptor agonists and antagonists appears to be blunted in old age partly, it is believed, through reduction in the number of receptors.
- Baroreceptor sensitivity is reduced leading to the potential for orthostatic hypotension with drugs that reduce blood pressure.

Rules of prescribing for the elderly[31]

1. Think about the necessity for drugs. Is the diagnosis correct and complete? Is the drug really necessary? Is there a better alternative?
2. Do not prescribe drugs that are not useful. Think carefully before giving an old person a drug that may have major side-effects, and consider alternatives.
3. Think about the dose. Is it appropriate to possible alterations in the patient's physiological state? Is it appropriate to the patient's renal and hepatic function at the time?
4. Think about drug formulation. Is a tablet the most appropriate form of drug or would an injection, a suppository or a syrup be better? Is the drug suitably packaged for the elderly patient, bearing in mind any disabilities?
5. Assume any new symptoms may be due to drug side-effects, or more rarely, to drug withdrawal. Rarely (if ever) treat a side-effect of one drug with another.
6. Take a careful drug history. Bear in mind the possibility of interaction with substances the patient may be taking without your knowledge, such as herbal or other non-prescribed remedies, old drugs taken from the medicine cabinet or drugs obtained from friends.
7. Use fixed-combinations of drugs only when they are logical and well studied and they either aid compliance or improve tolerance or efficacy. Few fixed-combinations meet this standard.
8. When adding a new drug to the therapeutic regimen, see whether another can be withdrawn.
9. Attempt to check whether the patient's compliance is adequate, e.g. by counting remaining tablets. Has the patient (or relatives) been properly instructed?
10. Remember that stopping a drug is as important as starting it.

Note. The old (80+ years) are particularly intolerant of neuroleptics (given for confusion) and of diuretics (given for ankle swelling that is postural and not due to heart failure) which cause adverse electrolyte changes. Both classes of drug may result in admission to hospital of semicomatose 'senior citizens' who deserve better treatment from their juniors.

PREGNANCY

As the pregnancy evolves, profound changes occur in physiology, including fluid and tissue composition.

Absorption. Gastrointestinal motility is decreased but there appears to be no major defect in drug absorption except that reduced gastric emptying delays the appearance in the plasma of orally administered drugs, especially during labour. Absorption from an intramuscular site is likely to be efficient because tissue perfusion is increased due to vasodilatation.

Distribution. Total body water increases by up to 8 litres creating a larger space within which water-soluble drugs may distribute. As a result of haemodilution, plasma albumin (normal 33–55 g/l) declines by some 10 g/l. Thus there is scope for increased free concentration of drugs that bind to albumin. Unbound drug, however, is free to distribute and to be metabolised and excreted; e.g. the free (and pharmacologically active) concentration of

---

[31] By permission from Caird F I (ed) 1985 Drugs for the elderly. WHO (Europe) Copenhagen.

phenytoin is unaltered, although the total plasma concentration is reduced. Therapeutic drug monitoring interpreted by concentrations appropriate for nonpregnant women thus may mislead. A useful general guide during pregnancy is to maintain concentrations at the lower end of the recommended range. Body fat increases by about 4 kg and provides a reservoir for lipid-soluble drugs.

Hepatic metabolism increases though not blood flow to the liver. Consequently, there is increased clearance of drugs such as phenytoin and theophylline, whose elimination rate depends on liver enzyme activity. Drugs that are so rapidly metabolised that their elimination rate depends on their delivery to the liver, i.e. on hepatic blood flow, have unaltered clearance, e.g. propranolol.

Elimination. Renal plasma flow almost doubles and there is more rapid loss of drugs that are excreted by the kidney, e.g. amoxycillin, whose dose should be doubled for systemic infections (but not for urinary tract infections as penicillins are highly concentrated in the urine).
  Placenta: see page 92.

DISEASE

Diseases can cause pharmacokinetic changes.

Absorption

- Surgery that involves resection and reconstruction of the gut may lead to malabsorption of iron, folic acid and fat-soluble vitamins after partial gastrectomy, and of vitamin B_{12} after ileal resection.
- Delayed gastric emptying and intestinal stasis during an attack of migraine interfere with absorption of drugs.
- Severe low output cardiac failure or shock (with peripheral vasoconstriction) delays absorption from subcutaneous or intramuscular sites; reduced hepatic blood flow prolongs the presence in the plasma of drugs that are so rapidly extracted by the liver that removal depends on their rate of presentation to it, e.g. lignocaine.

Distribution. Hypoalbuminaemia from any cause, e.g. burns, malnutrition, sepsis, allows a higher proportion of free (unbound) drug in plasma. Although free drug is available for metabolism and excretion, there remains a risk of enhanced or adverse responses especially with initial doses of those that are highly protein bound, e.g. phenytoin. Inflammation is associated with increase in the concentration of the acute-phase protein, α_1-acid glycoprotein, which binds a number of basic drugs, e.g. lignocaine, disopyramide, monitoring of which may thus give misleadingly high results.

Metabolism. Acute inflammatory disease of the liver (viral, alcoholic) and cirrhosis affect both the functioning of the hepatocytes and blood flow through the liver. Reduced extraction from the plasma of drugs that are normally highly cleared in first pass through the liver results in increased systemic availability of drugs such as propranolol, labetalol and chlormethiazole. Many other drugs exhibit prolonged $t^1/_2$ and reduced clearance in patients with chronic liver disease, e.g. diazepam, tolbutamide, rifampicin (see Drugs and the liver, p. 591). Thyroid disease has the expected effects, i.e. drug metabolism is accelerated in hyperthyroidism and diminished in hypothyroidism.

Elimination. Disease of the kidney (p. 496) has profound effects on the pharmacokinetics and thence the actions of drugs that are eliminated by that organ.

Pharmacodynamic changes occur, e.g.:

- Asthmatic attacks can be precipitated by beta-adrenoceptor blockers.
- Malfunctioning of the respiratory centre (raised intracranial pressure, severe pulmonary insufficiency) causes patients to be intolerant of opioids, and indeed any sedative may precipitate respiratory failure.
- Myocardial infarction predisposes to cardiac dysrhythmia with digitalis glycosides or sympathomimetics.
- Myasthenia gravis is made worse by quinine and quinidine and myasthenics are intolerant of competitive neuromuscular blocking agents and aminoglycoside antibiotics.

FOOD

- The presence of food in the stomach, especially

if it is fatty, delays gastric emptying and the absorption of certain drugs; the plasma concentration of ampicillin and rifampicin may be much reduced if they are taken on a full stomach. More specifically, calcium, e.g. in milk, interferes with absorption of tetracyclines and iron (by chelation).

- Substituting protein for fat or carbohydrate in the diet is associated with an increase in drug oxidation rates. Some specific dietary factors induce drug metabolising enzymes, e.g. alcohol, charcoal grilled (broiled) beef, cabbage and Brussels sprouts.

Protein malnutrition causes changes that are likely to influence pharmacokinetics, e.g. loss of body weight, reduced hepatic metabolising capacity, hypoproteinaemia.

Citrus flavinoids (in grapefruit but not orange juice) interact at the gut significantly to increase absorption of cyclosporin, calcium antagonists and probably other drugs.

Drug interactions

When a drug is administered, a response occurs; if a second drug is given and the response to the first drug is altered, a drug interaction is said to have occurred.[32] A drug interaction may be desired or undesired, i.e. beneficial or harmful. It is deliberately sought in multidrug treatment of tuberculosis and when naloxone is given to treat morphine overdose. It is an embarrassment when a woman taking a combined oestrogen/progestogen oral contraceptive for a desired interaction is prescribed a drug that is a metabolic enzyme inducer, with the result that she becomes pregnant.

Although dramatic unintended interactions attract most attention and are the principal subject of this section they should not distract attention from the many therapeutically useful interactions that are the basis of rational polypharmacy. These useful interactions are referred to throughout the book whenever it is relevant to do so.

---

[32] The term drug–drug interaction is also used, to make the distinction from drug–food interactions, and interaction with endogenous transmitters and hormones.

CLINICAL IMPORTANCE OF DRUG INTERACTIONS

If doctors were to limit their prescribing to the list in Use of Essential Drugs (WHO) (p. 29) and were to prescribe four drugs for any patient at any one time, the number of possible combinations would be more than 64 million. There can be no doubt that the number of drug interactions that might occur in this imagined situation would be too large to commit to memory or to paper. But the observation that one drug can be shown measurably to alter the disposition or effect of another drug does not mean that the interaction is necessarily of clinical importance. In this section we highlight the circumstances in which clinically important interactions can occur; we describe their pharmacological basis and provide a schematic framework to identify potential drug interactions during clinical practice.

Clinically important **adverse** drug interactions become likely with the following:

- Drugs that have a steep dose-response curve and a small therapeutic index (p. 82) so that relatively small quantitative changes at the target site, e.g. receptor or enzyme, will lead to substantial changes in effect, as with digoxin or lithium
- Drugs that are known enzyme inducers or inhibitors (pp 101, 102)
- Drugs that exhibit saturable metabolism (zero-order kinetics), when small interference with kinetics may lead to large alteration of plasma concentration, e.g. phenytoin, theophylline
- Drugs that are used longterm, where precise plasma concentrations are required, e.g. oral contraceptives, antiepilepsy drugs, cardiac antidysrhythmia drugs, lithium
- When drugs that may interact are used to treat the same disease, for this increases the chance of their being given concurrently, e.g. theophylline and salbutamol given for asthma may cause cardiac dysrhythmia
- In severely ill patients, for they may be receiving several drugs; signs of iatrogenic disease may be difficult to distinguish from those of existing disease and the patients' condition may be such that they cannot tolerate further adversity
- In patients with significantly impaired liver or

kidney function, for these are the principal organs that terminate drug action

- In the elderly, for they tend to have multiple pathology, may receive several drugs concurrently, and are specially susceptible to adverse drug effects (p. 113).

PHARMACOLOGICAL BASIS OF DRUG INTERACTIONS

Some knowledge of the pharmacological basis of how one drug may change the action of another is useful in obtaining those interactions that are wanted, as well as in recognising and preventing those that are not.

Drug interactions are of two principal kinds:

1. *Pharmacodynamic interaction*: both drugs act on the target site of clinical effect, exerting synergism (below) or antagonism. The drugs may act on the same or different receptors or processes, mediating similar biological consequences. Examples include: alcohol + benzodiazepine (to produce sedation), morphine + naloxone (to reverse opioid overdose), rifampicin + isoniazid (effective antituberculosis combination).
2. *Pharmacokinetic interaction*: the drugs interact remotely from the target site to alter plasma (and other tissue) concentrations so that the amount of the drug at the target site of clinical effect is altered, e.g. enzyme induction (rifampicin/warfarin), enzyme inhibition (ciprofloxacin/theophylline)

Interaction may result in antagonism or synergism.

Antagonism occurs when the action of one drug opposes the action of another. Two drugs simply have opposite pharmacodynamic effects, e.g. histamine and adrenaline on the bronchi exhibit physiological or functional antagonism; or they compete reversibly for the same drug receptor, e.g. isoprenaline (isoproterenol) and β-adrenoceptor blockers exhibit competitive antagonism.

Synergism.[33] The probability that pharmacologists will, in the foreseeable future, agree on the terminology to describe drug synergism is remote.

Therefore, the following will suffice. Synergism is of two sorts:

1. Summation or addition occurs when the effects of two drugs having the same action are additive, i.e. 2 + 2 = 4 (a β-adrenoceptor blocker plus a thiazide diuretic have an additive antihypertensive effect).
2. Potentiation (to make more powerful) occurs when one drug increases the action of another, i.e. 2 + 2 = 5. Sometimes the two drugs both have the action concerned (trimethoprim plus sulphonamide) and sometimes one drug lacks the action concerned (benserazide plus levodopa), i.e. 0 + 2 = 5.

IDENTIFYING POTENTIAL DRUG INTERACTIONS

Drugs can interact at any stage from when they are mixed with other drugs in a pharmaceutical formulation or by a clinician, e.g. in an i.v. infusion or syringe, to their final excretion either unchanged or as metabolites. When a drug is added to an existing regimen, a doctor can evaluate the possibility of an interaction by logically thinking through the usual sequence of processes to which a drug is subject and which are outlined earlier in this chapter, i.e. interactions may occur:

- outside the body
- at the site of absorption
- during distribution
- on receptors or body systems (pharmacodynamic interactions)
- during metabolism
- during excretion.

INTERACTIONS OUTSIDE THE BODY

Intravenous fluids offer special scope for interactions (incompatibilities) when drugs are added to the reservoir or syringe, for a number of reasons. Drugs commonly are weak organic acids or bases. They are often insoluble and to make them soluble it is necessary to prepare salts. Plainly, the mixing of solutions of salts can result in instability which may or may not be evident from visible change in the solution, i.e. precipitation. Furthermore, the

---

[33] Greek: *syn*, together; *ergos*, work.

solutions have little buffering capacity and pH readily changes with added drugs. Dilution of a drug in the reservoir fluid may also lead to loss of stability.

Serious loss of potency can result from incompatibility between an infusion fluid and a drug that is added to it. Issues of compatibility are complex but specific sources of information are available in manufacturers' package inserts, formularies or from the hospital pharmacy (where the addition ought to be made). The general rule must be to consult these sources before ever adding a drug to an infusion fluid or mixing in a syringe.

Mixing drugs formulated for injection in a syringe may cause interaction, e.g. protamine zinc insulin contains excess of protamine which binds with added soluble insulin and reduces the immediate effect of the dose.

INTERACTIONS AT SITE OF ABSORPTION

In the complex environment of the gut there are opportunities for drugs to interfere with each other both directly and indirectly via alteration of gut physiology. Usually the result is to impair absorption.

Direct chemical interaction in the gut is a significant cause of reduced absorption. Antacids that contain aluminium and magnesium form insoluble complexes with tetracyclines, iron and prednisolone. Milk contains sufficient calcium to warrant its avoidance as a major article of diet when tetracyclines are taken. Cholestyramine interferes with absorption of thyroxine, digoxin and some acidic drugs, e.g. warfarin. Sucralfate reduces the absorption of phenytoin. Interactions of this type depend on both drugs being in the stomach at the same time, and can be prevented if the doses are separated by at least 2 hours.

Gut motility may be altered by drugs. Those having antimuscarinic effects, e.g. some antidepressants, and opioid analgesics, reduce gastric emptying and delay absorption of other drugs. Purgatives reduce the time spent in the small intestine and give less opportunity for the absorption of poorly soluble substances such as adrenal steroids and digoxin.

Alterations in gut flora by antimicrobials may potentiate oral anticoagulant by reducing bacterial synthesis of vitamin K (usually only after antimicrobials are given orally in high dose, e.g. to treat *Helicobacter pylori*).

Interactions other than in the gut are exemplified by the use of hyaluronidase to promote dissipation of a s.c. injection, and by the addition of vasoconstrictors, e.g. adrenaline, felypressin, to local anaesthetics to delay absorption and usefully prolong local anaesthesia.

INTERACTIONS DURING DISTRIBUTION

1. Displacement from plasma protein binding sites may contribute to adverse reaction. A drug that is extensively protein bound can be displaced from its binding site by a competing drug, so raising the free (and pharmacologically active) concentration of the first drug. Unbound drug, however, is available for distribution away from the plasma and for metabolism and excretion. Commonly, the result is that the free concentration of the displaced drug quickly returns close to its original value and any extra effect is transient.

For a displacement interaction to become clinically important, a second mechanism usually operates: sodium valproate can cause phenytoin toxicity because it both displaces phenytoin from its binding site on plasma albumin and inhibits its metabolism. Similarly aspirin and probenecid (and possibly other nonsteroidal anti-inflammatory drugs) displace the folic acid antagonist methotrexate from its protein-binding site and reduce its rate of active secretion by the renal tubules; the result is serious methotrexate toxicity. Bilirubin is displaced from its binding protein by sulphonamides, vitamin K, X-ray contrast media or indomethacin; in the neonate this may cause a significant risk of kernicterus, for its capacity to metabolise bilirubin is immature.

Direct interaction between drugs may also take place in the plasma, e.g. protamine with heparin; desferrioxamine with iron; dimercaprol with arsenic (all useful).

2. Displacement from tissue binding may cause unwanted effects. When quinidine is given to patients who are receiving digoxin, the plasma concentration of free digoxin may double because quinidine displaces digoxin from binding sites in tissue (as well as plasma proteins). As with interaction due to displacement from plasma proteins, however, an additional mechanism contributes to the overall effect, for quinidine also impairs renal excretion of digoxin.

INTERACTIONS DIRECTLY ON RECEPTORS OR ON BODY SYSTEMS

This category of pharmacodynamic interactions comprises specific interactions between drugs on the same receptor, and includes less precise interactions involving the same body organ or system; whatever the precise location, the result is altered drug action.

1. Action on receptors provides numerous examples. Beneficial interactions are sought in overdose, as with the use of naloxone for morphine overdose (opioid receptor), of atropine for anticholinesterase, i.e. insecticide poisoning (acetylcholine receptor), of isoproterelol (isoprenaline) for overdose with a β-adrenoceptor blocker (β-adrenoceptor), of phentolamine for the monoamine oxidase inhibitor–sympathomimetic interaction (α-adrenoceptor).

Unwanted interactions include the loss of antihypertensive effect of β-blockers when common cold remedies containing ephedrine, phenylpropanolamine or phenylephrine are taken, usually unknown to the doctor; their α-adrenoceptor agonist action is unrestrained in the β-blocked patient.

2. Actions on body systems provide scope for a variety of interactions. The following list shows something of the range of possibilities; others may be found under accounts of individual drugs:

Beta-adrenoceptor blockers lose some antihypertensive efficacy when nonsteroidal anti-inflammatory drugs (NSAIDs), especially indomethacin, are co-administered; the effect involves inhibition of production of vasodilator prostaglandins by the kidney leading to sodium retention.

Diuretics, especially of the loop variety, lose efficacy if administered with NSAIDs; the mechanism may involve inhibition of prostaglandin synthesis, as above.

Potassium supplements, given with potassium-retaining diuretics, e.g. amiloride, spironolactone, or with ACE-inhibitors may cause dangerous hyperkalaemia.

Digoxin is more effective, but also more toxic in the presence of hypokalaemia, which may be caused by thiazide or loop diuretics.

Verapamil given i.v. with a β-blocker, e.g. atenolol, for supraventricular tachycardia may cause dangerous bradycardia since both drugs delay atrioventricular conduction.

Theophylline potentiates β-adrenergic effects, e.g. of salbutamol, and cardiac dysrhythmia may result during treatment of asthma.

Lithium toxicity may result if thiazide diuretic is co-administered; when there is sodium depletion, resorption of lithium by the proximal renal tubule is increased and plasma concentrations rise.

Central nervous system depressant drugs including benzodiazepines, several H_1-receptor antihistamines, alcohol, phenothiazines, antiepilepsy drugs interact to augment their sedative effects.

Loop diuretics and aminoglycoside antibiotics are both ototoxic in high dose; the chance of an adverse event is greater if they are administered together.

INTERACTIONS DURING METABOLISM

1. Enzyme induction by drugs and other substances (see p. 101) accelerates metabolism and is a cause of therapeutic failure. The following are examples:

Oral contraceptive steroids are metabolised more rapidly when an enzyme inducer, e.g. phenytoin, is added, and unplanned pregnancy has occurred (doctors have been successfully sued for negligence). In this circumstance an oral contraceptive of high oestrogen content may be substituted (or an alternative contraceptive method); if breakthrough bleeding occurs, the oestrogen content is not high enough. The metabolism of progestogens is also increased by enzyme induction.

Anticoagulant control with warfarin is dependent on a steady state of elimination by metabolism. Enzyme induction leads to accelerated metabolism of warfarin, loss of anticoagulant control and danger of thrombosis. Conversely, if a patient's anticoagulant control is stable on warfarin plus an inducing agent, there is a danger of haemorrhage if the inducing agent is discontinued because warfarin will be eliminated at a slower rate.

Chronic alcohol ingestion causing enzyme induction is a likely explanation of the tolerance shown by alcoholics to hydrocarbon anaesthetics and to tolbutamide.

Cyclosporin is extensively metabolised; its concentration in blood may be reduced due to enzyme induction by rifampicin, with danger of inadequate immunosuppression hazarding an organ or marrow transplant.

2. Enzyme inhibition by drugs (see p. 102) potentiates other drugs that are inactivated by metabolism, causing adverse reactions.

Examples appear below, and it will be noted that inhibitors of isoenzymes of cytochrome P450 figure prominently. The drugs with which they interact are also given but the list is not complete, and there should be a general awareness of the possibility of metabolic inhibition when the following drugs are used.

Cimetidine is an inhibitor of microsomal P450 and so potentiates a large number of drugs ordinarily metabolised by that system, notably propranolol, theophylline, warfarin and phenytoin. Depending on the interacting drug, up to 50% inhibition of metabolism may occur when cimetidine 2000 mg/d is taken.

Erythromycin inhibits a cytochrome P450 enzyme and impairs the metabolism of theophylline, warfarin, carbamazepine and methylprednisolone. The mean reduction in drug clearance is 20–25%.

Quinolone antimicrobials inhibit specific isoenzymes of P450 responsible for the metabolism of methylxanthines, notably theophylline, the clearance of which may be reduced by 50% by enoxacin; ciprofloxacin has a lesser inhibitory effect.

Monoamine oxidase inhibitors (MAOI) are not completely selective for MAO and impair the metabolism of tricyclic antidepressants, of some sympathomimetics, e.g. phenylpropanolamine, amphetamine, of opioid analgesics, especially pethidine, and of mercaptopurine.

Sodium valproate appears to be a nonspecific inhibitor and impairs the metabolism of phenytoin, phenobarbitone and primidone.

Allopurinol specifically inhibits xanthine oxidase and thus prevents metabolism of azathioprine to mercaptopurine (with potentially dangerous toxicity).

INTERACTIONS DURING EXCRETION

Clinically important interactions, both beneficial and potentially harmful, occur in the kidney.

Interference with passive diffusion (see p. 90). Reabsorption of a drug by the renal tubule can be reduced, and its excretion increased, by altering urine pH (see Drug overdose, p. 142).

Interference with active transport. Organic acids are passed from the blood into the urine by active transport across the renal tubular epithelium. Penicillin is mostly excreted in this way. Probenecid, an organic acid that competes successfully with penicillin for this transport system, may be used to prolong the action of penicillin when repeated administration is impracticable, e.g. in sexually transmitted diseases, where compliance is notoriously poor. Interference with renal excretion of methotrexate by aspirin, of zidovudine by probenecid and of digoxin by quinidine, contribute to the potentially harmful interactions with these combinations.

GUIDE TO FURTHER READING

Brown E M et al 1995 Calcium-ion-sensing cell-surface receptors. New England Journal of Medicine 333: 234

Lefkowitz R J 1995 G proteins in medicine. New England Journal of Medicine 332: 186

Montamat S C et al 1989 Management of drug therapy in the elderly. New England Journal of Medicine 321: 303

Partridge M, Woodcock A 1995 Metered dose inhalers free of fluorocarbons. British Medical Journal 310: 684

Rolf S, Harper N J N 1995 Ability of hospital doctors to calculate drug doses. British Medical Journal 310: 1173

Rubin P C 1986 Prescribing in pregnancy: general principles. British Medical Journal 293: 1415

Rylance G W 1988 Prescribing for infants and children. British Medical Journal 296: 984

8

Unwanted effects and adverse drug reactions

Background

Cur'd yesterday of my disease
I died last night of my physician.[1]

Nature is neutral, i.e. it has no 'intentions' towards humans, though it is often unfavourable to them. It is mankind, in its desire to avoid suffering and death, that decides that some of the biological effects of drugs are desirable (therapeutic) and others are undesirable (adverse). In addition to this arbitrary division, which has no fundamental biological basis, unwanted effects of drugs are promot-

[1] From, The remedy worse than the disease. Matthew Prior (1664–1721).

ed, or even caused, by numerous nondrug factors. Because of the variety of these factors, attempts to make a simple account of the unwanted effects of drugs must be imperfect.

There is general agreement that drugs prescribed for disease are themselves the cause of a serious amount of disease (adverse reactions), ranging from mere inconvenience to permanent disability and death.

Since drugs are intended to relieve suffering, patients find it peculiarly offensive that they can also cause disease (of which, frequently, they are not warned). Therefore it is important to know how much disease they do cause and why they cause it, so that preventive measures can be taken.

It is not enough to measure the incidence of adverse reactions to drugs, their nature and their severity, though accurate data are obviously useful. It is necessary to take, or to try to take, into account which effects are avoidable (by skilled choice and use) and which are unavoidable (inherent in drug or patient). Also, different adverse effects can matter to a different degree to different people.

Since there can be no hope of eliminating all adverse effects of drugs it is necessary to evaluate patterns of adverse reaction against each other. One drug may frequently cause minor ill-effects but pose no threat to life, though patients do not like it and may take it irregularly, to their own detriment. Another drug may be pleasant to take, so that patients take it consistently, with benefit, but it may rarely kill someone. It is not obvious which drug is to be preferred.

Some patients, e.g. those with a history of allergy or previous reactions to drugs, are up to four times more likely to have another adverse reaction, so that the incidence does not fall evenly.

It is also useful to discover the causes of adverse reactions, for such knowledge can be used to render avoidable what are at present unavoidable reactions.

Avoidable adverse effects will be reduced by more skilful prescribing and this means that doctors, amongst all the other claims on their time, must find time better to understand drugs, as well as to understand their patients and their diseases.

Estimates of the incidence and severity of adverse reactions to drugs are various, for reliable data are hard to get.

Definitions

Many unwanted effects of drugs are medically trivial, and in order to avoid inflating the figures of drug-induced disease, it is convenient to retain the term **side-effects** for minor effects of type A events/effects (p. 125).

The term **adverse reaction** should be confined to: harmful or seriously unpleasant effects occurring at doses intended for therapeutic (including prophylactic or diagnostic) effect and which call for reduction of dose or withdrawal of the drug and/or forecast hazard from future administration; it is effects of this order that are of importance in evaluating drug-induced disease in the community.

Toxicity implies a direct action of the drug, often at high dose, damaging cells, e.g. liver damage from paracetamol overdose, eighth cranial nerve damage from gentamicin. All drugs, for practical purposes, are toxic in overdose and overdose can be absolute or relative; in the latter case an ordinary dose may be administered but may be toxic due to an underlying abnormality in the patient, e.g. disease of the kidney. Mutagenicity, carcinogenicity and teratogenicity (see index) are special cases of toxicity.

Secondary effects are the indirect consequences of a primary drug action. Examples are: vitamin deficiency or opportunistic infection which may occur in patients whose normal bowel flora has been altered by antibiotics; diuretic-induced hypokalaemia causing digoxin intolerance.

Intolerance means a low threshold to the normal pharmacodynamic action of a drug. Individuals vary greatly in their susceptibility to drugs, those at one extreme of the normal distribution curve being intolerant of the drugs, those at the other, tolerant.

Idiosyncrasy (see Pharmacogenetics) implies an inherent qualitative abnormal reaction to a drug, usually due to genetic abnormality, e.g. porphyria.

Causation: degrees of certainty

Reliable attribution of a cause–effect relationship provides the biggest problem in this field. Karch and Lasagna[2] proposed the following degrees of certainty for attributing adverse events to drugs:

● *Definite:* time sequence from taking the drug is reasonable; event corresponds to what is known of the drug; event ceases on stopping the drug; event returns on restarting the drug (rarely advisable).

● *Probable:* time sequence is reasonable; event corresponds to what is known of the drug; event ceases on stopping the drug; event not reasonably explained by patient's disease.

● *Possible:* time sequence is reasonable; event corresponds to what is known of the drug; event could readily have been result of the patient's disease or other therapy.

● *Conditional:* time sequence is reasonable; event does not correspond to what is known of the drug; event could not reasonably be explained by the patient's disease.

● *Doubtful:* event not meeting the above criteria.

Recognition of adverse drug reactions. When an unexpected event, for which there is no obvious

---

[2] Journal of the American Medical Association (1975) 234: 1236.

cause, occurs in a patient already taking a drug, the possibility that it is drug-caused must always be considered. Distinguishing between natural progression of a disease and drug-induced deterioration is particularly challenging, e.g. sodium in antacid formulations may aggravate cardiac failure, tricyclic antidepressants may provoke epileptic seizures, bronchospasm may be caused by aspirin in some asthmatics.

Pharmacovigilance and pharmacoepidemiology

The principal methods of collecting data on adverse reactions are:

- *Experimental* studies, i.e. formal therapeutic trials of Phases I–III. These provide reliable data on only the commoner events as they involve relatively small numbers of patients (hundreds); they detect an incidence of up to about 1:200.
- *Observational* studies, where the drug is observed epidemiologically under conditions of normal use in the community, i.e. pharmacoepidemiology. Techniques used for post-marketing (Phase IV) studies include:
  — The observational cohort study
  — The case-control study (see p. 62).

Surveillance systems

Systems in operation for post-marketing studies include:

1. Prescription event monitoring, which is a form of observational cohort study. Prescriptions for a drug (say, 20 000) are collected (in the UK this is made practicable by the existence of a National Health Service in which prescriptions are sent to a single central authority for pricing and payment of the pharmacist). The prescriber is sent a questionnaire and asked to report all events that have occurred (not only suspected adverse reactions) without a judgement about causality. Thus 'a broken leg is an event. If more fractures were associated with this drug they could have been due to

hypotension, CNS effects or metabolic disease'.[3] By linking general practice and hospital records and death certificates, both prospective and retrospective studies can be done and unsuspected effects can be detected. Prescription event monitoring can be used routinely on newly licensed drugs, especially those likely to be widely prescribed in general practice, and it can also be implemented quickly in response to a suspicion raised, e.g. by spontaneous reports.

2. Voluntary reporting systems, e.g. the 'Yellow Card'[4] system in the UK, depend on doctors' intuitions and willingness to respond. They provide the first line in post-marketing surveillance and, having no limit of quantitative sensitivity, may detect the rarest events, e.g. those with an incidence of 1:5000–1:10 000. Voluntary systems are, however, plainly unreliable for quantification, and reporting is particularly low for reactions with long latency, e.g. tardive dyskinesia from chronic neuroleptic use.

It is recommended[5] that for:

- newer drugs: doctors should report all suspected reactions, i.e. any adverse or any unexpected event, however minor, which could conceivably be attributed to the drug
- established drugs: doctors should report all serious suspected reactions even if the effect is well recognised.

3. Record linkage schemes, see page 62.

4. Population statistics, e.g. birth defect registers and cancer registers. These are insensitive unless a drug-induced event is highly remarkable or very frequent. If suspicions are aroused then case-control and observational cohort studies will be initiated (see p. 62).

---

[3] Inman W H W et al 1986 Prescription-event monitoring. In: Inman W H W (ed) Monitoring for drug safety, 2nd edn. MTP, Lancaster, p. 217.

[4] Doctors and pharmacists are supplied with (yellow) cards on which to record suspected adverse reactions to drugs. The results are collated by the Committee on Safety of Medicines of the government's Medicines Control Agency.

[5] New England Journal of Medicine (1977) 296: 481.

DRUG-INDUCED ILLNESS

The discovery of drug-induced illness has been usefully analysed by Jick[6] thus:

- Drug commonly induces an otherwise rare illness: this effect is likely to be discovered by clinical observation in the licensing (premarketing) formal therapeutic trials and the drug will almost always be abandoned; but some patients are normally excluded from such trials, e.g. pregnant women, and detection will then occur later.
- Drug rarely induces an otherwise common illness: this effect is likely to remain undiscovered.
- Drug rarely induces an otherwise rare illness: this effect is likely to remain undiscovered before the drug is released for general prescribing; the effect should be detected by informal clinical observation or during any special post-registration surveillance and confirmed by a case-control study (see p. 62), e.g. chloramphenicol and aplastic anaemia; practolol and oculomucocutaneous syndrome.
- Drug commonly induces an otherwise common illness: this effect will not be discovered by informal clinical observation. If very common, it may be discovered in formal therapeutic trials and in case-control studies, but if only moderately common it may require observational cohort studies, e.g. sulphonylureas and cardiovascular mortality in diabetics.
- Drug adverse effects and illness incidence in intermediate range: both case-control and cohort studies may be needed.

PRACTICALITIES OF DETECTING RARE ADVERSE REACTIONS

For reactions with no background incidence the number of patients required to give a good (95%) chance of detecting the effect is given in Table 8.1. Assuming that three events are required before any regulatory or other action should be taken, it shows the large number of patients that must be monitored to detect even a relatively high incidence adverse effect. The problem can be many orders of magnitude worse if the adverse reactions

Table 8.1 Detecting rare adverse reactions[7]

Expected incidence of adverse reaction	Required number of patients for event		
	1 event	2 events	3 events
1 in 100	300	480	650
1 in 200	600	960	1300
1 in 1000	3000	4800	6500
1 in 2000	6000	9600	13 000
1 in 10 000	30 000	48 000	65 000

closely resemble spontaneous disease with a background incidence in the population.

- Adverse reactions cause 2–3% of consultations in general practice.
- Up to 3% of admissions to acute care hospital wards (and 0.3% of general hospital admissions) are due to adverse drug reactions.
- Death due to therapeutic use of drugs is uncommon. A review of records of a Coroner's Inquests for a district with a population of 1.19 million (UK) during the period 1986–91 found that of 3277 inquests on deaths, 10 were due to errors of prescribing and 36 were caused by adverse drug reactions.[8]
- Overall incidence in hospital in-patients is 10–20%, with possible prolongation of hospital stay in 2–10% of patients in acute medical wards.
- Predisposing factors: age over 60 years or under one month, female, previous history of adverse reaction, hepatic or renal disease.
- Adverse reactions most commonly occur early in therapy (days 1–10).

Caution. About 80% of well people not taking any drugs admit on questioning to symptoms (often several) such as are commonly experienced as lesser adverse reactions to drugs. These symptoms are

---

[6] New England Journal of Medicine (1977) 296: 481.

[7] By permission from, Safety requirements for the first use of new drugs and diagnostic agents in man. CIOMS (WHO) 1983. Geneva.

[8] Ferner R E, Whittington R M 1994 Journal of the Royal Society of Medicine 87: 145.

[9] On the other hand people may take drugs without realising they are doing so. A man presented with a seven-week history of tinnitus and hearing loss. He was diagnosed as

intensified (or diminished) by administration of a placebo. Thus, many (minor) symptoms may be wrongly attributed to drugs.[9]

It is important to avoid alarmist or defeatist extremes of attitude. Many treatments are dangerous, e.g. surgery, electroshock, drugs, and it is irrational to accept the risks of surgery for biliary stones or hernia and refuse to accept any risk at all from drugs for conditions of comparable seriousness.

Many patients whose death is deemed to be partly or wholly caused by drugs are dangerously ill already; justified risks may be taken in the hope of helping them; ill-informed criticism in such cases can act against the interest of the sick. On the other hand there is no doubt that some of these accidents are avoidable. Avoidability is often more obvious when reviewing the conduct of treatment after death, i.e. with hindsight, than it was at the time.

Sir Anthony Carlisle,[10] in the first half of the 19th century, said that 'medicine is an art founded on conjecture and improved by murder'. Although medicine has advanced so rapidly, there is still a ring of truth in that statement[11] to anyone who follows the introduction of new drugs and observes how, after the early enthusiasm, the reports of serious toxic effects appear.

Another cryptic remark of this therapeutic nihilist was 'digitalis kills people' and this is true. William Withering in 1785 laid down rules for the use of digitalis that would serve today. Neglect of these rules resulted in needless suffering for patients with heart failure for more than a century until the therapeutic criteria were rediscov-

ered. Any drug that is really worth using can do harm.

> It is an absolute obligation on doctors to use only drugs about which they have troubled to inform themselves.

Effective therapy depends not only on the correct choice of drugs but also on their correct use. This latter is sometimes forgotten and a drug is condemned as useless when it has been used in a dose or way which absolutely precluded a successful result; this can be regarded as a negative adverse effect.

Classification

Adverse reactions are of two principal kinds:

Type A (**A**ugmented) reactions will occur in everyone if enough of the drug is given because they are due to excess of normal, predictable, dose-related, pharmacodynamic effects. They are common and skilled management reduces their incidence, e.g. postural hypotension, hypoglycaemia, hypokalaemia.

Type B (**B**izarre) reactions will occur only in some people. They are not part of the normal pharmacology of the drug, are not dose-related and are due to unusual attributes of the patient interacting with the drug. These effects are predictable where the mechanism is known (though predictive tests may be expensive or impracticable), otherwise they are unpredictable for the individual, although the incidence may be known. The class includes unwanted effects due to inherited abnormalities (idiosyncrasy) (see Pharmacogenetics) and immunological processes (see Drug allergy). These account for most drug fatalities.

Three subordinate types may be recognised:

Type C (**C**ontinuous) reactions due to longterm use, e.g. analgesic nephropathy, tardive dyskinesia with neuroleptics.

Type D (**D**elayed) effects, e.g. teratogenesis, carcinogenesis.

Type E (**E**nding of use) reactions, where discontinuation is too abrupt, e.g. rebound adrenocortical insufficiency.

having bilateral meningiomas. He escaped craniotomy when an alert doctor discovered the man's enormous intake of 'tonic water', stopped it and the patient recovered. The quinine used as a flavour in 'tonic water' was responsible (cinchonism) (Yohalem S B 1953 Journal of the American Medical Association 153: 1304).

[10] Noted for his advocacy of the use of 'the simple carpenter's saw' in surgery.

[11] In the less candid language of our times the opinion has been repeated; 'The trend of greater risks for greater gain is likely to continue'. Royal Commission on Civil Liability and Compensation for Personal Injury. 1978 HMSO, London, Cmnd. 7045.

Causes

When an unusual or unexpected event, for which there is no evident natural explanation, occurs in a patient already taking a drug, the possibility that the event is drug-caused must always be considered, and may be categorised as follows:

- **The patient** may be predisposed by age, genetic constitution, tendency to allergy, disease, personality, habits.
- **The drug**. Anticancer agents are by their nature cytotoxic. Some drugs, e.g. digoxin, have steep dose-response curves and small increments of dose are more likely to induce augmented (type A) reactions. Other drugs, e.g. antimicrobials, have a tendency to cause allergy and may lead to bizarre (type B) reactions. Ingredients of a formulation, e.g. colouring, flavouring, sodium content,[12] rather than the active drug may also cause adverse reactions.
- **The prescriber**. Adverse reactions may occur because a drug is used for an inappropriately long time (type C), at a critical phase in pregnancy (type D), is abruptly discontinued (type E) or given with other drugs (interactions).

Aspects of the two sections above, Classification and Causes, appear throughout the book. Selected topics are discussed below.

AGE

The very old and the very young are liable to be intolerant of many drugs, largely because the mechanisms for disposing of them in the body are less efficient. The young, it has been aptly said, are not simply 'small adults'; 'respect for their pharmacokinetic variability should be added to the list of our senior citizens' rights'.[13] The old are also frequently exposed to multiple drug therapy which predisposes to adverse effects (see Prescribing for the elderly, p. 114).

---

[12] The sodium content (by weight) of certain formulations may exceed that of the drug it contains.

[13] Fogel B S 1983 New England Journal of Medicine 308: 1600.

GENETIC CONSTITUTION
(see also Pharmacogenetics, p. 109)

The *hepatic porphyrias* (acute intermittent porphyria, variegate porphyria, hereditary coproporphyria, porphyria cutanea tarda) are a rare group of genetically determined single enzyme defects. The greatest care in prescribing for these patients is required if serious illness is to be avoided. In healthy people, forming haemoglobin for their erythrocytes, the rate of *haem* synthesis is controlled by negative feedback according to the amount of haem present.

When more haem is needed there is increased production of the rate-controlling enzyme delta-aminolaevulinic acid (ALA) synthase which provides the basis of the formation of porphyrin precursors of haem. But in people with porphyria one or other of the enzymes that convert the various porphyrins to haem is deficient and so porphyrins accumulate.

A vicious cycle occurs: less haem → more ALA synthase → more porphobilinogen (in the case of acute intermittent porphyria), the metabolism of which is blocked, and a clinical attack occurs. The exact precipitating mechanism of the clinical features of an acute attack of porphyria is uncertain. Increase in the haem-containing hepatic oxidising enzymes of the cytochrome P450 group causes an increased demand for haem. Therefore drugs that induce these enzymes would be expected to precipitate acute attacks of porphyria and they do so; tobacco smoking may act by this mechanism.

It would be rational to use any safe means of depressing the formation of ALA-synthase. Fructose (laevulose) will do this; up to 400 g have been given i.v. per day in acute attacks with apparent benefit within 24 hours; glucose may be substituted. Haematin infusion (haem arginate), by replenishing haem and so removing the stimulus to ALA-synthase, has also been found effective if given early and may prevent chronic neuropathy.

It is of interest that those who inherited acute intermittent porphyria and variegate porphyria suffered no biological disadvantage from the natural environment and bred as well as the normal population until the introduction of barbiturates and sulphonamides. They are now at serious disadvantage, for many other drugs can precipitate fatal acute attacks.

Apparently unexplained attacks of porphyria should be an indication for close enquiry into all possible chemical intake, e.g. surreptitious ingestion of mouthwash containing alcohol, eucalyptol and menthol caused attacks in one patient (the eucalyptol induced hepatic ALA-synthase activity). Guaiphenesin is hazardous; it is included in a multitude of multi-ingredient cough medicines (often nonprescription). Patients must be educated to understand their condition and to protect themselves from themselves and from others, including prescribing doctors.

Patients (1 in 10 000 UK population) are so highly vulnerable that we provide a partial list of drugs known and believed to be hazardous (see Table 8.2, p. 128).

THE ENVIRONMENT

Significant environmental factors causing adverse reactions to drugs include simple pollution, e.g. halothane in the air of surgical operating theatres causing abortions amongst female staff; penicillin in the air of hospitals or in milk (see below), causing allergy.

Drug metabolism may also be increased by hepatic enzyme induction from insecticide accumulation, e.g. dicophane (DDT) and from alcohol and the tobacco habit, e.g. smokers require a higher dose of theophylline.

Antimicrobials used in feeds of animals for human consumption have given rise to concern in relation to the spread of resistant bacteria that may affect man.

DRUG INTERACTIONS
(see p. 116)

Allergy in response to drugs

Allergic reactions to drugs are the resultant of the interaction of drug or metabolite (or a nondrug element in the formulation) with patient and disease, and subsequent re-exposure.

Lack of previous exposure is not the same as lack of history of previous exposure, and 'first dose reactions' are among the most dramatic. Exposure is not necessarily medical, e.g. penicillins may occur in dairy products following treatment of mastitis in cows (despite laws to prevent this), and penicillin antibodies are commonly present in those who deny ever having received the drug.

Immune responses to drugs may be harmful (allergy) or harmless; the fact that antibodies are produced does not mean a patient will necessarily respond to re-exposure with clinical manifestations; most of our population has antibodies to penicillins but, fortunately, comparatively few react clinically to penicillin administration.

Whilst macromolecules (proteins, peptides, dextran polysaccharides) can act as complete antigens, most drugs are simple chemicals (mol. wt less than 1000) and act as incomplete antigens or haptens, which become complete antigens in combination with a body protein.

The chief target organs of drug allergy are the skin, respiratory tract, gastrointestinal tract, blood and blood vessels.

Drugs may elicit allergic reactions of all types.

Type I reactions: immediate or anaphylactic type. The drug causes formation of tissue-sensitising IgE antibodies that are fixed to mast cells or leucocytes; on subsequent administration the allergen (conjugate of drug or metabolite with tissue protein) reacts with these antibodies, activating but not damaging the cell to which they are fixed and causing release of pharmacologically active substances, e.g. histamine, leukotrienes, prostaglandins, platelet-activating factor, and causing effects such as urticaria, anaphylactic shock and asthma. Allergy develops within minutes and lasts 1–2 hours.

Type II reactions: antibody-dependent cytotoxic type. The drug or metabolite combines with a protein in the body so that the body no longer recognises the protein as self, treats it as a foreign protein and forms antibodies which combine with the antigen and activate complement which damages cells, e.g. methyldopa or penicillin-induced haemolytic anaemia.

Type III reactions: complex-mediated type. Antigen and antibody form large complexes and activate complement. Small blood vessels are damaged or blocked. Leucocytes attracted to the site of reaction engulf the immune complexes and release pharmacologically active substances (including lysosomal enzymes), starting an inflammatory process. These reactions include serum sickness, glomerulonephritis, vasculitis and pulmonary disease.

Table 8.2 Unsafe prescribing in acute porphyria

The drugs in this table have been shown to be porphorynogenic in humans, animals or in in vitro systems. Drugs in **bold** with an asterisk have been associated with acute attacks of porphyria in humans; drugs that are bracketed have conflicting evidence of porphyrnogenicity (positive and negative). Absence of a drug from this list does *not* mean that it is safe.

Alcuronium	Ergometrine tartarate	(Oxazepam)
*Alphaxalone	***Erythromycin**	Oxybutynin
*Alphadolone	Ethamsylate	Oxycodone
Alprazolam	***Ethanol**	***Oxymetazoline**
Aluminium preparations	Ethionamide	Oxyphenbutazone
Amidopyrine	Ethosuximide	Oxytetracycline
Aminoglutethimide	Etidocaine	Paramethadione
Aminophylline	Etomidate	Pargyline
Amiodarone	Fenfluramine	***Pentazocine**
(Amitriptyline)	***Flucloxacillin**	Perhexiline
(Amphetamines)	***Flufenamic acid**	Phenacetin
*Amylobarbitone	Flunitrazepam	Phenelzine
Antipyrine	Flupenthixol	***Phenobarbitone**
Auranofin	Flurazepam	Phenoxybenzamine
Aurothiomalate	***Frusemide**	Phensuximide
Azapropazone	***Glutethimide**	(Phenylbutazone)
Baclofen	Glipizide	Phenylhydrazine
*Barbituates	Gramicidin	***Phenytoin**
*Bemigride	***Griseofulvin**	Piretamide
Bendrofluazide	Haloperidol	***Piroxicam**
Benoxaprofen	***Halothane**	***Pivampicillin**
Bromocriptine	***Hydantoins**	Prazepam
Busulphan	Hydralazine	Prenylamine
Captopril	***Hydrochlorothiazide**	***Prilocaine**
*Carbamazepine	***Hydroxyzine**	***Primidone**
*Carbromal	Hyoscine	(Probenecid)
*Carisoprodol	***Imipramine**	***Progesterone** (ogens)
(Cefuroxime)	Iproniazid	Promethazine
(Cephalexin)	Isometheptene mucate	(Propanidid)
(Cephalosporins)	(Isoniazid)	***Pyrazinamide**
(Cefradine)	Ketoconazole	Quinalbarbitone
(Chlorambucil)	Lignocaine	Rifampicin
*Chloramphenicol	**Lisinopril**	Simvastatin
*Chlordiazepoxide	Loprazolam	(Sodium valproate) (has been used safely in
*Chlormezanone	Loxapine	seizure prophylaxis)
Chloroform	Lysuride	Spironolactone
*Chlorpropamide	Maprotiline	Stanozolol
Cimetidine	Mebeverine	Succinimides
Cinnarizine	(Mefenamic acid)	Sulphacetamide
Clemastine	Megestrol	***Sulphadimidine**
(Clobazam)	Mepivacaine	Sulphadoxine
(Clomipramine)	***Meprobamate**	Sulphamethoxazole
(Clonazepam) (has been used safely in	Mercaptopurine	***Sulphasalazine**
status epilepticus)	Mercury compounds	Sulphonylureas
Clonidine	Mestranol	Sulphinpyrazone
Clorazepate	(Metapramine)	Sulpiride
Cocaine	Methamphetamine	Sulthiame
(Colistin)	Methohexitone	***Tamoxifen**
Co-trimoxazole	Methotrexate	***Terfenadine**
Cyclophosphamide	Methoxyflurane	Tetrazepam
Cycloserine	Methsuximide	***Theophylline**
Cyclosporin	***Methyldopa**	***Thiopentone**
Danazol	***Methyprylone**	Thioridazine
Dapsone	Methysergide	Tilidate
Dexfenfluramine	***Metoclopramide**	Tinidazole
Dextropropoxyphene	Metyrapone	
(contd next page)	*(contd next page)*	*(contd next page)*

Table 8.2 *Cont'd*

(Diazepam) (has been used safely in status epilepticus)	Mianserin	Tolazamide
	Miconazole	Tolbutamide
*Dichloralphenzone	(Mifepristone)	Tranylcypromine
Diclofenac	Minoxidil	Trazodone
Dienostrol	Nalidixic acid	Trimethoprim
Diethylpropion	(Nandrolone)	(Trimipramine)
*Dihydroergotamine	Natamycin	Troxidone
*Dimenhydrinate	(Nicergoline)	Valpromide
*Diphenhydramine	*Nifedipine	*Verapamil
(Dothiepin)	*Nikethamide	*Vibramycin
Doxycycline	Nitrazepam	Viloxazine
(Dydrogesterone)	(Nitrofurantoin)	(Vinblastine)
*Econazole	Nordiazepam	(Vincristine)
*Enalapril	Norethynodrel	Zuclopenthixol
Enflurane	Nortriptyline	
*Ergot compounds	Novobiocin	
	*Oral contraceptives	
	*Orphenadrine	

We are grateful to Dr M R Moore for permission to base these lists on the more comprehensive data supplied by the Porphyria Research Unit, Western Infirmary, Glasgow, UK.

Type IV reactions: cell-mediated type. Antigen-specific receptors develop on T-lymphocytes. Subsequent administration leads to a local or tissue allergic reaction, e.g. contact dermatitis.

Distinctive features of allergic reactions[14]

- No correlation with known pharmacological properties of the drug
- No linear relation with drug dose (very small doses may cause very severe effects)
- Rashes, angioedema, serum sickness syndrome, anaphylaxis or asthma; characteristics of classic protein allergy
- Require an induction period on primary exposure, but not on re-exposure
- Disappear on cessation of administration and reappear on re-exposure
- Occur in a minority of patients receiving the drug
- May be a temporary condition
- Can respond to desensitisation.

Cross-allergy within a group of drugs is usual, e.g. the penicillins. When allergy to a particular drug is established, a substitute should be selected from a chemically different group. Patients with allergic diseases, e.g. eczema, are more likely to develop allergy to drugs.

PRINCIPAL CLINICAL MANIFESTATIONS AND TREATMENT

1. Urticarial rashes and angioedema (types I, III). These are probably the commonest type of drug allergy. Reactions may be generalised, but frequently are worst in and around the external area of administration of the drug. The eyelids, lips and face are usually most affected. They are usually accompanied by itching. Oedema of the larynx is rare but may be fatal if tracheostomy is not done. They respond to adrenaline (i.m. if urgent), ephedrine, H_1-receptor antihistamine and adrenal steroid.

2a. Nonurticarial rashes (types I, II, IV). These occur in great variety; frequently they are weeping exudative lesions. It is often difficult to be sure when a rash is due to a drug. Apart from stopping

---

[14] Assem E-S K 1992 In: Davies D M (ed) Textbook of adverse drug reactions. Oxford University Press, London.

the drug, treatment is nonspecific; in severe cases an adrenal steroid should be tried. Skin sensitisation to antimicrobials may be very troublesome, especially amongst those who handle them (see Drugs and the skin, p. 275, for more detail).

2b. Diseases of the lymphoid system. Infectious mononucleosis (and lymphoma, leukaemia) is associated with an increased incidence (40%+) of characteristic maculopapular, sometimes purpuric, rash which is probably allergic, when an aminopenicillin (ampicillin, amoxycillin) is taken; patients may not be allergic to other penicillins. Erythromycin may cause a similar reaction.

3. Anaphylactic shock (type I) occurs with penicillin, anaesthetics (i.v.), iodine-containing radiocontrast media and a huge variety of other drugs. A severe fall in blood pressure occurs, with bronchoconstriction, angioedema (including larynx) and sometimes death due to loss of fluid from the intravascular compartment. Anaphylactic shock usually occurs suddenly, in less than an hour after the drug, but within minutes if it has been given i.v.

Treatment is urgent, as follows:
- First 0.5–1.0 ml of adrenaline injection (1 mg/ml: 1 in 1000) should be given i.m. (s.c. is less effective) to raise the blood pressure and to dilate the bronchi. Up to 10% of patients may need a second injection 10–20 min later and subsequent injections may be given until the patient improves. Noradrenaline lacks any useful bronchodilator action (β-effect) (for adrenaline in cardiopulmonary resuscitation, see p. 471).
- If treatment is delayed and shock has developed, adrenaline should be given i.v. either by injection of 3–5 ml of adrenaline 1 in 10 000 over 5 min or by continuous infusion of 1 ml of adrenaline 1 in 1000 diluted in 500 ml of dextrose 5% at a rate 0.25–2.5 ml/min.[15]
- Note that preventive self-management is feasible where susceptibility to anaphylaxis is known, e.g. in patients with allergy to bee- or wasp-stings. The patient is taught to administer adrenaline either from prefilled syringes (Min-I-Jet Adrenaline, Epipen autoinjector) or by metered-dose aerosol inhaler (Medihaler-Epi).

- The adrenaline should be accompanied by an H_1-receptor antihistamine (say, chlorpheniramine 10 mg i.v.) and hydrocortisone (100 mg i.m. or i.v.). The adrenal steroid may act by reducing vascular permeability and by suppressing further response to the antigen–antibody reaction. Benefit from an adrenal steroid is not immediate; it is unlikely to begin for 30 minutes and takes hours to reach its maximum.

In severe anaphylaxis, hypotension is due to vasodilation and loss of circulating volume through leaky capillaries. Colloid is more effective at restoring blood volume than crystalloid and 1–2 l of plasma substitute should be infused rapidly. Oxygen and artificial ventilation may be necessary.

Any hospital ward or other place where anaphylaxis may be anticipated should have all the drugs and equipment necessary to deal with it in one convenient kit, for when they are needed there is little time to think and none to run about from place to place (see Pseudoallergic reactions, p. 132).

4a. Pulmonary reactions: asthma (type I). Aspirin and other nonsteroidal anti-inflammatory drugs may cause an asthmatic attack which can be fatal; 0.25–1.0 ml of adrenaline injection (1 mg/ml s.c.) will usually cut short an attack. The other treatments for asthma are also effective. Whether this is an allergic or pseudoallergic reaction or a mixture of the two is uncertain.

4b. Other types of pulmonary reaction (type III). include syndromes resembling acute and chronic lung infections, pneumonitis, fibrosis and eosinophilia.

5. The serum-sickness syndrome (type III). This occurs about 1–3 weeks after administration. Treatment is by an adrenal steroid, and as above if there is urticaria.

6. Blood disorders[16]

a. Thrombocytopenia (type II, but also pseudo-

---

[15] Drug and Therapeutics Bulletin (1994) 32(3): 19.

[16] Where cells are being destroyed in the periphery and production is normal, transfusion is useless or nearly so, as

allergic) may occur after exposure to any of a large number of drugs, including: gold, quinine, quinidine, rifampicin, heparin, thionamide derivatives, thiazide diuretics, sulphonamides, oestrogens, indomethacin. Adrenal steroid may help.

b. Granulocytopenia (type II, but also pseudo-allergic) sometimes leading to agranulocytosis, is a very serious allergy which may occur with many drugs, e.g. clozapine, carbamazepine, carbimazole, chloramphenicol, sulphonamides (including diuretic and hypoglycaemic derivatives), colchicine, gold.

The value of precautionary leucocyte counts for drugs having special risk remains uncertain.[17]

Weekly counts may detect presymptomatic granulocytopenia from antithyroid drugs[18] but onset can be sudden and an alternative view is to monitor only with drugs having special risk, e.g. clozapine. The chief clinical manifestation of agranulocytosis is sore throat or mouth ulcers and patients should be warned to report such events immediately and to stop taking the drug; but they should not be frightened into noncompliance with essential therapy. Treatment of agranulocytosis involves both stopping the drug responsible and giving a bactericidal drug, e.g. a penicillin, to prevent or treat infection.

c. Aplastic anaemia (type II, but not always allergic). Causal agents include chloramphenicol, sulphonamides and derivatives (diuretics, antidiabetics), gold, penicillamine, allopurinol, felbamate, phenothiazines and some insecticides, e.g. dicophane (DDT). In the case of chloramphenicol, bone marrow depression is a normal pharmacodynamic effect (type A reaction) although aplastic anaemia may also be due to idiosyncrasy or allergy (type B reaction).

Death occurs in about 50% of cases, and treat-

ment is as for agranulocytosis, with, obviously, blood transfusion.

d. Haemolysis of all kinds is included here for convenience. There are three principal categories:

- *Allergy (type II)* occurs with methyldopa, levodopa, penicillins, quinine, quinidine, sulphasalazine and organic antimony. It may be that in some of these cases a drug-protein-antigen / antibody interaction involves erythrocytes casually, i.e. a true 'innocent bystander' phenomenon.
- *Dose-related pharmacodynamic action on normal cells* e.g. lead, benzene, phenylhydrazine, chlorates (weed-killer), methyl chloride (refrigerant), some snake venoms.
- *Idiosyncrasy* (see Pharmacogenetics). Precipitation of a haemolytic crisis may also occur with the above drugs in the rare genetic haemoglobinopathies. Treatment is to withdraw the drug, and an adrenal steroid is useful in severe cases if the mechanism is immunological. Blood transfusion may be needed.

7. Fever is common; a mechanism is the release of interleukin-1 by leucocytes into the circulation which acts on receptors in the hypothalamic thermoregulatory centre, releasing prostaglandin-E_1.

8. Collagen diseases (type II) and syndromes resembling them, e.g. systemic lupus erythematosus are sometimes caused by drugs, e.g. hydralazine, procainamide, isoniazid, sulphonamides. Adrenal steroid is useful.

9. Hepatitis and cholestatic jaundice are sometimes allergic (type II, see Drugs and the liver). Adrenal steroid may be useful.

10. Nephropathy of various kinds (types II, III) occurs as does damage to other organs, e.g. myocarditis. Adrenal steroid may be useful.

DIAGNOSIS OF DRUG ALLERGY

This still depends largely on clinical criteria, history, type of reaction, response to withdrawal and systemic rechallenge (if thought safe to do so).

---

the transfused cells will be destroyed, though in an emergency even a short cell life (platelets, erythrocytes) may tip the balance usefully. Where the bone marrow is depressed, transfusion is useful and the transfused cells will survive normally.

[17] In contrast to the case of a drug causing bone marrow depression as a pharmacodynamic dose-related effect, when blood counts are part of the essential routine monitoring of therapy, e.g. cytotoxics.

[18] Tajiri N et al 1990 Archives of Internal Medicine 150: 621.

Simple patch skin testing is naturally most useful in diagnosing contact dermatitis, but it is unreliable for other allergies. Skin prick or intradermal injection tests (especially the latter) are more reliable in specialist hands, but they can cause anaphylactic shock. False negative and false positive results occur.

Development of reliable in vitro predictive tests, e.g. employing serum or lymphocytes, is a matter of considerable importance, not merely to remove hazard but to avoid depriving patients of a drug that may be useful. Detection of drug-specific circulating antibodies by the radioallergosorbent test (RAST) is best developed for penicillins and can virtually supplant skin tests for patients with type I allergy (see p. 199).

Drug allergy, once it has occurred, is not necessarily permanent, e.g. less than 50% of patients giving a history of allergy to penicillin have a reaction if it is given again.

DESENSITISATION

Once patients become allergic to a drug, it is better that they should never again come into contact with it. This can, however, be inconvenient, for instance an allergy to antituberculosis drugs in both patients and nurses. Such people can be desensitised by giving very small amounts of allergen, which are than gradually increased (usually every few hours) until a normal dose is tolerated. This may have been done under cover of a corticosteroid and a β-adrenoceptor agonist (both of which inhibit mediator synthesis and release). An H_1-receptor antihistamine may be added if an adverse reaction occurs. A full kit for treating anaphylactic shock should be at hand.

The ease and safety of desensitisation varies with different drugs; penicillin is troublesome and antituberculosis drugs generally less so. Desensitisation may only be temporary.

The mechanism underlying desensitisation may involve the production by the patient of blocking antibodies that compete successfully for the allergen but whose combination with it is innocuous; or the threshold of cells to the triggering antibodies may be raised. Sometimes allergy is to an ingredient of the preparation other than the essential drug and merely changing the preparation is sufficient.

Impurities are sometimes responsible and purified penicillins and insulins reduce the incidence of reactions.

PREVENTION OF ALLERGIC REACTIONS

Prevention is important since these reactions are unpleasant and may be fatal; it provides good reason for taking a drug history. Patients should always be told when they are thought to be allergic to a drug. *If a patient says he or she is allergic to some drug then that drug should not be given without careful enquiry that may include testing (as above); neglect of this has caused death.*

When looking for an alternative drug to avoid an adverse reaction it is important not to select one from the same chemical group, as may inadvertently occur because the proprietary name gives no indication of the nature of the drug. This is another good reason for using nonproprietary (generic) names as a matter of course.

PSEUDO-ALLERGIC REACTIONS

These are effects that mimic allergic reactions but have no immunological basis and are largely genetically determined. They are due to release of endogenous, biologically active substances, e.g. histamine and leukotrienes, by the drug. A variety of mechanisms is probably involved, direct and indirect, including complement activation leading to formation of polypeptides that affect mast cells, as in true immunological reactions. Some drugs may cause both allergic and pseudo-allergic reactions.

Pseudo-allergic effects mimicking type I reactions (above) are called anaphylactoid and they occur with aspirin and other nonsteroidal anti-inflammatory drugs (indirect action as above) (see also Pulmonary reactions, above); corticotrophin (direct histamine release); i.v. anaesthetics and a variety of other drugs i.v. (morphine, tubocurarine, dextran, radiographic contrast media) and inhaled (cromoglycate). Severe cases are treated as for true allergic anaphylactic shock (above) from which, at the time, they are not distinguishable.

Type II reactions are mimicked by the haemolysis induced by drugs (some antimalarials, sulphonamides and oxidising agents) and food (broad beans) in subjects with inherited abnormalities of erythrocyte enzymes or haemoglobin (see p. 111).

Type III reactions are mimicked by nitrofurantoin (pneumonitis) and penicillamine (nephropathy). Lupus erythematosus due to drugs (procainamide, isoniazid, phenytoin) may be pseudo-allergic.

Miscellaneous adverse reactions

Transient reactions to intravenous injections are fairly common, resulting in hypotension, renal pain, fever or rigors, especially if the injection is very rapid.

Effects of prolonged administration: chronic organ toxicity

Eye. Toxic cataract can be due to chloroquine and related drugs, adrenal steroids (topical and systemic), phenothiazines, naphthalene, carbromal, ergot, dinitrophenol, galactose, lactose, paradichlorobenzene and alkylating agents. Corneal opacities occur with amiodarone, phenothiazines and chloroquine. Retinal injury occurs with thioridazine (particularly, of the neuroleptics), chloroquine, ethambutol and indomethacin.

Kidney: see Analgesic nephropathy (p. 252).

Liver: see Alcohol, page 166.

Carcinogenesis: see also Preclinical testing (p. 43). Mechanisms of carcinogenesis are complex; prediction from animal tests is uncertain and causal attribution in man has finally to be based on epidemiological studies. The principal mechanisms are:

- *Alteration of DNA* (genotoxicity, mutagenicity). Many chemicals or their metabolites act by causing mutations, activating oncogenes; those substances that are used as medicines include griseofulvin and alkylating cytotoxics.

Leukaemias and lymphomas are the most common malignancies.

- *Immunosuppression.* The immune system has a role in suppressing cancers (immune surveillance). A wide range of cancers develop in immunosuppressed patients, e.g after organ transplantation and cancer chemotherapy.
- *Hormonal.* Longterm use of oestrogen replacement in postmenopausal women induces endometrial cancer.

Combined oestrogen/progestogen oral contraceptives may both suppress and enhance cancers (see p. 655).

Stilboestrol caused vaginal adenosis and cancer in the offspring of mothers who took it during pregnancy in the hope of preventing miscarriage. It was used for this purpose for decades after its introduction in the 1940s, on purely theoretical grounds. Controlled therapeutic trials were not done and there is no valid evidence of therapeutic efficacy. Male fetuses developed nonmalignant genital abnormalities.

Carcinogenesis due to medicines requires that drug exposure be prolonged,[19] i.e. months or years; the cancers develop most commonly over 3–5 years and often years after treatment has ceased.

Incidence of second cancers in patients treated for primary cancer can be as high as 15 times the normal rate. The use of immunosuppression in, e.g. rheumatoid arthritis and organ transplants, also increases the incidence of cancers.

Adverse effects on reproduction

Testing of new drugs on animals for their effects on reproduction has been mandatory since the thalidomide disaster even though the extrapolation of the findings to humans is uncertain (see Preclinical testing, p. 43). The placental transfer of drugs from the mother to the fetus is considered on page 92.

Drugs may act on the **embryo and fetus**:

Directly (thalidomide, cytotoxic drugs, anti-

---

[19] Carcinogens that are effective as a single dose in animals are known, e.g. nitrosamines.

thyroid drugs, aromatic retinoids, e.g. isotretinoin): any drug affecting cell division, enzymes, protein synthesis or DNA synthesis, is a potential teratogen, e.g. many antimicrobials.

Indirectly

- on the uterus (vasoconstrictors reduce blood supply and cause fetal anoxia, misoprostol causes uterine contraction leading to abortion)
- on the mother's hormone balance.

Early pregnancy. During the first week after fertilisation, exposure to antimetabolites, ergot alkaloids or stilboesterol can cause abortion which may not be recognised as such. The most vulnerable period for major anatomical abnormality is that of organogenesis which occurs during weeks 2–8 of intrauterine life (4–10 weeks after the first day of the last menstruation). After the organs are formed, abnormalities are less anatomically dramatic; thus the activity of a teratogen (*teratos:* monster) is most devastating soon after implantation, at doses which may not harm the mother and at a time when she may not know she is pregnant.

Drugs known to be teratogenic include cytotoxics, warfarin, alcohol, lithium, phenytoin, valproate, adrenocortical steroids and isotretinoin. Selective interference can produce characteristic anatomical abnormalities, and the phocomelia (flipper-like) limb defect was one factor that caused thalidomide to be so readily recognised. (For an account of thalidomide see p. 69.) Drugs which are probably teratogenic include cocaine, and sex hormones in general.

Innumerable drugs have come under suspicion, including gastric antacids, iron, neuroleptics, benzodiazepines, diuretics and aspirin. Naturally the subject is a highly emotional one for prospective parents. A definitive list of unsafe drugs is not practicable. Much depends on the dose taken and at what stage of pregnancy. The topic must be followed in the current literature.

Late pregnancy. Because the important organs are already formed, drugs will not cause the gross anatomical defects that can occur when they are given in early pregnancy. Administration of hormones, androgens or progestogens, can cause fetal masculinisation; iodide and antithyroid drugs in high dose can cause fetal goitre, as can lithium; tetracyclines can interfere with tooth and bone development, angiotensin-converting enzyme inhibitors are associated with hypoplasia of lungs and kidneys and a skull ossification defect. Tobacco smoking retards fetal growth; it does not cause anatomical abnormalities in man as far as is known.

Inhibitors of prostaglandin synthase (aspirin, indomethacin) may delay onset of labour and, in the fetus, cause closure of the ductus arteriosus, patency of which is dependent on prostaglandins.

It is probable that drug allergy in the mother can also occur in the fetus and it is possible that the fetus may be sensitised where the mother shows no effect, e.g. neonatal thrombocytopenia from thiazide diuretics.

The suggestion that congenital cataract (due to denaturation of lens protein) might be due to drugs has some support in man. Chloroquine and chlorpromazine are concentrated in the fetal eye. Since both can cause retinopathy it would seem wise to avoid them in pregnancy if possible.

Anticoagulants in pregnancy: see page 522.

Drugs given to the mother just prior to labour can cause postnatal effects: CNS depressants may persist in and affect the baby for days after birth; vasoconstrictors can cause fetal distress by reducing uterine blood supply; β-adrenoceptor blockers may impair fetal response to hypoxia; sulphonamides displace bilirubin from plasma protein (risk of kernicterus); anticoagulants can cause haemorrhage.

Babies born to mothers dependent on opioids may show a physical withdrawal syndrome.

Drugs given during labour. Any drug that depresses respiration in the mother can cause respiratory depression in the newborn; opioid analgesics are notorious in this respect, but there can also be difficulty with any sedatives and general anaesthetics; they may also cause fetal distress by reducing uterine blood flow, and prolong labour by depressing uterine muscle.

Drugs used to relax the uterus in premature labour, e.g. β-adrenoceptor agonists (isoxsuprine) may affect the fetal circulation at birth. Diazepam (and other depressants) in high doses may cause hypotonia in the baby and possibly interfere with suckling. There remains the possibility of later behavioural effects due to impaired development of the central nervous system due to psychotropic drugs used during pregnancy; such effects have been shown in animals including impaired ability to learn their way around mazes.

Detection of teratogens. Anatomical abnormalities are the easiest to detect. Nonanatomical (functional) effects can also occur, though it is not appropriate to use the term teratogenesis (see definition above). They include effects on brain biochemistry which may have late behavioural consequences.

There is a substantial spontaneous background incidence of birth defect in the community (up to 2%) so that the detection of a low-grade teratogen that increases the incidence of one of the commoner abnormalities presents an intimidating task. Also, most teratogenic effects are probably multifactorial.

In this emotionally charged area it is indeed hard for the public and especially for parents of an affected child to grasp that:

> The concept of absolute safety of drugs needs to be demolished. It has been suggested that a particular antinauseant used in pregnancy (Debendox, Bendectin)[20] should have been taken off the market until it could be proved to be safe. In real life it can never be shown that a drug (or anything else) has no teratogenic activity at all, in the sense of never being a contributory factor in anybody under any circumstances. This concept can neither be tested nor proved.
>
> Let us suppose for example, that some agent doubles the incidence of a condition that has natural incidence of 1 in 10 000 births. If the hypothesis is true, then studying 20 000 pregnant women who have taken the drug and 20 000 who have not may yield respectively two cases and one case of the abnormality. It does not take a statistician to realise that this signifies nothing, and it may need ten times as many pregnant women (almost half a million) to produce a statistically significant result. This would involve such an extensive multicentre study that hundreds of doctors and hospitals have to participate. The participants then each tend to bend the protocol to fit in with their clinical customs and in the end it is

difficult to assess the validity of the data. Alternatively, a limited geographical basis may be used, with the trial going on for many years. During this time other things in the environment change, so again the results would not command our confidence. If it were to be suggested that there was something slightly teratogenic in milk, the hypothesis would be virtually untestable.

In practice we have to make up our minds which drugs may reasonably be given to pregnant women. Do we start from a position of presumed guilt or from one of presumed innocence? If the former course is chosen then we cannot give any drugs to pregnant women because we can never prove that they are completely free of teratogenic influence. It therefore seems that we must start from a position of presumed innocence and then take all possible steps to find out if the presumption is correct.

Finally, we must put the matter in perspective by considering the benefit/risk ratio. The problem of prescription in pregnancy cannot be considered from the point of view of only one side of the equation. Drugs are primarily designed to do good, and if a pregnant woman is ill it is in the best interests of her baby and herself that she gets better as quickly as possible. This often means giving her drugs. We can argue about the necessity of giving drugs to prevent vomiting, but there is no argument about the need for treatment of women with meningitis, septicaemia or venereal disease.

What we must try to avoid is medication by the media or prescription by politicians. A public scare about a well-tried drug will lead to wider use of less-tried alternatives. We do not want to be forced to practise the kind of defensive medicine that is primarily designed to avoid litigation. The best decisions for patients are made by well-informed doctors.[21]

MALE REPRODUCTIVE FUNCTION

Impotence may occur with drugs affecting autonomic sympathetic function, e.g. antihypertensives.

Spermatogenesis is reduced by sulphasalazine

---

[20] A combination of an antimuscarinic (dicyclomine, later omitted), an antihistamine (doxylamine) and a vitamin (pyridoxine).

[21] By permission from Smithells R W 1983 In: Hawkins D F (ed) Drugs and pregnancy. Churchill Livingstone, Edinburgh.

and mesalazine (reversible) and by cytotoxic anti-cancer drugs (reversible and irreversible). Men are advised not to father children within 6 months of taking griseofulvin. There has been a global decline in sperm concentration[22] and an environmental cause, e.g. chemicals that possess oestrogenic activity, seems likely.

Causation of birth defects due to abnormal sperm remains uncertain.

GENERAL DISCUSSION

Human toxic effects not predicted from animal experiments are often reversible, but even the most optimistic enthusiasts for drugs must shrink from the thought that their hands wrote prescriptions resulting in deformed, surviving babies.

Clinical data are, at present, inevitably open to doubt, and any list of suspected drugs must, so slight is our knowledge, become obsolete and misleading very quickly. This topic must, therefore, be followed in the periodical press and manufacturers' up-to-date information.

The medical profession clearly has a grave duty to refrain from all unessential prescribing of drugs with, say, less than 10–15 years widespread use behind them, for all women of childbearing potential. It is not sufficient safeguard merely to ask a woman if she is or may be pregnant (the natural reluctance to broach this subject to unmarried women may, even in a permissive society, act as a salutary check to casual prescribing), but it will also be necessary to consider the possibility of a woman, who evidently is not pregnant at the time of prescribing, becoming so whilst taking the drug.

Since morning sickness of pregnancy occurs during the time when the fetus is vulnerable, it is specially important to restrict drug therapy of this symptom to a minimum; but severe vomiting with its accompanying biochemical changes may itself harm the fetus.

Thus, before a drug is condemned as a cause of fetal damage, it is necessary to consider whether the disease for which it was given, or other inter-current disease, might perhaps be responsible. Since the only way to be certain that a drug causes fetal damage in humans is to test it in humans, it is necessary that doctors should (a) suspect a drug-induced abnormality when it occurs and (b) report it to a central organisation (UK Committee on Safety of Medicines) or to a national register of all birth defects (such a register ideally should be kept plus a full drug history of the mother from prior to conception). Unfortunately, none of these requirements is easily satisfied. Minor congenital abnormalities are common in the absence of drug therapy and some may be virtually undetectable, e.g. reduced intelligence of learning ability. Human frailty also causes any reporting system based on voluntary cooperation to be less than perfect. For example, the UK Committee on Safety of Medicines has found that when a letter exhorting doctors to report drug reactions is sent out, there is a large, but very short-lived increase in reports.

In addition, the more cautiously a new drug is introduced, the more difficult it is going to be to detect, by epidemiological methods, a capacity to cause fetal abnormality. This is especially so if the abnormality produced is already fairly common.

The possibility of fetal abnormalities resulting from drugs taken by the father exists but has only begun to be explored.

GUIDE TO FURTHER READING

Bochner B S et al 1991 Anaphylaxis. New England Journal of Medicine 324: 1785

Brennan T A et al 1991 Incidence of adverse events and negligence in hospitalized patients. New England Journal of Medicine 324: 370 (also Leape L L et al Nature of adverse events: 377)

Editorial 1995 Male reproductive health and environmental oestrogens. Lancet 324: 933

Ferner R E 1992 Hazards, risks and reality. British Journal of Clinical Pharmacology 33: 125

Fisher M 1995 Treatment of acute anaphylaxis. British Medical Journal 311: 731

Herbst A L 1984 Diethylstilboestrol exposure — 1984 [effects of exposure during pregnancy on mother and daughters]. New England Journal of Medicine 311: 1433

Inman W H W et al 1993 Prescriber profile and post-marketing surveillance. Lancet 342: 658

---

[22] From 133 million per ml in 1938 to 66 million per ml in 1990. Carlsen B et al 1992 Lancet 305: 609.

Jick H 1974 Drugs — remarkably non-toxic. New England Journal of Medicine 291: 824

Kramer M S et al 1979 An algorithm for the operational assessment of adverse reactions. Journal of the American Medical Association 242: 623

Park B K et al 1988 The immunological basis of adverse drug reactions. British Journal of Clinical Pharmacology 26: 491

Rawlins M D 1988 Spontaneous reporting of adverse drug reactions. British Journal of Clinical Pharmacology 26: 1, 1, 7

Scott J L et al 1965 A controlled double-blind study of the haematologic toxicity of chloramphenicol. New England Journal of Medicine 272: 1137

Steenland K 1996 Chronic neurological effects of organophosphate pesticides. British Medical Journal 312: 1312

Poisoning, overdose, antidotes

SYNOPSIS

- Deliberate and accidental self-poisoning
- Principles of treatment
- Poison-specific measures
- General measures
- Specific poisonings: cyanide, methanol, ethylene glycol, hydrocarbons, volatile solvents, heavy metals, herbicides and pesticides, biological substances (Overdose of medicinal drugs is dealt with under individual agents)
- Incapacitating agents: drugs used for torture

Self-poisoning

Deliberate self-poisoning. A curious by-product of the modern 'drug and prescribing explosion' is the rise in the incidence of nonfatal deliberate self-harm. The majority of people who do this lack serious suicidal intent and are therefore termed parasuicides. In over 90% of instances in the UK, poisoning is the means chosen, usually by medicines taken in overdose and these amount to at least 100 000 per annum in England and Wales (population 51 million). Two or more drugs are taken in over 30% of episodes, not including alcohol which is also taken in over 50% of the instances. Repeated episodes are not rare.[1] Prescribed drugs are used in over 75% of episodes but teenagers tend to favour nonprescribed analgesics available by direct sale, e.g. paracetamol, which is important bearing in mind its potentially serious toxicity. The mortality rate of self-poisoning is very low (less than 1% of acute hospital admissions), but 'completed' suicides by poisoning still number 3500 per annum in England and Wales.

Accidental self-poisoning causing admission to hospital occurs predominantly amongst children under 5 years, usually with medicines left within reach or with domestic chemicals, e.g. bleach, detergents.

Principles of treatment

Successful treatment of acute poisoning depends on a combination of speed and common sense as well as on the nature of the poison, the amount taken and the time which has since elapsed. The majority of those admitted to hospital require only observation and medical and nursing supportive measures while they metabolise and eliminate the poison. Some require a specific antidote or a specific measure to increase elimination. Intensive care facilities

---

[1] An extreme example is that of a young man who, over a period of 6 years, was admitted to hospital following 82 episodes of self-poisoning, 31 employing paracetamol; he had had a disturbed, unhappy upbringing and had been expelled from both the Danish Navy and the British Army. Prescott L F et al 1978 British Medical Journal 2: 1399.

are needed by only a few. In the UK the centres of the National Poisons Information Service provide information and advice over the telephone throughout the day and night.[2]

> **Poison-specific measures**
> - Identification
> - Prevention of further absorption
> - Specific antidotes
> - Acceleration of elimination
>
> **General measures**
> - Initial assessment and resuscitation
>
> **Supportive measures**
> - Psychiatric and social assessment

Poison-specific measures

IDENTIFICATION OF THE POISON(S)

The key pieces of information are:

- the identity of the substance(s) taken
- the dose(s)
- the time that has since elapsed. Adults may be sufficiently conscious to give some indication of the poison or may have referred to it in a suicide note, or there may be other circumstantial evidence. Rapid (1–2 h) biochemical 'screens' of plasma or urine are available but are best reserved for seriously ill or unconscious patients in whom the cause of coma is unknown. Analysis of plasma for specific substances is essential in suspected cases of paracetamol or iron poisoning, to indicate which patients should receive antidotes; it is also required for salicylate, lithium and some sedative drugs, e.g. trichloroethanol derivatives, phenobarbitone, when a decision is needed about using urine alkalinisation, haemodialysis or haemoperfusion. Response to a specific antidote may provide a diagnosis, e.g. dilatation of constricted pupils and increased respiratory rate after i.v. naloxone (opioid poisoning) or

arousal from unconsciousness in response to i.v. flumazenil (benzodiazepine poisoning).

PREVENTION OF FURTHER ABSORPTION OF THE POISON

From the environment

When a poison has been inhaled or absorbed through the skin, the patient should be taken from the toxic environment, contaminated clothing removed and the skin cleansed.

From the gut

Oral adsorbents. *Activated charcoal* (Carbomix, Medicoal) reduces drug absorption better than syrup of ipecacuanha or gastric lavage, is easiest to administer and has fewest adverse effects. It consists of a very fine black powder prepared from vegetable matter, e.g. wood pulp, coconut shell, which is 'activated' by an oxidising gas flow at high temperature to create a network of fine (10–20 nm) pores to give it an enormous surface area in relation to weight (1000 m^2/g). This binds to, and thus inactivates, a wide variety of compounds in the gut. Thus it is simpler to list the exceptions, i.e. substances that are **not adsorbed** by charcoal which are: iron, lithium, cyanide, strong acids and alkalis, and organic solvents and corrosive agents.

Indeed, activated charcoal comes nearest to fulfilling the long-sought notion of a 'universal antidote'.[3] It should be given as soon as possible after a poison has been ingested, whilst a significant amount remains yet unabsorbed and, to be most effective, 5–10 times as much charcoal as poison, weight for weight, is needed; in the adult an initial dose of 50–100 g is usual. If the patient is vomiting, the charcoal should be given through a nasogastric tube. Activated charcoal also accelerates elimination of poison that has been absorbed (see p. 142).

Activated charcoal, although unpalatable,

---

[2] For telephone numbers see the British National Formulary (BNF).

[3] For centuries it was supposed not only that there could be, but that there actually was, a single antidote to all poisons. This was Theriaca Andromachi, a formulation of 72 (a magical number) ingredients amongst which particular importance was attached to the flesh of a snake (viper). The antidote was devised by Andromachus whose son was physician to the Roman Emperor, Nero (AD 37–68).

appears to be relatively safe but constipation or mechanical bowel obstruction may be caused by repeated use. Aspiration of charcoal into the lungs can cause hypoxia through obstruction and arteri-ovenous shunting. Charcoal adsorbs and so inactivates ipecacuanha but may be used after successful emesis with that substance; methionine, used for paracetamol poisoning, is also adsorbed.

Other oral adsorbents have specific uses. Fuller's earth and bentonite (both natural forms of aluminium silicate) bind and inactivate the herbicides, paraquat (activated charcoal is superior) and diquat; cholestyramine and colestipol adsorb warfarin.

Gastric lavage is best confined to the hospitalised adult who is believed to have taken a significant amount of a toxic substance within 4–6 h, or longer in the case of drugs that delay gastric emptying, e.g. aspirin, tricyclic antidepressants, sympathomimetics, theophylline, opioids. Lavage is probably worth undertaking in any unconscious patient, who is believed to have ingested poison, regardless of the interval after ingestion, and provided the airways are protected by a cuffed endotracheal tube. Paradoxically, lavage may wash an ingested substance into the small intestine, enhancing its absorption. Leaving activated charcoal in the stomach after lavage is appropriate to lessen this risk. Nevertheless, patients who have ingested tricyclic antidepressants or centrally depressant drugs must be continued after the lavage.

The passing of a gastric tube, naturally, takes second place to emergency resuscitative measures, institution of controlled respiration or suppression of convulsions. Nothing is gained by aspirating the stomach of a corpse.

Emesis, in fully conscious patients only, may be used for children and also for adults who refuse activated charcoal or gastric lavage. It may safely be given in the patient's home. Emesis is induced by Ipecacuanha Emetic Mixture, Pediatric (BNF), 10 ml for a child 6–18 months, 15 ml for an older child and 30 ml for an adult, i.e. all ages may receive the same preparation but in a different dose, which is followed by a tumblerful of water (250 ml); the dose may be repeated after 20 minutes. The active constituent of ipecacuanha is emetine; it can cause pro-longed vomiting, diarrhoea and drowsiness that may be confused with effects of the ingested poison. Even fully conscious patients may develop aspiration pneumonia after ipecacuanha.

Both emesis and lavage are contraindicated for corrosive poisons, because there is a risk of perforation of the gut, and for petroleum distillates as the danger of causing inhalational chemical pneumonia outweighs that of leaving the substance in the stomach.

Cathartics or whole-bowel irrigation[4] have been used for the removal of sustained-release formulations, e.g. theophylline, iron, aspirin. Evidence of benefit is conflicting. Activated charcoal in repeated doses is generally preferred. Sustained-release formulations are now common, and patients have died from failure to recognise the danger of continued release of drug from such products, after apparently successful gastric lavage.

SPECIFIC ANTIDOTES[5]

Specific antidotes reduce or abolish the effects of poisons through a variety of mechanisms, which may be categorised as follows:

- receptors, which may be activated, blocked or bypassed
- enzymes, which may be inhibited or reactivated
- displacement from tissue binding sites
- exchanging with the poison
- replenishment of an essential substance

---

[4] Magnesium sulphate may be used; alternatively, irrigation with large volumes of a polyethylene glycol-electrolyte solution, e.g. Klean-Prep, by mouth causes minimal fluid and electrolyte disturbance (it was developed for preparation for colonoscopy).

[5] Mithridates the Great (?132–63 BC) king of Pontus (in Asia Minor) was noted for 'ambition, cruelty and artifice'. 'He murdered his own mother . . . and fortified his constitution by drinking antidotes' to the poisons with which his domestic enemies sought to kill him (Lemprière). When his son also sought to kill him, Mithridates was so disappointed that he compelled his wife to poison herself. He then tried to poison himself, but in vain; the frequent antidotes which he had taken in the early part of his life had so strengthened his constitution that he was immune. He was obliged to stab himself, but had to seek the help of a slave to complete his task. Modern physicians have to be content with less comprehensively effective antidotes, some of which are listed in Table 9.1.

• binding to the poison (including chelation). Table 9.1 illustrates these mechanisms with antidotes that are of therapeutic value.

CHELATING AGENTS

Chelating agents are used for poisoning with heavy metals. They incorporate the metal ions into an inner ring structure in the molecule (Greek: *chele*, claw) by means of structural groups called ligands (Latin: *ligare*, to bind); effective agents form stable, biologically inert complexes that are excreted in the urine.

Dimercaprol (British Anti-Lewisite, BAL). Arsenic and other metal ions are toxic in low concentration because they combine with the -SH groups of essential enzymes, thus inactivating them. Dimercaprol provides -SH groups which combine with the metal

Table 9.1 Specific antidotes, indications and modes of action (see Index for fuller account of individual drugs)

Antidote	Indication	Mode of action
acetylcysteine	paracetamol, chloroform, carbon tetrachloride	Replenishes depleted glutathione stores
atropine	cholinesterase inhibitors, e.g. organophosphorus insecticides	Blocks muscarinic cholinoceptors
	β-blocker poisoning	Vagal block accelerates heart rate
benztropine	drug-induced movement disorders	Blocks muscarinic cholinoceptors
calcium gluconate	hydrofluoric acid, fluorides	Binds or precipitates fluoride ions
desferrioxamine	iron	Chelates ferrous ions
dicobalt edetate	cyanide and derivatives, e.g. acrylonitrile	Chelates to form nontoxic cobalti- and cobalto-cyanides
digoxin-specific antibody fragments (FAB)	digitalis glycosides	Binds free glycoside in plasma, complex excreted in urine
dimercaprol (BAL)	arsenic, copper, gold, lead, inorganic mercury	Chelates metal ions
ethanol	ethylene glycol, methanol	Competes for alcohol and acetaldehyde dehydrogenases, preventing formation of toxic metabolites
flumazenil	benzodiazepines	Competes for benzodiazepine receptors
glucagon	β-adrenoceptor antagonists	Bypasses blockade of the β-adrenoceptor; stimulates cyclic AMP formation with positive cardiac inotropic effect
isoprenaline (or prenalterol)	β-adrenoceptor antagonists	Competes for β-adrenoceptors
methionine	paracetamol	Replenishes depleted glutathione stores
naloxone	opioids	Competes for opioid receptors
neostigmine	antimuscarinic drugs	Inhibits acetylcholinesterase, causing acetylcholine to accumulate at cholinoceptors
oxygen	carbon monoxide	Competitively displaces carbon monoxide from binding sites on haemoglobin
penicillamine	copper, gold, lead, elemental mercury (vapour), zinc	Chelates metal ions
phenoxybenzamine	hypertension due to α-adrenoceptor agonists, e.g. with MAOI, clonidine, ergotamine	Competes for α-adrenoceptors (long-acting)
phentolamine	as above	Competes for α-adrenoceptors (short-acting)
phytomenadione (vitamin K₁)	coumarin (warfarin) and indandione anticoagulants	Replenishes vitamin K
pralidoxime	cholinesterase inhibitors, e.g. organophosphorus insecticides	Competitively reactivates cholinesterase
propranolol	β-adrenoceptor agonists, ephedrine, theophylline, thyroxine	Blocks β-adrenoceptors
protamine	heparin	Binds ionically to neutralise
Prussian blue (potassium ferric hexacyanoferrate)	thallium (in rodenticides)	Potassium exchanges for thallium
calciumedetate	lead	Chelates lead ions
unithiol	lead, elemental and organic mercury	Chelates metal ions

141

ions to form relatively harmless ring compounds which are excreted, mainly in the urine. As dimercaprol, itself, is oxidised in the body and renally excreted, repeated administration is necessary to ensure that an excess is available until all the metal has been eliminated.

Dimercaprol may be used for poisoning by antimony, arsenic, bismuth, gold and mercury (inorganic, e.g. $HgCl_2$).

Adverse effects are common, particularly with larger doses, and include nausea and vomiting, lachrymation and salivation, paraesthesiae, muscular aches and pains, urticarial rashes, tachycardia and a raised blood pressure. Gross overdosage may cause overbreathing, muscular tremors, convulsions and coma.

Unithiol (dimercaptopropanesulphonate, DMPS) effectively chelates lead and mercury; it appears to be well tolerated.

Sodium calciumedetate is the calcium chelate of the disodium salt of ethylenediaminetetra-acetic acid (calcium EDTA). It is effective in lead poisoning because of its capacity to exchange calcium for lead: the lead chelate is excreted in the urine, leaving behind a harmless amount of calcium. Dimercaprol may usefully be combined with sodium calciumedetate when lead poisoning is severe, e.g. with encephalopathy.

Adverse effects are fairly common, and include hypotension, lachrymation, nasal stuffiness, sneezing, muscle pains and chills. Renal damage can occur.

Dicobalt edetate. Cobalt forms stable, nontoxic complexes with cyanide. It is toxic (especially if the wrong diagnosis is made and no cyanide is present), causing hypertension, tachycardia and chest pain; consequent cobalt poisoning is treated by giving sodium calcium edetate and i.v. glucose.

Penicillamine (dimethylcysteine) is a metabolite of penicillin that contains -SH groups; it may be used to chelate lead and also copper (see Hepatolenticular degeneration). Its principal use is for rheumatoid arthritis (see Index).

Desferrioxamine: see Iron.

ACCELERATION OF ELIMINATION OF THE POISON

Techniques for eliminating poisons have a role that is limited, but important when applicable. Each method depends, directly or indirectly, on removing drug from the circulation and successful use requires that:

- The poison should be present in high concentration in the plasma relative to that in the rest of the body, i.e. it should have a small distribution volume
- The poison should dissociate readily from any plasma protein binding sites
- The effects of the poison should relate to its plasma concentration.

Methods used are:

Repeated doses of activated charcoal

Activated charcoal by mouth not only adsorbs ingested drug in the gut, preventing absorption into the body (see above), it also adsorbs drug that diffuses from the blood into the gut lumen when the concentration there is lower; because binding is irreversible the concentration gradient is maintained and drug is continuously removed; this has been called 'intestinal dialysis'. Charcoal also adsorbs drugs that are secreted into the bile, i.e. it can interrupt an enterohepatic cycle. Evidence shows that activated charcoal in repeated doses effectively adsorbs (shortens $t^{1}/2$ of) phenobarbitone (phenobarbitone), carbamazepine, theophylline, quinine, dapsone and salicylate.[6] Repeated-dose activated charcoal is increasingly preferred to alkalinisation of urine (below) for phenobarbitone and salicylate poisoning. Activated charcoal in an initial dose of 50–100 g should be followed by not less than 12.5 g/h; the regular hourly administration is more effective than larger amounts less often.

Alteration of urine pH and diuresis

By manipulation of the pH of the glomerular filtrate, a drug can be made to ionise, become less

---

[6] Bradberry S M, Vale A J 1995 Journal of Toxicology: Clinical Toxicology 33(5): 407.

lipid-soluble, remain in the renal tubular fluid, and so be eliminated in the urine (see p. 90). Maintenance of a good urine flow (e.g. 100 ml/h) helps this process but 'it is the alteration of tubular fluid pH that is important'.[7] The practice of forcing diuresis with frusemide and large volumes of i.v. fluid does not add significantly to drug clearance but may cause fluid overload; it is obsolete.

Alkalinisation may be used for salicylate (> 500 mg/l + metabolic acidosis, or in any case > 750 mg/l), phenobarbitone (75–150 mg/l) or phenoxy herbicides, e.g. 2,4-D, mecoprop, dichlorprop. The objective is to maintain a urine pH of 7.5–8.5 by an i.v. infusion of sodium bicarbonate. Available preparations of sodium bicarbonate vary between 1.2 and 8.4% (1 ml of the 8.4% preparation contains 1 mmol of sodium bicarbonate) and the concentration given will depend on the patient's fluid needs.

Acidification may be used for severe, acute amphetamine, dexfenfluramine or phencyclidine poisoning. The objective is to maintain a urine pH of 5.5–6.5 by giving i.v. infusion of arginine hydrochloride (10 g) or lysine hydrochloride (10 g) over 30 min, followed by ammonium chloride (4 g) 2-hourly by mouth. It is rarely necessary. Phenoxybenzamine should be adequate for amphetamine-like drugs (α-adrenoceptor block).

Peritoneal dialysis

Peritoneal dialysis involves instilling appropriate fluid into the peritoneal cavity. Poison in the blood diffuses into the dialysis fluid down the concentration gradient. The fluid is then drained and replaced. The technique requires little equipment but is one-half to one-third as effective as haemodialysis; it may be worth using for lithium and methanol poisoning.

Haemodialysis and haemoperfusion

A temporary extracorporeal circulation is established, usually from an artery to a vein in the arm. In haemodialysis, a semipermeable membrane separates blood from dialysis fluid and the poison passes passively from the blood, where it is present

in high concentration. The principle of haemoperfusion is that blood flows over activated charcoal or an appropriate ion-exchange resin which adsorbs the poison. Loss of blood cells and activation of the clotting mechanism are largely overcome by coating the charcoal with an acrylic hydrogel which does not reduce adsorbing capacity, though the patient must be anticoagulated with heparin.

Such artificial methods of removing poison from the body are invasive, demand skill and experience on the part of the operator and are expensive in manpower. Their use should therefore be confined to cases of severe, prolonged or progressive clinical intoxication, when high plasma concentration indicates a dangerous degree of poisoning, and when removal by haemoperfusion or dialysis constitutes a significant addition to natural methods of elimination.

- **Haemodialysis** is effective for: salicylate (> 750 mg/l + renal failure, or in any case > 900 mg/l), isopropanol (present in aftershave lotions and window-cleaning solutions), lithium and methanol.
- **Haemoperfusion** is effective for: phenobarbitone (> 100–150 mg/l, but repeat-dose activated charcoal by mouth appears to be as effective, see above) and other barbiturates, ethchlorvynol, glutethimide, meprobamate, methaqualone, theophylline, trichloroethanol derivatives.

General measures

INITIAL ASSESSMENT AND RESUSCITATION

The initial clinical review should include a search for known consequences of poisoning, which include: impaired consciousness with flaccidity (benzodiazepines, alcohol, trichloroethanol) or with hypertonia (tricyclic antidepressants, antimuscarinic agents), hypotension, shock, cardiac dysrhythmia, evidence of convulsions, behavioural disturbances (psychotropic drugs), hypothermia, aspiration pneumonia and cutaneous blisters, burns in the mouth (corrosives).

Maintenance of an adequate oxygen supply is the

---

[7] Prescott L F et al 1982 British Medical Journal 285: 1383.

first priority. A systolic blood pressure of 80 mmHg can be tolerated in a young person but a level below 90 mmHg will imperil the brain or kidney of the elderly. Expansion of the venous capacitance bed is the usual cause of shock in acute poisoning and blood pressure may be restored by placing the patient in the head-down position to encourage venous return to the heart, or by the use of a colloid plasma expander such as gelatin or etherified starch. External cardiac compression may be necessary and should be continued until the cardiac output is self-sustaining, which may be a long time when the patient is hypothermic or poisoned with cardiodepressant drugs, e.g. tricyclic antidepressants, β-adrenoceptor blockers. The airway must be sucked clear of oropharyngeal secretions or regurgitated matter.

Supportive treatment

The salient fact is that patients recover from most poisonings provided they are adequately oxygenated, hydrated and perfused, for, in the majority of cases, the most efficient mechanisms are the patients' own and, given time, they will inactivate and eliminate all the poison. Patients require the standard care of the unconscious, with special attention to the problems introduced by poisoning which are outlined below.

Airway maintenance is essential; some patients require a cuffed endotracheal tube but seldom for more than 24 h.

Ventilation needs should be assessed, if necessary supported by blood gas analysis. A mixed respiratory and metabolic acidosis is common. Hypoxia may be corrected by supplementing the inspired air with oxygen but mechanical ventilation is necessary if the Pa CO_2 exceeds 6.5 kPa.

Hypotension is common and in addition to the resuscitative measures indicated above, infusion of a combination of dopamine and dobutamine in low dose may be required to maintain renal perfusion.

Convulsions should be treated if they are persistent or protracted. Diazepam i.v. is the first choice.

Cardiac dysrhythmia frequently accompanies poisoning, e.g. with tricyclic antidepressants, theophylline, β-adrenoceptor blockers. Acidosis, hypoxia and electrolyte disturbance are often important contributory factors; the emphasis of therapy should be to correct these and to resist the temptation to resort to an antidysrhythmic drug. If dysrhythmia leads to persistent peripheral circulatory failure, then an appropriate drug ought to be used, e.g. a β-adrenoceptor blocker for poisoning with a sympathomimetic drug.

Hypothermia may occur if temperature regulation is impaired by CNS depression. Core temperature must be monitored by a low-reading rectal thermometer, while the patient is nursed in a heat retaining 'space blanket'.

Immobility may lead to pressure lesions of peripheral nerves, cutaneous blisters and necrosis over bony prominences.

Rhabdomyolysis may result from prolonged pressure on muscles, from agents that cause muscle spasm or convulsions (phencyclidine, theophylline) or be aggravated by hyperthermia due to muscle contraction, e.g. with MDMA ('ecstacy'). Aggressive volume repletion and correction of acid base abnormality may be needed, and urine alkalinisation may prevent acute tubular necrosis.

PSYCHIATRIC AND SOCIAL ASSESSMENT

Most cases of self-poisoning are precipitated by interpersonal or social problems, which should be addressed. Major psychiatric illness ought to be identified and treated.

Some poisonings

(for medicines: see individual drugs)

Common toxic syndromes[8]

Many substances used in accidental or self-poison-

[8] Based on Kulig K 1992 New England Journal of Medicine 326: 1677.

ing cause dysfunction of the central or autonomic nervous systems and produce a variety of effects which may be usefully grouped to aid the identification of the agent(s) responsible.

Antimuscarinic syndromes consist of tachycardia, dilated pupils, dry, flushed skin, urinary retention, decreased bowel sounds, mild elevation of body temperature, confusion, cardiac dysrhythmias and seizures. They are commonly caused by antipsychotics, tricyclic antidepressants, antihistamines, antispasmodics and many plants (see p. 147).

Cholinergic (muscarinic) syndromes comprise salivation, lachrymation, abdominal cramps, urinary and faecal incontinence, vomiting, sweating, miosis, muscle fasciculation and weakness, bradycardia, pulmonary oedema, confusion, CNS depression and fitting. Common causes include organophosphorus and carbamate insecticides, neostigmine and other anticholinesterase drugs, and some fungi (mushrooms).

Sympathomimetic syndromes include tachycardia, hypertension, hyperthermia, sweating, mydriasis, hyperreflexia, agitation, delusions, paranoia, seizures and cardiac dysrhythmias. These are commonly caused by amphetamine (and its derivatives), cocaine, proprietary decongestants, e.g. ephedrine, and theophylline (in the latter case, excluding psychiatric effects).

Sedatives, opioids and ethanol cause signs that may include respiratory depression, miosis, hyporeflexia, coma, hypotension and hypothermia.

Poisonings by (nondrug) chemicals

Cyanide causes tissue anoxia by chelating the ferric part of the intracellular respiratory enzyme, cytochrome oxidase. Poisoning may occur as a result of self-administration of hydrocyanic (prussic) acid, by accidental exposure in industry, through inhaling smoke from burning polyurethane foams in furniture, through ingesting amygdalin which is present in the kernels of several fruits including apricots, almonds and peaches

(constituents of the unlicensed anticancer agent, laetrile), or from excessive use of sodium nitroprusside for severe hypertension.[9] The symptoms of acute poisoning are due to tissue anoxia, with dizziness, palpitations, a feeling of chest constriction and anxiety; characteristically the breath smells of bitter almonds. In more severe cases there is acidosis and coma. Inhaled hydrogen cyanide may lead to death within minutes but when it is ingested as the salt several hours may elapse before the patient is seriously ill. Chronic exposure damages the nervous system causing peripheral neuropathy, optic atrophy and nerve deafness.

The principles of specific therapy are as follows:

- *Dicobalt edetate* (Kelocyanor) to chelate the cyanide is the treatment of choice when the diagnosis is certain. The dose is 300–600 mg given i.v. over one minute, followed by a further 300 ml if recovery is not evident within one minute.
- Alternatively, a two-stage procedure may be followed by i.v. administration of:
  (1) *sodium nitrite*, which rapidly converts haemoglobin to methaemoglobin, the ferric ion of which takes up cyanide as cyanmethaemoglobin (up to 40% methaemoglobin can be tolerated);
  (2) *sodium thiosulphate*, which more slowly detoxifies the cyanide by permitting the formation of thiocyanate. When the diagnosis is uncertain, administration of thiosulphate plus oxygen is a safe course.

There is evidence that oxygen, especially if at high pressure (hyperbaric), overcomes the cellular anoxia in cyanide poisoning; the mechanism is uncertain, but oxygen should be administered.

---

[9] Or in other more bizarre ways. 'A 23-year-old medical student saw his dog (a puppy) suddenly collapse. He started external cardiac massage and a mouth-to-nose ventilation effort. Moments later the dog died, and the student felt nauseated, vomited and lost consciousness. On the victim's arrival at hospital, an alert medical officer detected a bitter almonds odour on his breath and administered the accepted treatment for cyanide poisoning after which he recovered. It turned out that the dog had accidentally swallowed cyanide, and the poison eliminated through the lungs had been inhaled by the master during the mouth-to-nose resuscitation.' Journal of the American Medical Association (1983) 249: 353.

Carbon monoxide (CO) is formed when substances containing carbon and hydrogen are incompletely combusted; poisoning results from inhalation. Oxygen transport to cells is impaired and myocardial and neurological injury result; delayed (2–4 weeks) neurological sequelae include parkinsonism and cerebellar signs. The concentration of CO in the blood may confirm exposure (cigarette smoking alone may account for up to 10%) but is no guide to severity of poisoning. Patients with signs of cardiac ischaemia or neurological defect should be treated with hyperbaric oxygen.

Methanol is widely available as a solvent and in paints and antifreezes, and may be consumed as a cheap substitute for ethanol. As little as 10 ml may cause permanent blindness and 30 ml may kill, through its toxic metabolites. Methanol, like ethanol, is metabolised by zero-order processes that involve the hepatic alcohol and aldehyde dehydrogenases, but whereas ethanol forms acetaldehyde and acetic acid which are partly responsible for the unpleasant effects of 'hangover', methanol forms formaldehyde and formic acid. Blindness may be due to retinal aldehyde dehydrogenase (for the interconversion of retinol and retinene) allowing the local formation of formaldehyde. Acidosis is due to the formic acid, which itself enhances pH-dependent hepatic lactate production, so that lactic acidosis is added.

The clinical features are severe malaise, vomiting, abdominal pain and tachypnoea (due to the acidosis). Loss of visual acuity and scotomata indicate ocular damage and, if the pupils are dilated and nonreactive, permanent loss of sight is probable. Coma and circulatory collapse may follow.

Therapy is directed at:

- *Correcting the acidosis.* Achieving this largely determines the outcome; sodium bicarbonate is given i.v. in doses up to 2 mol in a few hours, carrying an excess of sodium which must be managed. Methanol is metabolised slowly and the patient may relapse if bicarbonate administration is discontinued too soon.
- *Inhibiting methanol metabolism.* Ethanol, which occupies the dehydrogenase enzymes in preference to methanol, competitively prevents metabolism of methanol to its toxic products. A single oral dose of ethanol 1 ml/kg (as a 50% solution or as the equivalent in gin or whisky) is followed by 0.25 ml/kg/h orally or i.v., aiming to maintain the blood ethanol at about 100 mg/100 ml until no methanol is detectable in the blood.
- *Eliminating methanol* and its metabolites by *dialysis.* Haemodialysis is 2–3 times more effective than is peritoneal dialysis. Folinic acid 30 mg i.v. 6-hourly may protect against retinal damage by enhancing formate metabolism.

Ethylene glycol is readily accessible as a constituent of antifreezes for car radiators. It has been used criminally to give 'body' and sweetness to white table wines. Metabolism to glycolate and oxalate causes acidosis and renal damage, and usually the situation is further complicated by lactic acidosis. In the first 12 hours after ingestion the patient appears as though intoxicated with alcohol but does not smell of that; subsequently there is increasing acidosis, pulmonary oedema and cardiac failure, and in 2–3 days renal pain and tubular necrosis develop because calcium oxalate crystals form in the urine. Acidosis is corrected with i.v. sodium bicarbonate and hypocalcaemia with calcium gluconate. As with methanol (above), ethanol is given competitively to inhibit the metabolism of ethylene glycol and haemodialysis is used to eliminate the poison.

Hydrocarbons, e.g. paraffin oil (kerosene), petrol (gasoline), benzene, chiefly cause CNS depression and pulmonary damage from inhalation. It is vital to avoid aspiration into the lungs during attempts to remove the poison or in spontaneous vomiting. Gastric aspiration should be performed only if a cuffed endotracheal tube is effectively in place, if necessary after anaesthetising the subject.

Volatile solvent abuse or 'glue sniffing', is common among teenagers, especially males. The success of the modern chemical industry provides easy access to these substances as adhesives, dry cleaners, air fresheners, deodorants, aerosols and other products. Various techniques of administration are employed: viscous products may be inhaled from a plastic bag, liquids from a handkerchief or plastic bottle. The immediate euphoriant and excitatory effects are replaced by confusion, hallucinations and

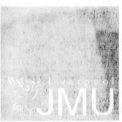

delusions as the dose is increased. Chronic abusers, notably of toluene, develop peripheral neuropathy, cerebellar disease and dementia; damage to the kidney, liver, heart and lungs also occurs with solvents. Over 50% of deaths from the practice follow cardiac dysrhythmia, probably caused by sensitisation of the myocardium to catecholamines and by vagal inhibition from laryngeal stimulation when aerosol propellants are sprayed into the throat.

Standard cardiorespiratory resuscitation and antidysrhythmia treatment are used for acute solvent poisoning. Toxicity from carbon tetrachloride and chloroform involves the generation of phosgene (a 1914–18 war gas) which is inactivated by cysteine, and by glutathione which is formed from cysteine; treatment with N-acetylcysteine, as for poisoning with paracetamol, is therefore recommended.

Poisoning by herbicides and pesticides

Organophosphorus pesticides are anticholinesterases; poisoning and its management are described on page 404. Organic carbamates are similar.

Dinitro-compounds. Dinitro-orthocresol (DNOC) and dinitrobutylphenol (DNBP) are used as selective weed killers and insecticides, and cases of poisoning occur accidentally, e.g. when safety precautions are ignored. These substances can be absorbed through the skin and the hands, face or hair are usually stained yellow. Symptoms and signs indicate a very high metabolic rate (due to uncoupling of oxidative phosphorylation); copious sweating and thirst proceed to dehydration and vomiting, weakness, restlessness, tachycardia and deep, rapid breathing, convulsions and coma. Treatment is urgent and consists of cooling the patient and attention to fluid and electrolyte balance. It is essential to differentiate this type of poisoning from that due to anticholinesterases because atropine given to patients poisoned with dinitrocompound will stop sweating and may cause death from hyperthermia.

Phenoxy herbicides (2,4-D, mecoprop, dichlorprop) are used to control broad-leaved weeds. Ingestion causes nausea, vomiting, pyrexia (due to uncoupling of oxidative phosphorylation), hyperventilation, hypoxia and coma. Their elimination is enhanced by urine alkalinisation.

Organochlorine pesticides, e.g. dicophane (DDT), may cause convulsions in acute overdose. Treat as for status epilepticus.

Rodenticides include warfarin and thallium (see Table 9.1); for strychnine, which causes convulsions, give diazepam.

Paraquat is a widely used herbicide which is extremely toxic if it is ingested; a mouthful of commercial solution taken and spat out may be enough to kill. Ulceration and sloughing of the oral and oesophageal mucosa are followed 5–10 days later by renal tubular necrosis and subsequently there is pulmonary oedema followed by pulmonary fibrosis; whether the patient lives or dies depends largely on the condition of the lung. Treatment is urgent and includes gastric lavage, activated charcoal or aluminium silicate (Fuller's earth) by mouth as adsorbents, and osmotic purgation (magnesium sulphate). Haemodialysis or haemoperfusion may have a role in the first 24 h, the rationale being that reducing the plasma concentration by these methods protects the kidney, failure of which allows the slow but relentless accumulation of paraquat in the lung.

Diquat is similar but the late pulmonary changes may not occur.

Poisoning by biological substances

Many plants form substances that are important for their survival either by enticing animals which disperse their spores, or by repelling potential predators. Poisoning occurs when children eat berries or chew flowers, attracted by their colour; adults may mistake nonedible for edible varieties of salad plants and fungi (mushrooms) for they may resemble each other closely and some are greatly prized by epicures.

The range of toxic substances which these plants produce is reflected in a diversity of symptoms which, however, may be grouped broadly thus:

- *Atropinic*, e.g. from deadly nightshade (*Atropa belladonna*) and thorn apple (*Datura*), causing dilated pupils, blurred vision, dry mouth, flushed skin, confusion and delirium.
- *Nicotinic*, e.g. from hemlock (*Conium*) and

Laburnum, causing salivation, dilated pupils, vomiting, convulsions and respiratory paralysis.

- *Muscarinic*, e.g. from *Inocybe* and *Clitocybe* fungi (mushrooms), causing salivation, lachrymation, miosis, perspiration, bradycardia and bronchoconstriction, also hallucinations.
- *Hallucinogenic*, e.g. from psilocybin-containing mushrooms (liberty cap), which may be taken specifically for this effect ('magic mushrooms').
- *Cardiovascular*, e.g. from foxglove (*Digitalis*), mistletoe (*Viscum album*) and lily-of-the-valley (*Convallaria*) which contain cardiac glycosides that cause vomiting, diarrhoea and cardiac dysrhythmia.
- *Hepatotoxic*, e.g. from *Amanita phalloides* (death cap mushroom), from *Senecio* (ragwort) and *Crotalatia* and from 'bush teas' prepared from these plants in the Caribbean. Aflatoxin, from *Aspergillus flavus*, a fungus which contaminates foods, is probably a cause of primary liver cancer.
- *Convulsant*, e.g. from water dropwort (*Oenanthe*) and cowbane (*Cicuta*), which contain the related and very dangerous substances, oenanthotoxin and cicutoxin.
- *Cutaneous irritation*, e.g. directly with nettle (*Urtica*), or dermatitis following sensitisation with *Primula*.
- *Gastrointestinal symptoms*, nausea, vomiting, diarrhoea and abdominal pain occur with numerous plants.

Treatment of plant poisonings consists mainly of activated charcoal to adsorb toxin in the gastrointestinal tract. Inducing emesis with ipecacuanha may make the diagnosis more difficult for vomiting is often the earliest sign of poisoning. Convulsions should be controlled with diazepam. In 'death cap' mushroom poisoning, penicillin may be used to displace toxin from plasma albumin, provided haemodialysis is being used, which latter may also benefit the renal failure.

Incapacitating agents

(harassing, disabling, antiriot agents)

Harassing agents may be defined as chemical substances that are capable when used in field conditions, of rapidly causing a temporary disablement that lasts for little longer than the period of exposure.[10]

The pharmacological requirements for a safe and effective harassing agent must be stringent (it is hardly appropriate to refer to benefit versus risk). As well as potency and rapid onset and offset of effect in open areas under any atmospheric condition, it must be safe in confined spaces where concentration may be very high and may affect an innocent, bedridden invalid should a projectile enter a window.

CS (chlorobenzylidene malononitrile, a tear 'gas') is a favoured substance at present. This is a solid that is disseminated as an aerosol (particles of 1 micron diameter) by including it in a pyrotechnic mixture. The spectacle of its dissemination has been rendered familiar by television. It is not a gas, it is an aerosol or smoke. The particles aggregate and settle to the ground in minutes so that the risk of prolonged exposure out of doors is not great.

According to the concentration of CS to which a person is exposed, the effects vary from a slight pricking or peppery sensation in the eyes and nasal passages up to the maximum symptoms of streaming from the eyes and nose, spasm of the eyelids, profuse lachrymation and salivation, retching and sometimes vomiting, burning of the mouth and throat, cough and gripping pain in the chest.[11]

The onset of symptoms occurs immediately on exposure (an important factor from the point of view of the user) and they disappear dramatically:

At one moment the exposed person is in their grip. Then he either stumbles away, or the smoke plume veers or the discharge from the grenade stops, and, immediately, the symptoms begin to roll away. Within a minute or two, the pain in the chest has gone and his eyes, although still streaming, are open. Five or so minutes later, the excessive

---

[10] Health aspects of chemical and biological weapons. 1970 WHO Geneva.

[11] Home Office Report (1971) of the enquiry into the medical and toxicological aspects of CS. pt II. HMSO, London: Cmnd 4775.

salivation and pouring tears stop and a quarter of an hour after exposure, the subject is essentially back to normal.[11]

Exposed subjects absorb small amounts only, and the plasma $t^{1/2}$ is about 5 seconds.

Investigations of the effects of CS are difficult in 'field use', but some have been done and at present there is no evidence that even the most persistent rioter will suffer any permanent effect. The hazard to the infirm or sick seems to be low, but plainly it would be prudent to assume that asthmatics or bronchitics could suffer an exacerbation from high concentrations, though bronchospasm does not occur in healthy people. Vomiting seems to be due to swallowing contaminated saliva. Transient looseness of the bowels may follow exposure. Hazard from CS is probably confined to situations where the missiles are projected into enclosed spaces.

CN (chloroacetophenone, a tear gas) is generally used as a solid aerosol or smoke; solutions (Mace) are used at close quarters.

CR (dibenzoxazepine) was put into production in 1973 after testing on army volunteers. In addition to the usual properties (above) it may induce a transient rise in intraocular pressure. Its solubility allows use in water 'cannons'.

'Authority' is reticent about the properties of all these substances and no further important information is readily available.

This brief account has been included, because, in addition to helping victims, even the most well-conducted and tractable students and doctors may find themselves exposed to CS smoke in our troubled world; and some may even feel it their duty to incur exposure. The following points are worth making:

- Wear disposable plastic gloves, for the object of treating the sufferer is frustrated if the physician becomes affected.
- Contaminated clothing should be put in plastic bags and skin should be washed with soap and water. Showering or bathing may cause symptoms to return by releasing the agent from contaminated hair. Cutaneous erythema is usual and blistering may occur with high

concentrations of CS and CN in warm, moist conditions.
- The eyes should be left to irrigate themselves; raised intraocular pressure may cause acute glaucoma in those over 40 years.

DRUGS USED FOR TORTURE, INTERROGATION AND JUDICIAL EXECUTION

Regrettably, drugs have been and are being used for torture, sometimes disguised as 'interrogation' or 'aversion therapy'. Facts are, not surprisingly, hard to obtain, but it seems that suxamethonium, hallucinogens, thiopentone, neuroleptics, amphetamines, apomorphine and cyclophosphamide have been employed to hurt, frighten, confuse or debilitate in such ways as callous ingenuity can devise. When the definition of criminal activity becomes perverted to include activities in defence of human liberty, the employment of drugs offers inducement to inhuman behaviour. Such use, and any doctors or others who engage in it, or who misguidedly allow themselves to believe that it can be in the interest of victims to monitor the activity by others, must surely be outlawed.

It might be urged that it is justifiable to use drugs to protect society by discovering serious crimes such as murder. There is no such thing as a 'truth drug' in the sense that it guarantees the truth of what the subject says. There always must be uncertainty of the truth of evidence obtained with drugs, e.g. thiopentone, that cannot be independently confirmed. But accused people, convinced of their own innocence, sometimes volunteer to undergo such tests. The problem of discerning truth from falsehood remains.

In some countries drugs are used for judicial execution, e.g. combinations of thiopentone, potassium, curare, given intravenously.

GUIDE TO FURTHER READING

Ashton C H 1990 Solvent abuse. Little progress after twenty years. British Medical Journal 300: 135

Flanagan R J et al 1990 Alkaline diuresis for acute poisoning with chlorophenoxy herbicides and ioxynil. Lancet 335: 454

Henry J A 1992 Ecstasy and the dance of death. British Medical Journal 305: 5

Kindwall E P 1993 Hyperbaric oxygen. British Medical Journal 307: 515

Kulig K 1991 Cyanide toxicity and fire toxicity. New England Journal of Medicine 325: 1801

MacLennan W J 1990 The challenge of fire effluents. Poisonous gases are potential killers. British Medical Journal 300: 696

Murray V S G, Volans G N 1991 Management of injuries due to chemical weapons. British Medical Journal 302: 129

Reisman R E 1994 Insect stings. New England Journal of Medicine 331: 523

Ridker P M, McDermott W V 1989 Comfrey herb tea and hepatic veno-occlusive disease. Lancet 1: 657

Vale J A, Proudfoot A T 1993 How useful is activated charcoal? British Medical Journal 306: 78

World Health Organization 1970 Health aspects of chemical and biological weapons. Geneva

Yih J-P 1995 CS gas injury to the eye. British Medical Journal 311: 276

Nonmedical use of drugs

Social aspects

The enormous social importance of this subject warrants discussion here.

> All the naturally occurring sedatives, narcotics, euphoriants, hallucinogens and excitants were discovered thousands of years ago, before the dawn of civilisation ... By the late Stone Age man was systematically poisoning himself. The presence of poppy heads in the kitchen middens of the Swiss Lake Dwellers shows how early in his history man discovered the techniques of self-transcendence through drugs. There were dope addicts long before there were farmers.[1]

The drives that induce a person more or less mentally healthy to resort to drugs to obtain chemical vacations from intolerable selfhood, will be briefly considered here, as well as some account of the pharmacological aspects of drug dependence.

> That humanity at large will ever be able to dispense with Artificial Paradises seems very unlikely. Most men and women lead lives at the worst so painful, at the best so monotonous, poor and limited that the urge to escape, the longing to transcend themselves if only for a few moments, is

---

[1] Huxley A 1957 Annals of the New York Academy of Sciences 67: 677.

and has always been one of the principal appetites of the soul.[2]

The dividing-line between legitimate use of drugs for social purposes and their abuse is indistinct for it is not only a matter of which drug, but of amount of drug and of whether the effect is directed antisocially or not. 'Normal' people seem to be able to use alcohol for their occasional purposes without harm but, given the appropriate personality and/or environmental adversity, many may turn to it for relief and become dependent on it, both psychologically and physically. But drug abuse is not primarily a pharmacological problem, it is a social problem with important pharmacological aspects.

SOME TERMS USED

Abuse potential of a drug is related to its capacity to produce immediate satisfaction, which may be a feature of the drug itself (amphetamine and heroin give rapid effect while tricyclic antidepressants do not) and its route of administration in descending order: inhalation/i.v.; i.m./s.c.; oral.

Drug abuse[3] implies excessive (in terms of social norms) nonmedical or social drug use.

Nonmedical drug use, i.e. all drug use that is not on generally accepted medical grounds, may be a term preferred to 'abuse'. Nonmedical use means the continuous or occasional use of drugs by individuals, whether of their own 'free' choice or under feelings of compulsion, to achieve their own well being, or what they conceive as their own well being (see motives below).

Drugs used for nonmedical purposes are often divided into two groups, hard and soft.

Hard drugs are those that are liable seriously to disable the individual as a functioning member of society by inducing severe psychological and, in the case of cerebral depressants, physical, dependence. The group includes heroin and cocaine.

Soft drugs are less dependence-producing. There may be psychological dependence, but there is little or no physical dependence except with heavy doses of depressants (alcohol, barbiturates). The group includes sedatives and tranquillisers, amphetamines, cannabis, hallucinogens, alcohol, tobacco and caffeine.

This classification fails to recognise individual variation in drug use. Alcohol can be used in heavy doses that are gravely disabling and induce severe physical dependence with convulsions on sudden withdrawal; i.e. for the individual the drug is 'hard'. But there are many people mildly psychologically dependent on it who retain their position in home and society.

Hard-use where the drug is central in the user's life and soft-use where it is merely incidental, are terms of assistance in making this distinction, i.e. what is classified is not the drug but the effect it has or the way it is used by the individual.

Drug dependence (see p. 155).

Addiction. The term 'addict' or 'addiction' has not been completely abandoned in this book because it remains convenient. It refers to the most severe forms of dependence where compulsive craving dominates the subject's daily life. Such cases pose problems as grave as dependence on tea-drinking is trivial. But the use of the term *drug dependence* is welcome, because it renders irrelevant arguments about whether some drugs, e.g. tobacco, are addictive or merely habit-forming.

Nonmedical drug use has two principal forms:

● *Continuous use*, when there is a true dependence, e.g. opioids, alcohol, benzodiazepines.
● *Intermittent or occasional use* to obtain a recreational experience, e.g. 'ecstasy' (tenamphetamine), LSD, cocaine, cannabis, solvents, or to relieve stress, e.g. alcohol.

Both uses commonly occur in the same subject, and some drugs, e.g. alcohol, are used in both ways, but others, e.g. 'ecstasy', LSD, cannabis, are virtually confined to the second use.

---

[2] Huxley A 1954 The doors of perception. Chatto and Windus, London.

[3] The World Health Organization adopts the definition of the United Nations Convention on Psychotropic Drugs (1971). Drug abuse means the use of psychotropic substances in a way that would 'constitute a public health and social problem'.

Drives to nonmedical (or nonprescription) drug use are:[4]

- *Relief of anxiety*, tension and depression; escape from personal psychological problems; detachment from harsh reality; ease of social intercourse.
- *Search for self-knowledge* and for meaning in life, including religion. The cult of 'experience' including aestheticism and artistic creation, sex and 'genuine', 'sincere' interpersonal relationships, to obtain a sense of 'belonging'.
- *Rebellion against* or *despair* about orthodox social values and the environment. Fear of missing something, and conformity with own social subgroup (the young, especially).
- *Fun*, amusement, recreation, excitement, curiosity (the young, especially).

Rewards for the individual

It is inherently unlikely that chemicals could be central to a constructive *culture* and no convincing support for the assertion has yet been produced. (That chemicals might be central to a destructive culture is another matter.) Certainly, like-minded people practising what are often illegal activities will gather into closely knit subgroups for mutual support, and will feel a sense of community, but that is hardly a 'culture'. Even when drug-using subgroups are accepted as representing a subculture, it may be doubted if drugs are sufficiently central to their ideology to justify using 'drug' in the title. But claims for value to the individual and to society of drug experience must surely be tested by the criterion of fruitfulness for both, and the judgement of the individual concerned alone is insufficient; it must be agreed by others. The results of both

legal and illegal drug use do not give encouragement to press for a large-scale experiment in this field.

It is claimed that drugs provide *mystical experience* and that this has valid religious content. Mystical experience may be defined as a combination of feelings of unity (oneness with nature and/or God), ineffability (experience beyond the subject's power to express), joy (peace, sacredness), knowledge (insight into truths of life and values, illuminations), and transcendence (of space and time).

When such states do occur there remains the question whether they tell us something about a reality outside the individual or merely something about the mind of the person having the experience. Mystical experience is not a normal dose-related pharmacodynamic effect of any drug, its occurrence depends on many factors such as the subject's personality, mood, environment, conditioning. The drug facilitates rather than induces the experience; and drugs can facilitate unpleasant as well as pleasant experiences. It is not surprising that mystical experience can occur with a wide range of drugs that alter consciousness:

> ... I seemed at first in a state of utter blankness ... with a keen vision of what was going on in the room around me, but no sensation of touch. I thought that I was near death; when, suddenly, my soul became aware of God, who was manifestly dealing with me, handling me, so to speak, in an intense personal, present reality ... I cannot describe the ecstasy I felt.[5]

This experience occurred in the 19th century with chloroform; a general anaesthetic obsolete because of cardiac depression and hepatotoxicity.

There is no good evidence that drugs can produce experience that passes the test of results, i.e. fruitfulness to the individual and to society. Plainly there is a risk of the experience becoming an end in itself rather than a means of development.

It is interesting that the double-blind controlled trial has been attempted in the field of spiritual experience and knowledge where, it has been pointed out, the passion with which a belief is

---

[4] Psychoactive drug use by medical professionals has been studied by questionnaire (USA). Responses by approx. 300 out of 500 approached in each group. Use for recreation, self-treatment or to assist work or athletic performance (caffeine and alcohol excluded) was: physicians 59%; pharmacists 46%; medical students 77%; pharmacy students 62%. The results do not differ substantially from those of general urban populations. The trend of such use is upwards; the authors express concern. McAuliffe et al 1986 New England Journal of Medicine 315: 805.

[5] Quoted in James W 1902 Varieties of religious experience. Longmans, Harlow, and many subsequent editions of this classic. See also Leary T 1970. The politics of ecstasy. MacGibbon and Kee, London. Other editions, USA.

defended is commonly in inverse proportion to the strength of the evidence that can be adduced for it.

Twenty well-prepared Christian theological students received, by random allocation, either psilocybin (a hallucinogen) or nicotinic acid (as an 'active' placebo). They attended a Good Friday church service lasting 2.5 h and wrote accounts of their feelings, completed questionnaires and were interviewed to elicit evidence of mystical experience. It was concluded that psilocybin facilitated mystical experience.[6] Whilst such work is of interest it may be remembered that religious experience

> ...means the whole of life interpreted, rather than isolated feelings. A religious man is not one who has 'experiences'...but one who takes all life in a religious way...religious experience...is not the isolated outbreak of abnormal phenomena in this or that individual (though to read some psychological treatments of religious experience one would suppose so).[7]

CONCLUSIONS

The value of nonmedical use of psychotropic drugs can be summed up thus.

- *For relaxation*, recreation, protection from and relief of stress and anxiety; relief of depression: moderate use of some 'soft' drugs may be accepted as part of our society.
- *For spiritually valuable experience*: justification is extremely doubtful.
- *As basis for a 'culture'* in the sense that drug experience (a) can be, and (b) should be central to an individually or socially constructive way of life: a claim without validity.
- *For acute excitement*: extremely dangerous.

GENERAL PATTERN OF USE

Divisions are not rigid and they change with fashion.

- Any age: alcohol; tobacco; mild dependence on hypnotics and tranquillisers; occasional use of LSD and cannabis.

---

[6] Pahnke W N 1970 In: Aaronson et al (eds) Psychedelics: the uses and implications of hallucinogenic drugs. Hogarth Press, London.

[7] Dodd C H 1960 The authority of the Bible. Fontana, London.

- Aged 16–35 years: hard-use drugs, chiefly heroin, cocaine and amphetamines (including 'ecstasy'). Surviving users tend to reduce or relinquish heavy use as they enter middle age.
- Under 16 years: volatile inhalants, e.g. solvents of glues, aerosol sprays, vaporised (by heat) paints, 'solvent or substance' abuse, 'glue-sniffing'.
- Miscellaneous: any drug or combination of drugs reputed to alter consciousness may have a local vogue, however brief, e.g. drugs used in parkinsonism and metered aerosols for asthma.

Decriminalisation and legalisation

The decision whether any drug is acceptable in medical practice is made after an evaluation of its safety in relation to its efficacy. The same principle should be used for drugs for nonmedical or social use. But the usual scientific criteria for evaluating efficacy are hardly applicable. The reasons why people choose to use drugs for nonmedical purposes are listed above. None of them carries serious weight if the drug is found to have serious risks to the individuals[8] or to society, with either acute or chronic use. Ordinary prudence dictates that any such risks should be carefully defined before a decision on legalisation is made.

There is no doubt that many individuals think, rightly or wrongly, that private use of cannabis, if not of 'harder' drugs, is their own business and that the law should permit this freedom. The likelihood that demand can be extinguished by education or by threats appears to be zero. The autocratic implementation of laws that are not widely accepted in the community leads to violent crime, corruption in the police, and alienation of reasonable people who would otherwise be an important stabilising influence in society.

But though written laws are so often inflexible and combine what would best be separated, informal judicial discretion under present law may be permitting more experimentation than would

---

[8] Hazard to the individual is not a matter for the individual alone if it also has consequences for society.

recurrent legislative debate. It is recognised that this untidy approach, which may be best for the time being, cannot satisfy the extravagant advocates either of licence or of repression.

A suggested intermediate course for cannabis, and perhaps even for heroin, is that penalties for possession of small amounts for personal consumption should be removed (decriminalisation as opposed to legalisation), whilst retaining criminal penalties for suppliers. Such an approach is increasingly and informally being implemented.

Nobody knows what would happen if the production, supply and use of the major drugs, cannabis, heroin and cocaine, were to be legalised, as tobacco and alcohol are legalised (with weak selling restrictions). There are those who, shocked by the evils of illegal trade, consider that legalisation could only make matters better. The debate continues about what kinds of evils affecting the individual and society can be tolerated and how they can be balanced against each other.

Dependence

> **Drug dependence** is a state arising from repeated, periodic or continuous administration of a drug, that results in harm to the individual and sometimes to society. The subject feels a desire, need or compulsion to continue using the drug and feels ill if abruptly deprived of it (abstinence or withdrawal syndrome).

For discussion of abrupt withdrawal of drugs in general see page 107.

Drug dependence is characterised by:

- Psychological dependence: the first to appear; there is emotional distress if the drug is withdrawn.
- Physical dependence: accompanies psychological dependence in some cases; there is a physical illness if the drug is withdrawn.
- Tolerance.

PSYCHOLOGICAL DEPENDENCE

This may occur with any drug that alters consciousness however bizarre, e.g. muscarine (see index) and to some that, in ordinary doses, do not, e.g. non-narcotic analgesics, purgatives, diuretics; these latter provide problems of psychopathology rather than of psychopharmacology.

Psychological dependence can occur merely on a tablet or injection, regardless of its content, as well as to drug substances. Mild dependence does not require that a drug should have important psychic effects; the subject's beliefs as to what it does are as important, e.g. purgative and diuretic dependence in people obsessed with dread of obesity. We are all physically dependent on food, and some develop a strong emotional dependence and eat too much (or the reverse); sexual activity, with its unique mix of arousal and relaxation, can for some become compulsive or addictive.

PHYSICAL DEPENDENCE AND TOLERANCE

Physical dependence and tolerance imply that adaptive changes have taken place in body tissues so that when the drug is abruptly withdrawn these adaptive changes are left unopposed, resulting generally in a rebound overactivity. The discovery that the CNS employs morphine-like substances (endorphins) as neurotransmitters offers the explanation that exogenously administered opioid may suppress endogenous production of endorphins by a feedback mechanism. When administration of opioid is suddenly stopped there is an immediate deficiency of endogenous opioid, which thus causes the withdrawal syndrome.

Tolerance may result from a compensatory biochemical cell response to continued exposure to opioid. In short, both physical dependence and tolerance may follow the operation of homeostatic adaptation to continued high occupancy of opioid receptors. Changes of similar type may occur with GABA transmission, involving benzodiazepines. Tolerance also results from metabolic changes (enzyme induction) and physiological/behavioural adaptation to drug effects, e.g. alcohol.

Physical dependence develops to a substantial degree with cerebral depressants, but is minor or absent with excitant drugs.

There is commonly cross-tolerance between drugs of similar, and sometimes even of dissimilar, chemical groups, e.g. alcohol and benzodi-azepines.

There is danger in personal experimentation; as an American addict has succinctly put it, 'They all think they can take just one joy-pop but it's the first one that hooks you'.[9]

Unfortunately subjects cannot decide for themselves that their dependence will remain mild.

TYPES OF DRUG DEPENDENCE

The World Health Organization recommends that drug dependence be specified by 'type' when under detailed discussion.

Morphine-type:

— psychological dependence severe
— physical dependence severe; develops quickly
— tolerance marked
— cross-tolerance with related drugs
— naloxone induces abstinence syndrome

Barbiturate-type:

— psychological dependence severe
— physical dependence very severe; develops slowly at high doses
— tolerance less marked than with morphine
— cross-tolerance with alcohol, chloral, meprobamate, glutethimide, chlordiazepoxide, diazepam, etc.

Amphetamine-type:

— psychological dependence severe
— physical dependence slight: psychoses occur during use
— tolerance occurs

Cannabis-type:

— psychological dependence
— physical dependence dubious (no characteristic abstinence syndrome)
— tolerance slight

Cocaine-type:

— psychological dependence severe
— physical dependence slight
— tolerance slight (to some actions)

Alcohol-type:

— psychological dependence severe
— physical dependence with prolonged heavy use
— cross-tolerance with other sedatives

Tobacco-type:

— psychological dependence strong
— physical dependence slight

Drug mixtures:

Barbiturate-amphetamine mixtures induce a characteristic alteration of mood that does not occur with either drug alone
— psychological dependence strong
— physical dependence occurs
— tolerance occurs
Heroin-cocaine mixtures: similar characteristics.

ROUTE OF ADMINISTRATION AND EFFECT

With the i.v. route or inhalation much higher peak plasma concentrations can be reached than with oral administration. This accounts for the 'kick' or 'flash' that abusers report and which many seek, likening it to sexual orgasm or better. As an addict said 'The ultimate high is death' and it has been reported that when hearing of someone dying of an overdose, some addicts will seek out the vendor since it is evident he is selling 'really good stuff'.[10] Addicts who rely on illegal sources are inevitably exposed to being supplied diluted or even inert preparations at high prices. North American addicts who have come to the UK believing themselves to be accustomed to high doses of heroin, have suffered acute poisoning when given, probably for the first time, pure heroin at an official UK drug dependence clinic.

SUPPLY OF DRUGS TO ADDICTS

In the UK, supply of officially listed drugs (a range of opioids and cocaine) *for the purpose of sustaining addiction* is permitted under strict legal limitations. Addicts must be notified by the physician to the

---

[9] Maurer D W, Vogel V H 1962 Narcotics and narcotic addiction. Thomas, Springfield.

[10] Bourne P 1976 Acute drug abuse emergencies. Academic Press, New York.

Home Office and in the case of some opioids and cocaine, the physician requires a special licence. By such procedure it is hoped to limit the expansion of the illicit market, and its accompanying crime and dangers to health, e.g. from infected needles and syringes. The object is to sustain young (usually) addicts, who cannot be weaned from drug use, in reasonable health until they relinquish their dependence (often over about 10 years).

When injectable drugs are prescribed there is currently no way of assessing the truth of an addict's statement that he/she needs x mg of heroin (or other drug), and the dose has to be assessed intuitively by the doctor. This has resulted in addicts obtaining more than they need and selling it, sometimes to initiate new users. The use of oral methadone or other opioid for maintenance by prescription is devised to mitigate this problem.

TREATMENT OF DEPENDENCE

Withdrawal of the drug. Whilst obviously important, this is only a step on what can be a long and often disappointing journey to psychological and social rehabilitation, e.g. in 'therapeutic communities'. In the case of drugs that cause physical dependence, withdrawal may be gradual (over about 10 days or more) or sudden, provided that in the latter case steps are taken to limit the abstinence syndrome.

This may be done by judicious use of the same drug, but some prefer to use alternative drugs, generally, though not always, of similar kind, having a longer duration of action. A *heroin* addict can be given methadone, an *alcoholic* may be given chlormethiazole or chlordiazepoxide, a *barbiturate* addict may be given phenobarbitone. If patients are in very poor physical condition, withdrawal should be postponed until they are better. Sympathetic autonomic overactivity can be treated with a β-adrenoceptor blocker (or clonidine) (see Abrupt withdrawal of drugs).

Maintenance and relapse. Relapsed addicts who live a fairly normal life are sometimes best treated by supplying drugs under supervision. There is no legal objection to doing this in the UK (see above) but naturally this course, which abandons hope of cure, should not be adopted until it is certain that cure is virtually impossible. A less harmful drug by a less harmful route may be substituted, e.g. oral methadone for i.v. heroin. Addicts are often particularly reluctant to abandon the i.v. route, which provides the 'immediate high' that they find, or originally found, so desirable.

Drugs are adjuvant only in the prevention of relapse, e.g. the use of an opioid antagonist so that if, in a moment of weakness, the subject takes a dose of heroin, the 'kick' is blocked. Such treatment requires on the part of the subject a strong will to succeed.

Severe pain in an opioid addict presents a special problem. High-efficacy opioid may be ineffective (tolerance) or overdose may result; low-efficacy opioids will not only be ineffective but may induce withdrawal symptoms, especially if they have some antagonist effect, e.g. pentazocine. This leaves as drugs of choice nonsteroidal anti-inflammatory drugs (NSAIDs), e.g. indomethacin, and nefopam (which is neither opioid nor NSAID).

Mortality

Young illicit users by i.v. injection (heroin, barbiturates, benzodiazepines, amphetamine) have a mortality up to $\times$ 40 normal. Either death follows overdose, or septicaemia, endocarditis, hepatitis, AIDS, gas gangrene, tetanus and pulmonary embolism ensue from the contaminated materials used without aseptic precautions (schemes to provide clean equipment mitigate this). Smugglers of illicit cocaine or heroin sometimes carry the drug in plastic bags concealed by swallowing or in the rectum ('body packing'). Leakage of the packages, not surprisingly, may have a fatal result.

Escalation

A variable proportion of subjects who start with cannabis eventually take heroin. This disposition to progress from occasional to frequent soft use of drugs through to hard drug use, when it occurs, is less likely to be due to pharmacological actions, than to psychosocial factors, although increased suggestibility induced by cannabis may contribute.

De-escalation also occurs as users become disillusioned with drugs over about 10 years.

'Designer drugs'

This unhappily chosen term means molecular modifications produced in secret for profit by skilled and criminally minded chemists. Manipulation of fentanyl has resulted in compounds of extraordinary potency.

In 1976 a too-clever 23-year-old addict seeking to manufacture his own pethidine 'took a synthetic shortcut and injected himself with what was later with his help proved to be two closely related byproducts; one was MPTP (methylphenyltetrahydropyridine).[11] Three days later he developed a severe parkinsonian syndrome that responded to levodopa. MPTP selectively destroys melanin-containing cells in the substantia nigra. Further such cases have occurred from use of supposed synthetic heroin. MPTP has since been used in experimental research on parkinsonism.

What the future holds for individuals and for society in this area can only be imagined.

Volatile substance abuse

Seekers of the 'self-gratifying high' also inhale any volatile substance that may affect the central nervous system. These include: adhesives ('glue-sniffing'), lacquer-paint solvents, petrol, nail varnish, any pressurised aerosol and butane liquid gas (which latter especially may 'freeze' the larynx, allowing fatal inhalation of food, drink, gastric contents, or even the liquid itself to flood the lungs). Even solids, e.g. paint scrapings, solid shoe polish, may be volatilised over a fire. These substances are particularly abused by the very young (schoolchildren), no doubt largely because they are accessible at home and in ordinary shops and they cannot easily buy alcohol or 'street' drugs (although this latter may be changing as dealers target the youngest). CNS effects include confusion and hallucinations, ataxia, dysarthria, coma, convulsions, respiratory failure. Liver, kidney, lung and heart damage occur. Sudden cardiac death may be due to sensitisation of the heart to endogenous catecholamines. If the substance is put in a plastic bag from which the user takes deep inhalations, or is sprayed in a confined space, e.g. cupboard, there is particularly high risk.

> A 17-year-old boy was offered the use of a plastic bag and a can of hair spray at a beach party. The hair spray was released into the plastic bag and the teenager put his mouth to the open end of the bag and inhaled . . . he exclaimed, 'God, this stuff hits ya fast!' He got up, ran 100 yards; and died.[12]

Signs of frequent volatile substance abuse include peri-oral eczema and inflammation of the upper respiratory tract.

Drugs and sport

The rewards of competitive sport, both financial and in personal and national prestige, are the cause of determination to win at (almost) any cost. Drugs are used to enhance performance though efficacy is largely undocumented. Detection can be difficult when the drugs or metabolites are closely related to or identical with endogenous substances, and when the drug can be stopped well before the event without apparent loss of efficacy, e.g. anabolic steroids (but suppression of endogenous trophic hormones can be measured, and can assist).

PERFORMANCE ENHANCEMENT

There follow illustrations of the mechanisms by which drugs can enhance performance in various sports; naturally, these are proscribed by the authorities (International Olympic Committee (IOC) Medical Commission, and the governing bodies of individual sports).

For **'strength sports'** in which body weight and brute strength are the principal determinants (weight lifting, rowing, wrestling): *anabolic agents*, e.g. clenbuterol (β-adrenoceptor agonist), methandienone, nandrolone, stanozolol, testosterone. Taken together with a high-protein diet and exer-

---

[11] Williams A 1984 British Medical Journal 289: 1402.
Davis G C et al 1979 Psychiatry Research 1: 249.

[12] Bass M 1970 Sudden sniffing death. Journal of the American Medical Association 212: 2075.

cise, these increase lean body weight (muscle) but not necessarily strength. It is claimed they allow more intensive training regimens (limiting cell injury in muscles). Rarely, there may be episodes of violent behaviour, known amongst athletes as 'roid [steroid] rage'.

High doses are used, with risk of liver damage (cholestatic, tumours) especially if the drug is taken longterm, which is certainly insufficient to deter 'sportsmen'. They may be more inclined to take more seriously the fact the anabolic steroids suppress pituitary gonadotrophin, and so testosterone production.

Growth hormone (somatrem, somatropin) and *corticotrophin* use may be combined with that of anabolic steroids. *Chorionic gonadotrophin* may be taken to stimulate testosterone production (and prevent testicular atrophy). Similarly, *tamoxifen* (an anti-oestrogen) may be used to attenuate some of the effects of anabolic steroids.

For events in which **output of energy** is explosive (100 m sprint): *stimulants*, e.g.amphetamine, cocaine, ephedrine and caffeine (>12 mg/l in urine). Death has probably occurred in bicycle racing (continuous hard exercise with short periods of sprint) due to hyperthermia and cardiac dysrhythmia in metabolically stimulated and vasoconstricted subjects exercising maximally under a hot sun.

For **endurance sports** to enhance the oxygen carrying capacity of the blood (bicycling, marathon running): *erythropoietin*, *'blood doping'* (the athlete has blood withdrawn and stored, then transfused once the deficit had been made up naturally, so raising the plasma haemoglobin above normal).

For events in which **steadiness of hand** is essential (pistol, rifle shooting): *β-adrenoceptor blockers*. Tremor is reduced by the β_2-adrenoceptor blocking effect, as are somatic symptoms of anxiety.

For events in which **body pliancy** is a major factor (gymnastics): *delaying puberty* in child gymnasts by endocrine techniques.

For **weight reduction**, e.g. boxers, jockeys: *diuretics*. These are also used to flush out other drugs in the hope of escaping detection; severe volume depletion can cause venous thrombosis and pulmonary embolism.

Generally, owing to recognition of natural biological differences most competitive events are sex-segregated. In many events men have a natural physical **biological advantage** and the (inevitable) consequence has been that women have been deliberately virilised (by administration of *androgens*) so that they may outperform their sisters.

It seems safe to assume that anything that can be thought up to gain advantage will be tried by competitors eager for immediate fame. Reliable data are difficult to obtain in these areas. No doubt placebo effects are important, i.e. beliefs as to what has been taken and what effects ought to follow.

The dividing line between what is and what is not acceptable practice is hard to draw. *Caffeine* can improve physical performance and illustrates the difficulty of deciding what is 'permissible' or 'impermissible'. A cup of coffee is part of a normal diet, but some consider taking the same amount of caffeine in a tablet, injection or suppository to be 'doping'.

For minor injuries sustained during athletic training *NSAIDs* and *corticosteroids* suppress symptoms and allow the training to proceed maximally. Their use is allowed subject to restrictions about route of administration, but strong opioids are disallowed. Similarly, the IOC Medical Code defines acceptable and unacceptable treatments for relief of cough, hay fever, diarrhoea, vomiting, pain and asthma. Doctors should remember that they may get their athlete patients into trouble with sports authorities by inadvertent prescribing of banned substances.[13]

Some of the isssues seem to be ethical rather than medical as witness the reported competition success of a swimmer who, it is alleged, had been persuaded under *hypnosis* into the belief that he was being pursued by a shark.

Tobacco

Tobacco was introduced to Europe from South America in the 16th century. Although its potential for harm was early recognised its use was taken up avidly in every society that met it.

---

[13] UK prescribers can find general advice in the British National Formulary.

COMPOSITION

The composition of tobacco smoke is complex (about 500 compounds have been identified) and varies with the type of tobacco and the way it is smoked. The chief pharmacologically active ingredients are *nicotine* (acute effects) and *tars* (chronic effects).

Smoke of cigars and pipes is *alkaline* (pH 8.5) and nicotine is relatively un-ionised and lipid-soluble so that it is readily absorbed in the mouth. Cigar and pipe smokers thus obtain nicotine without inhaling (they also have a lower death rate from lung cancer; which is caused by non-nicotine constituents).

Smoke of cigarettes is *acidic* (pH 5.3) and nicotine is relatively ionised and insoluble in lipids. Desired amounts are absorbed only if nicotine is taken into the lungs, where the enormous surface area for absorption compensates for the lower lipid solubility. Cigarette smokers therefore inhale (and have a high rate of death from tar-induced lung cancer). The amount of nicotine absorbed from tobacco smoke varies from 90% in those who inhale to 10% in those who do not.

Tobacco smoke contains 1–5% *carbon monoxide* and habitual smokers have 3–7% (heavy smokers as much as 15%) of their haemoglobin as carboxyhaemoglobin, which cannot carry oxygen. This is sufficient to reduce exercise capacity in patients with angina pectoris. Chronic carboxyhaemoglobinaemia causes polycythaemia (which increases the viscosity of the blood).

Substances *carcinogenic* to animals (polycyclic hydrocarbons and nicotine-derived N-nitrosamines) have been identified in tobacco smoke condensates from cigarettes, cigars and pipes. Polycyclic hydrocarbons are responsible for the hepatic enzyme induction that occurs in smokers.

Tobacco dependence

Psychoanalysts have made a characteristic contribution to the problem. 'Getting something orally', one asserts . . . , 'is the first great libidinous experience in life'; first the breast, then the bottle, then the comforter, then food and finally the cigarette.[14]

Sigmund Freud, inventor of psychoanalysis, was a life-long tobacco addict. He suggested that some children may be victims of a 'constitutional intensification of the erotogenic significance of the labial region', which, if it persists, will provide a powerful motive for smoking.[15]

The immediate satisfaction of smoking is due to nicotine and also to tars, which provide flavour. Initially the factors are psychosocial; pharmacodynamic effects are unpleasant. But under the psychosocial pressures the subject continues, learns to limit and adjust nicotine intake, so that the pleasant pharmacological effects of nicotine develop and tolerance to the adverse effects occurs. Thus to the psychosocial pressure is now added pharmacological pleasure. The extraordinary power of this 'pleasure-drug', nicotine, has been summed up,

'And a woman is only a woman, but a good cigar is a Smoke.'[16]

TYPES OF SMOKING: A SUMMARY

Nonpharmacological

● Psychosocial: uses symbolic value of the act to increase social confidence, status and self-esteem.
● Sensorimotor: to obtain oral, sensory and manipulatory satisfaction.

Pharmacological

● Indulgent, the commonest: to obtain pleasure or to enhance an already pleasurable situation.
● Stimulant: to get a 'lift', to aid thinking or concentration, help with stressful situation, or help performance of monotonous task.
● Addictive: to avoid withdrawal feelings that occur as plasma nicotine ($t\frac{1}{2}$ 2 h) concentration

---

[14] Scott R B 1957 British Medical Journal 1: 67 1.

[15] Quoted in Royal Collage of Physicians 1977 Smoking or health. Pitman, London. In 1929 Freud posed for a photograph holding a large cigar prominently. 'He was always a heavy smoker — twenty cigars a day were his usual allowance and he tolerated abstinence from it with the greatest difficulty'. Jones E 1953 Sigmund Freud: life and work. Hogarth Press, London.

[16] Rudyard Kipling, poet (1865–1936).

falls below a minimum, usually about 30 min after the end of the last smoke. (The plasma concentration of nicotine is sustained by changes in rate and depth of inhalation.)

CHARACTERISTICS OF TOBACCO DEPENDENCE

Psychological dependence is extremely strong and accounts largely for the difficulty of stopping smoking. Tolerance and some physical dependence occurs. Transient withdrawal effects include EEG and sleep changes, impaired performance in some psychomotor tests, disturbance of mood, and increased appetite (with weight gain), though it is difficult to disentangle psychological from physical effects in these last.

ACUTE EFFECTS OF SMOKING TOBACCO

- *Increased airways resistance* occurs due to the nonspecific effects of submicronic particles, e.g. carbon particles less than 1 μm across. The effect is reflex; even inert particles of this size cause bronchial narrowing sufficient to double airways resistance; this is insufficient to cause dyspnoea, though it might affect athletic performance. Pure nicotine inhalations of concentration comparable to that reached in smoking do not increase airways resistance.
- *Ciliary activity*, after transient stimulation, is depressed, and particles are removed from the lungs more slowly.
- *Carbon monoxide absorption* may be clinically important in the presence of coronary heart disease (see above) although it is physiologically insignificant in healthy young adults.

Nicotine pharmacology

Pharmacodynamics

Large doses.[17] Nicotine is an agonist to receptors at the ends of peripheral cholinergic nerves whose cell bodies lie in the central nervous system, i.e. it acts at autonomic ganglia and at the voluntary neuromus-

cular junction. This is what is meant by the term 'nicotine-like' or 'nicotinic' effect. Higher doses paralyse at the same points. The central nervous system is stimulated, including the vomiting centre, both directly and via chemoreceptors in the carotid body; tremors and convulsions may occur. As with the peripheral actions, depression follows stimulation.

Doses from/with smoking. Nicotine causes release of catecholamines in the CNS, also serotonin, and antidiuretic hormone, corticotrophin and growth hormone. The effects of nicotine on viscera are probably largely reflex, from stimulation of sensory receptors (chemoreceptors) in the carotid and aortic bodies, pulmonary circulation and left ventricle. Some of the results are mutually antagonistic.

The following account tells what generally happens after one cigarette, from which about 1 mg nicotine is absorbed, although much depends on the amount and depth of inhalation and on the duration of end-inspiratory breath-holding:

On the cardiovascular system the effects are those of sympathetic autonomic stimulation. There is vasoconstriction in the skin and vasodilatation in the muscles, tachycardia and a rise in blood pressure of about 15 mmHg systolic and 10 mmHg diastolic, and increased plasma noradrenaline. Ventricular extrasystoles may occur. Cardiac output, work and oxygen consumption increase. Increased demand for blood flow that is not met because coronary vessels are narrowed by atherosclerosis may be a mechanism of tobacco-induced angina pectoris. Nicotine increases platelet adhesiveness, an effect

---

[17] Fatal nicotine poisoning has been reported from smoking, from swallowing tobacco, from tobacco enemas, from topical application to the skin and from accidental drinking of nicotine insecticide preparations. In 1932 a florist sat down on a chair, on the seat of which a 40% free nicotine insecticide solution had been spilled. Fifteen minutes later he felt ill (vomiting, sweating, faintness, and respiratory difficulty, followed by loss of consciousness and cardiac irregularity). He recovered in hospital over about 24 h. On the fourth day he was deemed well enough to leave hospital and was given his clothes which had been kept in a paper bag. He noticed the trousers were still damp. Within one hour of leaving hospital he had to be readmitted suffering again from poisoning due to nicotine absorbed transdermally from his still contaminated trousers. He recovered over three weeks, apart from persistent ventricular extrasystoles [Faulkner J M 1933 JAMA 100: 1663].

that may be clinically significant in atheroma and thrombosis.

Metabolic rate. Nicotine increases the metabolic rate, only slightly at rest,[18] but approximately doubles it during light exercise (occupational tasks, housework). This may be due to increase in autonomic sympathetic activity. The effect declines over 24 h on stopping smoking and accounts for the characteristic weight gain that is so disliked and which is sometimes given as a reason for continuing or resuming smoking. Smokers weigh 2–4 kg less than nonsmokers (not enough to be a health issue).

Tolerance develops to some of the effects of nicotine, taken repeatedly over a few hours; a first experience commonly causes nausea and vomiting, which quickly ceases with repetition of smoking. Tolerance is usually rapidly lost; the first cigarette of the day has a greater effect on the cardiovascular system than do subsequent cigarettes.

Conclusion: the pleasurable effects of smoking are derived from a complex mixture of multiple pharmacological and nonpharmacological factors.

In this account nicotine is represented as being the major (but not the sole) determinant of tobacco dependence after the smoker has adapted to the usual initial unpleasant effects. But there remains some uncertainty as to its role, e.g. nicotine i.v. fails adequately to substitute the effects of smoking. An understanding of the full function of nicotine is important if less harmful alternatives to smoking, such as nicotine chewing gum, are to be exploited.

Pharmacokinetics

Nicotine is absorbed through mucous membranes in a highly pH-dependent fashion. The $t^{1/2}$ is 2 h. It is largely metabolised to inert substances, e.g. cotinine, though some is excreted unchanged in the urine (pH dependent, it is unionised at acid pH). Cotinine is used as a marker for nicotine intake in

smoking surveys because of its convenient $t^{1/2}$ (20 h).

Effects of chronic smoking

The Royal College of Physicians of London feels it has a duty to pronounce 'on a question of public health when action is required'. In 1725 it offered advice 'concerning the disastrous consequences of the rising consumption of cheap gin', and in 1962, 1977 and 1983, on the effects of smoking on health.[19] Its published reports are models of clarity and brevity.[20] The USA Public Health Service has published extensive reports.

The evidence for an association of smoking with various diseases consists of case-control and cohort studies. *To decide whether an observed association is causal*, several criteria, no one of which alone is sufficient, must be satisfied. These include:

● Consistency of association: diverse methods of approach should give the same answer.
● Specificity and strength of association: specificity means the precision with which the presence of, e.g. chronic bronchitis or lung cancer, can be used to predict that the victim smokes and vice versa; also the size of effect should be sufficient not to be obscured by any associated but noncausal factors, e.g. alcohol consumption.
● Temporal association: the supposed cause, smoking, must operate before any evidence of the disease appears.
● Coherence of association: the associated event should fit in with all known facts of the natural history of the disease.

MORTALITY

The importance of finding out just what smoking does or does not do is shown below:

---

[18] The metabolic rate at rest accounts for about 70% of daily energy expenditure.

[19] It is not intended to imply that the College was unconcerned about public health for over a century. This account relies heavily on these reports and on those of the USA Public Health Service.

[20] We are grateful to the College for permission to use its Reports in the account that follows.

Percentage of men aged 35 who may expect to die before the age of 65:	
Nonsmokers	15%
Smokers of 1–14 cigarettes a day	22%
Smokers of 15–24 cigarettes a day	25%
Smokers of 25 or more cigarettes a day	40%

- The average loss of life of a smoker of 25 cigarettes/day is about 5 years (UK and USA studies).
- The time by which a habitual smoker's life is shortened is about 5 min per cigarette smoked.
- The extra risk of death (compared with that of lifelong nonsmokers) declines after a smoker ceases to smoke and returns to about that of nonsmokers over 10–15 years.

The above applies to ordinary cigarettes.

SMOKING AND CANCER

Bronchial carcinoma

Between 1920 and 1950 an epidemic of bronchial carcinoma occurred (rate in men increased × 20). Cigarette smoking satisfies the criteria for determining causation of an association (above) (lesser causes include exposure to a variety of industrial chemicals and atmospheric pollution).

In men under 65 the death-rate is now falling, but it is still rising in women (except the youngest age group). These facts are compatible with the inevitable 20–40-year lag before changed habits affect the incidence of the disease. The risk of death from lung cancer is related to the number of cigarettes smoked and the age of starting. Giving up smoking reduces the risk of death.

Other cancers

The risk of smokers developing cancer of the mouth, throat and oesophagus is 5–10 times greater than that of nonsmokers. It is as great for pipe and cigar smokers as it is for cigarette smokers. Cancer of the pancreas, kidney and urinary tract is also commoner in smokers.

DISEASES OF THE HEART AND BLOOD VESSELS

Ischaemic heart disease (IHD) is now the leading cause of death in many developed countries. In the UK about 30% of these deaths can be attributed to smoking.

> Under the age of 65 years smokers are about twice as likely to die of ischaemic heart disease as are non-smokers, and heavy smokers about 3.5 times as likely.

Sudden death may be the first manifestation of IHD and, especially in young men, is related to cigarette smoking. Smoking is especially dangerous for people in whom other risk factors (increased blood cholesterol, high blood pressure) are present.

Atherosclerotic narrowing of the smallest coronary arteries is enormously increased in heavy and even in moderate smokers; the *increased platelet adhesiveness* caused by smoking increases the readiness with which thrombi form.

Stopping smoking reduces the excess risk of IHD in people under the age of 65, and after about 4 years of abstinence the risk approximates to that of nonsmokers.

Pipe and cigar smokers run little or no excess risk of IHD provided they are not heavy smokers and do not inhale. Heavy cigarette smokers who change over to pipe or cigar smoking often continue to inhale and thereby fail to reduce their risk.

Disease of the arteries of the leg is even more closely related to smoking, over 95% of patients with this condition being smokers.

Femoropopliteal vein grafts to coronary arteries survive less well in smokers.

Death from *aneurysm of the aorta* is about 5 times commoner in smokers.

SMOKING AND CHRONIC LUNG DISEASE

The adverse effects of cigarette smoke on the lungs may be separated into two distinct conditions.

- *Chronic mucus hypersecretion*, which causes persistent cough with sputum and fits with the original definition of simple chronic bronchitis. This condition arises chiefly in the large airways, usually clears up when the subject stops smoking and does not on its own carry any substantial risk of death.
- *Chronic obstructive lung disease*, which causes

difficulty in breathing due to narrowing of the air passages in the lungs. This condition originates chiefly in the small airways, includes a variable element of destruction of peripheral lung units (emphysema), is progressive and largely irreversible and may ultimately lead to disability and death.

Both conditions can coexist in one person and they predispose to recurrent acute infective illnesses.

The obstructive syndrome is as specifically related to smoking as is lung cancer. Despite this, in discussing the health effects of tobacco, there has generally been far more emphasis on lung cancer than on this more disabling, but equally fatal disorder.

INTERACTIONS WITH DRUG THERAPY

Induction of hepatic drug metabolising enzymes by non-nicotine constituents of smoke causes increased metabolism of a range of drugs, including oestrogens, theophylline, warfarin.

WOMEN AND SMOKING

Fertility. Women who smoke are more likely to be infertile or take longer to conceive than women who do not smoke. In addition, smokers are more liable to have an earlier menopause than are nonsmokers. Increased metabolism of oestrogens may not be the whole explanation.

Complications of pregnancy. Smokers have a small increased risk of spontaneous abortion, bleeding during pregnancy and the development of various placental abnormalities. On the other hand, women who smoke have a lowered incidence of toxaemia of pregnancy though the advantages of this do not offset the disadvantages of smoking during pregnancy. The placenta is heavier in smoking than nonsmoking women and its diameter larger. The enlarged placenta and placental abnormalities may represent adaptations to lack of oxygen due to smoking, secondary to raised concentrations of circulating carboxyhaemoglobin.

The child. The babies of women who smoke are approximately 200 g lighter than those of women who do not smoke. They have an increased risk of death in the perinatal period which is independent of other variables such as social class, level of education, age of mother, race or extent of antenatal care. The increased risk rises twofold or more in heavy smokers and appears to be entirely accounted for by the placental abnormalities and the consequences of low birthweight.

Ex-smokers and women who give up smoking in the first 20 weeks of pregnancy have offspring whose birthweight is similar to that of the children of women who have never smoked.

Contraception. The risk of myocardial infarction, stroke and other cardiovascular diseases in young women is increased slightly by the combined oral contraceptive or by smoking. But when the two are added the risks multiply to an approximately tenfold increase in risk overall. This effect is unacceptably high ($\times$ 100) in heavy smokers (15/day or more) over 40 years of age. Only a light smoker under age 30 has a risk approximating to that of a nonsmoking user.

Starting and stopping use

Contrary to popular belief it is not generally difficult to stop, only 14% finding it 'very difficult'. But ex-smoker status is unstable and the longterm success rate of a smoking withdrawal clinic is rarely above 30%. The situation is summed up by the witticism, 'Giving up smoking is easy, I've done it many times'. That persons in upper economic/social classes, and especially doctors, are most likely to stop suggests the importance of educated recognition of the health risks.

Though they are as aware of the risks of smoking as men, women find it harder to stop; they consistently have lower success rates. This trend crosses every age group and occupation. Women particularly dislike the weight gain.

Aids *to giving up* smoking include nicotine as chewing gum, transdermal patch or oral spray (it is better to take nicotine than tobacco smoke). When used casually without special attention to technique, nicotine formulations have proved no better than other aids but, if used carefully and withdrawn as recommended, results are two to three times better than in smokers who try to stop without this assistance. Restlessness during terminal illness may be due to nicotine withdrawal and go unrecognised; a nicotine patch may benefit a (deprived) heavy smoker. Nicotine transdermal patches may cause nightmares and abnormal dreaming, and skin reactions (rash, pruritus and 'burning' at the application site).

If the patient is heavily tobacco-dependent and severe anxiety, irritability, headache, insomnia and weight gain (about 3 kg) and tension are concomitants of attempts to stop smoking, an anxiolytic sedative (or β-adrenoceptor blocker) may be useful for a short time, but it is important to avoid substituting one drug-dependence for another.

There is ample evidence to warrant strong advice against starting to smoke but over-hasty and unreasonable prohibitions on patients' longstanding pleasures (or vices) do no good. The pliable patient is made wretched, but most are merely alienated.

> My doctor's issued his decree
> That too much wine is killing me,
> And furthermore his ban he hurls
> Against my touching naked girls.
> How then? Must I no longer share
> Good wine or beauties, dark and fair?
> Doctor, goodbye, my sail's unfurled,
> I'm off to try the other world.
>   D G Rossetti, poet (1828–82)

Passive (involuntary) smoking

Many nonsmokers are exposed to tobacco smoke. At home, at work, on public transport and in public places, they can scarcely avoid breathing air contaminated by other people's smoke. This mode of smoke inhalation is not actively sought; it is involuntary or passive smoking.

It is difficult to measure the extent of the risk to health from passive smoke exposure, but evidence is accumulating of actual harm.[21] Although the risks are, naturally, smaller, the number of people affected is large. Smoke drawn through the tobacco and taken in by the smoker is known as mainstream smoke. Smoke which arises from smouldering tobacco and passes directly into the surrounding air, whence it may be inhaled by smokers and nonsmokers alike, is known as sidestream smoke.

Mainstream and sidestream smoke differ in composition, partly because of the different temperatures at which they are produced. Substances found in greater concentrations in undiluted sidestream smoke than in undiluted mainstream smoke include: nicotine ($\times$ 2.7), carbon monoxide ($\times$ 2.5), ammonia ($\times$ 73), and some carcinogens (e.g. benzo-a-pyrene $\times$ 3.4). Sidestream smoke constitutes about 85% of smoke generated in an average room during cigarette smoking.

Smoke-free air contains about 2.0 parts per million (ppm) of carbon monoxide. Examples of concentrations found in smoky conditions include 7–9 ppm at parties, 8–33 ppm in a conference room, 40 ppm in a submarine, and 12–110 ppm in a car. The concentrations reached obviously depend on the degree of ventilation. Under ordinary social conditions with good ventilation, levels are usually below 10 ppm when smokers are present and below 3 ppm when they are not.

The balance of evidence on passive smoking in adults is that there are small causal effects on bronchial carcinoma, decrease in lung function tests and increased cardiovascular disease (relative risks 1.2–2.7).[22]

In *children*, especially those under 5 years and where the mother smokes, effects are greater. There is an increase in acute respiratory and in middle ear infections and effusions (glue ear), in chronic respiratory disease and a decrease in lung function.

---

[21] In 1992 the USA Environmental Protection Agency classified environmental tobacco smoke as a known human carcinogen (EPA 1992 A/600/6–90/006F).

[22] A remarkable legal action was conducted in the Federal Court of Australia. The Court sat for 90 days and heard international evidence. The judge concluded that there is compelling evidence that cigarette smoke causes in nonsmokers, cancer, asthma attacks and, in children, respiratory disease. This judgement was a 'major turning point in the worldwide efforts to reduce smoking related diseases' (Chapman S et al 1991 British Medical Journal 302: 943).

Some of these matters remain controversial; epidemiological studies measuring small risks are inevitably imprecise.

Medical students and smoking

Male students smoke about the same as the general public of the same age and social class, i.e. the incidence of smoking is related to social class and not to specialised knowledge or to any feeling of obligation to set an example to others in this serious health issue. But, amongst women medical students, the smoking rate is only 50% that of the female general public of the same age and social class.

Hospital nurses are the sole studied health professional group in which smoking prevalence is not very much lower than in the general population.

Ethyl alcohol (Ethanol)

The services rendered by intoxicating substances in the struggle for happiness and in warding off misery rank so highly as a benefit that both individuals and races have given them an established position within their libido-economy. It is not merely the immediate gain in pleasure which one owes to them, but also a measure of that independence of the outer world which is so sorely craved ... We are aware that it is just this property which constitutes the danger and injuriousness of intoxicating substances ...[23]

Alcohol is chiefly important in medicine because of the consequences of its misuse/abuse. Alcohol misuse is a social problem with pharmacological aspects, which latter are discussed here.

The history of alcohol is part of the history of civilisation 'ever since Noah made his epoch-making discovery'.[24]

---

[23] Freud S 1939 Civilisation, war and death, Psycho-analytic epitomes, No. 4. Hogarth Press, London.

[24] Genesis; 9:21; Huxley A 1957 Annals of the New York Academy of Sciences 67: 675.

Pharmacokinetics

Absorption of alcohol taken orally is rapid, for it is highly lipid-soluble and diffusible from the stomach and the small intestine. Solutions above 20% are absorbed more slowly because high concentrations of alcohol inhibit gastric peristalsis, thus delaying the arrival of the alcohol in the small intestine which is the major site of absorption.

Absorption is delayed by food, especially milk, the effect of which is probably due to the fat it contains. Carbohydrate also delays absorption of alcohol.

Alcohol is subject to *gastric first-pass metabolism* (by alcohol dehydrogenases in the gastric but not in the intestinal wall); the liver, unusually, plays little role in presystemic elimination although it has a major role in its subsequent metabolism. The stomach wall in **women** has less alcohol dehydrogenase and due to this, and to the lower volume of distribution (see below), alcohol attains higher concentration in systemic blood for the same dose, per kg, than in men.

Distribution of alcohol is rapidly and throughout the body water (dist. vol. 0.7 l/kg men: 0.6 l/kg women); it is not selectively stored in any tissue.

Maximum *blood concentrations* after oral alcohol therefore depend on numerous factors including the total dose, sex, the strength of the solution, the time over which it is taken, the presence or absence of food, the time relations of taking food and alcohol and the kind of food eaten, as well as on the speed of metabolism and excretion. A single dose of alcohol, say 60 ml (48 g) (equivalent to 145 ml of whisky, 5–6 measures, or units; see Fig. 10.1), taken over a few minutes on an empty stomach will probably produce maximal blood concentration at 30–90 min and will not all be disposed of for 6–8 h or even more. There are very great individual variations.

Metabolism. About 95% of absorbed alcohol is metabolised, the remainder being excreted in the breath, urine and sweat; convenient methods of estimation of alcohol in all these are available.

Alcohol in the systemic circulation is oxidised in the liver; principally (90%) by alcohol dehydrogenase to acetaldehyde and then by aldehyde dehydrogenase to products that enter the citric acid cycle or are utilised in various anabolic reactions. Other alcohol-metabolising enzymes are microsomal cytochrome P450 2E1 (which is also induced by alcohol) and catalase.

Alcohol metabolism by alcohol dehydrogenase follows first-order kinetics after the smallest doses. Once the blood concentration exceeds about 10 mg/100 ml the enzymatic processes are saturated and elimination rate no longer increases with increasing concentration but becomes steady at 10–15 ml per hour in occasional drinkers. Thus alcohol is subject to *dose-dependent kinetics*, i.e. saturation or zero-order kinetics, with potentially major consequences for the individual.

Induction of hepatic drug metabolising enzymes occurs with repeated exposure to alcohol and this contributes to tolerance in habitual users, and to toxicity. Increased formation of metabolites causes organ damage in chronic overconsumption (acetaldehyde in the liver and probably fatty ethyl esters in other organs) and increases susceptibility to liver injury when heavy drinkers are exposed to anaesthetics, industrial solvents and to drugs. But chronic use of large amounts reduces hepatic metabolic capacity by causing cellular damage. An acute substantial dose of alcohol (binge drinking) inhibits hepatic drug metabolism.

Inter-ethnic variation is recognised in the ability to metabolise alcohol (see p. 172).

Blood concentration of alcohol has great medico-legal importance. Alcohol in alveolar air is in equilibrium with that in pulmonary capillary blood and reliable, easily handled devices have been developed to measure it, for this avoids 'assaulting' the subject with a needle and can be used by police at the roadside on both drivers and pedestrians.

Pharmacodynamics

Central nervous system. Alcohol acts in the

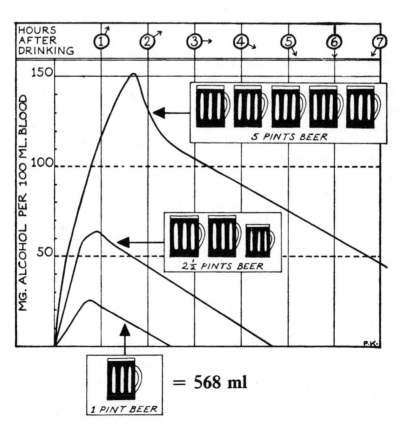

Fig. 10.1 Approximate blood concentrations after 3 doses of alcohol

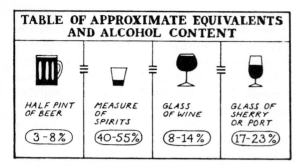

TABLE OF APPROXIMATE EQUIVALENTS AND ALCOHOL CONTENT

HALF PINT OF BEER	MEASURE OF SPIRITS	GLASS OF WINE	GLASS OF SHERRY OR PORT
3 - 8 %	40-55%	8 -14 %	17-23 %

Fig. 10.2 Four standard units of drink (in which social consumption is measured); a unit contains approx. 10 ml (8 g) of alcohol. Knowledge of blood alcohol concentration does not allow a reliable estimate of how much has been consumed

manner of general anaesthetics. It enhances GABA-stimulated flux of chloride through receptor-gated membrane ion channels, a receptor subtype effect that may be involved in the motor impairment caused by alcohol. It also enhances endorphin production.

It is not a stimulant; hyperactivity, when it occurs, is due to removal of inhibitory effects. The concept of higher levels of the central nervous system dominating lower levels is naive. There is a complex interdependence of various parts of the brain, so that changes at one 'level' affect function at other 'levels', 'higher' or 'lower'. Alcohol in ordinary doses may act chiefly on the arousal mechanisms of the brainstem reticular formation, inhibiting polysynaptic function and enhancing presynaptic inhibition. Direct cortical depression probably only occurs with high doses.

With increasing doses the subject passes through all the stages of general anaesthesia and may die of respiratory depression.[25] Psychic effects are the most important socially, and it is to obtain these that the drug is habitually used in so many societies, to make social intercourse not merely easy but even pleasant. They have been admirably described by Sollmann:

> The first functions to be lost are the finer grades of judgement, reflection, observation and attention —

the faculties largely acquired through education, which constitute the elements of the restraint and prudence that man usually imposes on his actions. The orator allows himself to be carried by the impulse of the moment, without reflecting on ultimate consequences, and as his expressions become freer, they acquire an appearance of warmth, of feeling, of inspiration. Not a little of this inspiration is contributed by the audience if they are in a similar condition of increased appreciation . . . Another characteristic feature, evidently resulting from paralysis of the higher functions, is the loss of power to control moods.[26]

Environment, personality, mood and dose of alcohol are all relevant to the final effect on the individual.[27] These and other effects that are characteristic of alcohol, have been celebrated in the following couplets:[28]

> Ho! Ho! Yes! Yes! It's very all well,
> You may drunk I am think, but I tell you I'm not,
> I'm as sound as a fiddle and fit as a bell,
> And stable quite ill to see what's what . . .
> And I've swallowed, I grant, a beer of lot —
> But I'm not so think as you drunk I am . . .
>
> I shall stralk quite weight and not yutter an ell,
> My feech will not spalter the least little jot:
> If you knownly had own! — well, I gave him a dot,
> And I said to him, 'Sergeant, I'll come like a lamb —
> The floor it seems like a storm in a yacht,
> But I'm not so think as you drunk I am.
>
> I'm sorry, I just chair over a fell —
> A trifle — this chap, on a very day hot —
> If I hadn't consumed that last whisky of tot!
> As I said now, this fellow, called Abraham —
> Ah? One more? Since it's you! just a do me will spot —
> But I'm not so think as you drunk I am.

There is a good reason to believe that, in general, efficiency, both mental and physical, is reduced by alcohol in any amount worth taking for social pur-

---

[25] Loss of consciousness occurs at blood concentrations around 300 mg/100 ml; death at about 400 mg/100 ml. But the usual cause of death in acute alcohol poisoning is inhalation of vomit.

[26] Sollmann T 1957 Manual of pharmacology, 8th edn. Saunders, Philadelphia.

[27] That which hath made them drunk hath made me bold. Lady Macbeth in Macbeth, Act 2, Scene 2. W. Shakespeare.

[28] By Sir J C Squire (1884–1958). Quoted, by permission, R H A Squire.

poses. There is an important exception; the person who is so disabled by anxiety or nervous tension that performance is gravely impaired may improve with the correct dose of alcohol. The alleviation of great anxiety may improve performance more than the alcohol depresses it. Such people, experiencing the immediate relief that alcohol brings, are more liable to become alcohol addicts. Another exception is a minority of introverted people.

Innumerable tests of physical and mental performance have been used to demonstrate the effects of alcohol. Results show that alcohol reduces visual acuity and delays recovery from visual dazzle; it impairs taste, smell and hearing, muscular coordination and steadiness and prolongs reaction time. It also causes nystagmus and vertigo. At the same time the subjects commonly have an increased confidence in their ability to perform well when tested and underestimate their errors, even after quite low doses. Attentiveness and ability to assimilate, sort and quickly take decisions on continuously changing information input, decline. This results particularly in inattentiveness to the periphery of the visual field, which is important in motoring. All these are evidently highly undesirable effects when a person is in a position where failure to perform well may be dangerous.

Car driving and alcohol

The effects of alcohol and psychotropic drugs on motor driving (Fig. 10.3) have been the subject of well-deserved attention, and many countries have made laws designed to prevent motor accidents caused by alcohol. The problem has nowhere been solved. In general it can be said that the weight of evidence points to a steady deterioration of driving skill and an increased liability to accidents beginning with the entry of alcohol into the blood and steadily increasing with blood concentration.

In one study on city bus drivers, all of whom were recipients of awards for safe driving, it was found that even with these experienced professionals there was no 'safe' blood-alcohol level below which it was certain that no impairment of judgement would occur. Drivers attempted to pass through gaps less than the width of the bus.[29]

Alcohol plays a huge part in causing motor accidents, being a factor in as many as 50%. For this reason, the compulsory use of a roadside breath test, followed if necessary by provision of a blood sample (or urine sample if the subject objects to blood being taken) is acknowledged to be in the public interest. But the breath test is now accurate enough to be sole evidence. In the UK a blood concentration exceeding 80 mg alcohol/100 ml blood (17.4 mmol/l)[30] whilst in charge of a car is a statutory offence. At this concentration, the liability to accident is about twice normal. Other countries set lower limits, e.g. Nordic countries,[31] some states of USA, Australia, Greece.

So clearly is it in the public interest that drunken driving be reduced that the privileges normally attaching to freedom of conscience as well as to personal eccentricity must take second place. In one instance, an ingenious driver, having provided a positive breath test, offered a blood sample on the condition it should be taken from his penis; the physician refused to take it; the police demanded a urine sample; the subject refused on the ground that he had offered blood and that his offer had been refused. He was acquitted, but a Court has since decided that the choice of site for blood-taking is for the physician, not for the subject, and that such transparent attempts to evade justice should be treated as unreasonable refusal to supply a specimen under the law. The subject is then treated as though he had provided a specimen that was above the statutory limit. Yet another trick is to take a dose of spirits after the accident and before the police arrive. The police are told it was taken as a remedy for nervous shock. This is known is the 'hip-flask' defence.

Where blood or breath analysis is not immediate-

---

[29] Cohen J et al 1958 British Medical Journal 1: 1938.

[30] Approximately equivalent to 35 μg alcohol in 100 ml expired air (or 107 mg in 100 ml urine). In practice, prosecutions are undertaken only when the concentration is significantly higher to avoid arguments about biological variability and instrumental error. Urine concentrations are little used since the urine is accumulated over time and does not provide the immediacy of blood and breath.

[31] In 1990 Sweden lowered the limit to 20 mg/100 ml, which has been approached by ingestion of glucose which becomes fermented by gut flora — the 'autobrewery' syndrome.

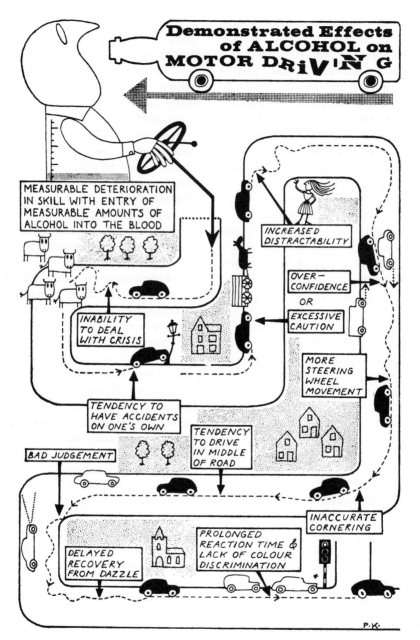

Fig. 10.3 Alcohol and driving

ly available after an accident it may be measured hours later and 'back calculated' to what it would have been at the time of the accident. It is usual to assume that the blood concentration falls at about 15 mg/100 ml/h. Naturally, the validity of such calculations leads to acrimonious disputes in the courts of law.

Prescribed medicines and driving

Ability to drive can be impaired by many prescribed drugs. In road traffic accident fatalities 7.4% of persons had taken a drug 'likely' to affect the CNS (chiefly older subjects). In addition cannabis was found in 2.6%. Unfortunately, accurate control figures are not available except in the case of epilepsy:

1.3% of fatalities had taken an antiepileptic drug and the incidence of the disease in the general population is 0.4%.[32] Apart from drugs that affect the CNS, driving may be influenced by antihistamines (drowsiness, but less commonly with newer nonsedative agents), mydriatics and antimicrobials for topical ocular use (blurred vision), antihypertensives (hypotension) and insulins and oral antidiabetic agents (hypoglycaemia).

FURTHER EFFECTS OF ALCOHOL CONSUMPTION

Peripheral vasodilatation. Alcohol depresses the vasomotor centre and this accounts for the feeling of warmth that follows taking the drug. Body heat loss is increased so that it is undesirable to take alcohol before going out into severe cold for any length of time, but it may be harmlessly employed on coming into a warm environment from the cold to provide quickly a pleasant feeling of warmth. In very cold places the overuse of alcohol can cause rapid hypothermia, e.g. drunks collapsed out of doors in winter.

Blood pressure. An acute dose of 4–5 units raises the blood pressure which parallels the blood concentration. The mechanism appears to involve centrally mediated sympathetic stimulation.

Diuretic effect. Alcohol acts by inhibiting secretion of antidiuretic hormone by the posterior pituitary gland. The reason it is useless as a diuretic in heart failure is that the diuresis is of water, not of salt. Labour is delayed by inhibition of oxytocin release from the posterior pituitary.

Gastric mucosa. Injury occurs because alcohol allows back diffusion of acid from the gastric lumen into the mucosa. After an acute binge the mucosa shows erosions and petechial haemorrhages (recovery may take 3 weeks) and up to 60% of chronic alcoholics show chronic gastritis.

Vomiting. This common accompaniment of acute

alcoholism seems to be partly a central effect, for the incidence of vomiting at equivalent blood alcohol concentrations is similar following oral or i.v. administration. This is not to deny that very strong solutions and dietary indiscretions accompanying acute and chronic alcoholism can cause vomiting by local gastric effects. That the emetic blood alcohol concentration is below that which induces coma may be one of the reasons for the rarity of deaths from acute alcoholism and for the fact that when death occurs, it is commonly due to suffocation from inhaled vomit.

Glucose tolerance. Alcohol initially increases the blood glucose, due to reduced uptake by the tissues. This leads to increased glucose metabolism.

But alcohol also inhibits gluconeogenesis and a person whose hepatic glycogen is already low, e.g. a person who is getting most of his calories from alcohol or who has not eaten adequately for 3 days, can experience *hypoglycaemia* that can be severe enough to cause irreversible brain damage. The hypoglycaemia is commonly at its maximum 6–18 h after taking the alcohol. It can be difficult to recognise clinically in a person who has been drunk, and this adds to the risk. Heavy drinking with a meal can enhance the normal insulin response to carbohydrate intake and lead to brisk hypoglycaemia.

Hyperuricaemia occurs (with precipitation of gout) due to accelerated degradation of adenine nucleotides resulting in increased production of uric acid and its precursors. Only at high alcohol concentrations does alcohol-induced high blood lactate compete for renal tubular elimination and so diminish excretion of urate. But heavy drinkers (>30 units / week) may stop having gout if they stop drinking alcohol.

Effects on sexual function. Nothing really new has been said since William Shakespeare wrote that alcohol 'provokes the desire, but it takes away the performance'. Performance in other forms of athletics is also impaired. Prolonged substantial consumption lowers plasma testosterone concentration at least partly as a result of hepatic enzyme induction; feminisation may be seen and men have been threatened with genital shrinkage.

---

[32] Advice to patients on prescribed medicines is contained in Medical Commission on Accident Prevention 1995 Medical Aspects of Fitness to Drive; HMSO, London.

Source of energy. Alcohol may be useful as an energy source (rather than a food) in debilitated patients. It is rapidly absorbed from the alimentary tract without requiring digestion and it supplies 7 calories[33] per gram as compared with 9 from fat and 4 from carbohydrate and protein. Heavy doses cause hyperlipidaemia in some people.

Tolerance to alcohol can be acquired and the point has been made that it costs the regular heavy drinker 2.5 times as much to get visibly drunk as it would cost the average abstainer. This is probably due both to enzyme induction and to adaptation of the central nervous system. *Inter-ethnic variation* in tolerance to alcohol is well recognised, for Oriental persons, particularly Japanese, develop flushing, headache and nausea after what are, by Caucasian standards, small amounts of the substance. Genetic deficiency of aldehyde dehydrogenase with slow metabolism of (toxic) acetaldehyde may explain these features (see p. 166).

Acute alcohol poisoning is a sufficiently familiar condition not to require detailed description. It is notorious that the characteristic behaviour changes, excitement, mental confusion (including 'blackouts'), incoordination and even coma, can be due to numerous other conditions and diagnosis can be extremely difficult if a sick or injured patient happens to have taken alcohol as well. Alcohol can cause severe hypoglycaemia (see above). Anyone who is liable to find himself called upon to make a clinical diagnosis of drunkenness, or rather perhaps to exclude other causes as responsible for a person's behaviour, should consider the procedure very carefully.

An arrested man was told, in a police station, by a doctor, that he was drunk. The man asked, 'Doctor, could a drunk man stand up in the middle of this room, jump into the air, turn a complete somersault, and land down on his feet?'

The doctor was injudicious enough to say, 'Certainly not' — and was then and there proved wrong'.[34] The introduction of the breathalyser, which has a statutory role only in road traffic situations, has largely eliminated such professional humiliations.

When a person is behaving in an excited or violent fashion due to alcohol it is dangerous to attempt control with sedatives or opioids because of the risk of inducing severe respiratory depression as a result of synergism of the drugs. But, if sedation is essential, chlorpromazine or diazepam in low dose are least hazardous. In patients who are comatose, the stomach may be emptied by tube; emesis, either therapeutic or due to the alcohol, is dangerous in any patient with impaired consciousness. Alcohol dialyses well, but dialysis will only be used in extreme cases.

Large doses of *fructose* (laevulose) i.v. enhance alcohol metabolism but also induce lactic acidosis. Claims that a dose of fructose swallowed during and/or at the end of an evening's drinking can render fit a subject who is unfit to drive, are dangerously misleading.

Acute hepatitis, which may be extremely severe, can occur with extraordinarily heavy acute drinking bouts. The serum transaminase rises after alcohol in alcoholics but not in others. The single case-report that after a binge the cerebrospinal fluid tasted of gin remains unconfirmed.

Chronic consumption

For *benefits* of chronic alcohol consumption, see page 176.

Malnutrition. With heavy continuous drinking, subjects take all the calories they need from alcohol, cease to eat adequately and develop deficiency of B group vitamins particularly. The malnutrition complicates the longterm effects of alcohol itself.

Organ damage. Chronic heavy alcohol use is associated with: hepatic cirrhosis, deteriorating brain function (psychotic states, dementia, seizures, Wernicke's encephalopathy, attacks of loss of memory); peripheral neuropathy and, separately, myopathy (including cardiomyopathy); cancer of the upper alimentary and respiratory tracts (many alcoholics also smoke heavily, and this contributes),

---

[33] 1 calorie = 4.2 joules.

[34] Worthing C L 1957 British Medical Journal 1: 643.

hepatic carcinoma and breast cancer in women; chronic pancreatitis; cardiomyopathy; bone marrow depression, including megaloblastosis (due to the alcohol and to alcohol-induced folate deficiency); deficiency of vitamin K-dependent blood clotting factors (due to liver injury); psoriasis; multiple effects on the hypothalamic/pituitary/endocrine system (endocrine investigations should be interpreted cautiously); Dupuytren's contracture.

Hypertension. Heavy chronic use of alcohol is an important cause of hypertension and this should always be considered in both diagnosis and management. Cessation of use may be sufficient to eliminate or reduce the need for drug therapy. But even social drinking can raise blood pressure, and hypertensives should be told this.

In general, **reversal** of all or most of the above effects is usual in early cases if alcohol is abandoned. In more advanced cases, the disease may be halted (except cancer) but in severe cases it may continue to progress. When wine rationing was introduced in Paris, France, in the 1939–45 war, deaths from hepatic cirrhosis dropped to about one-sixth the previous level; 5 years after the war they had regained their former level.

Blood lipoproteins. Moderate intake of alcoholic drinks may increase high density lipoprotein and diminish low density lipoprotein, which may account for the observed protective effect against ischaemic heart disease (see below).

Alcohol dependence syndrome[35]

General aspects of dependence are discussed earlier in this chapter. Dependence (chronic alcoholism) varies from social drinkers for whom companionship is the principal factor, through individuals who take a drink at the end of a working (or indeed any) day, who feel a need and who would be reluctant to give it up, to the person who is overcome by need, who cannot resist and whose whole life is dominated by the quest for alcohol. The major factors determining physical dependence are dose, frequency of dosing, and duration of abuse.

---

[35] A World Health Organization report prefers this term to 'alcoholism'.

Fluoxetine (serotonin antagonist) has been found to assist reduction of intake in problem drinkers.

Withdrawal of alcohol

Abrupt withdrawal of alcohol from an addict who has developed physical dependence, such as may occur when an ill or injured alcoholic is admitted to hospital, can precipitate withdrawal syndrome in 6 h and an acute psychotic attack (*delirium tremens*) and seizures (at 72 h), as well as agitation, anxiety and excess sympathetic autonomic activity.

Withdrawal should be supervised in hospital with the patient receiving a sedative (in substantial doses). Chlordiazepoxide (Librium) is given by mouth 100 mg initially, 100 mg 2–4 h later, 50 mg 4 h later, 50 mg 4 h later, 25 mg 4 h later, then further doses as is judged necessary. Alternatively, chlormethiazole (Heminevrin) (an anticonvulsant sedative) is given orally (1 capsule = 192 mg): first day, 9–12 capsules; second day, 6–8 capsules; third day, 4–6 capsules (the capsules being taken in 3–4 divided doses); then further doses as is judged necessary. Both drugs have potential for causing dependence.

A β-adrenoceptor blocker may be given for the symptoms of sympathetic overactivity, and butyrophenone neuroleptic for psychosis (not a phenothiazine, which may precipitate seizures). General aspects of care, e.g. attention to fluid and electrolyte balance, are important. It is usual to administer vitamins, especially thiamine, in which alcoholics are commonly deficient, and i.v. glucose unaccompanied by thiamine may precipitate Wernicke's encephalopathy.

Subsequent psychosocial therapy is more important than drugs, which are only of limited use. Naltrexone, a μopioid antagonist (that blocks euphoria and craving), may help some patients to maintain abstinence and diminish the severity and number of relapses in which endorphins play a part.

Knowledge of daily intake is valuable to allow prediction of disease and prevention, both by users and their medical advisers. Amounts suggested here relate to risk of *hepatic cirrhosis*, and not to acute effects. A daily consumption of 10 units (100 ml; 80 g) in men and 6 units (60 ml; 48 g) in women exposes the drinker to serious liver injury. But such injury may occur with 6 units (men) and as little as 2 units (women).[36]

SAFE LIMITS FOR CHRONIC CONSUMPTION

These cannot be accurately defined. But both patients and nonpatients justifiably expect some guidance, and doctors and government departments will wish to be helpful. They may reasonably advise as a 'safe' or prudent maximum (there being no particular individual contraindication): men 3–4 units/day, women 2–3 units/day.[37] Consistent drinking more than these amounts carries a progressive risk to health (see also Alcoholic drinks and mortality, p. 176). In other societies recommended maxima are higher or lower.

Alcoholics with established cirrhosis have usually consumed about 23 units (230 ml; 184 g) daily for 10 years. It has long been thought that total consumption accumulated over time was the crucial factor for cirrhosis. Heavy drinkers may develop hepatic cirrhosis at a rate of about 2% per annum. The type of drink (beer, wine, spirits) is not particularly relevant to the adverse health consequences.

A standard bottle of spirits (750 ml) contains 300 ml (240 g) of alcohol (i.e. 40% by volume). A standard human cannot metabolise more than about 170 g per day. People whose intake is concentrated at the weekend allow their livers time for repair and have a lower risk of liver injury than do those who consume the same total on an even daily basis.

Drinking amongst medical students. In a questionnaire survey (350 students, 260 replies) the mean consumption was: males 20 units/week; females 14 units/week. Male consumption was similar to the matched general population, female consumption was higher. Of males 23% exceeded 35 units/week and 22% of women exceeded 21 units/week. Smoking was positively associated with heavy drinking. 'The results suggest that some medical students are compromising their future health and their academic performance through excessive drinking.'[38]

Indicator of heavy drinking. 50% of men who admit to drinking above 450 g (56 units) a week have a raised plasma concentration of the enzyme gamma-glutamyl transferase (GGT >50 IU). The rise is due to hepatic enzyme induction by alcohol and perhaps also to cellular damage. The finding is not specific for alcohol, indicating only liver injury. Various other measures including aspartate aminotransferase, blood urate, triglyceride and raised mean red corpuscular volume have been used as markers, though they are all nonspecific. But taken together, these measures identify 75% of heavy drinkers; they return to normal rapidly on abstention (except mean corpuscular volume) which therefore can be misleading.

Pregnancy, the fetus and lactation

Pregnancy is unlikely to occur in severely alcoholic women (who have amenorrhoea secondary to liver injury). The spontaneous miscarriage rate in the second trimester is doubled by consumption of 1–2 units/day.

Fetal injury can occur in early pregnancy (fetal alcohol syndrome). It may be due to the metabolite, acetaldehyde, and so acute (binge) consumption is more hazardous than similar total intake on a daily basis. Plainly, disulfiram should not be used in a woman who is or might become pregnant.

The vulnerable period of pregnancy is at 4–10 weeks. Because of this, prevention cannot be reliably achieved after diagnosis of pregnancy (usually 3–8 weeks).

---

[36] Women appear to be more susceptible to liver injury than are men. This is not solely a matter of pharmacokinetics but may be also due to the greater occurrence of autoimmune reactivity that has been shown in women with alcoholic liver disease.

[37] Report of an Inter-Departmental Working Group, 1995 Sensible Drinking. Department of Health.

[38] Collier D J, Beales I L P 1989 British Medical Journal 299: 19.

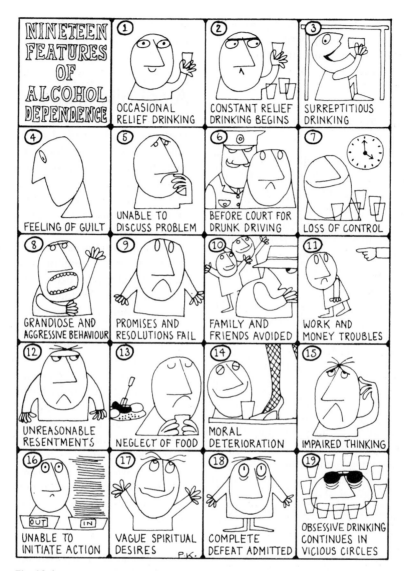

Fig. 10.4

There is no level of maternal consumption that can be guaranteed safe for the fetus. But it is plainly unrealistic to leave the matter there, and it has been suggested that if the ideal of total abstinence is unachievable then women who are pregnant or are thinking of becoming pregnant should not drink more than 1–2 units of alcohol per week and should avoid periods of intoxication.[37]

In addition to the fetal alcohol syndrome there is general fetal/embryonic growth retardation (1% for every 10 g alcohol per day) and this is not 'caught up' later.

Fetal alcohol syndrome includes the following characteristics: microcephaly, mental retardation with irritability in infancy, low body weight and length, poor coordination, hypotonia, small eyeballs and short palpebral fissures, lack of nasal bridge.[39]

Children of about 10% of alcohol abusers may show the syndrome. In women consuming 12 units of alcohol per day the incidence may be as much as 30%.

---

[39] For pictures see Streissguth A P et al 1985 Lancet 2: 85.

Lactation. Even small amounts of alcohol taken by the mother delay motor development in the child; an effect on mental development is uncertain.

Pharmacological deterrence

Disulfiram (Antabuse). In alcoholics who are well and motivated, an attempt may be made to discourage drinking by inducing immediate unpleasantness. Disulfiram inhibits the enzyme aldehyde dehydrogenase so that acetaldehyde (toxic metabolite of alcohol) accumulates. The objective of administering disulfiram is that patients will find the experience so unpleasant that they will avoid alcohol.

A typical reaction of medium severity comes on about 5 min after taking alcohol and consists of generalised vasodilatation and fall in blood pressure, sweating, dyspnoea, headache, chest pain, nausea and vomiting. Severe reactions include convulsions and circulatory collapse; they may last several hours. Some advocate the use of a test dose of alcohol under supervision (after the fifth day), so that patients can be taught what to expect and also to induce an aversion from alcohol. Such therapy is likely to play no more than a minor part in the treatment of alcoholism, a disease that is primarily a manifestation of psychological disorder.

The disulfiram – alcohol interaction came to therapeutics only by the chance experience of two Danish pharmacologists.[40]

> Dr. Hald suggested that disulfiram could be employed as an anthelmintic . . . The drug was tested on rabbits infected with worms and results were sufficiently encouraging to warrant clinical trial.
>
> According to the custom in this house we never give a new drug to patients before we have taken at least double the recommended dose ourselves. During this routine procedure Dr. Hald and I discovered that we had developed an intolerance to alcohol. We compared symptoms and found them identical. The only thing we had in common was the tablets.

---

[40] Dr Erik Jacobsen. Personal communication.

Further investigation disclosed the mechanism of the effect.

Alcoholic drinks

The pharmacology of alcoholic drinks is not the same as the pharmacology of alcohol. The drinks contain other ingredients that may reduce the rate of absorption of alcohol (carbohydrate in beer), act as a carminative (essential oils), or diuretic (juniper oil in gin) or inhibit enzymes that are concerned in some drug metabolism. There is no conclusive evidence on this point, but there is reason to believe that the effects of ethanol in some drinks are prolonged by the presence of other substances, e.g. propyl to octyl alcohols, ethers, aldehydes, which delay ethanol metabolism by occupying the same metabolic paths (competition). These other ingredients are themselves hardly more toxic than ethanol. It should be remembered that when enough alcoholic drink has been taken to cause 'hangover', subjects have commonly debauched themselves in other ways too. Dehydration (due to diuresis) is a prominent cause of 'hangover'; it may be usefully mitigated by drinking a substantial volume of water before going to bed.

Cardiovascular benefit (below) appears to be due mainly to ethanol itself but nonethanol ingredients (anti-oxidants, phenols, flavinoids) may contribute (see below).

ALCOHOLIC DRINKS AND MORTALITY

The curve that relates mortality (vertical axis) to alcoholic drink consumption (horizontal axis) is J-shaped; i.e. as consumption rises above zero the all-cause mortality declines, then levels off, and finally rises.

The benefit is largely a reduction of deaths due to cardio- and cerebrovascular disease for regular drinkers of 1–2 units/d for men over 40 years and postmenopausal women. Consumption over 2 units/d does not provide any major additional health benefit. The mechanism may be an improvement in lipoprotein (HDL/LDL) profiles and perhaps a reduction in platelet aggregation.

The rising (adverse) arm of the curve is associated with known harmful effects of alcohol (already described), but also, for example, with pneumonia (which may be secondary to direct alcohol effects, or with the increased smoking of alcohol users).

Whether the cardioprotective effect differs between classes of alcoholic drink remains an open issue. Suggestion that wine confers greater advantage than spirits was not supported by a review of 12 ecological, 3 case-control and 10 prospective cohort studies; a substantial proportion of the benefit appeared to derive from ethanol itself.[41] The social importance of alcohol combined with the very substantial scientific problems posed by these studies (including the problem of unreliably reported intakes) render the whole matter controversial. We recommend study of the references below.[42,43]

Alcohol and other drugs

All cerebral depressants (hypnotics, tranquillisers, antiepileptics, antihistamines) can either potentiate or synergise with alcohol, and this can be important at ordinary doses in relation to car driving. But, when supplies of hypnotics or tranquillisers are given to patients known to drink heavily, they should be warned to omit the drugs when they have been drinking. Deaths have occurred from these combinations.

Alcohol-dependent people with a physical tolerance are relatively tolerant of some other cerebral depressant drugs (hydrocarbon anaesthetics and barbiturates), but of course the synergism with these drugs still occurs. There is no significant acquired cross-tolerance with opioids.

[41] Rimm E B et al 1996 Review of moderate alcohol consumption and reduced risk of coronary heart disease: is the effect due to beer, wine or spirits? British Medical Journal 312: 731.

[42] Doll R et al 1994 Mortality in relation to the consumption of alcohol: 13 years' observations in British male doctors. British Medical Journal 309: 911.

[43] Grønbæk M et al 1995 Mortality associated with moderate intakes of beer and spirits. British Medical Journal 310: 1165.

Sulphonylureas (antidiabetics) cause a disulfiram-like reaction, as may metronidazole, griseofulvin, and chloral.

Oral anticoagulants. Control may be disturbed by alcohol inhibiting hepatic metabolism directly, or enhancing it by enzyme induction; moderate drinking is unlikely to cause trouble.

Antiepileptics can be metabolised faster due to enzyme induction and this contributes to its well-known adverse effect on epilepsy.

Monoamineoxidase inhibitors (MAOIs). Some alcoholic (and de-alcoholised) drinks contain tyramine, sufficient to cause a hypertensive crisis in a patient taking a MAOI.

Miscellaneous uses of alcohol. Alcohol precipitates protein and is used to harden the skin in bedridden patients. Local application also reduces sweating and may allay itching. As a skin antiseptic 70% by weight (76% by volume) is most effective. Stronger solutions are less effective. Alcohol injections are sometimes used to destroy nervous tissue in cases of intractable pain (trigeminal neuralgia, carcinoma involving nerves).

Opioids, heroin, etc.: see Chapter 17.

Psychodysleptics or hallucinogens

These substances produce mental changes that resemble those of some psychotic states. They are used by people seeking a new experience or escape.

Psychiatrists also have used these drugs in supervised therapeutic sessions to encourage the release and reliving of unconscious material in the hope that, assisted by appropriate psychotherapy, patients may gain insight and an improved ability to cope with their environment. Such use remains experimental and potentially dangerous (suicide, prolonged psychosis).

Experiences with these drugs vary greatly with the subject's expectations, existing frame of mind and personality and environment. Subjects can be prepared so that they are more likely to have a good 'trip' than a bad one.

Experiences with psychodysleptics

The following brief account of experiences with **LSD** (lysergic acid diethylamide, lysergide) in normal subjects will serve as a model. Experiences with **mescaline** and **psilocybin** are similar:

● Vision may become blurred and there may be hallucinations; these generally do not occur in the blind and are less if the subject is blind-folded. Objects appear distorted, and trivial things, e.g. a mark on a wall, may change shape and acquire special significance.

● Auditory acuity increases, but hallucinations are uncommon. Subjects who do not ordinarily appreciate music may suddenly come to do so.

● Foods may feel coarse and gritty in the mouth.

● Limbs may be left in uncomfortable positions.

● Time may seem to stop or to pass slowly, but usually it gets faster and thousands of years may seem suddenly to go by.

● The subject may feel relaxed and supremely happy, or may become fearful or depressed. Feelings of depersonalisation and dreamy states occur.

The experience lasts a few hours, depending on the dose; intervals of normality then occur and become progressively longer.

Somatic symptoms include nausea, dizziness, paraesthesiae, weakness, drowsiness, tremors, dilated pupils, ataxia. Effects on the cardiovascular system and respiration vary and probably reflect fluctuating anxiety.

So disrupting to the individual are some of these drugs, particularly in respect of thought processes, that legal control is needed, perhaps especially in view of the possibility of their use in a 'person in a position of high authority when faced with decisions of great importance'.[43]

There is no shortage of sensational accounts of experience with psychodysleptics, because there has been a vogue amongst intellectuals, begun by Mr Aldous Huxley,[44] for publishing their experiences. Subsequent accounts are tedious to most except their authors and to those who would do the same; they have little pharmacological importance and reveal more about the author's egocentricity than about pharmacology. The same applies to published accounts of what it is like to be a drug addict.

Individual substances

LYSERGIDE (LSD)

Lysergic acid provides the nucleus of the ergot alkaloids and it was during a study of derivatives of this in a search for an analeptic that in 1943 a Swiss worker investigating LSD (which structurally resembles nikethamide) felt peculiar and had visual hallucinations. This led him to take a dose of the substance and so to discover its remarkable potency, an effective oral dose being about 30 microgams. The $t^{1}/_{2}$ is 3 h. (See description of experience, above.) Mechanisms of action are complex and include agonist effect at presynaptic 5-HT receptors in the CNS.

Tachyphylaxis (acute tolerance) occurs to LSD. Psychological dependence may occur; physical dependence does not.

LSD has been used in the dying; it induces analgesia and indifference. Its effect on the brain may partly be due to antagonism of serotonin at autoreceptors.

Serious adverse effects include: psychotic reaction (which can be delayed in onset) with suicide; teratogenic and mutagenic effects are speculative and the risk is small at worst.

LSD has curious effects in animals: green sunfish become aggressive, Siamese fighting fish float nose up, tail down and goats walk in unaccustomed stereotyped patterns. The elephant exhibits episodically a form of sexual or delinquent behaviour known as 'musth'. LSD 100 μg/kg i.m. was given to an animal (the usual dose for man is up to about 2 μg/kg) to test whether this induced a similar state. The elephant developed laryngospasm and status epilepticus and died.[45] Badly planned experiments give useless results.

---

[43] Hoffer A 1965 Clin Pharmacology and Therapeutics 6: 183.

[44] Huxley A 1964 The doors of preception. Chatto and Windus, London.

[45] Cohen S 1967 Annual Review of Pharmacology 7: 30 1.

Mescaline is an alkaloid from a Mexican cactus (peyotl), the top of which is cut off and dried and used as 'peyote buttons' in religious ceremonies. Mescaline does not induce serious dependence and the drug has little importance except to members of some North and Central American societies and to psychiatrists and biochemists who are interested in the mechanism of induced psychotic states.

Tenamfetamine ('ecstasy', MDMA: methylene-dioxymethamphetamine) is structurally related to mescaline as well as to amphetamine. It was originally patented in 1914 as an appetite suppressant and has recently achieved widespread popularity as a dance drug at 'rave' parties (where it is deemed necessary to keep pace with the beat and duration of the music; popular names include White Dove, White Burger, Red and Black, Denis the Menace). Tenamfetamine stimulates central and peripheral α- and β-adrenoceptors; thus the pharmacological effects are compounded by those of physical exertion, dehydration and heat. In susceptible individuals a severe and fatal idiosyncratic reaction may occur with fulminant hyperthermia, convulsions, disseminated intravascular coagulation, rhabdomyolysis, and acute renal and hepatic failure. Treatment includes: oral activated charcoal, diazepam for convulsions, β-blockade (atenolol) for tachycardia, α-blockade (phentolamine) for hypertension, and dantrolene if the rectal temperature exceeds 39°C.

Phencyclidine ('angel dust') was made in a search for a better intravenous anaesthetic. It is structurally related to pethidine. Phencyclidine was found to induce analgesia without unconsciousness, but with amnesia, in man. The postoperative course, however, was complicated by psychiatric disturbance (agitation, abreactions, hallucinations). As the interest of anaesthetists waned, so that of psychiatrists grew and the drug has been used in experimental therapy. Ketamine originated from this work.

Psilocybin is derived from varieties of the fungus *Psilocybe* ('magic mushrooms') that grow in many countries. It is related to LSD.

CANNABIS

Cannabis is obtained from the annual plant *Cannabis sativa* (hemp) and its varieties *Cannabis indica* and *Cannabis americana*. The preparations that are smoked are called marihuana (grass, pot, weed, etc.) and consist of crushed leaves and flowers. There is a wide variety of regional names, e.g. ganja (India, Caribbean), kif (Morocco), dagga (Africa). The resin scraped off the plant is known as hashish (hash). The term cannabis is used to include all the above preparations. Since most preparations are illegally prepared it is not surprising that they are impure and of variable potency. The plant grows wild in the Americas,[46] Africa and Asia. It can also be grown successfully in the open in the warmer southern areas of Britain.

Pharmacokinetics

Of the scores of chemical compounds that the resin contains, the most important are the oily cannabinoids, including tetrahydrocannabinol (THC), which is the chief cause of the psychic action. Samples of resin vary greatly in the amounts and proportions of these cannabinoids according to their country of origin; as the sample ages, its THC content declines. As a result, the THC content of samples can vary from almost zero to 8%.

Smoke from a cannabis cigarette (the usual mode of use is to inhale and hold the breath to allow maximum absorption) delivers 25–50% of the THC content to the respiratory tract.

THC ($t^1/_2$ 4 d) and other cannabinoids undergo extensive biotransformation in the body, yielding scores of metabolites, several of which are themselves psychoactive. They are extremely lipid-soluble and are stored in body fat from which they are slowly released.[47] Hepatic drug metabolising

---

[46] The commonest pollen in the air of San Francisco, California is said to be that of the cannabis plant, illegally cultivated.

[47] When a chronic user discontinues, cannabinoids remain detectable in the urine for an average of 4 weeks and it can be as long as 11 weeks before 10 consecutive daily tests are negative (Ellis G M et al 1986 Clinical Pharmacology and Therapeutics 38: 572).

enzymes are inhibited acutely but may also be induced by chronic use of crude preparations.

Pharmacodynamics

The mechanisms of action are not yet defined.

Psychological reactions are very varied, being much influenced by the behaviour of the group. They commence within minutes of starting to smoke and last 2–3h. Euphoria is common, though not invariable, with giggling or laughter which can seem pointless to an observer. Sensations become more vivid, especially visual, and contrast and intensity of colour can increase, although no change in acuity occurs. Size of objects and distance are distorted. Sense of time can disappear altogether, leaving a sometimes distressing sense of timelessness. Recent memory and selective attention are impaired; the beginning of a sentence may be forgotten before it is finished, and the subject is very suggestible and easily distracted. Psychological tests such as mental arithmetic, digit-symbol substitution and pursuit meter tests show impairment. These effects may be accompanied by feelings of deep insight and truth. Memory defect may persist for weeks after abstinence.

Once memory is impaired, concentration becomes less effective, since the object of attention is less well remembered. With this may go an insensitivity to danger or the consequences of actions.

A striking phenomenon is the intermittent wave-like nature of these effects which affects mood, visual impressions, time sense, spatial sense, and other functions.

The desired effects of cannabis, as of other psychodysleptics, depend not only on the expectation of the user and the dose, but also on the environmental situation and personality. Genial or revelatory experiences may indeed occur, e.g. 'Haschich Fudge':[48]

> (which anyone can whip up on a rainy day). This is the food of Paradise ... euphoria and brilliant storms of laughter, ecstatic reveries and extension of one's personality on several simultaneous

planes are to be complacently expected. Almost anything St Teresa[49] did, you can do better ...

But this cannot be relied on.

The effects can be unpleasant, especially in inexperienced subjects, particularly timelessness and the feeling of loss of control of mental processes. Feelings of unease, sometimes amounting to anguish and acute panic occur as well as 'flashbacks' of previously experienced hallucinations, e.g. on LSD. There is also, especially in the habitual user, a tendency to paranoid thinking. High or habitual use can be followed by a psychotic state; this is usually reversible, quickly with brief periods of cannabis use, but more slowly after sustained exposures.

The effect of an acute dose usually ends in drowsiness and sleep. It is claimed that death has not occurred.

Tolerance, with continued heavy use, and a withdrawal syndrome occur (depression, anxiety, sleep disturbance, tremor and other symptoms), and many users find it very difficult to abandon cannabis. In studies of self-administration by monkeys, spontaneous use did not occur but, once use was initiated, drug-seeking behaviour developed. Subjects who have become tolerant to LSD or opioids as a result of repeated dosage respond normally to cannabis but there appears to be cross-tolerance between cannabis and alcohol.

'Amotivational syndrome'. This term dignifies an imprecisely characterised state, ranging from a feeling of unease and sense of not being fully effective, up to a gross lethargy, with social passivity and deterioration. It is difficult to assess, when personal traits and intellectual rejection of technological civilisation are also taken into account. Yet the reversibility of the state, its association with cannabis use, and its recognition by cannabis users make it impossible to ignore. (Escalation theory, see p. 157.)

Cannabis and skilled tasks, e.g. car driving. General performance in both motor and psycholog-

---

[48] From The Alice B Toklas cook book 1954 Michael Joseph, London. The author was companion to Gertrude ('rose is a rose is a rose') Stein (1874–1946).

[49] St Teresa of Avila (1515–82) was noted for her power of levitation.

ical tests deteriorates, more in naive than in experienced subjects. Effects may be similar to alcohol, but experiments in which the subjects are unaware that they are being tested (and so do not compensate voluntarily) are difficult to do, as with alcohol. Some scientists claim the effects are negligible but this view has been 'put in proper perspective' by a commentator[50] who asked how these scientists 'would feel if told that the pilot of their international jet taking them to a psychologists' conference, was just having a reefer or two before opening up the controls'.

Other effects. Cannabis smoked or taken by mouth produces reddening of the eyeballs (probably the forerunner of the general dilatation of blood vessels and fall of blood pressure with higher doses), unsteadiness (particularly for precise movements), and tachycardia. The smoke produces the usual smoker's cough, and the tar from reefer cigarettes is as carcinogenic in animal experiments as cigarette tobacco tar. Increase in appetite is commonly experienced.

Cannabis is teratogenic in animals, but effect in humans is unproved, although there is impaired fetal growth with repeated use.

MANAGEMENT OF ADVERSE REACTIONS

Mild and sometimes even severe episodes ('bad trips') can be managed by reassurance including talk, 'talking the patient down', and physical contact, e.g. hand holding (LSD and mescaline). The objective is to help patients relate their experience to reality and to appreciate that the mental experiences are drug-induced and will abate. Because short-term memory is disrupted the treatment can be very time-consuming since therapists cannot absent themselves without risking relapse. But with phencyclidine such intervention may have the opposite effect, i.e. overstimulation. It is therefore appropriate to sedate all anxious or excited subjects with diazepam (or chlorpromazine or haloperidol). With sedation the 'premorbid ego' may be rapidly re-established.

If the 'bad trip' is due to overdose of an antimus-

---

[50] Dr G Milner.

carinic drug, natural or synthetic, then diazepam is specially preferred, or a neuroleptic with no or minimal antimuscarinic effects, e.g. haloperidol. A dose of anticholinesterase that penetrates the central nervous system (physostigmine: tacrine) is effective in severe reaction to an antimuscarinic.

Stimulants

COCAINE

Cocaine (see also Local anaesthetics, p. 388) use is a widespread and ancient practice amongst South American peasants who chew coca leaves with lime to release the alkaloid. It is claimed to give relief from fatigue and hunger; from altitude sickness in the Andes, experienced even by natives when journeying by car or other 'fast' transportation; and also to induce a pleasant introverted mental state. Remarkable feats of endurance attributed to chewing coca leaves have been reported, but there is no sound scientific confirmation of them. A United Nations enquiry into coca-leaf chewing (1950) reported that there was psychological but no physical dependence. It also reported that its use caused physical exhaustion rather than the reverse, and advocated gradual suppression in the interest of the populations concerned. But what may have been (or even still may be) an acceptable feature of these ancient stable societies has now developed into a massive, criminal business, not for leaf chewing, but for the manufacture and export of purified cocaine to supply an eager and lucrative demand from unhappy but economically richer societies where its use constitutes an intractable social problem. These economically developed societies, which cannot control social demand and importation, seek to eliminate the drug at its source in peasant societies that have come to rely on it for economic subsistence. When coca plantations are destroyed great distress to local populations ensues by a combination of economic deprivation and removal of the coca leaf, which, when used in the traditional way, helps to make tolerable lives of deprivation.

Cocaine (snow) is used as snuff (snorting), swallowed, smoked (below) or injected i.v. It is taken to obtain the immediate characteristic intense euphoria which is often followed in a few minutes by dysphoria. This leads to repeated use (10–45 min) during 'runs' of usually about 12 h. After the 'run' there follows the 'crash' (dysphoria, irritability, hypersomnia) lasting hours to days. After the 'crash' there may be depression ('cocaine blues') and decreased capacity to experience pleasure (anhedonia) for days to weeks.

Psychological dependence with intense compulsive drug-seeking behaviour is characteristic of even short-term use, but physical dependence is arguably slight or absent. Tachyphylaxis, acute tolerance, occurs.

The psychotropic effects of cocaine are similar to those of amphetamine (euphoria and excitement) but briefer and are due to blockade of the reuptake of dopamine at central nervous system synapses, which increases its concentration at receptors and produces the characteristic 'high'.

Intranasal use causes mucosal vasoconstriction, anosmia and eventually necrosis and perforation of the nasal septum.

Smoking involves converting the nonvolatile HCl into the volatile 'free base' or 'crack' (by extracting the HCl with alkali); for use it is vaporised by heat (it pops or cracks) in a special glass 'pipe'; or mixed with tobacco in a cigarette. Inhalation with breath-holding allows pulmonary absorption that is about as rapid as an i.v. injection. It induces an intense euphoric state. The mouth and pharynx become anaesthetised.

Intravenous use gives the expected rapid effect (kick, flash, rush). Cocaine may be mixed with heroin (as 'speedball').

Cocaine is metabolised by plasma esterases; the $t^{1}/_{2}$ is 50 min.

Overdose is common amongst users (up to 22% of heavy users report losing consciousness). The desired euphoria and excitement turns to acute fear, with psychotic symptoms, convulsions, hypertension, tachycardia, dysrhythmias, hyperthermia; coronary vasospasm (sufficient to provoke chest pain and myocardial infarction) may occur. Treatment is chosen according to the clinical picture (and the known mode of action), from amongst, e.g. haloperidol (rather than chlorpromazine) for mental disturbance; diazepam for convulsions; a vasodilator, e.g. a calcium channel blocker, for

hypertension; glyceryl trinitrate for myocardial ischaemia (but **not** a β-blocker which aggravates cocaine-induced coronary vasospasm).

Fetal growth is retarded by maternal use, but teratogenicity is uncertain.

Amphetamine (p. 349) effects and use are similar to cocaine, but 'runs' are longer (see also tenamfetamine, 'ecstasy').

Caffeine: see page 351.

Khat. The leaves of the khat shrub (*Catha edulis*) contain an alkaloid (cathinone) structurally similar to amphetamine. They are chewed fresh (for maximum alkaloid content) so that the habit was confined to geographical areas favourable to the shrub (Arabia, E. Africa) until modern transportation allowed wider distribution. Khat chewers (mostly male) became euphoric, loquacious, excited, hyperactive and even manic. As with some other drug dependencies subjects may give priority to their drug needs above personal, family and other social and economic responsibilities. Cultivation takes up serious amounts of scarce arable land and irrigation water.

Drugs as adjuvants to crime

Since time immemorial drugs have been used to facilitate sexual excess and robbery, e.g. opium and plants containing antimuscarinics (hyoscine, etc.). All such acts constitute a criminal offence.

The advent of synthetic drugs widened the scope and ease of administration.

In 19th century Chicago (USA) the proprietor of the Lone Palm Saloon, Michael J Finn, employed girls to ensure his customers consumed drinks to which he had added chloral hydrate — the 'Mickey Finn' — they were robbed when unconscious.

Recently there has been a vogue for using clonidine for the same purpose (a doctor or pharmacist must surely have been responsible for this curious but, it seems, effective choice). Victims become confused and unresisting from sedation, bradycardia, other cardiac dysrhythmias, ataxia, hypothermia, hypo- or hypertension.

GUIDE TO FURTHER READING

Ashton C H 1990 Solvent abuse: little progress after 20 years. British Medical Journal 300: 135

Bardin C W 1996 The anabolic action of testosterone. New England Journal of Medicine 335: 52

Brewer R D et al 1994 The risk of dying in alcohol-related automobile crashes among habitual drunk drivers. New England Journal of Medicine 331: 513

Brookoff D et al 1994 Testing reckless drivers for cocaine and marijuana. New England Journal of Medicine 331: 518

Charness M E 1989 Ethanol and the nervous system. New England Journal of Medicine 321: 442

Criqui M H, Ringel B L 1994 Does diet explain the French paradox? Lancet 344: 1719 (A study of diet, alcohol and mortality from 21 affluent contries.)

Doll R et al 1994 Mortality in relation to smoking: 40 years' observations on male British doctors. British Medical Journal 309: 901

Gawin F H, Ellinwood E H 1988 Cocaine and other stimulants: actions, abuse, and treatment. New England Journal of Medicine 318: 1173

Green A R, Goodwin G M 1996 Ecstasy and neurodegeneration. British Medical Journal 312: 1493

Grunberg N E 1991 Smoking cessation and weight gain. New England Journal of Medicine 324: 768

Hallaghan J B et al 1989 Anabolic-androgenic steroid use by athletes. New England Journal of Medicine 321: 1042

Henningfield J E 1995 Nicotine medication for smoking cessation. New England Journal of Medicine 333: 1196

Hollander J E 1995 The management of cocaine-associated myocardial ischaemia. New England Journal of Medicine 333: 1267

Kaplan N M 1995 Alcohol and hypertension. Lancet 345: 1588

Lieber C S 1995 Medical disorders of alcoholism. New England Journal of Medicine 333: 1058

Marc B et al 1989 Managing drug dealers who swallow the evidence. British Medical Journal 299: 1082

Nutt D J 1996 Addiction: brain mechanisms and their treatment implications. Lancet 457: 31 (see also other articles in this series on pages 97, 162, 237, 301, 373)

Peto R 1994 Smoking and death: the past 40 years and the next 40. British Medical Journal 309: 937

Wynder E L et al 1959 Cancer and coronary artery disease in seventh day adventists. Cancer 12: 1016[51]

---

[51] This curious by-way is a study of lung cancer in Seventh Day Adventists, in the USA. It appears that members of this religious sect, which prohibits smoking, have an incidence of lung cancer one-eighth of that of non-members. Indeed the only two men with lung cancer were converts who had smoked cigarettes until middle-age. In respect of cancer of sites not associated with smoking there was no difference from the control group, so that Seventh Day Adventists evidently have no general immunity from cancer. Therefore, to accommodate this evidence to the hypothesis of a genetic cause of both smoking and lung cancer, it would be necessary to stipulate that those born into the sect, but not those converted to it, inherit a low susceptibility to lung cancer.

'To many it will come as no surprise to learn that the benefits of religious observances are by no means restricted to the future life. But not often before can the evidence have been put on such a sure statistical basis' (Editorial 1959 A new angle on smoking. British Medical Journal 2: 1465).

INFECTION AND INFLAMMATION

Chemotherapy of infections

SYNOPSIS

Infection is a major category of human disease and skilled management of antimicrobial drugs is of the first importance. The term *chemotherapy* is used for the drug treatment of parasitic infections in which the parasites (viruses, bacteria, protozoa, fungi, worms) are destroyed or removed without injuring the host. The use of the term to cover all drug or synthetic drug therapy needlessly removes a distinction which is convenient to the clinician and has the sanction of long usage. By convention the term is used to include therapy of cancer.

- Classification of antimicrobial drugs
- How antimicrobials act
- Principles of antimicrobial therapy
- Use of antimicrobial drugs: choice; combinations; chemoprophylaxis and pre-emptive suppressive therapy
- Problems with antimicrobial drugs: resistance; opportunistic infection; masking of infections
- Antimicrobial drugs of choice (Reference table)

HISTORY

Many substances that we now know to possess therapeutic efficacy have been used in the past. The Ancient Greeks used male fern, and the Aztecs chenopodium, as intestinal anthelminthics. The Ancient Hindus treated leprosy with chaulmoogra. For hundreds of years moulds have been applied to wounds, but, despite the introduction of mercury as a treatment for syphilis (16th century), and the use of cinchona bark against malaria (17th century), the history of modern rational chemotherapy did not begin until Ehrlich[1] developed the idea from his observation that aniline dyes selectively stained bacteria in tissue microscopic preparations and could selectively kill them. He invented the word 'chemotherapy' and in 1906 he wrote:

> In order to use chemotherapy successfully, we must search for substances which have an affinity for the cells of the parasites and a power of killing them greater than the damage such substances cause to the organism itself ... This means ... we must learn to aim, learn to aim with chemical substances.

The antimalarials pamaquin and mepacrine were developed from dyes and in 1935 the first sulphonamide, linked with a dye (Prontosil), was introduced as a result of systematic studies by Domagk.[2] The results obtained with sulphonamides

---

[1] Paul Ehrlich (1854–1915), the German scientist who was the pioneer of chemotherapy and discovered the first cure for syphilis (Salvarsan).

[2] Gerhard Domagk (1895–1964), bacteriologist and pathologist, who made his discovery while working in

in puerperal sepsis, pneumonia and meningitis were dramatic and caused a revolution in scientific and medical thinking.

In 1928, Fleming[3] accidentally rediscovered the long-known ability of penicillium fungi to suppress the growth of bacterial cultures but put the finding aside as a curiosity.

In 1939, principally as an academic exercise, Florey[4] and Chain[5] undertook an investigation of antibiotics, i.e. substances produced by microorganisms that are antagonistic to the growth or life of other microorganisms.[6] They prepared penicillin and confirmed its remarkable lack of toxicity.[7] When the preparation was administered to a policeman with combined staphylococcal and streptococcal septicaemia there was dramatic improvement; unfortunately the manufacture of penicillin (in the Pathology Laboratory) could not keep pace with the requirements (it was also

extracted from the patient's urine and re-injected); it ran out and the patient later succumbed to infection. Subsequent development amply demonstrated the remarkable therapeutic efficacy of penicillin.

Classification of antimicrobial drugs

Antimicrobial agents may be classified according to the type of organism against which they are active and in this book follow the sequence:

- Antibacterial drugs
- Antiviral drugs
- Antifungal drugs
- Antiprotozoal drugs
- Anthelminthic drugs.

Antimicrobial drugs may also be classified broadly into:

- *bacteriostatic*, i.e. those that act primarily by arresting bacterial growth, such as sulphonamides, tetracyclines and chloramphenicol
- *bactericidal*, i.e. those which act primarily by killing bacteria, such as penicillins, cephalosporins, aminoglycosides, isoniazid and rifampicin.

The classification is somewhat arbitrary because most bacteriostatic drugs can be shown to be bactericidal at high concentrations. It does retain a certain usefulness in that when a bacteriostatic drug is used, the defence mechanisms of the body are relied on to destroy the organisms whose multiplication has been stopped by the drug. When these mechanisms are inadequate, e.g. in the immunocompromised and in infective endocarditis, bactericidal drugs should be used.

Bactericidal drugs act most effectively on rapidly dividing organisms. Thus a bacteriostatic drug, by reducing multiplication, may protect the organism from a bactericidal drug. Such mutual antagonism of antimicrobials may be clinically important, but the matter is complex for drugs are not purely bactericidal or bacteriostatic at all concentrations.

Germany. Awarded the 1939 Nobel prize for Physiology or Medicine, he had to wait until 1947 to receive the gold medal because of Nazi policy at the time.

[3] Alexander Fleming (1881–1955). He researched for years on antibacterial substances that would not be harmful to humans. His findings on penicillin were made at St. Mary's Hospital, London.

[4] Howard Walter Florey (1898–1969), Professor of Pathology at Oxford University.

[5] Ernest Boris Chain (1906–79). Biochemist. Fleming, Florey and Chain shared the 1945 Nobel prize for Physiology or Medicine.

[6] Strictly, the definition should refer to substances that are antagonistic in dilute solution for it is necessary to exclude various metabolic products such as alcohol and hydrogen peroxide. The term *antibiotic* is now commonly used for antimicrobial drugs in general, and it would be pedantic to object to this.

[7] The importance of this discovery for a nation at war was obvious to these workers but the time, July 1940, was unpropitious, for invasion was feared. The mood of the time is shown by the decision to ensure that, by the time invaders reached Oxford, the essential records and apparatus for making penicillin would have been deliberately destroyed; the productive strain of *Penicillium* mould was to be secretly preserved by several of the principal workers smearing the spores of the mould into the linings of their ordinary clothes where it could remain dormant but alive for years; any member of the team who escaped (wearing the right clothes) could use it to start the work again (Macfarlane G 1979 Howard Florey, Oxford).

How antimicrobials act

It should always be remembered that drugs are seldom the sole instruments of cure but act together with the natural defences of the body.

Antimicrobials act at different sites in the target organism as follows:

The cell wall. This gives the bacterium its characteristic shape and provides protection against the much lower osmotic pressure of the environment. Bacterial multiplication involves breakdown and extension of the wall; interference with its function allows the cell to absorb water so that it bursts. As the cells of higher, e.g. human, organisms do not possess this type of wall, drugs that act here are especially selective; obviously, the drugs are effective only against growing cells. They include: penicillins, cephalosporins, vancomycin, bacitracin, cycloserine.

The cytoplasmic membrane inside the cell wall is the site of most of the microbial cell's biochemical activity. Drugs that interfere with its function include: polyenes (nystatin, amphotericin), polymyxins (colistin, polymyxin B).

Protein synthesis. Drugs that interfere at various points with the build-up of peptide chains on the ribosomes of the organism include: chloramphenicol, erythromycin, fusidic acid, tetracyclines, aminoglycosides.

Nucleic acid metabolism. Drugs may interfere

- directly with microbial DNA, e.g. quinolones, metronidazole, or with RNA, e.g. rifampicin
- indirectly, e.g. sulphonamides, trimethoprim.

Principles of antimicrobial chemotherapy

The following principles, many of which apply to drug therapy in general, are a guide to good practice with antimicrobial agents.

- *Make a diagnosis* as precisely as is possible, defining the site of infection, the organism(s) responsible and their sensitivity to drugs. This objective will be more readily achieved if all relevant biological samples for the laboratory are taken before treatment is begun.

- *Remove barriers to cure*, e.g. lack of free drainage of abscesses, obstruction in the urinary or respiratory tracts.

- *Decide whether chemotherapy is really necessary.* As a general rule, acute infections require chemotherapy whilst chronic infections may not. Chronic abscess or empyema respond poorly, although chemotherapeutic cover is essential if surgery is undertaken in order to avoid a flare-up of infection or its dissemination due to the breaking down of tissue barriers. Even some acute infections such as gastroenteritis are better managed symptomatically than by antimicrobials.

- *Select the best drug.* This involves consideration of:

  — *specificity*; ideally the antimicrobial activity of the drug should match that of the infecting organisms. Indiscriminate use of broad-spectrum drugs encourages opportunistic infections (see p. 193). There are, however, times when 'best guess' chemotherapy of reasonably broad spectrum must be given because of the absence of precise identification of the responsible microbe.
  — *pharmacokinetic factors*; to ensure that the chosen drug is capable of reaching the site of infection in adequate amounts, e.g. by crossing the blood–brain barrier.
  — *the patient*; who may previously have exhibited allergy to antimicrobials or whose routes of elimination may be impaired, e.g. by renal disease.

- *Administer the drug* in optimum *dose* and *frequency* and by the most appropriate *route(s)*. Inadequate dose may encourage the development of microbial resistance. In general, intermittent dosing is preferred to continuous infusion. Plasma concentration monitoring can be applied to optimise therapy.

- *Continue therapy* until apparent cure has been achieved; most acute infections are treated for 5–10 days. There are many exceptions to this, such as typhoid fever, tuberculosis and infective endocarditis, in which relapse is possible long after apparent clinical cure and so the drugs are continued for a longer time, determined by experience.

● *Test for cure.* In some infections, microbiological proof of cure is desirable because disappearance of symptoms and signs occurs before the organisms are eradicated, e.g. urinary tract infections. Microbiological examination must be done, of course, after withdrawal of chemotherapy.

● *Prophylactic chemotherapy* for surgical and dental procedures should be of very limited duration. It should start at the time of surgery to reduce the risk of producing resistant organisms prior to surgery (see p. 191).

● *Carriers of pathogenic organisms*, in general, should not be treated to remove the organisms for it is better to allow natural re-establishment of a normal flora.

Use of antimicrobial drugs

CHOICE

The general rule is that selection of antimicrobials should be based on identification of the microbe and sensitivity tests. All appropriate specimens (blood, pus, urine, sputum, cerebrospinal fluid) must therefore be taken for examination before administering any antimicrobial.

This process inevitably takes time and therapy must usually be started on the basis of the 'best guess', from which point of view infections may be categorised as those in which:

1. Choice of antimicrobial follows automatically from the clinical diagnosis because the causative organism is always the same, and is virtually always sensitive to the same drug, e.g. segmental pneumonia in a young person which is almost always caused by *Streptococcus pneumoniae* (benzylpenicillin), some haemolytic streptococcal infections, e.g. scarlet fever, erysipelas (benzylpenicillin), typhus (tetracycline), leprosy (dapsone with rifampicin).

2. The infecting organism is identified by the clinical diagnosis, but no assumption can be made as to its sensitivity to any one antimicrobial, e.g. tuberculosis.

3. The infecting organism is not identified by the clinical diagnosis, e.g. in urinary tract infection or meningitis.

In the second and third categories particularly, choice of an antimicrobial may be guided by:

Knowledge of the likely pathogens (and their current sensitivity to antimicrobials) in the clinical situation. Cephalexin is a reasonable first choice for lower urinary tract infection (coliform organisms), and benzylpenicillin for meningitis in the adult (meningococcal or pneumococcal).

Simple staining tests. The antimicrobial may be selected in the knowledge that the organism is a Gram-positive or Gram-negative coccus or bacillus. It is necessary to know the current sensitivities to antimicrobial drugs for organisms so classified; flucloxacillin may be indicated when clusters of Gram-positive cocci are found (indicating staphylococci), an aminoglycoside if Gram-negative bacilli are detected. Ziehl-Neelsen staining may reveal acid-fast tubercle bacilli.

Modification of treatment can be made later if necessary, in the light of culture and sensitivity tests. Treatment otherwise should be changed only after adequate trial, usually 3 days, for over-hasty alterations cause confusion and tend to produce resistant organisms.

COMBINATIONS

Treatment with a single antimicrobial is sufficient for most infections. The indications for use of two or more antimicrobials are:

● To avoid the development of drug resistance, especially in chronic infections, e.g. tuberculosis

● To broaden the spectrum of antibacterial activity: (1) in a known mixed infection, e.g. peritonitis following gut perforation or (2) where the infecting organism cannot be predicted but treatment is essential before a diagnosis has been reached, e.g. septicaemia complicating neutropenia or severe community-acquired pneumonia; full doses of each drug are needed

● To obtain potentiation, i.e. an effect unobtainable with either drug alone, e.g. penicillin plus gentamicin for enterococcal endocarditis.

Selection of agents. A bacteriostatic drug, by reducing multiplication, may protect the organism from a bactericidal drug (see above, Antagonism). When a combination must be used blind, it is preferable to use two bacteriostatic or two bactericidal drugs, lest there be antagonism.

CHEMOPROPHYLAXIS AND PRE-EMPTIVE SUPPRESSIVE THERAPY

It is sometimes assumed that what a drug can cure it will also prevent, but this is not necessarily so.

The basis of effective, true, chemoprophylaxis is the use of a drug in a healthy person to prevent infection by one organism of virtually uniform susceptibility, e.g. benzylpenicillin against a group A streptococcus. But the term chemoprophylaxis is commonly extended to include suppression of existing infection. The main categories of chemoprophylaxis may be summarised as follows:

● *True prevention of infection*: rheumatic fever,[8] recurrent urinary tract infection.

● *Prevention of opportunistic infections*, e.g. due to commensals getting into the wrong place (bacterial endocarditis after dentistry and peritonitis after bowel surgery). Note that these are both high risk situations of short duration; prolonged administration of drugs before surgery would result in the areas concerned (mouth and bowel) being colonised by drug-resistant organisms with potentially disastrous results (see below). Immunocompromised patients can benefit from chemoprophylaxis, e.g. prophylaxis of Gram-negative septicaemia complicating neutropenia or leukaemia with an oral quinolone.

● *Suppression* of existing infection before it causes overt disease, e.g. tuberculosis, malaria, animal bites, trauma.

● *Prevention of exacerbations* of a chronic infection, e.g. bronchitis, in cystic fibrosis.

---

[8] Rheumatic fever is caused by a large number of types of Group A streptococci and immunity is type-specific. Recurrent attacks are commonly due to infection with different strains of these, all of which are sensitive to penicillin and so chemoprophylaxis is effective. Acute glomerulonephritis is also due to group A streptococci. But only a few types cause it, so that natural immunity is more likely to protect and, in fact, second attacks are rare. Therefore, chemoprophylaxis is not used (see also p. 217).

● *Prevention of spread amongst contacts* (in epidemics and/or sporadic cases). Spread of influenza A can be partially prevented by amantadine; in an epidemic of meningitis, or when there is a case in the family, rifampicin may be used; very young and fragile non-immune child contacts of pertussis might benefit from erythromycin.

Prophylaxis of bacterial infection can be achieved often by doses that are inadequate for therapy. Details of the practice of chemoprophylaxis are given in the appropriate sections.

Attempts to use drugs routinely in groups specially at risk to prevent infection by a range of organisms, e.g. pneumonia in the unconscious or in patients with heart failure and in the newborn after prolonged labour, have not only failed but have sometimes permitted infections with less susceptible organisms. Attempts routinely to prevent bacterial infection secondary to virus infections, e.g. in respiratory tract infections, measles, have not been sufficiently successful to outweigh the disadvantages of drug allergy and infection with drug-resistant bacteria. In these situations it is generally better to be alert for complications and then to treat them vigorously, than to try to prevent them.

Chemoprophylaxis in surgery

The principles governing use of antimicrobials in this context are as follows.

● Chemoprophylaxis is justified:

1. when the risk of infection is high because of the presence of large numbers of bacteria in the viscus which is being operated on, e.g. the large bowel

2. when the risk of infection is low but the consequences of infection would be disastrous, e.g. insertion of prosthetic joints or prosthetic heart valves, or colonisation of abnormal heart valves following the transient bacteraemia of dentistry

3. when the patient is generally susceptible to infection, e.g. patients who are neutropenic due to treatment of leukaemia, or otherwise immunocompromised.

● Antimicrobials should be selected with a knowledge of the likely pathogens at the sites of surgery and their prevailing antimicrobial susceptibility.

● Antimicrobials should be given i.v., i.m. or occasionally rectally at the beginning of anaesthesia and for no more than 48 h. Specific instances are:

1. *Colorectal surgery*, because there is a high risk of infection with *Escherichia coli*, clostridia and bacteroides which inhabit the gut (a cephalosporin plus metronidazole is satisfactory)

2. *Gastroduodenal surgery*, for colonisation of the stomach with gut organisms occurs especially when acid secretion is low, e.g. in gastric malignancy, following use of a histamine H_2-receptor antagonist or following previous gastric surgery to reduce acid (usually a cephalosporin alone provides adequate chemoprophylaxis)

3. *Gynaecological surgery*, because the vagina contains bacteroides, streptococci, coliforms and anaerobes (metronidazole and a cephalosporin are used). Chemoprophylaxis is indicated for hysterectomy, by the vaginal and by the abdominal route, and for perineal floor repair but probably not for other elective procedures

4. *Leg amputation*, because there is a risk of gas gangrene in an ischaemic limb and the mortality is high (benzylpenicillin should be given, or metronidazole for the patient with allergy to penicillin)

5. *Insertion of prosthetic joints*. Chemoprophylaxis is justified because infection (*Staphylococcus aureus* and *Escherichia coli* are commonest) almost invariably means that the artificial joint, valve or vessel must be replaced.

Problems with antimicrobial drugs

RESISTANCE

Microbial resistance to antimicrobials is a matter of great importance; if sensitive strains are supplanted by resistant ones, then a valuable drug may become useless. Just as:

Some are born great, some achieve greatness, and some have greatness thrust upon them.[9]

so microorganisms may be naturally ('born') resistant, 'achieve' resistance by mutation or have resistance 'thrust upon them' by plasmids.

Mechanisms of resistance act as follows:

● *Naturally resistant strains*. In the course of therapy, the naturally sensitive strains are eliminated and those naturally resistant proliferate and occupy the biological space created by the drug.

● *Spontaneous mutation* brings about selective multiplication of the resistant strain so that it eventually dominates as above.

● *Transmission of genes from other organisms* is the commonest and most important mechanism. Genetic material may be transferred, e.g. in the form of *plasmids* which are strands of DNA that lie outwith the chromosomes and contain genes capable of controlling various metabolic processes including formation of β-lactamases (that destroy some penicillins and cephalosporins), and enzymes that inactivate aminoglycosides. Alternatively genetic transfer may occur through a bacteriophage (a virus which infects bacteria), particularly in the case of staphylococci.

Resistance is mediated most commonly by the production of enzymes that modify the drug, e.g. aminoglycosides are phosphorylated, β-lactamases inactivate penicillins. Other mechanisms include decreasing the passage into or increasing the efflux of drug from the bacterial cell, and modification of the target site so that the antimicrobial binds less effectively, e.g. methicillin resistance in staphylococci.

Limitation of resistance to antimicrobials may be achieved by:

● Avoidance of indiscriminate use by ensuring that the indication for, the dose and duration of treatment are appropriate

● Using antimicrobial combinations in appropriate circumstances, e.g. tuberculosis

● Constant monitoring of resistance patterns in a hospital or community, and outbreak control to prevent the spread of resistant bacteria

---

[9] Malvolio in Twelfth Night, Act 2 Scene 5, by William Shakespeare (1564–1616). We are grateful to C A Mims et al (1993 Medical Microbiology, Mosby, London) for drawing our attention to the aptness of this quotation.

● Restricting drug use, which involves agreement between clinicians and microbiologists, e.g. delaying the emergence of resistance by limiting the use of the newest member of a group of antimicrobials so long as the currently-used drugs are effective; restricting use of a drug may become necessary where it promotes the proliferation of resistant strains, as occurred when neurosurgical infections were caused by Klebsiella resistant to ampicillin used for prophylaxis.

OPPORTUNISTIC INFECTION

When any antimicrobial drug is used, there is usually suppression of part of the normal bacterial flora of the patient, according to the drug. Often, this causes no ill effects, but sometimes a drug-resistant organism, freed from competition, proliferates to an extent which allows an infection to be established. The principal organisms responsible are *Candida albicans* and pseudomonads. But careful assessment is essential, as the mere presence of such organisms in diagnostic specimens taken from a site in which they may be present as commensals, does not necessarily mean they are causing disease.

Antibiotic-associated colitis is an example of an opportunistic infection. Almost any antimicrobial that can alter bowel flora may initiate this condition but the drugs most commonly reported are clindamycin, amoxycillin, ampicillin and cephalosporins. It takes the form of an acute, nonspecific colitis (pseudomembranous colitis) with diarrhoeal stools containing blood or mucus, abdominal pain, leucocytosis and dehydration. A history of antibiotic use in the previous 3 weeks, even if the drug therapy has been stopped, should alert the physician to the diagnosis which is confirmed by typical appearances on proctosigmoidoscopy and the isolation of *Clostridium difficile* or its toxin from the stools; it is this toxin that causes the colitis. Mild cases usually respond to discontinuation of the offending antimicrobial allowing re-establishment of the patient's normal bowel flora. More severe cases merit treatment with oral metronidazole or vancomycin.

A special problem of opportunistic infection arises in patients whose immune systems are compromised by disease (e.g. AIDS, hypogammaglobulinaemia, leukaemia, cystic fibrosis) or drugs (e.g. cytotoxics, adrenal steroids). Treatment should be prompt, initiated before the results of bacteriological tests are known and usually involving combinations of bactericidal drugs administered parenterally.

MASKING OF INFECTIONS

Masking of infections by chemotherapy is an important possibility. The risk cannot be entirely avoided but it can be minimised by intelligent use of antimicrobials. For example, a course of penicillin adequate to cure gonorrhoea may prevent simultaneously contracted syphilis from showing primary and secondary stages without effecting a cure and a serological test for syphilis should be done 3 months after treatment for gonorrhoea.

Drugs of choice

Table 11.1 is provided for reference. It is a summary of the choice of antimicrobial drugs and owes its form and much of its contents to *Medical Letter on Drugs and Therapeutics* (USA) (1996).[10]

The table should be used to supplement the general text. Some differences will be noted between text and table for there may be no single correct procedure for each infection. Tables on drugs for viruses, fungi, protozoa and helminths are provided in Chapter 14.

GUIDE TO FURTHER READING

Bisno A L 1991 Group A Streptococcal infections and acute rheumatic fever. New England Journal of Medicine 325: 783
Colbridge M J et al 1995 Antibiotics carried in general practitioners' emergency bags: four years on. British Medical Journal 310: 29
Colebrook L, Kenny M 1939 Treatment with prontosil of puerperal infections. Lancet 2: 1319 (a classic paper)
Fletcher C 1984 First clinical use of penicillin. British Medical Journal 289: 1721 (a classic paper)

[10] We are grateful to the Chairman of the Editorial Board for permission to use this material. D R L, P N B, M J B.

Table 11.1   Reference data on antimicrobial drugs of choice

* Resistance may be a problem; sensitivity tests should be performed.
◊ Suggested alternatives do not necessarily comprise all options.

Infecting organism	Drug(s) of first choice	Alternative drugs◊
Gram-positive cocci		
Enterococcus		
endocarditis or other severe infection	benzylpenicillin or amoxycillin + gentamicin, or streptomycin	vancomycin + gentamicin or streptomycin
uncomplicated urinary tract infection	amoxycillin	trimethoprim or nitrofurantoin
Staphylococcus aureus or *epidermidis*		
nonpenicillinase-producing	benzylpenicillin or phenoxymethylpenicillin	a cephalosporin or vancomycin or imipenem or erythromycin
penicillinase-producing	cloxacillin or flucloxacillin	a cephalosporin or vancomycin or co-amoxiclav or imipenem or erythromycin or a quinolone
methicillin-resistant	vancomycin ± gentamicin ± rifampicin	co-trimoxazole or a tetracycline (minocycline) or a quinolone or sodium fusidate or rifampicin
Streptococcus pyogenes (Group A) and Groups C and G *Streptococcus*, Group B	benzylpenicillin or phenoxymethypenicillin or amoxycillin	erythromycin or a cephalosporin or vancomycin or clindamycin (the latter for necrotising fasciitis)
Streptococcus, viridans group (endocarditis)	benzylpenicillin ± gentamicin	vancomycin or a cephalosporin
Streptococcus, anaerobic	benzylpenicillin	metronidazole
Streptococcus pneumoniae (pneumococcus)	benzylpenicillin or phenoxymethylpenicillin or amoxycillin	erythromycin or a cephalosporin or vancomycin or rifampicin (or chloramphenicol for meningitis)
Gram-negative cocci		
Moraxella (Branhamella) catarrhalis	co-amoxiclav	erythromycin or a tetracycline
Neisseria gonorrhoeae (gonococcus)	amoxycillin (+ probenecid) or a quinolone or ceftriaxone	spectinomycin or cefixime or cefotaxime or a quinolone
Neisseria meningitidis (meningococcus)	benzylpenicillin	chloramphenicol or cefotaxime
Gram-positive bacilli		
Bacillus anthracis (anthrax)	benzylpenicillin	erythromycin or a tetracycline
Clostridium perfringens (gas gangrene)	benzylpenicillin	metronidazole or clindamycin
Clostridium tetani (tetanus)	benzylpenicillin	a tetracycline
Clostridium difficile (pseudomembraneous colitis)	metronidazole (oral)	vancomycin (oral)
Corynebacterium diphtheriae (diphtheria)	erythromycin	benzylpenicillin
Listeria monocytogenes (listeriosis)	amoxycillin ± gentamicin	erythromycin + gentamicin
Enteric Gram-negative bacilli		
Bacteroides oropharyngeal strains	benzylpenicillin	metronidazole or clindamycin
gastrointestinal strains	metronidazole	co-amoxiclav or clindamycin or imipenem
Campylobacter jejuni	erythromycin or a quinolone	tetracycline *(cont'd)*

Table 11.1 (cont'd)

* Resistance may be a problem; sensitivity tests should be performed.
◊ Suggested alternatives do not necessarily comprise all options.

Infecting organism	Drug(s) of first choice	Alternative drugs◊

*Enterobacteriaceae
e.g. *Enterobacter
   aerogenes
  *Escherichia coli
  *Klebsiella
   pneumoniae
  *Proteus spp.		

lower urinary tract	a quinolone or an oral cephalosporin	amoxycillin or trimethoprim
septicaemia	gentamicin or cefuroxime or cefotaxime	a quinolone or imipenem
*Helicobacter pylori	amoxycillin + clarithromycin + metronidazole (with omeprazole)	amoxycillin + metronidazole + bismuth chelate or tetracycline + clarithromycin + bismuth chelate
*Salmonella typhi (typhoid fever)	ceftriaxone or a quinolone	chloramphenicol or co-trimoxazole or amoxycillin
*other Salmonella	a quinolone	amoxycillin or co-trimoxazole or chloramphenicol
*Shigella	a quinolone	trimethoprim or ampicillin
*Yersinia enterocolitica	co-trimoxazole	a quinolone or gentamicin or tetracycline
Other Gram-negative bacilli		
*Bordetella pertussis (whooping cough)	erythromycin	ampicillin
*Brucella (brucellosis)	a tetracycline + streptomycin	co-trimoxazole or rifampicin + a tetracycline
Calymmatobacterium granulomatis (granuloma inguinale)	a tetracycline	streptomycin or gentamicin or co-trimoxazole
*Fusobacterium	benzylpenicillin	metronidazole or clindamycin
Gardnerella vaginalis (bacterial vaginosis)	oral metronidazole	topical clindamycin or metronidazole, or oral clindamycin
*Haemophilus ducreyi (chancroid)	erythromycin	a quinolone
*Haemophilus influenzae		
meningitis, epiglottitis, arthritis or other serious infections	cefotaxime or ceftriaxone or amoxycillin	cefuroxime (but not for meningitis) or chloramphenicol
upper respiratory infections and bronchitis	amoxycillin	co-amoxiclav or cefuroxime
Legionella pneumophila (legionnaire's disease)	erythromycin ± rifampicin	
Pasteurella multocida (from animal bites)	benzylpenicillin	co-amoxiclav or a cephalosporin
*Pseudomonas aeruginosa		
urinary tract infection	a quinolone	ticarcillin or piperacillin or mezlocillin
other infections	ticarcillin or mezlocillin, or piperacillin or gentamicin or amikacin	ceftazidime or imipenem
Vibrio cholerae (cholera)	tetracycline	a quinolone
Acid-fast bacilli		
*Mycobacterium tuberculosis	isoniazid + rifampicin + pyrazinamide ± ethambutol or streptomycin	a quinolone or cycloserine or capreomycin or kanamycin or ethionamide *(cont'd)*

Table 11.1 (cont'd)

* Resistance may be a problem; sensitivity tests should be performed.
◊ Suggested alternatives do not necessarily comprise all options.

Infecting organism	Drug(s) of first choice	Alternative drugs◊
Mycobacterium leprae (leprosy)	dapsone +rifampicin ± clofazimine	ethionamide or cycloserine
Actinomycetes		
Actinomyces israelii (actinomycosis)	benzylpenicillin	a tetracycline
Nocardia	co-trimoxazole	amikacin or minocycline or imipenem
Chlamydiae		
Chlamydia psittaci (psittacosis, ornithosis)	tetracycline	chloramphenicol
Chlamydia trachomatis		
trachoma	azithromycin	tetracycline (topical plus oral) or a sulphonamide (topical plus oral)
inclusion conjunctivitis	erythromycin (oral or i.v.)	a sulphonamide
pneumonia	erythromycin	a sulphonamide
urethritis, cervicitis	doxycycline or azithromycin	erythromycin or ofloxacin
lymphogranuloma venereum	tetracycline	erythromycin
Chlamydia pneumoniae (TWAR strain)	tetracycline	erythromycin
Ehrlichia		
Ehrlichia chaffeensis	a tetracycline	
Mycoplasma		
Mycoplasma pneumoniae	erythromycin or tetracycline	clarithromycin or azithromycin
Ureaplasma urealyticum	erythromycin	tetracycline or clarithromycin
Rickettsia		
Q fever, typhus	tetracycline	chloramphenicol or a quinolone
Spirochaetes		
Borrelia burgdorferi (Lyme disease)	doxycycline or amoxycillin	cefuroxime or ceftriaxone or cefotaxime or benzylpenicillin
Borrelia recurrentis (relapsing fever)	tetracycline	benzylpenicillin
Leptospira (leptospirosis)	benzylpenicillin	tetracycline
Treponema pallidum (syphilis)	benzylpenicillin	tetracycline or ceftriaxone
Treponema pertenue (yaws)	benzylpenicillin	tetracycline

GUIDE TO FURTHER READING (cont'd)

Jacoby G A, Archer G L 1991 New mechanisms of bacterial resistance to antimicrobial agents. New England Journal of Medicine 324: 601

Loudon I 1987 Puerperal fever, the streptococcus, and the sulphonamides, 1911–1945. British Medical Journal 295: 485

Mackowiak P A 1982 The normal microbiological flora. New England Journal of Medicine 307: 83

Murray B E 1994 Can antibiotic resistance be controlled? New England Journal of Medicine 330: 1229

O'Brien T F 1992 Preoperative antibiotic prophylaxis. New England Journal of Medicine 326: 337

Report 1994 Multiple-antibiotic-resistant pathogenic bacteria. New England Journal of Medicine 330: 1247

Antibacterial drugs

SYNOPSIS

The range of antibacterial drugs is wide and affords the clinician scope to select with a knowledge of the likely or proved pathogen(s) and of factors relevant to the patient, e.g. allergy, renal disease.

Antibacterial drugs are here discussed in groups primarily by their site of antibacterial action and secondly by molecular structure, for members of each structural group are usually handled by the body in a similar way and have the same range of adverse effects.

Table 11.1 is a general reference for this chapter.

Classification

INHIBITION OF CELL WALL SYNTHESIS

- **Beta-lactams**, the structure of which contains a β-lactam ring.

The major subdivisions are:
  (a) *penicillins* whose official names include or end in 'cillin'
  (b) *cephalosporins* and *cephamycins* which are recognised by the inclusion of 'cef' or 'ceph' in their official names.

Lesser categories of β-lactams include
  (c) *carbapenems* and (d) *monobactams*.

- Other inhibitors of cell wall synthesis include vancomycin and teicoplanin.

INHIBITION OF PROTEIN SYNTHESIS

- **Aminoglycosides.** The names of those that are derived from streptomyces end in 'mycin', e.g. tobramycin. Others include gentamicin (from *Micromonospora purpurea* which is not a fungus, hence the spelling as 'micin') and semisynthetic drugs, e.g. amikacin.
- **Tetracyclines** as the name suggests are four-ringed structures and their names end in '-cycline'.
- **Macrolides:** e.g. erythromycin. *Clindamycin*, structurally a lincosamide, has a similar action and overlapping antibacterial activity.
- Other drugs that act by inhibiting protein synthesis include *chloramphenicol* and *sodium fusidate*.

INHIBITION OF NUCLEIC ACID SYNTHESIS

- **Sulphonamides.** Usually their names contain 'sulpha' or 'sulfa'. These drugs, and *trimethoprim*, with which they may be combined, inhibit synthesis of nucleic acid precursors.
- **Quinolones** are structurally related to nalidixic acid; the names of the most recently introduced members of the group end in '-oxacin', e.g. ciprofloxacin. They act by preventing DNA replication.
- **Azoles** all contain an azole ring and the names end in '-azole', e.g. metronidazole. They act by the

production of short-lived intermediate compounds which are toxic to DNA.

Antimicrobials that are restricted to certain specific uses, i.e. tuberculosis, urinary tract infections, are described with the treatment of these conditions in Chapter 13.

Inhibition of cell wall synthesis

Beta-lactams

Penicillins

Benzylpenicillin (1942) is produced by growing one of the penicillium moulds in deep tanks. In 1957 the penicillin nucleus (6-amino-penicillanic acid) was synthesised and it became possible to add various side-chains and so to make semisynthetic penicillins with different properties.

It is important to recognise that not all penicillins have the same antibacterial spectrum and that it is necessary to choose between a number of penicillins just as between antimicrobials of different structural groups, as is shown below.

A general account of the penicillins follows and then of the individual drugs in so far as they differ.

Mode of action is by inhibiting the enzymes that are involved in the formation of the peptidoglycan layer of the cell wall which protects the bacterium from its environment; incapable of withstanding the osmotic gradient between its interior and its environment the cell swells and ruptures. Penicillins are thus bactericidal and are effective only against multiplying organisms, as resting organisms are not making new cell wall. The main defence of bacteria against penicillins is to produce enzymes, β-lactamases, which open the β-lactam ring and terminate their activity. The remarkable safety of the penicillins is due to the fact that human cell walls have a different structure that is unaffected by penicillin.

PENICILLINS	
Narrow spectrum (natural penicillins)	benzylpenicillin phenoxymethylpenicillin
Antistaphylococcal penicillins (β-lactamase resistant)	cloxacillin, flucloxacillin
Broad spectrum	ampicillin, amoxycillin, bacampicillin, pivampicillin
Mecillinam	temocillin
Monobactam (active against Gram-negative bacteria excluding *Pseudomonas aeruginosa*)	aztreonam[1]
Antipseudomonal *Carboxypenicillins*	carbenicillin, ticarcillin
Ureidopenicillins	azlocillin, piperacillin

Pharmacokinetics. Benzylpenicillin is destroyed by gastric acid and is unsuitable for oral use. Others, e.g. phenoxymethylpenicillin, resist acid and are absorbed in the upper small bowel. The plasma $t\frac{1}{2}$ of penicillins is usually <2 h. They are distributed mainly in the body water and enter well into the CSF if the meninges are inflamed. Penicillins are organic acids and their rapid clearance from plasma is due to secretion into renal tubular fluid by the anion transport mechanism in the kidney. Renal clearance therefore greatly exceeds the glomerular filtration rate (127 ml/min). The excretion rate of penicillin can be usefully delayed by concurrently giving probenecid which competes successfully for the transport mechanism. Dosage of penicillins may need to be reduced for patients with severely impaired renal function.

Adverse effects. The main hazard with the penicillins is *allergic reactions*. These include itching, rashes (eczematous or urticarial), fever and angioneurotic oedema. Rarely (about 1 in 10 000) there is anaphylactic shock which can be fatal (about 1 in 50 000–100 000 treatment courses). Allergies are least likely when penicillins are given

---

[1] While not strictly a penicillin, it has a similar spectrum of action including some antipseudomonal activity.

orally and most likely with local application or with procaine penicillin i.m. Metabolic opening of the β-lactam ring creates a highly reactive penicilloyl group which binds with tissue proteins to form the major antigenic determinant. The anaphylactic reaction involves specific IgE antibodies which can be detected in the plasma of susceptible persons.

There is *cross-allergy* between all the various forms of penicillin, probably due in part to their common structure, and in part to the degradation products common to them all. *Partial cross-allergy* exists between penicillins and cephalosporins (10%) which is of particular concern when the reaction to either group of antimicrobials has been angioneurotic oedema or anaphylactic shock.

When attempting to predict whether a patient will have an allergic reaction, a reliable history of a previous adverse response to penicillin is valuable. Immediate-type reactions such as urticaria, angio-oedema and anaphylactic shock can be taken to indicate allergy, but interpretation of maculopapular rashes is more difficult. Since an alternative drug can usually be found, a penicillin is best avoided if there is suspicion of allergy, although the condition is undoubtedly overdiagnosed and may be transient (see below).

When the history of allergy is not clear-cut and it is necessary to prescribe a penicillin, the presence of *IgE antibodies* in serum is a useful indicator of reactions mediated by these antibodies, i.e. immediate (type 1) reactions. Additionally, an *intradermal test* for allergy may be performed using standard amounts of a mixture of a major determinant (metabolite) (benzylpenicilloyl polylysine) and minor determinants (such as benzylpenicillin), of the allergic reaction; appearance of a flare and weal reaction indicates a positive response. The fact that only about 10% of patients with a history of 'penicillin allergy' respond suggests that many who are so labelled are not, or are no longer, allergic to penicillin.

Other (non-allergic) adverse effects include diarrhoea due to alteration in normal intestinal flora which may lead to opportunist infection with pseudomonads or *Candida albicans*, although this is uncommon. Neutropenia is a risk if penicillins (or other β-lactam antibiotics) are used in high dose and usually for a period of longer than 10 days.

Rarely the penicillins cause anaemia, sometimes haemolytic. Penicillins are presented as their sodium or potassium salts which are inevitably taken in significant amounts if high dose of antimicrobial is used. Physicians should be aware of this unexpected source of sodium or potassium especially in patients with renal or cardiac disease. Extremely high plasma penicillin concentrations cause convulsions.

NARROW SPECTRUM PENICILLINS

Benzylpenicillin (penicillin G) ($t^{1\!/}_{2}$ 0.5 h)

Benzylpenicillin is used when high plasma concentration is required. The short $t^{1\!/}_{2}$ means that reasonably spaced doses have to be large to maintain a therapeutic concentration. Only the extraordinary lack of dose-related toxicity of penicillin allows the resulting fluctuations to be acceptable. Benzylpenicillin is eliminated by the kidney, about 80% being actively secreted by the renal tubule and this can be blocked usefully by probenecid, e.g. to reduce the frequency of injection for small children or for single dose therapy as in gonorrhoea.

Uses (see Table 11.1). Benzylpenicillin is highly active against *Streptococcus pneumoniae* and the Lancefield group A, β-haemolytic streptococci. Viridans streptococci are usually sensitive unless the patient has recently received penicillin. *Enterococcus* (formerly *streptococcus*) *faecalis* is less susceptible and, especially for endocarditis, penicillin should be combined with an aminoglycoside, usually gentamicin. Benzylpenicillin is the drug of choice for infections due to *Neisseria meningitidis* (meningococcal meningitis), *Bacillus anthracis* (anthrax), *Clostridium perfringens* (gas gangrene) and *Clostridium tetani* (tetanus), *Corynebacterium diphtheriae* (diphtheria), *Treponema pallidum* (syphilis), *Leptospira* spp. (leptospirosis) and *Actinomyces israelii* (actinomycosis). It is also the drug of choice for *Borrelia burgdorferi* (Lyme disease) in children. The sensitivity of *Neisseria gonorrhoeae* varies in different parts of the world, and in some resistance is rife.

Adverse effects are in general uncommon, apart from allergy (above). It is salutary to reflect that the first clinically useful true antibiotic (1942) still in use and is also amongst the least toxic.

Preparations and dosage for injection. Benzylpenicillin may be given i.m. or i.v. (by bolus injection or by continuous infusion). For a sensitive infection, benzylpenicillin[2] 300–600 mg × 6 h is enough. This is obviously inconvenient in domiciliary practice where a mixture of benzylpenicillin and one of its long-acting variants may be preferred (see below).

For relatively insensitive infections and where sensitive organisms are in avascular tissue (infective endocarditis) 7.2–14.4 g are given daily i.v. in divided doses. When an infection is controlled, a change may be made to the oral route using phenoxymethylpenicillin, or amoxycillin which is better absorbed.

Procaine penicillin, given i.m. only, is a stable salt and liberates benzylpenicillin over 12–24 h, according to the dose administered, on average 360 mg × 12–24 h. There is no general agreement on its place in therapy. It is probably best to use benzylpenicillin in the most severe infections, especially at the outset, as procaine penicillin will not give therapeutic blood concentrations for some hours after injection.

Preparations and dosage for oral use. Phenoxymethylpenicillin (penicillin V), is resistant to gastric acid and so reaches the small intestine intact where it is moderately well absorbed. It is less active than benzylpenicillin against *Neisseria gonorrhoeae* and *Neisseria meningitidis*, and so is unsuitable for use in gonorrhoea and meningococcal meningitis. It is a satisfactory substitute for benzylpenicillin against *Streptococcus pneumoniae*, *Streptococcus pyogenes* and *Staphylococcus aureus*, especially after the acute infection has been brought under control. The dose is 250–500 mg × 6 h.

All oral penicillins are best given on an empty stomach to avoid the absorption delay caused by food.

Antistaphylococcal penicillins

Certain bacteria produce β-lactamases which open

the β-lactam ring that is common to all penicillins, and thus terminate the antibacterial activity. Drugs that resist the action of staphylococcal β-lactamase do so by their possession of an acyl side-chain which protects the β-lactam bond by preventing the enzyme getting access to it. The drugs do have activity against other bacteria for which penicillin is indicated, but benzylpenicillin is substantially more active against these organisms — up to 20 times more so in the cases of pneumococci, β-haemolytic streptococci and *Neisseria*. Hence, when infection is mixed, it may be necessary to give benzylpenicillin as well as a β-lactamase-resistant drug. These include:

Cloxacillin ($t^{1}/_{2}$ 0.5 h) resists degradation by gastric acid and is absorbed from the gut, but food markedly interferes with absorption.

Flucloxacillin ($t^{1}/_{2}$ 1 h) is better absorbed and so gives higher blood concentration than does cloxacillin. It may cause cholestatic jaundice, particularly when used for more than 2 weeks or to patients > 55 years.

Methicillin: its use is now confined to laboratory sensitivity tests. Identification of methicillin-resistant *Staphylococcus aureus* (MRSA) in patients indicates the organisms are resistant to flucloxacillin and cloxacillin and often to other antibacterial drugs, and demands special infection-control measures.

BROAD SPECTRUM PENICILLINS

The activity of these semisynthetic penicillins extends beyond the Gram-positive and Gram-negative cocci which are susceptible to benzylpenicillin, and includes many Gram-negative bacilli. They do not resist β-lactamases and are therefore ineffective against organisms that produce these enzymes.

As a general rule these agents are rather less active than benzylpenicillin against Gram-positive cocci, but more active than the β-lactamase-resistant penicillins (above). They have very useful activity against *Enterococcus faecalis* and many strains of *Haemophilus influenzae*. *Enterobacteriaceae* are variably sensitive and laboratory testing for sensitivity is important in infections with these organisms. The differences between the members of this group are pharmacological rather than bacteriological.

---

[2] 600 mg = 1 000 000 units, 1 mega-unit

Amoxycillin (t½ 1 h) is a structural analogue of ampicillin (below) and is better absorbed from the gut (especially after food), and for the same dose achieves approximately double the plasma concentration. Diarrhoea is less frequent with amoxycillin than with ampicillin. The oral dose is 250 mg × 8 h; a parenteral form is available but offers no advantage over ampicillin. For oral use, however, amoxycillin is preferred because of its greater bioavailability and fewer adverse effects.

Co-amoxiclav (Augmentin). *Clavulanic acid* is a β-lactam compound which has little intrinsic antibacterial activity but is important because it binds to β-lactamases and thereby competitively protects the penicillin, so potentiating it against bacteria which owe their resistance to production of β-lactamases, i.e. clavulanic acid acts as a 'suicide' inhibitor. It is formulated in tablets as its potassium salt (equivalent to 125 mg of clavulanic acid) in combination with amoxycillin (250 or 500 mg), as co-amoxiclav, and is a satisfactory oral treatment for infections due to β-lactamase-producing organisms, notably in the respiratory or urinary tracts. It should be used when β-lactamase-producing amoxycillin resistant organisms are either suspected or proven by culture. These include most strains of *Staphyloccocus aureus*, many strains of *Escherichia coli* and an increasing number of strains of *Haemophilus influenzae*. The dose is one tablet × 8 h.

Ampicillin (t½ 1 h) is acid-stable and is moderately well absorbed when swallowed. The oral dose is 0.25–1 g × 6–8 h; or i.m. or i.v. 250–1000 mg × 4–6 h. Approximately one-third of a dose appears unchanged in the urine. The drug is concentrated in the bile.

Pivampicillin and *bacampicillin* are esters of ampicillin which are de-esterified in the gut mucosa or liver to release ampicillin to the systemic circulation. The esters are better absorbed than ampicillin itself, give higher blood concentrations for equivalent doses, are less affected by food in the gut and cause less diarrhoea.

Adverse effects. Ampicillin may cause diarrhoea but the incidence (12%) is less with prodrugs of ampicillin or with amoxycillin. Ampicillin and its analogues have a peculiar capacity to cause a macular rash resembling measles or rubella, usually unaccompanied by other signs of allergy. These rashes are very common in patients with disease of the lymphoid system, notably infectious mononucleosis (use of ampicillin or its analogues may declare this diagnosis when given for sore throat), and in lymphoid leukaemia. A macular rash should not be taken to imply allergy to other penicillins which tend to cause a true urticarial reaction. Patients with renal failure and those taking allopurinol for hyperuricaemia also seem more prone to ampicillin rashes. Cholestatic jaundice has been associated with use of co-amoxiclav even up to 6 weeks after cessation of the drug; the clavulanic acid may be responsible.

MECILLINAM

Temocillin (t½ 5 h) is closely related to the broad spectrum penicillins but has different antibacterial activity: it is active against Gram-negative organisms including β-lactamase-producing *Enterobacteriaceae* but is inactive against *Pseudomonas aeruginosa*, and against Gram-positive organisms. Temocillin has been used to treat urinary infection and septicaemia but a cephalosporin is usually preferred. Diarrhoea, rash and pain at the site of i.m. injection may occur.

MONOBACTAM

Aztreonam is the first member of this class of β-lactam antibiotics. It is active against Gram-negative organisms including *Pseudomonas aeruginosa*, *Haemophilus influenzae* and *Neisseria meningitidis* and *gonorrhoeae*. Aztreonam is used to treat septicaemia and complicated urinary tract infections, Gram-negative lower urinary tract infections and gonorrhoea. Adverse effects include reactions at the site of infusion, rashes, gastrointestinal upset, hepatitis, thrombocytopenia and neutropenia.

ANTIPSEUDOMONAL PENICILLINS

Carboxypenicillins

These in general have the same antibacterial spectrum as ampicillin (and are susceptible to β-lactamases), but have the additional capacity to destroy *Pseudomonas aeruginosa* and indole positive *Proteus* spp.

Carbenicillin (t½ 1 h) was the first penicillin with

activity against *Pseudomonas aeruginosa*: it is given parenterally. Ticarcillin (below) or a ureidopenicillin is now preferred for severe infection.

Ticarcillin ($t^{1/2}$ 1 h) is 4 times more active against *Pseudomonas aeruginosa* than is carbenicillin. It is given by i.m. or slow i.v. injection or by rapid i.v. infusion. Combination with clavulanic acid (Timentin) provides greater activity against β-lactamase-producing organisms.

Notes. 1. Both carbenicillin and ticarcillin are presented as disodium salts and each 1 g delivers about 5.4 mmol of sodium; this source of sodium should be borne in mind when treating patients with impaired cardiac or renal function.

2. Carboxypenicillins inactivate aminoglycosides if both drugs are administered in the same syringe or intravenous infusion system.

Ureidopenicillins

These are adapted from the ampicillin molecule, with a side-chain derived from urea. Their major advantage over the carboxypenicillins is higher efficacy against *Pseudomonas aeruginosa* and the fact that as **mono**sodium salts they deliver on average about 2 mmol of sodium per gram of antimicrobial (see Note 1, above) and are thus safer where sodium overload should particularly be avoided. They are degraded by β-lactamases. Ureidopenicillins must be administered parenterally and are eliminated in the urine. Accumulation in patients with poor renal function however, is less than with other penicillins because 25% is excreted in the bile. An unusual feature of their kinetics is that, as dose is increased, plasma concentration rises disproportionately, i.e they exhibit *saturation (zero-order) kinetics*.

For pseudomonas septicaemia, a ureidopenicillin plus an aminoglycoside provides a synergistic effect but the co-administration in the same fluid results in inactivation of the aminoglycoside (as with carboxypenicillins, above).

Azlocillin ($t^{1/2}$ 1 h), highly effective against *Pseudomonas aeruginosa* infections, is less so than the other ureidopenicillins against other common Gram-negative organisms.

Piperacillin ($t^{1/2}$ 1 h) has the same or slightly greater activity as azlocillin against *Pseudomonas aeruginosa* but is more effective against the common

Gram-negative organisms. It is also available as a combination with the β-lactamase inhibitor tazobactam (Tazocin).

Cephalosporins

Cephalosporins were first obtained from a fungus *Cephalosporium* cultured from the sea near a Sardinian sewage outfall in 1945; their molecular structure is closely related to that of penicillin, and many semisynthetic forms have been introduced. They now comprise a group of antibiotics having a wide range of activity and low toxicity. The term cephalosporins will be used here in a general sense although some are strictly cephamycins, e.g. cefoxitin and cefotetan.

Mode of action is that of the β-lactams, i.e. cephalosporins impair bacterial cell wall synthesis and hence are bactericidal.

Addition of various side-chains on the cephalosporin molecule confers variety in pharmacokinetic and antibacterial activities. The β-lactam ring can be protected by such structural manoeuvring, which results in compounds with improved activity against Gram-negative organisms. Cephalosporins resist attack by β-lactamases but bacteria develop resistance to them by other means. Methicillin-resistant *Staphylococcus aureus* (MRSA) should be considered resistant to all cephalosporins.

Pharmacokinetics. Usually, cephalosporins are excreted unchanged in the urine, but some, including cefotaxime, form a desacetyl metabolite. Many are actively secreted by the renal tubule, a process which can be blocked with probenecid. In general, the dose of cephalosporins should be reduced in patients with poor renal function. Cephalosporins in general have a $t^{1/2}$ of 1–4 h. Wide distribution in the body allows treatment of infection at most sites, including bone, soft tissue and muscle. Data on individual cephalosporins appear in Table 12.1.

Classification and uses. The cephalosporins are conventionally categorised by generations having broadly similar antibacterial and pharmacokinetic properties; newer agents have rendered this clas-

sification less precise but it retains sufficient usefulness to be presented in Table 12.1.

Adverse effects. Cephalosporins have a low incidence of adverse effects. The most usual are allergic
reactions of the penicillin type. *There is cross-allergy*
between penicillins and cephalosporins involving
about 10% of patients; if a patient has had a severe
or immediate allergic reaction or if serum or skin
testing for penicillin allergy is positive (see p. 199),
then a cephalosporin should not be used. Pain may
be experienced at the sites of i.v. or i.m. injection. If
cephalosporins are continued for more than 2
weeks, thrombocytopenia, neutropenia, interstitial
nephritis or abnormal liver function tests may
occur; these reverse on stopping the drug. The
broad spectrum of activity of the third generation
cephalosporins may predispose to opportunist
infection with resistant bacteria or *Candida albicans*.
Ceftriaxone achieves high concentrations in bile
and, as the calcium salt, may precipitate to cause
symptoms resembling cholelithiasis (biliary
pseudolithiasis). Cefamandole may cause prothrombin deficiency and a disulfiram-like reaction
after ingestion of alcohol.

Other β-lactam antibacterials

CARBAPENEMS

Imipenem

Imipenem (t$\frac{1}{2}$ 1 h) is the most important member of
this class of β-lactam antibacterials. It has the
widest spectrum of all currently available antimicrobials, being bactericidal against most Gram-positive and Gram-negative aerobic and anaerobic
pathogenic bacteria.

Imipenem is inactivated by metabolism in the
kidney to products that are potentially toxic to renal
tubules; combining imipenem with cilastatin (as
Primaxin), a specific inhibitor of dihydropeptidase
— the enzyme responsible for its renal metabolism
— prevents both inactivation and toxicity.

Imipenem is used to treat septicaemia, particularly of renal origin, intra-abdominal infection and
nosocomial pneumonia. In terms of imipenem,

1–2 g/d is given by i.v. infusion in 3–4 doses;
reduced doses are recommended when renal function is impaired.

Adverse effects. It may cause gastrointestinal
upset, blood disorders, allergic reactions, confusion
and convulsions.

Meropenem is similar to imipenem but is stable to
renal dihydropeptidase and can therefore be given
without cilastatin. It penetrates into the CSF.

Other inhibitors of cell wall synthesis

Vancomycin (t$\frac{1}{2}$ 8 h)

Vancomycin acts on multiplying organisms by
inhibiting cell wall formation at a site different from
the β-lactam antibacterials. It is bactericidal against
most strains of clostridia, including *Clostridium
difficile*, almost all strains of *Staphyloccocus aureus*,
including those that produce β-lactamase and
methicillin-resistant strains, and *Streptococcus viridans* and enterococci (organisms that cause endocarditis).

Vancomycin is poorly absorbed from the gut and,
there being no satisfactory intramuscular preparation, is given i.v. for systemic infections. It distributes effectively into body tissues and is eliminated
by the kidney.

Uses. Vancomycin is the drug of choice for antibiotic-
associated pseudomembranous colitis (due to
Clostridium difficile or less commonly to staphylococci) in a dose of 125 mg × 6 h by mouth. Combined
with an aminoglycoside, it may be given i.v. for
streptococcal endocarditis in patients who are allergic to benzylpenicillin. It may also be used for serious infection with multiply-resistant staphylococci.
It is necessary to monitor plasma concentration.

Adverse effects. The main disadvantage to vancomycin is auditory damage. Tinnitus and deafness
may improve if the drug is stopped. Nephrotoxicity
and allergic reactions also occur. Rapid i.v. infusion
may cause a maculopapular rash possibly due to
histamine release (the 'red man' syndrome).

Table 12.1 The cephalosporins

Drug	$t^{1}/_{2}$ (h)	Excretion in urine (%)	Comment
First generation			
Parenteral			
Cephazolin	2	90	May be used for staphylococcal infections but generally have been replaced by the newer cephalosporins
Cephradine (also oral)	1	86	
Oral			
Cefaclor	1	86	All very similar. Effective against the common respiratory pathogens *Streptococcus pneumoniae* and *Moraxella catarrhalis* but (excepting cefaclor) have poor activity against *Haemophilus influenzae*. Also active against *Escherichia coli* which, increasingly, is demonstrating resistance to amoxycillin and trimethoprim. May be used for uncomplicated upper and lower respiratory tract, urinary tract and soft tissue infections, and also as follow-on treatment once parenteral drugs have brought an infection under control
Cefadroxil	2	88	
Cephalexin	1	88	
Second generation			
Parenteral			
Cefoxitin (a cephamycin) (Cefotetan is similar)	1	90	More resistant to β-lactamases than the first generation drugs and active against *Staphylococcus aureus*, *Streptococcus pyogenes*, *Streptococcus pneumoniae*, *Neisseria* spp., *Haemophilus influenzae* and many *Enterobacteriaceae*. Cefoxitin also kills *Bacteroides fragilis* and is effective in abdominal and pelvic infections. Cefuroxime may be given for community-acquired pneumonia, commonly due to *Strep. pneumoniae* (not when causal organism is *Mycoplasma pneumoniae*, *Legionella* or *Chlamydia*). The *oral* form, *cefuroxime axetil*, is also used for the range of infections listed for the first generation oral cephalosporins (above)
Cefuroxime (also oral)	1	80	
Cephamandole	1	75	
Third generation			
Parenteral			
Cefodizime	3	80	More effective than the second generation drugs against Gram-negative organisms whilst retaining useful activity against Gram-positive bacteria. Cefotaxime, ceftizoxime and ceftriaxone are used for serious infections such as septicaemia, pneumonia, and for meningitis. Ceftriaxone also used for gonorrhoea and Lyme disease
Cefotaxime	1	60	
Ceftazidime	2	88	
Ceftizoxime	1	90	
Ceftriaxone	8	56 (44 bile)	
Oral			
Cefixime	4	23 (77 bile)	Active against a range of Gram-positive and Gram-negative organisms including *Staphylococcus aureus* (excepting cefixime), *Streptococcus pyogenes*, *Streptococcus pneumoniae*, *Neisseria* spp., *Haemophilus influenzae* and (excepting cefpodoxime) many *Enterobacteriaceae*. Used to treat urinary, upper and lower respiratory tract infections
Ceftibuten	2	65	
Cefpodoxime proxetil	2	80	

Teicoplanin is structurally related to vancomycin and is active against Gram-positive bacteria. The $t^{1}/_{2}$ of 50 h allows once daily i.v. or i.m. administration. It is used for serious infection with Gram-positive bacteria including endocarditis, and peritonitis in patients undergoing chronic ambulatory peritoneal dialysis.

Cycloserine is used for drug-resistant tuberculosis (see p. 229).

Inhibition of protein synthesis

Aminoglycosides

In the purposeful search that followed the demonstration of the clinical efficacy of penicillin, streptomycin was obtained from *Streptomyces griseus* in 1944, cultured from a heavily manured field, and also from a chicken's throat. Aminoglycosides resemble each other in their mode of action, and their pharmacokinetic, therapeutic and toxic properties. The main differences in usage reflect variation in their range of antibacterial activity; cross-resistance is variable.

Mode of action. The aminoglycosides are bactericidal. They act inside the cell by binding to the ribosomes in such a way that incorrect amino acid sequences are entered into peptide chains. The abnormal proteins which result are fatal to the microbe.

Pharmacokinetics. Aminoglycosides are water-soluble and do not readily cross cell membranes. Poor absorption from the intestine necessitates their administration i.v. or i.m. for systemic use and they distribute mainly to the extracellular fluid; transfer into the cerebrospinal fluid is poor even when the meninges are inflamed.

Their $t^{1}/_{2}$ is 2–5h and they are eliminated unchanged mainly by glomerular filtration and attain high concentrations in the urine. Significant accumulation occurs in the renal cortex unless there is severe renal parenchymal disease. Dose reduction is necessary to compensate for varying degrees of renal impairment, including that of normal ageing, and dosage schemes are available to assist such prescribing. Plasma concentration should be measured regularly and frequently in renally impaired patients, and indeed it is good practice to monitor it even if renal function is normal. With prolonged high-dose therapy, e.g. endocarditis (gentamicin), monitoring must be meticulous, and may have to comprise both peak and trough plasma concentrations. Numerous successful legal actions by patients against doctors for negligence in this area have resulted in large compensation payments, especially for ototoxicity.

Antibacterial activity. Aminoglycosides are in general active against staphylococci and aerobic Gram-negative organisms including almost all the *Enterobacteriaceae*; individual differences in activity are given below. Bacterial resistance to aminoglycosides is an increasing problem, notably by acquisition of *plasmids* (see p. 192) which mediate the formation of drug-destroying enzymes.

Uses include:

● *Gram-negative bacillary infection*, particularly septicaemia, pelvic and abdominal sepsis. Gentamicin remains the drug of choice but tobramycin should be preferred for infections caused by *Pseudomonas aeruginosa*. Amikacin has the widest antibacterial spectrum of the aminoglycosides but is best reserved for infection caused by gentamicin-resistant organisms. An aminoglycoside may be included in the initial best-guess regimen for treatment of serious septicaemia before the causative organism(s) is identified.

● *Bacterial endocarditis*. An aminoglycoside, usually gentamicin, should comprise part of the antimicrobial combination for enterococcal, streptococcal or staphylococcal infection of the heart valves, and for the therapy of clinical endocarditis which fails to yield a positive blood culture.

● *Other infections*: tuberculosis, tularaemia, plague, brucellosis.

● *Topical uses*. Neomycin and framycetin, whilst

too toxic for systemic use, are effective for topical treatment of infections of the conjunctiva or external ear. They are used in antimicrobial combinations to sterilise the bowel of patients who are to receive intense immunosuppressive therapy.

Adverse effects. Aminoglycoside toxicity is a risk when the dose administered is high or of long duration, renal clearance is inefficient (because of disease or age), or the patient is dehydrated. It may take the following forms:

- *Ototoxicity*. Both vestibular and auditory damage may occur, causing hearing loss, vertigo and tinnitus which may be permanent (see above). Tinnitus may give warning of auditory nerve damage. Early signs of vestibular toxicity include motion-related headache, dizziness or nausea. Serious ototoxicity can occur with topical application, including ear drops.

- *Nephrotoxicity*. Dose-related changes, which are usually reversible, occur in renal tubular cells, where aminoglycosides accumulate. Low blood pressure, loop diuretics and advanced age are recognised as added risk factors.

- *Neuromuscular blockade*. Aminoglycosides may impair neuromuscular transmission and aggravate (or reveal) myasthenia gravis, or cause a transient myasthenic syndrome in patients whose neuromuscular transmission is normal.

- *Other* reactions include rashes, and haematological abnormalities, including marrow depression, haemolytic anaemia and bleeding due to antagonism of factor V.

INDIVIDUAL AMINOGLYCOSIDES

Gentamicin is active against aerobic Gram-negative bacilli including *Escherichia coli*, *Enterobacter*, *Klebsiella pneumoniae*, *Proteus* (indole positive) and *Pseudomonas aeruginosa*. In the best-guess treatment of septicaemia, gentamicin should be combined with a β-lactam antibiotic or an anti-anaerobic agent, e.g. metronidazole, or with both. Gentamicin is a drug of choice for serious Gram-negative septicaemia and it is effective for abdominal and pelvic sepsis, when combined with an agent effective against *Bacteroides fragilis*, e.g. metronidazole. In streptococcal and enterococcal endocarditis gentamicin is combined with benzylpenicillin, in staphylococcal endocarditis with an antistaphylo-

coccal penicillin, and in enterococcal endocarditis with ampicillin.

Dose is 2–5 mg/kg body weight per day (the highest dose for more serious infections) either in 3 equally divided doses or as a single dose. The rationale behind single dose administration is to achieve higher peak plasma concentrations (10–14 mg/l) which correlate with therapeutic efficacy and more time at lower trough concentrations (16 h at <1 mg/l) which are associated with reduced risk of toxicity. Therapy should rarely exceed 7 days. Gentamicin applied to the eye gives effective corneal and aqueous humour concentrations.

Tobramycin is similar to gentamicin; in particular, it is more active against most strains of *Pseudomonas aeruginosa* and may be less nephrotoxic.

Amikacin is mainly of value because it is resistant to more of the aminoglycoside-inactivating bacterial enzymes than is gentamicin. Amikacin is therefore normally reserved for treatment of infections with gentamicin-resistant organisms. Peak plasma concentrations should be kept between 20–30 mg/l and trough concentrations below 10 mg/l.

Netilmicin is a semisynthetic aminoglycoside which is active against some strains of bacteria that resist gentamicin and tobramycin; evidence suggests that it may be less ototoxic and nephrotoxic.

Neomycin is principally used topically for skin, eye and ear infections and, by some, to reduce the bacterial load in the colon in preparation for bowel surgery, or in hepatic failure. Enough absorption can occur from both oral and topical use to cause eighth cranial nerve damage, especially if there is renal impairment.

Framycetin is similar to neomycin in use and in toxicity.

Streptomycin and *kanamycin*, superseded as first-line choices for tuberculosis, may be used to kill resistant strains of the organism.

Spectinomycin is active against Gram-negative organisms but its clinical use is confined to gonorrhoea in patients allergic to penicillin, or to infection with gonococci that are β-lactam drug resistant. The steady growth of resistant gonococci, particularly the β-lactamase-producing type, suggests that spectinomycin will continue to have a significant role in this disease, although resistance to it is reported.

Tetracyclines

Tetracyclines have a broad range of antimicrobial activity and differences between individual members are in general small.

Mode of action. Tetracyclines interfere with protein synthesis by binding to bacterial ribosomes and their selective action is due to higher uptake by bacterial than by human cells. They are bacteriostatic.

Pharmacokinetics. Most tetracyclines are only partially absorbed from the alimentary tract, enough remaining in the intestine to alter the flora and cause diarrhoea. They are distributed throughout the body and cross the placenta. Tetracyclines are excreted mainly unchanged in the urine and should be avoided when renal function is severely impaired. Exceptionally among the tetracyclines, doxycycline and minocycline are eliminated by nonrenal routes and may be used in patients with impaired renal function because of this property.

Uses. Tetracyclines are active against nearly all Gram-positive and Gram-negative pathogenic bacteria but increasing bacterial resistance limits their use. They remain drugs of first choice, however, for infection with chlamydiae (psittacosis, trachoma, pelvic inflammatory disease, lymphogranuloma venereum), mycoplasma (pneumonia), rickettsiae (Q fever, typhus), *Vibrio cholerae* (cholera) and borreliae (Lyme disease, relapsing fever) (for use in acne, see p. 280).

An unexpected use for a tetracycline occurs in the treatment of chronic hyponatraemia due to the syndrome of inappropriate antidiuretic hormone secretion (SIADH) for which demeclocycline is effective when water restriction has failed. Demeclocycline produces a state of unresponsiveness to ADH, probably by inhibiting the formation and action of cyclic AMP in the renal tubule. It is convenient to use in SIADH because this action is both dose-dependent and reversible.

Adverse reactions. Heartburn, nausea and vomiting due to gastric irritation are common, and attempts to reduce this with milk or antacids impair absorption of tetracyclines (see below). Loose bowel movements occur, due to alteration of the bowel flora, and this sometimes develops into diarrhoea and opportunistic infection (antibiotic associated or pseudomembranous colitis) may supervene. Disorders of epithelial surfaces, perhaps due partly to vitamin B complex deficiency and partly due to mild opportunistic infection with yeasts and moulds, lead to sore mouth and throat, black hairy tongue, dysphagia and perianal soreness. Vitamin B preparations may prevent or arrest alimentary tract symptoms.

Tetracyclines are selectively taken up in the teeth and growing bones of the fetus and of children, due to their chelating properties with calcium phosphate. This causes dental enamel hypoplasia with pitting, cusp malformation, yellow or brown pigmentation and increased susceptibility to caries. After the fourteenth week of pregnancy and in the first few months of life, even short courses can be damaging. Prevention of discolouration of the permanent front teeth requires that tetracyclines be avoided from the last 2 months of pregnancy to 4 years, and of other teeth to 8 years of age (or 12 years if the third molars are valued). Prolonged tetracycline therapy can also stain the fingernails at all ages.

The effects on the bones after they are formed in the fetus are of less clinical importance because pigmentation has no cosmetic disadvantage and a short exposure to tetracycline is unlikely significantly to delay growth.

Since tetracyclines act by inhibiting bacterial protein synthesis, the same effect occurring in man causes blood urea to rise (the antianabolic effect). The increased nitrogen load can be clinically important in renal failure and in the elderly.

Tetracyclines also induce photosensitisation and other rashes. Liver and pancreatic damage can occur, especially in pregnancy and with renal disease, when the drugs have been given i.v. Rarely tetracyclines cause benign intracranial hypertension.

Interactions. Dairy products reduce absorption to a degree but antacids and iron preparations do so much more, by chelation to calcium, aluminium and iron.

INDIVIDUAL TETRACYCLINES

Tetracycline (t$\frac{1}{2}$ 6 h) may be taken as representative of most tetracyclines. Because of incomplete absorption from the gut i.v. doses need be less than half of the oral dose to be similarly effective. Tetracycline is eliminated by the kidney and in the bile. The dose is 250–500 mg 6-hourly by mouth, 500 mg twice daily by i.v. infusion (maximum 2 g/d).

Doxycycline (t$\frac{1}{2}$ 16 h) is well absorbed from the gut, even after food. It is excreted in the bile, in the faeces which it re-enters by diffusing across the small intestinal wall and, to some extent, in the urine. These nonrenal mechanisms compensate effectively when renal function is impaired and no reduction of dose is necessary: 200 mg is given on the first day, then 100 mg/d.

Minocycline (t$\frac{1}{2}$ 15 h) differs from other tetracyclines in that its antibacterial spectrum includes *Neisseria meningitidis* and it has been used for meningococcal prophylaxis. It is well absorbed from the gut, even after a meal, partly metabolised in the liver and partly excreted in the bile and urine. Dose reduction is not necessary when renal function is impaired; 200 mg initially is followed by 100 mg twice daily. Minocycline but not other tetracyclines may cause a reversible vestibular disturbance with dizziness, tinnitus and impaired balance, especially in women.

Other tetracyclines include demeclocycline (see above), lymecycline and oxytetracycline.

Macrolides

Erythromycin (t$\frac{1}{2}$ 2 h)

Erythromycin binds to bacterial ribosomes and interferes with protein synthesis; it is bacteriostatic. It is effective against Gram-positive organisms because these accumulate the drug more efficiently than Gram-negative organisms, and its antibacterial spectrum is similar to but not identical with that of penicillin.

Absorption after oral administration is best with erythromycin estolate, even if there is food in the stomach. Hydrolysis of the estolate in the body releases the active erythromycin which diffuses readily into most tissues; the t$\frac{1}{2}$ is dose-dependent and elimination is almost exclusively in the bile and faeces.

Uses. Erythromycin is the drug of choice for:

- *Mycoplasma pneumoniae* in children, although in adults a tetracycline may be preferred
- *Legionella* spp. (including Legionnaires' disease), with or without rifampicin
- Diphtheria (including carriers), pertussis and for some chlamydial infections.

In gastroenteritis caused by *Campylobacter jejuni*, erythromycin is effective in eliminating the organism from the faeces, although it does not necessarily reduce the duration of the symptoms.

Erythromycin is an effective alternative choice for penicillin-allergic patients infected with *Staphyloccocus pyogenes*, *Streptococcus pneumoniae* or *Treponema pallidum*.

Acne: see page 280.

Dose is 250 mg × 6 h or twice this in serious infection. The ethylsuccinate and stearate esters of erythromycin produce lower plasma concentrations of the active drug than does the same dose of the estolate.

Adverse reactions. Erythromycin is remarkably nontoxic, but the estolate can cause cholestatic hepatitis with abdominal pain and fever which may be confused with viral hepatitis, acute cholecystitis or acute pancreatitis. This is probably an allergy, and recovery is usual but the estolate should not be given to a patient with liver disease. Other allergies are rare. Gastrointestinal disturbances occur (up to 28%), particularly diarrhoea, but, the antibacterial spectrum being narrower than with tetracycline, opportunistic infection is less troublesome.

Interactions. Erythromycin and the other macrolides are enzyme inhibitors and interfere with the metabolic inactivation of some drugs, e.g. warfarin, carbamazepine, theophylline, disopyramide, increasing their effects. Reduced inactivation of astemizole and terfenadine may lead to serious cardiac dysrhythmias, and of ergot alkaloids may cause ergotism.

Clarithromycin ($t^{1/2}$ 3 h after 250 mg, 9 h after 1200 mg) acts like erythromycin and has a similar spectrum of antibacterial activity, i.e. mainly against Gram-positive organisms. It is rapidly and completely absorbed from the gastrointestinal tract, 60% of a dose is inactivated by metabolism which is saturable (note that the $t^{1/2}$, above, increases with dose) and the remainder is eliminated in the urine. Clarithromycin is used for respiratory tract infections including atypical pneumonias and soft tissue infections. It causes fewer gastrointestinal tract adverse effects (7%) than erythromycin. Interactions: see erythromycin (above).

Azithromycin ($t^{1/2}$ 50 h) interferes with bacterial ribosomal function and inhibits protein formation. It is active against a number of important Gram-negative organisms including *Haemophilus influenzae* and *Neisseria gonorrhoeae*, and also against *Chlamydiae*, but is less effective against Gram-positive organisms than erythromycin.

Azithromycin achieves high concentrations in tissues relative to those in plasma. It remains largely unmetabolised and is excreted in the bile and faeces. It is used to treat respiratory tract and soft tissue infections, and sexually transmitted diseases, especially genital *Chlamydia* infections. Gastrointestinal effects (9%) are less than with erythromycin but diarrhoea, nausea and abdominal pain occur. In view of its high hepatic excretion use in patients with liver disease should be avoided. Interactions: see erythromycin (above).

Clindamycin ($t^{1/2}$ 3 h), structurally a lincosamide rather than a macrolide, binds to bacterial ribosomes to inhibit protein synthesis. Its antibacterial spectrum is similar to that of erythromycin (with which there is partial cross-resistance) and benzylpenicillin (but including penicillin-resistant staphylococci); it has the useful additional property of efficacy against *Bacteroides fragilis*, an anaerobe that is involved in gut-associated sepsis. Clindamycin is well absorbed from the gut and distributes to most body tissues including bone. The drug is metabolised by the liver and enterohepatic cycling occurs with bile concentrations 2–5 times those of plasma. Significant excretion of metabolites occurs via the gut.

Clindamycin is used for staphylococcal bone and joint infections, dental infections, serious intra-abdominal sepsis and non-sexually transmitted infection of the genital tract in women (both of the latter usually involve anaerobes resistant to penicillins and, for these, clindamycin is usually combined with an aminoglycoside).

The most serious **adverse effect** is antibiotic-associated (pseudomembranous) colitis (see p. 193) usually due to opportunistic infection of the bowel with *Clostridium difficile* which produces an enterotoxin; clindamycin should be stopped if any diarrhoea occurs.

Other inhibitors of protein synthesis

Chloramphenicol ($t^{1/2}$ 5 h in adults)

Chloramphenicol is primarily bacteriostatic but also may be bactericidal against *Haemophilus influenzae*, *Neisseria meningitidis* and *Streptococcus pneumoniae*.

Pharmacokinetics. For oral use, chloramphenicol is available as the base in capsules to reduce the bitter taste and for i.v. or i.m. use as the succinate ester which is soluble. Chloramphenicol succinate is hydrolysed to the active chloramphenicol and there is much individual variation in the capacity to perform this reaction. Chloramphenicol is inactivated by conjugation with glucuronic acid in the liver. In the *neonate*, the process of glucuronidation is slow, and plasma concentrations are extremely variable (see below). Monitoring of plasma concentration is therefore essential in the neonate and infant, and in the adult with serious infection. Chloramphenicol penetrates well into all tissues including the CSF and brain.

Uses. The decision to use chloramphenicol is influenced by its rare but serious toxic effects (see below). There is a case for initiating treatment of bacterial meningitis with chloramphenicol plus benzylpenicillin, until the causal organism is identified. When the organism is *Haemophilus influenzae*, type B, chloramphenicol should be continued and the benzylpenicillin stopped. Similarly, in the initial empirical treatment of brain abscess, chloramphениcol may be given with penicillin. Chloramphenicol may be used for salmonella infections (typhoid fever, salmonella septicaemia) but ciprofloxacin is preferred. Topical administration is effective for bacterial conjunctivitis.

Adverse effects include gastrointestinal upset which tends to be mild. Optic and peripheral neuritis occur with prolonged use (which should be avoided) but are uncommon. The systemic use of chloramphenicol is dominated by the fact that it can cause rare (about 1:18 000–50 000 courses) though serious bone marrow damage. This is of two types:

1. a dose-dependent, reversible depression of erythrocyte, platelet and leucocyte formation that occurs early in treatment (type A adverse drug reaction);
2. an idiosyncratic (probably genetically determined), non-dose-related, and usually fatal aplastic anaemia which tends to develop during, or even weeks after, prolonged treatment, and sometimes on re-exposure to the drug (type B reaction) (avoid repeated courses); it has also occurred with eye drops.

Marrow depression may be detected at an early and recoverable stage by frequent examination of the blood.

The 'grey baby' syndrome occurs in neonates as circulatory collapse in which the skin develops a cyanotic grey colour. It is caused by high chloramphenicol plasma concentration due to failure of the liver to conjugate, and of the kidney to excrete the drug.

Sodium fusidate

Sodium fusidate is a steroid antimicrobial which is used almost exclusively against β-lactamase-producing staphylococci. As these bacteria fairly rapidly become resistant, the drug should be combined with another antistaphylococcal drug, e.g. flucloxacillin. Sodium fusidate is readily absorbed from the gut and distributes widely in body tissues including bone. It is metabolised and very little is excreted unchanged in the urine; the t½ is 5 h.

Uses. Sodium fusidate is a valuable drug for treating severe staphylococcal infections, including osteomyelitis and is available as i.v. and oral prepa-

rations. In an ointment or gel, sodium fusidate is used topically for staphylococcal skin infection and as a cream is applied to eradicate the staphylococcal nasal carrier state.

Adverse effects. It is well tolerated but mild gastrointestinal upset occurs. Jaundice may develop, particularly with high doses.

Inhibition of nucleic acid synthesis

Sulphonamides and sulphonamide combinations

Sulphonamides, amongst the first successful chemotherapeutic agents, now have their place in medicine mainly as combinations with trimethoprim.

The enzyme dihydrofolic acid (DHF) synthase (see below) converts *p*-aminobenzoic acid (PABA) to DHF which is subsequently converted to tetrahydric folic acid (THF), purines and DNA. Sulphonamides are structurally similar to PABA, successfully compete with it for DHF synthase and so ultimately impair DNA formation. Bacteria do not use preformed folate, but humans derive DHF from dietary folate and their cells are unharmed by the metabolic effect of sulphonamides. Trimethoprim acts at the subsequent step by inhibiting DHF reductase which converts DHF to THF. The drug is relatively safe because bacterial DHF reductase is much more sensitive to trimethoprim than is the human form of the enzyme. Both sulphonamides and trimethoprim are bacteriostatic.

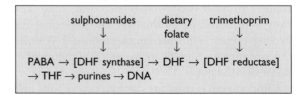

Pharmacokinetics. Sulphonamides for systemic use are absorbed rapidly from the gut. Sulphadiazine enters CSF more readily than others. The principal metabolic path is acetylation and the capacity to acetylate is genetically determined in a bimodal form, i.e. there are slow and fast acetylators (see Pharmacogenetics) but the differences are of limited practical importance in therapy. Both the parent drug and its microbiologically inactive acetylated form enter the glomerular filtrate and the urine is the principal mode of excretion.

Classification and uses. Sulphonamides may be classified as follows:

Systemic use

Sulphonamide-trimethoprim combination. Co-trimoxazole (sulphamethoxazole plus trimethoprim); the optimum synergistic effect against most susceptible bacteria is achieved with 5:1 ratio of sulphamethoxazole to trimethoprim. Each drug is well absorbed from the gut, has a $t^{1/2}$ of 10 h and is 80% excreted by the kidney; consequently, the dose of co-trimoxazole should be reduced when renal function is impaired.

Co-trimoxazole, at first, very largely replaced the use of a sulphonamide alone. In turn, trimethoprim on its own has emerged as effective in many conditions for which the combination was originally recommended (principally respiratory and urinary tract infections), and it causes fewer adverse reactions. The combination is, however, retained for:

- Prevention and treatment of pneumonia due to *Pneumocystis carinii*, a life-threatening infection in immunosuppressed patients
- Prevention and treatment of toxoplasmosis and treatment of nocardiasis
- Urinary tract infections and acute exacerbations of chronic bronchitis only where there is bacteriological evidence of infection with a susceptible organism and good reason to prefer co-trimoxazole to a single antimicrobial
- Otitis media in children only where there is positive reason to prefer the combination.

Sulphadiazine ($t^{1/2}$ 10 h) and *sulphadimidine* (sulphamethazine) ($t^{1/2}$ approx. 6 h, dose dependent) may be used for urinary tract infections and meningococcal meningitis but are not drugs of first choice.

Topical application

Silver sulphadiazine is used for prophylaxis and treatment of infected burns, leg ulcers and pressure sores because of its wide antibacterial spectrum (which includes pseudomonads).

Miscellaneous

Sulphasalazine (salicylazosulphapyridine) is used in inflammatory bowel disease (see p. 587); in effect the sulphapyridine component acts as a carrier to release the active 5-aminosalicylic acid in the colon.

Adverse effects of sulphonamides include malaise, diarrhoea, mental depression and rarely cyanosis, which latter is due to methaemoglobinaemia. These may all be transient and are not necessarily indications for stopping the drug. Crystalluria may rarely occur.

Allergic reactions include: rash, fever, hepatitis, agranulocytosis, purpura, aplastic anaemia, peripheral neuritis and polyarteritis nodosa. Rarely, severe skin reactions including erythema multiforme bullosa (Stevens–Johnson syndrome) and toxic epidermal necrolysis (Lyell's syndrome) occur. Haemolysis may occur in glucose-6-phosphate dehydrogenase-deficient subjects. Co-trimoxazole in high dose may cause macrocytic anaemia due to interference with conversion of DHF to THF. Co-trimoxazole should not be used in pregnancy because of the possible *teratogenic effects* of inducing folate deficiency.

Trimethoprim ($t^{1/2}$ 10 h)

Subsequent to its extensive use in combination with sulphonamides, trimethoprim has emerged as a broad spectrum antimicrobial of considerable efficacy on its own. It is active against many Gram-positive and Gram-negative aerobic organisms excepting *Pseudomonas aeruginosa*; the emergence of resistant organisms is becoming a problem. The drug is rapidly and completely absorbed from the gastrointestinal tract and is largely excreted unchanged in the urine. Trimethoprim is effective as sole therapy in treating urinary and respiratory tract infections due to susceptible organisms and for prophylaxis of urinary tract infections.

Adverse effects are fewer than with co-trimoxazole and include: skin rash, anorexia, nausea, vomiting, abdominal pain and diarrhoea.

Quinolones

(4-quinolones, fluoroquinolones)

The first widely used quinolone was nalidixic acid which was effective for urinary tract infections because it concentrated in the urine, but had little systemic activity. It was subsequently found that fluorination of the quinolone structure produced compounds that were up to 60 times more active than nalidixic acid and killed a wider range of organisms. They act principally by inhibiting bacterial (but not human) DNA gyrase, so preventing the supercoiling of DNA, a process that is necessary for compacting chromosomes into the bacterial cell; they are bactericidal. In general quinolones are particularly active against Gram-negative organisms including *Escherichia coli*, *Salmonella* sp., *Shigella* sp., *Neisseria* sp., *Pseudomonas aeruginosa*, *Haemophilus influenzae* and *Legionella pneumophila*. They are less active against Gram-positive organisms and are not effective against anaerobes.

Pharmacokinetics. Quinolones are well absorbed from the gut, and widely distributed in body tissue. Mechanisms of inactivation (hepatic metabolism, renal and biliary excretion) are detailed for individual members (see below).

Uses vary between individual drugs (see below).

Adverse effects include gastrointestinal upset and allergic reactions (rash, pruritus, arthralgia, photosensitivity and anaphylaxis). CNS effects may develop with dizziness, headache and confusion, and are sufficient to require cautioning the patient against driving a motor vehicle. Convulsions have occurred during treatment (avoid or use with caution where there is a history of epilepsy or concurrent use of NSAIDs which potentiate this effect). Reversible arthropathy has developed in weight-bearing joints in immature animals exposed to quinolones. While the significance for humans is uncertain quinolones should be used with caution in children and adolescents. Rupture of tendons, notably the Achilles tendon, has occurred, more in the elderly and those taking corticosteroids concurrently.

Some quinolones are potent enzyme inhibitors and impair the metabolic inactivation of other drugs including warfarin, theophylline and sulphonylureas, increasing their effect. Magnesium- and aluminium-containing antacids impair the absorption of quinolones from the gastrointestinal tract probably through forming a chelate complex; ferrous sulphate and sucralfate also reduce quinolone absorption.

Individual members of the group include the following:

Ciprofloxacin ($t^{1/2}$ 3 h) is effective against a range of bacteria but particularly the Gram-negative organisms (see above); it has less activity against Gram-positive bacteria such as *Streptococcus pneumoniae* and *Enterococcus faecalis*. Chlamydia and mycoplasma are sensitive but most anaerobes are not. Ciprofloxacin is indicated for infections of the urinary, gastrointestinal and respiratory tracts, tissue infections, gonorrhoea and septicaemia caused by sensitive organisms. The dose is 250–750 mg × 2/d by mouth, 200 mg × 2/d i.v. but should be halved when the glomerular filtration rate is <20 ml/min. To discourage the emergence of resistant strains, it is a good policy to reserve ciprofloxacin for infections caused by organisms that are resistant to other drugs. Ciprofloxacin impairs the metabolism of theophylline and of warfarin, both of which should be monitored carefully when co-administered.

Acrosoxacin ($t^{1/2}$ 7 h) is effective as a single 300 mg oral dose for gonorrhoea; it is usually reserved for patients who are allergic to penicillin or for organisms that are resistant to that drug.

Cinoxacin ($t^{1/2}$ 2 h) is used for urinary tract infections, but not when renal function is impaired.

Norfloxacin ($t^{1/2}$ 3 h) is used for acute or chronic recurrent urinary tract infections.

Ofloxacin ($t^{1/2}$ 4 h) is indicated for urinary and respiratory tract infections and gonorrhoea.

Nalidixic acid ($t^{1/2}$ 6 h) is now used principally for the prevention of urinary tract infection. It may cause haemolysis in glucose-6-phosphate dehydrogenase deficient subjects.

Azoles

This group includes:

- Metronidazole and tinidazole (antibacterial and antiprotozoal) which are described here.
- Fluconazole, itraconazole, clotrimazole, econazole, ketoconazole, isoconazole and miconazole which are described under Antifungal drugs (p. 235).
- Albendazole, mebendazole and thiabendazole which are described under Anthelminthic drugs (p. 246).

Metronidazole

In anaerobic microorganisms (but not in aerobic microorganisms which it also enters) metronidazole is converted into an active form by reduction of its nitro group: this binds to DNA and prevents nucleic acid formation; it is bacteriostatic.

Pharmacokinetics. Metronidazole is well absorbed after either oral or rectal administration and distributed to achieve sufficient concentration to eradicate infection in liver, gut wall and pelvic tissues. It is eliminated in the urine, partly unchanged and partly as metabolites. The $t^{1/2}$ is 8 h.

Uses. Metronidazole is active against a wide range of anaerobic bacteria and also protozoa. Its clinical indications are:

- Treatment of sepsis to which anaerobic organisms, e.g. *Bacteroides* spp. and anaerobic cocci, are contributing, notably postsurgical infection, intra-abdominal infection and septicaemia, but also wound and pelvic infection, osteomyelitis and abscesses of brain or lung
  - Pseudomembraneous colitis
  - Trichomoniasis of the urogenital tract in both sexes
  - Amoebiasis (*Entamoeba histolytica*), whether symptomless carriers of cysts or intestinal and extra-intestinal infection
    - Giardiasis (*Giardia lamblia*)
    - Acute ulcerative gingivitis and dental infections (*Fusobacterium* spp.)
    - Anaerobic vaginosis (*Gardnerella vaginalis*).

Dose. Established anaerobic infection is treated with metronidazole by mouth 400 mg $\times$ 8 h; by rectum 1 g $\times$ 8 h for 3 days followed by 1 g $\times$ 12 h; or by i.v. injection 0.5 g $\times$ 8 h; treatment should continue for up to 7 days.

Adverse effects include nausea, vomiting, diarrhoea, furred tongue and an unpleasant metallic taste in the mouth; also headache, dizziness and ataxia. Rashes, urticaria and angioedema occur. Peripheral neuropathy occurs if treatment is prolonged and epileptiform seizures if the dose is high. Large doses of metronidazole are carcinogenic in rodents and the drug is mutagenic in bacteria; however, longterm studies have failed to discover oncogenic effects in humans.

A disulfiram-like effect occurs with alcohol because metronidazole inhibits alcohol and aldehyde dehydrogenase; patients should be warned appropriately.

Tinidazole is similar to metronidazole but has a longer $t^{1/2}$ (13 h). It is excreted mainly unchanged in the urine. The indications for use and adverse effects are essentially those of metronidazole. The longer duration of action of tinidazole may be an advantage, e.g. in giardiasis, trichomoniasis and acute ulcerative gingivitis, in which tinidazole 2 g by mouth in a single dose is as effective as a course of metronidazole.

MINOR ANTIMICROBIALS

These are included because they are effective topically without serious risk of allergy, although toxicity limits or precludes their systemic use.

Mupirocin is active against both Gram-positive and Gram-negative organisms including those commonly associated with skin infections. It is available as an ointment for use, e.g. in folliculitis and impetigo, and to eradicate nasal staphylococci, e.g. in carriers of resistant organisms.

POLYPEPTIDE ANTIBIOTICS

Colistin is effective against Gram-negative organisms particularly *Pseudomonas aeruginosa*. It is used for bowel sterilisation in neutropenic patients and topically is applied to skin, including external ear infections.

Polymyxin B is also active against Gram-negative organisms, particularly *Pseudomonas aeruginosa*. Its principal use now is topical application for skin, eye and external ear infections.

Gramicidin is used in various topical applications as eye- and ear-drops, combined with neomycin and framycetin.

GUIDE TO FURTHER READING

Aronson J K, Reynolds D J M 1992 ABC of monitoring drug therapy. Aminoglycoside antibiotics. British Medical Journal 305: 1421

Barza M et al 1996 Single or multiple doses of aminoglycosides: a meta-analysis. British Medical Journal 312: 338

Brumfitt W, Hamilton-Miller J 1989 Methicillin-resistant *Staphylococcus aureus*. New England Journal of Medicine 320: 1188

Holgate S 1988 Penicillin allergy: how to diagnose and when to treat. British Medical Journal 296: 1213

Hooper D C, Wolfson J S 1991 Fluoroquinolone antimicrobial agents. New England Journal of Medicine 324: 384

Parker S E, Davey P G 1993 Once-daily aminoglycoside dosing. Lancet 341: 346

Chemotherapy of bacterial infections

SYNOPSIS

We live in a world heavily populated by microorganisms of astonishing diversity. Most of these exist in our external environment but certain classes are normally harboured within our bodies. Depending on the circumstances, infectious disease can arise from organisms living exogenously or endogenously, and a knowledge of common pathogens at specific sites often provides a good basis for rational initial therapy.

This chapter considers the bacteria that cause disease in individual body systems, the drugs that are used to combat them, and how they are best used. It discusses infection of:

- Blood
- Paranasal sinuses and ears
- Throat
- Bronchi, lungs and pleura
- Endocardium
- Meninges
- Intestines
- Urinary tract
- Genital tract
- Eye
- Also mycobacteria, that infect many sites

Table 11.1 (p. 194) is a general reference for this chapter.

Infection of the blood

Septicaemia is a medical emergency. Accurate microbiological diagnosis is of the first importance and blood cultures should be taken before starting antimicrobial therapy. Usually, the infecting organism(s) is not known and treatment must be instituted on the basis of a 'best guess'. The clinical circumstances may provide some clues.

- When septicaemia follows gastrointestinal or genital tract surgery, *Escherichia coli* (or other Gram-negative bacteria), anaerobic bacteria, e.g. *Bacteroides*, streptococci or enterococci are likely pathogens and the following combinations are effective: cefuroxime plus metronidazole or gentamicin plus amoxycillin plus metronidazole.
- Septicaemia related to urinary tract infection usually involves *Escherichia coli* (or other Gram-negative bacteria), enterococci: gentamicin plus amoxycillin are indicated or gentamicin plus ceftazidime where *Pseudomonas aeruginosa* is a suspected pathogen.
- Neonatal septicaemia is usually due to streptococci or coliforms, occasionally to *Pseudomonas aeruginosa*: cefotaxime alone, or with netilmicin, is used.
- Staphylococcal septicaemia may be suspected where there is an abscess, e.g. of bone or lung: flucloxacillin is indicated.

● Toxic shock syndrome occurs in circumstances that include healthy women using vaginal tampons, abortion or childbirth, cutaneous or subcutaneous infection. The clinical problem is due to toxins produced by staphylococci: while this is not strictly an infection of the blood, flucloxacillin is used to eliminate the source.

Antimicrobials should be given i.v. in septicaemia.

Infection of paranasal sinuses and ears

SINUSITIS

Infection of the paranasal sinuses causes significant morbidity. Since oedema of the mucous membrane hinders the drainage of pus, a logical first step is to open the obstructed passage with a sympathomimetic vasoconstrictor, e.g. ephedrine nasal drops. The common infecting organisms (*Streptococcus pneumoniae*, *Haemophilus influenzae*, *Streptococcus pyogenes*, *Moraxella* (*Branhamella*) *catarrhalis*) usually respond to oral amoxycillin (with or without clavulanic acid) or to doxycycline.

In chronic sinusitis, correction of the anatomical abnormalities (polypi, nasal septum deviation) is often important. Very diverse organisms, many of them normal inhabitants of the upper respiratory tract, may be cultured, e.g. anaerobic streptococci, *Bacteroides* spp., and a judgement is required as to whether any particular organism is acting as a pathogen. Choice of antibiotic should be guided by culture and sensitivity testing; therapy may need to be prolonged.

OTITIS MEDIA

Mild cases, characterised by pinkness or infection of the eardrum, often resolve spontaneously and need only analgesia and observation. They are normally viral. A bulging, inflamed eardrum indicates bacterial otitis media usually due to *Streptococcus pneumoniae*, *Haemophilus influenzae*, *Moraxella* (*Branhamella*) *catarrhalis*, *Streptococcus pyogenes* (Group A) or *Staphylococcus aureus*.

Amoxycillin is satisfactory. Chemotherapy has not removed the need for myringotomy when pain is very severe, and also for later cases, as sterilised pus may not be completely absorbed and may leave adhesions that impair hearing. Chronic infection presents a similar problem to that of chronic sinus infection, above.

Infection of the throat

Pharyngitis is usually viral but the more serious cases may be caused by *Streptococcus pyogenes* (Group A) which is always sensitive to benzylpenicillin. *Streptococcus pneumoniae* and *Haemophilus influenzae* may be secondary invaders. Unfortunately, streptococcal sore throats cannot be clinically differentiated from the nonstreptococcal with any certainty. Prevention of complications is more important than relief of the symptoms which seldom last long.

There is no general agreement whether chemotherapy should be employed in mild sporadic sore throat; the disease usually subsides in a few days, septic complications are uncommon and rheumatic fever rarely follows. It is reasonable to withhold penicillin unless streptococci are cultured or the patient develops a high fever. Severe sopradic or epidemic sore throat is likely to be streptococcal and phenoxymethylpenicillin by mouth (or erythromycin in the penicillin allergic) should be given to prevent these complications. Ideally, it should be continued for 10 days but compliance is bad once the symptoms have subsided and 5 days should be the minimum objective. If there is a possibility that the pharyngitis is due to infectious mononucleosis, amoxycillin must not be used as the patient is very likely to develop a rash (see p. 210). In a closed community, chemoprophylaxis of unaffected people to stop an epidemic may be considered, for instance with phenoxymethylpenicillin 125 mg × 2/d orally, for a period depending on the course of the epidemic, or a single intramuscular injection of benzathine penicillin 900 mg.

In *scarlet fever* and *erysipelas*, the infection is invariably streptococcal (Group A) and benzylpenicillin should be used even in mild cases, to prevent rheumatic fever and nephritis.

Chemoprophylaxis

Chemoprophylaxis of streptococcal (Group A) infection with phenoxymethylpenicillin should be undertaken in patients who have had one attack of rheumatic fever. It is continued for at least 5 years, or until aged 20, whichever is the longer period, although some hold that it should continue for life, for histological study of atrial biopsies shows that the cardiac lesions may progress despite absence of clinical activity. Chemoprophylaxis should be continued for life after a second attack of rheumatic fever. A single attack of acute nephritis is not an indication for chemoprophylaxis but in the rare cases of nephritis in which recurrent haematuria occurs after sore throats, chemoprophylaxis should be used. Ideally, chemoprophylaxis should continue throughout the year but, if the patient is unwilling to submit to this, at least the colder months should be covered (see also p. 191).

Adverse effects are uncommon. Patients taking penicillin prophylaxis are liable to have penicillin resistant viridans type streptococci in the mouth, so that during even minor dentistry, e.g. scaling, there is a risk of bacteraemia and thus of infective endocarditis with a penicillin-resistant organism in those with any residual rheumatic heart lesion. The same risk applies to urinary, abdominal and chest surgery, and patients need special chemoprophylaxis (see Endocarditis). Patients taking penicillins are also liable to carry resistant staphylococci.

Other causes of pharyngitis

Vincent's infection (microbiologically complex, includes anaerobes, spirochaetes) responds readily to benzylpenicillin; a single i.m. dose of 600 mg is often enough except in a mouth needing dental treatment, when relapse may follow. Metronidazole 200 mg × 8 h by mouth for 3 days is also effective.

Diphtheria (*Corynebacterium diphtheriae*). Antitoxin 10 000–30 000 units i.m. or 40 000–100 000 units i.v. in 2 divided doses 0.5–2 h apart is given to neu-

tralise toxin already formed according to the severity of the disease. Erythromycin or benzylpenicillin is also used, to prevent the production of more toxin by destroying the bacteria.

Whooping-cough (*Bordetella pertussis*). Chemotherapy is needed in children who are weak, have damaged lungs or are under 3 years old. Erythromycin is usually recommended at the catarrhal stage and should be continued for 14 days (also as prophylaxis in cases of special need). It may curtail an attack if given early enough (before paroxysms have begun) but is not dramatically effective; it also reduces infectivity to others. A corticosteroid, salbutamol, and physiotherapy may be helpful for relief of symptoms, but reliable evidence of efficacy is lacking.

Infection of the bronchi, lungs and pleura

BRONCHITIS

Most cases of acute bronchitis are viral; where bacteria are responsible the usual organisms are *Streptococcus pneumoniae* or *Haemophilus influenzae*. It is questionable if there is role for antimicrobials in uncomplicated acute bronchitis but amoxycillin or trimethoprim are appropriate if treatment is considered necessary.

In chronic bronchitis, suppressive chemotherapy, generally needed only during the colder months (in temperate, colder regions), should be considered for patients with symptoms of pulmonary insufficiency, recurrent acute exacerbations or permanently purulent sputum. Amoxycillin or trimethoprim are suitable.

For intermittent therapy, the patient is given a supply of the drug and is told to take it in full dose at the first sign of a 'chest' cold, e.g. purulent sputum, and to stop it after 3 days if there is rapid improvement. Otherwise, the patient should continue the drug until recovery takes place. If the exacerbation lasts for more than 10 days, there is a need for clinical reassessment.

Occasionally, *continuous longterm therapy* may be deemed necessary; this reduces the duration of acute exacerbations rather than their number, perhaps because the exacerbations are initiated by virus infection which promotes secondary bacterial invasion.

PNEUMONIAS

The clinical setting is a useful guide to the causal organism and hence to the 'best guess' early choice of antimicrobial.

Pneumonia in previously healthy people (community acquired)

● Disease that is segmental or lobar in distribution is almost certainly caused by *Streptococcus pneumoniae* (pneumococcus). *Haemophilus influenzae* is also a cause, although it more often leads to exacerbations of chronic bronchitis. Benzylpenicillin i.v. is the treatment of choice if pneumococcal pneumonia can be diagnosed with certainty; alternatively, amoxycillin is used, or erythromycin in a penicillin-allergic patient.

● Pneumonia following influenza is often caused by *Staphylococcus aureus*, and sodium fusidate and flucloxacillin i.v. are used in combination.

● Atypical cases of pneumonia may be caused by *Mycoplasma pneumoniae* which may be epidemic, or more rarely *Chlamydia psittaci* (psittacosis/ ornithosis) or *Coxiella burnetii* (Q fever) and a tetracycline should be given by mouth. Treatment of ornithosis should continue for 10 days after the fever has settled and in mycoplasma pneumonia and Q fever a total of 3 weeks treatment may be needed to prevent relapse.

Pneumonia acquired in hospital

● Pneumonia is defined as nosocomial (Greek: *nosokomeian*, hospital) if it is acquired after at least 3 days in hospital. It occurs primarily among patients admitted with medical problems or recovering from abdominal or thoracic surgery. The common pathogens are *Staphylococcus aureus*, *Streptococcus pneumoniae*, *Pseudomonas aeruginosa*, *Enterobacteriaceae* and *Haemophilus influenzae*. It is reasonable to initiate therapy with ciprofloxacin or ceftazidime until the results of sputum culture and bacterial sensitivity are known.

Pneumonia in people with chronic lung disease

● Normal commensals of the upper respiratory tract proliferate in damaged lungs especially following viral infections, pulmonary congestion or pulmonary infarction. Mixed infection is therefore common, and since *Haemophilus influenzae* and *Streptococcus pneumoniae* are often the pathogens, amoxycillin or trimethoprim are reasonable choices, but if response is inadequate co-amoxiclav or a quinolone should be substituted.

● *Klebsiella pneumoniae* tends to cause lung infection in the debilitated elderly and abscesses form, particularly in the upper lobes: cefotaxime possibly with an aminoglycoside is recommended.

● *Moraxella* (previously *Branhamella*) *catarrhalis*, a commensal of the oropharynx, may be a pathogen; as many strains produce β-lactamase co-amoxiclav or erythromycin should be used.

Pneumonia in immunocompromised patients. Pneumonia is common, e.g. in acquired immunodeficiency syndrome (AIDS) or in those who are receiving immunosuppressive drugs.

Common pathogenic bacteria may be responsible (*Staphylococcus aureus*, *Streptococcus pneumoniae*) but often organisms of lower natural virulence (viruses, fungi) are causal and strenuous efforts should be made to identify the microbe including, if feasible, bronchial washings or lung biopsy.

● Until the pathogen is known the patient should receive broad-spectrum antimicrobial treatment, such as an aminoglycoside plus amoxycillin.

● Aerobic Gram-negative bacilli, e.g. *Enterobacteriaceae*, *Klebsiella* spp., are pathogens in half of the cases and respond to cefotaxime or ceftazidime.

● An important respiratory pathogen in this group is the protozoon *Pneumocystis carinii*, which should be treated with co-trimoxazole 120 mg/kg/d by mouth or i.v. in 2 divided doses for 14 days, or with pentamidine (see p. 246).

● *Pseudomonas aeruginosa* may cause pneumonia in these patients; for treatment see Reference data on antimicrobial drugs of choice, page 194, Table 11.1.

Legionnaires' disease

Legionella pneumophila responds to erythromycin

2–4 g/d i.v. in divided doses but rifampicin may be added in more severe infections.

PNEUMONIA DUE TO ANAEROBIC MICROORGANISMS

Pneumonia is often caused by aspiration of material from the oropharynx, or due to the presence of other lung pathology such as pulmonary infarction or bronchogenic carcinoma. The pathogens include anaerobic streptococci, *Bacteroides* spp. and *Fusobacterium*, and the diagnosis may be missed unless anaerobic cultures of fresh material are taken. Treatment for several weeks with cefuroxime plus metronidazole may be needed to prevent relapse.

Pulmonary abscess is treated according to the organism identified and with surgery if necessary.

Empyema is treated according to the organism isolated and with aspiration and drainage.

Endocarditis

When suspicion is high enough, three blood cultures should be taken over a few hours and antimicrobial treatment commenced; it can be adjusted later in the light of the results. Delay in treating only exposes the patient to the risk of grave cardiac damage or systemic embolism.

Streptococci and staphylococci are causal in 80% of cases with viridans group streptococci, the most common pathogen. In intravenous drug abusers, *Staphylococcus aureus* is the most likely organism. Culture-negative endocarditis (up to 20% of cases) is usually due to prior antimicrobial therapy or to special culture requirements of the microbe; it is best regarded as being due to streptococci and treated accordingly.

PRINCIPLES FOR TREATMENT

● High doses of bactericidal drugs are needed because the organisms are difficult to access in avascular vegetations on valves and the protective host reaction is negligible.

● Drugs should be given parenterally at least initially and preferably by intravenous bolus injection which achieves the necessary high peak concentration to penetrate the relatively avascular vegetations. The antimicrobial should never be added to the infusion reservoir where its only function is to keep open the route into the vein.

● The infusion site should be changed every 2–3 days to prevent opportunistic infection, which is usually with staphylococci or fungi. Alternatively, use may be made of a central subclavian venous line sited with meticulous attention to aseptic technique.

● Prolonged therapy is needed, usually 4 weeks, and in the case of infected prosthetic valves at least 6 weeks. The patient should be reviewed one month after completing the antimicrobial treatment. Valve replacement may be needed.

● Dosage must be adjusted according to the sensitivity of the infecting organism and therapy may be regarded as adequate if a 1:8 dilution of the patient's plasma kills it (serum bactericidal titration test).

DOSE REGIMENS

The following regimens will serve:

1. Initial (best guess) treatment should comprise benzylpenicillin 1.2–2.4 g 4 hourly, plus gentamicin in low dose, e.g. 80 mg × 2/d, by i.v. injection (synergy allows this dose of gentamicin and minimises risk of adverse effects); if *Staphylococcus aureus* is suspected, flucloxacillin plus either gentamicin or sodium fusidate should be used. Patients allergic to penicillin should be treated with vancomycin.

2. When an organism has been identified and its sensitivity to drugs determined:

Viridans group streptococci: benzylpenicillin plus gentamicin i.v. for at least 4 weeks or, if the organism is very sensitive, for 2 weeks followed by amoxycillin i.v. for 2 weeks.

Enterococcus faecalis (Group D): benzylpenicillin plus gentamicin i.v. for at least 4 weeks.

Staphylococcus aureus: flucloxacillin by i.v. injection plus either gentamicin by i.v. injection or sodium fusidate by mouth.

Staphylococcus epidermidis has a predilection for prosthetic valves and should be managed as for

Staphylococcus aureus if the organism is sensitive but, even if this is so, valve replacement may be needed.

Coxiella or Chlamydia: tetracycline by mouth for at least 4–6 weeks. Valve replacement is advised in most cases but some may continue indefinitely on tetracycline.

Fungal endocarditis: amphotericin plus flucytosine are used.

Culture-negative endocarditis: benzylpenicillin plus gentamicin i.v. are given for 6 weeks.

PROPHYLAXIS

Transient bacteraemia is provoked by dental procedures, surgical incision of the skin, instrumentation of the urinary tract, parturition and even seemingly innocent activities such as brushing the teeth or chewing toffee. Experience shows that people with *acquired* or *congenital* heart defects are at risk from bacteraemia and are protected by antimicrobials used prophylactically. The drugs are given as a short course in high dose at the time of the procedure to coincide with the bacteraemia and avoid emergence of resistant organisms. There follow general recommendations[1] on antimicrobial prophylaxis; not every contingency is covered because prophylaxis may be needed for patients with cardiac defects whenever surgery or instrumentation is undertaken on tissue that is heavily colonised or infected, e.g. in surgery or instrumentation of the upper respiratory or genitourinary tracts, or obstetric, gynaecological or gastrointestinal procedures. The physician should consult special sources and exercise a clinical judgement that relates to individual circumstances. All oral drugs should be taken under supervision.

Dental procedures

Under local or no anaesthesia

● Adults who are not allergic to penicillins and who have not taken penicillin more than once in the previous month should receive amoxycillin 3 g by mouth 1 h before the procedure.

● Patients **allergic** to penicillins or who have taken penicillin more than once in the previous

month should receive clindamycin 600 mg by mouth 1 h before the procedure.

Under general anaesthesia

● Patients who are not allergic to penicillins and who have not taken penicillin more than once in the previous month should receive amoxycillin 1 g i.m. or i.v. at induction then 0.5 g by mouth 6 h later. Alternatively amoxycillin 3 g may be taken by mouth together with probenecid 1 g by mouth 4 h before the procedure (probenecid delays renal excretion and thus maintains a high blood concentration of amoxycillin).

● **Special risk** patients, i.e. with prosthetic valves or with previous endocarditis should receive amoxycillin 1 g i.m. or i.v. and gentamicin 120 mg at induction then amoxycillin 0.5 g by mouth 6 h later. Patients who are penicillin-allergic or have received penicillin more that once in the previous month should receive vancomycin 1 g i.v. over 100 min then gentamicin 120 mg i.v. at induction or 15 min before the procedure; *or* teicoplanin 400 mg i.v. plus gentamicin 120 mg i.v. at induction or 15 min before the procedure; *or* clindamycin 300 mg over at least 10 min at induction or 15 min before the procedure then clindamycin 150 mg i.v. or by mouth 6 h later.

Meningitis

Speed of initiating treatment and accurate bacteriological diagnosis are the major factors determining the fate of the patient. When meningococcal disease is suspected (and unless the patient has a history of penicillin anaphylaxis) treatment with benzylpenicillin should be started by the general practitioner before transfer to hospital; benefit to the patient outweighs the reduced chance of identifying the causative organism.

Drugs must be given i.v.; the regimens below provide the recommended therapy, with alternatives for patients allergic to first choices. Intrathecal therapy is now considered unnecessary, and can be dangerous, e.g. encephalopathy with penicillin.

Initial therapy should be sufficient to kill all pathogens, which are likely to be:

---

[1] Simmons N A 1993 Recommendations for endocarditis prophylaxis. Journal of Antimicrobial Chemotherapy 31: 437.

- All ages over 5 years.

For *Neisseria meningitidis* and *Streptococcus pneumoniae* benzylpenicillin should be given, followed, in the case of *Neisseria meningitidis*, by rifampicin for 2 days prior to discharge from hospital (to eradicate persisting organisms, lest a carrier state develop). *Haemophilus influenzae* is much less common but if it is suspected, e.g. in a patient with head injury, cefotaxime or ceftriaxone should be used instead of benzylpenicillin.

- Children under 5 years.

Neisseria meningitidis is now commonest and *Haemophilus influenzae*, formerly a frequent pathogen, is much less often isolated (as a result of immunisation programmes). *Streptococcus pneumoniae* is also less commonly found.

Give a cephalosporin, e.g. cefotaxime or chloramphenicol; where *Haemophilus influenzae* is isolated give rifampicin for 4 days before discharge from hospital.

- Neonates. For *Escherichia coli* or Group B streptococci: give cefotaxime or ceftazidime.

Ampicillin must be added if *Listeria monocytogenes* is suspected.

Dexamethasone given i.v. and early appears to reduce longterm neurological sequelae, especially sensorineural deafness, in infants and children. There is not, however, general agreement about the use of dexamethasone for meningitis in adults.

Subsequent therapy. When the infecting organism has been identified, specific therapy is chosen as follows. Intravenous administration should continue until the patient is capable of taking drugs by mouth. Antimicrobials (except aminoglycosides) enter well into the CSF when the meninges are inflamed; relapse may be due to restoration of the blood–CSF barrier as inflammation is reduced.

Neisseria meningitidis: benzylpenicillin 2.4 g 4–6 hourly or cefotaxime 2–3 g 8 hourly is given. Hydrocortisone should be added if there is evidence of adrenocortical insufficiency (Waterhouse–Friderichsen syndrome). Treatment should continue for 5 days after the patient has become afebrile.

Streptococcus pneumoniae: cefotaxime 2–3 g 8 hourly is given or benzylpenicillin 2.4 g 4–6 hourly if the organism is penicillin-sensitive. Treatment should continue for 10 days after the patient has

become afebrile and the physician should be aware of the possibility of relapse.

Haemophilus influenzae: chloramphenicol 100 mg/kg/d or cefotaxime 2–3 g 8 hourly is given. Treatment should continue for 10 days after the temperature has settled.

Chemoprophylaxis. The three common pathogens (below) are spread by respiratory secretions. Asymptomatic nasopharyngeal carriers seldom develop meningitis but they may transmit the pathogens to close personal contacts. Rifampicin by mouth is effective at reducing carriage rates.

Meningococcal meningitis often occurs in epidemics, in closed communities but also in isolated cases. Close personal contacts should receive rifampicin 600 mg × 12 h for 2 days.

Haemophilus influenzae type b has an infectivity similar to that of the meningococcus. Rifampicin 600 mg × 1/d may be given for 4 days.

Pneumococcal meningitis tends to occur in isolated cases and chemoprophylaxis of contacts is not at present recommended.

Infection of the intestines

(For stomach see p. 572.) Antimicrobial therapy should be reserved for specific conditions with identified pathogens where benefit has been shown; not all acute diarrhoea is infective for it can be caused by bacterial toxins in food, dietary indiscretions, anxiety and by drugs. Even if diarrhoea is infective, it may be due to viruses; or, if it is bacterial, antimicrobial agents may not reduce the duration of symptoms and may aggravate the condition by permitting opportunistic infection. Maintenance of water and electrolyte balance, either by i.v. infusion or orally with a glucose-electrolyte solution together with an antimotility drug (except in small children) are the mainstays of therapy in such cases (see Oral rehydration therapy, p. 584).

Some specific intestinal infections do benefit from chemotherapy:

Campylobacter jejuni. Erythromycin or ciprofloxacin by mouth will eliminate the organism from the stools and a 5-day course is worth giving if the illness is severe or turns out to be protracted.

Shigella. Mild disease requires no specific antimicrobial therapy but toxic shigellosis with high fever should be treated with ciprofloxacin or amoxycillin by mouth.

Salmonella. An antimicrobial should be used for severe salmonella gastroenteritis, or for bacteraemia or salmonella enteritis in an immunocompromised patient. The choice lies between ciprofloxacin, amoxycillin or co-trimoxazole, according to the sensitivity of the pathogen.

Typhoid fever is a generalised infection and requires treatment with ciprofloxacin, amoxycillin or co-trimoxazole; the i.v. route should be used at least initially, followed by oral administration. A longer period of treatment may be required for those who develop complications such as osteomyelitis or abscess.

A carrier state develops in a few individuals who have no symptoms of disease but who can infect others.[2] Organisms reside in the biliary or urinary tracts. Amoxycillin in high dose by mouth for 3 months may be successful for what can be a very difficult problem. Cholecystectomy may be needed.

Escherichia coli is a normal inhabitant of the bowel but some enterotoxigenic strains are pathogenic and are a frequent cause of travellers' diarrhoea. A quinolone, e.g. ciprofloxacin, is the drug of choice in most high-risk parts of the world for a severe attack (see Travellers' diarrhoea, p. 585). Antimicrobials are not generally given for prophylaxis but, when it is indicated, a quinolone should be used.

Staphylococcus aureus. Staphylococcal enteritis, although rare may complicate abdominal surgery, shock or antimicrobial therapy. Dehydration, shock and electrolyte imbalance should be treated vigorously. Vancomycin by mouth or flucloxacillin by mouth or i.v. is effective.

Vibrio cholerae. The cause of death in cholera is electrolyte and fluid loss in the stools which may exceed 1 l/h. The most important aim of treatment is prompt replacement and maintenance of water and electrolytes with oral or intravenous electrolyte solutions. Doxycycline, *given early*, significantly reduces the amount and duration of diarrhoea and eliminates the organism from the faeces (thus lessening the contamination of the environment). Carriers may be treated by doxycycline by mouth in high dose for 3 days. Ciprofloxacin may be given for resistant organisms.

Suppression of bowel flora is useful in *hepatic insufficiency*. Here, absorption of products of bacterial breakdown of protein (ammonium, amines) in the intestine lead to cerebral symptoms and even to coma. In acute coma, neomycin 6 g/d should be given by gastric tube; as prophylactic, 1–4 g/d may be given to patients with protein intolerance who fail to respond to dietary protein restriction (see also lactulose, p. 580).

Selective decontamination of the gut reduces the risk of nosocomial infection from gut organisms (including fungi) in patients who are immunocompromised or receiving intensive care (notably mechanical ventilation). Combinations of nonabsorbable (framycetin, colistin, nystatin and amphotericin) and i.v. (cefotaxime) antimicrobials are used to reduce the number of Gram-negative bacilli and yeasts while maintaining normal anaerobic flora.

Peritonitis is usually a mixed infection and antimicrobial choice must take account of coliforms, anaerobes and streptococci; a combination of gentamicin, amoxycillin plus metronidazole or of cefuroxime plus metronidazole is usually effective.

Chemoprophylaxis in surgery: see page 191.

Antibiotic-associated colitis: see page 193.

Infection of the urinary tract

(excluding sexually transmitted infections)

Common pathogens include:

- *Escherichia coli*
- *Proteus* spp.
- *Klebsiella pneumoniae*
- *Pseudomonas aeruginosa*
- *Enterobacteriaceae*
- *Staphylococcus saprophyticus*.

Identification of the causative organism and of its

---

[2] The most famous carrier was Mary Mallon ('Typhoid Mary') who worked as a cook in New York City, USA, using various assumed names and moving through several different households. She caused at least 10 outbreaks with 51 cases of typhoid fever and 3 deaths. To protect the public, she was kept in detention for 23 years.

sensitivity to drugs are important because of the range of organisms and the prevalence of resistant strains.

For infection of the lower urinary tract a low dose may be effective, as many antimicrobials are concentrated in the urine. Infections of the substance of the kidney require the doses needed for any systemic infection. Elimination of infection is hastened by a large urine volume (over 1.5 l/d) and by frequent micturition.

Drug treatment of urinary tract infection falls into several categories:

Lower urinary tract infection

Initial treatment with an oral cephalosporin, e.g. cephalexin, trimethoprim or ampicillin is usually satisfactory. Therapy should normally last 5 days and may need to be altered once the results of bacterial sensitivity are known. Single dose therapy with *amoxycillin* 3 g by mouth may be sufficient to cure uncomplicated lower urinary tract infection.

Upper urinary tract infection

Acute pyelonephritis may be accompanied by septicaemia and it is advisable to start with gentamicin plus amoxycillin i.v. or alternatively cefotaxime i.v. alone. This is an infection of the kidney substance and needs adequate blood as well as urine concentrations.

Recurrent urinary tract infection

Attacks following rapidly with the same organism may be relapses and indicate a failure to eliminate the original infection. Attacks with a longer interval between them and produced by differing bacterial types may be regarded as due to reinfection, presumably from a source outside the urinary tract. In treating a relapse it is wise to use a drug capable of achieving high tissue concentrations, e.g. trimethoprim. Repeated short courses of antimicrobials should overcome most recurrent infections but, if these fail, 7–14 days of high dose treatment may be given, following which continuous low-dose prophylaxis may be needed.

Asymptomatic infection

This may be found by routine urine testing of pregnant women or patients with known structural abnormality of the urinary tract. Such infection may explain micturition frequency or incontinence in the elderly. Appropriate antimicrobial therapy should be given. Amoxycillin or a cephalosporin is preferred in pregnancy.

Prostatitis

The commonest pathogens are Gram-negative aerobic bacilli. Trimethoprim or ciprofloxacin or erythromycin are effective and, being lipid soluble, penetrate the prostate in adequate concentration; they may usefully be combined. Response to a single, short course is often good, but recurrence is common and a patient can be regarded as cured only if he has been symptom-free and off antimicrobials for a year.

Chemoprophylaxis

Chemoprophylaxis is sometimes undertaken in patients liable to recurrent attacks or acute exacerbations of ineradicable infection. It may prevent subclinical renal damage in girls who are found to have asymptomatic bacteriuria on routine screening. Nitrofurantoin (50–100 mg/d), nalidixic acid (0.5–1.0 g/d) or trimethoprim (100 mg/d) are satisfactory. The drugs are best given as a single oral dose at night.

Tuberculosis of the genitourinary tract is treated on the principles described for pulmonary infection (p. 225).

SPECIAL DRUGS FOR URINARY TRACT INFECTIONS

General antimicrobials are used for urinary tract infections and described elsewhere. A few agents are used solely for infection of the urinary tract:

Nitrofurantoin ($t^{1}/_2$ 30 min), a synthetic antimicrobial, is active against the majority of urinary pathogens except pseudomonads. It is well absorbed from the gastrointestinal tract and is concentrated in the urine; but plasma concentrations are too low to treat infection of kidney tissue. Excretion is reduced when there is renal insufficiency, rendering the drug both more toxic and less effective. The main use of nitrofurantoin is now for prophylaxis. Adverse effects include nausea and vomiting and diarrhoea. Polyneuritis occurs especially in patients with significant renal impairment, in whom the drug is contraindicated. Allergic reactions include rashes, generalised urticaria and pulmonary infiltration with lung consolidation or pleural effusion.

Fosfomycin ($t^{1}/_2$ 5 h) is a member of the phosphonic acid class of antimicrobials which use a bacterial phosphate transport system to gain entry to the cell, whereupon they inhibit cell wall synthesis by blocking enol pyruvyltransferase. Fosfomycin is rapidly bactericidal. Fosfomycin is active against a broad spectrum of bacteria isolated in urinary tract infections including beta-lactamase producers, e.g. *Escherichia coli*, *Proteus* spp., *Klebsiella pneumoniae*, staphylococci and streptococci. It is administered orally, <3% bound to plasma proteins, not metabolised and eliminated in the urine. Fosfomycin is used to treat uncomplicated urinary tract infections, given as a single 3 g oral dose which maintains bactericidal urine concentrations for 36 h. It is generally well tolerated but gastrointestinal upsets including diarrhoea (2–8%), nausea and vomiting are the commonest adverse effects. Co-administration with metoclopramide should be avoided as lower urine concentrations result.

Nalidixic acid: see page 212.

Genital tract infections

A general account of orthodox literature is given below, but treatment is increasingly the prerogative of specialists, who, as is so often the case, get the best results.

GONORRHOEA

The problem of resistant *Neisseria gonorrhoeae* is increasing, and selection of a particular drug will depend on sensitivity testing and a knowledge of resistance patterns in different geographical locations. Effective treatment requires exposure of the organism briefly to a high concentration of the drug. Single dose regimens are practicable as well as being obviously desirable for social reasons, including compliance. The following schedules are effective:

Uncomplicated anogenital infections: amoxycillin with probenecid by mouth; spectinomycin i.v. or ciprofloxacin by mouth may be used for penicillin-allergic patients.

Pharyngeal gonorrhoea responds less well to the single dose regimen, and tetracycline in high dose by mouth is needed for 7 days.

Coexistent infection. *Chlamydia trachomatis* is frequently present with *Neisseria gonorrhoeae*; tetracycline by mouth for 7 days will limit chlamydial urethritis (if it is suspected).

Nongonococcal urethritis

The vast majority of cases of urethritis with pus in which gonococci cannot be identified, are due to sexually-transmitted organisms, usually *Chlamydia trachomatis* and sometimes *Ureaplasma urealyticum*. Tetracycline or erythromycin by mouth is effective.

Pelvic inflammatory disease

Several pathogens are involved including *Chlamydia trachomatis*, *Neisseria gonorrhoeae* and *Mycoplasma hominis*. A combination of antimicrobials is usually required, e.g. metronidazole plus doxycycline by mouth.

SYPHILIS

Treponema pallidum is invariably sensitive to penicillin.

Primary and secondary syphilis are effectively treated by procaine penicillin i.m. daily for 10–21 days. Tetracycline or erythromycin orally may be used for penicillin-allergic patients.

Tertiary syphilis should have the same treatment, ensuring that it continues for 3 weeks.

Congenital syphilis in the newborn should be treated with benzylpenicillin for 10 days at least.

A pregnant woman with syphilis should be treated as for primary syphilis, in each pregnancy, some advocate, in order to avoid all danger to children. Therapy is best given between the third and sixth month, as there may be a risk of abortion if it is given earlier.

Results of treatment of syphilis with penicillin are excellent; virtually 100% cure is achieved in seronegative cases, but the cure rate is lower in seropositive cases. Follow-up of all cases is essential, for 5 years if possible.

The Herxheimer (or Jarisch–Herxheimer) *reaction* is probably caused by cytokine (mainly tumour necrosis factor) release following massive slaughter of spirochaetes. Presenting as pyrexia, it is common during the few hours after the first penicillin injection; other features include tachycardia, headache, myalgia and malaise which last up to a day. It cannot be prevented by giving graduated doses of penicillin. Prednisolone may prevent it and should probably be given if a reaction is specially to be feared, e.g. in a patient with syphilitic aortitis.

CHANCROID

The causal agent, *Haemophilus ducreyi*, normally responds to erythromycin for 7 days or a single dose of ceftriaxone or azithromycin.

GRANULOMA INGUINALE

Calymmatobacterium granulomatis infection is treated with ampicillin or co-trimoxazole or a tetracycline for 2 weeks.

NONSPECIFIC VAGINITIS

Anaerobic vaginosis is a common form of vaginal inflammation in which neither *Trichomonas vaginalis* nor *Candida albicans* can be isolated. There is evidence to associate the condition with *Gardnerella vaginalis*, and anaerobic organisms, especially of the *Bacteroides* species, the latter being responsible for the characteristic odour of the vaginal discharge. The condition responds well to a single 2 g oral dose of metronidazole.

SPECIFIC VAGINITIS

Candida vaginitis: see page 235.
    Trichomonas vaginitis: see pages 213, 246.

Eye infections

Superficial infections, caused by a variety of organisms, are treated by chloramphenicol, framycetin, gentamicin, ciprofloxacin or neomycin in drops (or ointments where drops are inconvenient), e.g. at night. Gentamicin or tobramycin are used for *Pseudomonas aeruginosa*, and fusidic acid for *Staphylococcus aureus*. Preparations often contain hydrocortisone or prednisolone, but the steroid masks the progress of the infection, and should it be applied with an antimicrobial to which the organism is resistant (bacterium or virus), it may make the disease worse by suppressing protective inflammation. Local chemoprophylaxis without corticosteroid is used to prevent secondary bacterial infection in viral conjunctivitis.

Chlamydial conjunctivitis. In the developed world, the genital (D-K) serotypes of the organism are responsible and the reservoir and transmission is maintained by sexual contact. Endemic trachoma in developing countries is usually caused by serotypes A, B and C. In either case, tetracycline is effective. Alternatively, pregnant or lactating women may receive erythromycin.

Herpes keratitis (see p. 271). It is essential that a corticosteroid should **never** be put on the eye; the disease is exacerbated and permanent blindness can result.

Mycobacterial infections

PULMONARY TUBERCULOSIS

Drug therapy has transformed tuberculosis from a disabling and often fatal disease into one in which almost 100% cure is obtainable. Chemotherapy was formerly protracted, but a better understanding of the mode of action of antituberculosis drugs has allowed the development of effective short-course regimens.

> ### Principles of antituberculosis therapy
>
> - A large number of actively multiplying bacilli must be killed: isoniazid achieves this.
> - Treat persisters, i.e. semidormant bacilli that metabolise slowly or intermittently: rifampicin and pyrazinamide are the most efficacious.
> - Prevent the emergence of drug resistance by multiple therapy to suppress drug-resistant mutants that exist in all large bacterial populations: isoniazid and rifampicin are best.
> - Combined formulations are used to ensure that poor compliance does not result in monotherapy with consequent drug resistance.

All short-course regimens include isoniazid, pyrazinamide and rifampicin. After extensive clinical trials, the following have been found satisfactory:

1. An *unsupervised* regimen of *daily* dosing comprising isoniazid and rifampicin for 6 months, plus pyrazinamide for the first 2 months.

2. A *supervised* (*directly observed*) regimen for patients who cannot be relied upon to comply with treatment, comprising thrice-weekly dosing with isoniazid and rifampicin for 6 months, plus pyrazinamide for the first 2 months (isoniazid and pyrazinamide are given in higher dose than in the unsupervised regimen).

With both the above regimens, ethambutol by mouth or streptomycin i.m. should be added for the first 2 months if there is a likelihood of drug-resistant organisms, or if the patient is severely ill with extensive active lesions.

3. A *less costly*, yet still effective, regimen favoured by some countries comprises *supervised* daily administration of isoniazid, rifampicin, pyrazinamide and either ethambutol or streptomycin for 2 months followed by 6 months of unsupervised daily isoniazid and thiacetazone.

All the regimens are highly effective, with relapse rates of 1–2% in those who continue for 6 months; even if patients default after, say, 4 months, tuberculosis can be expected to recur in only 10–15%. Drug resistance seldom develops with any of these regimens.

Special problems

Resistant organisms. Initial resistance occurs in about 4% of isolates, usually to isoniazid. Multiple-drug-resistant tuberculosis, i.e. resistant to rifampicin and isoniazid at least, should be treated with 3 or 4 drugs to which the organisms are sensitive and should extend for 12–24 months after cultures become negative. Atypical mycobacteria are often resistant to standard drugs; their virulence is low but they can produce serious infection in immunocompromised patients which may respond, e.g. to erythromycin or a quinolone or a tetracycline, often in combination.

Chemoprophylaxis may be either

- primary, i.e. the giving of antituberculosis drugs to uninfected individuals, which is seldom justified; or
- secondary, which is the treatment of infected but symptom-free individuals, e.g. those known to be in contact with the disease and who develop a positive tuberculin reaction. Secondary chemoprophylaxis may be justified in children under the age of 3 because they have a high risk of disseminated disease; isoniazid alone for 6 months may be used since there is little risk of resistant organisms emerging.

Pregnancy. Drug treatment should never be interrupted or postponed during pregnancy. On the general principle of limiting exposure of the fetus, the standard 3-drug, 6-month course (1 above) is best. Streptomycin should be excluded from any regimen (danger of fetal eighth cranial nerve damage).

Nonrespiratory tuberculosis. The principles of treatment, i.e. multiple therapy and prolonged follow-up, are the same as for respiratory tuberculosis. In only a few cases is surgery now necessary. It should always be *preceded* and *followed* by chemotherapy. Many chronic tuberculous lesions may be relatively inaccessible to drugs as a result of avascularity of surrounding tissues; treatment frequently has to be prolonged and dosage high, especially if damaged tissue cannot be removed by surgery, e.g. tuberculosis of bones.

Meningeal tuberculosis. It is essential to use isoniazid and pyrazinamide which penetrate well into the CSF. Rifampicin enters inflamed meninges well but noninflamed meninges less so. An effective regimen is isoniazid, rifampicin, pyrazinamide and streptomycin. Treatment may need to continue for much longer than modern short course chemotherapy for pulmonary tuberculosis.

Adrenal steroid and tuberculosis. In pulmonary tuberculosis a corticosteroid may be given to severely ill patients. It reduces the injurious reaction of the body to tuberculoprotein and buys time for the chemotherapy to take effect. It also causes the patient to feel better much more quickly.

> In the absence of effective chemotherapy, an adrenal steroid will cause tuberculosis to extend and it should never be used alone, e.g. for another disease, if tuberculosis is suspected.

ANTITUBERCULOSIS DRUGS

Isoniazid

Isoniazid ($t^{1/2}$ see below) (INH, INAH, isonicotinic acid hydrazide) is selectively effective against *Mycobacterium tuberculosis* because it prevents the synthesis of components that are unique to mycobacterial cell walls. Hence it is bactericidal against actively multiplying bacilli (whether within macrophages or at extracellular sites) but is bacteriostatic against nondividing bacilli; it has little or no activity against other bacteria. Isoniazid is well absorbed from the alimentary tract and is distributed throughout the body water, readily crossing tissue barriers and entering cells and cerebrospinal fluid. It should always be given in cases where there is special risk of meningitis (miliary tuberculosis and primary infection). Isoniazid is inactivated by conjugation with an acetyl group and the rate of the reaction is bimodally distributed (see Pharmacogenetics, p. 109). The $t^{1/2}$ is 1 h in fast and 4 h in slow acetylators; steady state plasma concentration in fast acetylators is less than half that in slow acetylators but standard oral doses (5 mg/kg/d) on daily regimens give adequate tuberculocidal concentrations in both groups.

Adverse effects. Isoniazid is in general well tolerated. The most severe adverse effect is liver damage which may range from moderate elevation of hepatic enzymes to severe hepatitis and death. It is probably caused by a chemically reactive metabolite(s), e.g. acetylhydrazine. Most cases develop within the first 8 weeks of therapy and liver function tests should be monitored monthly during this period at least.

Isoniazid is a structural analogue of pyridoxine and accelerates its excretion, the principal result of which is peripheral neuropathy with numbness and tingling of the feet, motor involvement being less common. Neuropathy is more frequent in slow acetylators, malnourished people, the elderly and those with liver disease and alcoholism. Such patients should receive pyridoxine 10 mg/d by mouth, which prevents neuropathy and does not interfere with the therapeutic effect; some prefer simply to give pyridoxine to all patients. Other adverse effects include mental disturbances, incoordination, optic neuritis and convulsions.

Isoniazid inhibits the metabolism of phenytoin, carbamazepine and ethosuximide, increasing their effect.

Rifampicin

Rifampicin (Rifampin) ($t^{1/2}$ 4 h) has bactericidal activity against the tubercle bacillus, comparable to that of isoniazid. It is also used in leprosy.

It acts by inhibiting RNA synthesis, bacteria being sensitive to this effect at much lower concentrations than mammalian cells; it is particularly effective against mycobacteria that lie semidormant within cells. Rifampicin has a wide range of antimicrobial activity. Other uses include leprosy, severe Legionnaires' disease (with erythromycin), and the chemoprophylaxis of meningococcal meningitis.

Rifampicin is well absorbed from the gastrointestinal tract. It penetrates well into most tissues. Entry into the CSF when meninges are inflamed is sufficient to maintain therapeutic concentrations at normal oral doses but transfer is reduced as inflammation subsides in 1 or 2 months. Enterohepatic recycling takes place, and eventually about 60% of a single dose is eliminated in the faeces; urinary excretion of unchanged drug also occurs. The $t^{1/2}$ is 4 h after initial doses, but shortens on repeated dosing because rifampicin is a very effective enzyme inducer and increases its own metabolism (as well as that of several other drugs, see below).

Adverse reactions. Rifampicin rarely causes serious toxicity. Adverse reactions include flushing and itching with or without a rash, and thrombocytopenia. Rises in plasma bilirubin and hepatic enzymes may occur when treatment starts but are often transient and are not necessarily an indication for stopping the drug; fatal hepatitis, however, has occurred. *Intermittent* dosing, i.e. less than twice weekly, either as part of a regimen or through poor compliance, promotes certain effects that probably have an immunological basis, namely, an influenza-like syndrome (malaise, headache and fever, shortness of breath and wheezing), acute haemolytic anaemia and acute renal failure sometimes with haemolysis, sometimes without. Red discolouration of urine, tears and sputum is a useful indication that the patient is taking the drug. Rifampicin also causes an orange discolouration of soft contact lenses.

Other uses. Rifampicin is a powerful *enzyme inducer* and speeds the metabolism of numerous drugs, including warfarin, steroid contraceptives, narcotic analgesics, oral antidiabetic agents, phenytoin and dapsone. Appropriate increase in dosage is required to compensate for increased drug metabolism.

Pyrazinamide

Pyrazinamide ($t\frac{1}{2}$ 9 h) is a derivative of nicotinamide and is included in first-choice combination regimens because of its particular ability to kill persisters, i.e. mycobacteria that are semidormant, often within cells. Its action is dependent on the activity of intrabacterial pyrazinamidase which converts pyrazinamide to the active pyrazinoic acid; this enzyme is most effective in an acidic environment such as the interior of cells. Pyrazinamide is well absorbed from the gastrointestinal tract and metabolised in the liver, very little unchanged drug appearing in the urine.

Adverse effects include hyperuricaemia and arthralgia, which is relatively frequent with daily

but less so with intermittent dosing and, unlike gout, affects both large and small joints. Pyrazinoic acid, the principal metabolite of pyrazinamide, inhibits renal tubular secretion of urate. Symptomatic treatment with an NSAID is usually sufficient and it is rarely necessary to discontinue pyrazinamide because of arthralgia. Hepatitis, which was particularly associated with high doses, is not a problem with modern short-course schedules. Sideroblastic anaemia and urticaria also occur.

Ethambutol

Ethambutol ($t\frac{1}{2}$ 4 h), being bacteriostatic, is used in conjunction with other antituberculosis drugs to delay or prevent the emergence of resistant bacilli. It is well absorbed from the gastrointestinal tract and effective concentrations occur in most body tissues including the lung; in tuberculous meningitis, sufficient may reach the CSF to inhibit mycobacterial growth but insignificant amounts cross into the CSF if the meninges are not inflamed. Excretion is mainly by the kidney, by tubular secretion as well as by glomerular filtration; the dose should be reduced when renal function is impaired.

Adverse effects. In recommended oral doses (15 mg/kg per day) (taking account of reduced renal function), ethambutol is relatively nontoxic. The main problem is *optic neuritis* (unilateral or bilateral) causing loss of visual acuity, central scotomata, occasionally also peripheral vision loss and red–green colour blindness. The changes reverse if treatment is stopped promptly; if not, the patient may go blind. It is prudent to note any history of eye disease and to get baseline tests of vision before starting treatment with ethambutol. The drug should not be given to a patient whose vision is much reduced and who may not notice further minor deterioration. Patients should be told to make a point of reading small print in newspapers (with each eye separately) and if there is any deterioration to stop the drug immediately and seek advice. Patients who cannot understand and comply should be given **alternative therapy**, if possible. The need for repeated specialist ophthalmological monitoring is controversial. Peripheral neuritis occurs but is rare.

Streptomycin: see page 206.

Thiacetazone

Thiacetazone ($t^1/2$ 13 h) is tuberculostatic and is used with isoniazid to inhibit the emergence of resistance to the latter drug. It is absorbed from the gastrointestinal tract, partly metabolised and partly excreted in the urine.

Adverse reactions include gastrointestinal symptoms, conjunctivitis and vertigo. More serious effects are erythema multiforme, haemolytic anaemia, agranulocytosis, cerebral oedema and hepatitis.

Alternative or reserve drugs are used where there are problems of drug intolerance and bacterial resistance. They are in this class because of either greater toxicity or of lesser efficacy and include: *ethionamide* (gastrointestinal irritation, allergic reactions), *capreomycin* (nephrotoxic), *cycloserine* (effective but neurotoxic), and *kanamycin* (see Aminoglycosides).

LEPROSY

Effective treatment of leprosy is complex and requires much experience to obtain the best results. Problems of resistant leprosy now requires that multiple drug therapy be used and involve:

● *for paucibacillary* disease: dapsone and rifampicin for 6 months
● *for multibacillary* disease: dapsone, rifampicin and clofazimine for 2 years. Follow-up for 4–8 years may be necessary.

Dapsone ($t^1/2$ 27 h), a bacteriostatic sulphone (related to sulphonamides, and acting by the same mechanism, see p. 210), has for many years been the standard drug for the treatment of all forms of leprosy but irregular and inadequate duration of treatment with a single drug have allowed the emergence of resistance, both primary and secondary, to become a major problem. Dapsone is also used to treat dermatitis herpetiformis and (with pyrimethamine) is given for malaria prophylaxis. Adverse effects range from gastrointestinal symptoms to agranulocytosis, haemolytic anaemia and generalised allergic reactions that include exfoliative dermatitis.

Rifampicin (see above) is bactericidal, and is safe and effective when given once monthly. This long interval renders feasible the directly observed administration of rifampicin which the above regimens require.

Clofazimine ($t^1/2$ 70 days) has a leprostatic action and an anti-inflammatory effect that prevents erythema nodosum leprosum. It causes gastrointestinal symptoms. Reddish discolouration of the skin and other cutaneous lesions also occur, and may persist for months after the drug has been stopped.

Other antileprotics include ethionamide and prothionamide. Thalidomide (see Index) despite its notorious past still finds a use in the control of allergic lepromatous reactions.

OTHER BACTERIAL INFECTIONS

Burns. Infection may be substantially reduced by application of silver sulphadiazine cream. Substantial absorption can occur from any raw surface and use of an aminoglycoside, e.g. neomycin, preparations can cause ototoxicity.

Gas gangrene. The skin between the waist and the knees is normally contaminated with anaerobic faecal organisms. However assiduous the skin preparation for orthopaedic operations or thigh amputations, this will not kill the spores. Surgery done for vascular insufficiency where tissue oxygenation may be poor is likely to be followed by infection. Gas gangrene (*Clostridium perfringens*) may occur; it may be prevented by benzlypenicillin which should be used in such operations.

Wounds. Systemic chemoprophylaxis is necessary for several days at least in dirty wounds where sutures have to be left below the skin, and in penetrating wounds of body cavities. Benzylpenicillin is probably best, but in the case of penetrating abdominal wounds, metronidazole should be added, intravenously (see also Tetanus). Weak iodine solution is an effective skin antiseptic where the patient is not allergic. It is, however, inactivated by serum so that its painful application to wounds is pointless; povidone-iodine is preferred.

Abscesses and infections in bone and serous cavities are treated according to the antimicrobial sensitivity of the organism concerned but require high doses because of poor penetration. Local instillation of the drug may be needed.

In osteomyelitis, early treatment is urgent to prevent bone necrosis. Bacteriological identification is of great importance and blood for culture (50% of cases are positive) should be taken before therapy begins; indeed, aspiration of the bone to get to the organism has been advocated. As the organism is commonly *Staphylococcus aureus*, flucloxacillin and sodium fusidate should be used. Treatment is required for weeks. Surgery is often needed in late cases.

Actinomycosis. *Actinomyces israelii* is sensitive to several drugs but access is poor because of granulomatous fibrosis. High doses of benzylpenicillin are given for several weeks. Surgery is likely to be needed.

Leptospirosis. To be maximally effective, chemotherapy should be started within 4 days of the onset of symptoms. Benzylpenicillin is recommended; a Herxheimer reaction may be induced (see Syphilis). General supportive management is important, including attention to fluid balance and observation for signs of hepatic, renal or cardiac failure.

Lyme disease. Keeping the skin covered and use of insect repellants are effective to prevent tick bites. In most manifestations of the disease, *Borrelia burgdorferi* responds to amoxycillin or doxycycline orally for up to 21 days but when the central nervous system is invaded large doses of benzylpenicillin or cefotaxime should be given i.v. for 14 days.

Berman S 1995 Otitis media in children. New England Journal of Medicine 332: 1560

Bignell C 1994 The eradication of gonorrhoea. British Medical Journal 309: 1103

Bourke S J 1993 Chlamydial respiratory infections. British Medical Journal 306: 1219

Conference report 1995 The challenge of tuberculosis: statements on global control and prevention. Lancet 346: 809

Dupont H L, Ericsson C D 1993 Prevention and treatment of traveller's diarrhoea. New England Journal of Medicine 328: 1821

Durack D T 1995 Prevention of infective endocarditis. New England Journal of Medicine 332: 38

Durand M L et al 1993 Acute bacterial meningitis in adults. A review of 493 episodes. New England Journal of Medicine 328: 21

Gonzales R, Sande M 1995 What will it take to stop physicians from prescribing antibiotics in acute bronchitis? Lancet 345: 665

Iseman M D 1993 Treatment of multidrug-resistant tuberculosis. New England Journal of Medicine 329: 784

McCormack W M 1994 Pelvic inflammatory disease. New England Journal of Medicine 330: 115

O'Connell S 1995 Lyme disease in the United Kingdom. British Medical Journal 310: 303

Parrillo J E 1993 Pathogenic mechanisms of septic shock. New England Journal of Medicine 328: 1471

Reid M M 1994 Splenectomy, sepsis, immunisation, and guidelines. Lancet 344: 970

Tabaqchali S, Jumaa P 1995 Diagnosis and management of *Clostridium difficile* infection. British Medical Journal 310: 1375

Tunkel A R, Scheld W M 1995 Acute bacterial meningitis. Lancet 346: 1675

Tuomanen E L et al 1995 Pathogenesis of pneumococcal infection. New England Journal of Medicine 332: 1280

GUIDE TO FURTHER READING

Bartlett J G, Mundy L M 1995 Community acquired pneumonia. New England Journal of Medicine 333: 1618

14

Viral, fungal, protozoal and helminthic infections

SYNOPSIS

- **Viruses** present a more difficult problem of chemotherapy than do higher organisms, e.g. bacteria, for they are intracellular parasites that use the metabolism of host cells. Identification of differences between viral and human metabolism, however, has led to the development of effective antiviral agents, whose roles are increasingly well defined.
- **Fungus infections** range from inconvenient skin conditions to life-threatening systemic diseases; the latter have become more frequent as opportunistic infections in patients immunocompromised by drugs or AIDS.
- **Protozoal infections**. Malaria is the major transmissible parasitic disease. The life cycle of the plasmodium that is relevant to prophylaxis and therapy is described. Drug resistance is an increasing problem and differs with geographical location, and type of plasmodium.
- **Helminthic infestations** cause considerable morbidity. The drugs that are effective against these organisms are summarised.

Viral infections

Antiviral agents are most active when viruses are replicating. The earlier that treatment is given, therefore, the better the result. An important difficulty is that a substantial amount of viral multiplication has often taken place before symptoms occur. Apart from primary infection, viral illness is often the consequence of reactivation of latent virus in the body. In both cases patients whose immune systems are compromised may suffer particularly severe illness.

CLASSIFICATION OF ANTIVIRAL DRUGS

Drugs that directly impair virus replication:
See Table 14.1

Drugs that modulate the host immune system:
alfa interferons, inosine pranobex

An overview of the place of antiviral agents in therapy is given in Table 14.1.

Viruses are as capable of developing resistance to antimicrobial drugs as bacteria, with similar implications for the individual patient, for the community and for drug development.

Table 14.1 Drugs of choice for virus infections

Organism	Drug of choice	Alternative
Varicella-zoster		
chickenpox	aciclovir	
zoster	aciclovir, famciclovir	
Herpes simplex		
keratitis	aciclovir (topical)	
labial	aciclovir (topical and/or oral)	
genital	aciclovir (topical and/or oral) famciclovir (oral)	
encephalitis	aciclovir	
disseminated	aciclovir	
Human immuno-deficiency virus (HIV)	zidovudine, didanosine, ritonavir indinavir saquinavir	zalcitabine stavudine
Hepatitis B, C or D	interferon alfa-2a and -2b	
Influenza A	amantadine	
Cytomegalovirus (CMV)	ganciclovir	foscarnet(for retinitis in HIV patients)
Respiratory syncytial virus	tribavirin	

Drugs that directly impair virus replication

HERPES SIMPLEX AND VARICELLA-ZOSTER

Aciclovir ($t^{1/2}$ 3 h)

Aciclovir (Zovirax) inhibits viral DNA synthesis only after phosphorylation by virus-specific thymidine kinase, which accounts for its high therapeutic index; phosphorylated aciclovir inhibits DNA polymerase and so prevents viral DNA being formed. Taken orally about 20% is absorbed from the gut, but this is sufficient for the systemic treatment of some infections. It distributes widely in the body; the concentration in CSF is approximately half that of plasma, and the brain concentration may be even less. These differences are taken into account in dosing for viral encephalitis (for which aciclovir

must be given i.v.). The drug is excreted in the urine. Oral and topical use are $\times 5/d$.

Indications for aciclovir include:

Herpes simplex virus:

● skin infections, including initial and recurrent labial and genital herpes (as a cream), most effectively when new lesions are forming; skin and mucous membrane infections (as tablets or oral suspension)
● ocular keratitis (as an ointment)
● prophylaxis and treatment in the immunocompromised (oral, as tablets or suspension)
● encephalitis, disseminated disease (i.v.).

Aciclovir-resistant herpes simplex virus has been reported in patients with AIDS; foscarnet has been used in these cases.

Varicella-zoster virus:

● chickenpox, particularly in the immunocompromised (i.v.) or in the immunocompetent with pneumonitis or hepatitis (i.v.)
● shingles in immunocompetent persons (as tablets or suspension, and best within 48 h of the appearance of the rash). Immunocompromised persons will often have more severe symptoms and require i.v. administration.

Adverse reactions are remarkably few. The ophthalmic ointment causes a mild transient stinging sensation and a diffuse superficial punctate keratopathy which clears when the drug is stopped. Oral or i.v. use may cause gastrointestinal symptoms, headache and neuropsychiatric reactions. Extravasation with i.v. use causes severe local inflammation.

Valaciclovir is a prodrug (ester) of aciclovir, i.e. after oral administration the parent aciclovir is released. The higher bioavailability of valaciclovir (about 60%) allows dosing only $\times 3/d$. It is used for treating herper-zoster infections.

Famciclovir is a prodrug of penciclovir which is similar to aciclovir; it is used for herpes zoster and herpes simplex infections. It need be given only $\times 3/d$.

Idoxuridine

Idoxuridine was the first widely used antivirus

drug. It is superseded by aciclovir but is effective topically for ocular and cutaneous herpes simplex with few adverse reactions.

HUMAN IMMUNODEFICIENCY VIRUS (HIV)

Zidovudine (Retrovir) ($t^1/_2$ 1 h)

Human immunodeficiency virus replicates by converting its single-stranded RNA into double-stranded DNA which is incorporated into host DNA; this crucial conversion, the *reverse* of the normal cellular transcription of nucleic acids, is accomplished by the enzyme *reverse transcriptase*, i.e. it is a reverse transcriptase inhibitor (RTI). Zidovudine, as the triphosphate, has a high affinity for reverse transcriptase and is integrated by it into the viral DNA chain, causing premature chain termination. The drug must be present continuously to prevent viral alteration of the host DNA, which is permanent once it occurs.

Pharmacokinetics. Zidovudine is well absorbed from the gastrointestinal tract (it is available as capsules and syrup) and is rapidly cleared from the plasma; concentrations in CSF are approximately half those in plasma. The drug is inactivated mainly by metabolism but 20% is excreted unchanged by the kidney.

Uses. Zidovudine is indicated for serious manifestations of human immunodeficiency virus infection in patients with acquired immunodeficiency syndrome (AIDS) or AIDS-related complex, i.e. those with opportunistic infection, constitutional or neurological symptoms; treatment reduces the frequency of opportunistic infections and may prolong survival. It is also indicated for early symptomatic and asymptomatic HIV infection when blood markers indicate risk of disease progression.

Adverse reactions early in treatment may include anorexia, nausea, vomiting, headache, dizziness, malaise and myalgia, but tolerance develops to these and usually the dose need not be altered. More serious are anaemia and neutropenia which develop when the dose is high, and with advanced disease. A toxic myopathy (not easily distinguish-able from HIV-associated myopathy) may develop with longterm use.

Didanosine (DDI) ($t^1/_2$ 1 h), is a reverse transcriptase inhibitor like zidovudine but has a much longer intracellular duration and thus prolonged antiretroviral activity. Didanosine is rapidly but incompletely absorbed from the gastrointestinal tract, is widely distributed in body water; 30–65% is recovered unchanged in the urine which it enters both by glomerular filtraton and tubular secretion. Didanosine may cause pancreatitis with an incidence of 7% at a dose of 500 mg/d; other adverse effects include peripheral neuropathy, hyperuricaemia and diarrhoea, any of which may give reason to reduce the dose or discontinue the drug.

Zalcitabine (DDC) is a reverse transcriptase inhibitor; its adverse effects include peripheral neuropathy and pancreatitis which are reason to discontinue the drug.

Lamivudine (3Tc) is a reverse transcriptase inhibitor with a relatively long intracellular half-life (12–15 h). In combination with zidovudine (see below), lamivudine appears to reduce viral load effectively and to be well tolerated.

Protease inhibitors (ritonavir, indinavir, saquinavir) constitute a new class of agent for HIV infection. In its process of replication, HIV produces protein and also a protease which cleaves the protein into component parts that are subsequently reassembled into virus particles; protease inhibitors disrupt this essential process. Protease inhibitors have been shown to reduce viral RNA, increase CD4 counts and improve survival, when compared with placebo.

Stavudine is a nucleotide analogue that may be used in HIV patients in whom zidovudine is no longer indicated.

Uses. Viral reverse transcriptase inhibitors (RTI) are central to current specific therapy against HIV, i.e. apart from the prevention and treatment of opportunist infection. In this evolving scene there is evidence that combination therapy, e.g. with zidovudine plus didanosine, or zidovudine plus lamivudine, is superior to monotherapy, i.e. any of these drugs alone. Issues that must be clarified include:

- when to introduce RTI, e.g. in symptomatic or unsymptomatic patients

- their optimal dose
- the most efficacious combinations
- their use in advanced disease when benefits may outweigh the risk of toxicity.

INFLUENZA A

Amantadine

Amantadine ($t^{1}/_{2}$ 3 h) is effective only against influenza A; it acts by interfering with the uncoating and release of viral genome into the host cell. It is well absorbed from the gastrointestinal tract and is eliminated in the urine. Amantadine may be used orally for the prevention and treatment of infection with influenza A (but not influenza B) virus. Those most likely to benefit include the debilitated, persons with respiratory disability and people living in crowded conditions, especially during an influenza epidemic.

Adverse reactions include dizziness, nervousness, lightheadedness and insomnia. Drowsiness, hallucinations, delirium and coma may occur in patients with impaired renal function. Convulsions may be induced, and amantadine should be avoided in epileptic patients.

Amantadine for Parkinson's disease: see page 366.

CYTOMEGALOVIRUS

Ganciclovir

Ganciclovir ($t^{1}/_{2}$ 4 h) is similar to aciclovir in its mode of action. It is given i.v. or orally and is eliminated in the urine, mainly unchanged. Ganciclovir is active against several types of virus but because of toxicity, its use is limited to life- or sight-threatening cytomegalovirus (CMV) infection in immunocompromised patients, and to prevent CMV disease in patients receiving immunosuppressive therapy following organ transplantation. Ganciclovir-resistant cytomegalovirus isolates have been reported.

Adverse reactions include neutropenia and thrombocytopenia which are usually but not always reversible after withdrawal. Concomitant use of potential marrow-depressant drugs, e.g. co-trimoxazole, amphotericin B, zidovudine, should be avoided. Other reactions are fever, rash, gastrointestinal symptoms, confusion and seizure (the last especially if imipenem is coadministered).

Foscarnet is used for retinitis due to CMV in patients with HIV infection when ganciclovir is contraindicated; it has also been used to treat aciclovir-resistant herpes simplex virus infection. It causes numerous adverse effects, including renal toxicity.

RESPIRATORY SYNCYTIAL VIRUS

Tribavirin is a synthetic nucleoside which is administered by inhalation as an aerosol or nebulised solution for severe respiratory syncytial virus bronchiolitis in infants and children. Systemic absorption by this route is negligible. It is also effective in treating Lassa fever.

Coryza (common cold). Recent evidence suggests that lozenges containing zinc shorten the duration of symptoms.[1]

DRUGS THAT MODULATE THE HOST IMMUNE SYSTEM

Interferons

Virus infection stimulates the production of protective glycoproteins (interferons) which act: (1) directly on uninfected cells to induce enzymes that degrade viral RNA; (2) indirectly by stimulating the immune system. Interferons also modify cell regulatory mechanisms and inhibit neoplastic growth. They are classified as alfa, beta or gamma according to their antigenic and physical properties. Alfa interferons (subclassified -2a, -2b and -N1) are effective against conditions that include hairy cell leukaemia, chronic myelogenous leukaemia, recurrent or metastatic renal cell carcinoma, Kaposi's sarcoma in AIDS patients (an effect that may be partly due to its activity against HIV) and *condylomata acuminata* (genital warts). Interferon alfa-2a and -2b also improve the manifestations of viral hepatitis but responses differ according to the infecting agent. Whereas both hepatitis B and C patients may respond to interferon alfa, those with hepatitis C

---

[1] Maknin M L et al 1996 Annals of Internal Medicine 125: 81.

have a higher rate of relapse and may need pro-longed therapy. Hepatitis D requires a much larger dose of interferon to obtain a response and yet may relapse if the drug is withdrawn.

Adverse reactions are common and include an influenza-like syndrome (naturally-produced inter-feron may cause symptoms in natural influenza infection), fatigue and depression which respond to lowering the dose. Other effects are anorexia (sufficient to induce weight loss), convulsions, hypotension, hypertension, cardiac dysrhythmias and bone marrow depression. Interferons inhibit the metabolism of theophylline, increasing its effect.

Inosine pranobex

This drug is reported to stimulate the host immune response to virus infection and has been used for mucocutaneous herpes simplex and genital warts (but aciclovir is superior). It is administered by mouth and metabolised to uric acid, so should be used with caution in patients with hyperuricaemia or gout.

Fungal infections

Widespread use of immunosuppressive chemo-therapy and the emergence of AIDS have con-tributed to a rise in the incidence of opportunistic infection ranging from comparatively trivial cuta-neous infections to systemic disease that demands prolonged treatment with potentially toxic agents.

CLASSIFICATION OF ANTIFUNGAL AGENTS

- Drugs that disrupt the fungal cell membrane
  polyenes: e.g. amphotericin
  azoles: imidazoles, e.g. ketoconazole
         triazoles, e.g. fluconazole
  allylamine: terbinafine
- Drug that inhibits mitosis: griseofulvin
- Drug that inhibits DNA synthesis: flucytosine

Treatment

SUPERFICIAL MYCOSES

Dermatophyte infections (ringworm, tinea)

Longstanding remedies such as Compound Benzoic Acid Ointment (Whitfield's ointment) are still acceptable for mild infections but a topical imi-dazole (clotrimazole, econazole, miconazole, sul-conazole), which is also effective against candida, is now usually preferred. Tioconazole is effective topically for nail infections. Griseofulvin orally should be used for extensive scalp or nail tinea infection.

Candida infections

Cutaneous infection is generally treated with topi-cal amphotericin, clotrimazole, econazole, micona-zole or nystatin. Local hygiene is also important. An underlying explanation should be sought if a patient fails to respond to these measures, e.g. dia-betes, the use of a broad-spectrum antibiotic or of immunosuppressive drugs.

Candidiasis of alimentary tract mucosa responds to amphotericin, fluconazole, ketoconazole, miconazole or nystatin as lozenges (to suck, for oral infection), gel (held in the mouth before swallow-ing), suspension or tablets.

Vaginal candidiasis is treated by clotrimazole, econazole, isoconazole, ketoconazole, miconazole or nystatin as pessaries or vaginal tablets or cream inserted once or twice a day with cream or ointment on surrounding skin. Failure may be due to a concurrent intestinal infection causing reinfection and nystatin tablets may be given by mouth 8-hourly with the local treatment. The male sexual partner may use a similar anti-fungal ointment for his benefit and for hers (rein-fection).

SYSTEMIC MYCOSES

The principal treatment options are summarised in Table 14.2.

Table 14.2 Drugs of choice for fungal infections

Infection	Drug of first choice	Alternative
Aspergillosis	amphotericin	itraconazole
Blastomycosis[1]	ketoconazole[2] or amphotericin	itraconazole
Candidiasis		
systemic	amphotericin ± flucytosine	fluconazole
Chromomycosis	flucytosine	itraconazole
Coccidioidomycosis[1]	ketoconazole[2] or amphotericin	itraconazole or fluconazole
Cryptococcosis	amphotericin ± flucytosine	fluconazole or itraconazole
chronic suppression[3]	fluconazole	amphotericin
Histoplasmosis	ketoconazole[2] or amphotericin	itraconazole
chronic suppression[3]	amphotericin	itraconazole
Mucormycosis	amphotericin	no dependable alternative
Paracoccidioido-mycosis[1]	ketoconazole[2] or miconazole	itraconazole or a sulphonamide[4]
Sporotrichosis		
cutaneous	potassium iodide	local heat itraconazole
deep	amphotericin	itraconazole

[1]Patients with severe illness, meningitis, AIDS or some other causes of immunosuppression should receive amphotericin.
[2]Continue treatment for 6-12 months.
[3]For patients with AIDS.
[4]Sulphadiazine or sulphamethoxypyridazine for 3-5 y.
(This Table is drawn substantially from the Medical Letter on Drugs and Therapeutics (1992, USA). We are grateful to the Chairman of the Editorial Board for permission to publish the material. DRL, PNB, MJB)

Individual drugs

POLYENE ANTIBIOTICS

These act by binding tightly to sterols present in cell membranes. The resulting deformity of the membrane allows leakage of intracellular ions and enzymes, causing cell death. Those polyenes that have useful antifungal activity bind selectively to ergosterol, the most important sterol in fungal (but not mammalian) cell walls.

Amphotericin ($t^{1/2}$ 15 d)

Amphotericin is negligibly absorbed from the gut and must be given by i.v. infusion for systemic infection; about 10% remains in the blood and the fate of the remainder is not known but it is probably bound to tissues. The $t^{1/2}$ is 15 d, i.e. after stopping treatment, drug persists in the body for several weeks.

Amphotericin is at present the *drug of choice* for most systemic fungal infections (see Table 14.2). The diagnosis of systemic infection ought to be firmly established because toxicity to amphotericin is significant; tissue biopsy and culture may be necessary. A conventional course of treatment lasts 6–12 weeks during which at least 2 g of amphotericin is given. Lipid-associated formulations of amphotericin offer the prospect of reduced risk of toxicity while retaining therapeutic efficacy.[2]

Adverse reactions. Although gradual escalation of the dose limits toxic effects, they may have to be tolerated in life-threatening infection. Renal impairment is invariable, although amphotericin need not be stopped until serum creatinine has risen to 200 μmol/l; the same dose may then be resumed after 3–5 days. Hypokalaemia (due to distal renal tubular acidosis) may necessitate replacement therapy. Other adverse effects include: anorexia, nausea, vomiting, malaise, abdominal, muscle and joint pains, loss of weight, anaemia, hypomagnesaemia and fever. Symptoms may be alleviated by aspirin, an antihistamine (H_1) or an antiemetic. Severe febrile reactions are mitigated by hydrocortisone 25–50 mg before each infusion.

Nystatin (named after *New York State* Health Laboratory)

Nystatin is too toxic for systemic use. It is not absorbed from the alimentary canal and is used to prevent or treat superficial *candidiasis* of the mouth, oesophagus or intestinal tract (as suspension,

---

[2] In an aqueous medium, a lipid with hydrophilic and hydrophobic properties will form vesicles (*liposomes*) comprising an outer lipid bilayer surrounding an aqueous centre. The *AmBisome* formulation incorporates amphotericin in a lipid bilayer of phosphatidylcholine, distearoylphosphatidylglycerol and cholesterol (diameter 55–75 nm) from which the drug is released. Amphotericin is also formulated as other lipid-associated complexes, e.g. Abelcet, Amphocil.

tablets or pastilles), for vaginal candidiasis (pessaries) and cutaneous infection (cream, ointment or powder).

AZOLES

The antibacterial, antiprotozoal and anthelminthic members of this group are described in the appropriate sections. Antifungal azoles comprise the following:

- *Imidazoles* (ketoconazole, miconazole, clotrimazole, isoconazole, tioconazole) interfere with fungal oxidative enzymes to cause lethal accumulation of hydrogen peroxide; they also reduce the formation of ergosterol, an important constituent of the fungal cell wall which thus becomes permeable to intracellular constituents. Lack of selectivity in these actions results in important adverse effects.
- *Triazoles* (fluconazole, itraconazole) damage the fungal cell membrane by inhibiting a demethylase enzyme; they have greater selectivity against fungi, better penetration of the CNS, resistance to degradation and cause less endocrine disturbance than do the imidazoles.

Ketoconazole $(t^{1/2}\, 8\, h)$

Ketoconazole is well absorbed from the gut (poorly where there is gastric hypoacidity, see below); it is widely distributed in tissues but concentrations in CSF and urine are low; its action is terminated by metabolism. Ketoconazole is effective by mouth for systemic mycoses (see Table 14.2). It is less toxic but less effective than amphotericin, which may be preferred where the illness is severe, e.g. meningitis or AIDS. Impairment of steroid synthesis by ketoconazole has been put to other uses, e.g. inhibition of testosterone synthesis lessens bone pain in patients with advanced androgen-dependent prostatic cancer.

Adverse reactions include nausea, giddiness, headache, pruritus and photophobia. Impairment of testosterone synthesis may cause gynaecomastia and decreased libido in men. Of particular concern is impairment of liver function, ranging from tran-

sient elevation of hepatic transaminases and alkaline phosphatase to severe injury and death. Liver damage may progress despite discontinuing ketoconazole.

Drugs that lower gastric acidity, e.g. antacids, histamine H_2-receptor antagonists, impair the absorption of ketoconazole from the gastrointestinal tract. Inhibition of drug metabolism by ketoconazole leads to increased effects of oral anticoagulants, phenytoin and cyclosporin, and increases the risk of cardiac dysrhythmias with astemizole and terfenadine. A disulfiram-like reaction occurs with alcohol. Concurrent use of rifampicin, by enzyme induction, markedly reduces the plasma concentration of ketoconazole.

Miconazole is an alternative. *Clotrimazole* is an effective topical agent for dermatophyte, yeast, and other fungal infections (intertrigo, athlete's foot, ringworm, pityriasis versicolor, fungal nappy rash). *Econazole* and *sulconazole* are similar. *Tioconazole* is used for fungal nail infections and *isoconazole* for vaginal candidiasis.

Fluconazole

Fluconazole $(t^{1/2}\, 30\, h)$ is absorbed from the gastrointestinal tract and is excreted largely unchanged by the kidney. It is effective by mouth for oropharyngeal and oesophageal candidiasis, and i.v. for systemic candidiasis and cryptococcosis (including cryptococcal meningitis). It may cause gastrointestinal discomfort, headaches, elevation of liver enzymes and allergic rash. Animal studies demonstrate embryotoxicity and fluconazole ought not to be given to pregnant women. High doses increase the effects of phenytoin, cyclosporin and warfarin.

Itraconazole is an alternative (see Table 14.2).

ALLYLAMINE

Terbinafine

Terbinafine $(t^{1/2}\, 14\, h)$ interferes with ergosterol biosynthesis, and thereby with the formation of the fungal cell membrane. It is absorbed from the gastrointestinal tract and undergoes extensive metabolism in the liver. Terbinafine is used *topically* for dermatophyte infections of the skin and *orally* for infections of hair and nails where the site (e.g. hair), severity or extent of the infection render topical use inappropriate (see p. 282). Treatment (250 mg/d) may need to continue for several weeks. It may cause nausea, diarrhoea, dyspepsia, headaches and cutaneous reactions.

OTHER ANTIFUNGAL DRUGS

Griseofulvin

Griseofulvin ($t^{1}/2$ 15 h) prevents fungal growth by inhibiting mitosis. The therapeutic efficacy of griseofulvin depends on its capacity to bind to keratin as it is being formed in the cells of the nail bed, hair follicles and skin, for dermatophytes specifically infect keratinous tissues. Griseofulvin does not kill fungus already established, it merely prevents infection of new keratin so that the duration of treatment is governed by the time that it takes for infected keratin to be shed; on average, hair and skin infection should be treated for 4–6 weeks while toenails may need a year or more. Treatment must continue for a few weeks after both visual and microscopic evidence have disappeared.

Fat in a meal enhances absorption of griseofulvin; it is metabolised in the liver and induces hepatic enzymes.

Griseofulvin is effective against all superficial ringworm (dermatophyte) infections but is ineffective against pityriasis versicolor, superficial candidiasis and all systemic mycoses.

Adverse reactions include gastrointestinal upset, rashes, photosensitivity, headache, and various central nervous system disturbances (see porphyria).

Flucytosine

Flucytosine (5-fluorocytosine) ($t^{1}/2$ 4 h) is metabolised in the fungal cell to 5-fluorouracil which inhibits nucleic acid synthesis. It is well absorbed from the gut, penetrates effectively into tissues and almost all is excreted unchanged in the urine. The dose should be reduced for patients with impaired renal function, and the plasma concentration should be monitored. The drug is well tolerated when renal function is normal. *Candida albicans*

rapidly becomes resistant to flucytosine which ought not to be used alone; it may be combined with amphotericin (see Table 14.2) but this increases the risk of adverse effects (leucopenia, thrombocytopenia, enterocolitis).

Potassium iodide is given by mouth to treat cutaneous sporotrichosis.

Protozoal infections[3]

Malaria

Over 90 million cases of malaria occur each year; in socioeconomic impact, it is the most important of the transmissible parasitic diseases.

Quinine as cinchona bark was introduced into Europe from South America in 1633. It was used for all fevers, amongst them malaria. Further advance in the chemotherapy of malaria was delayed until 1880, when Laveran[4] finally identified the parasites in the blood.

LIFE CYCLE OF THE MALARIA PARASITE AND SITES OF DRUG ACTION (Fig. 14.1)

The incubation period of malaria is 10–35 days. The principal features of the life cycle of the malaria parasite must be known in order to understand its therapy. Female anopheles mosquitoes require a blood meal for egg production and in the process of feeding they inject salivary fluid containing *sporozoites* into humans. Since no drugs are effective against sporozoites, infection with the malaria parasite cannot be prevented.

---

[3] Material for this section is drawn substantially from WHO Model Prescribing Information 1990. Drugs used in parasitic diseases. World Health Organization, Geneva. We are very grateful to the World Health Organization for their permission to use this source. DRL, PNB, MJB.

[4] Charles Louis Alphonse Laveran (1845–1922), Professor of Medicine, Paris (France); Nobel prize winner.

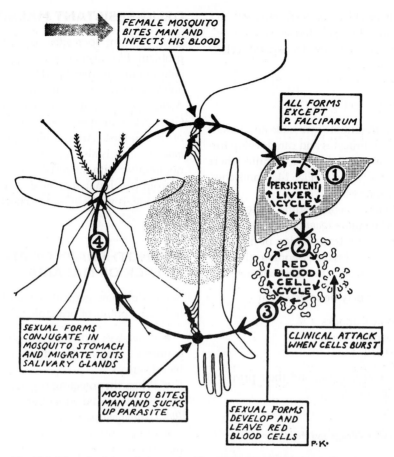

Fig. 14.1 Life cycle of the malaria parasite. The numbers are referred to in the text

Hepatic cycle (site 1 in Fig. 14.1)

Sporozoites enter liver cells where they develop into *schizonts* which form large numbers of *merozoites* which, usually after 5-16 days but sometimes after months or years, are released into the circulation. *Plasmodium falciparum* differs in that it has no persistent hepatic cycle.

Primaquine, proguanil and tetracyclines (*tissue schizontocides*) act at this site and are used for:

● *Radical cure*, i.e. an attack on persisting hepatic forms (*hypnozoites*, i.e. sleeping) once the parasite has been cleared from the blood; this is most effectively accomplished with primaquine; proguanil is only weakly effective

● *Preventing* the *initial* hepatic cycle. This is also called *causal prophylaxis*. Primaquine has long been regarded as too toxic for prolonged use but evidence now suggests it may be used safely, and it is inexpensive; proguanil is weakly effective. Doxycycline may be used short-term.

Erythrocyte cycle (site 2 in Fig. 14.1)

Merozoites enter red cells where they develop into *schizonts* which form more merozoites which are released when the cells burst giving rise to the features of the clinical attack. The merozoites re-enter red cells and the cycle is repeated.

Chloroquine, quinine, mefloquine, halofantrine, proguanil, pyrimethamine, and tetracyclines (*blood schizontocides*) kill these asexual forms. Drugs which act on this stage in the cycle of the parasite may be used for:

● *Treatment* of acute attacks of malaria.

● *Prevention* of attacks by early destruction of the erythrocytic forms. This is called *suppressive prophylaxis* as it does not cure the hepatic cycle (above).

Sexual forms (site 3 in Fig. 14.1)

Some merozoites differentiate into male and female *gametocytes* in the erythrocytes and can develop further only if they are ingested by a mosquito where they form *sporozoites* (site 4 in Fig. 14.1) and complete the transmission cycle.

Quinine, mefloquine, chloroquine, artesunate, artemether and primaquine (*gametocytocides*) act on sexual forms and prevent transmission of the infection because the patient becomes noninfective and the parasite fails to develop in the mosquito (site 4).

In summary, drugs may be selected for:

● treatment of clinical attacks
● prevention of clinical attacks
● radical cure.

Drugs used to treat malaria, and their principal actions are classified in Table 14.3.

Table 14.3 Antimalarial drugs and their locus of action

Drug	Biological activity	
	Blood schizontocide	Tissue schizontocide
4-Aminoquinolone		
chloroquine	++	0
Arylaminoalcohols		
quinine	++	0
mefloquine	++	0
Phenanthrene methanol		
halofantrine	++	0
Antimetabolites		
proguanil	+	+
pyrimethamine	+	0
sulfadoxine	+	0
dapsone	+	0
Antibiotics		
tetracycline	+	+
doxycycline	+	+
minocycline	+	+
8-Aminoquinolone		
primaquine	0	+
Sesquiterpenes		
artesunate	+	0
artemether		

DRUG-RESISTANT MALARIA

Drug-resistant parasites constitute a persistent problem. *Plasmodium falciparum* is now resistant to chloroquine in many parts of the world. Areas of *high risk* for resistant parasites include Sub-Saharan Africa, Latin America, Oceania (Papua New Guinea, Solomon Islands, Vanuatu) and some parts of South-East Asia. Chloroquine-resistant *Plasmodium vivax* is also reported. The physician who is not familiar with the resistance pattern in the locality from which patients have come or to which they are going, is well advised to check the current position.

CHEMOTHERAPY OF AN ACUTE ATTACK OF MALARIA[5]

Successful management demands attention to the following points of principle:

● Whenever possible, the diagnosis should be confirmed before treatment by examination of blood smears.
● When the infecting organism is not known or infection is mixed, treatment should begin as for *Plasmodium falciparum* (below).
● Drugs used to treat *Plasmodium falciparum* malaria must always be selected with regard to the prevalence of local patterns of drug resistance.
● Patients not at risk of reinfection should be re-examined several weeks after treatment for signs of recrudescence which may result from inadequate chemotherapy or survival of persistent hepatic forms.

Falciparum malaria

The regimen depends on the condition of the patient; the doses quoted are for adults. Chloroquine resistance is now usual.

If the patient can swallow and there are no serious complications such as impairment of consciousness, treatment may be with quinine, mefloquine **or** halofantrine as follows:

---

[5] Treatment regimens vary in detail; those quoted here accord with the recommendations in the British National Formulary 1996.

- A quinine salt[6] 600 mg × 8 h by mouth for 7 days followed by pyrimethamine plus sulfadoxine (Fansidar) 3 tablets as a single dose. Where there is resistance to Fansidar, tetracycline 250 mg × 6 h, should be given **after** the quinine for 7 days. This additional therapy is necessary as quinine alone tends to be associated with a higher rate of relapse.
- Mefloquine 20 mg/kg (base) by mouth may be given as 2 divided doses 6–8 h apart.
- Halofantrine 1.5 g given as 3 doses of 500 mg 6h apart on an empty stomach; the course should be repeated after one week.

It is not necessary to add Fansidar or tetracycline after mefloquine or halofantrine.

Seriously ill patients should be treated with

- a quinine salt 20 mg/kg as a loading dose[7] (maximum 1.4 g) infused i.v. over 4 h
- followed 8 h later by a maintenance infusion of 10 mg/kg (maximum 700 mg) infused over 4 h
- repeated every 8 h,[8] until the patient can swallow tablets to complete the 7-day course. Fansidar or (when renal function is normal) tetracycline should be given subsequently, as above.

Benign malarias

These are usually due to *Plasmodium vivax* or less commonly to *Plasmodium ovale* or *Plasmodium malariae*; the drug of choice is *chloroquine*, which should be given by mouth as follows:

- initial dose: 600 mg (base),[9] then 300 mg as a single dose 6–8 h later
- second day, 300 mg as a single dose
- third day, 300 mg as a single dose.

The total dose of chloroquine base over 3 days should be approximately 25 mg/kg base. This is sufficient for *Plasmodium malariae* infection but, for

Plasmodium vivax and *Plasmodium ovale*, eradication of the hepatic parasites is necessary to prevent relapse, by giving:

- primaquine, 15 mg/d for 14–21 days started after the chloroquine course has been completed (30 mg once weekly for 8 weeks will suffice without undue risk of haemolysis).

CHEMOPROPHYLAXIS OF MALARIA

Geographically variable plasmodial drug resistance has become a major factor in malaria. The World Health Organization publishes advice in its annually revised booklet, Vaccination Certificate Requirements and Health Advice for International Travel; and national bodies publish advice (e.g. British National Formulary) that applies particularly to their own residents. These or other appropriate sources ought to be consulted before specific advice is given.

The following general principles apply:

- Chemoprophylaxis is part of a broader regimen; travellers should protect against bites by using mosquito nets and repellents.
- Mefloquine, chloroquine, proguanil, and pyrimethamine plus dapsone (Maloprim), alone or in combination are most commonly advised for prophylaxis regimens; and doxycycline for special cases (drug resistance or intolerance); primaquine is being re-evaluated.
- Effective chemoprophylaxis requires that there be a plasmodicidal concentration of drug in the blood when the first infected mosquito bites, and that it be sustained safely for long periods.
- Prompt achievement of efficacy and safety by one (or two) doses is plainly important for travellers, who cannot wait on dosage schedules to deliver both only when steady-state blood concen-

---

[6] Acceptable as quinine hydrochloride, dihydrochloride or sulphate, but not quinine bisulphate which contains less quinine.

[7] The loading dose should not be given if the patient has received quinine, quinidine or mefloquine in the previous 24 h; see also warnings about halofantrine (below).

[8] Reduced to 5–7 mg/kg if the infusion lasts for >72 h.

[9] The active component of many drugs, whether acid or base, is relatively insoluble and may present a problem in formulation. This is overcome by adding an acid to a base or vice versa; the weight of the salt differs according to the acid or base component, i.e. chloroquine base 150 mg = chloroquine sulphate 200 mg = chloroquine phosphate 250 mg (approximately). Where there may be variation, therefore, the amount of drug prescribed is expressed as the weight of the active component, in the case of chloroquine, the base.

trations are attained (after $t^{1/2} \times 5$), especially with long $t^{1/2}$ drugs such as mefloquine and chloroquine (see below). The progressive rise in plasma concentration to steady state, sometimes attained only after weeks, allows that unwanted effects that will impair compliance or be unsafe may occur after a subject has entered a malarial area. Thus it is advised that prophylaxis be begun long enough before travel to reveal acute intolerance and to impress on the subject the importance of compliance (to relate drug-taking to a specific daily or weekly event).

All these factors contribute to conventional advice to travellers.

Examples of standard regimens

— chloroquine 300 mg (base) once weekly (start one week before travel)
— proguanil 200 mg once daily (start 2–3 days before travel)
— chloroquine plus proguanil in the above doses
— mefloquine 250 mg once weekly (start one week before travel).

For 'last minute' travellers. The standard regimens normally provide immediate protection but for special assurance a priming/loading dose may be considered, e.g. the standard prophylactic dose daily for 2–3 days (this has been suggested for mefloquine).

Drug interactions. Where subjects are already taking other drugs, e.g. antiepileptics, some cardiovascular drugs, it is desirable to start prophylaxis as much as 2–3 weeks in advance to establish safety.

● Prophylaxis should continue for at least 4 weeks after leaving an endemic area to kill parasites that are acquired about the time of departure, are still incubating in the liver and will develop into the erythrocyte phase. The traveller should be aware that any illness occurring within a year, and especially within 3 months, of return may be malaria.

● *Naturally acquired immunity* offers the most reliable protection for people living permanently in endemic areas (below). Repeated attacks of malaria confer partial immunity and the disease often becomes no more than an occasional inconve-

nience. Vaccines to confer active immunity are under development.

● *The partially immune* as a rule should not take a prophylactic. The reasoning is that immunity is sustained by the red cell cycle, loss of which through prophylaxis diminishes their resistance and leaves them highly vulnerable to the disease. There are however **exceptions** to this general advice and the partially immune may or should use a prophylactic:
— if it is virtually certain that they will never abandon its use
— if they go to another malarial area where the strains of parasite may differ
— during the last few months of pregnancy in areas where *Plasmodium falciparum* is prevalent, to avert the risk of miscarriage.

Antimalarial drugs and pregnancy

Women living in endemic areas in which *Plasmodium falciparum* remains sensitive to chloroquine should take chloroquine prophylactically throughout pregnancy. Proguanil (an 'antifol', see below) may be taken for prophylaxis provided it is accompanied by folic acid 5 mg/d. Chloroquine may be used in full dose to treat chloroquine-sensitive infections. Quinine is the only widely available drug that is acceptable as suitable for treating chloroquine-resistant infections during pregnancy. Mefloquine is teratogenic in animals and a woman should avoid pregnancy whilst taking it, and for 3 months after; pyrimethamine plus dapsone (Maloprim) should not be given in the first trimester, but may be given in the second and third trimesters with a folate supplement.

INDIVIDUAL ANTIMALARIAL DRUGS

Chloroquine

Chloroquine ($t^{1/2}$ 50 d) is concentrated within parasitised red cells and forms complexes with plasmodial DNA. It is active against the blood forms and also the gametocytes (formed in the mosquito) of *Plasmodium vivax*, *Plasmodium ovale* and *Plasmodium malariae*; it is ineffective against many strains of *Plasmodium falciparum* and also its immature gametocytes. Chloroquine is readily absorbed from the gastrointestinal tract and is concentrated several-fold in various tissues, e.g. erythrocytes, liver, spleen, heart, kidney, cornea and retina; the $t^{1}/_{2}$ of 50 days reflects slow release from these sites. A priming dose is used in order to achieve adequate free plasma concentration (see acute attack, above). Chloroquine is partly inactivated by metabolism and the remainder is excreted unchanged in the urine.

Adverse effects are infrequent at doses normally used for malaria treatment and prophylaxis, but are more common with the higher or prolonged doses given for resistant malaria or for rheumatoid arthritis or lupus erythematosus (see Index).

Corneal deposits of chloroquine may be asymptomatic or may cause halos around lights or photophobia. These are not a threat to vision and reverse when the drug is stopped. Retinal toxicity is more serious, however, and may be irreversible. In the early stage it takes the form of visual field defects; late retinopathy classically gives the picture of macular pigmentation surrounded by a ring of pigment (the 'bull's-eye' macula). The functional defect can take the form of scotomas, photophobia, defective colour vision and decreased visual acuity resulting, in the extreme case, in blindness.

Other reactions include pruritus, which may be intolerable and is common in Africans, headaches, gastrointestinal disturbance, precipitation of acute intermittent porphyria in susceptible individuals, mental disturbances and interference with cardiac rhythm, the latter especially if the drug is given intravenously in high dose (it has a quinidine-like action).

Acute overdose may be rapidly fatal without treatment and indeed has even been described as a means of suicide.[10] (Chloroquine may now be bought from pharmacies in the UK without a prescription.) Pulmonary oedema is followed by convulsions, cardiac dysrhythmias and coma; as little as 50 mg/kg can be fatal. These effects are principally due to the profound negative inotropic action of chloroquine. Diazepam was found fortuitously to protect the heart and adrenaline reduces intraventricular conduction time; this combination of

---

[10] Report 1993 Chloroquine poisoning. Lancet 307: 49.

drugs, given by separate i.v. infusions, improves survival.

Halofantrine

Halofantrine ($t^{1}/_{2}$ 1–4 d) is active against the erythrocytic forms of all four *Plasmodium* species, especially *Plasmodium falciparum* and *Plasmodium vivax*, and at the schizont stage. Its mechanism of action is not fully understood. Absorption of halofantrine from the gastrointestinal tract is variable, incomplete and substantially increased ($\times$ 6–10) by taking the drug with food (see below). It is metabolised to an active metabolite and no unchanged drug is recovered in the urine. Halofantrine is used for the treatment of uncomplicated chloroquine-resistant *Plasmodium falciparum* and *Plasmodium vivax* malaria. It should not be given for prophylaxis.

Adverse effects. Halofantrine may cause gastrointestinal symptoms; pruritis occurs but to a lesser extent than with chloroquine which may be reason for it to be preferred. It prolongs the cardiac QT interval and may predispose to hazardous dysrhythmia. The drug should therefore **not** be taken

- with food
- with other potentially dysrhythmic drugs, e.g. antimalarials, tricyclic antidepressants, antipsychotics, astemizole, terfenadine
- with drugs causing electrolyte disturbance
- by patients with cardiac disease associated with prolonged QT interval.

Mefloquine

Mefloquine ($t^{1}/_{2}$ 21 d) is similar in several respects to quinine although it does not intercalate with plasmodial DNA. It is used for malaria chemoprophylaxis, to treat uncomplicated *Plasmodium falciparum*, (both chloroquine-sensitive and chloroquine-resistant) and chloroquine-resistant *Plasmodium vivax* malaria. Mefloquine is rapidly absorbed from the gastrointestinal tract and its action is terminated by metabolism. When used for prophylaxis, the normal dose of 250 mg (base)/week may be reduced after 3 weeks to 125 mg (base)/week to reduce the risk of toxicity. It should not be given to patients with hepatic or renal impairment.

Adverse effects include nausea, dizziness, disturbance of balance, vomiting, abdominal pain, diarrhoea and loss of appetite. More rarely, hallucinations, seizures and psychoses occur. Mefloquine should be avoided in patients taking β-adrenoceptor and calcium channel antagonists for it causes sinus bradycardia; quinine can potentiate these and other dose-related effects of mefloquine. Use of mefloquine is contraindicated in those whose activities require fine coordination or spatial performance, e.g. airline crews.

Primaquine

Primaquine ($t^{1/2}$ 6 h) acts at several stages in the development of the plasmodial parasite, possibly by interfering with its mitochondrial function. Its unique effect is to eliminate the hepatic forms of *Plasmodium vivax* and *Plasmodium ovale* after standard chloroquine therapy, but only when the risk of reinfection is absent or slight. Primaquine is well absorbed from the gastrointestinal tract, is only moderately concentrated in the tissues and is rapidly metabolised.

Adverse effects include anorexia, nausea, abdominal cramps, methaemoglobinaemia and haemolytic anaemia, especially in patients with genetic deficiency of erythrocyte glucose-6-phosphate dehydrogenase (G-6-PD). Subjects should be tested for G-6-PD and in those that are deficient, the risk of haemolytic anaemia is greatly reduced by giving primaquine in reduced dose.

Proguanil (chloroguanide)

Proguanil ($t^{1/2}$ 17 h) inhibits dihydrofolate reductase which converts folic to folinic acid, deficiency of which inhibits plasmodial cell division. Plasmodia, like some bacteria and unlike humans, cannot make use of preformed folic acid. Pyrimethamine and trimethoprim, which share this mode of action, are collectively known as the '*antifols*'. Their plasmodicidal action is markedly enhanced by combination with sulphonamides or sulphones because there is inhibition of sequential steps in folate synthesis (see Sulphonamide combinations, p. 210).

Proguanil is moderately well absorbed from the gut and is excreted in the urine either unchanged or as an active metabolite. Being little stored in the tissues, proguanil must be used daily when given for prophylaxis, its main use, particularly in pregnant women (with folic acid 5 mg/d, which does not antagonise therapeutic efficacy) and nonimmune individuals. In prophylactic doses, it is well tolerated.

Pyrimethamine

Pyrimethamine ($t^{1/2}$ 4 d) inhibits plasmodial dihydrofolate reductase, for which it has a high affinity. It is well absorbed from the gastrointestinal tract and is extensively metabolised. It is seldom used alone (see below). Pregnant women should receive supplementary folic acid when taking pyrimethamine.

Adverse effects include anorexia, abdominal cramps, vomiting, ataxia, tremor, seizures and megaloblastic anaemia.

Pyrimethamine with sulfadoxine

Pyrimethamine ($t^{1/2}$ 8 d) acts synergistically with sulfadoxine (as Fansidar) to inhibit folic acid metabolism (see 'antifols', above); sulfadoxine is excreted in the urine. The combination is chiefly used with quinine to treat acute attacks of malaria caused by susceptible strains of *Plasmodium falciparum*; a single dose of pyrimethamine 75 mg plus sulfadoxine 1.5 g (3 tablets) usually suffices.

Sulphonamide-induced allergic reactions can be severe, e.g. erythema multiforme, Stevens–Johnson syndrome and toxic epidermal necrolysis. Because of its 'antifol' action the combination should not be used by pregnant women unless they take a folate supplement.

Pyrimethamine with dapsone

Pyrimethamine is combined with dapsone (Maloprim) (see p. 241) for prophylaxis of *Plasmodium falciparum* malaria.

Quinine

Quinine ($t^{1/2}$ 9–18 h) is obtained from the bark of the South American Cinchona tree. It binds to plasmodial DNA to prevent protein synthesis but its exact mode of action remains uncertain. It is used to treat *Plasmodium falciparum* malaria in areas of multiple-drug resistance. Apart from its antiplasmodial effect, quinine is used for myotonia and muscle cramps because it prolongs the muscle refractory period. Quinine is included in dilute concentration in tonics and aperitifs for its desired bitter taste.

Quinine is well absorbed from the gastrointestinal tract and is almost completely metabolised in the liver. The t½ of 9 h is 18 h in severe malaria.

Adverse effects include tinnitus, diminished auditory acuity, headache, blurred vision, nausea and diarrhoea (common to quinine, quinidine, salicylates and called cinchonism). Idiosyncratic reactions include pruritus, urticaria and rashes. Hypoglycaemia may be significant when quinine is given by i.v. infusion and supplementary glucose may be required.

When large amounts are taken, e.g. (unreliably) to induce abortion or in attempted suicide, ocular disturbances, notably constriction of the visual fields, may occur and even complete blindness, the onset of which may be very sudden. Vomiting, abdominal pain and diarrhoea result from local irritation of the gastrointestinal tract. Quinidine-like effects include hypotension, disturbance of atrioventricular conduction and cardiac arrest. Emesis or gastric lavage should be undertaken and activated charcoal given. Supportive measures are employed thereafter as no specific therapy has proven benefit.

Quinidine, the dextrorotatory-isomer of quinine, has antimalarial activity, but is used mainly as a cardiac antidysrhythmic (see p. 461).

Artesunate, artemether, from the Chinese herb qinghao (*Artemisia annua*) act against the blood, including sexual forms, of the plasmodium and may also reduce its transmissibility. They are rapidly effective and well tolerated in severe, and multi-drug resistant, malaria. Their place in therapy is being evaluated.

Amoebiasis

Infection occurs when mature cysts are ingested

and pass into the colon where they divide into trophozoites; these forms either enter the tissues or reform cysts. Amoebiasis occurs in two forms, both of which need treatment.

- *Bowel lumen amoebiasis* is asymptomatic and trophozoites (noninfective) and cysts (infective) are passed into the faeces. Treatment is directed at eradicating cysts with a luminal amoebicide; diloxanide, *iodoquinol* or *paromomycin* are used.
- *Tissue-invading amoebiasis* gives rise to dysentery, hepatic amoebiasis and liver abscess. A systemically active drug (tissue amoebicide) effective against trophozoites must be used, e.g. metronidazole, tinidazole. Parenteral forms of these are available for patients too ill to take drugs by mouth. In severe cases of amoebic dysentery, tetracycline lessens the risk of opportunistic infection, perforation and peritonitis when it is given in addition to the systemic amoebicide.

Treatment with tissue amoebicides should always be followed by a course of a luminal amoebicide to eradicate the source of the infection.

Dehydroemetine (from ipecacuanha), less toxic than the parent emetine, is claimed by some authorities to be the most effective tissue amoebicide. It is reserved for dangerously ill patients, but these are more likely to be vulnerable to its cardiotoxic effects. When dehydroemetine is used to treat amoebic liver abscess, chloroquine should also be given.

The drug treatment of other protozoal infections is summarised in Table 14.4.

Some drugs for protozoal infections

Benznidazole is rapidly absorbed from the alimentary tract. Adverse effects include rashes which, if severe and accompanied by fever and purpura, are reason to stop the drug. Peripheral neuritis, leucopenia and agranulocytosis also occur.

Diloxanide may cause troublesome flatulence and pruritus and urticaria may occur.

Dehydroemetine inhibits protein synthesis; it may cause pain at the site of injection, weakness and muscular pain, hypotension, praecordial pain and cardiac dysrhythmias.

Table 14.4 Drugs for some protozoal infections

Infection	Drug Comment
Giardiasis	Metronidazole, mepacrine or tinidazole; family and institutional contacts should also be treated
Leishmaniasis visceral	Sodium stibogluconate or meglumine antimoniate; resistant cases may benefit from combining antimonials with allopurinol, pentamidine or amphotericin
cutaneous	Mild lesions heal spontaneously; antimonials may be injected intralesionally
Pneumocystosis (*Pneumocystis carinii*)	Co-trimoxazole in high dose; intolerant or resistant cases may benefit from pentamidine. Atovaquone for mild to moderate cases intolerant of co-trimoxazole
Toxoplasmosis	Pyrimethamine with sulphadiazine for chorioretinitis, and active toxoplasmosis in immunodeficient patients; folinic acid is used to counteract the inevitable megaloblastic anaemia. Spiramycin for primary toxoplasmosis in pregnant women
Trichomoniasis	Metronidazole or tinidazole is effective
Trypanosomiasis African (sleeping sickness)	Suramin or pentamidine is effective during the early stages but are ineffective for the later neurological manifestations for which melarsoprol should be used. Eflornithine is effective for both early and late stages
American (Chagas' disease)	Nifurtimox or benznidazole is effective in the early stages

Eflornithine inhibits protozoal DNA synthesis; it may cause anaemia, leucopenia and thrombocytopenia, and seizures.

Melarsoprol, a trivalent organic arsenical, acts through its high affinity for sulphydryl groups of enzymes. Adverse effects include encephalopathy, myocardial damage, proteinuria and hypertension.

Pentamidine must be administered parenterally as it is unreliably absorbed from the gastrointestinal tract; it does not enter the CSF. It frequently causes nephrotoxicity, which is reversible; acute hypotension and syncope are common after rapid i.v. injection. Pancreatic damage may cause hypoglycaemia due to insulin release.

Mepacrine (quinacrine) was formerly used as an antimalarial. It may cause gastrointestinal upset, occasional acute toxic psychosis, hepatitis and aplastic anaemia.

Nifurtimox. Adverse effects include: anorexia,

nausea, vomiting, gastric pain, insomnia, headache, vertigo, excitability, myalgia, arthralgia and convulsions. Peripheral neuropathy may necessitate stopping treatment.

Sodium stibogluconate is an organic pentavalent antimony compound; it may cause anorexia, vomiting, coughing and substernal pain. *Meglumine antimoniate* is similar.

Suramin does not cross the blood–brain barrier; it forms stable complexes with plasma protein and is detectable in urine for up to 3 months after the last injection. It may cause tiredness, anorexia, malaise, polyuria, thirst and tenderness of the palms and soles.

Helminthic infections

Helminths have complex life-cycles, special knowledge of which is required by those who treat infections. Table 14.5 will suffice here. Drug resistance has not so far proved to be a clinical problem, though it has occurred in animals on continuous chemoprophylaxis.

Drugs for helminth infections

Diethylcarbamazine kills both microfilariae and adult worms. Fever, headache, anorexia, malaise, urticaria, vomiting and asthmatic attacks following the first dose are due to products of destruction of the parasite.

Ivermectin may cause immediate reactions due to the death of the microfilaria (see diethylcarbamazine). It can be effective in a single dose.

Levamisole paralyses the musculature of sensitive nematodes which, unable to maintain their anchorage, are expelled by normal peristalsis. It may cause abdominal pain, nausea, vomiting, headache and dizziness.

Mebendazole blocks glucose uptake by nematodes. Mild gastrointestinal discomfort may be caused. *Albendazole* is similar.

Metriphonate is an organophosphorus anticholinesterase compound that was originally used as an insecticide. Adverse effects include abdominal pain, nausea, vomiting, diarrhoea, headache and vertigo.

Table 14.5 Drugs for helminthic infections

Infection	Drug	Comment
Cestodes (tapeworms)		
Beef tapeworm *Taenia saginata*	niclosamide or praziquantel	Praziquantel cures with single dose
Pork tapeworm *Taenia solium*	niclosamide or praziquantel	Praziquantel cures with single dose
Cysticercosis *Taenia solium*	albendazole or praziquantel	Treat in hospital as dying and disintegrating cysts may cause cerebral oedema
Fish tapeworm *Diphyllobothrium latum*	niclosamide or praziquantel	
Hydatid disease *Echinococcus granulosus*	albendazole	Surgery for operable cyst disease
Nematodes (intestinal)		
Ascariasis *Ascaris lumbricoides*	mebendazole, levamisole, pyrantel, piperazine or albendazole	
Hookworm *Ancylostoma duodenale Necator americanus*	mebendazole, pyrantel or albendazole	Anaemic patients require iron
Strongyloidiasis *Strongyloides stercoralis*	thiabendazole or ivermectin	Alternatively, albendazole is better tolerated
Threadworm (pinworm) *Enterobius vermicularis*	pyrantel, mebendazole, albendazole or piperazine salts	
Whipworm *Trichuris trichiuria*	mebendazole or albendazole	
Nematodes (tissue)		
Cutaneous larva migrans *Ancylostoma braziliense Ancylostoma caninum*	thiabendazole	Calamine lotion for symptom relief
Guinea worm *Dracunculus medinensis*	metronidazole, mebendazole	Rapid symptom relief
Trichinellosis *Trichinella spiralis*	mebendazole	Prednisolone may be needed to suppress allergic and inflammatory symptoms
Visceral larva migrans *Toxocara canis Toxocara cati*	diethylcarbamazine, albendazole or mebendazole	Progressive escalation of dose lessens allergic reactions to dying larvae; prednisolone suppresses

Table 14.5 (cont'd)

Infection	Drug	Comment
		inflammatory response in ophthalmic disease
Lymphatic filariasis *Wuchereria bancrofti Brugia malayi Brugia timori*	diethylcarbamazine	Destruction of microfilia may cause an immunological reaction (see below)
Onchocerciasis (river blindness) *Onchocerca volvulus*	ivermectin	Cures with single dose. Suppressive treatment; a single annual dose prevents significant complications
Schistosomiasis		
Intestinal *Schistosoma mansoni Schistosoma japonicum*	praziquantel	Oxamniquine only for *Schistosoma mansoni*
Urinary *Schistosoma haematobium*	praziquantel	Metriphonate only for *Schistosoma haematobium*
Flukes Intestinal) Lung) Liver)	praziquantel	Alternatives: niclosamide for intestinal fluke, bithionol for lung fluke

Niclosamide blocks glucose uptake by intestinal tapeworms. It may cause mild gastrointestinal symptoms.

Piperazine may cause hypersensitivity reactions, neurological symptoms and may precipitate epilepsy.

Praziquantel paralyses both adult worms and larvae. It is extensively metabolised. Praziquantel may cause nausea, headache, dizziness and drowsiness; it cures with a single dose (or divided doses in one day).

Pyrantel depolarises neuromuscular junctions of susceptible nematodes which are expelled in the faeces. It cures with a single dose. It may induce gastrointestinal disturbance, headache, dizziness, drowsiness and insomnia.

Thiabendazole inhibits cellular enzymes of susceptible helminths. Gastrointestinal, neurological and hypersensitivity reactions, and crystalluria may be induced.

GUIDE TO FURTHER READING

Bruce-Chwatt L J 1988 Three hundred and fifty years of the Peruvian fever bark. British Medical Journal 296: 1486

Como J A, Dismukes W E 1994 Oral azole drugs as systemic antifungal therapy. New England Journal of Medicine 330: 263

Di Bisceglie A M 1994 Interferon therapy for chronic viral hepatitis. New England Journal of Medicine 330: 137

Dunne D W et al 1995 Prospects for immunological control of schistosomiasis. Lancet 345: 1488

Gerberding J L 1995 Management of occupational exposures to blood-borne viruses. New England Journal of Medicine 332: 444

Gil-Grande L A et al 1993 Randomised controlled trial of efficacy of albendazole in intra-abdominal hydatid disease. Lancet 342: 1269

Graham B S, Wright P F 1995 Candidate AIDS vaccines. New England Journal of Medicine 333: 1331

Hay J, Dutton G N 1995 Toxoplasma and the eye. British Medical Journal 310: 1021.

Liu L X, Weller P F 1996 Antiparasitic drugs. New England Journal of Medicine 334: 1178

Mabey D 1993 Onchocerciasis: ivermectin and onchocercal optic nerve lesions. Lancet 341: 153

Moradpour D, Wands J R 1995 Understanding hepatitis B virus infection. New England Journal of Medicine 332: 1092

Stevens D A 1995 Coccidioidomycosis. New England Journal of Medicine 332: 1077

van der Poel C L et al 1994 Hepatitis C virus six years on. Lancet 344: 1475

Inflammation, arthritis and nonsteroidal anti-inflammatory drugs (NSAIDs)

SYNOPSIS

Everyone has personal experience of tissue injury causing inflammation and pain and there are many longterm sufferers from rheumatoid arthritis and osteoarthritis. The processes that underlie the phenomenon of inflammation are now increasingly understood, and so are the modes of action of drugs that are used to treat it.

- Inflammation and arthritis
- Nonsteroidal anti-inflammatory drugs (NSAIDs) and their effects
- Classification of NSAIDs
- Drug treatment of rheumatoid diseases
- Gout and drugs

Inflammation

In acute inflammation the tissues become red, swollen, tender or painful, there is local heat and the patient may be febrile. At a cellular level the capillaries become more permeable and fluid and other elements from the blood leak into the tissue spaces. Phagocytic cells including leucocytes migrate into the area and rupture of cell lysosomes releases lytic enzymes into the tissues.

Inflammation may also be chronic, as in rheumatoid arthritis. Macrophages in the hypertrophied synovial tissue are stimulated to produce proteases and collagenases which are involved in the destruction of collagen and bone. In addition, an inflammatory exudate of neutrophil leucocytes takes place into the synovial space apparently in response to an antigen–antibody interaction with complement. In phagocytosing the antigen–antibody complement complexes the leucocytes liberate lysosomal enzymes that may contribute to damage of tissues including cartilage.

Advances in understanding the dauntingly complex mechanisms of inflammation have led to the introduction of new agents that selectively modify its components. An outline of the mediators and cells of inflammation in general is therefore presented below as a framework for explaining the relationship of existing, new and potential drugs to each other. Inflammation is of such fundamental biological importance to the organism that substances that modify the process are found to achieve therapeutic usefulness not only in arthritis but also in diverse conditions including pain, neoplasia, neutropenia and liver disease.

The description above shows that inflammation entails both humoral and cellular factors. Humoral inflammation involves the triggering of enzyme cascades that activate the coagulation, fibrinolytic (see Ch. 29), complement and kinin systems.

CELLULAR INFLAMMATION

Neutrophils and monocytes play a vital part in

defence against invading organisms and in the removal of debris from the sites of inflammation. These cells act in part through release of *cytokines* which are peptides that regulate cell growth, differentiation and activation; certain of these have been found to be therapeutically valuable.

Cytokines

These include:

- *Interleukins*. These are produced by a variety of cells including T cells, monocytes and macrophages. Recombinant interleukin-2 (aldesleukin) is used to treat metastatic renal cell carcinoma and malignant melanoma. Interleukin-1 may play a part in conditions such as the sepsis syndrome and rheumatoid arthritis, and successful blockade of its receptor offers a therapeutic approach for these conditions.
- *Cytotoxic factors*. These include tumour necrosis factor-α (TNF-α) which is similar to interleukin-1. Monoclonal antibody to TNF-α has been shown to improve clinical and laboratory parameters in patients with rheumatoid arthritis which suggests that specific cytokine blockade offers scope for treatment of this condition.
- *Interferons*. These are so named because they were found to interfere with replication of live virus in tissue culture. Interferon alfa is used for a variety of neoplastic conditions (see p. 566) and for chronic active hepatitis.
- *Colony-stimulating factors*. These have been developed to treat neutropenic conditions, e.g. filgrastim (recombinant human granulocyte colony stimulating factor, G-CSF) and molgramostim (recombinant human granulocyte macrophage-colony stimulating factor, GM-CSF) (see p. 558).

Eicosanoids

Eicosanoids (prostaglandins, thromboxanes, leukotrienes) is the name given a group of 20-carbon[1] unsaturated fatty acids derived principally from arachidonic acid in cell walls. They are short-lived, extremely potent and formed in almost every tissue

in the body. Eicosanoids are involved in most types of inflammation and it is on manipulation of their biosynthesis that most present anti-inflammatory therapy is based. Their biosynthetic paths are shown in Figure 15.1.

Arachidonic acid is stored mainly in phospholipids of cell walls, from which it is mobilised largely by the action of phospholipaseA$_2$. Glucocorticoids prevent the formation of *arachidonic acid* by inducing the synthesis of an inhibitory polypeptide called *lipocortin-1*; inhibiting the subsequent formation of both prostaglandins and leukotrienes, explains part of the powerful anti-inflammatory effect of glucocorticoids (for other actions, see p. 616).

Arachidonic acid is further metabolised:

- *by cyclo-oxygenase* (now termed prostaglandin G/H synthase), which changes the linear fatty acids into the cyclical structures of the *prostaglandins*. Nonsteroidal anti-inflammatory

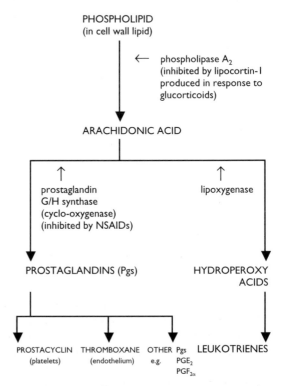

Fig. 15.1 Biosynthetic paths of eicosanoids (see text for description). Prostaglandins are found in virtually all tissues of the body

---

[1] The Greek word for 20 is *eicosa*, hence the term eicosanoid.

drugs (NSAIDs) exert their anti-inflammatory effects by inhibiting prostaglandin G/H synthase. The latter is present in at least two forms: cyclo-oxygenase-1 (COX-1) which is noninducible and present in many tissues including platelets, stomach and kidney; and COX-2 which is induced by cytokines and endotoxins at sites of inflammation, e.g. joints.

• *by lipoxygenase* to straight-chain hydroperoxy acids and then to *leukotrienes* which cause increased vascular permeability, vasoconstriction, bronchoconstriction, as well as chemotactic activity for leucocytes (whence their name). Inhibitors of lipoxygenase, and leukotriene receptor antagonists, are being evaluated and are likely to find uses in inflammatory and allergic conditions.

Synthetic analogues of prostaglandins are being used in medicine.

• PGI_2: *epoprostenol* (inhibits platelet aggregation, used for extracorporeal circulation and primary pulmonary hypertension).

• PGE_1: *alprostadil* (used to maintain the patency of the ductus arteriosus in neonates with congenital heart defects, and for erectile dysfunction by injection into the corpus cavernosum of the penis); *misoprostol* (used for prophylaxis of peptic ulcer associated with NSAIDs); *gemeprost* (used as pessaries to soften the uterine cervix and dilate the cervical canal prior to vacuum aspiration for termination of pregnancy).

• PGE_2: *dinoprostone* (used as cervical and vaginal gel to induce labour and for late therapeutic abortion).

• $PGF_{2\alpha}$: *dinoprost* (termination of pregnancy).

NSAIDs and their effects

The class of drug described here, of which aspirin is the prototype, is worthy of separate consideration for its members, although structurally heterogeneous, possess a single common mode of action which is to block *prostaglandin G/H synthase* (above). Various NSAIDs possess other actions that are related to inflammation, e.g. inhibition of lipoxygenases (diclofenac, indomethacin), superoxide production and leucocyte migration which may contribute to differences between the drugs, but their key action of inhibiting prostaglandin formation is reflected in the range of effects both beneficial and adverse which all the members share, to varying degrees, as follows:

EFFECTS

Analgesia: NSAIDs are effective against pain of mild to moderate intensity. Their maximum therapeutic efficacy is much lower than that of the opioids but they do not cause dependence (but see Analgesic nephropathy, below).

Anti-inflammatory action: this is useful in several conditions including rheumatoid arthritis, osteoarthritis, musculoskeletal disorders and pericarditis. In general, the greater the anti-inflammatory action, the greater the capacity to cause adverse effects.

Antipyretic action: cytokines, e.g. interleukins -Iβ and -6, produced at sites of inflammation stimulate prostaglandin synthesis in the hypothalamus, and this is blocked by NSAIDs.

Platelet function is reduced because formation of thromboxane is prevented; this action is used to protect against vascular occlusion (see p. 531).

Prolongation of gestation and labour: prostaglandin synthesis by the uterus increases substantially in the hours before parturition. Inhibition of prostaglandin synthesis, e.g. by indomethacin, prolongs labour. Indeed, indomethacin has been used to prevent premature labour but it causes transient constriction of the ductus arteriosus in some fetuses (below) and a β_2-adrenoceptor agonist, e.g. ritodrine, salbutamol, terbutaline, is preferred.

Patency of the ductus arteriosus is maintained by prostaglandins and, when the ductus remains patent after birth, an attempt may be made to close it by giving indomethacin, to escape the alternative of surgical ligation.

Primary dysmenorrhoea is associated with the production of large quantities of prostaglandins in the uterus and with uterine hypercontractility; this is the rationale for its treatment with an NSAID, e.g. mefenamic acid.

Gastric or intestinal mucosal damage is the commonest adverse effect of the NSAIDs. Mucosal prostaglandins inhibit acid secretion and further appear to exert a cytoprotective effect by promoting the secretion of mucus and by strengthening resistance of the mucosal barrier to back-diffusion of acid from the gastric lumen into the submucosal tissues where it causes damage. Inhibition of prostaglandin biosynthesis is believed to account for the erosions, ulceration and bleeding caused by NSAIDs; toxicity relates to anti-inflammatory efficacy, i.e. it is least with paracetamol and greatest with drugs such as azapropazone and piroxicam. Prophylactic use of a prostaglandin analogue, misoprostol, may be justified in some patients with NSAID-caused peptic ulcer. The development of selective inhibitors for the inducible form of prostaglandin G/H synthase (COX-2, see above) offers the prospect of reducing prostaglandin formation in inflamed joints while avoiding this action against the noninducible form (COX-1). Ulceration and stricture of the small bowel may also be caused by NSAIDs, and in some patients there is occult blood loss, diarrhoea and malabsorption, i.e. a clinical syndrome indistinguishable from Crohn's disease.

Urticaria, severe rhinitis and asthma occur in susceptible individuals, e.g. with nasal polyposis, who are exposed to NSAIDs, notably aspirin; the mechanism may involve inhibition of synthesis of bronchodilator prostaglandins, notably PGE_2 (see Index: Pseudoallergic reactions).

Renal effects. Renal blood flow is reduced because the synthesis of vasodilator renal prostaglandins is inhibited; the result is sodium and fluid retention and arterial blood pressure may rise. Renal failure may occur when glomerular filtration is dependent on the vasodilator action of prostaglandins, e.g. in the elderly, those with pre-existing renal disease, hepatic cirrhosis, cardiac failure, or on diuretic therapy sufficient to reduce intravascular volume.

Analgesic nephropathy. Mixtures of NSAIDs (rather than single agents) taken repeatedly cause grave and often irreversible renal damage, notably chronic interstitial nephritis, renal papillary necrosis and acute renal failure; these effects appear to be due at least in part to ischaemia through inhibition of formation of locally produced vasodilator prostaglandins. The condition is most common in people who take high doses over years, e.g. for severe chronic rheumatism and patients with personality disorder. Whilst analgesic nephropathy appears to be associated with longterm abuse of NSAID mixtures, strong evidence that phenacetin was particularly responsible has rendered this drug obsolete.[2]

Abuse of phenacetin and possibly of paracetamol may also lead to the development of cancer of the renal pelvis and ureters.

Pharmacokinetic characteristics

In general, NSAIDs are absorbed almost completely from the gastrointestinal tract, tend not to

---

[2] During the influenza pandemic of 1918 a physician to a big factory in a Swedish town prescribed an antipyretic powder containing phenacetin, phenazone (both NSAIDs) and caffeine. Survivors of the epidemic thought they felt fitter and reinvigorated during convalescence if they took the powder and they continued to take it after recovery. Consumption increased and many families 'could not think of beginning the day without a powder. Attractively wrapped packages of powder were often given as birthday presents'. Deaths from renal insufficiency rose in the 'phenacetin town', but not in a similar Swedish town, and in the decade of 1952–61 they were more than 3 times as many. An investigation was resisted by the factory workers to the extent that there was an organised burning of a questionnaire on powder-taking. It was eventually discovered that most of those who used the powders did so, not for pain, but to maintain a high working pace, from 'habit', or to counter fatigue (an effect probably due to the caffeine).

Eventually the rising death rate brought home to the consumers the gravity of the matter, something that has yet to be achieved for tobacco smoking or alcohol drinking (Grimlund K 1964 Acta Medica Scandinavica 174: suppl. 405).

Another NSAID, amidopyrine, was rendered obsolete because of the frequency with which it caused agranulocytosis. It is surely a matter of concern that the sodium sulphonate of amidopyrine, dipyrone, is still widely prescribed.

undergo first-pass (presystemic) elimination, are highly bound to plasma albumin and have small volumes of distribution. Their $t^{1}/_{2}$ s in plasma tend to group into those that are short (1–5 h) or long (10–60 h). Differences in $t^{1}/_{2}$ are not necessarily reflected proportionately in duration of effect, however, for peak and trough drug concentrations at their intended site of action in *synovial* (joint) *fluid* at steady-state dosing are much less than those in plasma. The vast majority of NSAIDs are weakly acidic drugs that localise preferentially in the synovial tissue of inflamed joints (see pH partition hypothesis, p. 91).

Interactions

● Renal impairment: there is increased risk that renal function will deteriorate when NSAIDs, e.g. indomethacin, are administered with diuretics, e.g. triamterene, and with ACE inhibitors. The nephrotoxic effect of cyclosporin is aggravated by NSAIDs.

● Renal tubular excretion: elimination of the cytotoxic drug methotrexate is impaired by NSAIDs and co-administration may cause toxicity. NSAIDs also delay the excretion of lithium by the kidney and may cause lithium toxicity. Probenecid delays the excretion of NSAIDs and raises their plasma concentration.

● Hyperkalaemia may result if indomethacin and possibly other NSAIDs are administered with ACE inhibitors and potassium retaining diuretics.

● Inhibition of metabolism by azapropazone and phenylbutazone increases the plasma concentration of phenytoin, sodium valproate, sulphonylurea hypoglycaemics and oral anticoagulants, increasing the risk of toxicity from these drugs.

● Hypertension: antihypertensive drugs and diuretics may be rendered less effective (see Renal effects, above).

● Bleeding: the risk from using anticoagulants is increased by the antiplatelet action of NSAIDs and effects on gastrointestinal mucosa (except paracetamol). All NSAIDs are extensively protein-bound and may displace warfarin from its binding protein, transiently increasing its anticoagulant effect.

● Convulsions may occur if NSAIDs are administered with 4-aminoquinolone antimicrobials.

Individual NSAIDs

The currently available NSAIDs exhibit a variety of molecular structures and it is usual to classify these drugs by their structural groups. Clinical trials in rheumatoid arthritis and osteoarthritis, however, rarely find substantial differences in response to average doses of NSAIDs whatever their structure, and this no doubt reflects their common mode of action. A structural classification is nevertheless used here as it provides a convenient framework, and toxicity profiles may relate to chemical group.

Classification of NSAIDs

● Para-aminophenol group: paracetamol
● Propionic acids: fenbufen, fenoprofen, flurbiprofen, ibuprofen, ketoprofen, naproxen, tiaprofenic acid
● Fenamic acids: mefenamic acid
● Salicylic acids: aspirin, benorylate, choline magnesium, trisalicylate, diflunisal, salsalate
● Acetic acids: acemetacin, diclofenac, etodolac, indomethacin (indometacin), ketorolac, sulindac, tiaprofenic acid, tolmetin
● Enolic acids: piroxicam, tenoxicam, azapropazone, oxyphenbutazone, phenylbutazone
● Nonacidic drug: nabumetone

PARA-AMINOPHENOL

Paracetamol (acetaminophen) (Panadol)

This is a popular domestic analgesic and antipyretic for adults and children. It is a major metabolite of the now obsolete phenacetin (see above). Its analgesic efficacy is equal to that of aspirin but in therapeutic doses it has only weak anti-inflammatory effects (for this reason it is sometimes deemed not to be an NSAID). Paracetamol inhibits prostaglandin synthesis in the brain but hardly at all in the periphery; it does not affect platelet function. Paracetamol (Panadol) is effective in mild to moderate pain such as that of headache or dysmenorrhoea and it is also useful in patients who should avoid aspirin because of gastric intolerance, a bleeding tendency or allergy, or because they are aged <12 years.

Pharmacokinetics. Paracetamol ($t^{1}/_{2}$ 2h) is well absorbed from the alimentary tract and is inactivated in the liver principally by conjugation as glucuronide and sulphate. Minor metabolites of paracetamol are also formed of which one oxidation product, N-acetyl-p-benzoquinoneimine (NABQI), is highly reactive chemically. This substance is normally rendered harmless by conjugation with glutathione. But the supply of hepatic glutathione is limited and if the amount of NABQI formed is greater than the glutathione available, then the metabolite oxidises thiol (SH-) groups of key enzymes, which causes cell death. This explains why a normally safe drug can, in overdose, give rise to hepatic and renal tubular necrosis (the kidneys also contain drug oxidising enzymes).

The oral dose is 0.5–1 g × 4–6 h to a maximum of 4 g in a day.

Adverse effects with occasional use are few. The drug may rarely cause skin rash and allergy. It is well tolerated by the stomach because its inhibition of prostaglandin synthesis in the periphery is weak. But heavy, longterm daily use may predispose to chronic renal disease.[3]

Acute paracetamol overdose. Severe hepatic and renal damage can result from taking 150 mg/kg (about 10 g or 20 tablets) in one dose, which is only 2.5 times the recommended maximum daily clinical dose. Patients specially at risk are:

* those whose enzymes are induced as a result of taking drugs or alcohol for their livers and kidneys form more NABQI
* those who are malnourished (chronic alcohol abuse, HIV infection) to the extent that their livers and kidneys are depleted of glutathione to conjugate with NABQI (see above).

The INR (prothrombin time) is preferred to plasma bilirubin and hepatic enzymes as a monitor of liver damage, and renal impairment is better assessed by plasma creatinine than urea (which is

metabolised by the liver). The clinical signs (jaundice, abdominal pain, hepatic tenderness) do not become apparent for 24–48 h and liver failure, when it occurs, does so between 2 and 7 days after the overdose. It is vital that this delay be remembered for lives can be saved only by effective anticipatory action (see below). The plasma concentration of paracetamol is of predictive value; if it lies above a semilogarithmic graph joining points between 200 mg/l (1.32 mmol/l) at 4 h after ingestion to 50 mg/l (0.33 mmol/l) at 12 h, then serious hepatic damage is likely. Patients who are enzyme induced or malnourished (see above) are regarded as being at risk at 50% of these plasma concentrations (plasma concentrations measured earlier than 4 h are unreliable because of incomplete absorption).

The general principles for limiting drug absorption apply (Ch. 9) if the patient is seen within 4 h. Activated charcoal by mouth is effective but the decision to use it must take into account its capacity to bind an oral antidote (methionine). Specific therapy is directed at replenishing the store of liver glutathione which combines with and so diminishes the amount of toxic metabolite available to do harm. Glutathione itself cannot be used as it penetrates cells poorly but N-acetylcysteine (NAC) (Parvolex) and methionine are effective as they are precursors for the synthesis of glutathione. NAC is more effective because its conversion into glutathione requires fewer enzymes; also, it is administered by i.v. infusion which is an advantage if the patient is vomiting. Methionine alone may be used to initiate treatment when facilities for infusing NAC are not immediately available.

The earlier such therapy is instituted the better and it should be started if:

* a patient is estimated to have taken >150 mg/kg, without waiting for the measurement of the plasma concentration
* plasma concentration indicates the likelihood of liver damage (above)
* there is any uncertainty about the the amount taken or its timing.

NAC is administered i.v. 150 mg/kg in dextrose 5% (200 ml) over 15 min; then 50 mg/kg in dextrose 5% (500 ml) over 4 h; then 100 mg/kg in dextrose 5% (1000 ml) over 16 h, to a total of about 300 mg/kg in

---

[3] Sandler D P et al 1989 New England Journal of Medicine 320: 1238.

20 h. While it is most effective if administered within 8 h of the overdose, evidence shows that treatment continuing up to 72 h yet provides benefit.

The INR and serum creatinine should be measured daily. If the INR exceeds 2 there is risk of infection and gastric bleeding, and an antimicrobial plus either sucralfate or a histamine H_2-receptor antagonist should be given prophylactically. The patient should be kept well hydrated; falling urine output may necessitate i.v. infusion of a colloid, e.g. albumin, or dopamine 2–3 µg/kg/min.

A *paracetamol-methionine combination* (co-methiamol; Pameton) has been marketed, the methionine content ensuring that hepatic glutathione concentrations are maintained when the drug is used in therapeutic (and over-) dose. But the problem of ensuring that this is used by the people most likely to benefit from such prophylaxis has not been solved since paracetamol is on direct sale to the public and this proprietary preparation is more expensive than generic paracetamol.

PROPIONIC ACIDS

Ibuprofen (Brufen) ($t^1/_2$ 2 h) is typical of the group. It is well absorbed after an oral dose and is inactivated by metabolism.

Others include fenbufen ($t^1/_2$ 10 h), fenoprofen ($t^1/_2$ 3 h), flurbiprofen ($t^1/_2$ 4 h), ketoprofen ($t^1/_2$ 1 h), naproxen ($t^1/_2$ 14 h) and tiaprofenic acid ($t^1/_2$ 2 h). They all have similar properties and are most useful in painful conditions such as mild rheumatoid disease and musculoskeletal disorders. Patients often prefer one to another. Naproxen and fenbufen are suitable for twice-daily dosing because of their long duration of action.

The main advantage over aspirin is a lower incidence of adverse effects particularly in the gastrointestinal tract, and especially with ibuprofen at low dose. Nevertheless epigastric discomfort, activation of peptic ulcer and bleeding may occur. Other effects include headaches, dizziness, fever and rashes.

FENAMIC ACIDS

Mefenamic acid (Ponstan) ($t^1/_2$ 3 h) is slowly absorbed from the small intestine and is eliminated mainly as metabolites in the urine and faeces. It is used for mild to moderate pain where inflammation is not marked, e.g. muscular, dental and traumatic pain and headache, and also for dysmenorrhoea and menorrhagia due to uterine dysfunction. The principal adverse effects are diarrhoea, upper abdominal discomfort, peptic ulcer and haemolytic anaemia. Elderly patients who take mefenamic acid may develop nonoliguric renal failure especially if they become dehydrated, e.g. by diarrhoea; the drug should be avoided or used with close supervision in the elderly.

SALICYLIC ACIDS

Aspirin

Aspirin (acetylsalicylic acid) was introduced in 1899 and remains the prototype NSAID; it is by far the commonest form in which salicylate is taken. The bark of the willow tree (Salix) contains salicin from which salicylic acid is derived; it was used for fevers in the 18th century as a cheap substitute for imported cinchona (quinine) bark.

Mode of action. Acetylsalicylic acid is unique among NSAIDs in that it also irreversibly inhibits prostaglandin G/H synthase by acylating the active site of the enzyme, so preventing the formation of products including thromboxane, prostacyclin and other prostaglandins; recovery of enzyme action requires resynthesis. Acetylsalicylic acid is rapidly hydrolysed to salicylic acid in the plasma. Salicylic acid also has an anti-inflammatory action but additionally exerts important effects on respiration, intermediary metabolism and acid-base balance, and it is highly irritant to the stomach. This account refers generally to aspirin.

Principal effects:

- *Anti-inflammatory effect* (see above).
- *Analgesic effect* is mild (less than that of codeine) because prostaglandin G/H synthase is readily regenerated. It seems to be due to both central and peripheral action. Aspirin is most effective against mild pain of somatic as opposed to visceral origin.
- *Antiplatelet effect* is due to permanent inactiva-

tion of prostaglandin G/H synthase in platelets (which prevents thromboxane synthesis). Being non-nucleated, platelets cannnot regenerate the enzyme as can nucleated cells, and the resumption of thromboxane production is dependent on the entry of new platelets into the circulation (platelet life-span 8 days). Thus continuous antiplatelet effect is readily achieved with low doses.

• *Antipyresis.* Aspirin acts in the hypothalamus to place at a lower level the set point of temperature regulation which is controlled by prostaglandin synthesis (see above). It does not affect temperature raised by exercise or heat and does not lower normal temperature.

• *Respiratory stimulation* is a characteristic of aspirin intoxication and occurs both directly by stimulation of the respiratory centre and indirectly through increased CO_2 production (see below).

• *Metabolic effects* including increased O_2 consumption and CO_2 production are important and understanding them aids the management of poisoning (see below).

• *Large doses* of aspirin (>5 g/d) cause *hypoprothrombinaemia* possibly due to competition between salicylate and vitamin K, for it is preventable and reversible by vitamin K_1. High doses also reduce *renal tubular reabsorption of urate* (both substances are transported by the same mechanism), but other treatments for hyperuricaemia are preferred. Indeed aspirin should be avoided in gout as low doses (<2 g/day) inhibit urate secretion, causing urate retention and on balance its effects on urate elimination are adverse.

Pharmacokinetics. Aspirin (acetylsalicylic acid) ($t^1/_2$ 15 min) is well absorbed from the stomach and upper intestinal tract (for pH-dependent absorption and gastric toxicity, see below and p. 91). Hydrolysis removes the acetyl group, and the resulting salicylate ion is inactivated largely by conjugation with glycine. At low therapeutic doses this reaction proceeds by first-order kinetics with a $t^1/_2$ of about 4 h but at higher therapeutic doses and in overdose the process becomes progressively saturated, i.e. kinetics become zero-order, and most of the drug in the body is present as the salicylate. The problem in overdose therefore is to remove salicylate.

A reasonably steady plasma concentration can be maintained if aspirin is given 6-hourly by mouth but if a high dose is given repeatedly there is risk of accumulation to toxic amounts; tinnitus is a useful warning sign.

Uses. Aspirin relieves mild to moderate pain of nonvisceral origin, e.g. headache, dysmenorrhoea, osteoarthritis, myalgia and painful bony metastases. The anti-inflammatory action is valuable for conditions in which an inflammatory reaction is prominent, e.g. rheumatoid disease, Still's disease and acute rheumatic fever (for cardiovascular uses, see p. 531).

Preparations and dosages. There is a plethora of commercial preparations, plain, buffered, soluble, effervescent, enteric-coated, sustained-release. A properly compounded Aspirin Tablet, Dispersible (single dose 300–900 mg) and a reliable enteric-coated preparation will suffice for most patients. Forms made for the purpose, e.g. dispersible, effervescent, should be dissolved in water and drunk. Low dose tablets, 75 mg, or 150 mg sustained release, are used for prevention of thrombosis.

Adverse reactions to aspirin

These are in general those described earlier for NSAIDs, but some aspects merit further comment.

Gastrointestinal effects. About 1 in 15 of the population cannot take aspirin without symptoms (heartburn, epigastric distress, vomiting). The characteristic lesion is a superficial gastric erosion and bleeding from this is enhanced by the antiplatelet effect (see above). Occult blood loss (usually 5 ml/d above control value of 0.7 ml/d) occurs in most people taking aspirin long term, sometimes sufficient to cause iron-deficiency anaemia. The site of bleeding is predominantly the stomach and anything that reduces the concentration of aspirin applied to the mucous membrane or increases ionisation, e.g. sodium bicarbonate (so that it is less lipid-soluble and less will penetrate gastric mucosal cells), decreases the liability to erosion and blood loss. A rapidly dispersing tablet that is swallowed as a liquid is less likely to cause trouble.[4] Enteric-coated aspirin causes less blood loss, for the small intestine is less affected than the stomach, but absorption is delayed for 6 or more hours, so that this preparation is unsuitable for occasional analgesia, though well suited for longterm medication, as in rheumatoid arthritis.

A history of taking aspirin recently is more common in patients with overt gastroduodenal haemorrhage, particularly those with acute erosions. The risk seems to be greatest in those who take aspirin frequently or in large dose but some patients suffer profuse gastric haemorrhage as a result of taking a single dose of aspirin. The latter appears to be an idiosyncratic response, possibly in individuals who have a minor haemostatic abnormality.

Salicylism (the symptoms of too high dose) is expressed as tinnitus and hearing difficulty, dizziness, headache and confusion.

Allergy. Aspirin is a common cause of allergic or pseudo-allergic symptoms and signs. Patients exhibit severe rhinitis, urticaria, angioedema, asthma or shock. Those who already suffer from recurrent urticaria, nasal polyps or asthma are more susceptible.

Reye's syndrome. Epidemiological evidence relates aspirin use to the development of the rare Reye's syndrome (encephalopathy, liver injury) in children recovering from febrile viral infections (respiratory, varicella). Acknowledging this, paracetamol is preferred for such febrile illnesses in children under 12 years, and parents should be educated not to use aspirin as most such administration is on their initiative, not prescribed.

Overdose

The typical clinical picture of moderate overdose

---

[4] Alka-Seltzer contains aspirin 324 mg, citric acid 965 mg, Na bicarbonate 1625 mg; the tablet is big. In water it forms a solution of Na acetylsalicylate, Na citrate and Na bicarbonate. The reaction also takes place if the tablets are stored in damp conditions.

(plasma salicylate 500–750 mg/l) includes nausea, vomiting, epigastric discomfort, tinnitus, deafness, hyperpnoea, headache, sweating, pyrexia, hypokalaemia and restlessness. With a large overdose (plasma salicylate >750 mg/l) these symptoms may be followed by pulmonary oedema, convulsions and coma with severe dehydration and ketosis. Despite the fact that aspirin reduces platelet activity and salicylates cause hypoprothrombinaemia and adverse effects on the stomach, gastric erosions and bleeding are uncommon after acute salicylate overdose.

Metabolic changes are important and understanding them aids the management of poisoning. As the plasma salicylate concentration rises the following occur:

- *Respiratory alkalosis* develops, directly due to stimulation of the respiratory centre, and indirectly by increased CO_2 production (from increased peripheral O_2 consumption due to uncoupling of oxidative phosphorylation).

- *Blood pH* thus rises, and is compensated by renal loss of bicarbonate which is necessarily accompanied by sodium and potassium ions as well as water; dehydration and hypokalaemia result. The reduction of plasma bicarbonate deprives the body of one of its buffering systems so that it becomes particularly vulnerable to metabolic acidosis.

- *Metabolic acidosis* is the outcome of several factors including accumulation of lactic and pyruvic acids due to toxic interference with citric acid cycle enzymes, and stimulation of lipid metabolism causing increased production of ketone bodies. Late toxic respiratory depression may also cause CO_2 retention.

Adults who have taken a single large quantity usually develop a respiratory alkalosis but when poisoning is severe a metabolic acidosis follows; commonly a mixed acid-base disturbance is found.

Children under 4 years may not show the respiratory alkalosis, but they readily develop severe metabolic acidosis, perhaps because mistaken ingestion as sweets may take place over hours.

Serial measurements of plasma salicylate are necessary to monitor the course of the overdose, for the concentration may rise over the early hours.

The general measures described in Chapter 9

apply to management but the following are relevant specifically for salicylate.

- *Gastric lavage* (or therapeutic emesis with syrup of ipecacuanha in children) is worth undertaking at least up to 12 h after overdose for tablets may lie as an insoluble mass in the stomach. Activated charcoal is worth giving as it adsorbs both salicylate that has not been absorbed from the gut and also drug that diffuses back from the blood into the gut.
- *Correction of dehydration* due to sweating, vomiting and overbreathing, is of the first importance. As hypokalaemia is usual and hypoglycaemia is common, dextrose 5% given i.v. with added potassium will often be indicated.
- *Acid-base disturbance.* Patients showing alkalosis or mixed alkalosis/acidosis with normal blood pH need no therapy directed to changing the blood acid-base balance. Sodium bicarbonate is used to correct metabolic acidosis (blood pH < 7.2) and to alkalinise the urine to remove salicylate (below).
- *Removal of salicylate* from the body. Activated charcoal, given in repeated doses is effective (see p. 142). Alternatively, maintaining alkalinity the urine (pH >7.5) is rational (see p. 142). A high urine flow rate produced by infusing fluid i.v. assists this process but forcing a diuresis, e.g. with a loop diuretic in high dose, does not improve salicylate clearance; the high pH of the urine is of far greater importance than its volume.[5]
- *Haemodialysis* can be undertaken in specially equipped centres when the plasma salicylate exceeds 750 mg/l and there is renal failure, or in any event exceeds 900 mg/l. The decision to haemodialyse should not be left until the victim is moribund.

Salicylic acid derivatives

Benorylate (Benoral) is an ester of aspirin and paracetamol which, being nonionic and lipid soluble, is well absorbed from the gut; it is also less irritant to the stomach and causes less blood loss from

it than does aspirin. When benorylate is hydrolysed in the liver and plasma, paracetamol and aspirin are released.

Diflunisal (Dolobid) is a fluorophenyl derivative of salicylic acid. Its elimination is saturable (zero-order) and the $t^{1}/_{2}$ increases from 7 h when the dose is 250 mg/d to 15 h when it is 500 mg/d. Diflunisal compares favourably with aspirin in the treatment of osteoarthritis and it may cause fewer gastric adverse effects, although diarrhoea is more common; it is also uricosuric. There may be cross allergy with aspirin.

Methyl salicylate (oil of wintergreen) is too irritant to be used internally but it is included in counterirritant liniments. Its smell sometimes attracts children; if they drink it, treatment is urgent.

ACETIC ACIDS

Indomethacin (indometacin) (Indocid)

This is a highly effective anti-inflammatory, analgesic and antipyretic agent. Absorption from the gut is rapid and almost complete, it is inactivated by metabolism ($t^{1}/_{2}$ 4 h). Indomethacin is used to relieve moderate to severe pain and the inflammation of rheumatoid disease, acute musculoskeletal disorders and gout. It is also effective for pain due to pleuritic and pericardial inflammation, for pain following minor operations, and to reduce opioid requirements for pain after major surgery. The oral dose is 50–200 mg/d in divided doses with food; a suppository of 100 mg at night is effective for relief of morning stiffness.

Adverse effects of indomethacin include gastric irritation with ulcer formation, bleeding and perforation. So effective is the anti-inflammatory action that signs of infection may be masked. Indomethacin may cause salt and fluid retention. It reduces the effectiveness of diuretic drugs (and may cause renal failure with triamterene); it antagonises the antihypertensive action of β-adrenoceptor antagonists. Headache is common, often similar to migraine, and is attributed to cerebral oedema; it can be limited by starting at a low dose and increasing slowly. Vomiting, dizziness and ataxia

---

[5] Prescott L F et al 1982 British Medical Journal 285: 1383.

occur. Indomethacin may aggravate pre-existing renal disease. Thus the drug is best avoided where there is gastroduodenal, renal or central nervous system disease or in the presence of infection. Allergic reactions occur and there is cross-reactivity with aspirin.

Acemetacin ($t^{1}/_{2}$ 3 h) also has anti-inflammatory and analgesic actions due to its metabolism in the liver (50–90%) to indomethacin.

Sulindac (Clinoril) ($t^{1}/_{2}$ 8 h) is structurally related to indomethacin. It is a prodrug, i.e. the substance itself is inactive or very weak but it is converted into a highly active sulphide metabolite ($t^{1}/_{2}$ 16 h) in the body and by the gut flora. Sulindac is used for pain and inflammation in rheumatoid disease, musculoskeletal disorders and in gout. Its anti-inflammatory action is less than that of indomethacin, but so is its gastric and central nervous system toxicity. Adverse effects on the kidney may be less likely as, unusually among the NSAIDs, the active (sulphide) metabolite of sulindac appears not to inhibit renal prostaglandin synthesis.

Diclofenac (Voltarol) ($t^{1}/_{2}$ 2 h) is used for moderate pain and inflammation due to rheumatoid disease, musculoskeletal disorders, renal colic and postoperative pain. Gastrointestinal and central nervous system and other adverse effects occur in common with other members of this group.

Tolmetin (Tolectin) ($t^{1}/_{2}$ 1 h) is used to relieve pain and inflammation in rheumatoid disease and musculoskeletal disorders. Allergic (anaphylactic) reactions appear to be more common with tolmetin and may occur in those who are not allergic to aspirin or other NSAIDs.

Etodolac (Lodine) ($t^{1}/_{2}$ 7 h) for rheumatoid and osteoarthritis appears to be well tolerated.

Ketorolac ($t^{1}/_{2}$ 5 h) is given by i.m. injection to provide short-term relief of acute postoperative pain.

ENOLIC ACIDS

Piroxicam (Feldene) ($t^{1}/_{2}$ 45 h) is completely absorbed from the gastrointestinal tract and a proportion undergoes enterohepatic cycling which helps to maintain the plasma concentration. Steady-state plasma concentrations appear not to alter significantly with age. Piroxicam is used for rheumatoid disease, musculoskeletal disorders and gout in a dose of 10–30 mg/d in single or divided amounts. Adverse effects are those to be expected with NSAIDs, gastrointestinal and central nervous system complaints being the commonest.

Tenoxicam is similar, except that its $t^{1}/_{2}$ of 72 h indicates that steady state will only be reached after at least 2 weeks.

Azapropazone (Rheumox) has anti-inflammatory, analgesic, antipyretic and uricosuric actions. Adverse reactions are relatively frequent and it should be used only in rheumatoid arthritis, ankylosing spondylitis and acute gout when other drugs have failed.

Phenylbutazone is also relatively toxic (gastrointestinal, hepatic, renal, bone marrow); it is rarely indicated except in ankylosing spondylitis under specialist supervision.

NONACIDIC DRUG

Nabumetone ($t^{1}/_{2}$ 22 h), while itself nonacidic (unlike most other NSAIDs), is largely metabolised to an active metabolite which is an acid and a potent inhibitor of prostaglandin synthesis. In rheumatoid arthritis and osteoarthritis, nabumetone 1000 mg once daily is as effective as aspirin 3600 mg in divided doses, and it is used for these conditions. The commonest adverse effects are dyspepsia with or without epigastric pain, diarrhoea and rash.

TOPICAL USE OF NSAIDs

Salicylates, diclofenac, piroxicam, felbinac (a metabolite of fenbufen), ketoprofen and ibuprofen are available as gels and creams for topical use on the skin for relief of symptoms caused by soft tissue trauma. The objective is to produce therapeutic local concentrations without (undesirable) systemic effects. They have less therapeutic efficacy.

POSTOPERATIVE PAIN

NSAIDs are used to relieve pain after minor surgery and, commenced on the first day after major operations, reduce by about 30% the requirement of opioid (reducing risk of sedation, respiratory depression and gastrointestinal stasis). Ketorolac and diclofenac may be given i.m. and ibuprofen and indomethacin by rectal suppository for this purpose.

Drug treatment of rheumatoid diseases

Rheumatoid disease affects 1–3% of the population of Europe and North America. Best results are obtained with early treatment and a multidisciplinary approach involving drugs, appropriate counselling, joint protection and exercise.

Drug therapy is used:

- To relieve pain, inflammation and muscle stiffness with NSAIDs.
- To modify the course of the disease or induce remission.

Choice of drugs in rheumatoid arthritis

- NSAIDs are often used: usually a propionic acid derivative to control the symptoms of inflammation. The choice of drug will depend on the amount of pain or inflammation present and on patient tolerance. When inflammation is prominent, an NSAID with strong anti-inflammatory action (and more risk of adverse effects), e.g. indomethacin or piroxicam, is appropriate.
- Intra-articular injections of corticosteroid are valuable for individual joints that are more severely affected.
- Slow-acting antirheumatic drugs (SAARDs) are now introduced early, once the diagnosis of rheumatoid arthritis is confirmed. The former approach of adding a SAARD only when NSAIDs have failed is outmoded. Evidence suggests that these drugs slow the progress of the disease although they may not reduce the ultimate degree of deformity and disability. Gold, penicillamine and sulphasalazine appear to have a similar therapeutic efficacy, but sulphasalazine is significantly the least toxic; the immunosuppressives are more effective and generally more toxic; the antimalarials are less effective and less toxic.
- Systemic corticosteroids are reserved for cases with inflammation so severe that it cannot be controlled by SAARDs.

RELIEF OF PAIN AND MUSCLE STIFFNESS AND SUPPRESSION OF INFLAMMATION

NSAIDs improve clinical indicators of disease activity such as joint swelling, but have no effect on laboratory indices, e.g. plasma viscosity, or on its outcome, e.g. joint destruction. When the disease is mild, a reasonable course is to start with ibuprofen or diclofenac, since these drugs are less toxic to the stomach. It may be necessary to try several within the group to find one which suits an individual patient; any drug selected should be used for 1–2 weeks before abandoning it (unless adverse effects are substantial). Paracetamol may be added if additional analgesia is required.

When inflammation is more severe an NSAID with more pronounced anti-inflammatory effect (and more risk of adverse effects) is needed. Some prefer aspirin (2–6 g/d) but the high dose required (just below that which induces tinnitus) means that gastric intolerance is common. Alternatively, indomethacin or piroxicam may be used. If nocturnal pain or morning stiffness is a problem, indomethacin given either orally or as a suppository the night before may benefit because its duration of action is sufficiently long. Gastric intolerance and peptic ulceration may be reduced by concurrent administration of a histamine H_2-receptor antagonist or misoprostol and their prophylactic use may be justified in patients deemed to be at particularly risk, e.g. those with a history of bleeding from peptic ulcer.

MODIFICATION OF THE DISEASE PROCESS

Certain drugs improve both the clinical and laboratory indices of inflammation, and probably also the course of the disease, i.e. retard structural damage to joints; these are known as **slow acting antirheumatic drugs** (SAARDs), namely:

- gold salts
- hydroxychloroquine
- penicillamine
- methotrexate
- sulphasalazine.

The decision to embark on the treatment with

such agents should be undertaken only by a physician with special experience of their use. Evidence indicates that radiographic progression of the disease is slowed. They appear to be of similar therapeutic efficacy and the choice may be dictated by their profile of adverse effects, e.g. penicillamine or gold would be avoided in a patient with proteinuria or leucopenia.

Gold salts

These exert analgesic, anti-inflammatory and immunomodulating actions by modifying a variety of cellular and humoral immune responses; their effects include reduction in the serum immune globulins and in the titre of rheumatoid factor. *Sodium aurothiomalate* by deep i.m. injection or *auranofin* by mouth are most commonly used. The oral form appears to be marginally less effective but causes fewer and less severe adverse reactions.

Disposition of gold is complex; it binds extensively to plasma albumin and is also distributed to inflamed synovium, kidney and liver. Gold is excreted mainly by the kidney and to a lesser extent in the faeces which it probably enters via the bile. The $t^{1/2}$ of elimination from plasma is 22 days, consistent with which steady-state concentrations are reached only after about 3 months.

Gold is used in patients in whom the diagnosis of rheumatoid arthritis has been made, ideally before deformities or radiological bone changes have occurred, usually in conjunction with anti-inflammatory analgesics; those with high titres of rheumatoid factor appear to respond better. If there is no response within 4 months, it is probably best to change to another drug.

Adverse effects occur in about one-third of patients and in some gold may have to be discontinued. They include pruritus, dermatitis, glossitis and stomatitis, most commonly, and also leucopenia and thrombocytopenia (which may threaten life), hepatic and renal damage, peripheral neuritis and encephalopathy. Serious toxicity is rare when observation is careful (monthly blood counts and urinalysis) and the drug stopped at the earliest sign of harm. Any serious effect, or one which does not subside rapidly, should be treated with a chelating agent; dimercaprol is probably preferable to peni-

cillamine. Because of its toxicity, gold is used less commonly than sulphasalazine or methotrexate as the first choice SAARD.

Hydroxychloroquine

Hydroxychloroquine ($t^{1/2}$ 18 days) (and also chloroquine) in addition to their antimalarial actions (see Ch. 14) exert anti-inflammatory and immunomodulating effects that are useful in rheumatoid disease. Its action is terminated by metabolism.

Hydroxychloroquine is best used for mild disease as it is relatively nontoxic and achieves a useful response in about 50% of patients after 4 weeks.

Hydroxychloroquine accumulates in many organs, including the eye where it can cause retinal damage that may be irreversible. In practice this complication is rare in the doses that are used to treat rheumatoid arthritis, even longterm, e.g. below 6.5 mg/kg/d, but it is prudent for patients over 60 years of age to have an ophthalmological examination before starting, and every 6 months during therapy.

Methotrexate ($t^{1/2}$ 9 h)

This folic acid antagonist is increasingly used in rheumatoid disease for its immunosuppressing properties despite concern about its potential longterm adverse effects. Methotrexate is absorbed from the gastrointestinal tract by an active process also used by folates and its distribution volume is approximately that of total body water. It is eliminated by the kidney. Methotrexate is effective in a dose of 7.5 mg once weekly by mouth increasing to a maximum of 20 mg per week. The toxicity profile of methotrexate used in a longterm regimen for rheumatoid disease includes chronic liver disease, pneumonitis, and opportunistic infections. Note also the use of methotrexate as a cytotoxic (p. 547) and for psoriasis (p. 280).

Penicillamine

The mode of action of penicillamine in rheumatoid arthritis is unclear but it reduces rheumatoid factor and also the concentration of immune complexes in plasma and synovial fluid. Its action as a chelator of a number of metals (including gold), is valuable in poisoning (see Ch. 9 and hepatolenticular degeneration). Penicillamine is incompletely but adequately absorbed following administration by mouth and undergoes metabolism by the liver, the products being excreted in the urine and faeces. After a single oral dose the $t\frac{1}{2}$ is 3 h.

Adverse effects are frequent. Patients may experience gastrointestinal upset, and dose-related impairment of taste is common. Thrombocytopenia is frequent but resolves when the drug is withdrawn unless it indicates the more serious aplastic anaemia which may also occur. Allergic reactions (rashes, fever) tend to occur during the early stages of treatment. Proteinuria, if it is heavy, is a reason for stopping penicillamine for it may herald the development of the nephrotic syndrome.

Sulphasalazine

Radiographic evidence indicates that sulphasalazine delays the progression of rheumatoid arthritis, but its mode of action is unclear. The doses necessary to achieve this are greater than those normally used for ulcerative colitis and adverse effects, notably dyspepsia, can be troublesome. The safety profile of sulphasalazine is similar to that established from experience in inflammatory bowel disease and treatment of rheumatoid disease (usually of more severe disease) can be continued longterm.

Tenidap[6]

This drug ($t\frac{1}{2}$ 23 h) has little structural resemblance to any of the above classes of antirheumatic drug. Its diverse anti-inflammatory actions include inhibition of cyclo-oxygenase (prostaglandin G/H synthase) and 5-lipoxygenase and it appears to combine properties of both the NSAIDs and the slow acting antirheumatic drugs (e.g. reducing the concentration of C-reactive protein). Tenidap is 85% absorbed from the gastrointestinal tract. Its place in therapy is being evaluated.

Other immunosuppressants. Azathioprine, cyclos-

porin and cyclophosphamide may be used for patients with resistant disease and as steroid-sparing agents, i.e. to escape corticosteroid toxicity. Cytotoxic immunosuppressants are carcinogenic and the magnitude of this risk, particularly important in younger patients with a long life expectancy, is uncertain; they are also mutagenic and teratogenic, which hazards have also to be judged when they are used.

ADRENAL CORTICOSTEROIDS

Although symptom relief is dramatic, there is reluctance to use systemic corticosteroid for rheumatoid disease because of adverse effects but this course is justified in some circumstances.

● To provide interim relief of inflammatory symptoms during the weeks that it takes slow-acting antirheumatic drugs (SAARDs) to act.

● Spaced single enormous doses (pulse treatment), e.g. methylprednisolone 1 g monthly for 1–3 months, are sometimes used for rapid and sustained relief of flares of the disease.

● In extreme severity, high dose prednisolone (20–40 mg/d) will very effectively suppress inflammation, e.g. with vasculitis or rheumatoid lung.

● Where SAARDs have failed or have produced intolerable adverse effects. The object is to control inflammation in affected joints whilst minimising adverse effects, e.g. prednisolone 7.5 mg or its equivalent of other steroid given once daily (at 08:00 h to reduce adrenal-pituitary suppression).

● There is some evidence that prednisolone 7.5 mg/day added to standard treatment may reduce the rate of joint destruction in moderate or severe disease of less than 2 years duration.[7]

Intra-articular injection of corticosteroid (triamcinolone, hydrocortisone, prednisolone or dexamethasone) is very effective when one joint is more affected than others. Benefit from one injection may last many weeks. Aseptic precautions must be extreme, for any introduced infection may spread dramatically. Too frequent resort to corticosteroid injection may actually promote joint damage by removing the protective limitation conferred by pain; such injections in a single joint should not exceed 3 per year.

---

[6] Madhok R 1995 Lancet 346: 481.

[7] Kirwan R 1995 New England Journal of Medicine 333: 142.

Other aspects of the treatment of this disease are important but are outside the scope of this book.

RHEUMATIC FEVER

In the acute stage, oral Aspirin Tabs, Dispersible (a soluble form) in a dose of about 100 mg/kg/d is effective and failure to respond casts doubt on the diagnosis. In the adult a plasma salicylate of 250 mg/l is usually sufficient but, in children, up to 350 mg/l may be required (but see Reye's syndrome).

When there is evidence of carditis (cardiac enlargement or pericarditis), a corticosteroid should be used instead of aspirin since the latter may precipitate cardiac failure. Prednisolone 10–15 mg/d (adult dose) is usually sufficient and specific therapy for cardiac failure may also be necessary.

Neither aspirin nor adrenal steroids prevents the development of late cardiac complications.

A 10-day course of benzylpenicillin should be given to kill any streptococci (for prophylaxis see p. 217).

OSTEOARTHRITIS

An NSAID is used, the choice being appropriate to the amount of pain and inflammation experienced by the patient, and on the tolerance of adverse effects. Evidence suggests that use of powerful anti-inflammatory drugs may accelerate destruction of some joints, e.g. the hip, by inhibiting the synthesis of vasodilator prostaglandins which are essential for adequate perfusion with blood for the natural repair of joint structures. NSAID needs should be regularly reviewed; exposure to other NSAIDs may be limited by use of paracetamol, an opioid-containing compound analgesic or an antidepressant in low dose (see p. 297).

There is no general case for using intra-articular corticosteroid in osteoarthritis but local injection of triamcinolone can provide relief for a single periarticular tender spot or for a knee joint that is acutely inflamed.

ANKYLOSING SPONDYLITIS

Indomethacin is effective and may also be needed at night to treat stiffness the next morning. Adrenal steroids are rarely used (low therapeutic efficacy in relation to adverse effects). Phenylbutazone is very effective, but toxic. The value of radiotherapy is controversial. Physical methods of treatment including active exercises are of the first importance to prevent deformity.

Gout and Drugs

Gout affects about 0.25% of the population of Europe and North America. Drugs are effective in management and some drugs can precipitate attacks. Patients with gout but no visible tophi have a urate pool that is 2 or 3 times normal and since this exceeds the amount that can be carried in solution in the extracellular fluid, microcrystalline deposits form; patients with tophi have a urate pool that may be 15–26 times normal.

Urate is freely filtered by the glomerulus and then reabsorbed from the tubule fluid. It is also secreted from the blood into the tubular fluid. The urate that appears in the urine represents the excess of secretion over reabsorption; these are both active, energy-requiring processes that can be affected by drugs.

Hyperuricaemia and gout from whatever cause (e.g. metabolic, renal disease, neoplasia) depend essentially on two processes, (1) overproduction and (2) underexcretion of urate. Both mechanisms may operate in the same patient but *decreased renal clearance* contributes to hyperuricaemia in most patients with gout. Drugs may influence these processes as follows:

Overproduction of urate, due to excessive cell destruction releasing nucleic acids, occurs when myeloproliferative or lympho-proliferative disorders are treated by drugs.

Underexcretion of urate is caused by all diuretics (except spironolactone), aspirin (in low dose, see p. 256), ethambutol, pyrazinamide, nicotinic acid, and alcohol (which increases urate synthesis and also causes a rise in blood lactic acid that inhibits tubular secretion of urate).

DRUG MANAGEMENT

Aims are to:

● *suppress the symptoms* (anti-inflammatory drugs),

i.e. indomethacin, diclofenac, naproxen, piroxicam and sulindac; azapropazone; colchicine; adrenal steroids
- *prevent urate synthesis*, i.e. allopurinol
- *promote elimination of urate* (uricosurics), i.e. probenecid, sulphinpyrazone.

Anti-inflammatory drugs

Except for colchicine, those listed above are described earlier in the chapter or elsewhere.

Colchicine $(t^{1/2} 1 \text{ h})$

This is an alkaloid from the autumn crocus (*Colchicum*). Colchicine rapidly relieves pain and inflammation, most effectively if it is used within 24 h of onset of an acute attack. Such swift relief is considered to confirm the diagnosis because non-gouty arthritis is unaffected, though failure does not prove the patient is free of gout. The curious specificity of colchicine in alleviating the pain of gout is not fully explained but may be due to its binding to the microtubular system of cells which is necessary for mitosis, and for cellular (leucocyte) migration to the inflamed area. A similar mechanism operates in its use in recurrent hereditary polyserositis (familial Mediterranean fever), including amyloid formation.

Colchicine is absorbed from the gut; some is metabolised in the liver and some is excreted unchanged in the bile and reabsorbed from the gut. This enhances its gut toxicity.

In acute gout colchicine 1 mg may be given by mouth, followed by 0.5–1 mg 2-hourly until either relief or adverse effects ensue. Benefit is usually felt in 2 or 3 h and is marked within 12 h. The total needed is usually 3–6 mg and it is unwise to exceed 10 mg. Once the effective dose is known, patients can take this total at once when they feel an attack coming on, and then 0.5 mg hourly.

Adverse effects may be severe, with abdominal pain, vomiting and diarrhoea which may be bloody, and probably due to inhibition of mitosis in the rapidly reproducing cells of the intestinal mucosa. Renal damage can occur, and, rarely, blood disorders. Large doses cause muscular paralysis.

Prevention of uric acid synthesis

Allopurinol (Zyloric) inhibits xanthine oxidase, the enzyme that converts xanthine and hypoxanthine to uric acid. Patients taking allopurinol excrete less uric acid and more xanthine and hypoxanthine in the urine; these compounds are both more readily excreted in renal failure and are more soluble than uric acid so that xanthine stones rarely form.

Allopurinol $(t^{1/2} 2 \text{ h})$ is readily absorbed from the gut, it is metabolised in the liver to alloxanthine $(t^{1/2} 25 \text{ h})$ which is also a xanthine oxidase inhibitor; it is excreted unchanged and as alloxanthine by the kidney.

Allopurinol is indicated in recurrent gout, in blood diseases where there is spontaneous hyperuricaemia, and during treatment of myeloproliferative disorders when cell destruction creates a high urate load. Allopurinol prevents hyperuricaemia due to diuretics. It can be combined with a uricosuric agent. A single dose of 300 mg/d by mouth is usually adequate but up to 600 mg or even more in total may be given in severe cases.

Adverse effects apart from the precipitation of acute gout (below) are uncommon but include allergies, e.g. exfoliative skin reactions, arthralgia, fever, lymphadenopathy, vasculitis and hepatitis, which may necessitate withdrawal of the drug. Allopurinol prevents the oxidation of the active drug mercaptopurine to an inactive metabolite; if an ordinary dose of mercaptopurine be given to a patient whose gout is being treated with allopurinol, dangerous potentiation occurs.

Uricosurics

Probenecid (Benemid) competitively inhibits the active transport of organic anions across the kidney tubule, preventing both reabsorption from the tubular fluid and secretion into it; inhibition of urate reabsorption increases its excretion in the urine. (Inhibition of tubular secretion of penicillin by probenecid is utilised when high plasma penicillin concentrations must be maintained after a single dose, e.g. in treating gonorrhoea.)

Probenecid is partly metabolised and partly excreted unchanged in the urine. The $t^{1/2}$ depends on dose and varies from 6–12 h.

To prevent gout, probenecid 0.5 g/d is taken by

mouth for the first week, rising to 1–2 g/d total. As the initial loss is high, crystals of urate may appear in the urine unless it is maintained at pH 6 or above for the first month of probenecid (or any other uricosuric) administration, e.g. with Potassium Citrate Mixture 12–24 g/d with water or sodium bicarbonate powder 5–10 g/d with water. A high fluid intake (2 l/d) should also be taken to avoid the dangers of mechanical obstruction or stone formation. Probenecid should not be used if there is severe renal impairment: it may be ineffective and may worsen renal damage.

Probenecid causes gastrointestinal upset in a few patients and occasionally allergy. It blocks renal tubular excretion of and thus prolongs the effect of organic acids including penicillins, cephalosporins, zidovudine, acyclovir, naproxen, indomethacin, methotrexate and sulphonylureas. Its uricosuric effect is blocked by aspirin.

Sulphinpyrazone (Anturan) is structurally related to phenylbutazone and acts like probenecid. It is a potent uricosuric and alkalinisation of the urine and high fluid intake (see above) are necessary at first to avoid crystalluria. Sulphinpyrazone causes gastric upset and is contraindicated in peptic ulcer.

Fenofibrate is an antihyperlipidaemic drug with added uricosuric action.

DRUG TREATMENT

Acute gout

NSAIDs (but not aspirin which in low dose causes urate retention) are highly effective, terminating the attack in a few hours. Early treatment is important. Indomethacin is a first choice and 25–50 mg may be given orally 3 times a day with a fourth (sometimes larger) dose at night, possibly taken as a suppository (100 mg). Naproxen, diclofenac, sulindac, piroxicam and azapropazone are effective alternatives. Colchicine is traditional and may be used when patients cannot tolerate NSAIDs or in a first attack of severe monarticular arthritis, as a good response helps make the diagnosis. If these drugs fail, prednisolone 40 mg/d may be used, reducing as quickly as symptoms allow. It requires only a moment's thought to appreciate that uricosurics and allopurinol will not relieve an acute attack of gout.

Recurrent and progressive gout

In principle it would seem reasonable that overproducers of urate be treated with allopurinol and underexcreters with a uricosuric drug. In practice most patients respond well to *allopurinol*, which is the drug of choice, especially if renal function is impaired (see above). Treatment is initiated if the serum urate consistently exceeds 0.6 mmol/l and the patient has had 3 or more attacks of acute gout. Persuading the patient to avoid chronic dietary excess or acute debauchery is also relevant (see below).

Therapy with allopurinol should begin in a quiescent period. It may be combined with a uricosuric. Aspirin must not be taken concurrently with other uricosurics as it interferes with their action (tell the patient). Paracetamol may be used as an analgesic without interfering with therapy.

Colchicine or indomethacin may be used if an acute attack is expected, e.g. immediately after surgery.

Rapid lowering of plasma urate by any means may precipitate acute gout, probably by causing the dissolution of tophi. It is therefore usual to give prophylactic suppressive treatment with indomethacin or colchicine during the first 2 months of allopurinol or uricosuric treatment. It can create an unfavourable impression if the patient, who has been told only that a drug will prevent gout, promptly has a severe attack.

Benefit from the lowered plasma urate will not be noticeable for some weeks. Medication should be adjusted to keep the plasma urate in the normal range. It can seldom be abandoned.

Chronic tophaceous gout. Tophi can sometimes be reduced in size and even removed by the prolonged use of allopurinol and uricosuric agents.

Precipitation of gout by diuretics. Any vigorous diuresis may precipitate acute gout by causing volume depletion which results in increased reabsorption of all substances that are normally only partially reabsorbed in the proximal renal tubule, including urate. Furthermore, most diuretics are organic acids that may compete with urate for secretion by the renal tubule. Diuretic-induced gout is of special importance in the elderly, in whom the presentation may be atypical. Spironolactone probably alone amongst the diuretics does not induce hyperuricaemia.

Aspirin and salicylic acid derivatives should be avoided in gout (the patient should be warned of the ubiquity of aspirin in proprietary preparations) because small doses competitively inhibit urate secretion, causing urate to be retained.

Acute calcium pyrophosphate arthropathy (pseudogout) responds similarly to acute gout; colchicine can be an effective prophylactic agent.

DIET, ALCOHOL AND GOUT

Dietary purines can be a significant contributory cause of hyperuricaemia and patients should avoid excesses of foods that contain purines, e.g. sweetbread (pancreas, thymus), kidney, liver. Gouty patients tend also to be overweight and loss of weight lowers the plasma urate. Knowledge that alcohol induces acute gout is of long standing, and has been celebrated in verse:

A taste for drink, combined with gout,
Had doubled him up for ever.
Of that there is no manner of doubt —
No probable, possible shadow of doubt —
No possible doubt whatever.[8]

GUIDE TO FURTHER READING

Allison M C et al 1992 Gastrointestinal damage associated with the use of nonsteroidal anti-inflammatory drugs. New England Journal of Medicine 327: 749

Cash J M, Kippel J H 1994 Second-line drug therapy for rheumatoid arthritis. New England Journal of Medicine 330: 1368

Dieppe P A et al 1993 Is research into the treatment of osteoarthritis with nonsteroidal anti-inflammatory drugs misdirected? Lancet 341: 353

Dinarello C A, Wolff S M 1993 The role of interleukin in disease. New England Journal of Medicine 328: 106

Emerson B T 1996 The management of gout. New England Journal of Medicine 334: 445

Glasgow J F T, Moore R 1993 Reye's syndrome 30 years on. British Medical Journal 307: 950

Hamerman D 1989 The biology of osteoarthritis. New England Journal of Medicine 320: 1322

Henry D et al 1996 Variability in risk of gastrointestinal complications with individual non-steroidal anti-inflammatory drugs: results of a collaborative meta-analysis. British Medical Journal 3012: 1563

Kirwan J R et al 1995 The effect of glucocorticoids on joint destruction in rheumatoid arthritis. New England Journal of Medicine 333: 142

Langman M J S et al 1994 Risks of bleeding peptic ulcer associated with individual nonsteroidal anti-inflammatory drugs. Lancet 343: 1075

Maiden N, Madhok R 1995 Misoprostol in patients taking non-steroidal anti-inflammatory drugs. British Medical Journal 311: 1518

Marcus A J 1995 Aspirin as prophylaxis against colorectal cancer. New England Journal of Medicine 333: 656

O'Callaghan C A et al 1994 Renal disease and the use of topical nonsteroidal anti-inflammatory drugs. British Medical Journal 308: 110

Porter D R, Sturrock R D 1993 Medical management of rheumatoid arthritis. British Medical Journal 307: 425

Ronco P M, Flahault A 1994 Drug-induced end-stage renal disease. New England Journal of Medicine 331: 1711

Saper C B, Breder C D 1994 The neurogenic basis of fever. New England Journal of Medicine 330: 1880

Scott J T 1989 Alcohol and gout. British Medical Journal 298: 1054

---

[8] Don Alhambra's song in Act 1 of the Savoy opera, The Gondoliers or the King of Barataria. W S Gilbert (1836–1911).

Drugs and the skin

SYNOPSIS

This account is confined to therapy directed primarily at the skin. It is well-established that the skin may react to emotion, e.g. in atopic eczema, and sedatives or tranquillisers may be useful adjuvant therapy of skin diseases. These aspects are addressed in other chapters.

- Dermal pharmacokinetics
- Dermal preparations: Vehicles for presenting drugs to the skin; Emollients, barrier preparations and dusting powders; Topical analgesics; Antipruritics; Adreno-cortical steroids; Sunscreens
- Dermal adverse drug reactions
- Individual disorders: Psoriasis, Acne, Urticaria, Skin infections

It is easy to do more harm than good with potent drugs, and this is particularly true in skin diseases. Many skin lesions are caused by systemic or topical use of drugs, often taking the form of immediate or delayed hypersensitivity.

Dermal pharmacokinetics

The stratum corneum (superficial keratin layer) is both the principal barrier to penetration of drugs into the skin and a reservoir for drugs; a cortico-steroid may be detectable even 4 weeks after a single application.

Drugs are presented in *vehicles*, e.g. cream, ointment, and their entry into the skin is determined by:

- the rate of diffusion of drug from the vehicle to the surface of the skin (this depends on the type of vehicle, see below)
- the partitioning of the drug between the vehicle and the stratum corneum (a physicochemical feature of the individual drug) and
- the degree of hydration of the stratum corneum (hydration reduces resistance to diffusion of drug).

Vehicles are designed to vary in the extent to which they increase the hydration of the stratum corneum; e.g. oil-in-water creams promote hydration (see below). Some vehicles contain substances intended to enhance penetration, e.g. squalane (p. 274).

Absorption through normal skin varies with site; from the sole of the foot and the palm of the hand it is relatively low, and increases progressively on the forearm, the scalp, the face until on the scrotum and vulva absorption is very high.

Where the skin is damaged by inflammation, burn or exfoliation, absorption is further increased.

If an *occlusive dressing* (impermeable plastic membrane) is used, absorption increases by as much as tenfold (plastic pants for babies are occlusive, and some ointments are partially occlusive). Serious systemic toxicity can result from use of occlusive dressing over large areas.

Drug readily diffuses from the stratum corneum into the epidermis and then into the dermis, where it enters the capillary microcirculation of the skin, and thus the systemic circulation. There may be a degree of presystemic (first-pass) metabolism in the epidermis and dermis, a desirable feature to the extent that it limits systemic effects.

Transdermal delivery systems are used to administer drugs via the skin for systemic effect (see p. 97).

Dermal preparations

It is convenient to think of these under the following headings:

- Vehicles for presenting drugs to the skin
- Emollients, barrier preparations and dusting powders
- Topical analgesics
- Antipruritics
- Adrenocortical steroids
- Sunscreens
- Miscellaneous substances.

VEHICLES FOR PRESENTING DRUG TO THE SKIN

The formulations are described in order of decreasing water content. Water-based formulations must contain preservatives, e.g. chlorocresol, but these rarely cause allergic contact dermatitis.

Lotions or wet dressings

Water is the most important component. Wet dressings are generally used to cleanse, cool and relieve pruritus in acutely inflamed lesions, especially where there is much exudation and on hairy areas. The frequent reapplication and the cooling effect of evaporation of the water reduces the inflammatory response by inducing superficial vasoconstriction. Sodium chloride solution 0.9%, or solutions of *astringent*[1] and weakly antimicrobial substances, e.g. aluminium acetate lotion, are often used. Soaks or compresses of approximately 0.05% potassium

permanganate are satisfactory if the lesion is on the limbs. Lotions containing more active ingredients are sometimes used on subacute lesions, but occasionally these irritate the skin further. The use of lotions or wet dressings over very large areas can reduce body temperature dangerously in the old or the very ill.

Shake lotions, e.g. calamine lotion, are essentially a convenient way of applying a powder to the skin (see Dusting powders, p. 270) with additional cooling due to evaporation of the water. They are contraindicated when there is much exudate because crusts form. Lotions, after evaporation, sometimes produce excessive drying of the skin, but this can be reduced if oils are included, as in oily calamine lotion.

Creams

These are emulsions either of oil-in-water (washable; cosmetic 'vanishing' creams) or water-in-oil. The water content allows the cream to rub in well. A cooling effect (cold creams) is obtained with both groups as the water evaporates.

Oil-in-water creams, e.g. aqueous cream (see emulsifying ointment, below), mix with serous discharges and are especially useful as vehicles for water-soluble active drugs. They may contain a wetting (surface tension reducing) agent (cetomacrogol). Aqueous cream is also used as an emollient (see below), i.e. as well as hydrating the skin it soothes and smooths scaly conditions. Various other ingredients, e.g. calamine, zinc, may be added to it.

Water-in-oil creams, e.g. oily cream, zinc cream, behave like oils in that they do not mix with serous discharges, but their chief advantage over ointments (below) is that the water content makes them easier to spread and they give a better cosmetic effect. They are useful as barrier preparations for protecting the skin, e.g. when it is chapped or dried, or on babies' buttocks, and can be used on hairy parts. They can be used as vehicles for *lipid-soluble* substances. A dry skin is mainly short of water, and

---

[1] Astringents are weak protein precipitants, e.g. tannins, salts of aluminium and zinc.

oily substances are needed to provide a barrier that reduces evaporation of water, i.e. the presence of oils contributes to epidermal hydration.

Ointments

Ointments are greasy and are thicker than creams. Some preparations are both *lipophilic* and *hydrophilic*, i.e. by occlusion they promote dermal hydration, and are also water miscible. Other ointment bases are composed largely of *lipid*; by preventing water loss they have a hydrating effect on skin and are used in chronic dry conditions. Ointments contain fewer preservatives and are less likely to sensitise. There are three kinds:

Water-soluble ointments are mixtures of macrogols and polyethylene glycols; their consistency can be varied readily. They are easily washed off and are used in burn dressings, as lubricants and as vehicles that readily allow passage of drugs into the skin, e.g. hydrocortisone.

Emulsifying ointments are emulsions that allow evaporation as they mix with water and skin exudate; they are useful as vehicles for drugs. Emulsifying ointment is made from emulsifying wax (cetostearyl alcohol and sodium lauryl sulphate) and paraffins. Aqueous cream is an oil-in-water emulsion of emulsifying ointment.

Nonemulsifying ointments do not mix with water. They adhere to the skin to prevent evaporation and heat loss, i.e. they can be considered a form of occlusive dressing (with increased systemic absorption of active ingredients); skin maceration may occur. Nonemulsifying ointments are helpful in chronic conditions, such as atopic eczema to soften crusts, and as vehicles; they are not appropriate where there is significant exudation. They are difficult to remove except with oil or detergents and are messy and inconvenient, especially on hairy skin. Paraffin ointment contains beeswax, paraffins and cetostearyl alcohol.

Collodions

Collodions are preparations of cellulose nitrate (pyroxylin) dissolved in an organic solvent. The solvent evaporates rapidly and the resultant flexible film is used to hold a medicament, e.g. salicylic acid, in contact with the skin. They are irritant and inflammable and are used to treat only small areas of skin.

Pastes

Pastes, e.g. zinc compound paste, are stiff, semi-occlusive ointments containing insoluble powders. They are very adhesive and give good protection to circumscribed lesions, preventing spread of active ingredients to surrounding skin. Their powder content enables them to absorb a moderate amount of discharge. They can be used as vehicles, e.g. coal tar paste, which is zinc compound paste with 7.5% coal tar. Lassar's paste is used a vehicle for dithranol in the treatment of plaque psoriasis.

EMOLLIENTS, BARRIER PREPARATIONS AND DUSTING POWDERS

Emollients hydrate the skin and soothe and smooth dry scaly conditions. They need to be applied frequently as their effects are short-lived. There is a variety of preparations but aqueous cream in addition to its use as a vehicle (above) is effective when used as a soap substitute. Various other ingredients may be added to emollients, e.g. menthol, camphor or phenol for its mild antipruritic effect and zinc and titanium dioxide as astringents.

Barrier preparations. Many different kinds have been devised for use in medicine, in industry and in the home to reduce dermatitis. They rely on water-repellent substances, e.g. silicones (dimethicone cream), and on soaps, as well as on substances that form an impermeable deposit (titanium, zinc, calamine). They are more useful in protecting skin from discharges and secretions (colostomies, napkin rash) than when used under industrial working conditions. The objective is difficult to achieve, i.e. to maintain a complete barrier that is also easily removed by ordinary washing when no longer needed. If it is not readily removable, complications due to blockage of sweat glands and follicles and skin irritation follow. Allergic reactions can occur.

Barrier creams may make the cleansing of the skin more easy after dirty work but a simple emollient is probably as effective.

Silicone sprays and occlusives, e.g. hydrocolloid dressings, may be effective in preventing and treating pressure sores.

Masking creams (camouflaging preparations) for obscuring unpleasant blemishes from view are greatly valued by the victims.[2] They may consist of the inert titanium oxide in an ointment base with colouring appropriate to the site and the patient.

Dusting powders, e.g. zinc starch and talc,[3] may cool by increasing the effective surface area of the skin and they reduce friction between skin surfaces by their lubricating action. Though usefully absorbent, they cause crusting if applied to exudative lesions. They may be used alone or as a vehicle for, e.g. fungicides.

Gels or jellies are semisolid colloidal solutions or suspensions used as lubricants and as vehicles for drugs. They are sometimes useful for treating the scalp.

TOPICAL ANALGESICS

Counterirritants and rubefacients are irritants that stimulate nerve endings in intact skin to relieve pain in skin, e.g. postherpetic, viscera or muscle supplied by the same nerve root. All produce inflammation of the skin which becomes flushed, hence rubefacients. They are often effective though their precise mode of action is unknown.

The best counterirritants are physical agents, especially heat. Many drugs, however, have been used for this purpose and suitable preparations containing salicylates, nicotinates, menthol, camphor, capsaicin (depletes skin substance P) and turpentine are also available.

---

[2] In the UK the Red Cross offers a free cosmetic camouflage service through hospital dermatology departments.

[3] Talc is magnesium silicate. It must not be used for dusting surgical gloves as it causes granulomas if it gets into wounds or body cavities.

Topical NSAIDs (see p. 259) are used to relieve musculoskeletal pain.

Local anaesthetics. Lignocaine, prilocaine are available as gels, ointments and sprays to provide reversible block of conduction along cutaneous nerves (see p. 388). Benzocaine and amethocaine carry a high risk of sensitisation.

Volatile aerosol sprays, beloved by sportspeople, produce analgesia by cooling and by placebo effect.

ANTIPRURITICS

Mechanisms of itch are both peripheral and central. Impulses pass along the same nerve fibres as those of pain, but the sensation experienced differs qualitatively as well as quantitatively from pain. In the CNS endogenous opioid peptides are released and naloxone can relieve some cases of intractable itch. Local liberation of histamine and other autacoids in the skin also contributes and may be responsible for much of the itch of urticarial allergic reactions. Histamine release by bile salts may explain some, but not all, of the itch of obstructive jaundice. It is likely that other chemical mediators, e.g. serotonin and prostaglandins, are involved.

Generalised pruritus

Treatment of the underlying cause is obviously required, e.g. parasites, iron deficiency, liver or renal failure and reticulosis, but there remain patients in whom the cause either cannot be removed or is not known.

Antihistamines (H$_1$) especially hydroxyzine (Atarax) orally are used but probably act by their sedative or anxiolytic effect (except in urticarial conditions); they should not be applied topically over a prolonged period for risk of allergy.

In severe pruritus, sedation during the day and a hypnotic at night is sometimes helpful. In chronic cases a sedative antidepressant may help. *Chlorpromazine* or a related drug, e.g. trimeprazine (Vallergan), may also provide relief, probably by altering the patient's attitude to the itching.

The itching of obstructive jaundice may be

relieved by androgens but they may increase the jaundice. If obstruction is only partial, *cholestyramine* and *phototherapy* can be useful.

Localised pruritus

Scratching or rubbing seems to give relief by converting the intolerable persistent itch into a more bearable pain, and may even cure the itch at the cost of removing the epidermis. A vicious cycle can be set up in which itching provokes scratching and scratching leads to skin lesions which itch, as in neurodermatitis. Covering the lesion or enclosing it in a medicated bandage so as to prevent any further scratching or rubbing may help.

Topical hydrocortisone or fluorinated steroid preparations are probably the most effective antipruritics in local inflammatory conditions, e.g. eczema. Obviously they should not be used for generalised pruritus due to systemic disease (see below).

Any cooling application has some antipruritic effect, but a variety of substances, such as menthol or camphor, is often added because they have a reputation as antipruritics probably by weak local anaesthetic action.

Calamine and astringents (aluminium acetate, tannic acid) may help. Local anaesthetics do not offer any longterm solution and since they are liable to sensitise the skin they are best avoided; lignocaine is least troublesome in this respect.

Crotamiton, an acaricide, is reputed to have a specific but unexplained antipruritic action, although it may exacerbate an already inflamed skin; convenient proprietary preparations (Eurax) are available.

Pruritus ani is managed by attention to hygiene, emollients and a weak corticosteroid with antiseptic/anticandida application used as briefly as practicable (some cases are a form of neurodermatitis). Secondary contact sensitivity, e.g. to local anaesthetics, is common. Emollients, e.g. washing with aqueous cream, can help.

ADRENOCORTICAL STEROIDS

Actions. Adrenal steroids possess a range of actions

(see p. 600) of which the following are relevant to topical use:

● Inflammation is suppressed, particularly when there is an allergic factor, and immune responses are reduced

● Antimitotic activity suppresses proliferation of keratinocytes, fibroblasts and lymphocytes (useful in psoriasis, but also causes skin thinning)

● Vasoconstriction reduces ingress of inflammatory cells and humoral factors to the inflamed area; this action (blanching effect on human skin) has been used to measure the potency of individual topical corticosteroids (see below).

Penetration into the dermal layers is governed by the factors outlined at the beginning of this chapter. The vehicle should be appropriate to the condition being treated: an ointment for dry, scaly conditions, a water-based cream for weeping eczema.

Uses. Adrenal steroids should be considered a symptomatic, and sometimes curative but not preventive treatment. Ideally a potent steroid (see below) should be given only as a short course and reduced as soon as the response allows. Corticosteroids are most useful for *eczematous disorders* (atopic, discoid, contact) and other inflammatory conditions save those due to infection. Psoriasis of the scalp or flexures or inflamed (uninfected) psoriasis may be treated with a preparation of mild potency, e.g. hydrocortisone not exceeding 1%. Use for other forms of psoriasis is a matter for those with special experience, for short-term response may be followed by relapse and even rebound of the disease. Adrenal steroids of highest potency are reserved for recalcitrant dermatoses, e.g. lichen simplex, lichen planus, nodular prurigo and discoid lupus erythematosus.

Topical corticosteroids are of no use for urticarial conditions and are *contraindicated* in infection, e.g. fungal, herpes, impetigo, scabies, because the infection will exacerbate and spread. Where appropriate, an adrenal steroid formulation may include an antimicrobial, e.g. miconazole, fusidic acid, in infected eczema.

The difficulties and dangers of *systemic* adrenal steroid therapy are sufficient to restrict such use to serious conditions (such as pemphigus and generalised exfoliative dermatitis) not responsive to other forms of therapy.

- Use for symptom relief and never prophylactically
- Choose the appropriate therapeutic potency (see Table 16.1), i.e. mild for the face. In cases likely to be resistant, use a very potent preparation, e.g. for 3 weeks, to gain control, after which change to a less potent preparation.
- Choose the appropriate vehicle, i.e. a water-based cream for weeping eczema, an ointment for dry scaly conditions.
- Use a combined adrenal steroid/antimicrobial formulation if infection is present.
- Advise the patient to apply the formulation very thinly, just enough to make the skin surface shine slightly.
- Prescribe in small amounts so that serious overuse is unlikely to occur without the doctor knowing, e.g. weekly quantity by group (Table 16.1): very potent 15 g; potent 30 g; others 50 g.
- Occlusive dressing should be used only briefly. NB. Babies' plastic pants are an occlusive dressing as well as being a social amenity.

Table 16.1 Topical corticosteroid formulations conventionally ranked according to therapeutic potency

Very potent	Clobetasol (0.05%) [also formulations of diflucortolone (0.3%), halcinonide]
Potent	Beclomethasone (0.025%) [also formulations of betamethasone, budesonide, desonide, desoxymethasone, diflucortolone (0.1%), fluclorolone, fluocinolone (0.025%), fluocinonide, fluticasone, hydrocortisone butyrate, mometasone (once daily), triamcinolone]
Moderately potent	Clobetasone (0.05%) [also formulations of alclometasone, clobetasone, desoxymethasone, fluocinolone (0.00625%), fluocortolone, fluandrenolone, hydrocortisone plus urea (see p. 275)
Mildly potent	Hydrocortisone (0.1-1.0%) [also formulations of alclomethasone, fluocinolone (0.0025%), methylprednisolone]

Important note: the ranking is based on agent and its concentration: the same drug appears in more than one rank.

Choice. Corticosteroids are classified according to their *therapeutic potency* (efficacy), i.e. according to both drug and % concentration (see Table 16.1). Choice of preparation relates both to the disease and the site of intended use. High potency preparations are commonly needed for lichen planus and discoid lupus erythematosus; weaker preparations (hydrocortisone 0.5–2.5%) are usually adequate for eczema, use on the face and in childhood.

When a skin disorder requiring a corticosteroid is already infected, a preparation containing an antimicrobial is added, e.g. neomycin, clotrimazole, nystatin. When the infection is eliminated the corticosteroid may be continued alone.

It is inappropriate to use corticosteroid/antimicrobial preparations in the absence of initial infection.

Intralesional injections are occasionally used to provide high local concentrations without systemic effects in chronic dermatoses, e.g. hypertrophic lichen planus and discoid lupus erythematosus.

Adverse effects. Used with restraint topical corticosteroids are effective and safe. Adverse effects are more likely with formulations ranked therapeutically as very potent or potent in Table 16.1.

- *Short-term use.* Infection may spread.
- *Longterm use.* Skin atrophy can occur within 4 weeks and may or may not be fully reversible. It reflects loss of connective tissue which also causes striae (irreversible) and generally occurs at sites where dermal penetration is high (face, groins, axillae).

Other effects include: local hirsutism; perioral dermatitis (especially in young women) responds to steroid withdrawal and may be mitigated by tetracycline by mouth for 4–6 weeks; depigmentation (local); acne (local). Potent corticosteroids should not be used on the face unless this is unavoidable. Systemic absorption can lead to all the adverse effects of systemic corticosteroid use. Suppression of the hypothalamic/pituitary axis readily occurs with overuse of the very potent agents, and when 20% of the body is under an *occlusive dressing* with mildly potent agents. Other complications of occlusive dressings include infections (bacterial, candidial) and even heat stroke when large areas are occluded.

---

[4] Adapted from Munro D D 1977 Prescribers' Journal 17: 84.

Applications to the eyelids may get into the eye and cause glaucoma.

Rebound exacerbation of the disease can occur after abrupt cessation of therapy. This can lead the patient to reapply the steroid and so create a vicious cycle.

Allergy. Corticosteroids, particularly hydrocortisone and budesonide, or other ingredients in the formulation, may cause allergic contact dermatitis and the possibility of this should be considered where expected benefit fails to occur.

SUNSCREENS
(Sunburn and Photosensitivity)

Ultraviolet (UV) solar radiation consists of:

- UVA (320–400 nanometres): causes skin ageing (damage to collagen) and probably skin cancer
- UVB (290–320 nm): is × 1000 more active than UVA, acutely causes sunburn and tanning, and chronically skin cancer and skin ageing
- UVC (200–290 nm) is prevented, at present, from reaching the earth at sea level by the stratospheric ozone layer, though it can cause skin injury at high altitude.

Protection of the skin

Protection from UV radiation is effected by:

Absorbent sunscreens. These organic chemicals absorb UVB and UVA at the surface of the skin (generally more effective for UVB).

UVB protection: aminobenzoic acid and aminobenzoates (padimate-O), cinnamates, salicylates, camphors.

UVA protection: benzophenones (mexenone, oxybenzone), dibenzoylmethanes.

Reflectant sunscreens. Inert minerals such as titanium dioxide, zinc oxide and calamine act as a physical barrier to UVB and UVA: they are cosmetically unattractive but newer micronised preparations are more acceptable.

The performance of a sunscreen is expressed as the *sun protective factor* (SPF) which refers to UVB (UVA is more troublesome to measure and protec-tion is indicated by a star rating system with 4 stars providing the greatest). A SPF of 10 means that the dose of UVB required to cause erythema must be 10 times greater on protected than on unprotected skin. Sunscreens should protect against both UVB and UVA. Absorbent and reflectant components are combined in some preparations. The washability of the preparation (including removal by sweat and swimming) is also relevant to efficacy and frequency of application; some penetrate the stratum corneum (padimate-O) and are more persistent than others.

Uses. Apart from protecting against effects of incidental UV radiation on normal skin, sunscreens are used by people having *photosensitivity* due to drugs (below) or to disease, i.e. photodermatoses such as photosensitivity dermatitis, polymorphic light eruptions, cutaneous porphyrias, lupus erythematosus.

Sunburn

Subjects who burn easily should use a preparation with SPF 15-20; it will reduce or prevent tanning as well as burn. The lower lip receives a substantial dose of UV but may be neglected when a sunscreen is applied (specific lip-blocks are available). Sunscreens can cause allergic dermatitis or photodermatitis (but not titanium dioxide, though its vehicle may).

Treatment of mild sunburn is usually with a lotion such as oily calamine lotion. Severe cases are helped by hydrocortisone cream (1%). NSAIDs can help if given early, by preventing the formation of prostaglandins, e.g. indomethacin.

Photosensitivity

Drug photosensitivity means that an adverse effect occurs as a result of drug plus light, usually UVA; sometimes even the amount of ultraviolet radiation from fluorescent light tubes is sufficient.

Systemically taken drugs that induce photosensitivity are many. Of the drug groups given below, those most commonly reported are:[5]

---

[5] Data from The Medical Letter (1995) 37: 35.

antimicrobials: demeclocycline, doxycycline, nalidixic acid, sulphonamides
antipsychotics: chlorpromazine, prochlorperazine
cardiac dysrhythmic: amiodarone
diuretics: frusemide, chlorothiazide, hydrochlorothiazide
hypoglycaemic: tolbutamide
nonsteroidal anti-inflammatory: piroxicam.

Topically applied substances that can produce photosensitivity include:

para-aminobenzoic acid and its esters (used as sunscreens)
coal tar derivatives
psoralens from juices of various plants (e.g. bergamot oil)
6-methylcoumarin (used in perfumes, shaving lotions, sunscreens)
musk ambrette (used in perfumes).

There are two forms of photosensitivity:

Phototoxicity, like drug toxicity, is a normal effect of too high a dose of UV in a subject who has been exposed to the drug. The reaction is like severe sunburn. *The threshold returns to normal when the drug is stopped.*

Photoallergy, like drug allergy, is a cell-mediated immunological effect that occurs only in some people, and which may be severe with a small dose. Photoallergy due to drugs is the result of a photochemical reaction caused by UVA in which the drug combines with tissue protein to form an antigen. *Reactions may persist for years after the drug is withdrawn*; they are usually eczematous.

Systemic protection, as opposed to application of drug to exposed areas, should be considered when topical measures fail. Antimalarials such as *chloroquine* for short periods may be effective in polymorphic light eruption and in cutaneous lupus erythematosus.

Psoralens (obtained from citrus fruits and other plants), e.g. methoxsalen, are used to *induce* photochemical reactions in the skin. After topical or systemic administration of the psoralen and

subsequent exposure to UVA there is an erythematous reaction that goes deeper than ordinary sunburn and that may reach its maximum only after 48 h (sunburn maximum is 12–24 h). Melanocytes are activated and pigmentation occurs over the following week. This action is used to repigment areas of disfiguring depigmentation, e.g. vitiligo in black-skinned persons.

In the presence of UVA the psoralen interacts with DNA, forms thymine dimers, and inhibits DNA synthesis. Psoralen plus UVA (PUVA) treatment is used chiefly in severe psoriasis (a disease characterised by increased epidermal proliferation), and cutaneous T cell lymphoma.

Severe adverse reactions can occur with psoralens and ultraviolet radiation, including increased risk of skin cancer (due to mutagenicity inherent in their action), cancer of the male genitalia, cataracts and accelerated skin ageing; the treatment is used only by specialists.

Miscellaneous substances

Keratolytics are used to destroy unwanted tissue, including warts and corns. Great care is obviously necessary to avoid ulceration. They include trichloracetic acid, silver nitrate sticks, salicylic acid and many others. Resorcinol and sulphur are mild keratolytics used in acne.

Squalane is a saturated hydrocarbon insoluble in water but soluble in sebum. It therefore penetrates the skin and is a vehicle for delivery of agents; it is water repellent and is used for incontinence and prevention of bed sores. It appears in mixed formulations.

Tars are mildly antiseptic, antipruritic and they inhibit keratinisation in an ill-understood way. They are safe in low concentrations. Tars are used in chronic conditions associated with parakeratosis, e.g. psoriasis. Photosensitivity occurs. There are very many preparations, which usually contain other substances, e.g. calamine and coal tar ointment, or coal tar and salicylic acid ointment; it is sometimes useful to add an adrenal steroid.

Ichthammol is a sulphurous tarry distillation product of fossilised fish (obtained in the Austrian Tyrol); it has a weaker effect than coal tar.

Zinc oxide provides mild astringent, barrier and occlusive actions.

Calamine is basic zinc carbonate that owes its pink colour to added ferric oxide. It has a mild astringent action and is used as a dusting powder and in shake and oily lotions.

Urea is used topically to assist skin hydration, e.g. in ichthyosis.

Insect repellents, e.g. against mosquitoes, ticks, fleas, such as deet (diethyl toluamide), dimethyl phthalate. These are applied to the skin and repel insects principally by vaporisation. They must be applied to all exposed skin, and sometimes also to clothes if their objective is to be achieved (some damage plastic fabrics and spectacle frames). Their duration of effect is limited by the rate at which they vaporise (skin and ambient temperature), by washing off (sweat, rain, immersion) and by mechanical factors causing rubbing (physical activity). They can cause allergic and toxic effects, especially with prolonged use. About 10% is absorbed. Plainly the vehicle in which they are applied is also important, and an acceptable substance achieving persistence of effect beyond a few hours has yet to be developed. But the alternative of spreading insecticide in the environment causing general pollution and indiscriminate insect kill is unacceptable. Selective environmental measures against some insects, e.g. mosquitoes, are sometimes feasible.

Benzyl benzoate may be used on clothes; it resists one or two washings.

Dermal adverse drug reactions

Drugs taken systemically or applied locally often cause rashes. These take many different forms and the same drug may produce different rashes in different people.

Irritant or *allergic contact dermatitis* is eczematous and is often caused by antimicrobials, local anaesthetics, topical antihistamines, and increasingly commonly by topical corticosteroids. It is often due to the vehicle in which the active drug is applied, particularly a cream.

Reactions to *systemically administered* drugs are commonly erythematous, like those of measles, scarlatina or erythema multiforme. They give no useful clue to the cause. They commonly occur during the first 2 weeks of therapy, but some immunological reactions may be delayed for months.

> Though drugs may change, the clinical problems remain depressingly the same: a patient develops a rash; he is taking many different tablets; which, if any, of these caused his eruption, and what should be done about it? It is no answer simply to stop all drugs, though the fact that this can often be done casts some doubt on the patient's need for them in the first place. All too often potentially valuable drugs are excluded from further use on totally inadequate grounds. Clearly some guidelines are needed but no simple set of rules exists that can cover this complex subject . . . [6]

The following questions should be asked in every case:

- Can other skin diseases be excluded?
- Are the skin changes compatible with a drug cause?
- Which drug is most likely to be responsible?
- Are any further tests worthwhile?
- Is any treatment needed?

These questions are deceptively simple but the answers are often difficult.[6]

DRUG-SPECIFIC RASHES

Despite great variability, some hints at drug-specific or characteristic rashes from drugs taken *systemically*, can be discerned, as follows:

Acne: e.g. corticosteroids, androgens.

Toxic erythema commonly occurs at about the ninth day of treatment (or day 2–3 in previously exposed patients); causes include antimicrobials,

---

[6] Hardie R A, Savin J A 1979 British Medical Journal 1: 935, to whom we are grateful for this quotation and classification.

especially ampicillin, sulphonamides and derivatives (sulphonylureas, frusemide and thiazide diuretics). It may begin even after the course of treatment had been completed.

Erythema multiforme: e.g. NSAIDs, sulphonamides, barbiturates, phenytoin.

Erythema nodosum: e.g. sulphonamides, oral contraceptives, prazosin.

Allergic vasculitis: e.g. sulphonamides, NSAIDs, thiazides, chlorpropamide, phenytoin, penicillin, retinoids.

Purpura: e.g. thiazides, sulphonamides, sulphonylureas, phenylbutazone, quinine.

Eczema: e.g. penicillins, phenothiazines.

Exfoliative dermatitis and erythroderma: gold, phenytoin carbamazepine, allopurinol, penicillins, neuroleptics, isoniazid.

Photosensitivity: see above.

Lupus erythematosus: e.g. hydralazine, isoniazid, procainamide, phenytoin, oral contraceptives.

Lichenoid eruption: e.g. β-adrenoceptor blockers, chloroquine, thiazides, frusemide, captopril, gold, phenothiazines.

Pemphigus: e.g. penicillamine, captopril, piroxicam, penicillin, rifampicin.

Bullous pemphigoid: frusemide (and other sulphonamide-related drugs), penicillamine, penicillin, PUVA therapy.

Fixed eruptions are eruptions that recur at the same site, often circumoral, with each administration of the drug: e.g. phenolphthalein (laxative self-medication), sulphonamides, quinine (in tonic water), tetracycline, barbiturates, naproxen, nifedipine.

Stevens–Johnson syndrome and toxic epidermal necrolysis:[7] e.g. anticonvulsants, sulphonamides, aminopenicillins, oxicam NSAIDs, allopurinol, chlormezanone, corticosteroids.

Urticaria and angioedema: e.g. penicillins, enalapril, gold, NSAIDs, e.g. aspirin.

Psoriasis may be aggravated by lithium and antimalarials.

Pruritus unassociated with rash: e.g. oral contraceptives, phenothiazines, rifampicin (cholestatic reaction).

Hair loss: e.g. cytotoxic anticancer drugs, acitretin, oral contraceptives, heparin, androgenic steroids (women), sodium valproate, gold.

Pigmentation: e.g. oral contraceptives (in photosensitive distribution), phenothiazines, heavy metals, amiodarone, chloroquine (pigmentations of nails and palate, depigmentation of the hair), minocycline.

Recovery after withdrawal of the causative drug generally begins in a few days, but lichenoid reactions may not improve for weeks.

Diagnosis. The patient's drug history may give clues. Reactions are commoner during early therapy (days) than after the drug has been given for months. Diagnosis by readministration of the drug (challenge) is safe with fixed eruptions, but not with others, particularly those that may be part of a generalised effect, e.g. vasculitis.

Patch and photopatch tests are useful in contact dermatitis, for they reproduce the causative process but should be performed only by those with special experience. Intradermal tests introduce all the problems of allergy to drugs, e.g. metabolism, combination with protein, fatal anaphylaxis (see pp 127, 199).

Treatment. Remove the cause; use cooling applications and antipruritics; use a histamine H_1-receptor blocker systemically for acute urticaria; give an adrenal steroid for severe cases.

---

[7] Roujeau C-J et al 1995 New England Journal of Medicine 333: 1600.

Table 16.2 Summary of treatment of skin disorders

Condition	Treatment	Remarks
Acne	see p. 280	
Alopecia:		
(1) male pattern baldness:	(1) Topical minoxidil is worth trying if the patient is embarrassed by baldness. Some hair regrowth can be detected in up to 50% but it is rarely cosmetically significant	Most patients who take minoxidil orally for hypertension experience some increased hair growth. It may act by a mitogenic effect on hair follicles. The response occurs in 4–12 months: stop treatment if no result in 1 year
(2) alopecia areata	(2) Although distressing, the condition is often self-limiting. A few individuals have responded to PUVA or contact sensitisation induced by diphencyprone	
Dermatitis herpetiformis	Dapsone is typically effective in 24 h, or sulphapyridine. Prolonged therapy necessary. A gluten-free diet can help	Antipruritics locally as required. Not other sulphonamides; beneficial effect not due to antimicrobial action. Methaemoglobinaemia may complicate dapsone therapy
Eczema		
Acute weeping	Lotions (aluminium acetate, calamine), wet dressings or soaks (sodium chloride, potassium permanganate); topical corticosteroid cream or lotion with antimicrobial if infected	Remove the cause where possible. Often exacerbated by soap and water. Antipruritics (not antihistamines or local anaesthetics) may be added to lotions, creams or pastes
Subacute	Zinc oxide cream or paste, with mild keratolytic if skin thickening present (salicylic acid or coal tar added); topical corticosteroid ointment	Gamolenic acid (Epogam, evening primrose oil) an essential fatty acid which is one of the cell wall precursors of immunomodulatory and anti-inflammatory prostaglandins; use is controversial. Taken longterm, it may benefit atopic eczema, especially itch and scaling. Possibility of benefit in a variety of other diseases is being explored
Chronic, with dry scaly lesions	Keratolytics and moisturising creams and emollients; topical corticosteroid	For severe chronic dermatitis consider phototherapy (PUVA), azathioprine or even cyclosporin
Exfoliative dermatitis	Chelating agent if due to a heavy metal. Cooling creams and powders locally. Adrenal steroid systemically when severe	
Hirsutism in women	*In severe cases*: combined oestrogen/progestogen contraceptive pill: or cyproterone plus ethinyloestradiol (Dianette). Spironolactone, cimetidine have been used	Local cosmetic approaches: epilation by wax or electrolysis: depilation (chemical), e.g. thioglycollic acid, barium sulphide
Hyperhidrosis	Astringents reduce sweat production, especially aluminium chloride hexahydrate (20%) in ethyl alcohol (95%). Antimuscarinics (topical) may help and high local concentrations can be obtained with iontophoresis. Surgery, cryotherapy or radiation in extreme cases	Treatment better in theory than in practice; the volume of sweat dilutes the topical application; the characteristic smell is produced by bacterial action, so cosmetic deodorants contain antibacterials rather than substances that reduce sweat production
Ichthyosis or xeroderma	Emollients to hydrate and smooth the skin, e.g. emulsifying ointment. Very severe variants may need acitretin	Avoid degreasing skin, e.g. by domestic detergents
Infections	see p. 281	
Intertrigo	Cleansing lotions, powders. A dilute corticosteroid with anticandida cream is often helpful	To cleanse, lubricate and reduce friction

(Cont'd)

Table 16.2 *(Cont'd)*

Condition	Treatment	Remarks
Lichen planus	Antipruritics; potent topical corticosteroid (rarely systemic)	May be drug caused, e.g. a phenothiazine or antimalarial
Lichen simplex (neurodermatitis)	Antipruritics; topical corticosteroid; explain scratch–itch cycle to patient	Covering the lesion so as to prevent scratching, e.g. with a medicated bandage, sometimes breaks the vicious cycle
Lupus erythematosus affecting the skin	Potent adrenal steroid topically or intralesionally. Hydroxychloroquine or mepacrine. Monitor for retinal toxicity when treatment is longterm	A systemic disease
Marginal blepharitis (various organisms)	Ointment containing adrenal steroid and an antimicrobial	Undue persistence can be due to allergy to treatment
Nappy rash	*Prevention*: rid reusable nappies of soaps, detergents and ammonia by rinsing. Change frequently and use an emollient cream, e.g. aqueous cream, to protect skin. Costly disposable nappies are useful. *Cure*: mild: Zn cream or calamine lotion, plus above measures. Severe: adrenal steroid topically, plus antimicrobial	
Pediculosis (lice) (head, body, genitals)	Malathion or carbaryl; (anticholinesterases, with safety depending on more rapid metabolism in man than in insects, and on low absorption). Alternatively, phenothrin or permethrin[8]	Ritual of application is important
Pemphigus and pemphigoid	Adrenal steroids topically and systemically: other immunosuppressives, e.g. azathioprine as an adrenal sparing agent; gold	Oral hygiene and general nutrition very important
Photosensitivity	see p. 273	
Pityriasis rosea	Antipruritics as appropriate	The disease is self-limiting
Pruritus	see p. 270	
Psoriasis	see p. 279	
Rosacea	Tetracycline; metronidazole, orally or topically	Corticosteroid exacerbates. Flushing makes it worse. Oestrogens for menopausal flushing
Scabies (*Sarcoptes scabiei*)	Permethrin dermal cream or lindane. In resistant cases consider monosulfiram or benzyl benzoate. Alternative: ivermectin (single dose). Crotamiton or calamine for residual itch	Apply to all members of the household, immediate family or partner. Change underclothes and bedclothes
Seborrhoeic dermatitis: dandruff (*Pityriasis capitis*)	A proprietary shampoo with pyrithione, selenium sulphide or coal tar; ketoconazole shampoo in more severe cases. Occasionally a corticosteroid lotion may be necessary. Keratolytics, e.g. Cocois are helpful if there is much scaling	
Sunburn	(see p. 273)	
Urticaria	(see p. 281)	
Vitiligo	No safe and reliable treatment. Methoxsalen or other psoralen, topically or systemically, plus daily exposure to UVA (PUVA) is toxic, and ineffective in Caucasians. Sunscreens to protect the depigmented areas and reduce pigmentation of surrounding skin	Probably an autoimmune disease. Note: dose-dependent risk of squamous cell cancer with PUVA

(Cont'd)

Table 16.2 *(Cont'd)*

Condition	Treatment	Remarks
Warts	All treatments are *destructive* and should be applied with precision. Cryotherapy (liquid nitrogen, solid CO_2). Salicylic acid 12% in collodion daily. Many other caustic (keratolytic) preparations exist, e.g. salicylic and lactic acid paint or gel. For plantar warts formaldehyde or glutaraldehyde; podophyllin (antimitotic) for plantar or anogenital warts. Follow the manufacturer's instructions meticulously. If one topical therapy fails it is worth trying a different type	Nonsurgical remedies may act by disrupting the wart so that virus is absorbed, antibodies develop and the wart is rejected immunologically. Warts often disappear spontaneously
X-ray dermatitis	Emollient and dilute topical corticosteroid	

Individual disorders

> **If it's wet, dry it; if it's dry, wet it**. The traditional advice contains enough truth to be worth repeating. One or two applications a day are all that is usually necessary unless common sense dictates otherwise.

Table 16.2 is not intended to give the complete treatment of even the commoner skin conditions but merely to indicate a reasonable approach.

Secondary infections of ordinarily uninfected lesions may require added topical or systemic antimicrobials.

Analgesics, sedatives or tranquillisers may be needed in painful or uncomfortable conditions, or where the disease is intensified by emotion or anxiety. Antidepressants may be helpful even where clinical depression is not apparent, particularly in chronic diseases.

Formulations for use on the skin. At the time of writing there are in the UK about 280 preparations for medical prescription (excluding minor variants and many of those on direct sale to the public). It is not practicable to give other than general guidance on choice. Physicians will select a modest range of products and get to know these well.

---

[8] Stichele R H V et al 1995 British Medical Journal 311: 604. This review of 28 *randomised* trials of treatment of *head lice* found evidence of efficacy only for permethrin; more evidence of efficacy was deemed necessary for malthion and carbaryl.

PSORIASIS

In psoriasis there is increased ($\times$ 10) epidermal undifferentiated cell proliferation and inflammation of the epidermis and dermis. The consequence of increased numbers of horn cells containing abnormal keratin is that no normal stratum corneum is formed. Drugs are used

- to *dissolve keratin* (keratolysis)
- *to inhibit cell division*.

An emollient such as aqueous cream reduces the inflammation. The proliferated cells may be eliminated by a *dithranol* (antimitotic) preparation applied accurately to the lesions (but not on the face) for 1 hour and removed; begin with 0.1% and increase to 1%. Dithranol is available in cream bases or in Lassar's paste (the preparations are not interchangeable). It is used daily until the lesions have disappeared; it is irritant to normal skin and stains skin and fabrics. Tar preparations are less effective alternatives, and are commonly used for psoriasis of the scalp.[9]

Topical adrenal steroid reduces epidermal cell division, and application, especially under occlu-

---

[9] But are not without risk. A 46-year-old man whose psoriasis was treated with topical corticosteroids, UV light and tar was seen in the hospital courtyard bursting into flames. A small ring of fire began several centimeters above the sternal notch and encircled his neck. The patient promptly put out the fire. He admitted to lighting a cigarette just before the fire, the path of which corresponded to the distribution of the tar on his body. Fader D J et al 1994 New England Journal of Medicine 330: 1541.

sive dressings, can be very effective, but increasing doses (concentrations) become necessary and rebound, which may be severe, follows withdrawal. Potent corticosteroid should never be used except for lesions on the scalp, palms and soles. *Systemic* corticosteroid administration should be avoided if at all possible (except for very brief use in very severe exacerbations), for high doses are needed to suppress the disease, which is liable to recur when treatment is withdrawn, as it must be if complications of longterm steroid therapy are to be avoided.

Calcipotriol is an analogue of calcitriol, the most active natural form of vitamin D (p. 670). Used topically it appears to be about as effective as dithranol and corticosteroid. It inhibits cell proliferation and encourages cell differentiation. Although it has less effect on calcium metabolism than does calcitriol, excessive use (greater than 100 g/week) can raise the plasma calcium concentration.

Vitamin A (retinols) plays a role in epithelial function and the retinoic acid derivative, *acitretin* (Neotigason, orally), inhibits psoriatic hyperkeratosis over 4–6 weeks. Acitretin should be used in courses (6–9 months) with intervals (3–4 months). It is **teratogenic**, like other vitamin A derivatives. Rigorous precautions for use in women of childbearing potential are laid down by the manufacturer and must be followed, including contraception for 2 years after cessation, because the drug is stored in the liver and in fat and released over many months. The plasma $t^{1/2}$ is 3 months. It can cause other serious toxicity (see Vitamin A).

A psoralen followed by ultraviolet light (PUVA) is used in severe cases (see Psoralens, p. 274).

Folic acid antagonists, e.g. methotrexate, also suppress epidermal activity temporarily, as does *cyclosporin*, but they are too toxic for use unless the psoriasis is life-threatening or severely disabling and, preferably, the patients are past their reproductive years.

It is plain from this brief outline that treatment of psoriasis requires considerable judgement and choice will depend on the patient's sex, age and the severity of the condition. The combination of UVB and dithranol is probably the safest. When psoriasis is moderate-to-severe a strategy of rotation of treat-

ments, e.g. UVB plus dithranol → PUVA → acitretin → UVB plus dithranol and so on may help to reduce the unwanted effects of any one therapy.

ACNE

Acne results from disordered function of the pilosebaceous follicle whereby abnormal keratin and sebum (the production of which is androgen driven), form debris which plugs the mouth of the follicle. *Propionibacterium acnes* colonises the debris. Bacterial action releases inflammatory fatty acids from the sebum.

The following measures are used progressively and selectively as the disease is more severe; they may need to be applied for up to 6 months:

- *Abrasive agents:* aluminium salt particles.
- *Mild keratolytic* (exfoliating, peeling) formulations unblock pilosebaceous ducts, e.g. benzoyl peroxide, sulphur, salicylic acid, azelaic acid.
- *Systemic or topical antimicrobial therapy* (tetracycline, minocycline, erythromycin, at low dose) is used over months (response begins after 2 months). Bacterial resistance is not a problem; benefit is due to suppression of bacterial lipolysis of sebum, which generates inflammatory fatty acids. Raised intracranial pressure with loss of vision has occurred with tetracycline used thus.
- A topical *adrenal steroid* reduces inflammation.
- *Vitamin A* (retinoic acid) *derivatives* reduce sebum production and keratinisation. Vitamin A is a teratogen.

Tretinoin (Retin-A) is applied topically (**not** in combination with other keratolytics). It may promote UV-induced skin cancer. Tretinoin should be avoided in sunny weather, and in pregnancy. Benefit is seen in about 10 weeks.

Isotretinoin (Roaccutane) ($t^{1/2}$ 15 h) orally is highly effective (in a course of 12–16 weeks), but is known to be a serious teratogen; its use should be confined to the *most severe cystic* and *conglobate cases*, and requires the utmost informed care and supervision. Fasting blood lipids should be measured before and during therapy (cholesterol and triglycerides may rise). Women of child-bearing potential should be carefully informed on this risk, should be pregnancy-tested before commencement and should use contraception for 4 weeks before, during and for 4 weeks after cessation.[10]

- *Hormone therapy.* The objective is to reduce androgen production or effect by using, (1) oestrogen, to suppress hypothalamic/pituitary gonadotrophin production, or (2) an antiandrogen (cyproterone). An oestrogen alone as initial therapy to get the acne under control or, in women, the cyclical use of an oral contraceptive containing 50 µg of oestrogen diminishes sebum secretion by 40%. A combination of ethinyloestradiol and cyproterone (Dianette) orally is also effective in women (it has a contraceptive effect, which is desirable as the cyproterone may feminise a male fetus).
- Topical corticosteroid should **not** be used.

URTICARIA

Acute urticaria (named after its similarity to the sting of a nettle, *Urtica*) and *angioedema* usually respond well to H_1-receptor antihistamines, although severe cases are relieved more quickly by adrenaline (adrenaline injection 1 mg/ml: 0.1–0.3 ml, s.c.). A systemic corticosteroid may be needed in severe cases.

Cold urticaria is due to release of autacoids on exposure to cold. It may respond to combined H_1- and H_2-receptor antagonists; the combination is needed to block fully the vascular effects of histamine, which cause flush and hypotension. Cyproheptadine is usually preferred as the H_1-antihistamine.

Chronic urticaria may respond to an H_1-antihistamine plus ephedrine or terbutaline, or to an H_1- plus an H_2-antihistamine.

Hereditary angioedema, with deficiency of C_1-esterase (a complement inhibitor), does not respond to antihistamines or corticosteroid but only to *fresh frozen plasma*. Delay in initiating treatment may lead to death from laryngeal oedema (try adrenaline i.m. in severe cases). For longterm prophylaxis androgen (stanozolol, danazol) is effective.

SKIN INFECTIONS

Superficial bacterial infections, e.g. impetigo, eczema, are commonly staphylococcal or streptococcal. They are treated by a topical antimicrobial for less than 2 weeks and applied twice daily after removal of crusts that prevent access of the drug, e.g. by a povidone-iodine preparation. Very extensive cases need systemic treatment.

Topical *neomycin* and *mupirocin* are preferred (as they are not ordinarily used for systemic infections and therefore development of drug resistant strains is less likely to have serious consequences). Framycetin and polymyxins are also used. Absorption of neomycin from all topical preparations can cause *serious injury* to the eighth cranial nerve.

Fusidic acid may be used, but only outside hospital where there is less risk of spread of resistant organisms, as the drug may be needed for systemic infection.

When prolonged treatment is required, topical antiseptics (hexachlorophane, povidone-iodine, cetrimide, chlorhexidine) are preferred and bacterial resistance is less of a problem.

Combination of antimicrobial with a *corticosteroid* (to suppress inflammation) is not generally useful but, if employed, there **must** be effective antimicrobial treatment or the infection may spread.

The **disadvantages** of antimicrobials are *contact allergy* and developments of *resistant organisms* (which may cause systemic, as well as local, infection). Failure to respond may be due to development of contact allergy (which may be masked by corticosteroid).

Infected leg ulcers generally do not benefit from antimicrobials. An antiseptic (plus a protective dressing with compression) is preferred if antimicrobial therapy is needed.

Nasal carriers of staphylococci may be cured (often temporarily) by topical mupirocin or neomycin plus chlorhexidine.

Formulations of antibacterials with and without corticosteroid are numerous.

---

[10] The risk of serious birth defect in a child of a woman who has taken isotretinoin when pregnant is estimated at 25%. Thousands of abortions have been done in such women in the USA. It is probable that hundreds of damaged children have been born. There can be no doubt that there has been irresponsible prescribing of this drug, e.g. in less severe cases. The fact that a drug having such a grave effect is yet permitted to be available is a tribute to its high efficacy.

Deep bacterial infections, e.g. boils, generally do not require antimicrobial therapy; but if they do it should be systemic. Cellulitis requires systemic chemotherapy.

Infected burns are treated with a variety of antimicrobials, including silver-sulphadiazine and mupirocin.

Topical antifungals include: imidazoles (e.g. clotrimazole, miconazole), Whitfield's ointment (benzoic acid ointment), nystatin (anticandidal), terbinafine or amorolfine for nail infections.

Systemic antifungals for dermal fungal and dermatophyte infections: itraconazole, griseofulvin, terbinafine.

Topical antivirals: aciclovir (acyclovir), idoxuridine (see p. 232).

Topical parasiticides (best as lotions): benzyl benzoate, carbaryl, lindane, malathion, permethrin, phenothrin.

Disinfection and cleansing of the skin. Numerous substances are used according to circumstances: ethanol or isopropyl alcohol (70%), chlorhexidine, cationic surfactants (benzalkonium, cetrimide), povidone-iodine (iodine complexed with polyvinylpyrolidone), phenol derivatives (chloroxylenol, hexachlorophane, triclosan).

GUIDE TO FURTHER READING

Barker J N W N 1991 The pathophysiology of psoriasis. Lancet 338: 227

Barker J N W N 1991 Keratinocytes as initiators of inflammation. Lancet 337: 211

Bos J D et al 1994: Pathogenesis of atopic eczema. Lancet 343: 1338

Fine J-D 1995 Management of acquired bullous skin diseases. New England Journal of Medicine 333: 1475

Gilchrest B A 1993 Sunscreens — the public health opportunity. New England Journal of Medicine 329: 1193

Greaves M W 1995 Chronic urticaria. New England Journal of Medicine 333: 1767

Greaves M W et al 1995 Treatment of psoriasis. New England Journal of Medicine 332: 581

Harper J 1994 Traditional Chinese medicine for eczema. British Medical Journal 308: 489

Healy E et al 1994 Acne vulgaris. British Medical Journal 309: 831

James M 1996 Isotretinoin for severe acne. (A patient's experience.) Lancet 347: 1749

Lowitt M H, Lowitt N R 1995 Recent advances: dermatology. British Medical Journal 311:1615

Marks R et al 1994 Sunburn and melanoma: how strong is the evidence? British Medical Journal 308: 75

Przybilla P et al 1994 Practical management of atopic eczema. Lancet 343: 1342

Roujeau J C, Stern R S 1994 Severe adverse cutaneous reactions to drugs. New England Journal of Medicine 331: 1272

Shuttleworth D 1993 Sunbeds and the pursuit of the year round tan. British Medical Journal 307: 1508

Simpson N 1988 Treating hyperhidrosis. British Medical Journal 296: 1345

NERVOUS SYSTEM

Pain and analgesics

> But pain is perfect misery, the worst
> Of evils, and, excessive, overturns
> All patience.
> (John Milton, 1608–1674, Paradise Lost)

Pain

Pain is an unpleasant sensory and emotional experience associated with actual or potential tissue damage, or described in terms of such damage.[1]

The word 'unpleasant' comprises the whole range of disagreeable feelings from being merely inconvenienced to misery, anguish, anxiety, depression and desperation, to the ultimate cure of suicide.[2]

- **Analgesic drug**: a drug that relieves pain due to multiple causes, e.g. aspirin, paracetamol, morphine. Drugs that relieve pain due to a single cause or specific pain syndrome only, e.g. ergotamine (migraine), carbamazepine (neuralgias), glyceryl trinitrate (angina pectoris), are not classed as analgesics; nor are adrenocortical steroids that suppress pain of inflammation of any cause.
- Analgesics are classed as **narcotic** (which act in the central nervous system and cause drowsiness, i.e. opioids) and **non-narcotic** (which act chiefly peripherally, e.g. aspirin).
- **Adjuvant drugs** are those used alongside analgesics in the management of pain. They are not

---

[1] Merskey H et al 1979 Pain terms: a list with definitions and notes on usage. Pain 6: 249.

[2] Melzack R, Wall P 1982 The challenge of pain. Penguin, London.

themselves analgesics, though they may modify the perception or the concomitants of pain that make it worse (anxiety, fear, depression),[3] e.g. psychotropic drugs, or they may modify underlying causes, e.g. spasm of smooth or of voluntary muscle.

The general principle that the best treatment of a symptom is removal of its cause applies. But this is often impossible to achieve and symptom relief of pain by analgesic drug is required.

Pain is the commonest symptom that takes patients to doctors, but the complaint does not mean that an analgesic is needed.

Optimal management of pain requires that the clinician should have a conceptual framework for what is happening to the patient in mind and body.

- *Acute* pain is managed primarily (but not invariably) by analgesic drugs.
- *Chronic* pain often requires adjuvant drugs in addition as well as nondrug measures.

Analgesics are chosen according to the cause of pain and its severity.

Phenomenon of pain

An understanding of the phenomenon of pain ought to accommodate the following points:

- Pain can occur without tissue injury or evident disease and can persist after injury has healed.
- Serious tissue injury can occur without pain.
- Emotion (anxiety, fear, depression) is an inseparable concomitant of pain and can modify both its intensity and the victim's behavioural response.
- There is important processing of afferent nociceptive (see below) and other impulses in the spinal cord and brain.

Appreciation that pain is both a sensory and an

emotional (affective) experience has allowed clinicians to realise that to meet a complaint of pain automatically with a prescription alone is not an appropriate response, for 'There is always more to analgesia than analgesics'.[4] Pain that is not the subject of an analysis by the clinician (and explanation to the patient) may be inadequately relieved because of lack of understanding. That doctors often do not provide adequate relief of severe pain (postsurgical, palliative care of advanced cancer) by bad choice and by overusing and, also important, underusing drugs, and by defective relations with their patients, has been, and still is, a justified and shaming criticism.

THE VARIOUS ASPECTS OF PAIN

Pain is not simply a perception, it is a complex phenomenon or syndrome, only one component of which is the sensation actually reported as pain.

Pain has 4 major aspects present to varying extent in any one case:

Nociception[5] is a consequence of tissue injury (trauma, inflammation) causing the release of chemical mediators (p. 288) which activate nociceptors (chemosensitive nerve endings) in the tissue. Nociceptors are specialised nerve endings serving their own afferent fibres (A-delta and C); nociception is not due to overstimulation of touch or other receptors.

Pain sensation is a result of nociceptive input *plus* a pattern of impulses of different frequency and intensity from other peripheral receptors, e.g. heat, and mechanoreceptors whose threshold of response is reduced by the chemical mediators. These are processed in the brain whence modulating inhibitory impulses pass down to regulate the continuing afferent input. But pain can occur without nociception (some neuralgias)[6] and nociception

---

[3] Tricyclic antidepressants may reduce morphine requirement in terminal care without noticeably altering mood.

[4] Twycross R G 1984 Journal of the Royal College of Physicians of London 18: 32.

[5] Latin: *noxa*: injury.

[6] *Neuralgia* is pain felt in the distribution of a peripheral nerve.

does not invariably cause pain; pain is a psychological state though most pain has an immediately antecedent physical cause.

Suffering is a consequence of pain and of lack of understanding by patients of the meaning of the pain; it comprises anxiety and fear (particularly in acute pain) and depression (particularly in chronic pain), which will be affected by patients' personalities, and their beliefs about the significance of the pain, e.g. whether merely a postponed holiday, or death, or a future of disability with loss of independence. Depression makes a major contribution to suffering; it is treatable, as are the other affective concomitants of pain.

Pain behaviour comprises consequences of the other three aspects (above); it includes behaviour that is interpreted by others as signifying pain in the victim, e.g. such immediate and obvious aspects as facial expression, restlessness, seeking isolation (or company), medicine-taking, as well as, in chronic pain, the development of querulousness, depression, despair and social withdrawal.

The clinician's task is to determine the significance of these items for each patient and to direct therapy accordingly. Analgesics may, but not necessarily will, be the mainstay of therapy; adjuvant (nonanalgesic) drugs may be needed, as well as nondrug therapy (radiation, surgery).

It is also useful to distinguish between acute pain (an event whose end can be predicted) and chronic pain (a situation whose end is commonly unpredictable, or will only end with life itself).

Acute pain (transmitted by fast conducting A-delta fibres) with major nociceptive input (physical trauma, pleurisy, myocardial infarct, perforated peptic ulcer) is seen by patients as a transient, though sometimes severe threat and they react accordingly. It is a symptom that may be dealt with unhesitatingly and effectively with drugs, by injection if necessary, at the same time as the causative disease is addressed. The accompanying anxiety will vary according to the severity of the pain, and particularly according to its meaning for the patient, whether termination with recovery will soon occur, major surgery is threatened, or there is prospect of death or invalidism. The choice of drug will depend on the clinician's assessment of these factors. Morphine by injection has retained a pre-eminent place for over 100 years because it has highly effective antinociceptive and anti-anxiety effects; modern opioids have not rendered morphine obsolete.

Acute pain without nociceptive (afferent) *input* (some neuralgias) is less susceptible to drugs unless consciousness is also depressed, and any frequently recurrent acute pain, e.g. trigeminal neuralgia, poses management problems that are more akin to chronic pain.

Chronic pain (transmitted by slow conducting type C fibres) is better regarded as a syndrome[7] rather than as a symptom (see above). It presents a depressing future to the victim who sees no prospect of release from suffering, and poses for that reason longterm management problems that differ from acute pain. Suffering and affective disorders can be of over-riding importance and the consequences of poor management may be prolonged and serious for the patient. Analgesics alone are often insufficient and adjuvant drugs as well as nondrug therapy gain increasing importance. Even when they are effective in chronic pain, the high-efficacy opioids (morphine, pethidine) alter mood and carry a substantial risk of dependence that will have adverse consequences in the long term. Continuous use of these drugs is best avoided in chronic pain, except that of palliative care. But the lower efficacy opioids (codeine, dextropropoxyphene) may often be needed and used. Sedation should be avoided and therapy should be oral if possible; regimens should be planned to avoid breakthrough pain. Antidepressants can often be useful.

Sedative-hypnotic drugs, e.g. benzodiazepines, may be needed for anxiety but may induce depression.

Chronic pain syndrome is a term used for persistence of pain when detectable disease has disappeared, e.g. after an attack of low back pain. It characteristically does not respond to standard treatment with analgesics. Whether the basis is neurogenic, psychogenic or sociocultural it should not be managed by intensi-

---

[7] A set of symptoms and signs that are characteristic of a condition though they may not always have the same cause (Greek: *syn:* together, *dramein:* to run).

fying drug treatment. Opioid analgesics, which may be producing dependence, should be withdrawn and the use of psychotropic drugs, e.g. antidepressants or neuroleptics, and nondrug therapy, including psychotherapy, should be considered.

MECHANISMS OF ANALGESIA

Endogenous opioid neurotransmitters (endorphins, dynorphins, enkephalins) in the spinal cord and brain constitute a pain inhibitory system that is activated by nociceptive and other input, including treatments such as transcutaneous nerve stimulation and acupuncture. Administered opioids produce analgesia via the specific opioid receptors of this system. The fact that there are several types of receptor — μ(mu), δ(delta), κ(kappa), ϵ(epsilon), σ(sigma) — explains the differing patterns of actions of opioids. Analgesia is associated with μ- and κ-, dysphoria or psychomimetic effects with σ-, and alteration in affective behaviour with δ-receptors. Receptor subtypes are also recognised, analgesia, euphoria and dependence being associated with effects on the μ_1; and respiratory depression and inhibition of gut motility with actions on the μ_2-receptor. Thus there is hope that new selective high-efficacy analgesics free from the disadvantages of the existing opioids may be designed.

Naloxone, the competitive opioid antagonist, binds to and blocks all opioid receptors but exerts no activating effect. Naloxone has particularly high affinity for the μ-receptor; it has been found to worsen (dental) pain, an effect that may be explained by blocking access of endogenous opioids to their receptor(s).[8] Naloxone does not induce hyperalgesia or spontaneous pain because the opioid paths are quiescent until activated by nociceptive and other afferent input.

In addition to these opioid mechanisms, nonopioid mediated pathways, e.g. serotonin, are important in pain. There is suggestion that opioid mechanisms are more important in acute severe pain, and nonopioid mechanisms in chronic pain, and that this may be relevant to choice of drugs.

NSAIDs. When a tissue is injured (any cause), or even merely stimulated, *prostaglandin synthesis* in that tissue increases. Prostaglandins have two major actions: they are mediators of inflammation and they also sensitise nerve endings, lowering their threshold of response to stimuli, mechanical (the tenderness of inflammation) and chemical, allowing the other mediators of inflammation, e.g. histamine, serotonin, bradykinin, to intensify the activation of the sensory endings.

Plainly, a drug that prevents the synthesis of prostaglandins is likely to be effective in relieving pain due to inflammation of any kind, and this is indeed how aspirin and other nonsteroidal anti-inflammatory drugs (NSAIDs) act. This discovery was made in 1971, aspirin having been extensively used in medicine since 1899.[9] NSAIDs act by inhibiting cyclo-oxygenase (prostaglandin G/H synthase). Thus it is evident that NSAIDs will relieve pain when there is some tissue injury with consequent inflammation, as there almost always is with pain. They also act in the central nervous system (prostaglandins, despite their name, are synthesised in all cells except erythrocytes) and there is probably some central component to the analgesic effect of NSAIDs.

But, analgesic and anti-inflammatory effects are not parallel, e.g. aspirin relieves pain rapidly at doses that do not significantly reduce inflammation and the onset of its anti-inflammatory effect at higher doses may be slow. Paracetamol is an effective analgesic for mild pain but has little anti-inflammation effect in arthritis, though substantial effect on post-dental extraction swelling. Other NSAIDs show a different mix of action against pain and inflammation (see Ch. 15).

Corticosteroids diminish inflammation of all kinds by preventing prostaglandin synthesis (the phospholipase A_2 that releases arachidonic acid for such synthesis is inhibited by lipocortin-1 which is produced in response to glucosteroids). Short-term use may be valuable; longterm use poses many problems

---

[8] Naloxone also appears to cause *pyrovats* (practitioners of religious firewalking ceremonies) to quicken their pace over the hot coals.

[9] Propagandists for complementary (alternative) medicine allege that conventional scientific medicine will not recognise any therapy, e.g. complementary medicine, unless its mode of action is known. This is untrue. Validated empirical observation, i.e. scientific evidence, is and always has been accepted.

(see Ch. 35); in general the corticosteroid should be withdrawn after one week if there is no benefit.

The pain threshold is lowered by anxiety, fear, depression, anger, sadness, fatigue, or insomnia, and is raised by relief of these (by drug or nondrug measures) and by successful relief of pain.

Since emotion is such an important factor in pain, it is no surprise that placebo tablets or injections alleviate pain, usually in about 35% of cases, but with the added disadvantage that they rapidly lose effect with repetition.

The importance of the meaning of pain to its victim is illustrated by injuries of war and of civilian life:

> To the wounded soldier who had been under unremitting shell fire for weeks, his wound was a good thing (it meant the end of the war for him) and was associated with far less pain than was the case of the civilians who considered their need for surgery a disaster.[10]

The desire for analgesics has been found to be less amongst victims of battle injuries than amongst comparable civilian injuries. On the other hand, morphine has been found to be relatively ineffective against experimental pain in man, probably because it acts best against pain that has emotional significance for the patient.

New analgesics have been successfully developed by animal testing, possibly because the emotional response to experimental pain in an animal is akin to the human response to disease or accidental injury. This emotional response does not generally occur in a subject who has volunteered to undergo laboratory experiments that can be stopped at any time, and it probably accounts for the fact that a placebo gives relief in only 3% of these cases.

Clinical evaluation of analgesics

Therapeutic trials in acute pain are often conducted on patients who have undergone abdominal surgery or third molar tooth extraction, and in chronic pain on chronic rheumatic conditions. Only the patients can say what they feel and pain is best measured by a questionnaire or by a visual analogue scale; this is a line, 10 or 20 cm long, one end of which represents pain 'as bad as it could possibly be' (which patients identify as 'agonising') and the other end 'no pain'; patients mark the line at the point they feel represents their pain between these two extremes. Such techniques are highly reproducible.

Adverse effects are, of course, simultaneously recorded and taken into account when deciding clinical utility. Since what is being measured is how patients say they feel, the trial must be double-blind. Observers who interrogate the patients for relief (intensity and duration) and adverse effects must be constant and trained. If asked by a personable young woman, a higher proportion of patients (of both sexes) admit to pain relief than if the same question is put by a man.

Choice of analgesics

RANKED BY CLINICAL EFFICACY[11]
(see also ranking of opioids, p. 304)

Mild pain

- Non-narcotic (nonopioid) analgesics or NSAIDs, e.g. aspirin, ibuprofen, paracetamol.[12] (Ch. 15)

Where these fail after using the full dose range, proceed to:

Moderate pain

- Narcotic (opioid) analgesics, low-efficacy opioids, e.g. codeine, dihydrocodeine, dextropropoxyphene, pentazocine.
- Combined therapy of NSAIDs plus low-

---

[10] Beecher H K 1957 Pharmacological Review 9: 59.

[11] Based on Twycross R G 1978 In: Saunders Cicely M (ed) The management of terminal disease. Arnold, London. The work of this author contributes much to this chapter.

[12] Paracetamol is sometimes not classed as an NSAID because its anti-inflammatory pattern differs substantially from most, i.e. its anti-inflammatory efficacy is weak in rheumatoid arthritis.

efficacy opioid, not necessarily as a fixed-dose formulation, many of which have an inadequate dose of one or other ingredient (see below) so that separate administration is commonly preferable though less convenient.

Where these fail proceed to:

Severe pain

● High-efficacy opioids, e.g. morphine, diamorphine, pethidine, buprenorphine. An added NSAID is useful if there is a substantial tissue injury component, e.g. gout, bone metastasis.

Overwhelming acute pain

● High efficacy opioid plus a sedative/anxiolytic (diazepam) or a phenothiazine tranquilliser, e.g. chlorpromazine, methotrimeprazine (which also has analgesic effect).

Note: adjuvant drugs (p. 297) may be useful in all grades of pain.

'KEEPING IT SIMPLE'[13]

The three basic analgesics are aspirin, codeine and morphine. Appreciating this helps to prevent the doctor 'kangarooing' from analgesic to analgesic in a desperate search for some drug that will suit the patient better. If non-narcotic or weak narcotic preparations such as aspirin-codeine, paracetamol-dextropropoxyphene, fail to relieve, it is usually best to move directly to a small dose of morphine [the quoted author refers to chronic cancer pain] than, for example, to prescribe dihydrocodeine, i.e. change to an analgesic of higher efficacy rather than to another of similar efficacy.

It is necessary to be familiar with one or two alternatives for use in patients who cannot tolerate the standard preparation. The individual doctor's basic analgesic ladder, with alternatives, should comprise no more than nine or ten drugs in total. It is better to know and understand a few drugs well than to have a passing acquaintance with the whole range.

[13] Twycross R G 1984 Journal of the Royal College of Physicians of London 18: 32. The author is a leading authority on pain control and the management of terminal disease.

USING TWO ANALGESICS

Simultaneous use of two analgesics of different modes of action is rational, but two drugs of the same class/mechanism of action are unlikely to benefit unless there is a difference in emphasis, e.g. analgesia and anti-inflammatory action (paracetamol plus aspirin), or in duration of action; a patient taking an NSAID with a long duration, e.g. naproxen (used once or twice a day), is benefited by an additional drug of shorter duration for an acute exacerbation, e.g. ibuprofen, aspirin.

A low-efficacy opioid can reduce the effectiveness of a high-efficacy opioid by successfully competing with the latter for receptors. Partial agonist (agonist/antagonist) opioids, e.g. pentazocine, will also antagonise the action of other opioids, e.g. heroin, and may even induce the withdrawal syndrome in dependent subjects.

FIXED-RATIO (COMPOUND) COMBINATIONS

Large numbers of these are offered particularly to bridge the efficacy gap between aspirin or paracetamol and morphine. Many have an inadequate dose of one or other ingredient, e.g. codeine 5 mg, caffeine 10 mg. Doctors should consider the formulae of these preparations before using them.

Caffeine has been shown to enhance the analgesic effect of aspirin and of paracetamol and to accelerate the onset of effect, but at least 30 mg and probably 60 mg are needed (a cup of coffee averages about 80 mg and of tea averages about 30 mg).

Tablets containing paracetamol (325 mg) plus dextropropoxyphene (32.5 mg) (co-proxamol, Distalgesic), in a dose of 1–2 tablets, provide an effective dose of both drugs and have been extremely popular with both prescribers and patients; its popularity may be influenced by a mild euphoriant effect of the opioid, to which dependence can occur. A major concern is that in (deliberate) overdose death may occur within one hour due to the rapid absorption of the dextropropoxyphene, and combination with alcohol appears seriously to add to the hazard.

We do not attempt to rank the many preparations available because comparative evidence is lacking.

Treatment of pain syndromes

In general, pain (acute or chronic) arising from *somatic structures* (skin, muscles, bones, joints) responds to analgesics such as aspirin and paracetamol (non-narcotic), which do not alter psychic function and do not induce serious dependence (addiction). But pain arising from *the viscera* is most readily reduced by morphine[14] (narcotic), which alters both the pain threshold and the psychic reaction to pain and induces dependence with prolonged use. This distinction is not, of course, absolute and a high-efficacy opioid is needed for severe somatic pain. Mild pain from any source may respond to the non-narcotic analgesics and these should always be tried first.

SPASM OF VISCERAL SMOOTH MUSCLE

Pain due to spasm of visceral smooth muscle, e.g. biliary, renal colic, when severe, requires a substantial dose of morphine, pethidine or buprenorphine. These drugs themselves cause spasm of visceral smooth muscle and so have a simultaneous action tending to increase the pain. Phenazocine and buprenorphine are less liable to cause spasm. An antimuscarinic drug such as atropine or hyoscine may be given simultaneously to antagonise this effect.

Prostaglandins are involved in control of smooth muscle and colic can be treated with NSAIDs, e.g. diclofenac, indomethacin (i.m., suppository or oral).

SPASM OF STRIATED MUSCLE

This is often a cause of pain, including chronic tension headache. Treatment is directed at reduction of the spasm in a variety of ways, including psychotherapy, sedation and the use of a centrally-acting muscle relaxant as well as non-narcotic analgesics, e.g. chlormezanone plus paracetamol

(Lobak), baclofen, diazepam, meprobamate; clinical efficacy is variable (see Other muscle relaxants, p. 387). Local infiltration with lignocaine is sometimes appropriate.

NEURALGIAS

Postherpetic neuralgia, trigeminal neuralgia, causalgia can present the most challenging problems. Analgesics may play only a subsidiary part in their management. In severe cases very high doses of non-narcotic analgesics with low-efficacy opioid are often reached with little benefit and an almost inevitable demand for high-efficacy opioid follows, with the risk of serious dependence as well as of inefficacy at doses that leave consciousness unimpaired. Psychotropic drugs may be useful adjuvants.

The antiepilepsy drug, carbamazepine (p. 361), was accidentally discovered to be effective in trigeminal neuralgia, probably by reducing excitability of the trigeminal nucleus. The initial dose should be low, and individuals generally soon learn to alter it themselves during remissions and exacerbations (200–1600 mg/d). It is not used for prophylaxis.

In resistant neuralgias phenytoin (which raises the threshold of nerve cells to electrical stimulation), baclofen and antidepressants or neuroleptics (which may potentiate analgesics and also have an independent effect) may be tried.

- *Herpes zoster*. The pain of the acute condition is mitigated by NSAIDs and opioids (as well as by oral aciclovir started within 48 h of the rash).
- *Postherpetic neuralgia*. Whether the incidence of this complication is reliably reduced by early treatment with antivirus drugs has yet to be proved. The established condition may be helped by drugs used for trigeminal neuralgia, including antidepressants. Conventional analgesics are ineffective. Transcutaneous nerve stimulation (TENS) helps some sufferers; it may act by promoting the release of endorphins.
- *Phantom limb pain* is commonly resistant to analgesics; clonazepam is worth trying. Prolonged relief may follow transient changes in sensory input, i.e. a decrease (local anaesthetic to sensitive spots in the stump) or an increase (vibration).

---

[14] Surgeons are rightly concerned that diagnosis of the acute abdomen be not hindered by a large dose of morphine administered with humane intent by the primary care doctor who first sees the patient.

- *Thalamic pain*, e.g. following a stroke, commonly fails to respond to analgesics. Chlorpromazine, carbamazepine and other adjuvant drugs may help.

OTHER PAIN SYNDROMES

- Inflammation responds to NSAIDs but may need support from a low-efficacy opioid.
  - Arthritis: see Chapter 15.
- Minor trauma, e.g. many sports injuries, is commonly treated by local skin cooling (spray of chlorofluoromethanes), counterirritants (see Index) and NSAIDs systemically or topically.
- Severe trauma including postsurgical pain (p. 377) usually needs narcotic analgesics.
- Peripheral vascular insufficiency should be treated with non-narcotic analgesics but may eventually require low efficacy opioids; vasodilator drugs may, but equally may not, provide benefit.
- Malignant disease requires the full range of analgesics and adjuvant drugs and procedures (see Palliative care, below).
- Bone pain, including cancer metastases, requires NSAIDs alone and with opioids.
- Nerve compression can be relieved by corticosteroid (prednisolone) or nerve block (local anaesthetic); nerve destruction can be achieved by alcohol, phenol.
  - Dysmenorrhoea, see page 662.
- Mastalgia may benefit from gamolenic acid (in evening primrose oil), danazol and bromocriptine; or from a combined contraceptive pill.
- In sickle cell anaemia crises avoid pethidine as the metabolite norpethidine may accumulate; hydroxyurea reduces the frequency.[15]

HEADACHE

Headache originating inside the skull may be due to traction on or distension of arteries arising from the circle of Willis, or to traction on the dura mater. Headache originating outside the skull may be due to local striated muscle spasm;[16] an anatomical connection, only recently identified, between an extracranial muscle and the cervical dura mater may help to explain headache of cervical origin. Treatment by drugs is directed to relieving the muscle spasm, producing vasoconstriction or simply administering analgesics, beginning, of course, with the non-narcotics, e.g. paracetamol and aspirin.

MIGRAINE

Migraine (classic and common) is triggered by a variety of factors, including stress (exertion, excitement, anxiety, fatigue, anger) and by food containing vasoactive amines (chocolate, cheese), by food allergy and also by hormonal changes (menstruation and oral contraceptives) and hypoglycaemia. These precipitants may initiate release of vasoactive substances stored in nerve endings and blood platelets. Attention to triggering factors is crucial to management.

The acute migraine attack appears to begin in serotonergic (5-HT) and noradrenergic neurons in the brain. These monoamines affect the cerebral and extracerebral vasculature (which may have developed abnormal responses) and they also cause release of further vasoactive substances such as histamine, prostaglandins and neuropeptides involved in pain, i.e. there is neurogenic inflammation that can be inhibited by specific antimigraine drugs (below).

The migraine aura of visual or sensory disturbance probably originates in the occipital or sensory cortex; the throbbing headache is due to dilatation of pain-sensitive arteries outside the brain, including scalp arteries.

The numerous known facts cannot yet be arranged in a coherent aetiological scheme, but the basis of rational treatment and prophylaxis is emerging; drugs with a variety of actions play an important part as is shown below.

Acute attacks. The acute migraine attack should be treated as early as possible with an oral dispersible (soluble) analgesic formulation so that it may be absorbed before there is vomiting and accompanying gastric stasis with slow and erratic drug absorption. Aspirin (600 mg) is effective and its anti-aggregatory action on the platelets may add to its advantage; paracetamol, ibuprofen and naproxen are alternatives.

---

[15] Charache S et al 1995 New England Journal of Medicine 332: 1317.

[16] As in tension headache or frontal headache from 'eyestrain'.

Metoclopramide, a dopamine agonist, is a useful antiemetic that also promotes gastric emptying and has been shown to enhance aspirin absorption. But plainly, if vomiting and gastric stasis already exist, it may not be absorbed and should be given i.m. (10 mg). Prochlorperazine (rectally), cyclizine and buclizine are alternative antiemetics.

A benzodiazepine, e.g. diazepam, is useful especially if the attack has been triggered by emotional stress, and sleep is an important remedy in migraine.

Efficient use of an analgesic, an antiemetic[17] and a sedative is adequate for 90% of acute attacks. The remaining 10% need ergotamine.

Severe migraine attacks require ergotamine (below), which, given early after the onset of headache, will benefit about 60% of those treated; or sumatriptan.

Ergotamine

Ergotamine ($t^{1}/_2$ 2 h) is a partial agonist at α-adrenoceptors (vasoconstrictor) and also a partial agonist at serotonergic receptors. It must be used with special care.

Ergotamine constricts all peripheral arteries (an effect potentiated by concomitant β-adrenoceptor block), not just those affected by the migraine process and overdose can cause peripheral gangrene; paraesthesiae in hands or feet give warning. Due to tissue binding, its effect on arteries persists as long as 24 h and repeated doses lead to cumulative effects long outlasting the migraine attack. Due to its complex actions on receptors, vasoconstriction due to overdose is best antagonised by a nonselective vasodilator such as sodium nitroprusside (rather than by an α-adrenoceptor blocker). Patients with vascular disease, coronary and peripheral, are particularly at risk.

Ergotamine is incompletely absorbed from the gastrointestinal tract and also after i.m. injection; altenative routes of administration may be preferred in the acute attack of migraine. It is extensively metabolised in the liver.

Ergotamine may be given orally (to be swallowed: crush the tablets), sublingually (bypassing gastric stasis), rectally, or by inhalation.

With *enteral* forms of ergotamine, total dosage in an acute attack should not exceed 6 mg (if there is no benefit from the first 2 mg, see below, the likelihood of higher dose being effective is small) and the maximum in one week should not exceed 10 mg.

By inhalation (360 µg per puff of metered aerosol), a puff may be given every 5 min for up to 6 puffs (2.2 mg in an attack) and in one week 15 puffs (5.4 mg) are maximum.

Mild overdose causes nausea and vomiting and can worsen headache (ergot has the complex agonist/antagonist action characteristic of ergot derivatives, p. 662) and this can lead patients and incautious doctors to think the migraine is uncontrolled and to increase the dose, with disastrous consequences. In one case of overdose a doctor overprescribed ergotamine and the dispensing pharmacist did not query the prescription. A court of law found both doctor and pharmacist to have been negligent and ordered doctor and pharmacist to share a payment of compensation to the patient, who had suffered peripheral gangrene.

Ergotamine is a powerful oxytocic and is dangerous in pregnancy. It may precipitate angina pectoris, probably by increasing cardiac pre- and afterload (venous and arterial constriction) rather than by constricting coronary arteries.

Ergotamine should not be used within 6 h of the last dose of sumatriptan (below); similarly sumatriptan should not be given until 24 h have elapsed after stopping ergotamine.

Caffeine enhances absorption of ergotamine (both speed and peak blood concentration) and is often combined with it (though it may prevent sleep). Ergotamine should not be used for prophylaxis of migraine.

Dihydroergotamine is less effective than ergotamine.

Sumatriptan

Sumatriptan (Imigran) ($t^{1}/_2$ 2 h) selectively stimulates a subtype of 5-hydroxytryptamine$_1$ receptors (called '5-HT$_1$-like' receptors) which are found in cranial blood vesssels, causing them to constrict. It is rapidly absorbed after oral administration and

---

[17] Patients report benefit from combinations of antiemetic (metoclopramide or buclizine) plus aspirin or paracetamol, sometimes with small amounts of codeine or docusate sodium, e.g. Migraleve, Migravess, Paramax.

undergoes extensive (84%) presystemic metabolism; but bioavailability by the s.c. route is 96%.

For acute migraine sumatriptan 6 mg is given s.c. as early as possible in the attack, the dose to be repeated once if necessary after 1 h but the total should not exceed 12 mg in 24 h. The oral dose is 100 mg, the 24 h total not to exceed 300 mg. Sumatriptan is also effective for the acute treatment of cluster headaches.

Sumatriptan is generally well tolerated. Malaise, fatigue, dizziness, vertigo and sedation are associated with oral use. Nausea and vomiting may follow oral or s.c. administration. The most important adverse effects are feelings of chest pressure, tightness and pain in about 5% of cases; these may be accompanied by cardiac dysrhythmia and myocardial infarction and appear to be due to coronary artery spasm. Patients with ischaemic heart disease, unstable angina or previous myocardial infarction should not be given sumatriptan; use after ergotamine (see above).

Drug prophylaxis of migraine

This should be considered when, after adjustment of lifestyle, there are still two or more attacks per month. Benefit may be delayed for several weeks.

Options (which may help up to 60% of patients) include:

- *β-adrenoceptor block* by propranolol(dl); (the d-isomer, which lacks β-blocking action though it has membrane stabilising effect, also prevents migraine), as do other pure antagonists (atenolol, metoprolol) but not partial (ant)agonists, see page 437. It seems that β-adrenoceptor block is not the prime therapeutic action. Note that if ergotamine (for an acute attack) is given to a patient taking propranolol for prophylaxis there is risk of additive vasoconstriction (block of β-receptor mediated dilatation with added α-receptor constriction).
- *Calcium entry blockers*, e.g. verapamil, flunarizine, may provide benefit.
- *Pizotifen and cyproheptadine block* serotonin (5-HT) receptors as well as having some H_1-antihistamine action; they can be effective.
- *A tricyclic antidepressant*, e.g. amitriptyline in low dose; start with 10 mg at night and increase to 50–75 mg.

- *Methysergide* (an ergot derivative) blocks serotonin receptors but it has a grave rare adverse effect, an inflammatory fibrosis, retroperitoneal (causing obstruction to the ureters), subendocardial, pericardial and pleural. Drug 'holidays', i.e. withdrawal for 1–2 months each 6 months, are a prudent safeguard. Because of this risk, methysergide cannot be a drug of first choice though it may be justified for a patient who is experiencing a sequence of severe attacks.

Premenstrual migraine may respond to mefenamic acid or to a diuretic.

After six months it is worth trying slow withdrawal of the prophylactic drug.

Cluster headaches may be treated as for migraine, but use of ergotamine may need to be more prolonged. If used over weeks, 2 days in each week should be ergot-free to avoid toxicity. Sumatriptan can be beneficial. Since bouts of headache tend to be of limited duration, e.g. a few weeks, short courses of methysergide are justified in intractable cases.

Headache of intracranial pressure (cerebral oedema) responds to dexamethasone (10 mg i.v.; 4 mg 6-hourly, 2–10 d) which reduces the pressure; and to nonopioid analgesics (see also Palliative care).

Patient-controlled analgesia

The attractions of enabling patients to manage their own analgesics rather than be dependent on others are obvious. In mild and moderate pain it is easy to provide tablets for this purpose, but in severe chronic and acute recurrent pain, e.g. terminal illness, postsurgical, obstetric, other routes are needed to provide speedy relief just when it is needed. Drug delivery systems range from inhalation devices to patient-controlled pumps for i.v., i.m., s.c. and epidural routes.

Despite the obvious problems, e.g. training patients, supervision, preventing overdose, these can achieve the objectives of satisfying the patient while reducing demand on nurses' time, especially when the aim is to allow the patient to die comfortably at home.

Inhalation via a demand valve of nitrous oxide and oxygen, as in obstetrics, may be used temporarily in other situations: e.g. urinary lithiasis, trigeminal neuralgia, during postoperative chest physiotherapy, for changing painful dressings and in emergency ambulances.

Drugs in palliative care

Symptom control

It is a general truth that we are all dying; the difference between individuals is the length and quality of the time that remains.[18] Terminal illness means that period (generally weeks) when active treatment of disease is no longer appropriate and the emphasis of care is palliative, i.e. to provide the maximum quality of life during these final weeks. This means that symptom control becomes the priority because,

> One cannot adequately help a man to come to accept his impending death if he remains in severe pain, one cannot give spiritual counsel to a woman who is vomiting, or help a wife and children say their goodbyes to a father who is so drugged that he cannot respond.[19]

As the scope of life contracts, so the quality of what remains becomes more precious. Symptoms should not be allowed to destroy it. Drugs are pre-eminent in symptom control.

An illustrative instance of success in palliative care is provided here by:

> an elderly gentleman with obstructing carcinoma of the oesophagus who was a keen gardener. He remained at home, free from pain, attended a

garden show on Saturday, worked in his garden on Sunday, and died on Monday.[20]

He was treated with continuous subcutaneous heroin (diamorphine) infusion. Whilst the randomised controlled trial provides a major basis for therapeutic advance, telling us what generally does happen, the clinical anecdote yet has value, telling us what can happen, and providing examples for us to emulate. With intelligent use of drugs, which follows from informed analyses of objectives, doctors can enable their patients to depart from life in peace[21] and with dignity, i.e. *true euthanasia*.[22]

Whilst the skilful use of drugs can provide incalculable relief and deserves careful study, this must not hide the fact that the manner, attentiveness and human feeling of the attendants are dominant factors once any grosser physical and mental aberrations have been controlled by drugs. The needs of the dying have been summarised as security, companionship, symptomatic treatment, and medical nursing and domestic care. Nearly half of the deaths in England and Wales occur in the patient's own home.

Pain

Analgesics should be given regularly, adjusted to the patient's need to *prevent* pain and not only to

---

[18] Mack R M 1984 Lessons from living with cancer. New England Journal of Medicine 311: 1640. Recommended reading: a personal account by a surgeon who had lung cancer with metastases.

[19] Dr Mary Baines, St Christopher's Hospice, London.

[20] Russell P S B 1984 New England Journal of Medicine 311: 1634.

[21] '...; and for many a time
I have been half in love with easeful Death,
Call'd him soft names in many a mused rhyme,
To take into the air my quiet breath;
 Now more than ever seems it rich to die,
To cease upon the midnight with no pain.'
(John Keats: 1795–1821).

[22] Euthanasia (Greek: *eu*: gentle, easy; *thanatos*: death) is the objective of all. It does not mean deliberately killing people peacefully, which is voluntary euthanasia. That giving increasing doses of opioids and sedative drugs may also shorten life (the 'double effect') 'is not in our view a reason for withholding treatment that would give relief, as long as a doctor acts in accordance with responsible medical practice with the objective of relieving pain or distress, and with no intention to kill'. Report of the select committee on medical ethics. House of Lords, January 1994. HMSO, London.

suppress it. Suppression of existent pain requires larger doses, particularly where the pain has generated anxiety and fear. When it is certain that pain will return, it is callous to allow it to do so when the means of prevention exist.

A dose of analgesic should be left accessible to the patient, especially at night, when unnecessary suffering may result from reluctance to call a nurse or disturb a relative. In terminal illness, the question of whether or not the patient will become dependent on opioids ceases to be of importance (but see below) and the ordinary precautions against dependence — low, widely-spaced doses — need not be rigorously applied.

Control of severe pain without objectionable sedation can be achieved in palliative care by morphine with adjuvant drugs (given orally) in up to 80% of patients. Oral use preserves patients' independence as well as reducing the unpleasantness of frequent injections.

Full relief can be achieved only by attention to detail. We therefore provide an account of morphine use in this most important area of medical care.

ORAL MORPHINE FOR PAIN IN PALLIATIVE CARE

Oral treatment allows independence and can be provided at home where most patients will prefer to die.

- A simple aqueous solution[23] may be used initially, the strength being adjusted to give a volume of 5–10 ml per dose, e.g. begin with 1 or 2 mg/ml.
- Alternatively, sustained-release tablets (MST Continus, Oramorph SR: 10, 30, 60, 100 mg, coloured differently) may be preferred.
- The usual oral starting dose to replace a weaker analgesic, e.g. co-proxamol, is 5–10 mg 4-hourly (2.5 mg in the frail elderly) of the aqueous solution or 10–30 mg 12-hourly of the sustained-release for-

mulations. Alternatively, use suppositories or buccal (sublingual) formulations (the latter route bypasses the first-pass or presystemic elimination and does not require such high doses as when swallowed).

- If the first dose is not more effective than previous medication, increase the second dose (aqueous solution) or third dose (sustained-release preparation).
- If the pain is not more than 90% controlled in the first 24 h increase the dose by 50%. After that adjust dose 24-hourly as below.
- **Dose.** Arbitrary fixed dosage is inappropriate; doses and frequency should be adjusted to meet the patients' need. Most patients get satisfactory pain control on 5–30 mg of the aqueous solution 4-hourly (a few will need more than 200 mg, rarely up to 500 mg is required). Dosage increments (4-hourly use) are:

below 15 mg, add 5 mg
up to 30 mg, add 10 mg
up to 90 mg, add 15 mg
up to 180 mg, add 30 mg
above 180 mg, add 60 mg until the desired effect is attained.

The dose of sustained-release tablets may be increased to 60 mg but the dose-interval should remain unaltered, i.e. 12-hourly.

- Breakthrough pain when the patient is taking a sustained-release preparation may be controlled by an additional dose of the aqueous solution; it gives the patient confidence. An NSAID can also be used.
- Change to morphine from other high-efficacy opioids; higher starting doses of oral morphine will be needed.
- A larger dose at night (1.5–2 × daytime dose) or an added hypnotic may allow the patient to pass the night without waking in pain (and so to omit one night dose).
- Constipation will occur, see below; it is essential to manage it.
- Initial drowsiness (a few days) and confusion (in the elderly) are common and usually pass off. This should be explained to the patient ('You may feel sleepy or a little muddled'): if unpleasant sedation persists then small doses of amphetamine may be added.

---

[23] Solutions of morphine deteriorate once they are exposed to air, and if exposed to light (keep in dark) and heat, they lose potency over as few as 2–4 weeks; competent pharmaceutical advice and preparation is required; stable formulations have been developed (Oramorph). The taste of morphine is bitter and patients may choose an accompanying drink to mask it. Tablets may be used.

- Initial nausea and vomiting may occur: an antiemetic controls it (e.g. prochlorperazine 2.5–5 mg, orally, 6–8-hourly), and can generally be withdrawn after 4–5 days.
- Myoclonus may occur, perhaps promoted by concurrent use of antidepressants or neuroleptics.
- Respiratory depression is seldom a problem with morphine dose escalated in this way.
- Dependence need not be feared. Both physical and psychological dependence occurs, but the latter to only a small degree compared with drug abuse or other chronic pain syndromes. The social, psychological and medical aspects of morphine use in palliative care are so different from that of drug abuse that comparisons are inappropriate. Dose reduction, when required, e.g. after relief of pain by palliative radiotherapy or nerve block, should, of course, be gradual; abrupt withdrawal (accidental) has been found to cause only a mild withdrawal syndrome.
- Acquired tolerance is dealt with by increasing the dose. There is no need for an arbitrary maximum dose.
- Transfer from the oral to the subcutaneous route may become necessary, e.g. due to difficult swallowing, vomiting. Diamorphine (heroin, preferred because it is more soluble than morphine) can be delivered by a portable syringe driver with minimal discomfort. The dose should be one-third the oral dose (4-hourly swallowed).
- A self-adhesive skin patch formulation which releases the opioid fentanyl (25 μg/h for 72 h) transdermally is also available for pain relief in palliative care.

ADJUVANT DRUGS

Phenothiazines are antiemetic, antianxiety and sedative agents and they may change the affective response to pain (particularly methotrimeprazine).

Tricyclic antidepressants (and perhaps others) have a morphine-sparing effect even in the absence of an effect or mood.

Amphetamine elevates mood and enhances analgesia.

In selected cases the full range of techniques of local and regional anaesthesia may be used, including extradural and intrathecal morphine (p. 390).

OTHER SYMPTOMS

- *Anorexia* is common in patients with widespread cancer; prednisolone 15–30 mg daily and/or alcohol (in the patient's preferred form) before meals, may help, or carbonated or other drink for which the patient has a taste.
- *Confusion* may not need treatment unless it is accompanied by restlessness. Useful in an emergency is haloperidol, or thioridazine (does not cause much sedation) or chlorpromazine (if sedation is desired). Chlormethiazole is helpful for insomnia.
- *Constipation* is usual in dying patients, whether due to opioid analgesic (see above) or to inadequate intake of food and fluid,[24] and physical inactivity. It can be exceedingly troublesome and management should begin early to forestall the need for the major unpleasantness and humiliations of manual removal of faeces and the lesser ones of enemas. Dietary measures should be used where practicable. A stimulant laxative and faecal softener (danthron plus poloxamer: co-danthramer) is commonly effective. Suppositories, e.g. glycerol or bisacodyl, should be used if the bowels have not been opened for three days and the rectum is found to be loaded.
- *Convulsions*. Sodium valproate orally is preferred to phenytoin as the latter interacts extensively with other drugs; where oral use is impracticable use phenobarbitone i.m. (for status epilepticus see p. 359).
- *Cough*: see page 500.
- *Diarrhoea*: see page 584.
- *Dyspnoea*. Chronic dyspnoea (not due to respiratory failure) may be relieved by an opioid (causing respiratory centre depression and reducing its sensitivity to chemical stimuli) but, when there is respiratory failure due to pulmonary disease, any sedation may be life-threatening. Oxygen is used as appropriate; a benzodiazepine reduces the anxiety of dyspnoea; dexamethasone reduces inflammation around obstructive tumours that cause dyspnoea.

---

[24] It is normal and comfortable to die slightly dehydrated; full hydration leads to full urinary bladder (with discomfort, restlessness, incontinence), salivary drooling and death rattle; it also increases heart failure (with dyspnoea which enhances death rattle); intravenous tubes make final embraces almost impossible (Lamerton R 1991 Lancet 337: 981).

Accumulations of mucus that the patient is too weak to expel cause 'death rattle'; this terminal event, often more distressing to others than to the patient may be eliminated by drying up secretions with an antimuscarinic drug (hyoscine or atropine 4- to 8-hourly).

- *Emergencies* such as major haemorrhage, pulmonary embolus, severe choking, fracture of large bone: give morphine 10 mg plus hyoscine 0.4 mg i.m.; this combination provides acute relief and some desirable short-term retrograde amnesia which may extend to the whole unpleasant episode.

- *Hiccup* (due to diaphragmatic spasm). Where this is intractable and exhausting, chlorpromazine (or other phenothiazine) or metoclopramide may help; also baclofen, nifedipine or sodium valproate.

- *Insomnia.* Use temazepam, or chlormethiazole (which may be less prone to cause confusion in the elderly).

- *Intestinal obstruction* can be managed without surgery[25] which only adds to the distress of dying. Give loperamide (or diphenoxylate) and/or hyoscine (or atropine) sublingually or s.c., for colic; antiemetics (sometimes combining two having different sites of action); and a faecal softener (without added laxative, which would increase peristalsis) for as long as obstruction is incomplete; there may be an inflammatory element in tumour obstruction, which can be relieved by substantial doses of corticosteroid (prednisolone 15–30 mg/day). When obstruction is complete the patient may vomit once or twice a day without great distress, but oral therapy may become impracticable; to avoid injections in an emaciated patient, drugs may be given by suppository (opioid plus antiemetic). Octreotide plus diamorphine administered s.c. by syringe driver may be effective.[26]

- *Itch*: see page 270.

- *Lymphoedema*, e.g. due to pelvic cancer, that causes pain may be helped by prednisolone (15–30 mg/day).

- *Mental distress* may be helped by an antidepressant or tranquilliser, according to circumstances. Patients may too easily be drugged into uncomplaining silence, but it does not follow that they are not still in deep distress:

... the grief that does not speak
Whispers the o'er-fraught heart, and bids it break.[27]

And this unpleasant way of ending life can be avoided by discerning choice and, particularly, careful dosage of drugs.

- *A mouth* that is dry and painful may be due to candidiasis (treat with nystatin), to dehydration (rehydrate the patient judiciously[24] where this can be done orally); the symptom can be managed by frequent small drinks or crushed ice to suck (plus assiduous mouth hygiene to prevent unpleasant infection); if due to antimuscarinic drugs, including some antidepressants, withdraw the drug or adjust its dose.

- *Nausea and vomiting*, whether due to disease or to opioid drug, cause great distress and can be more difficult to manage than pain; two drugs acting by different mechanisms may be needed when a single agent fails, e.g. metoclopramide (dopamine D_2-receptor antagonist) or ondansetron (5-HT$_3$-receptor antagonist) or hyoscine (antimuscarinic). For vomiting of *hypercalcaemia*: use an antiemetic and treat the cause (p. 672).

- *Night sweats* can be distressing and cause insomnia: indomethacin helps.

- *Restlessness* in terminal illness that has no obvious cause, e.g. pain, full bladder, may be treated with methotrimeprazine (a phenothiazine tranquilliser with analgesic effect) by injection. It may be combined with morphine (or diamorphine), which are tranquillisers as well as being analgesics; diazepam is useful for muscle twitching.

- *Swallowing* of solid-dose forms may be difficult and these may stick in the oesophagus in weak recumbent patients, especially if inadequate fluid is taken with the dose (at least two big gulps or 100 ml with the patient's trunk vertical).

- *Urinary frequency*, urgency and incontinence: flavoxate, terodiline, oxybutynin (antimuscarinics) may be useful; they may cause retention of urine if there is anatomical obstruction. The pain (with reflex muscle spasm) of an indwelling catheter may be alleviated by diazepam.

- *Raised intracranial pressure* (see p. 294): dexam-

---

[25] A detailed account is given by Baines M et al 1985 Lancet 2: 90.

[26] Steadman K, Franks A 1966 Lancet 347: 944.

[27] William Shakespeare (1564–1616). Macbeth, Act 4, Scene 3.

ethasone may be used indefinitely; reduce dose to 5 mg/d if practicable.

- *Fungating tumours* and ulcers may smell distressingly due to anaerobic bacterial growth. Benefit may be gained by topical providone-iodine or metronidazole gel.

Narcotic or opioid[28] analgesics

Agonists, partial agonists, antagonists

Among the remedies which it has pleased Almighty God to give to man to relieve his sufferings, none is so universal and so efficacious as opium (Thomas Sydenham, physician, 1680).

Opium (the dried juice of the seed head of the opium poppy) was certainly used in prehistoric times, and medical practice still leans heavily on its alkaloids, using them as analgesic, tranquilliser, antitussive and in diarrhoea.

The principal active ingredient in crude opium was isolated in 1806 by Friedrich Sertürner, who tested pure morphine on himself and three young men. He observed that the drug caused cerebral depression and relieved toothache, and named it after Morpheus.[29]

Opium contains many alkaloids, but the only important ones are *morphine* (10%) and *codeine*; *papaverine* is occasionally used as a vasodilator. Purified preparations of mixtures of opium alkaloids, e.g. papaveretum (Omnopon), are available; minus noscapine which is suspected of genotoxicity.

MODE OF ACTION

Endogenous opioid peptides (endorphins, dynorphins, enkephalins), have been termed 'the brain's own morphine'. Their discovery in 1975 explained why the brain had opioid receptors when there were no opioids in the body. These peptides are neurotransmitters in complex pain-inhibitory systems. They attach to specific opioid receptors, mainly μ (mu), κ (kappa), δ (delta), σ (sigma), and it is on these receptors that administered opioids also act (via neuronal K and Ca channels).

Pure morphine-like opioid agonists in general act on μ-, κ- and perhaps δ-receptors.

Mixed agonist-antagonists. Opioid drugs may be agonist to one class of opioid receptor, and antagonist to another, which explains the differing patterns of action seen. A single opioid may also have dual agonist/antagonist effect on a single receptor; these are known as partial agonists. Buprenorphine is a partial agonist at the σ- and a partial antagonist at the κ-receptor. Pentazocine probably produces anaesthesia by activating κ-receptors, dysphoria by activating σ-receptors and is a weak antagonist of μ-receptors. Partial agonists have a limited ceiling of therapeutic efficacy and by antagonism will precipitate a withdrawal syndrome if given to subjects dependent on morphine or heroin (high efficacy agonists). In addition, a weak (low-efficacy) agonist (codeine) will compete with a high-efficacy opioid for receptors and so reduce the receptor occupancy, and therefore the therapeutic efficacy of the latter, i.e. a weak agonist partially antagonises a strong agonist. It is thus no surprise that there are differences between opioids in both emphasis and the pattern of their many actions.

Pure competitive opioid antagonists, e.g. naloxone, naltrexone block all opioid receptors while exerting no activating effect.

Some of the endorphins, dynorphins and enkephalins are about as active as morphine and some have higher efficacy; some are short- and some are long-acting. The discovery of the role of natural

---

[28] The term opiate has been used for the natural alkaloids of opium, and opioid for other agents having similar action. The distinction is neither generally observed nor particularly useful. We here use opioid for all receptor-specific substances.

[29] In classical mythology Morpheus was son of Somnus, the infernal deity who presided over sleep. He was generally represented as a corpulent, winged boy holding opium poppies in his hand. His principal function seems to have been to stand by his sleeping father's black-curtained bed of feathers, on watch to prevent his being awakened by noise.

opioid mechanisms in physiology and pathology opens up possibilities for major developments in pain management, and indeed, wider, for endogenous opioid mechanisms may play a role, e.g. in shock.

Morphine and other opioids

Morphine will be described in detail and other opioid analgesics principally in so far as they differ. Morphine acts mainly on the opioid μ_1-receptors (analgesia, euphoria, dependence) and μ_2-receptors (respiratory depression, reduced gut motility).

The principal actions of morphine may be summarised:

On the central nervous system:

- *Depression*, leading to:

analgesia
respiratory depression
depression of cough reflex
sleep

- *Excitation*, leading to:

vomiting
miosis
hyperactive spinal cord reflexes (some only)
convulsions (very rare)

- *Changes of mood*: euphoria or dysphoria
- *Dependence*; affects other systems too.

Peripheral nervous system:
analgesia, some anti-inflammatory effect

Smooth muscle stimulation:
Gastrointestinal muscle spasm (delayed passage of contents with constipation)
Biliary tract spasm
Bronchospasm

Cardiovascular system:
Dilatation of resistance (arterioles) and capacitance (veins) vessels.

MORPHINE ON THE CENTRAL NERVOUS SYSTEM

Morphine is the most generally useful high-efficacy opioid analgesic; it eliminates pain and also allows subjects to tolerate pain, i.e. the sensation is felt but is no longer unpleasant. It both stimulates and depresses the central nervous system. It induces a state of relaxation, tranquillity, detachment and well-being (euphoria), or occasionally of unpleasantness (dysphoria), and causes sleepiness, inability to concentrate and lethargy, always supposing that this pleasant state is not destroyed by nausea and vomiting, more common if the patient is ambulant. Excitement can occur but is unusual. Morphine excites cats and horses, though it is illegal to put this to practical use. Generally, morphine has useful hypnotic and tranquillising actions and there should be no hesitation in using it in full dose in appropriate circumstances, e.g. acute pain and fear, as in myocardial infarction or road traffic accidents.

Morphine *depresses respiration*, principally by reducing sensitivity of the respiratory centre to rise in blood pCO_2. With therapeutic doses there is a reduced minute volume due to diminished rate and tidal volume. With higher doses carbon dioxide narcosis may develop. In overdose the patient may present with a respiratory rate as low as 2/min.

Morphine is *dangerous* when the respiratory drive is impaired by disease, including CO_2 retention from any cause, e.g. chronic obstructive lung disease, asthma or raised intracranial pressure.

In *asthmatics*, in addition to the effect on the respiratory centre, it may increase viscosity of bronchial secretions, which, with depression of cough and bronchospasm (see below) will increase small airways resistance.

Morphine also suppresses *cough* by a central action. It stimulates the third nerve nucleus causing miosis (pin-point pupils are characteristic of poisoning, acute or chronic; at therapeutic doses the pupil is merely smaller).

The chemoreceptor trigger zone of the *vomiting centre* is stimulated, causing nausea (10%) and vomiting (15%), an effect which, in addition to being unpleasant, can be dangerous to patients soon after abdominal operations or cataract surgery. A preparation of morphine plus an antiemetic, e.g. cyclizine (Cyclimorph) reduces this liability. Some spinal cord reflexes are also stimulated, causing myoclonus and so morphine is unsuitable for use in tetanus and convulsant poisoning; indeed, morphine can itself cause convulsions.

Morphine causes *antidiuresis* by releasing antidiuretic hormone, and this can be clinically important.

Appetite is lost with chronic use.

Peripheral nervous system. The discovery of opioid receptors in sensory nerves and their inhibiting effect on inflammatory mediators may lead to advances in pain control.

MORPHINE ON SMOOTH MUSCLE

Alimentary tract. Morphine activates receptors on the smooth muscle of the stomach (antrum) and of both large and small bowel, causing it to contract. Peristalsis (propulsion) is reduced and segmentation increased. Thus, although morphine 'stimulates' smooth muscle, delayed gastric emptying and constipation occur, with gut muscle in a state of tonic contraction. The central action of the drug probably also leads to neglect of the urge to defaecate. Delay in the passage of the intestinal contents results in greater absorption of water and increased viscosity of faeces, which contribute to the constipation. The management of opioid-induced constipation is an important aspect of palliative care.

Morphine increases pressure in the sigmoid colon and colonic diverticula may become obstructed and fail to drain into the colon. Pethidine neither produces these high pressures nor prevents drainage, and so is preferable if the pain of acute diverticulitis is severe enough to demand a narcotic analgesic. Morphine may also endanger anastomoses of the bowel immediately postoperatively and it should not be given in intestinal obstruction (excepting in palliative care).

Intrabiliary pressure may rise substantially after morphine (as much as 10 times in 10 minutes), due to spasm of the sphincter of Oddi. Sometimes biliary colic is made worse by morphine, presumably in a patient in whom the dose happens to be adequate to increase intrabiliary pressure, but insufficient to produce more than slight analgesia. In patients who have had a cholecystectomy this can produce a syndrome sufficiently like a myocardial infarction to cause diagnostic confusion. Naloxone may give dramatic symptomatic relief as may glyceryl trinitrate. Another result of this action of morphine is to dam back the pancreatic juice and so cause a rise in the serum amylase concentration. Morphine is therefore best avoided in pancreatitis; but buprenorphine has less of this effect.

Urinary tract. Any contraction of the ureters is probably clinically unimportant. Retention of urine may occur (particularly in prostatic hypertrophy) due to a mix of spasm of the bladder sphincter and to the central sedation causing the patient to ignore afferent messages from a full bladder.

Bronchial muscle is constricted, partly due to histamine release, but so slightly as to be of no importance, except in *asthmatics* in whom morphine is best avoided anyway because of its respiratory depressant effect. If given in a severe attack of asthma, *morphine may kill* by this action plus respiratory depression.

When morphine is used and the smooth muscle effects are objectionable, atropine may be given simultaneously to antagonise spasm. Unfortunately it does not always effectively oppose the rise of pressure induced in the biliary system, nor does it restore bowel peristalsis. Glyceryl trinitrate will relax morphine-induced spasm.

Uterus. Labour is prolonged, but this may be the result of central psychological effects reducing patient cooperation rather than to an action on the uterus.

CARDIOVASCULAR SYSTEM

Morphine, by a central action, impairs sympathetic vascular reflexes (causing veno- and arteriolar dilatation) and stimulates the vagal centre (bradycardia); it also releases histamine (vasodilatation). These effects are ordinarily unimportant, but they can be beneficial in acute left ventricular failure, relieving mental distress by tranquillising, cardiac distress by reduction of sympathetic drive and respiratory distress by rendering the centre insensitive to afferent stimuli from the congested lungs. The effect can sometimes be harmful in patients taking antihypertensives, in acute myocardial infarction and with low blood volume; excessive bradycardia can be blocked by atropine.

Other effects of morphine include sweating, histamine release, pruritus and piloerection.

TOLERANCE

Chronic use of morphine and other opioids is marked by acquired tolerance to the depressant agonist effects, e.g. analgesic action and respiratory depression (the fatal dose becomes higher), but not to some stimulant agonist effects, e.g. constipation and miosis, which persist.

Opioids that have mixed agonist/antagonist actions (partial agonists) induce tolerance to the agonist but not to the antagonist effects; naloxone (a pure antagonist) induces no tolerance to itself. There is a cross-tolerance between opioids (for dependence and withdrawal see below).

Acquired tolerance develops over days with continued frequent use and passes off (variably for different actions) over a few days to weeks.

PHARMACOKINETICS

Given s.c. (particularly) or i.m., morphine is rapidly absorbed when the circulation is normal, but in circulatory shock absorption will be delayed and it is best given i.v. Oral morphine is subject to extensive presystemic or first-pass metabolism (mainly conjugation in gut wall and liver) and only about 20% of a dose reaches the systemic circulation; the initial oral dose is about twice the injected dose. The buccal or the sublingual route are also practicable and there is no first-pass metabolism; these routes are comparable to i.m. injection.

Morphine in the systemic circulation is metabolised by both liver and kidney; the conjugated metabolites include the pharmacologically active morphine-6-glucuronide. Elimination of morphine (10%) and metabolites is largely renal; data conflict on whether action is prolonged in renal failure but are suffient to warrant care in choosing morphine and deciding its dose and dose interval for such patients.

The $t^{1}\!/_{2}$ is 2 h (active metabolites slightly longer) and the duration of useful analgesia is 3–6 h (shorter in younger than in older subjects).

Morphine crosses the placenta and depresses respiration in the fetus at birth.

Other routes of administration used by specialists are epidural (obstetrics) and intrathecal; very low doses are used.

Dosage. Given s.c., i.m. morphine 10 mg is usually adequate; with 15 mg unwanted effects increase more than does analgesia; i.v. give (slowly) $^{1}\!/_{4}$–$^{1}\!/_{2}$ of the i.m. dose. For oral dosage see Palliative care, page 296. Continuous pain suppression can be achieved by morphine orally 4-hourly and s.c. 3-hourly.

Intrathecal opioids, see page 390.

PRINCIPAL USES OF MORPHINE AND ITS ANALOGUES

- Relief of moderate to severe acute pain (or chronic pain often in terminal illness)
- Brief relief of anxiety in serious and frightening disease accompanied by pain, e.g. trauma
- Relief of dyspnoea in acute left ventricular failure, and in terminal cancer
- Premedication for surgery
- Symptomatic control of acute nonserious diarrhoea, e.g. travellers' diarrhoea (codeine)
- Suppression of cough (codeine)
- Production of euphoria as well as pain relief in the dying.

Any of the desired effects may be interfered with by opioid-induced nausea, vomiting and dysphoria.

Morphine and disease. When intense peripheral vasoconstriction accompanies, e.g. trauma, morphine administered s.c. or i.m. may appear to be ineffective because it fails quickly to enter the systemic circulation; repeating the dose before the first has been absorbed may lead to poisoning when the vasoconstriction passes off. In such circumstances morphine should be given slowly i.v. (2.5 mg every 5 min). If the blood volume is low morphine may cause serious hypotension.

In hepatic failure small doses can cause coma (see Drugs and the liver), and it may be dangerous in *hypothyroidism* (slow metabolism).

In an *acute asthmatic attack*, morphine is *dangerous*.

Adverse effects (type A) have been discussed. Dependence and overdose are treated below. Opioid use in obstetrics requires special care (p. 392).

Interactions. Morphine is potentiated by

monoamine oxidase inhibitors. Any central nervous system depressant (including alcohol) will have additive effects. Patients recently exposed to neuromuscular blocking agents (unless this is adequately reversed, e.g. by neostigmine) are particularly at risk from the respiratory depressant effects of morphine. The effect of diuretic drugs may be reduced by release of antidiuretic hormone by morphine. *Useful interactions* include the potientating effect on pain relief of tricyclic antidepressants and of dexamphetamine.

OPIOID DEPENDENCE

Physical dependence begins to occur within 24 h if morphine is given 4-hourly, and after surgery some patients may be unwittingly subjected to a withdrawal syndrome that passes for general postoperative discomfort.

Acquired tolerance may rapidly reach a high degree, and an addict may take morphine 600 mg (heroin equivalent 400 mg) or even more several times a day. An average addict is more likely to take about 300 mg. Duration of tolerance after cessation of administration is variable for different actions, from a few days to weeks. Thus, addicts who have undergone withdrawal and lost tolerance, and who later resume their opioid careers may overdose themselves inadvertently.

Morphine or heroin dependence is more disabling physically and socially than is opium dependence (treatment of pain in opioid dependent subjects, see p. 309). Chronic exposure to opioids leads to adaptive changes in the endogenous opioid system and no doubt in receptor numbers, sensitivity and cellular response. The abrupt withdrawal of administered opioid usually provokes rebound or a withdrawal syndrome. This consists largely of the opposite of the normal actions of opioids. Also, noradrenergic mechanisms are modulated by endogenous opioids and these mechanisms are depressed by continuous opioid administration. Abrupt withdrawal rebound can be described as 'noradrenergic storm'.

ACUTE WITHDRAWAL SYNDROME
(morphine, heroin)

When an addict misses his first shot, he senses mild withdrawal distress ('feels his habit coming on') but this is probably more psychological than physiological, for fear plays a considerable role in the withdrawal syndrome. At this stage a placebo may give relief. During the first 8–16 h of abstinence the addict becomes increasingly nervous, restless and anxious; close confinement tends to intensify these symptoms. Within 14 h (usually less) he will begin to yawn frequently; he sweats profusely and develops running of the eyes and nose comparable to that accompanying a severe head cold. These symptoms increase in intensity for the first 24 h, after which the pupils dilate and recurring waves of goose-flesh occur. Severe twitching of the muscles (the origin of the term 'kick the habit') occurs within 36 h and painful cramps develop in the backs of the legs and in the abdomen; all the body fluids are released copiously; vomiting and diarrhoea are acute; there is little appetite for food and the subject is unable to sleep. The respiratory rate rises steeply. Both systolic and diastolic blood pressure increase moderately to a maximum between the third and fourth day; temperature rises an average of about 0.5°C, subsiding after the third day; the blood sugar content rises sharply until the third day or after; the basal metabolic rate increases sharply during the first 48 h. These are the objective signs of withdrawal distress which can be measured; the subjective indications are equally severe and the illness reaches its peak within 48–72 h after the last dose of the opioid, gradually subsiding thereafter for the next 5–10 days. Complete recovery requires from 3–6 months with rehabilitation and, if needed, psychological treatment. The withdrawal syndrome proper is self-limiting and most addicts will survive it with no medical assistance whatever (this is known as kicking the habit, 'cold turkey'). Abrupt withdrawal is inhumane, but with the use of such drugs as methadone, it is possible to reduce the distress of withdrawal very considerably.[30]

It is usual to cover the acute withdrawal period (about 10 days) of injected morphine or heroin with an opioid taken orally and having a long half-life, e.g. methadone $t\frac{1}{2}$ 48 h, perhaps supplemented

---

[30] From Maurer D W, Vogel V H 1962 Narcotics and narcotic addiction. Thomas, Springfield, Illinois. Courtesy of the authors and publisher.

with a benzodiazepine. Clonidine (0.1 mg $\times$ 4/d, reducing over about 4 days) can reduce the effects of noradrenergic hyperactivity by its agonist action on central presynaptic α_2-adrenoceptors that results in inhibition of sympathetic autonomic outflow; hypotension may occur. Lofexidine, a structural analogue of clonidine, may also aid opioid detoxification.

A withdrawal syndrome occurs in the *newborn* of dependent mothers.

Opioids with partial agonist actions precipitate a withdrawal syndrome in dependent subjects, as do the antagonists naltrexone and naloxone (it is unkind, because it is unnecessary, to use an antagonist as a diagnostic test in suspected addicts).

Pharmacological aids to prevention of relapse of addicts: see methadone and naltrexone.

Therapeutic addiction. There is a risk of making patients seriously dependent if prolonged or frequent treatment of pain with a high-efficacy opioid is undertaken (the more widely the doses are spaced, the less the risk), e.g. for trigeminal neuralgia, sickle cell crises, migraine or recurrent urinary colic. Palliative care is an exception (see above). It is impossible to rule on how quickly a patient can become seriously dependent, but it is generally a matter of weeks or months, though detectable physical dependence can occur in a day if the drug is given intensively. Dependence is less severe with partial agonists.

OVERDOSE

Death (from all opioids, low and high efficacy; agonist or partial agonist) is due to respiratory failure. Blood pressure is usually well maintained, if the patient is supine, until cerebral anoxia causes circulatory failure. At this stage the (pinpoint) pupils may dilate (also if there is hypothermia). The combination of miosis and bradypnoea gives the diagnosis which is vital, for naloxone, a selective competitive antagonist, is life-saving. Naloxone, having none of the agonist effects of morphine (respiratory depression, miosis, coma), is safe to give as a diagnostic test in an unconscious or drowsy patient suspected of opioid overdose. The $t\frac{1}{2}$ of naloxone (1 h) is shorter than most opioids and repeated doses or infusion will be needed. The

guide to therapy is the state of respiration, not of consciousness. Patients with opioid overdose should be monitored for recurrence of ventilatory depression, which is an indication for further naloxone (for details of naloxone use see p. 308). Apart from naloxone the general treatment is the same as for overdose by any cerebral depressant.

Addicts often take overdoses, whether accidentally or not, and naloxone, as well as reversing the life-endangering respiratory depression, will induce an acute (noradrenergic) withdrawal syndrome. Close cardiovascular monitoring is necessary, with use of peripheral adrenoceptor blocking agents or perhaps clonidine (see above), according to need.

Classification of opioids by analgesic efficacy

The opioids discussed below are considered in relation to morphine ($t\frac{1}{2}$ does not necessarily indicate duration of useful analgesia, which is also related to affinity of the opioid for receptors: but $t\frac{1}{2}$ gives useful information on accumulation).

Opioid efficacy	
Low efficacy for mild and moderate pain	**High efficacy for severe pain**
codeine	*buprenorphine
dihydrocodeine	dextromoramide
dextropropoxyphene	diamorphine (heroin)
*nalbuphine	dipipanone
*pentazocine	*meptazinol
	methadone
	morphine
	papaveretum
	pethidine (meperidine)
	phenazocine
	tramadol

*Partial agonist
Notes:

- The division into two classes is not absolute and some drugs listed for moderate pain can be effective in severe pain by injection.
- Fentanyl, alfentanil and phenoperidine are high-efficacy opioids used for surgery/anaesthesia.

Etorphine is a high-efficacy opioid which, combined with a neuroleptic, is used to immobilise animals in veterinary practice. The doses used in large animals are enough to kill an adult human if, in a struggle, the drug is splashed on skin or mucous membrane, or there is a needle scratch. A competitive antagonist, naloxone (or diprenorphine which accompanies veterinary formulations, and is labelled for use in animals only) should be used at once in man in this urgent situation (do not delay to fetch an official human formulation; death has occurred where this was done).

Wash a splashed site copiously *at once*.

Partial agonists were developed in the unrealised hope of eliminating the potential for abuse whilst retaining analgesic efficacy; they may induce psychotomimetic reactions. They are indeed less liable to induce dependence and to cause respiratory depression than are the pure agonists, though they do have these effects. Their antagonist action is chiefly evident against large doses of agonist, e.g. in addicts.

Other opioids

(see also general account above)

CODEINE (methylmorphine)

Codeine ($t\frac{1}{2}$ 3 h) is a low-efficacy opioid that binds to μ-receptors; 10% is converted to morphine. It lacks efficacy for severe pain and most of its actions are about one-tenth those of morphine. A qualitative difference from morphine is that large doses cause excitement. Dependence occurs but much less than with morphine.

Its principal uses are for mild and moderate pain and cough (longterm use is accompanied by chronic constipation) and for the short-term symptomatic control of the milder acute diarrhoeas. There are numerous formulations for cough, e.g. Codeine Linctus, and for pain, in which it is commonly combined with aspirin and/or paracetamol (Aspirin and Codeine Tabs, co-codaprin; Aspirin, Paracetamol and Codeine Tabs).

PETHIDINE (meperidine, Demerol)

Pethidine ($t\frac{1}{2}$ 5 h) attracted attention as a possible analgesic because it caused the tails of laboratory mice to stand erect (Straub phenomenon), a characteristic of morphine-like drugs caused by spasm of the anal sphincter.

Pethidine binds to μ- and κ-receptors; it cannot relieve such severe pain as can morphine, i.e. it has lower therapeutic efficacy, but is effective against pain beyond the reach of codeine. Despite its substantial structural dissimilarity to morphine, pethidine has many similar properties including that of being antagonised by naloxone.

Pethidine differs from morphine in that it:

- does not suppress cough usefully
- does not constipate; but its effect in the upper small intestine is similar to morphine and there is spasm of the sphincter of Oddi
- is less likely to cause urinary retention and to prolong childbirth
- has little hypnotic effect
- has a shorter duration of analgesia (2–3 h).

Pethidine is extensively metabolised in the liver and the parent drug and metabolites are excreted in the urine; norpethidine retains pharmacological activity and accumulates when renal function in impaired.

Pethidine causes vomiting about as often as does morphine; it has atropine-like effects, including dry mouth and blurred vision (cycloplegia and sometimes mydriasis, though usually miosis). Overdose or use in renal failure can cause central nervous system stimulation (myoclonus, convulsions) due to norpethidine.

There is disagreement on the extent to which pethidine depresses respiration. It is probable that in equianalgesic doses it is as depressant as morphine.

Pethidine dependence occurs, with some tolerance, especially to the side-effects, but its psychic effects are less constant and less marked than those of morphine. Pethidine has evident advantages over morphine for pain that is not very intense, and it is widely used. It is usually given orally (50–100 mg) or i.m. (25–100 mg), when its effects last 2–3 h. The solution is irritant and so it is not given s.c. It is widely used in obstetrics because it does not delay labour like morphine; but it enters the fetus and can depress respiration at birth.

METHADONE (Physeptone)

Methadone ($t^{1}/_{2}$ 8 h) is a synthetic drug structurally and pharmacologically similar to morphine; it acts mainly at the μ-receptor. Methadone is largely metabolised to products that are excreted in the urine. The principal feature of methadone is its duration of action. Analgesia may last for as long as 24 h. If used for chronic pain in palliative care (12-hourly) an opioid of short $t^{1}/_{2}$ should be provided for breakthrough pain rather than an extra dose of methadone.

The long duration of action also favours its use to cover opioid withdrawal. Occupancy of opioid receptors by methadone reduces the desire for other opioids, and their effects, should any be taken; the slow offset diminishes the severity of the withdrawal. Addicts who are cooperative enough to take oral methadone feel reduced craving and less 'kick/buzz/rush' from i.v. heroin or morphine because their opioid receptors are already occupied by methadone and the i.v. drug must compete. Dependence occurs but this is less severe than with morphine or heroin.[31] Reports of deaths in addicts entering prescribed methadone substitution programmes have been attributed to the cardiovascular effects of a membrane stabilising action, unlike morphine (see naltrexone).

Vomiting is fairly common with methadone (though somewhat less than with morphine) especially if the patient is ambulant, and sedation is less.

Methadone is also useful for severe cough.

DIAMORPHINE (heroin)

This semisynthetic drug was first made from morphine at St. Mary's Hospital, London in 1874. It was introduced in 1898 as a remedy for cough and for morphine addiction; later it was appreciated that it 'cured' morphine addiction by substituting itself as the addicting agent.

Pharmacokinetics. Diamorphine (diacetylmorphine) is converted in the body within minutes to morphine and 6-monoacetylmorphine, a metabolite of both drugs; the effects of diamorphine are principally due to the actions of morphine and 6-monoacetylmorphine on the μ- and to a lesser extent the κ-receptors. Diamorphine given parenterally has a $t^{1}/_{2}$ of 3 min. When given orally it is subject to complete presystemic or first-pass metabolism and only morphine ($t^{1}/_{2}$ 3 h) and metabolites reach the systemic circulation. Thus oral diamorphine is essentially a prodrug. The greater potency of diamorphine (diamorphine 1 mg = morphine 1.5 mg) may be due to the metabolite 6-acetylmorphine and to the common use of morphine as sulphate and diamorphine as hydrochloride.

Use. Diamorphine is used medicinally for acute pain, e.g. myocardial infarction and chronic pain, e.g. in palliative care. Diamorphine provides a more rapid onset of pain relief than morphine because it is more lipid soluble and enters the brain more readily, and its duration of action is about the same.[32] Diamorphine is more *soluble* than morphine to a useful degree.[32] This, together with its greater potency (greater efficacy in relation to weight and therefore requiring a smaller volume) makes diamorphine suitable to deliver by s.c. infusion through a syringe driver when continuous pain control is required in palliative care and can no longer be achieved by enteral morphine (oral, buccal, suppository) (see Patient-controlled analgesia, p. 294).

Diamorphine is also used for severe *cough* (Diamorphine Linctus).

Abuse. It is commonly stated that diamorphine (heroin) is the 'most potent' of all dependence-producing opioids. Weight-for-weight it is certainly more effective than morphine, and this is of importance in illicit traffic as diamorphine takes up less space, but in so far as efficacy in inducing dependence is concerned, there is doubt.

---

[31] In the UK a special Methadone Mixture 1 mg/ml (the concentration is part of the official title) is specially provided for the management of opioid addicts; it is coloured green and formulated to prevent injection. It has × $2^{1}/_{2}$ the strength of Methadone Linctus, for cough (yellow or brown); they must not be confused.

---

[32] Solubility in water: morphine sulphate 1 in 21; diamorphine hydrochloride 1 in 1.6.

In almost every country the manufacture of diamorphine, even for use in medicine, is now illegal. The first to try this prohibition as a remedy for widespread drug addiction was the USA, which banned diamorphine manufacture in 1924, provoked by the magnitude of the addiction problem and not yet discouraged by the experience of this type of approach with alcohol prohibition (1919–1933).

An effort was made in 1953 to achieve a worldwide ban on diamorphine in medicine (so that any diamorphine, wherever it was found *must* be illegal) and most countries agreed. The UK did not agree because legitimate supplies for medicine were not then getting into illicit channels (it has since remained available for medicinal use but is not exported). A ban now would be pointless since illegal diamorphine is readily available worldwide.

PENTAZOCINE (Fortral)

Pentazocine ($t^1/_2$ 5 h) provides a type of analgesia that is different from morphine. Its analgesic effect is probably due to an agonist action at κ-receptors and its dysphoric action to activation of σ-receptors; it is a weak antagonist of μ-receptors (through which morphine produces analgesia). Thus pentazocine can cause a withdrawal syndrome in addicts (antagonist effect); it can also induce psychological and physical dependence (agonist effect), and this can be severe. It has not proved to be the solution to separating the property of analgesia from that of producing dependence, as was hoped for initially. Its *analgesic efficacy* approximates to that of morphine, but its *potency* (weight for weight) is about one-third of morphine. Compared to morphine pentazocine produces shorter duration of pain relief, less dependence (but this definitely occurs), more psychotomimetic effects, and less sedation and respiratory depression (naloxone can reverse the respiratory depression in overdose).

Pharmacokinetics. Pentazocine is extensively metabolised in the liver and less that 10% is excreted unchanged in the urine.

Uses. Pentazocine is given to relieve moderate to severe pain, and also for chronic pain, for its liability to induce dependence is less than morphine. Its *dysphoric* effect limits its usefulness. Avoid in myocardial infarction (hypertension).

Adverse effects of this partial agonist include: nausea, vomiting, dizziness, sweating, hypertension, palpitations, tachycardia, central nervous system disturbances (euphoria, dysphoria, psychotomimesis).

Phenazocine (Narphen) is a high-efficacy agonist used particularly in biliary colic for it has less capacity than other opioids to cause spasm of the sphincter of Oddi. It may be administered sublingually if the patient is vomiting.

Buprenorphine (Temgesic) ($t^1/_2$ 5 h) is a high-efficacy partial agonist at the μ-receptor and an antagonist at the κ-receptor. Its high receptor affinity (tenacity of binding) may explain why respiratory depression is only partially reversed by naloxone; a respiratory stimulant (doxapram) may be needed in overdose, or assisted respiration. It has less liability to induce dependence and respiratory depression than pure agonists, little effect on the cardiovascular system and may spare the sphincter of Oddi (from induced spasm). Duration of action is about 6 h. Because of extensive presystemic elimination when swallowed, buprenorphine is given by the buccal (sublingual) route (200–400 micrograms) or by i.m., or slow i.v., injection (300–600 micrograms). It is a useful analgesic because of the length and strength of its action, its low liability to cause dependence and the fact that administration by injection can be avoided, e.g. for children, patients with bleeding disorder.

Dextropropoxyphene (Doloxene) ($t^1/_2$ 5 h) is structurally similar to methadone and differs in that it is less analgesic, antitussive, and less dependence-producing. Its analgesic usefulness approximates to that of codeine. Dextropropoxyphene is rapidly absorbed from the gastrointestinal tract. In overdose the rapidity of absorption is such that respiratory arrest may occur within one hour and also hypotension (probably due to a membrane-stabilising or quinidine-like action causing cardiac dysrhythmia), so that many subjects die before reaching hospital. Combination with alcohol (common with self-poisoning) enhances respiratory depression. Dextropropoxyphene is commonly combined with paracetamol (co-proxamol, Distalgesic) and with aspirin (Doloxene Cpd). Dextropropoxyphene interacts with warfarin, enhancing its anticoagulant effect.

Dihydrocodeine (DFI18) is a low-efficacy opioid with an analgesic efficacy similar to that of codeine. It is used to relieve moderate acute and chronic pain on its own or as a compound tablet (co-dydramol; dihydrocodeine 10 mg plus paracetamol 500 mg). Dihydrocodeine caues histamine release and should not be used in patients with hyper-reactive airways.

Meptazinol (Meptid) is a high-efficacy partial agonist; it also has central cholinergic activity which adds to its analgesic effect. It is used to relieve acute or chronic pain of moderate intensity, e.g. postoperatively and in obstetrics. Meptazinol does not cause euphoria and withdrawal effects seem not to occur when it is discontinued. It appears not to induce a withdrawal syndrome in opioid-dependent subjects.

Tramadol (t$^{1/2}$ 6 h) is an opioid with additional actions; the basis of its analgesic effects appears to derive from its binding to opioid μ-receptors, but also to inhibition of neuronal noradrenaline uptake and serotonin release. It is rapidly absorbed from the gastrointestinal tract, 20% of an oral dose undergoes first-pass metabolism and less than 31% dose is excreted unchanged in the urine. Tramadol is approximately as effective as pethidine for post-operative pain and as morphine for moderate chronic pain.

Tramadol is claimed to be less likely to constipate, depress respiration and addict. Confusion, convulsions, hallucinations and anaphylaxis have been reported with its use.

Dipipanone (Diconal is dipipanone plus cyclizine, an antiemetic) is less sedating and shorter acting than morphine; it is suitable for acute attacks of pain, e.g. breakthrough pain in terminal illness. *Dextromethorphan*, the dextroisomer of the opioid levomethorphan is used as an antitussive, e.g. in Actifed; the latter is sought as a drug of abuse by addicts.

Opioids during and after surgery

Fentanyl (Sublimaze) (t$^{1/2}$ 3 h) has higher efficacy than morphine, analgesia lasts 30–60 min (single dose) and is used i.v.; when combined with droperidol it gives neuroleptanalgesia (see Index). Fentanyl is also given for chronic and intractable cancer pain as self-adhesive patches which release the drug at approximately 25 μg/h for 72 h. Fentanyl is so potent that discarded patches may yet contain sufficient drug to be dangerous.

Phenoperidine (Operidine) (t$^{1/2}$ 30 min) is similar.

Alfenatil (Rapifen) (t$^{1/2}$ 1.5 h), given i.v., provides maximum analgesia in 90 s, which lasts about 5–10 min from a single dose; it is used for brief (painful) operations.

Nalbuphine (Nubain) is a partial agonist given by injection.

Opioids (nonanalgesic) for antimotility effect on the gut include loperamide and diphenoxylate (p. 585).

Opioid antagonists

NALOXONE (Narcan)

Naloxone (t$^{1/2}$ 75 min) is a pure competitive antagonist at all opioid receptors, notably the μ-, κ- and σ-receptors; it has no agonist activity. Naloxone antagonises both agonist and partial agonist opioids (although it may not be sufficient to reverse the effects of buprenorphine in overdose, so tenaciously does the latter drug bind to receptors). It induces an acute withdrawal syndrome in opioid-dependent subjects.

Naloxone undergoes high presystemic elimination when swallowed and is not used by this route; some 70% of a dose appears in the urine as metabolites.

Given i.v., it causes reversal of opioid-induced respiratory depression in 1–2 min; reversal of analgesia and depressed consciousness can be slower. A prompt marked improvement in respiration has diagnostic value in opioid overdose, but poor or no response may occur because insufficient has been given, or with buprenorphine (above), or due to cerebral hypoxia or severe hypothermia.

Naloxone acts for about one hour after an i.v. injection of 100–200 micrograms, though the peak effect on depressed respiration may be as brief as 10 min. As opioid analgesics in general act for much longer than this, further i.v. boluses of 100 micrograms should be given at 2 min intervals until changes in respiration, pupils or consciousness indicate response; subsequent doses may be given by i.m. injection. A continuous i.v. infusion commencing with 2.5 micrograms/kg/h may be required for days with opioids having a long $t^{1/2}$ (methadone). Naloxone is also used to counter excess opioid effects after surgical analgesia or childbirth.

Naltrexone ($t^{1/2}$ 4 h: active metabolite 13 h) is similar to naloxone but longer-acting, with duration of effect 1–3 days according to dose. It can be used orally to assist in the rehabilitation of ex-opioid abusers who are *fully* withdrawn (otherwise it will induce an acute withdrawal syndrome). A patient who then takes an opioid fails to experience the 'kick' or euphoria, although naltrexone does not reduce craving as does the agonist methadone. This use of naltrexone requires careful selection and supervision of subjects.

Pain in opioid addicts

A non-opioid analgesic useful for pain in opioid addicts is *nefopam* (Acupan), being neither an opioid nor an NSAID. Its mode of action is not fully understood but may involve adrenergic and serotonergic mechanisms. It is effective against moderate pain. Since it lacks the disadvantages of opioids (constipation, respiratory depression) and has greater efficacy than NSAIDs, it provides an alternative. It is useful for pain in opioid addicts as are NSAIDs (see Ch. 15).

GUIDE TO FURTHER READING

Atkinson S W, Bihari D J 1993 Pre-emptive analgesia. British Medical Journal 306: 285

Davis C I, Hardy J R 1994 Palliative care. British Medical Journal 308: 1359

Expert Working Group of the European Association of Palliative Care 1996 Morphine in cancer pain: modes of administration. British Medical Journal 312: 823

Farrell M et al 1995 Methadone maintenance treatment in opioid dependence: a review. British Medical Journal 309: 997

Hockley J M et al 1988 Survey of distressing symptoms in dying patients and their families in hospital and the response to a symptom control team. British Medical Journal 296: 1715

Murphy D F 1993 NSAIDs and postoperative pain. British Medical Journal 306: 1493

Portenoy R K 1992 Cancer pain: pathophysiology and syndromes. Lancet 339: 1026

Seymour R A et al 1982 Dihydrocodeine-induced hyperalgesia in postoperative dental pain. Lancet 1: 1425

Stein C 1995 The control of pain in peripheral tissue by opioids. New England Journal of Medicine 332: 1685

Wanzer S H et al 1989 The physician's responsibility towards hopelessly ill patients. New England Journal of Medicine 320: 844

Sleep and anxiety

SYNOPSIS

- Sleep and hypnotics (drugs that induce sleep). About 30% of adults have difficulty sleeping and half of them consider the problem to be serious
- Insomnia: Management involves detailed analysis of the particular circumstances. A drug is not always appropriate but, if required, should be chosen for its suitable pharmacokinetics and used briefly
- Anxiety afflicts about 30% of the population. Drugs are only an appropriate treatment for disabling symptoms
- Hypnotics and anxiolytic sedatives: benzodiazepines, trichloroethanol derivatives, barbiturates
- Drugs can affect driving and skilled tasks

Sleep and hypnotics

Sleep is an active (not merely a passive) circadian, physiological depression of consciousness. It is characterised by cyclical electroencephalographic (EEG) and eye movement changes, measures of which are used to describe sleep stages because they are convenient and seem to correlate with the fundamental physiological changes in neurotransmitter (noradrenaline, dopamine, serotonin, acetylcholine) functions that are inaccessible to measurement in clinical situations. Since these neurotransmitters are involved in psychiatric disorders it is no surprise that sleep disturbances are associated with mental disease.

Normal sleep (categorised by eye movements) is of two kinds, alternating during the night:

- NREM (nonrapid eye movement) (orthodox) or slow-wave EEG sleep; awakened subjects state they were 'thinking': heart rate, blood pressure and respiration are steady or decline and muscles are relaxed; growth hormone secretion is maximal; sleep is 'restful'.
- REM (rapid eye movement) (paradoxical) or fast-wave EEG sleep; awakened subjects state they were dreaming: heart rate, blood pressure and respiration are fluctuant, cerebral blood flow increases above that during wakefulness, the penis is erect (unless there is dream anxiety), skeletal muscles are profoundly relaxed though body movements are more pronounced; the brain is 'active'.

A normal night begins with a sleep latency period as the subject passes from wakefulness into NREM sleep. An initial hour of NREM sleep is followed by about 20 min REM sleep, after which cycles of NREM sleep (about 90 min) abruptly alternate with REM sleep (about 20 min) for the rest of the night (i.e. about 4 cycles). Both kinds of sleep seem to be necessary for health (REM sleep especially to alleviate fatigue).

Hypnotics in full doses can disrupt the normal sleep pattern, suppressing REM sleep, though tolerance may develop. Benzodiazepines and chloral do this least. No hypnotic can be said to induce natural sleep.

On *abrupt withdrawal* of a drug that has suppressed REM sleep there is a rebound increase as though the body requires to recover what has been lost; nightmares occur with severe rebound; abnormal sleep patterns may persist for weeks after withdrawal. It has not been conclusively shown that the kind of abnormality induced by hypnotics is harmful. But there is some evidence that deprivation of REM sleep may be responsible for emotional disorder so that hypnotics should not be used without good reason. That hypnotics are extensively prescribed, and indeed overprescribed, is 'not disputed'.[1]

NONHYPNOTIC DRUGS AND SLEEP

A range of other drugs has effects on eye movement pattern similar to hypnotics, when given in sufficient dose, e.g. heroin, morphine, alcohol, tricyclic and MAOI antidepressants, amphetamine and other appetite suppressants (though not dexfenfluramine). But effects on onset and duration of sleep differ.

CLINICAL EVALUATION OF THE EFFECTS OF HYPNOTICS

Details of effects of hypnotics that will concern prescribers are illustrated by guidelines (WHO Europe[2]) for clinical evaluation. Evaluation begins with single dose studies in healthy volunteers in the morning, after a normal night's sleep. Tests to evaluate alertness, cognitive function, manual dexterity, coordination, reaction time, memory, etc. are administered. Then the drug is given at night to assess nocturnal effects, and residual effects the next day (hangover). The drug is then used in patients suffering insomnia (this presents particular ethical problems since the most suitable patients are those with chronic insomnia, in whom the clinical objective is to get them off all drugs rather than to encourage them to take new drugs).

Assessment is by questionnaires, with particular interest in sleep latency (time taken to go to sleep), number of nocturnal awakenings, time of final awakening and quality of sleep (including dreaming); subsequent daytime effects (hangover) are of particular concern.

Sleep laboratory studies with EEG, eye movement and electromyographic (under the jaw) recording are conducted on a small number of subjects.

It is also desirable to determine whether tolerance, and / or dependence occur, whether the drug is safe in longterm use, interactions with other drugs (including alcohol) and dosage in the old and in subjects with impaired elimination.

HANGOVER

The effects of hypnotics, including ordinary doses of some benzodiazepines (e.g. nitrazepam) taken at ordinary bedtime, carry over into the afternoon of the following day. Often patients are aware of drowsiness, but even when they are not, impaired psychomotor performance occurs as shown by reaction time, tapping speed, attentiveness, ability speedily to cross out all examples of a single letter on a printed page, and ocular flicker fusion. This is not surprising since the $t\frac{1}{2}$ of nitrazepam is about 30 h. Discussion of drug effects on skilled tasks, especially car driving, is on page 325. Patients who have accidents and who have not been warned of the hazards of sedation during the day are likely to have a valid claim for compensation for any injury due to the negligence of the prescriber.

Termination of action of a *single dose* of a drug having a long $t\frac{1}{2}$ is often determined by distribution into tissues where it has no action, e.g. fat, muscle, rather than by metabolism or elimination, so that the duration of action of a single dose may be satisfactorily free from hangover despite a long $t\frac{1}{2}$, e.g. nitrazepam. But when a drug with a long $t\frac{1}{2}$ is used *nightly*, there will be accumulation (of drug or of active metabolites) until a steady state is reached (at about $5 \times t\frac{1}{2}$) and daytime impairment of performance may then become unacceptable. Thus, knowledge of the $t\frac{1}{2}$ is useful, but is not the only

---

[1] '... many times, reaching for the prescription pad and writing something out is a way the doctor says "Get lost! I don't want to hear you". It is a way of terminating the encounter.' Leo Hollister, Professor of Medicine, Psychiatry and Pharmacology, Stanford University, USA.

[2] Guidelines for the clinical investigation of hypnotic drugs 1983 WHO Regional Office for Europe, Copenhagen.

factor in determining duration of action; tissue concentrations and receptor binding (affinity) are also important.

As a general guide, nightly use of drugs with a $t^{1/2} < 8$ h may, and those with a $t^{1/2} > 16$ h will, still have effects the following day.

But next-day amnesia occurs, particularly with triazolam although it has a short $t^{1/2}$.

TIMING OF HYPNOTIC ADMINISTRATION

Patients should be advised. Generally a hypnotic is best taken on going to bed or a few minutes before. If the hypnotic was taken on an empty stomach, sleep latency will commonly be about 20 min. Some people are suited by taking the hypnotic, e.g. a slowly absorbed benzodiazepine, one hour before going to bed, but for others this can carry a risk of going to sleep prematurely and even in a potentially hazardous or unpleasant situation, e.g. in the bath.

Occasionally it is appropriate to advise a patient who suffers intermittent insomnia or is being weaned from chronic drug use, to go to bed, read a suitable book and to take a short half-life drug, e.g. lormetazepam, if still wakeful after 1 or 2 hours; the availability of a single dose at the bedside, for use if needed, gives confidence and may itself increase the ability to do without it. (Availability of a bottle of tablets at the bedside traditionally carries risk of inadvertent repeated self-administration; the hazard of this is one reason why benzodiazepines replaced barbiturates.)

DEPENDENCE

It can be assumed that all hypnotics induce tolerance and dependence, with abrupt withdrawal consequences ranging from insomnia even to convulsions (where dosage has been high and prolonged). Withdrawal from chronic users should always be gradual (see Benzodiazepine dependence); the longer the use the slower should be the withdrawal (over weeks, reducing both dose and frequency); if symptoms (anxiety, insomnia, nightmares) occur then consumption should be stabilised until the symptoms disappear (a β-adrenoceptor blocker may assist by allaying

somatic symptoms of anxiety); obviously, withdrawal symptoms are less acute with drugs (and active metabolites) having a long $t^{1/2}$ (slow fall in drug concentration giving time for adaptation). The subject should be warned of the possibility of symptoms and counselled that they will pass away; if confidence is lost, withdrawal will be unsuccessful.

Overdose. A single heavy overdose of a hypnotic may be followed by disturbed sleep for weeks even in subjects not habitually taking hypnotics.

Insomnia

Insomnia deserves special attention because it is common and causes much distress to its subjects. Its successful management involves much more than merely prescribing drugs, which should be regarded as temporary expedients only (see also above). Insomnia is defined as a belief of patients that they are not getting enough sleep despite opportunity to sleep. It comprises:

● failure to fall asleep within 45 min or
● difficulty in staying asleep (6 or more awakenings per night, or less than 6 h sleep)
● either of these at least 4 nights a week.[3]

Poor sleepers tend to overestimate the time it takes them to fall asleep (sleep latency) and to underestimate the time they stay asleep. When awakened during NREM (orthodox) sleep, subjects who complain of insomnia may claim they were not asleep. But some studies have found that nurses are liable to overestimate patients' sleep.

Clinical types of insomnia

● Tense people who lie awake in bed for hours unable to relax, and then sleep well.
● Exhausted people who, because they sleep early in the evening, wake early in the morning. They probably need no drug, but a midday rest.

---

[3] Kales J et al 1971 Clinical Pharmacology and Therapeutics 12: 691.

- People who wake repeatedly throughout the night, for no obvious reason.
- People who wake repeatedly from physical discomfort or pain and who need treatment of that condition plus a hypnotic (temporarily).
- Depressed people in whom sleep is shorter (early waking), less sound, interrupted and restless; patients need treatment for depression, not hypnotics.
- Those whose difficulty getting to sleep is caused by caffeine, which increases with age; alcohol, though it can help people to get to sleep, can cause early waking (rebound).
- Those suffering from overuse of hypnotics with development of tolerance (3–14 days) and rebound insomnia when attempts to abstain are made.

PRESCRIBING HYPNOTICS

Recognition that it is much easier to start than to stop longterm treatment with a hypnotic has been followed by formalised advice to doctors how to advise their patients about nonpharmacological approaches to insomnia. Leaflets have been circulated to all British general practitioners for issue to insomniac patients. Much advice is no more than common sense and seeks to reassure the patient. The proscription of all reading in bed (some leaflets) seems harsh, and not in keeping with our own experience. Perhaps a pharmacology book is preferable to a whodunit.

A hypnotic is most often needed in:

- Short-term, transient and situational insomnia that is severe and distressing, e.g. acute emotional disturbance, bereavement, domestic conflict, noisy hotel, to help the patient cope with brief episodes.
- Longterm (>3 weeks) persistent insomnia, which may have no apparent cause or may follow on after the passing of an acute situation (conditioned insomnia); it also occurs in states of chronic anxiety and unhappiness. A detailed analysis of the pattern and the potential causes is required. If it is decided that a hypnotic is required, then the objective is to restore the sleep habit by brief use of a drug. Where use is prolonged beyond a few days, insomnia due to withdrawal may be interpreted by patients as demonstrating a need to continue the

drug, which can cause great difficulty, especially if the doctors have not adequately counselled the patients and got their own objectives clear. It is all too easy to follow the indulgent path of repeat prescriptions.

Thus in both the above situations there is danger that emotional and physical dependence on the drug will occur. It is important not to allow prescription of hypnotics and sedatives to become a means of evading the patient's real problem. 'Unfortunately, some patients use the sedative hypnotics as a crutch to help them in the struggle against the everyday pressure of living',[4] and sadly, even the best doctor sometimes surrenders to patient demand, though believing that continued use of a hypnotic is not in the patient's interest.

A prescription for a hypnotic is justified for a few nights or up to 4 weeks to combat insomnia due to *anxiety*, provided there is good reason to expect the cause to be removed either by changes in environment or by treatment[5] (e.g. sedative antidepressant drug or electric convulsions or other nondrug treatment). But where there is persistent insomnia or a longstanding personality disorder a prescription is not justified because: tolerance develops, dependence is likely, sleep is not natural.

> At a very rough reckoning about one night's sleep in every ten in this country (UK) is hypnotic induced .... People seem to want to turn consciousness on and off like a tap .... While it is time-consuming to take a careful clinical history, to conduct a full clinical examination and to give wise advice, it takes only a moment to write a prescription and this does please and often satisfies the patient .... We do not always draw a clear distinction between the patients' wants and what we think are their *needs*, and it is regrettable how much we accede to the patients' demands in order to placate them and to save ourselves time and trouble.[6]

[4] Friend D G 1960 Clinical Pharmacology and Therapeutics 1: 5.

[5] Oswald I 1968 Pharmacological Reviews 20: 274.

[6] Dunlop D 1970 British Medical Bulletin 26: 236.

Jet lag (loss of well-being and insomnia after trans-meridian flights) is related to the need to adapt to new circadian rhythms; it is more difficult to adapt after an eastward flight (shorter day) than after a westward flight (longer day). Where subjects have a substantial problem it can be appropriate to provide a medium $t^{1/2}$ hypnotic to enable them to get to sleep and stay asleep.

Melatonin is the pineal gland hormone, synthesised (by consecutive acetylation and methylation of serotonin) and secreted only during the night. Lack of light causes adrenergic stimulation of the pineal β-receptors, and melatonin secretion is abolished by β-blockade. The impressive nature of the diurnal rhythm in melatonin secretion has stimulated interest in its use therapeutically to reset biological clocks, with a number of reports from placebo-controlled studies that melatonin ameliorates jet lag on long haul flights.[7] However, the optimal timing of melatonin administration is uncertain and in most countries pharmaceutical preparations are not generally available.

CHOICE OF A HYPNOTIC

The benzodiazepines are now overwhelmingly the first choice because they:

- alter sleep pattern least
- are safer than other drugs in overdose
- do not significantly induce drug metabolising enzymes that cause unwanted interactions.

There are numerous members to choose from. The principal factors that determine selection are pharmacokinetic:

- speed of absorption and passage into the central nervous system, i.e. lipid-solubility
- half-life of the drug
- presence of active metabolites
- half-life of any active metabolites.

[7] Petrie K, Dawson A G, Thompson L et al 1993 A double blind trial of melatonin as a treatment for jet lag in international cabin crew. Biological Psychiatry 33: 526–530 (Abstract). Claustrat B, Brun J, David M et al 1992 Melatonin and jet lag: confirmatory result using a simplified protocol. Biological Psychiatry 32: 705–711.

Taking these factors into account, a choice may be offered as follows:

temazepam: ($t^{1/2}$ 13 h) inactive metabolites; insignificant accumulation with repeated daily use, but may sometimes be too short-acting for subjects of early waking; next-day amnesia is little or absent.

lormetazepam: ($t^{1/2}$ 9 h) with inactive metabolites; insignificant accumulation with daily use.

The above are *absorbed* reasonably fast: lorazepam and oxazepam are absorbed rather too slowly for use when rapid onset is important.

Benzodiazepines with long $t^{1/2}$ and/or with metabolites of long $t^{1/2}$, e.g. diazepam, nitrazepam, flurazepam, are satisfactory as hypnotics for single, but not for daily doses. The long $t^{1/2}$ drugs (and active metabolites) may be used if there is daytime anxiety. Speed of onset, duration of effect and incidence of hangover depend on the dose and on the patient almost as much as on the choice of drug. Benzodiazepines are numerous. Those not discussed here may give satisfactory results, but clinicians should decide what they want to achieve and consider the kinetics of the drug and its metabolites before prescribing.

Barbiturates are obsolete as hypnotics.

Warning. If insomnia is due to pain an analgesic is essential. A hypnotic alone may result in mental confusion and restlessness.

Safety of hypnotics

Benzodiazepines are the safest, i.e. they cause minimal enzyme induction and minimal hazard in overdose, including hazard to inquisitive children imitating their parents'/grandparents' pill-swallowing proclivities. Other hypnotics are more hazardous in overdose.

Irritant drugs (chloral hydrate) are obviously unsuitable for peptic ulcer patients. In cases where it is especially desired to avoid any *respiratory depression*, e.g. in severe asthmatics or in head injury, even benzodiazepines in ordinary doses can impair ventilation.

Interactions. All hypnotics synergise with alcohol and other cerebral depressants.

Many nonbenzodiazepine hypnotics are hepatic enzyme inducers. Benzodiazepines are hypnotics of first choice in patients taking warfarin (a drug with a narrow therapeutic range and particularly prone to pharmacokinetic interaction).

AGE AND HYPNOTICS

In the *elderly* it is normal for sleep requirement to become less, and nocturnal awakenings to become more frequent. An ageing person who complains of this should obviously not be treated with a hypnotic; any persistent demands should be resisted for the most likely result will be that they will spend the rest of their lives taking a hypnotic to no advantage and to potential disadvantage.

The elderly are less tolerant of hypnotics. They should generally not receive long t½ drugs, and should start with half the usual dose.

The old, particularly those with organic brain failure, may become confused with hypnotics and an occasional patient becomes excited or has nightmares on a particular drug; a neuroleptic (promazine) may be used alone, or even cautiously with a hypnotic. Confusion is more likely if a patient who has taken a full dose of hypnotic is kept awake by pain; adequate analgesia should accompany the hypnotic. The need to micturate may result in drugged old people hazardously wandering around the house, and there is evidence of increased incidence of falls with fractured hip.

Children should only rarely be given a hypnotic (e.g. occasional use for night terrors): a benzodiazepine, chloral hydrate, or phenothiazine (promethazine, trimeprazine or promazine) is used.

MISCELLANEOUS

Food as an aid to sleep.[8] A small meal of milk and cereal promotes less restless sleep and there is experimental support for the popular belief that milk-cereal drinks do the same. The effect persists into the later night, suggesting that the cause is not only psychological expectation resulting from folklore and advertising, though these doubtless assist. Since broken sleep increases with age it may be worth recommending the adoption of a prebed snack or drink before prescribing hypnotics to older patients with mild insomnia.

Snoring implies a risk of obstructive sleep

apnoea, from which the subject needs to wake up, and is usually caused by collapsing of the epiglottis. Hypnotics are contraindicated. Physical measures can help, including continuous positive airways pressure.

Anxiety

Anxiety in moderation is a normal, appropriate and even useful response to life events and situations provided it stimulates achievement that may mitigate or remove the cause. But inappropriate or excessive or chronic anxiety is disabling, especially where the cause cannot be removed.

Yet anxiety may also occur without apparent exogenous cause, and subjects of this free-floating anxiety need and deserve help. Nondrug therapy may be best for many, but drugs are often useful for patients having a high level of anxiety. Doctors should not be over-ready to prescribe drugs, but neither should they be over-timid, for anxiety can be a curse that destroys the quality of life.

Benzodiazepines now dominate anti-anxiety medication. But anxiety does not manifest itself only as a psychic or mental state, there are also somatic or physical concomitants, e.g. consciousness of the action of the heart (palpitations), tremor, diarrhoea, which are associated with increased activity of the sympathetic autonomic system. These symptoms are not only caused by anxiety, they also add to the feeling of anxiety (positive feedback loop). In patients whose complaints are primarily of somatic or autonomic symptoms of anxiety rather than of anxiety itself a *β-adrenoceptor blocking drug* can give benefit; but it will generally not help where there is, e.g. tachycardia that is not causing symptoms, although it will reduce this.

Somatic symptoms of sympathetic overactivity accompany the performance of stressful tasks such as car driving in busy traffic, public speaking, playing a musical instrument, surgery and sports requiring calm skill without maximum output of work, bowling, shooting and sitting examinations; β-adrenoceptor block allows the subject to feel calmer and so can improve performance.

Even in experienced surgeons a rise in heart rate

---

[8] Brezinova V et al 1972 British Medical Journal 2: 431.

begins as soon as scrubbing-up for an operating session is begun. In one study (8 operating surgeons) mean maximum heart rates were 137/min with mean heart rate 121/min (peak rates above 150/min were reached by 2 surgeons) regardless of the nature of the operation and regardless of seniority. Tachycardia of this degree corresponds to physical work that cannot be sustained for more than 10 min without extreme fatigue. Those people who cannot conceal their emotional state will be interested to know that 'if anything, those surgeons who were outwardly the most calm experienced the highest heart-rates'.[9] The mean heart-rate of surgeons operating after taking a β-adrenoceptor blocking drug (oxprenolol 40 mg orally) was 84/min. But it has not been shown that the surgeons actually operated better or were less fatigued.

The principal disadvantages of drug therapy are dependence and the 'medicalising' of what is essentially a matter of interpersonal relationships or an environmental problem.[10]

CHOICE AND MODE OF USE OF ANXIOLYTIC AGENTS

- Benzodiazepines, e.g. diazepam, oxazepam, are a first choice.
- A beta-adrenoceptor blocker, e.g. propranolol, where there are somatic symptoms.
- A sedative antidepressant where there is depression with anxiety, e.g. amitriptyline.
- Buspirone may be considered where a two-week delay in effect is acceptable.
- Other agents, e.g. chlormethiazole, may particularly suit the aged and alcoholics.

Recurrent panic attacks may be prevented, sometimes completely, by antidepressant or buspirone (with the expected delay in onset of effect). The antidepressant benzodiazepine, alprazolam, is quickly effective but has a particular risk of dependence with difficult withdrawal.

Use of low doses of neuroleptics, e.g. chlorpro-

mazine, for anxiety, has been superseded by benzodiazepines. Neuroleptics can be effective but are liable to have too many autonomic side-effects.

> **Benzodiazepine use** should be limited to 2–4 weeks in anxiety that is severe, disabling or seriously distressing (i.e. these drugs should **not** be used for short-term mild anxiety).

Benzodiazepines are liable to induce dependence and patients in acute high-level anxiety states should be counselled that treatment will be brief, even only a few days. But where chronic anxiety seriously impairs social coping capacities, particularly where the causes can be seen to be irremovable, longterm therapy may seem inescapable although there is evidence that brief nonspecialised counselling is as effective. After the drug has been taken for 4–6 months, a serious effort should be made to withdraw it; but this can be impossible and indefinitely prolonged therapy sometimes becomes obligatory as the lesser of two evils. This is why counselling should be preferred to the use of a drug at the outset.

Some **tolerance** to benzodiazepines occurs but anxiolytic efficacy has been claimed to last 6 months, although it is hard to distinguish between resurgence of the condition and a rebound or withdrawal syndrome.

Benzodiazepines with a long $t\frac{1}{2}$ (of parent drug and/or active metabolite) are preferred for smooth effect: either a single nocturnal dose (where there is also insomnia), which will give anxiolytic effect the next day, or small divided doses (to minimise peaks of effects) during the day. The less lipid-soluble oxazepam and lorazepam give particularly smooth effect (slower absorption and slower entry into the CNS).

Where there are somatic symptoms, a β-adrenoceptor blocker may be effective alone or in combination with a benzodiazepine.

Bereavement. In an unexpected bereavement it would be harsh to deprive a seriously distressed person of sedation and sleep. But drugs should not be necessary for less acute distress and there is reason to think that benzodiazepines may inhibit psychological adjustment to the loss.

---

[9] Foster S E et al 1987 Lancet 1: 1323.

[10] Lader M H 1987 Rational Drug Therapy 21: 9.

Hypnotics and anxiolytic sedatives[11]

BENZODIAZEPINES

Benzodiazepines were discovered by serendipity (p. 43). In the mid-1950s the clinical successes of chlorpromazine suggested that tranquillisers were more than just general cerebral depressants. Industrial chemists of Hoffman-LaRoche were encouraged to produce novel compounds that might have selective tranquillising effect and that would lend themselves to molecular manipulation. Chlordiazepoxide was synthesised, but, other problems seeming more important, the project lost priority and chlordiazepoxide was left untested for 2 years. When it was eventually studied in animals it was found to be superior to existing tranquillisers, having a marked taming effect in monkeys. Some 16 000 patients were soon treated and the drug was licensed for general use in 1960. Since then thousands of benzodiazepines have been synthesised, hundreds tested and many tens have been marketed.

Actions

Benzodiazepines have hypnotic, sedative, anxiolytic, anticonvulsant and (central) muscle relaxant actions. They attach to a specific site on the GABA receptor/chloride channel complex, potentiating the effect of GABA (gamma-aminobutyric acid), an important inhibitory transmitter in the CNS which acts by opening chloride ion channels into cells. There are three subtypes of benzodiazepine receptor, which raises the possibility of separating the various actions of the benzodiazepines by molecular manipulation so that, for example, anxiolytic effect may be achieved without concomitant seda-

---

[11] Sedative: a drug (or dose of a drug) that calms or soothes without inducing sleep though it may cause sleepiness: a small dose of a hypnotic or *tranquilliser* often suffices for this. The imprecise term tranquilliser implies a drug that will quieten a patient without significantly impairing consciousness. The ideal tranquilliser would allay pathological anxiety, i.e. be *anxiolytic*, and allay nervous tension without altering any other cerebral functions; especially it would not cause sleepiness; it would suppress mania and psychotic overactivity.

tion, which would be an important advance. Existing benzodiazepines bind to all three subtypes, but some of the newer, nonbenzodiazepine drugs, zolpidem and zopiclone, to only one or two of these, respectively.

Benzodiazepines may act chiefly on the brain reticular activating system (reducing sensory input), the limbic system (affect), the median forebrain bundle (reward and punishment systems) and the hypothalamus.

Once receptor *agonists* have been made, *antagonists* follow, e.g. flumazenil, used for termination of agonist effect after use, e.g. endoscopies and to diagnose overdose (p. 321).

There are also benzodiazepines that have opposite (not merely blocking) actions, i.e. excitation, and these are called *inverse agonists* (see p. 79). The full possibilities for scientific discovery and therapeutic use of benzodiazepines in behaviour modification have yet to be explored.

Occasionally the agonist (sedative) compounds in current use cause *paradoxical effects*, e.g. excitement, aggression and antisocial acts. Alteration of dose, up or down, may eliminate these (as may chlorpromazine in an acute severe situation).

Benzodiazepines shorten the time taken to go to sleep (sleep latency), decrease intermittent awakening and increase total sleep duration. Choice of drug as hypnotic is determined by *pharmacokinetic properties* (see Choice of a hypnotic, above). The choice as anxiolytic sedative is also largely determined by pharmacokinetic properties (see Table 18.1, p. 318); slow absorption and long t½ give smooth effect. Selectivity between anxiolytic and sedative effect is low, though some trials suggest it, e.g. clorazepate (Tranxene) may be less sedative than diazepam for equal anxiolytic effect, but no definitive recommendations can be made. Diazepam remains the standard member of the group, having a t½ of 30 h with an active metabolite (desmethyldiazepam) with a t½ of 80 h. A single dose before going to bed provides quick hypnotic effect and repeated doses give anxiolytic effect with some sedation throughout the next day. If a dose is needed during the day the rapid absorption of diazepam may cause undesirable sedation (which can be mitigated by using several small doses though that adds inconvenience). The more slowly absorbed oxazepam may be preferred.

As well as causing sedation and drowsiness, ben-

Table 18.1 Data on some benzodiazepines (Long t$\frac{1}{2}$ drugs/metabolites are appropriate for anxiety. Short t$\frac{1}{2}$ drugs/metabolites are appropriate hypnotics)

Name	Plasma (t$\frac{1}{2}$ h)	Metabolites (t$\frac{1}{2}$ h)	Remarks
Alprazolam (Xanax)	16	inactive	Has antidepressant activity
Bromazepam (Lexotan)	12	inactive	—
Chlordiazepoxide (Librium)	20	active (14 40) desmethyldiazepam (80) [see note 5]	Steady-state of effect about 3 days
Clobazam (Frisium)	35	active (42)	Used in epilepsy as well as anxiety
Clonazepam (Rivotril)	25	inactive	Used in epilepsy
Clorazepate (Tranxene)	prodrug	desmethyldiazepam (80)	
Diazepam (Valium)	30	active (10) desmethyldiazepam (80)	High lipid solubility so quickly effective (orally): but slow in i.m.
Flunitrazepam (Rohypnol)	29	active (minor)	—
Flurazepam (Dalmane)	prodrug (1)	active (6) desmethyldiazepam (80)	Effect depends on metabolites
Ketazolam (Anxon)	prodrug (1.5)	active (30) desmethyldiazepam (80)	Partly metabolised to diazepam
Loprazolam (Dormonoct)	7	active (7)	Insignificant accumulation
Lorazepam (Ativan)	20	inactive	Slowly absorbed and distributed (lower lipid solubility)
Lormetazepam (Lobramet, Noctamid)	9	inactive	Insignificant accumulation
Medazepam (Nobrium)	prodrug (1.5)	desmethyldiazepam (80)	—
Midazolam (Hypnovel)	3	inactive	Injected as adjunct in anaesthesia for endoscopies, dentistry, etc.
Nitrazepam (Mogadon)	30	inactive	Superseded because of long t$\frac{1}{2}$
Oxazepam (Serenid)	7	inactive	Slowly absorbed and distributed (lower lipid solubility)
Prazepam (Centrax)	prodrug (1.5)	desmethyldiazepam (80)	Effect depends on metabolites
Temazepam (Euhypnos)	13	inactive	Insignificant accumulation
Triazolam (Halcion)	3	active (7)	Amnesia; excess of psychiatric reactions

1. The use of official (generic) names to stress *similarity* and proprietary names to stress *difference* is well shown.
2. The t$\frac{1}{2}$ variability in individuals is very wide indeed though only a single figure is given in the table.
3. Formation of active metabolites does not necessarily mean they play a major role, especially with single doses.
4. Steady state will be reached in about t$\frac{1}{2}$ × 5 of parent drug and active metabolites when present (but some active metabolites have only a minor role in clinical effect).
5. The principal active metabolite having a long t$\frac{1}{2}$ (80 h, but with range 30–200) and common to many members is *desmethyldiazepam* (nordiazepam); drugs having this metabolite are suitable as anxiolytics. There is no point in changing a patient from one agent having desmethyldiazepam as a major metabolite to another drug of the same kind. Generally agents that are conjugated have inactive metabolites, and those that are oxidised have active metabolites.
6. Liver disease may prolong t$\frac{1}{2}$ up to × 3.
7. Duration of action is prolonged in the elderly (initial dose should be low) and additive effects with alcohol are important.

zodiazepines impair memory (see below) and intellectual and psychomotor function.

Uses

Benzodiazepines are used to treat: anxiety (without or with psychotic states), panic attacks, insomnia, alcohol withdrawal states, night terrors and somnambulism (children), muscle spasm due to a variety of causes, including tetanus and cerebral spasticity; epilepsy; anaesthesia and sedation for endoscopies and cardioversion.

Curiously, perhaps, benzodiazepines are extensively prescribed by primary care doctors for depression; but they are not antidepressant (except perhaps alprazolam when anxiety is dominant in a mixed anxiety/depression). The reason is obscure but may be related to complaints of side-effects from the usual antidepressants.

Benzodiazepines are not appropriate for phobic and obsessional states.

Tolerance occurs with chronic use and there is cross-tolerance within the group.

Amnesia for events subsequent to administration occurs with high doses, i.v. for endoscopy, dental surgery (with local anaesthetic), cardioversion, and in these situations it can be regarded as a blessing.[12] But embarrassing amnesia can also occur with oral use: it is wise to warn travellers of this. High doses of triazolam particularly may cause amnesia.

Elderly and/or troubled people arrested for shoplifting frequently claim that their crime was caused by chronic benzodiazepine (or other) therapy. Whilst it is natural to regard such claims with suspicion, those of us (not taking a benzodiazepine) who have nearly walked out of a self-service shop carrying goods we have neglected to present for payment will not be over-ready to dismiss the possibility (though amnesia selective for payment must arouse scepticism). A useful way of looking at the matter is to consider, not whether the drug caused an involuntary act of shoplifting (which is unlikely), but whether it might have made a contribution to absentmindedness so that the necessary conscious intent to steal (required by criminal law) was not formed. When the circumstances of the particular case are known, the question may be asked whether it is safe to convict the person, i.e. that it is beyond reasonable doubt[13] that the drug was irrelevant. Many doubtful and pathetic instances are recorded in the newspapers; doctors are often asked to given evidence in Court; they will seek to be neither credulous nor callous.

Benzodiazepine doses as hypnotic (oral)

Temazepam Tabs[14]	10–30 mg orally
Lormetazepam Tabs	500 micrograms–1 mg orally

The elderly should be started on half the above doses. Sudden withdrawal can cause confusion.

Doses as anxiolytic sedative

- Diazepam Tabs 2 mg × 3/d increasing to a total daily dose of 30 mg if really necessary (it may take 2 weeks to reach a steady state at each dose) or use 5–30 mg at night if there is insomnia and take advantage of anxiolytic effect the next day.
- Oxazepam Tabs 15–30 mg × 3/d.
- Suppositories are available, e.g. diazepam (10 mg).

Injectable preparations

- *Intravenous* formulations, e.g. diazepam 10–20 mg, given at 5 mg/min into a large vein (antecubital fossa) to minimise thrombosis: the dose may be repeated in 30–60 min for status epilepticus or in 4 h for severe acute anxiety or agitation: midazolam is a shorter acting alternative, e.g. for endoscopies. The dose should be titrated according to response, e.g. drooping eyelids, speech, response to commands.
- *Intramuscular* injection of diazepam is absorbed erratically and may be slower in acting than an oral dose: lorazepam and midazolam i.m. are absorbed rapidly.

The elderly should receive half doses.

Dependence, as shown by occurrence of *withdrawal symptoms*, is usual with therapeutic doses used beyond a few weeks, though it is commonly mild. Dependence occurs earlier with the short $t\frac{1}{2}$ members but rebound or withdrawal symptoms are not so well correlated with $t\frac{1}{2}$. Withdrawal symptoms begin after 2–3 days with alprazolam and lorazepam but may be delayed for 2–3 weeks with diazepam. They pass off over 2–4 weeks and are

---

[12] Although one patient, normally a gentle man, believed he was being lied to when told his endoscopy had been performed. 'He assaulted his physician and was calmed only by a second endoscopy.' Later he was very embarrassed and apologised repeatedly (Lurie Y et al 1990 Lancet 336: 576). Another post-dental surgery patient purchased a bone china teaset and later condemned his wife for extravagance.

[13] The criterion of proof used in English Courts of Law is:
Civil cases — balance of probabilities
Criminal cases — beyond reasonable doubt
Shoplifting is theft and is a criminal arrestable offence.

[14] Temazepam gel filled capsules have been withdrawn in some countries because of their potential for abuse by self-injection of melted gel with serious thromboembolic complications.

greatly affected by expectation and personality, i.e. the symptoms are passive dependent traits.[15]

Symptoms include anxiety, agitation, irritability, confusion, delirium, depersonalisation, sleep disturbance, tremor, headache, muscle twitching or aches, sweating and diarrhoea. But patients have commonly been prescribed a benzodiazepine for similar symptoms and there is doubt in many cases just how much is a recrudescence of previous disorder and how much is evidence of true pharmacological dependence. After prolonged high doses abrupt withdrawal may cause confusion, delirium, psychosis and convulsions. Accounts of supposed withdrawal symptoms lasting for several months should be interpreted with caution.

Withdrawal of benzodiazepines should be gradual after as little as 3 weeks' use, but for longterm users it should be very slow, e.g. about 0.125 ($\frac{1}{8}$) of the dose every 2 weeks, aiming to complete it in 6–12 weeks. Withdrawal should be slowed if marked symptoms occur (milder symptoms may be controlled by β-adrenoceptor block). Towards the end of the withdrawal of a short t½ drug it may be useful to substitute a long t½ drug (diazepam) to minimise rapid fluctuations in plasma concentrations.[16] Abandonment of the final dose may be particularly distressing. In difficult cases withdrawal may be assisted by concomitant use of a sedative antidepressant.

> The occurrence of **dependence** will be minimised by critical prescribing using low doses for short periods or intermittently. Only in exceptional cases should use exceed a few weeks.

Interactions. There are additive effects with CNS

depressants, including alcohol, which also speeds benzodiazepine absorption. Cimetidine may increase plasma concentrations of diazepam and chlordiazepoxide by as much as 50% (delayed metabolism and clearance), this does not happen with oxazepam and lorazepam. High caffeine intake reduces the anxiolytic effect.

Overdose. Benzodiazepines are remarkably safe in acute overdose and the therapeutic dose × 10 induces sleep from which the subject is easily aroused. It is said that there is no reliably recorded case of death from a benzodiazepine taken alone by a person in good physical (particularly respiratory) health, which is a remarkable tribute to their safety (high therapeutic index); even if the statement is not absolutely true, death must be extremely rare. But deaths have occurred in combination with alcohol (which combination is quite usual in those seeking to end their own lives).

Flumazenil (p. 321) selectively reverses benzodiazepine effects and is useful in diagnosis, but is not generally used in treatment since its t½ (1 h) is so short, and life-endangering CNS depression is so rare.

Benzodiazepines in pregnancy. The drugs are not certainly known to be safe, and indeed diazepam is teratogenic in mice.[17] The drugs should be avoided in early pregnancy as far as possible. It should be remembered that safety in pregnancy is not only a matter of avoiding prescription after a pregnancy has occurred, but that individuals on longterm therapy may become pregnant. Benzodiazepines cross the placenta and can cause fetal cardiac dysrhythmia, and muscular hypotonia and poor suckling in the newborn.

Adverse effects of benzodiazepines include sleepiness and impaired psychomotor function and amnesia, causing hazard with car driving or operating any machinery (warn the patient). Dependence (see above).

Additive effects occur with alcohol, which is best avoided, though this will be a counsel of perfection

---

[15] The difficulty of assessing symptoms is shown by a study in which patients on longterm diazepam therapy experienced symptoms when they thought the drug was being withdrawn but in fact dosage remained the same. (Tyrer P et al 1983 Lancet 2: 1402).

[16] The BNF advises transferring the patient to diazepam at the start of withdrawal and gives the following equivalents. Diazepam 5 mg ≡ chlordiazepoxide 15 mg: loprazolam 0.5–1 mg: lorazepam 0.5 mg: lormetazepam 0.5–1 mg: nitrazepam 5 mg: oxazepam 15 mg: temazepam 10 mg: (triazolam 250 micrograms).

[17] Determined investigators can devise experiments in animals so that either fetal hazard or fetal safety is implied and it may not be obvious which predicts to man.

in habitual alcohol users. Paradoxical behaviour effects (see above) and perceptual disorders, e.g. hallucinations, occur occasionally. Headache, giddiness, alimentary tract upset, skin rashes and reduced libido can occur. Extrapyramidal reactions, reversible by flumazenil, are rare.

Suggestions that longterm use can cause organic brain damage are not firmly substantiated.

Women, perhaps as many as 1 in 200, may experience sexual fantasies, including sexual assault, after *large doses* of benzodiazepine as used in some dental surgery, and have brought charges in law against male attendants. Plainly a court of law has, in the absence of a witness, great difficulty in deciding who to believe. No such charges have yet been brought, it seems, by a man against a woman.

Other benzodiazepines include brotizolam, camazepam, clotiazepam, cloxazolam, delorazepam, estazolam, etizolam, halazepam, haloxazolam, mexazolam, nimetazepam, oxazolam, pinazepam, quazepam, tetrazepam.

It is such profusion that gives rise to criticism of both the pharmaceutical industry which produces the drugs (each company hoping that its product will indeed be an advance, but marketing it all the same if it is not), and regulatory bodies which permit this. It is good to have a choice, but there is such a thing as too much.

Three special benzodiazepines

Lorazepam differs from other members sufficiently to warrant description. It has a plasma $t^{1/2}$ of about 20 h which means that it is not seriously accumulative. It is less lipid-soluble than others (diazepam) and penetrates and leaves the CNS more slowly so that onset and offset of effect are smoother. Lorazepam is metabolised (conjugated) to inactive metabolites, a process that is less influenced by age than is the oxidation of other members, e.g. diazepam. These properties render it more suitable as an anxiolytic than as a hypnotic. Unfortunately it appears to have a peculiar capacity to induce dependence and withdrawal of the drug can be particularly difficult, a substantial disadvantage.

Given i.v. as a sedative, e.g. in intensive care, and as premedication for surgery and endoscopies, the onset of effect (15 min) is slower than with diazepam and midazolam (2 min), which are more lipid-soluble; but it acts for longer and may induce more amnesia, for which many patients may be thankful.

Given i.m. it is absorbed more speedily than diazepam, which means that it is more suitable than diazepam for status epilepticus, when i.v. injection is impracticable.

Alprazolam (Xanax) may have useful antidepressant action as well as sedation in depression where anxiety is prominent; it also can benefit panic attacks, but it may be particularly difficult to withdraw completely.

Triazolam (Halcion) (see Table 18.1, p. 318). Some regulatory bodies think the risks of adverse psychiatric effects and illicit i.v. abuse outweigh its benefits.

Benzodiazepine antagonist

Flumazenil (Anexate) is a competitive antagonist at benzodiazepine receptors, and it may have some agonist actions, i.e. it is a partial agonist. It has a $t^{1/2}$ of 1 h (see Table 18.1 for $t^{1/2}$ of agonists) so that repeated i.v. doses or infusion may be needed in the clinical situation. Heavily sedated patients become alert within 5 minutes.

Clinical uses include reversal of benzodiazepine sedation after endoscopies, dentistry and in intensive care (recovery period needs supervision lest sedation recurs; if used in day surgery it is important to tell patients that they may *not* drive a car home). In self-poisoning flumazenil is chiefly useful in diagnosis; it does not oppose depression due to nonbenzodiazepines. *Adverse effects* of flumazenil include vomiting, brief anxiety, seizures in epileptics treated with a benzodiazepine and precipitation of withdrawal syndrome in dependent subjects.

Buspirone (Buspar)

Buspirone is structurally unrelated to other anxiolytics. It is a partial agonist at serotonin and dopamine receptors. Probably its main function is to suppress 5HT neurotransmission through a selective activation of the inhibitory presynaptic $5HT_{1A}$ receptor. It has no hypnotic, muscle relaxant or antiepileptic effect and it does not benefit benzodiazepine withdrawal symptoms.

Buspirone has a $t\frac{1}{2}$ of 7 h and is metabolised in the liver; it has an active metabolite that may accumulate over weeks.

Anxiolytic efficacy is similar to or rather less than benzodiazepines. A disadvantage is that useful anxiolytic effect is delayed for 2 or more weeks. Buspirone causes little, if any, depression of psychomotor function (unlike benzodiazepines) and does not, in modest doses, potentiate the effects of alcohol (unlike benzodiazepines).

Adverse effects include dizziness, headache, nervousness, excitement, nausea, tachycardia and drowsiness.

Nefazodone (see p. 344) is a newer sedating antidepressant.

TRICHLOROETHANOL DERIVATIVES

Chloral hydrate (1869)

The first synthetic hypnotic to be introduced was a welcome alternative to opium and alcohol. Chloral hydrate is a solid and is usually given orally in solution because it is so irritant to the stomach; it tastes horrible; a capsule is available.

Chloral induces sleep in about half an hour, lasting 6–8 h with little hangover. Chloral is a prodrug; it is rapidly metabolised by alcohol dehydrogenase into the active hypnotic trichloroethanol ($t\frac{1}{2}$ 8 h). This is conjugated with glucuronic acid to an inert form. The ultimate metabolites are excreted in the urine and give a positive result in urine tests for reducing substances, but not, of course, for the specific glucose oxidase (enzyme) tests. Chloral is dangerous in serious hepatic or renal failure, and aggravates peptic ulcer.

Interaction with ethanol is to be expected since chloral shares the same metabolic enzyme (alcohol dehydrogenase). Trichloroethanol is a competitive inhibitor of the conversion of ethanol to acetaldehyde so that plasma ethanol concentration is higher than it would otherwise be; thus ethanol is potentiated by chloral. If chloral has been taken for several days, ingestion of alcohol may induce vasodilata-

tion, hypotension and tachycardia that cannot be explained by a simple potentiation.

Interaction with warfarin gives enhanced anticoagulant effect.

Triclofos (Tricloryl) and *chloral betaine* (Welldorm) are alternatives.

OTHER HYPNOTICS

Paraldehyde (1882) has had long use as a safe (little respiratory depression), oral hypnotic and by injection, for control of mania, alcohol withdrawal, tetanus and status epilepticus. Except for this last use (see p. 359), however, the drug can now be deemed obsolete. This is because of several major disadvantages: it smells and tastes unpleasant and is partly excreted unchanged via the lungs (75% is metabolised; $t\frac{1}{2}$ 5 h); it is an irritant (avoid in peptic ulcer) and causes painful muscle necrosis when injected i.m. It dissolves plastic syringes.

Chlormethiazole (Heminevrin) is structurally related to vitamin B_1 (thiamine). It may act by altering dopamine function in the brain. It is particularly used during withdrawal from severe alcohol abuse (started at a high dose and withdrawn over 6 or 7 days; but not for patients who continue to drink) and in senile psychosis and confusion; it is a hypnotic, sedative and anticonvulsant (used in status epilepticus). It is comparatively free from hangover; it can cause nasal irritation and sneezing. Dependence occurs and use should always be brief. When taken orally, it is subject to extensive hepatic first-pass metabolism (which is defective in the old and in liver damaged alcoholics who get higher, as much as × 5, peak plasma concentrations), and the usual $t\frac{1}{2}$ is 4 h (with more variation in the old than the young); it may also be given i.v.

Phenothiazines. Promethazine (Phenergan) is a useful long-lasting hypnotic ($t\frac{1}{2}$ 12 h) especially in children. It is also an antihistamine (H_1-receptor); other antihistamines having sedative action are also used as hypnotics. Trimeprazine (Vallergan) is used for short-term sedation and hypnosis in children.

Zopiclone (Zimovane) is a cyclopyrrolone with a

t½ of 5 h. Like the benzodiazepines its target is the benzodiazepine/GABA receptor complex. Its efficacy is similar to benzodiazepines, but it causes less reduction in the proportion of REM sleep, less hangover effects the next day and less dependence. Withdrawal may therefore be easier. The recommended dose is 7.5 mg.

Zolpidem (Stilnoct), an imidazopyridine, is the newest hypnotic. It acts selectively on one of the 3 benzodiazepine receptor subtypes, and is distinguished from most other widely available benzodiazepines by its short t½ of 2 hours. In controlled studies, it is as effective as flunitrazepam, without any demonstrable reduction in cognitive or psychomotor function the next morning. It has not yet been compared with temazepam or zopiclone. The recommended dosing schedule is 10 mg every 3 or 4 nights for a maximum of 2–4 weeks.

Hypnotics and anxiolytic sedatives of no particular merit include: meprobamate (Miltown), chlormezanone (Trancopal); they are centrally acting muscle relaxants.

BARBITURATES[18] (1903)

There is an increasing consensus that barbiturates are unsuitable as hypnotics because:

- Barbiturates have a low therapeutic index, i.e. relatively small overdose ($\times$ 10 therapeutic dose) endangers life, with unconsciousness and respiratory depression
- Barbiturates illicitly obtained have been popular drugs of social abuse
- Physical dependence occurs, with severe withdrawal syndrome sometimes including convulsions
- Barbiturates are potent inducers of hepatic drug metabolising enzymes and so are a source of unintended drug interactions.

But use, and abuse, continues. Therefore a general account is retained here. Knowledge of how to handle overdose remains important.

---

[18] Derivatives of barbituric acid, reputedly named by the original synthesiser after 'a charming lady named Barbara'. Miller L C 1961 JAMA 127: 27.

Actions

Barbiturates provide depression of the **central nervous system** ranging from mild sedation to surgical anaesthesia (see Ch. 21). For use as hypnotics and sedatives, depressant barbiturates have qualitatively similar actions; but they differ in the rate and method of disposal in the body, which has a bearing on their clinical use, and phenobarbitone and methylphenobarbitone have a greater anticonvulsant effect relative to the hypnotic effect. The mode of action may be similar to benzodiazepines, but with much less selectivity.

Pain. There is also evidence that barbiturates can antagonise analgesics and this may be borne in mind when they are used in patients with pain.

Respiration. A hypnotic dose of a barbiturate in a patient with marked respiratory insufficiency, e.g. severe pulmonary emphysema or asthma, will depress respiratory minute volume and arterial oxygen saturation. Benzodiazepines, paraldehyde and chloral are less objectionable in this respect.

Cardiovascular function. Barbiturates lower blood pressure at hypnotic and anaesthetic doses by reducing cardiac output; venous return to the heart is reduced due to peripheral venous pooling. Compensatory vascular reflexes are depressed.

Toxic doses may depress the myocardium and also reduce the peripheral resistance by blocking the sympathetic nerves (hypotension).

Tolerance. When 18 former addicts were given 0.4 g pentobarbitone or quinalbarbitone daily for 90 days, tolerance began to develop within 14 days. They showed significant decrease in hours of sleep, in signs of clinical intoxication and in performance in psychomotor tests. Tolerance probably occurs to all hypnotics, but it is less marked than with opioids. With barbiturates and meprobamate the tolerance is at least partly due to enzyme induction.

Psychological and physical dependence occur with regular dosage of 0.4 g/day, or more, of barbiturate. If the dose exceeds 0.6 g/day the subject generally shows clinical signs of intoxication: impairment of mental ability, regression, confusion, emotional instability, nystagmus, dysarthria, ataxia and depressed somatic reflexes.

The withdrawal syndrome begins in 8–36 h and passes off over 8–14 days. It comprises, in approximate order of appearance: anxiety, twitching, intention tremor, weakness, dizziness, distorted vision, nausea; delirium and convulsions occur in severe cases.

Pharmacokinetics. Absorption after oral administration is rapid: plasma protein binding is variable, those with longer half-lives being less protein bound than those with shorter half-lives. Half-lives are the result of renal excretion and of metabolism in those used as hypnotics and sedatives.

Plasma t½

85 h: phenobarbitone

20–40 h: pentobarbitone, quinalbarbitone (secobarbital), amylobarbitone, butobarbitone

For those used as i.v. anaesthetics (see Index), redistribution is a major factor in plasma half-life of initial doses.

Barbiturates distribute throughout the body.

Metabolism. For most barbiturates metabolism is chiefly hepatic. Barbiturates induce drug metabolising hepatic enzymes.

Excretion. The reason why there is little urinary excretion of unchanged barbiturate (except phenobarbitone, 25%) is not that they do not appear in the glomerular filtrate, but because barbiturate that appears in the glomerular filtrate, if un-ionised, diffuses back into the circulation through the renal tubule. This diffusion will be less if the drug is ionised (see pKa variation and kinetics, p. 90). This has been used successfully in the *treatment of overdose by phenobarbitone*, which has a pKa of 7.2, and raising the urine pH to 7.5–8.5 (by sodium bicarbonate) achieves a substantial shift of un-ionised drug to the ionised and lipid-insoluble state. Urinary elimination may be more than doubled. Other barbiturates have higher pKa (nearer 8) and so alkalinisation of the urine does not have useful effect.

Severe overdose. Important features such as occur with acute abuse, often i.v., include:

- prolongation of t½ of the barbiturate with prolonged coma (days).
- hypotension due to CNS and cardiac depression leading to renal failure. This is treated by restoring central venous pressure and so cardiac output, by use of i.v. fluid and, if that fails, using a drug with cardiac inotropic effect (dobutamine).
- Elimination of the drug is promoted by ensuring a good urine volume (e.g. 200 ml/h) and rendering it alkaline for phenobarbitone (see above).
- Active elimination by haemoperfusion or dialysis may be needed in particularly severe and complicated cases.
- The use of a diuretic to enhance elimination makes management more difficult and risky without adequate benefit to compensate for this.
- Respiratory stimulation (doxapram) is only useful to sustain respiration until mechanical assistance can be set up.

After overdose sleep pattern may be abnormal for weeks even in unhabituated subjects.

Contraindications to barbiturates. In severe pulmonary insufficiency, e.g. emphysema, even hypnotic doses of barbiturates depress respiration (see general account above). Hepatic failure potentiates barbiturates. Attacks of porphyria (see Index) are induced in predisposed people.

The principal barbiturates have been listed under half-life (above) (see also Anaesthesia for i.v. barbiturates, and Epilepsy).

Uses. Barbiturates are obsolete as hypnotics and sedatives (see above). For oral use the barbiturate or its more soluble sodium salt can be used; it matters little; but for parenteral administration a sodium salt is required. Soluble barbiturates may be injected i.m. when the dose is similar to that given orally. For i.v. injection the drug is given slowly (except thiopentone for anaesthesia) and the dose judged by results. It is dangerous to give i.v. the more slowly metabolised and excreted drugs.

Acute adverse effects of barbiturates are almost

entirely those of overdose: coma and respiratory and circulatory failure, leading to renal failure. Allergic reactions occur occasionally, particularly with phenobarbitone, rashes being the most common, but severe and fatal reactions have rarely been recorded (see also Contraindications and Metabolism, above).

Dependence and acute abuse with overdose has been a serious social and medical problem (see above), but other drugs are now displacing barbiturates.

Bromides (1875) are handled in the body like chloride. They are now obsolete (not particularly effective and $t^1/2$ of 4 weeks) not only for epilepsy and as general sedatives but also for night screaming in children, townswomen who are going out of their minds, 'frightful imaginings' in late pregnancy, seasickness, somnambulism, nymphomania, and spermatorrhoea consequent on 'undue indulgence in bed'.[19]

Drugs and skilled tasks

Drugs can affect skilled tasks and car driving.

Many medicines affect performance, not only the obvious examples, psychotropic drugs of all kinds, but also: antihistamines, antimuscarinics, analgesics including some NSAIDs, e.g. indomethacin, antiepileptics, antidiabetics (hypoglycaemia), some antihypertensives. *Alcohol and cannabis* are discussed on pages 166 and 179.

It is plain that prescribers have a major responsibility here, both to warn patients and, in the case of those who need to drive for their work, to choose medicines having minimal liability to cause impairment. One example must suffice. In a study[20] of two histamine H_1-receptor blockers, terfenadine did not impair car driving tests (weaving amongst bollards and 'gap acceptance') whereas triprolidine did. Subjects who were aware of drowsiness were yet unable to compensate, so that it is not enough to warn drivers to be more careful if they feel drowsy; **they should not drive**.

Patients who must drive when taking a drug of known risk (e.g. benzodiazepine) should be specially warned of times of peak impairment.

A patient who has an accident and who was not warned of drug hazard, whether orally or by labelling, may successfully sue the doctor in law. It is also necessary that patients be advised of the **additive effect of alcohol with prescribed medicines**.[21]

Car driving is a complex multifunction task that includes[22]

- visual search and recognition
- vigilance
- information processing under variable demand
- decision-making and risk-taking
- sensorimotor control.

It is evident that drivers may be more than usually accident prone without any subjective feeling of sedation or dysphoria: the fact that they feel OK does not mean that they are OK.

The criteria for safety in air-crew are more stringent than those for car drivers.

Little is known of impairment and risk in skilled tasks other than driving. Concentration on psychomotor and physical aspects (injury) should not distract from the possibility that those who live by their intellect and imagination (politicians and even journalists may be included here) may suffer cognitive disability from thoughtless prescribing.

Resumption of car driving or other skilled activity after anaesthesia is a special case, and an extremely variable one. The following suggestions may serve.

---

[19] Ringer S, Sainsbury H 1897 A handbook of therapeutics. H K Lewis, London.

[20] Betts T et al 1984 British Medical Journal 288: 281.

[21] Nordic countries require that medicines liable to impair ability to drive or to operate machinery be labelled with a red triangle on a white background. The scheme covers antidepressants, benzodiazepines, hypnotics, drugs for motion sickness and allergy, cerebral stimulants, antiepileptics and hypotensive agents. In the UK there are some standard labels that pharmacists are recommended to apply, e.g. 'Warning. May cause drowsiness. If affected do not drive or operate machinery. Avoid alcoholic drink'. They are offered as 'a carefully considered balance between the unintelligibly short and the inconveniently long' (see BNF).

[22] In: Willett R E et al (eds) 1983 Drugs, driving and traffic safety. WHO, Geneva.

- After dentistry under local anaesthesia: drive alone after 2 h.
- Where a sedative (e.g. i.v. benzodiazepine, opioid or neuroleptic), or any general anaesthetic has been used: after 24 h at least.
- How the patient feels is **not** a reliable guide to recovery of skills.

SUMMARY

- The apparent ability of the benzodiazepine drugs to sedate, non addictively, led to their use more than any other type of drug.
- Belated appreciation of the development of benzodiazepine dependence has led to a reversal of such widespread prescription.
- In most patients, insomnia and anxiety need good advice, not bad medicine. Pharmacological treatment should be limited in most patients to a few weeks.
- Benzodiazepines with a range of $t_{1/2}$ are available, e.g. midazolam for use in endoscopies, temazepam for night-time sedation, and diazepam for daytime anxiolytic effect.
- Alternative hypnotic drugs, zopiclone and zolpidem, may have lower risk of dependence.
- Alternatives to benzodiazepines for their anxiolytic effect is β-adrenoceptor blockade in some patients, sedative antidepressants (amitriptyline) or newer drugs which reduce 5HT transmission, buspirone or nefazodone.
- There is still a role, especially in children, for older drugs such as sedative antihistamines. Barbiturates are rarely indicated, except as single doses to cover semi-invasive procedures in children.

GUIDE TO FURTHER READING

Anonymous 1990 Zopiclone: another carriage in the tranquilliser train. Lancet 335: 507–8

Bixler E O et al 1991 Next-day memory impairment with triazolam use. Lancet 337: 827

Brahams D 1990 Benzodiazepine and sexual fantasies. Lancet 335: 157

Controversies in therapeutics 1989 Risks of dependence on benzodiazepine drugs. British Medical Journal: (1) Tyrer P The importance of patient selection 298: 102 (2) Ashton H A major problem of long term treatment 298: 103

Gillin J C 1990 The diagnosis and management of insomnia. New England Journal of Medicine 322: 239; 324: 1735

Greenblatt D J et al 1989 Effect of gradual withdrawal on the rebound sleep disorder after discontinuation of triazolam. New England Journal of Medicine 317: 722

Shapiro C M, Devins G M, Hussain M R 1993 ABC of sleep disorders. Sleep problems in patients with medical illness. British Medical Journal 306: 1532–1535

Swift C G, Shapiro C 1993 ABC of sleep disorders. Sleep and sleep problems in elderly people. British Medical Journal 306: 1468–1471

Tyrer P 1993 ABC of sleep disorders. Withdrawal from hypnotic drugs. British Medical Journal 306: 706–708

19

Drugs and mental disorder

SYNOPSIS

Drugs are sometimes paramount in treatment but are often secondary to nondrug approaches.

In schizophrenia, neuroleptic drugs whose principal effect is to block dopamine receptors are used but they can exact a high price in adverse effects.

In depression, the monoamine hypothesis proposes that there is deficiency of noradrenaline and serotonin in the brain which can be modified by antidepressants.

Mania is associated with overactivity of brain noradrenergic transmission; it may be controlled and prevented by drugs.

- Drugs in mental disorder
- Schizophrenic syndrome and neuroleptics
- Affective disorders: depression, mania and other psychological conditions
- Psychotropic drugs
- Neuroleptics, antidepressants, SSRIs, MAOIs, lithium
- Psychostimulants, appetite control: amphetamines, methylxanthines, ginseng

Drugs in mental disorder

> Writing prescriptions is easy, understanding people is hard. (Franz Kafka, 1883–1924)

In the debate whether the basis for mental disorders is primarily physical or psychological it might seem that the two hypotheses are irreconcilable. But the ultimate experience of mental activity involves biochemical changes in transmission in the brain, and, whether the initiating factors are primarily psychological or physical (biochemical), the use of a chemical to alter function beneficially can be appropriate. Most psychiatrists would seek for precipitating psychological and social events and endeavour to modify these as a part of therapy. They would do this despite their knowledge that there are important biochemical changes in the brain, but they would also seek to modify these with drugs.

Overreliance on drugs could lead to an undesirable reduction in the vital role of trained staff operating in a positive therapeutic environment, but neuroleptics can be a valuable means of enabling these staff to make psychological contact with and work alongside disturbed patients.

Drugs are easier and cheaper to supply than are trained staff. But drugs are not a substitute for trained staff.

With the increasing recognition of mental illness as a major cause of unhappiness and disability, interest in the possibilities of drug therapy has increased. Medicinal chemists have responded by making analogues of endogenous neurotransmitters in the expectation that some of them will prove to be medicines. One snag is the difficulty of predicting therapeutic efficacy from the animal experiments that must necessarily precede clinical trial; another is how to determine by clinical trial whether a genuine therapeutic effect has occurred and, if so, whether it was in fact due to the drug or to environmental changes or to behavioural therapy, including any extra care by the physician.

Paul Ehrlich wrote that 'we must learn to aim, learn to aim with chemical substances'. But in order to aim we must have targets to aim at and, if benefits are to be obtained without unwanted effects, the targets must be precisely defined. In mental disorder the targets are increasingly being defined.

> Though there have been many apparent breakthroughs, time and again they have been like elephants' footprints in the mud, making a large initial impression but quickly fading into the background.[1]

There is greater likelihood of therapeutic success from drugs in the psychoses in which behaviour differs from normal in kind, than in psychoneuroses in which it differs from normal mainly in amount.

Psychotropic drugs (drugs that alter mental function) act by altering endogenous chemotransmitter systems that pass nerve impulses at synapses, i.e. from the ending of one neuron across the synaptic cleft to the next neuron, e.g. noradrenaline, dopamine, serotonin, acetylcholine, gamma-aminobutyric acid (GABA), histamine, endorphins. Plainly the formation, storage, release and the occupation of receptors and postreceptor events caused by these active substances offer opportunities for intervention with appropriately designed chemicals (drugs). Research concentrates on these aspects.

Sites of action

Localisation of function (via these transmitters) within the brain, suggests three main anatomical sites of action[2] of drugs in mental disease:

- *Reticular activating system*: attention, arousal, anxiety
- *Limbic system*: affect or emotional content
- *Hypothalamus*: control of autonomic nervous system; pituitary–endocrine control.

There is a complex range of interrelationships, e.g. the locus coeruleus interconnects the reticular formation, hypothalamus and cortex, also utilising these transmitters. But the transmitters are not confined to these sites, and so nonselective drugs will be expected to cause unwanted (adverse) effects, as indeed they do.

Schemes of drug action

Enough is now known to allow the formulation of provisional schemes of drug action and adverse reaction that begin to give the kind of understanding that may help clinicians to use psychotropic drugs more effectively than would be the case if they merely followed routine instructions as they do in cooking. The special difficulties with assessing or systematising psychotropic drugs arise because the physical basis, and therefore therapeutic targets, in psychiatric illness are not firmly established, and because the semiquantitative 'instruments' used to measure depression and anxiety in drug trials are hard to relate to the everyday clinical pictures which doctors are wanting to assess and treat. What follows, therefore, is not a definitive account, but is offered to show the kind of approaches and interpretations that are currently being made.

CLINICAL EVALUATION

Clinical evaluation is done by recording changes in behaviour, performance of tasks and psychomotor tests, and opinions of patients as well as of their families, nurses and doctors. There is a large number of rating scales, inventories, questionnaires and check lists to measure anxiety, depression, guilt, adverse effects, and they can be applied by observers or by the patients themselves. The final court of appeal for efficacy and acceptability must always be the patient's clinical condition.

---

[1] Editorial. 1978 Lancet 1: 422.

[2] After Hollister L E 1983 Clinical pharmacology of psychotherapeutic drugs, 2nd edn. Churchill Livingstone, Edinburgh.

Controlled trials in psychiatry also require to take into account important environmental factors and life events, e.g. attitudes of relatives, bereavement.

Some of the hazards of uncontrolled studies have been demonstrated. In one case patients and hospital staff were told that two new drugs were to be tried, an 'energiser' and a 'tranquilliser'. The tablets were orange and yellow respectively, and were available in two sizes. Improvement was reported in 53% of patients taking the 'energiser' and in 80% of those taking the 'tranquilliser'. In fact both 'drugs' were lactose, made to taste bitter with quinine.[3]

Even where a careful double-blind technique is used successfully, bias due to the personality and beliefs of the physicians about the remedies can still affect the result. In a study on relief of anxiety by two active drugs and a placebo, the results varied according to which of two physicians was treating the patients.

Dr A was youngish in appearance, he expected no difference between the three treatments and his attitude to the patients was noncommittal. No difference between the treatments was found.

Dr B had greying hair and a fatherly appearance and he expected that the pharmacologically active substances would prove superior to the placebo. Patients reported that he was 'helpful' and 'dependable'. A difference in favour of one of the active drugs appeared in his patients.

When both groups were added there was no significant difference.[4]

It is probable that effects of doctors' personalities and opinions can influence even the best conducted studies, and this may be more likely to happen where the drug is an adjuvant and not the mainstay of therapy. The fact that endeavours to eliminate bias are not invariably successful has been used as an argument against attempting controlled techniques in psychiatric comparisons. The logic of this is obscure.

CHOICE OF DRUGS IN MENTAL AND BEHAVIOURAL DISORDERS

Nondrug therapies are not discussed here. This is not because they are unimportant, but because they are outside the scope of a book on pharmacology.

Patients often get better without drugs, and sometimes in spite of them.

A patient with endogenous depression became very much better during 3 or 4 weeks following prescription of an antidepressant drug. The physician reminded her of the importance of continuing therapy despite the improvement. The patient smiled and said 'Oh, doctor, the tablets did not agree with me, so I stopped taking them after the first two or three days'.[5]

- Antidepressants require about 10 days to produce benefit
- There is a great deal more to treatment than simply prescribing drugs
- When a patient improves following a prescription, it cannot be assumed that it is because of the prescription.

Psychotropic drugs provide symptomatic or suppressive treatment only; they do not eliminate the disease but ameliorate the condition until recovery occurs. But it is possible that by reducing a symptom a vicious cycle may be broken so that recovery occurs sooner, and in severe cases drugs may allow the patient to re-establish contact with his environment and thus to become accessible to social and psychotherapy.

The effects of all drugs acting on mental processes vary greatly with the circumstances and the dose and the attitude of the prescriber.

In psychotic states (severe manic or depressive illness and schizophrenia) neuroleptics or antidepressants (tricyclic or allies) are given in rapidly increasing doses at first, with longer intervals between increases later. Once the maximum longterm benefit is achieved the dose may be reduced gradually, even by as much as half, without loss of benefit; frequency of administration may sometimes be reduced to the convenient once a day.

Eventual withdrawal should also be gradual to avoid sudden and dangerous relapse. Duration of treatment is impossible to predict; no attempt at withdrawal should be made until 6–8 weeks after

---

[3] Loranger A W et al 1961 JAMA 176: 920.

[4] Uhlenhuth E H et al 1959 American Journal of Psychiatry 115: 905.

[5] Merry J 1962 Lancet 1: 1175.

apparent recovery from an acute episode and two-thirds of chronic cases need treatment for 3–4 years, in which case a long-acting i.m. formulation may be preferred.

The minimum effective dose should always be used, especially in patients in the community, and the need to continue therapy reviewed at least twice a year.

Resistant cases may be admitted to hospital to receive high doses. Severe intercurrent illness may reduce drug requirement.

In psychoneuroses (anxiety, phobias, reactive depression, obsessive-compulsive disorders), the environment is relatively more important; drugs are best confined to short periods, to help patients over a bad phase of illness. Prolonged drug therapy is seldom rewarding. It must be admitted that this view is not unanimously held, some physicians believing that drug therapy is of great value in the routine treatment of psychoneuroses.

Combinations of psychotropic drugs are sometimes useful. Initially at least, the drugs should be given separately, e.g. first an anti-anxiety agent and then a neuroleptic added and the dose adjusted to suit the patient. Fixed-dose combinations are unsatisfactory, chiefly because of this need to adjust the dose; but patients are less likely to take separate drugs reliably. Mild-to-moderate mixed anxiety-depression (such as is seen in general practice and seldom finds a way to a psychiatrist) may benefit from a mix of tricyclic + neuroleptic (Motival, Triptafen).

Schizophrenic syndrome and neuroleptics[6]

Schizophrenia is associated with increased dopaminergic activity in the limbic structures of the brain. There is an increased number of dopamine-D_2 receptors in the brain and there may be receptor supersensitivity and overproduction of dopamine,

or reduced destruction due to enzyme abnormalities or deficiencies. It is not proved whether this is the primary defect in schizophrenia or whether it is a secondary or epiphenomenon.

Neuroleptic[6] drugs that benefit schizophrenia, e.g. phenothiazines, butyrophenones, thioxanthenes, are competitive antagonists of dopamine (dopamine-D_2 receptor blockers) and a precursor of dopamine, levodopa, predictably exacerbates symptoms of schizophrenia. D_1 receptors, postsynaptic and presynaptic (autoreceptors), are also involved but it is not yet possible to present a coherent, clinically useful account.

Dopaminergic neurons are not confined to the limbic system. Dopamine-D_2 receptors, for example, also occur in the nigrostriatal (extrapyramidal) system and elsewhere, e.g. controlling hypothalamic hormone-releasing factors. Thus a dopamine antagonist, e.g. chlorpromazine, would be expected to benefit schizophrenia but also to cause extrapyramidal movement disorders and endocrine changes, e.g. prolactin release. And this is indeed the case; all these effects occur with chlorpromazine. It also blocks *serotonin receptors* which may be relevant to its therapeutic effect. It has in addition alpha-adrenoceptor and cholinergic blocking activity. Indeed it was given the proprietary name 'Largactil' because it has such a large number of actions. Despite this lack of selectivity, chlorpromazine, the first (1951) neuroleptic or antipsychotic drug, was a major advance in therapeutics and it remains useful.

TREATMENT

Neuroleptics are the most effective drugs and can greatly reduce positive symptoms, e.g. aggression, hyperactivity, delusions and hallucinations. But negative symptoms, e.g. apathy, respond less well.

Acute episodes may respond at once, but in chronic states response may be delayed for 3 weeks or more. Additional treatments, e.g. an antidepressant (tricyclic) or electroconvulsive therapy (ECT), may be needed.

Maintenance therapy may be necessary to prevent relapse, especially if the patient's family is critical

---

[6] Neuroleptic: an imprecise term comprising the more powerful (major) tranquillisers used for antipsychotic effect. For definition of tranquilliser, see footnote on page 317.

or otherwise unsupportive, as it often is, understandably.

The choice of drug is wide and may be illustrated as follows:

- Acute schizophrenic state: chlorpromazine or haloperidol
- Maintenance therapy: chlorpromazine or alternative phenothiazine or pimozide
- Longterm maintenance where patient compliance needs to be known with certainty: sustained-release or depot i.m. injection, e.g. fluphenazine decanoate 2–6 weekly.

Unfortunately neuroleptics have a capacity (variable between groups and members of groups) to induce serious extrapyramidal neuromuscular adverse effects, in particular a late onset (tardive) dyskinesia which may be irreversible (see below). But sulpiride and clozapine are relatively free from this.

MECHANISM OF ADVERSE EFFECTS AND TREATMENT

Enough is now known to begin to explain the mechanism of the troublesome adverse effects of dopamine-receptor blocking neuroleptics (and antiemetics) and such knowledge is useful in management of patients. It may be summarised:

Neurological effects

Extrapyramidal motor disorders: tremor, dystonia, akinesia and/or a parkinsonian oculogyric crisis syndrome are to be expected. Idiopathic parkinsonism is due to underactivity or deficiency in dopaminergic neurons causing imbalance between dopaminergic and cholinergic systems (see Parkinson's disease). Evidently a dopamine receptor blocker will mimic this disease. Occurrence of the above effects may predict liability to tardive dyskinesia.

It is generally best to withdraw, or reduce the dose of, the drug. But this may not be practicable since valuable benefit may be lost. In such cases it is necessary to treat the motor disorder with another drug. An antimuscarinic drug (procyclidine, benztropine) should be used, but routine prophylactic use is not justified. Many phenothiazines also have antimuscarinic effects and these are less liable to cause extrapyramidal disorders because they mitigate the dopaminergic/cholinergic imbalance.

Levodopa (converted to dopamine in the brain) is inappropriate because it will either be ineffective in the presence of a dopamine receptor blocker or if it is effective it will also antagonise the therapeutic effect in the limbic system.

Akathisia (extreme restlessness) occurs in about 20% of patients. It may respond to propranolol (a β-adrenoceptor blocker that enters the CNS); antimuscarinics are generally ineffective.

The above effects generally occur early in the course of treatment, but also may be tardive (late onset). Of the latter, one form is particularly prominent, as follows.

Tardive dyskinesia

Tardive dyskinesia is a disorder of involuntary movements (choreoathetoid movements of lips, tongue, face, jaws, and of limbs and sometimes trunk). It occurs generally after 2–5 years use of a dopamine receptor blocker, though occasionally after a few months. It is due, paradoxically, to increased dopamine-sensitivity or activity due to changes in the receptors themselves and to up-regulation (increase in numbers) of receptors characteristic of exposure to any blocking drugs. It is still difficult to explain exactly how excessive dopamine receptor activation can occur in the presence of their blockade. Since multiple (at least 5) subtypes of dopamine receptor have been recognised, the explanation for the paradox may be that the dopamine antagonists in use do not block all of these equally, with heterologous sensitisation occurring of some of these. Some evidence for this explanation is the infrequency of the syndrome with clozapine, which selectively blocks the D_4 receptor subtype.

Tardive dyskinesia particularly affects patients with organic brain disease and the elderly who should not be given these drugs if it can be avoided. It occurs in about 20% of treated schizophrenic patients, but in up to 40% of longterm institutionalised patients. Though generally mild, it may be severe and permanent.

Patients pass from a state of drug-induced reduction of dopaminergic activity to an indirectly drug-induced excess of dopaminergic activity. If this state continues then damage to the presynaptic membrane may result so that the presynaptic autoreceptors become supersensitive and the condition is irreversible.

If the neuroleptic is suddenly withdrawn, tardive dyskinesia may become worse because of the sudden accessibility to transmitter of the previously blocked but now more numerous receptors.

Also, antimuscarinics which are useful where there is a deficiency of dopaminergic activity (extrapyramidal disorders, above, and parkinsonism), since they restore the dopaminergic/cholinergic balance, will exacerbate tardive dyskinesia by increasing the imbalance that has already risen.

Rational management of tardive dyskinesia, if the dopamine sensitivity hypothesis is correct, implies:

- Use of minimum effective dose of neuroleptic
- Alteration of neuroleptic dose (increase may, by blocking more dopamine receptors, cause transient improvement but may ultimately worsen the condition). Slow withdrawal of the drug is likely to be followed by recovery in early cases (occurring in the first year of therapy) but only half of later onset cases, who remain permanently affected. This is a serious matter
- Changing to a neuroleptic less likely to cause the condition, e.g. sulpiride, risperidone, clozapine
- Depletion of dopamine (catecholamine) stores, e.g. by tetrabenazine (p. 370).
- Increasing cholinergic activity by withdrawing any antimuscarinic drug being given against extrapyramidal reactions. Enhancement of cholinergic activity by giving precursors of acetylcholine, e.g. lecithin, has been only marginally effective; anticholinesterases have transiently modified the condition
- Increasing GABA-inhibitory action by using a benzodiazepine, baclofen or sodium valproate; there is a complex interrelation of GABA with dopaminergic/cholinergic balance
- Miscellaneous: lithium and diltiazem may have benefited individuals
- Drug holidays (1 month in 6) carry risk of

therapeutic relapse; they may not help and there is even suspicion they may increase the risk
- Early detection (by watching for developing tongue movements) when the condition is reversible is plainly important.

Other effects

Endocrine effects. Hyperprolactinaemia due to block of the dopamine-mediated prolactin-inhibiting path in the hypothalamus, leading to galactorrhoea with amenorrhoea; also false positive pregnancy test. Increased libido may occur perhaps due to interference with normal conversion of androgens to oestrogens. But defective sexual function (impotence, amenorrhoea) can occur and constitute a hidden source of noncompliance.

Sedation is common. *Antimuscarinic effects* include dry mouth and blurred vision. *Alpha-adrenoceptor block* causes hypotension. Hepatitis, blood disorders, corneal or lens opacities also occur.

Neuroleptic malignant syndrome is a rare condition of uncertain cause but clinically similar to the genetically determined anaesthetic malignant hyperthermia. It usually occurs early in therapy, developing over about 2 days; it can be fatal. The clinical state may not be distinguishable from a severe parkinsonian reaction, at least early in its development. Treatment is urgent: withdrawal of the drug and administration of dantrolene and a centrally active dopamine agonist, e.g. bromocriptine. In extreme cases a competitive neuromuscular blocking agent is effective (unlike malignant hyperthermia). The syndrome may recur if neuroleptic administration is resumed.

The commonest precipitants may be fluphenazine and haloperidol, but it can also occur with antidepressants.

Affective disorders

DEPRESSION AND ANTIDEPRESSANTS

The first drug to be found effective in elevating

mood in endogenous depression was amphetamine (developed in the late 1930s). But it was soon recognised as useful only in mild cases and to be prone to abuse. Amphetamines release noradrenaline stored in nerve endings and prevent its re-uptake into those same nerve endings by inhibiting the monoamine pump mechanism (see below).

In 1951, iproniazid (developed as an antituberculosis agent) was noticed to elevate mood, an effect associated with inhibition of the enzyme monoamine oxidase (MAOI). It was soon replaced in tuberculosis by isoniazid which did not inhibit MAO.

In 1954 reserpine (p. 444) was found to cause depression and to prevent the normal storage of noradrenaline (a substrate for MAO) in nerve endings.

Thus a drug that inhibited metabolism of monoamines (noradrenaline and serotonin) and allowed them to accumulate in nerve endings (iproniazid) relieved some cases of depression, and a drug that depleted nerve endings of their catecholamine stores (reserpine) was known to cause depression.

Research consequently was directed to monoamine metabolism, storage and release.

At about this time (1957) the development of further tricyclic neuroleptics derived from chlorpromazine led to the synthesis of a tricyclic iminodibenzyl derivative (imipramine) which, though it differed structurally only slightly from chlorpromazine, had no useful neuroleptic (dopamine receptor blocking) action but was found in clinical trials to have a useful antidepressant effect. When noradrenaline is released from a nerve ending into the synaptic cleft, its action on postsynaptic receptors is terminated not by destruction, as is the case with acetylcholine, but by diffusion away from the synaptic cleft and by re-uptake (by amine pump) into the nerve ending, where it is stored; its metabolism is regulated by MAO (which is wholly inside the nerve ending). Tricyclics block the amine uptake pump.

The monoamine hypothesis

Thus drugs affecting depression are concerned with amine storage, release, or uptake. These observations are the basis of the monoamine hypothesis of depression, which proposes that endogenous depression is due to deficiency of CNS noradrenergic or serotonergic (5-HT) (monoamine) activity or transmission; MAOIs rectify this by preventing amine destruction, and tricyclics by preventing re-uptake (by inhibition of amine pump). Thus the concentration in nerve endings and/or at postsynaptic receptors is enhanced. Differences in clinical effect are attributed to differences in pattern of MAO inhibition (MAO-A or MAO-B) or by differences in the ratio of inhibition of noradrenaline to serotonin re-uptake.

But this monoamine hypothesis in its simplest form must be inadequate, for there are now in use antidepressants that inhibit the amine pump (cell uptake) for noradrenaline only (viloxazine), for serotonin only (e.g. paroxetine) and for neither (mianserin). But some drugs, e.g. mianserin and trazodone, may block a negative feedback effect mediated by presynaptic adrenoceptors (autoreceptors),[7] so causing an increased release of transmitter.

Pharmacodynamic effect is immediate and the delay in onset of antidepressant effect (7–14 days) may represent the time needed to overcome compensatory feedback changes (if it is not due to inadequate initial dosage). Severe depression requires electroconvulsive therapy, which works quickly and may forestall suicide; it may work by increasing postsynaptic receptor response.

Treatment

Most cases of depression eventually recover spontaneously and most drugs take a week or two to act, so that careful controls are needed if credit for recovery is to be correctly attributed. Antidepressants can precipitate epilepsy in those with a family history of epilepsy, who have had previous ECT, or organic brain damage.

Endogenous depression: the tricyclic or an allied group is the first choice, and a sedative or stimulant member is chosen according to individual need (see

---

[7] An autoreceptor is a receptor anywhere on a neuron that responds to the transmitter released by that neuron. It usually mediates negative feedback. Presynaptic receptors are autoreceptors.

Table 19.3, p. 342). But ECT may be needed if depression is severe or if a quick effect is needed. A combination of a tricyclic and ECT may be ideal in severe cases, and the drug may reduce the number of shocks needed. Lithium may be added in resistant cases.

In very agitated depression a phenothiazine (chlorpromazine) may be a useful adjunct to a tricyclic antidepressant. Benzodiazepines are contraindicated (but see alprazolam).

It is important not to withhold ECT when a tricyclic fails. In one trial half the patients who failed to respond to imipramine in 4 weeks benefited from ECT.

At the first sign of overdose of antidepressant, the drug should be withdrawn and chlorpromazine given; but see mianserin.

Insomnia of depression (characteristically, early waking) may be relieved by an antidepressant drug and not require a hypnotic (though this may be kind in the period before the antidepressant effect occurs).

Reactive depression (exogenous), where drug therapy is necessary, is commonly associated with anxiety and is best treated by an anxiolytic sedative (though these are not antidepressants, except perhaps alprazolam), or a tricyclic antidepressant. An MAO inhibitor may be used if these fail.

Seasonal affective disorder (SAD) (winter depression) may respond to phototherapy (after 4 days); drug therapy (antidepressant, dexfenfluramine) is of uncertain benefit.

MANIA

Mania may be accompanied by overactivity of noradrenergic transmission, i.e. the opposite of depression, and drugs that enhance transmission can cause mania (MAOIs, tricyclics, levodopa). Lithium is effective; its exact mode of action remains uncertain. Because benefit is slow to develop (2–3 weeks) it is not suitable sole treatment of severe acute mania which will require a neuroleptic for control. Lithium is adequate for mild cases, but its chief use is prevention of relapse. Carbamazepine and valproate are alternatives for prophylaxis and treatment.

Acute severe mania may be controlled by either promazine orally or by haloperidol (5–10 mg i.m.) repeated as necessary; lower doses are used for less urgent cases, and transfer to oral therapy for longer-term management.

If the patient is in a single room, accompanied by a suitable nurse, smaller doses of neuroleptic drug will be needed, for excitement tends to subside sooner under these circumstances than it does in the presence of other patients, or if the patient is left entirely alone. Some manic patients are not quietened even by large doses of neuroleptic until they suddenly collapse with respiratory depression. Lithium can be used in milder cases where there is no haste.

Prevention of manic-depressive disorder. In this condition oscillation is between states both above and below normal mood (bipolar) and lithium is effective in prophylaxis of both the manic and depressive phases. Carbamazepine is used where lithium fails.

ANXIETY AND TENSION
see Chapter 18.

OBSESSIVE-COMPULSIVE DISORDER

Behavioural therapy may usefully be supplemented by an antidepressant that inhibits serotonin reuptake into neurons (clomipramine, fluoxetine); sometimes by an anxiolytic sedative.

Severe chronic phobic anxiety that has resisted other treatment sometimes responds to an MAOI or to a tricyclic antidepressant despite the absence of overt depression.

OTHER PSYCHOLOGICAL CONDITIONS

Acute behavioural disturbances: a neuroleptic or a benzodiazepine orally or i.m.

Appetite disorders: anorexia and bulimia. Drugs are adjuvant to behaviour therapy. In anorexia nervosa chlorpromazine is useful, and cyproheptadine may be tried as an appetite stimulant if there is no bulimia.

In bulimia dexfenfluramine and fluoxetine may benefit. An antidepressant may sometimes help either condition even if there is no clinical depression; benefit may be transient.

Obesity: see page 340.

Narcolepsy is benefited by activating noradrenergic mechanisms with amphetamine, dexamphetamine, methylphenidate, mazindol or caffeine. A tricyclic antidepressant may be tried.

Attention deficit disorder (hyperkinetic disorder) in children responds to adrenergic activation by dexamphetamine (or methylphenidate or pemoline). The child becomes more able to sustain attention and so less active. If these drugs fail, an antidepressant may be tried. Drug therapy should be as brief as possible (3 weeks–3 months) and confined to children above 5 years. There is risk that growth may be diminished by disruption of the sleep pattern and so of the circadian rhythm of growth hormone secretion. This is especially important at the period of closure of the epiphyses, when drugs should be withheld if possible.

There have been complaints, with seeming justification, that merely naughty active children who are a nuisance at school or in the home or whose behaviour is the result of parental problems are being misdiagnosed and made into drugged family scapegoats. There is virtually no situation in which an aggressive child or adolescent should be treated only with drugs.

Nocturnal enuresis in children can often be controlled by a tricyclic antidepressant (imipramine), but relapse on ceasing its use is usual. There is a very real hazard of accidental poisoning and parents must be made to understand the risk of leaving the drug accessible in the home of small children. Attractively tasty syrups are hazardous; tablets should be used, but only after nondrug approaches have failed, say after 7 years of age, not before.

Desmopressin (antidiuretic hormone) by intranasal metered aerosol has similar efficiency (15–40% completely dry during use). It has the advantage of being safer than an antidepressant. Short-term use, e.g. for a holiday, is acceptable. Children above 9 years respond best.

Organic brain syndromes and senile dementias of Alzheimer type where patients are seriously uncooperative and disturbed are sometimes helped by a neuroleptic, promazine, thioridazine or haloperidol. Anxiolytic sedatives (benzodiazepines) are best avoided lest slightly agitated patients who can conduct their personal toilet are converted to tranquil patients who cannot, or who fall down. These patients are commonly intolerant of drugs and a low dose should be used initially. Nocturnal delirium may be made worse by hypnotics and helped by caffeine taken as strong tea.

Some benefit may occur with agents that enhance cholinergic function, e.g. the centrally-acting anticholinesterase tacrine (tetrahydroaminoacridine, THA) and the acetylcholine precursor lecithin. Benefit is confined to the equivalent of the deterioration which could be expected over a few months. Concern about hepatic toxicity has led to variation in the response of national regulatory authorities in licensing tacrine. Although there is little evidence that the reported biochemical and histological changes lead to hepatic failure, the new generation of less toxic cholinomimetics will need to complete extensive trials before their place in therapy of Alzheimer's is certain. Antimuscarinic drugs (as used in parkinsonism) aggravate the condition. Some apathetic patients have obtained a little benefit from selegiline.

Intellectual or cognitive function (nootropic[8] drugs: cognition enhancers). With ageing populations becoming more and more forgetful, investigators and drug developers are turning to the possibilities of improving cognitive function, especially age-associated memory impairment. Experiments on memory in rats are easy to do and numerous drugs appear to have some effect, e.g. endorphins and naloxone, corticotrophin and vasopressin (peptides), adrenergic and cholinergic agents. The locus coeruleus of the brain is known to be concerned with memory regulation, and these drugs can be shown to increase its neuronal firing.

No drugs have been shown reliably and substantially to improve impaired or normal memory in man over long periods.

---

[8] Drugs affecting the intellect (Greek: mind turning).

But there is evidence of some effect for meclofenoxate, pemoline and co-dergocrine. It is unlikely that vasodilatation has any effect, and any benefit of such drugs is likely to be due to brain cell actions.

Prescribers who seek to help their senile or other patients' memories with drugs will do well to remember that whilst benefits will be limited at best, it is quite easy to impair the fragile intellectual function of the old with ill-chosen, uncritical, unmonitored prescribing.

Learning. Studies in animals have shown that drugs that modify cholinergic and adrenergic mechanisms in the central nervous system or alter the synthesis of RNA can enhance learning. It will be time to take this topic seriously in medicine when efficacy has been demonstrated in a resistant human population such as medical students.

Toxic confusional states, e.g. delirium tremens or postsurgical confusion, may be benefited by diazepam, chlorpromazine or chlormethiazole. Paraldehyde is also often satisfactory. Correction of any accessible biochemical, toxic or anoxic abnormality is of the first importance.

Behaviour control. The fact that drugs can be used to quell inconvenient behaviour of the mentally handicapped, the demented and psychotics, and as a cheap substitute for skilled staff in institutions, including prisons, is a matter for concern. Similar use on persons deemed by authority to be social or political deviants is also something to be feared; there is no doubt that it has occurred. Use of psychotropic drugs for 'problem children' is an area of particular concern, e.g. imipramine for school phobia.

Excessive sex drive in men may be reduced by oestrogen or by antiandrogen (cyproterone). The breasts may enlarge sufficiently to require surgical removal. These treatments may be indicated in abnormal personalities with pronounced sexual aggression. They raise particularly powerful ethical issues where the choice is between therapy with liberty, or loss of liberty, e.g. repeated sexual assaults on children. Benperidol (a butyrophenone) can also be effective.

Suicide and prescribed drugs. Sometimes it is necessary to prescribe drugs for potentially suicidal patients living at home. In such cases it is usual to prescribe minimal doses for short periods and, when the danger seems serious, to hand over the supply of drugs to a responsible person rather than to the patient. Benzodiazepines are the sedatives and hypnotics of choice in such patients as heavy overdose is most unlikely to kill the patient.

Some antidepressants, e.g. mianserin, may be less cardiotoxic in overdose than others.

An ingenious formulation of paracetamol containing enough methionine to protect the liver in overdose has been devised (Pameton).

Drug-induced suicide: see reserpine and Table 19.3 (Note 1).

Psychotropic[9] drugs

CLASSIFICATION

So little is known about the biochemical basis of mental disorder that no definitive classification based on mechanisms of action can yet be offered. Drugs are classified provisionally according to the symptoms they are used to relieve and by chemical group.

1. Neuroleptics (antipsychotics) are drugs with therapeutic effect on schizophrenia and some other psychoses. All are dopamine antagonists, with various admixtures of other actions. They cause emotional quietening, indifference and psychomotor slowing; they also cause movement disorders.

- *Phenothiazines*: see Table 19.1
- *Butyrophenones* are similar to class 3 phenothiazines (see Table 19.1). The group includes: benperidol (Anquil), droperidol (Droleptan), haloperidol (Serenace), trifluperidol (Triperidol)
- *Diphenylbutylpiperidines* are closely related to the butyrophenones: fluspirilene (Redeptin), pimozide (Orap)
- *Benzamide*: sulpiride (Dolmatil), remoxipride (Roxiam)

---

[9] Psychotropic (Greek): affecting the mind.

- *Dibenzodiazepine*: clozapine (Clozaril)
- *Thioxanthenes*: flupenthixol (Depixol), zuclopenthixol (Clopixol)
- *Indole derivative*: oxypertine (Integrin)
- *Benzisoxazole derivative*: risperidone

2. Anxiolytic sedatives and other drugs used in anxiety, see Chapter 18.

3. Antidepressants

- *Tricyclic* and related agents (see Table 19.3)
- *Selective serotonin re-uptake inhibitors (SSRIs)*: fluoxetine (Prozac), paroxetine, citalopram, sertraline, fluvoxamine
- *Selective noradrenaline and serotonin uptake inhibitor*: venlafaxine
- *Monoamine oxidase inhibitors (MAOIs):*
  - *Irreversible, non-selective*: phenelzine (Nardil), isocarboxazid (Marplan), tranylcypromine (Parnate)
  - *Reversible, selective MAO-A*: moclobemide
- *Miscellaneous:* L-tryptophan is a precursor of serotonin (5-HT); alprazolam is an antidepressant benzodiazepine.

4. Lithium and carbamazepine for mania and manic-depressive psychosis.

5. Psychostimulants increase the level of alertness and / or motivation.

- Amphetamines: methylphenidate (Ritalin), pemoline (Volital). This group is obsolete except for occasional use under specialist guidance, mainly in children with hyperkinesia or attention disorders.
- Caffeine.

6. Psychodysleptics (hallucinogens, psychedelics, psychotomimetics) produce mental phenomena, particularly cognitive and perceptual (see Nonmedical drug use).

DOSAGE

Because of the difficulty in measuring responses in psychiatry, and the variability caused by environmental factors, drugs are commonly given in arbitrarily fixed or at least crudely adjusted doses. This militates substantially against precise clinical evaluation and against achievement of optimum therapeutic effect, unless plasma concentrations are measured and can be related to therapeutic effect.

In the case of *tricyclic antidepressants*, standard doses may produce steady-state plasma concentrations varying by a factor of 10 or more. The ideal therapeutic response may occur at intermediate plasma concentrations, falling off as the concentration rises above an optimum, i.e. there is a *therapeutic window*. It is plain that when a patient does not respond, knowledge of plasma concentration will be valuable in order to allow a decision whether this is a true therapeutic failure, whether the dosage is wrong — or (if no drug is detectable) the patient is not taking the drug. However, such information is at present seldom available.

Once-daily dosage (at night) is commonly satisfactory, with increments at intervals appropriate to the plasma $t^{1/2}$ which indicates when a steady state will have been reached, i.e. about $5 \times t^{1/2}$.

For neuroleptics (which are difficult to measure chemically) also, individual variation is great and drug $t^{1/2}$ ranges from 10 to 50 h. Injectable depot formulations, given at intervals of weeks, are widely used.

Neuroleptics (see Table 19.1)

CHLORPROMAZINE

As a result of investigation of phenothiazine compounds for possible anthelminthic effect, first promethazine, the useful sedative and antihistamine, was discovered, and then chlorpromazine (1951).

Actions

Chlorpromazine has a large number of actions. It blocks dopamine, α-adreno-, muscarinic (cholinergic), serotonin and histamine-H_1 receptors. It has a quinidine-like effect on the heart and can cause cardiac dysrhythmias. Practical therapeutics might be better served if they were distributed amongst 3 or 4 drugs instead of being concentrated in one. They include:

Table 19.1 Phenothiazines classed by clinical effects

Name	Sedation	Anti-muscarinic effects	Extra-pyramidal effects
Class 1 (aliphatic compounds)			
Chlorpromazine (Largactil)			
Methotrimeprazine (*Veractil*)	strong	moderate	moderate
Promazine (Sparine)			
Class 2 (piperidines)			
Pericyazine (Neulactil)			
Pipothiazine (*Piportil*)	moderate	pronounced	slight
Thioridazine (Melleril)			
Class 3 (piperazines)			
Fluphenazine (Modecate)			
Perphenazine (Fentazin)			
Prochlorperazine (Stemetil)	slight	slight	pronounced
Thiethylperazine (Torecan)			
Thiopropazate (Dartalan)			
Trifluoperazine (Stelazine)			

Note. Antimuscarinic action protects against extrapyramidal effects.

Central nervous system. The term *neuroleptic* was introduced to describe the characteristic emotional quietening, indifference and psychomotor slowing induced by chlorpromazine.

There is evidence that chlorpromazine acts in the hypothalamus and brain-stem reticular formation. In animals chlorpromazine quietens wild and angry monkeys. Chlorpromazine has a remarkable ability to control hyperactive and hypomanic states without seriously impairing consciousness, and it modifies abnormal behaviour in schizophrenic states. It is ineffective against depression unless this is accompanied by agitation, and indeed may make it worse. Normal people often feel sleepy, apathetic and indifferent to the environment after taking chlorpromazine and it also induces some indifference to pain. In large doses chlorpromazine causes dystonias. In moderate doses it controls the muscle spasm of tetanus, but very large doses may make it

worse. This is probably an effect on the reticular formation where stimulation of one area activates, and of another depresses, spinal reflexes. Chlorpromazine also reduces muscle spasticity due to other neurological lesions. Epilepsy may be precipitated in predisposed people, but the drug has been used with success in epileptics with schizophrenic illness.

Chlorpromazine is an *antiemetic* effective against both drug and disease-induced vomiting, but ineffective against motion sickness.

The *peripheral α-adrenoceptor blocking effect* is moderately strong, and postural hypotension may occur. The peripheral vasodilatation induced by this action of chlorpromazine causes heat loss, and body temperature may fall, as with other long-acting vasodilators, especially if the patient is anaesthetised or is old. Some central effect on the temperature regulating mechanism is also probable.

Potentiation of other drugs. Chlorpromazine potentiates all cerebral depressants including alcohol, analgesics, hypnotics and anaesthetics. These effects can have clinical importance, but usually only if the drugs are being used in large doses.

Miscellaneous actions. Chlorpromazine has weak antihistamine, ganglion-blocking and quinidine-like actions (it can produce ECG changes) (see also above). It is a local anaesthetic, but in solution it is very irritant.

Pharmacokinetics. Chlorpromazine has a $t^{1/2}$ of about 35 h; there is substantial hepatic first-pass effect and drug action is terminated by metabolism. However, therapeutic effect on behaviour may be delayed for as long as 4 weeks; benefit may last months after cessation, and hepatic metabolites may be excreted for months.

Uses. Chlorpromazine's principal use is in mental disorders; its other indications are better met by alternative drugs. These other indications are still worth listing for the occasions when alternatives are not available, or have been tried and fail. Chlorpromazine is antiemetic and can aid the production of hypothermia in anaesthesia. It may be used in severe pain, both to potentiate other drugs and to induce indifference to pain by altering the emotional response. It is worth trying in persistent pruritis. It can be effective against intractable *hiccup*. Phenothiazine neuroleptics should not be used for minor conditions.

Dosage varies widely. Starting doses may be 25 mg orally (preferably not i.m: local toxicity) 4- to 6-hourly; dosage may be increased every 3–4 days (see Table 19.2).

Adverse reactions include: drowsiness and lethargy (though the patient remains rousable), postural hypotension, hypothermia in the elderly, dry mouth; weight gain; disturbance of male sexual function.

For important neurological effects see page 331.

Galactorrhoea (with amenorrhoea) is due to block of the dopamine-mediated prolactin-inhibiting path in the hypothalamus (plasma prolactin concentration is raised).

Blood disorders and rashes, sometimes photosensitive, occur, and with prolonged use there may be permanent pigmentation. Fits may occur and, rarely, lens opacities.

The most serious effect is cholestatic (obstructive) jaundice, in which cellular damage is generally trivial, the principal impact being on the bile canaliculi, which show cellular infiltration and biliary stasis. Jaundice most commonly occurs 2–4 weeks after starting therapy but relapse can occur at once on restarting it in a patient who has had chlorpromazine jaundice. This and its irregular occurrence

suggest that it is an allergic reaction. Recovery is almost invariably complete within a few weeks, but permanent liver damage has been reported. Hepatic biopsy has revealed lesions in patients taking chlorpromazine who are free from jaundice. The possibility of liver damage or blood disorder is sufficiently high to make casual use of chlorpromazine particularly reprehensible. The danger is particularly great if there is a history of alcoholism.

Cardiac dysrhythmias can occur. Chlorpromazine causes *contact dermatitis* and staff who inject it should take care; tablets should not be crushed.

Other phenothiazines. There is a great variety available. Although most of those advocated in psychiatry represent attempts to improve on chlorpromazine, none has been shown definitely to be an all-round improvement; but piperazine derivatives cause less hypotension. Their effects are similar to those of chlorpromazine although they differ in emphasis (see Table 19.1). They are classed by structural side chain (see Table 19.2).

Butyrophenones. Haloperidol ($t\frac{1}{2}$ 18 h) is pharmacodynamically similar to phenothiazines (class 3 in Table 19.1).

Thioxanthenes are also pharmacodynamically similar to the phenothiazines. Flupenthixol particularly is used, often as a depot i.m. injection of the

Table 19.2 Some neuroleptics, summarised by class

Class	Example	Dose (usual starting and maintenance dose)*	Extra-pyramidal effects	Anti-muscarinic effects	Drowsiness	Hypotension
aliphatic phenothiazine	chlorpromazine	25–300 mg	++	+++	+++	+++
piperidine phenothiazine	thioridazine	150–600 mg	+	+++	+++	+++
piperazine phenothiazine	fluphenazine trifluperazine	2–20 mg 5–20 mg	+++	++	++	++
butyrophenone	haloperidol	10–80 mg	+++	+	++	++
thioxanthene	flupenthixol	3–9 mg	+++	+	++	++
dibenzodiazepine	clozapine	12.5–300 mg		++	+++	+++
benzamide	sulpiride	50–400 mg	+	+		+
benzisoxazole	risperidone	1–8 mg	+	+	+	++

*Milder cases treated as out-patients generally received dosage at the lower end of this range. A single nightly dose may suffice sometimes. For agitation and restlessness in the elderly or debilitated: $\frac{1}{4}$–$\frac{1}{2}$ dose.

decanoate (in oil) every 2–4 weeks. It also has anti-depressant action. Zuclopenthixol belongs to this class.

Benzamide: sulpiride (Dolmatil) benefits negative symptoms of schizophrenia when used at low dose. Extrapyramidal effects are less than with other neuroleptics. The alternative in this class, remoxipride, has been associated with aplastic anaemia in a few cases, and blood counts therefore need to be monitored before and during therapy.

Dibenzoxazine: loxapine (Loxapac) has not been demonstrated to differ pharmacologically from the phenothiazines, but may have a lower incidence of extrapyramidal effects.

Dibenzodiazepine: clozapine (Clozaril) has shown efficacy in both positive and negative symptoms of schizophrenia resistant to other neuroleptics; it is selective for the D_4 dopamine receptor subtype. It has the particular advantage that extrapyramidal effects are ordinarily mild and transient. But it has the particular disadvantage that it causes agranulocytosis in 1–2% of patients. For this reason its use is confined to patients resistant to other neuroleptics or where benefit from these is marred by severe extrapyramidal effects, including tardive dyskinesia. Precautionary leucocyte counts are mandatory. Previously clozapine could be prescribed only by recognised specialists in psychiatry, who participated in the monitoring scheme organised by the manufacturer, and even now treatment needs to be initiated by specialists. Clozapine therapy is considered responsible for enabling large scale discharge of schizophrenics from mental hospitals to the community. On the other hand, only a third of schizophrenics are responsive, and it is important to discontinue this potentially toxic (and expensive) drug if it is not actually working.

Benzisoxazole: risperidone (Risperdal) is an antagonist at both D_2 and $5\text{-}HT_2$ receptors. These properties may contribute to risperidone's efficacy in treating the negative symptoms of schizophrenia, and to its freedom from extrapyramidal adverse effects. It may have slightly higher efficacy than phenothiazines or butyrophenones (at doses which avoid the extrapyramidal effects), but more evaluation is required to establish whether risperidone is

an alternative to clozapine for treatment of resistant schizophrenia.

Sertindole is similarly selective for $5HT_2$ and dopamine D_2 with some selectivity also for those in the limbic system rather than substantia nigra. Consequently sentindole causes fewer extrapyramidal adverse effects than other neuroleptic agents.

INJECTABLE DEPOT (SUSTAINED-RELEASE) NEUROLEPTICS

Since about 40% of schizophrenics do not take tablets prescribed and even in hospital 20% of patients may not actually swallow the tablet given to them, it is useful to have neuroleptics that can be given i.m. at long intervals (1–4 weeks) for maintenance therapy. Use of these preparations has three advantages. The default rate is halved, defaulters are identifiable, absence of hepatic first-pass metabolism (that accompanies oral use) may allow control that is unobtainable with the oral route.

The decanoates of fluphenazine (Modecate) flupenthixol (Depixol) and haloperidol (Haldol decanoate) are used.

A small test dose should precede regular use because response is variable and adverse effects, when they occur, will be prolonged.

Extrapyramidal syndromes are common (2 days after injection and lasting for 5 days) and can be controlled by antimuscarinic antiparkinsonian drugs, e.g. benzhexol, orphenadrine. Severe depression can occur, and sometimes excitement (flupenthixol).

Flupenthixol (Depixol) has been shown to have less depressant effects and in small doses is used as an antidepressant.

Antidepressants[10]

TRICYCLICS AND ALLIED AMINE PUMP INHIBITORS

Structurally related to the phenothiazines, tricyclics

---

[10] Classification of drugs by therapeutic use can be misleading, e.g. antidepressants can be useful in some cases of anxiety, panic attacks, chronic pain and nocturnal enuresis.

prevent the active re-uptake into neuronal stores of released noradrenaline (chiefly), and serotonin at high doses. This action probably contributes to their potentiating effect on injected adrenaline and noradrenaline (negligible with isoprenaline), and to their cardiotoxicity in overdose. They also have antimuscarinic effects. Therapeutic effect is delayed for 7–14 days, and this has been taken to imply a necessary change in receptors activated by the potentiated amines, e.g. downregulation of CNS β-adrenoreceptors. Because of the multiplicity of amines potentiated by re-uptake inhibitors, however, it is unlikely that the explanation for their efficacy is as simple as a change in one receptor population. Allied drugs inhibit re-uptake of both monoamines in varying proportions (see Table 19.3). One recent drug, *tianeptine* (an atypical tricyclic agent) enhances serotonin re-uptake. While this appears contradictory to the general amine theory of depression, the lesson is probably not to oversimplify the complex compensatory responses to changing synaptic concentrations of a single amine.

Pharmacokinetics. Tricyclic antidepressants, given orally, are well absorbed and have a high apparent volume of distribution implying that they preferentially enter some tissues and indeed they have been found to be concentrated in the myocardium. Steady-state plasma concentrations show great individual variation but are correlated with therapeutic effect and so measurement of plasma concentration can be useful (though it is often not available), especially if there is apparent failure of response. Tricyclics are metabolised in the liver. The $t^1/2$ varies from 15 to 100 h, with imipramine at the lower end and protriptyline at the upper.

Adverse effects include those characteristic of antimuscarinic action (dry mouth, raised intraocular pressure, blurred vision, bladder neck obstruction in older males). Male sexual function may be impaired. There also occur: postural hypotension, tremors, hallucinations, confusion, excitement, and violence to others and to self; precipitation of mania and epilepsy (avoid if there is a history of these); there may be cardiac hazard (sudden death) in using tricyclics in patients with any cardiac disease and perhaps even in those with apparently healthy hearts (but see mianserin).

Overdose causes cardiac dysrhythmias, hypotension and convulsions, which are treated by antidysrhythmic drugs, α- or β-adrenoceptor block and anticonvulsants, e.g. diazepam. Acidosis may occur and can be treated with sodium bicarbonate. Overdose should be taken extremely seriously, especially in children.

Physicians may find themselves in the curious position of giving warning of these hazards to patients who have expressed a desire to end their own lives, i.e. of the importance of keeping them in a place safe from children and of refraining from overdose to themselves. Nevertheless, the common antimuscarinic effects should be mentioned because they almost always occur and add to the burden of worry and so promote noncompliance in depressed patients if they are unaware of their origin and that they do not herald disaster.

Abuse is not a problem with tricyclics since their immediate effects are not noticeably pleasant, but some *dependence* does occur (see below).

Interactions. Catecholamines and other sympathomimetics are potentiated (but not β₂-receptor agonists used in asthma). This is important and even the amounts of adrenaline or noradrenaline in dental local anaesthetics may produce a serious rise in blood pressure. Severe toxicity, resembling atropine overdose, can occur if full doses of tricyclic are combined with an MAO inhibitor. Such combination is sometimes used clinically, but great caution is needed.

The interactions of tricyclics with antihypertensives are less of a problem with those in current use than with methyldopa, which is potentiated, or with the obsolescent adrenergic-neuron-blocking drugs, which the tricyclics antagonise by preventing their uptake into the adrenergic nerve ending.

Neuroleptics inhibit metabolism of tricyclics. Enzyme induction, e.g. antiepileptics, can even halve plasma concentration of tricyclics, though the clinical importance of this is diminished by the activity of some of the metabolites.

Effects of alcohol may be increased.

Choice of tricyclic or allied antidepressant. Choice is largely made on secondary psychotropic actions: sedative, less sedative or stimulant members (see Table 19.3).

In the presence of cardiac disease and old age, mianserin or trazodone may be preferred as safer than others.

Table 19.3 Tricyclic and other antidepressants

Name	Class	Remarks
Amitriptyline (Tryptizol)	tricyclic	Sedative: may be cardiotoxic (sudden death) rather more than other tricyclics
Amoxapine (Asendis)	tri-	Onset of effect may be quicker
Clomipramine (Anaframil)	tri-	Less sedative: serotonin uptake inhibitor
Desipramine (Pertofran)	tri-	Less sedative
Dothiepin (Prothiaden)	tri-	Sedative
Doxepin (Sinequan)	tri-	Sedative
Fluoxetine (Prozac)	other	Nonsedative: serotonin uptake inhibitor
Flupenthixol (Fluanxol Depixol)	thioxanthene	Antidepressant neuroleptic
Fluvoxamine (Faverin)	other	Nonsedative: serotonin uptake inhibitor
Imipramine (Tofranil)	tri-	Less sedative
Iprindole (Prondol)	tri-	Less sedative: does not inhibit amine pump
Lofepramine (Gamanil)	tetra-	Less sedative
Maprotiline (Ludiomil)	tetra-	Inhibits noradrenaline uptake: less sedative
Mianserin (Bolvidon)	tetra-	Sedative: does not inhibit amine pump: less cardiac risk: agranulocytosis
Nefazodone (Dutonin)	phenylpiperazine	serotonin uptake inhibitor and 5-HT$_2$ blocker
Nortriptyline (Aventyl)	tri-	Less sedative
Paroxetine (Seroxat)	other	Serotonin uptake inhibitor
Protriptyline (Concordin)	tri-	Stimulant
Sertraline (Lustral)	other	Serotonin uptake inhibitor
Trazodone (Molipaxin)	other	Weak noradrenaline and serotonin uptake inhibitor; sedative
Trimipramine (Surmontil)	tri-	Sedative
Venlafaxine (Efexor)	other	Noradrenaline and serotonin uptake inhibitor
Viloxazine (Vivalan)	bi-	Less sedative

1. **Warning**: abnormal behaviour, including violence to others and to self, can occur with antidepressants. Plainly, to distinguish between drug-caused and disease-caused events can be impossible.
2. Tolerance to sedation may occur.
3. Hypnotics and anxiolytic sedatives may be combined.
4. Another antidepressant or neuroleptic should not be combined without special reason.
5. Antimuscarinic side-effects are common and tolerance may develop with continued treatment.

Use. Antidepressants are commonly given 2 or 3 times a day. But it is often satisfactory, particularly for the sedative drugs, to give a single evening dose; the half-lives of most are long enough to render this appropriate, and peak plasma concentrations occur during the night; the stimulant drugs may increase insomnia.

Dose. A general scheme[11] that takes account of the need for quick response as well as the accumulative properties (long $t^1/2$) of some tricyclics is as follows:

- **Amitriptyline** single daily dose 3 h before bedtime, or
- Imipramine in the morning:

Day 1   50 mg
Day 2   75 mg
Day 3   100 mg
Day 4   150 mg

After 14 days, if response is inadequate: add 25 mg increment every 2–3 days up to a maximum daily dose of 200 mg.
Day 28: re-evaluate; if no response, reconsider diagnosis or change to different drug.

There may be some accumulation of drug and once therapeutic effect is established the dose may be gradually lowered to the minimum that will maintain benefit.

There is evidence that tricyclic antidepressants have a therapeutic range of concentration both below and above which efficacy is lost. Thus if a patient does not respond, or loses response, it may be because the plasma concentration is too high or too low. This need not astonish, for drugs at high concentrations may antagonise their own actions by a variety of mechanisms, e.g. activating or blocking receptors for which affinity is low at low concentrations. This therapeutic window is of clinical importance, and plainly will complicate patient management.

Duration and withdrawal. Therapy may be continued for 3–6 months and the drug withdrawn over about 6 weeks (to avoid an unpleasant acute

withdrawal syndrome of headache, nausea, anxiety and bad dreams) or else, if there is established cyclic (unipolar) depression, it may be continued at low dose for longterm prophylaxis (25–50 mg daily). Relapse of depression may be delayed for about 2 months, so follow-up of patients is essential.

Other uses include nocturnal enuresis and chronic pain. Pathological laughing and weeping such as occurs with bilateral forebrain disease, e.g. multiple sclerosis, may respond to low dose amitriptyline.

Other drugs listed in Table 19.3, page 342, can give satisfactory results. They vary in minor respects and some may be less cardiotoxic in overdose, e.g. mianserin (below).

Warnings. Benefit from antidepressants may be delayed for 7–14 days and patients should be told this for it is quite time enough for a person who is already minded to end his life to take a firm decision and to act on it. Electroconvulsive therapy acts quicker and may be needed as initial therapy, and there need be no delay in starting the drug.

Epilepsy. Drugs of this group are liable to precipitate fits in people with a family history of epilepsy, or who have had previous electroconvulsive therapy or who have organic brain damage. Treated epileptics are likely to require higher doses to compensate for hepatic enzyme induction by the anticonvulsants.

Atypical antidepressants. Mianserin ($t^1/2$ 30 h) does not inhibit the amine pump; it may act via central α_2-adrenoceptors. It is a sedative, has little antimuscarinic effect and is less cardiotoxic than are tricyclics, especially in acute overdose, properties that render it particularly suitable for use in the elderly. But it has a greater capacity to cause allergic blood disorders, agranulocytosis and aplastic anaemia (type B adverse reaction) especially during early weeks of treatment when the blood count should be monitored (monthly for 3 months). Hepatitis occurs. The role of mianserin as a second line agent has now been assumed by the SSRIs (see below) which have been used in sufficient patients to exclude any comparable major adverse effect.

Flupenthixol (Depixol) is an antidepressant neuroleptic (thioxanthene).

---

[11] Based on Hollister L E 1978, 1983 Clinical pharmacology of psychotherapeutic drugs. Churchill Livingstone, Edinburgh.

Selective serotonin re-uptake inhibitors (SSRIs)

Although covered under the heading of amine re-uptake inhibitors, this subclass is now sufficiently numerous and widely used to merit separate discussion. It includes fluoxetine (Prozac), fluvoxamine, paroxetine and sertraline. The older drug, clomipramine, was also to some extent selective for serotonin (5-HT) rather than noradrenaline. There is little evidence that the SSRIs offer greater efficacy in any patients than older drugs, either in relief of symptoms or in prevention of suicide. On the other hand, there has also been no substantiation for the scare early in their use that suicide risk might actually be increased. (Such scares are not uncommon, partly because of news mongering, partly because new drugs tend to be used first in 'difficult' patients who have failed on treatment with the older alternative.) The main advantage of SSRIs is their lack of antimuscarinic adverse effects. Lack of adverse effects can indirectly also permit an increase in efficacy, since the maximum tolerated dose in a patient is less likely to be limited by the undesired antimuscarinic effects. While in theory a selective agent should not have new adverse effects (absent from the older less-selective agents), idiosyncratic reactions can occur. Symptoms in psychiatric patients are particularly difficult to evaluate; the symptom of spontaneous orgasm during yawning in patients receiving clomipramine or fluoxetine was put out for 'peer review' on the Internet by one patient. We offer no explanation, but note that this is not an isolated case report.[12]

Nefazodone (Dutonin), as well as blocking serotonin uptake, blocks one of the postsynaptic receptors, the $5-HT_2$ receptor, with a presumed selective increase in stimulation of the $5-HT_{1A}$ receptor. This combination may contribute to an anxiolytic as well as antidepressant action of the drug, and it has also been claimed to cause less sexual dysfunction than the other SSRIs.

Monoamine oxidase inhibitors (MAOIs)

In 1951 iproniazid (related to isoniazid) was tested for clinical antituberculosis activity and it was noticed that it induced euphoria. Early trials in psychiatry proved negative, but in 1958 a favourable report of its effect in chronically regressed and withdrawn patients precipitated a flood of therapeutic trials.

Iproniazid inhibits monoamine oxidases, a group of enzymes present inside cells of the brain, in peripheral adrenergic and dopaminergic nerve endings, and in the liver and gut wall, and which is concerned in the breakdown of serotonin and catecholamines (adrenaline, noradrenaline, dopamine). Many compounds with this effect and less toxicity have since been made; the structure of nonhydrazines resembles that of amphetamine.

The group includes:

Hydrazine: phenelzine (Nardil); isocarboxazid (Marplan)

Nonhydrazine: tranylcypromine (Parnate), the member most likely to cause hypertension; moclobemide (Manerix); selegiline (Eldepryl) for parkinsonism.

Actions. Drugs of this group have been found to have, to varying degrees, the following actions.

- MAO inhibition (other enzymes too). In most cases, inhibition is irreversible, i.e. new enzyme needs to be synthesised for recovery of enzyme activity, so that the inhibition is cumulative over several doses, and lasts long after the drug itself has disappeared from the tissues. Sometimes, such drugs are called 'hit and run' or 'suicide' drugs, which is true only when chemical modification of the enzyme requires also chemical modification of the drug. An exception to this account is moclobemide
- Sympathomimetic effect by inhibiting noradrenaline re-uptake (tranylcypromine) (some only, see below)

---

[12] Such reports stem in part from the wide acceptance and use of SSRIs, particularly fluoxetine, increasingly among people who do not suffer from any clinically definable form of depression. The 'Prozac phenomenon' of taking a pill to improve, supposedly, healthy people's quality of life seems as much a comment on society as on the drug.

- Sympathetic ganglion blocking effect
- Selectivity for one of the two principal enzymes (MAO-A, MAO-B) (see discussion under parkinsonism). Except currently for moclobemide (selective inhibitor of MAO-A), nonselective inhibitors are used for depression.

When monoamine oxidases are nonselectively inhibited, there is an increase of serotonin and catecholamines (noradrenaline, dopamine) in the CNS. In man such increases have powerful mental effects, ranging from feelings of well-being and increased energy to frank psychosis.

The increase in catecholamine stores in adrenergic and dopaminergic nerve endings means that there will be *potentiation of sympathomimetics* that act *indirectly*, i.e. by releasing stored noradrenaline, and of orally administered sympathomimetics that are substrates for MAO (present in the gut wall and liver). But important potentiation of administered adrenaline, noradrenaline and isoprenaline is not to be expected since these substances are chiefly destroyed by catechol-O-methyltransferase in the blood and liver.

It is plain, both from experimental pharmacological studies and from fatal accidents during therapy, that sympathomimetics can be highly dangerous to patients taking MAO inhibitors. *Severe hypertension occurs* if levodopa (p. 364) is given in the presence of nonselective MAO inhibition (see p. 367).

Some MAO inhibitors (tranylcypromine) also have sympathomimetic activity similar to that of amphetamine, i.e. releasing stored noradrenaline, unrelated to enzyme inhibition and inhibition of noradrenaline re-uptake into the nerve endings. Thus, *hypertensive attacks are to be expected*; when they occur, they resemble the hypertensive attacks of phaeochromocytoma.

MAO inhibitors can, by themselves, also cause hypotension by sympathetic ganglion block. The hypertensive interactions mentioned above will still take place in the presence of hypotensive effect, so that a patient might suffer from postural hypotension, eat a meal of cheese (see below) and die in a hypertensive crisis.

Symptoms and treatment of hypertensive crisis. Severe throbbing headache occurs with slow palpitation. If headache occurs without hypertension it may be due to histamine release. The hypertension is due both to vasoconstriction from activation of α-adrenoceptors and to increased cardiac output consequent on activation of cardiac β-adrenoceptors. The mechanism is thus similar to that of the episodic hypertension in a patient with phaeochromocytoma. The rational and effective treatment is an α-adrenoceptor blocker (phentolamine, 5 mg i.v.).

Should excessive tachycardia occur after the phentolamine, a β-adrenoceptor blocker may be added (given initially it may further raise the blood pressure by blocking the peripheral vasodilator β2-receptors). A vasodilator is also effective, e.g. nifedipine (a reliable patient may be instructed in self diagnosis and use, as for an attack of angina pectoris).

Pharmacokinetics. MAO inhibitors are taken orally; they are *hit and run* drugs, i.e. their effects greatly outlast their detectable presence in the body because they inhibit the enzyme irreversibly and termination of effect is dependent on synthesis of fresh enzyme, which takes weeks. Thus *adverse interactions* may occur as long as 2–3 weeks after therapy has been withdrawn.

The hydrazine group (see above) is acetylated (like isoniazid) and the population is divided into slow and fast acetylators.

Warning patients. Patients must be warned not to indulge in *self-medication* of any kind for many trivial remedies sold direct to the public, e.g. for nasal congestion, coughs and colds, contain sympathomimetics (ephedrine, phenylpropanolamine). Unfortunately some foods contain substantial amounts of sympathomimetics, largely tyramine, which act by releasing tissue-stored noradrenaline. These substances are normally inactivated by MAO in the intestine wall and liver (presystemic elimination), where large amounts of enzyme occur. Patients taking an MAOI are therefore deprived of this protection, so that, as well as having larger stores in nerve endings (waiting to be released), they absorb more of the sympathomimetics.

The first food interaction with MAO inhibitors was reported in 1963 and concerned cheese. It might be thought that, as cheese has been known to contain tyramine for at least 60 years, the danger might have been predicted, but it was not, and the association of hypertensive headache with evening meals of cheese was made by clinical acumen of a pharmacist whose wife was taking an MAOI.

Responses are variable, but any food subjected to *autolysis* or *microbial decomposition* during preparation or storage may contain pressor amines resulting from decarboxylation of amino acids.

Foods likely to produce hypertensive effects

The following foods either can produce, or may be expected to be capable of producing, dangerous hypertensive effects:

- cheese, especially if well matured (the amines are produced from the amino acids of casein by bacteria, e.g. tyramine from tyrosine; the concentration is higher just beneath the rind and around fermentation cavities); 'cheese' reaction;
- some pickled herrings;
- broad bean pods (contain dopa, a precursor of adrenaline);
- hydrolysed protein (Marmite, Bovril);
- Wines (red or white) and beer including non- or low-alcohol varieties contain very variable but generally low amounts of tyramine;
- over-ripe bananas, avocados, figs;
- fermented bean curds including soy sauce;
- fermented sausage, e.g. salami, shrimp paste;
- flavoured textured vegetable protein.

This list may be incomplete and there is a large number of anecdotal case reports supposedly implicating a wide range of foods. Any partially decomposed food may cause a reaction. Milk and yoghurt appear safe. It is plain that patients must receive detailed instructions about their diet. They may cautiously try some of the above items to discover whether they are safe for themselves and, if they are, they should not assume that the same food from different sources is harmless.

Selective MAO-A inhibition (moclobemide) should in theory avoid the 'cheese' reaction by sparing the intestinal MAO, which is mainly MAO-B. However, the relative safety of the newer drugs may be due also to their being competitive, *reversible* inhibitors. Because reversible, MAO inhibition is incomplete except during peak plasma concentrations; because competitive, tyramine can then displace the inhibitor from the active site of the MAO enzyme.[13] However, hypertensive reactions have been reported.

Interactions with other drugs. The following

substances that are *not metabolised by MAO* may be potentiated:

Antidepressants: excitement with tricyclics and allied drugs, especially with those that act by inhibiting serotonin re-uptake (clomipramine, fluvoxamine, fluoxetine) when a life-threatening 'serotonin syndrome' may occur (hyperthermia, tremor, convulsions).

Narcotic analgesics: if pethidine is given to a patient taking an MAO inhibitor there is liable to be respiratory depression, restlessness, even coma, and hypo or hypertension. This is probably due to inhibition of the hepatic enzyme that demethylates pethidine. Interaction with other opioids occurs but is milder. If an opioid analgesic is essential, start with one-tenth of the usual dose.

Central nervous system depressants: barbiturates, anxiolytic sedatives, antihistamines, alcohol (probably), antiparkinsonian drugs; but not inhalation anaesthetics, carbamazepine, buspirone. Because of the use of numerous drugs during and around surgery, an MAOI is best withdrawn 2 weeks before, if practicable.

Interactions with antihypertensives acting on the sympathetic system refer mainly to older drugs acting via noradrenaline release. The interaction can increase or reduce the antihypertensive response, depending on whether noradrenaline release is affected more in the CNS (where it is hypotensive) or in the periphery (where it is hypertensive). Hypertension and excitement may occur with methyldopa. (See also levodopa above.)

Insulin and oral hypoglycaemics are potentiated. *Bee venom* (perhaps) is an environmental hazard.

The mechanisms of many of these interactions are obscure, and some are probably due to inhibition of other drug metabolising enzymes (than MAO). Reactions can be very severe and even fatal.

Use of MAO inhibitors. It is plain that patients taking these drugs are at risk in a number of ways and

---

[13] No severe cheese reactions have been reported with moclobemide. If a patient is supersensitive to tyramine, as occurs in some forms of central autonomic degeneration, moclobemide can still cause a pressor response to tyramine, and this has been put to controlled therapeutic use in such a patient. Karet F E et al 1994 Bovril and moclobemide: a novel therapeutic strategy for central autonomic failure. Lancet 344: 1263–1265.

that, in the absence of specific indications for them, as well as of any evidence that they are superior to tricyclic and allied antidepressants, they are not drugs of first choice, though they may be found to suit some patients best. They are more effective in reactive and atypical than in endogenous depression and have a place as adjuvants in severe phobic states (claustrophobia, agoraphobia) resistant to other forms of treatment, e.g. behaviour therapy. So numerous are the necessary precautions that patients taking an MAO inhibitor should be supplied with a printed card with appropriate warnings.

The *therapeutic effects* of MAO inhibitors occur in from 1–2 days to 2 weeks, and may persist for as long as 2–3 weeks after stopping treatment (as does the capacity for adverse drug reactions).

Anxiety and agitation may be made worse and depressed patients may even become hypomanic. Chlorpromazine can reduce this, monitored carefully in low dose.

Adverse effects in addition to the vascular effects (above) include: irritability, apathy, sadness, insomnia, fatigue, ataxia, tremulousness, restlessness, impotence, difficult micturition, sweating, hyperthermia, gastrointestinal disturbances, leucopenia, oedema, rashes, convulsions, jaundice. Optic nerve damage occurs with some. Appetite may increase.

Overdose can cause hypomania, coma and hypotension or hypertension. General measures are used as appropriate with minimal administration of drugs: chlorpromazine for restlessness and excitement; phentolamine for hypertension, no vasopressor drugs for hypotension, because of risk of hypertension (use posture and plasma volume expansion).

L-TRYPTOPHAN

L-tryptophan is an essential amino acid precursor of serotonin; some efficacy in depression has been shown; it can be toxic (eosinophilia/myalgia syndrome), though this may be due to an impurity; its place in therapy, if any, is uncertain.

Lithium

In 1949, during a search for biologically active substances in the urine of manic patients by injecting it into guinea pigs, it was found that the animals were affected by the accompanying large amounts of urea. Lithium urate, which is highly soluble, was selected to conduct investigations into urate toxicity. It was found to be sedative and to protect against manic urine toxicity. The carbonate was tried in manic patients, was found to be effective in the acute state and, later, to prevent recurrent attacks.[14]

The mode of action of lithium is interesting. Its probable main effect is to inhibit hydrolysis of myoinositol phosphate, thereby reducing recycling of free myoinositol for synthesis of phosphatidylinositides, which are important intracellular signalling molecules which regulate intracellullar Ca^{++}-ion concentration. Lithium modifies some receptor responses mediated via cyclic AMP, and this may also account for its capacity to affect adversely both thyroid and kidney function (below).

Pharmacokinetics. Knowledge of pharmacokinetics of lithium is important for successful use since the therapeutic plasma concentration is close to the toxic concentration (low therapeutic index). Lithium is a small ion that, given orally, is rapidly absorbed throughout the gut. High peak plasma concentration can be avoided by using sustained-release formulations. At first the distribution is throughout the extracellular water, but with continued administration it enters the cells and is eventually distributed throughout the total body water with a somewhat higher concentration in brain, bones and thyroid gland. The apparent volume of distribution is about 50 l in a 70 kg person (whose total body water is about 40 l) which is compatible with the above. Lithium is not bound to plasma or other proteins.

Lithium is easily dialysable from the blood but the concentration gradient from cell to blood is not great and intracellular concentration (which determines toxicity) falls slowly. Lithium enters cells about as readily as does sodium but does not leave as readily (mechanism uncertain).

[14] Cade J F J 1970 The story of lithium. In: Ayd F J, Blackwell B (eds) Biological psychiatry. Lippincott, Philadelphia.

Lithium ion is filtered at the glomerulus and reabsorbed in the renal tubule by diffusion at the same site as sodium. Intake of sodium and water are the principal determinants of lithium elimination. In sodium deficiency lithium is retained in the body, thus *concomitant use of a diuretic can* reduce lithium clearance by as much as 50%, and precipitate toxicity. Lithium toxicity is treated by giving sodium chloride and water.

With chronic use the $t\frac{1}{2}$ of lithium is 15–30 h. With such a $t\frac{1}{2}$ and the need to maintain a plasma concentration close to the toxic level it is important to avoid unnecessary fluctuation (peak and trough concentrations). Lithium is therefore usually given 12-hourly and reliable sustained-release formulations are welcome.

A steady-state plasma concentration will be attained after about $5 \times t\frac{1}{2}$, i.e. about 5–6 days in patients with normal renal function. Old people and patients with impaired renal function will have a longer $t\frac{1}{2}$ so that steady state will be reached later and dose increments must be adjusted accordingly.

Dose[15] **of lithium:** initially 0.2.–2.0 g daily, adjusted to achieve a plasma concentration of 0.4–1.0 mmol Li$^+$/l by measuring samples taken 12 h after the preceding dose on day 4 or 7 of treatment, then weekly until dosage has remained constant for 4 weeks; thereafter 1 to 3 monthly. Sustained-release formulations are usually given once a day.

Because of variations in pharmaceutical bioavailability patients should always take a formulation made by the same manufacturer. If change must be made then weekly monitoring of plasma concentration should be reinstituted.

It is evident that lithium therapy requires as much attention as insulin. Patients should be given a special information card.

Uses. Lithium may be used alone to control mild mania, but benefit is delayed for days and in severe cases a neuroleptic will be needed for immediate effect.

Lithium is the most effective drug in prophylaxis of manic depressive disorder. It should not be used unless monitoring of plasma concentration

can be done. Duration of use should best not exceed 3–5 years (renal toxicity) but indefinite use may be unavoidable. Criteria for safe, i.e. slow, withdrawal without relapse have not been precisely defined.

Adverse effects. Adverse effects become common as the plasma concentration exceeds 1.5 mmol/l. Over 2.0 mmol/l urgent treatment including dialysis should be considered. Maximum toxicity is delayed for 1–2 days after the toxic concentration is reached, though it will be earlier in acute overdose.

Early effects that may not interfere with treatment include nausea and mild diarrhoea. But diarrhoea that is severe enough to cause significant sodium loss increases the risk of toxicity.

As the plasma concentration rises, central nervous system effects become prominent (coarse tremor, drowsiness, giddiness, ataxia, tinnitus, blurred vision, dysarthria, muscle twitching) and now intervention is required. Oedema can occur. In severe overdose the patient may be unconscious and develop cardiac dysrhythmias, hypotension and renal failure.

Nephrogenic diabetes insipidus (at therapeutic plasma concentrations) can occur with even brief use; the distal renal tubule becomes refractory to antidiuretic hormone. Renal cellular injury may occur with use prolonged beyond 3–5 years and so may hypothyroidism due to interference with thyroxine synthesis.

Overdose is treated by diuresis with NaCl and water (alkalinisation with sodium bicarbonate adds somewhat to elimination); an osmotic diuretic is added as judgement counsels; dialysis is effective. Because lithium leaves cells slowly, plasma concentration may rise again after acute reduction; also due to continued absorption from sustained-release formulation. Sodium depletion during treatment must be avoided.

Precautions. Knowledge of renal and thyroid function is desirable before starting therapy. Patients should be warned of the common first symptoms of overdose, i.e. nausea, vomiting, diarrhoea, coarse tremor. They can then stop taking lithium immediately, and usually long before there is an oppor-

---

[15] Lithium carbonate 400 mg = 10.8 mmol Li$^+$.

tunity to measure the plasma concentration. Abrupt withdrawal may be followed by relapse into mania in about 2 weeks. Prolonged use (years) should only be practised if it is certain that benefit warrants it. Patients should always use the same formulation. Plasma concentration monitoring is essential (see Dosage, above). The minimum dose that is effective should be used.

Lithium toxicity may be precipitated by water and sodium loss as by diuretics, diarrhoea, vomiting and renal disease.

Interactions. Neuroleptics are potentiated as are other CNS active drugs; diuretics (see above); prostaglandin synthase inhibitors (NSAIDs) potentiate lithium (reduced elimination).

Pregnancy. Lithium may cause fetal cardiac abnormality. If lithium must be used, close monitoring of plasma concentration is needed because of the physiological pregnancy changes in body water and electrolytes. The newborn infant may be hypotonic and have a goitre; breast feeding is best avoided.

SUMMARY — schizophrenia and depression

- Treatment of schizophrenia is by blockade of dopamine receptors in the CNS.
- The phenothiazines and butyrophenones, nonselective antagonists of dopamine receptors, are first-line therapy for both acute and maintenance therapy.
- The choice of agent among these is governed by patient compliance and tolerance.
- The principal cause of intolerance, after prolonged therapy, is tardive dyskinesia (paradoxical dopamine receptor hypersensitivity). Such patients can be switched to more selective antagonists of the dopamine D_2 or D_4 receptors, e.g. sulpiride, risperidone or clozapine.
- The therapy of depression aims to increase amine concentration in the CNS.
- First-line treatment is the tricyclics which nonspecifically inhibit neuronal re-uptake of noradrenaline (norepinephrine) and serotonin (5-HT).
- Alternatives are selective inhibitors of serotonin uptake, or monoamine oxidase inhibitors.
- Available antidepressants differ in adverse effect profiles, rather than in efficacy.
- Lithium is the preferred treatment of bipolar depression, but requires careful monitoring.

Psychostimulants, appetite control

AMPHETAMINES

Amphetamine (racemic) and dexamphetamine (dextro: the laevo-form is relatively inactive) are the principal medicinal psychostimulants (caffeine can be regarded as the social psychostimulant); the use of amphetamines in depression is obsolete. Amphetamine will be described, and its allies only in the ways in which they differ.

Mode of action. Amphetamine acts by releasing noradrenaline stored in nerve endings in both the CNS and the periphery. As with all drugs acting on the central nervous system, the psychological effects vary with mood, personality and environment as well as with dose.

Subjects become euphoric and fatigue is postponed. Although physical and mental performance may improve, this cannot be relied on; subjects may be more confident and show more initiative, and be better satisfied with a more speedy performance that has deteriorated in accuracy. On the other hand there may be anxiety and a feeling of nervous and physical tension, especially with large doses, and subjects develop tremors and confusion, and feel dizzy. Time seems to pass with greater rapidity. The sympathomimetic effect on the heart, causing palpitations, may intensify discomfort or alarm.

Amphetamine increases peripheral oxygen consumption and this, together with vasoconstriction and restlessness, leads to hyperthermia in overdose, especially if the subject exercises.

Dependence on amphetamine and similar sympathomimetics occurs; it is chiefly psychological, but there is a withdrawal syndrome, suggesting physical dependence; tolerance occurs.

Mild dependence on prescribed amphetamines became common, particularly amongst people with unstable personalities, depressives and tired, lonely housewives. In the 1960s, adolescents began to turn to amphetamines for occasional use to keep awake to have 'fun' and then as an aid to the challenges normal to that stage of life. Unfortunately, drugs provide only the temporary solution of avoidance and postponement of such challenges, retarding rather than assisting progress to maturity.

As well as oral use, i.v. administration (with the pleasurable 'flash' as with opioids) is employed. Severe dependence induces behaviour disorders, hallucinations and even florid psychosis which can be controlled by haloperidol. Withdrawal is accompanied by lethargy, sleep, desire for food and sometimes severe depression, which leads to an urge to resume the drug.

Pharmacokinetics. Amphetamine ($t^1/2$ 12 h) is readily absorbed by any usual route and is largely eliminated unchanged in the urine. Urinary excretion is pH dependent; being a basic substance, elimination will be greater in an acid urine.

Uses. Amphetamine has had multifarious uses, but its potential for abuse is such that it should only be used where essential, and this is rare:

- Narcolepsy: patients pass directly into REM sleep; amphetamine delays onset of REM sleep
- In some hyperactive children with attention deficit disorder; also methylphenidate (Ritalin)
- Against fatigue: seldom justified
- Appetite suppression: alternatives are preferable (below)
- Use in sport is abuse

Interactions are as expected from mode of action, e.g. antagonism of antihypertensives; severe hypertension with MAOIs and β-adrenoceptor blocking drugs.

Acute poisoning is manifested by excitement and peripheral sympathomimetic effects; convulsions may occur; also, in acute or chronic overuse, a state resembling hyperactive paranoid schizophrenia with hallucinations develops. Hyperthermia occurs (see above), with cardiac dysrhythmias, vascular collapse and death. Treatment is chlorpromazine with added antihypertensive, e.g. labetalol, if necessary; these provide sedation and α- and β-adrenoceptor blockade (not a β-blocker alone), rendering unnecessary the enhancement of elimination by urinary acidification.

Chronic overdose can cause a psychotic state mim-

icking schizophrenia. A vasculitis of the cerebral and/or renal vessels can occur, possibly due to release of vasoconstrictor amines from both platelets and nerve endings. Severe hypertension can result from the renal vasculitis. Dexamphetamine, phentermine, diethylpropion, methylphenidate and pemoline are similar to amphetamine; for tenamphetamine (Ecstasy) see page 179.

Appetite suppression

It was noticed casually in 1937 that patients receiving amphetamine tended to lose weight. This was investigated in animals and man and found to be due to a reduction in voluntary food intake. Dogs would starve in the presence of food when given amphetamine, although they still showed interest in being fed and jealousy of the dog being fed before them. It was only when food was actually placed in their cage that enthusiasm abated.

Amphetamine-type sympathomimetics with pronounced psychostimulant effects (diethylpropion, phentermine) suppress appetite (hunger), but the effect is transient, being as short as 2–3 weeks; dependence occurs. *They should only be used briefly, if at all*; they do not improve the longterm outlook.

Dexfenfluramine

Dexfenfluramine (Adifax) replaces the racemic fenfluramine (Ponderax); it is structurally related to amphetamine, but it causes release of serotonin from nerve stores, rather than noradrenaline. It is sedative rather than stimulant to the CNS and it may induce satiety, i.e. the subject eats as frequently, but amount is less. There may be some elevation of mood at the outset of therapy; in overdose amphetamine-like stimulant effects occur. Blood pressure is reduced.

Dexfenfluramine also has some peripheral effects on carbohydrate and lipid metabolism and it is uncertain whether these promote weight reduction.

Use. Dexfenfluramine is probably the drug of choice for obesity (when a drug is needed), and certainly so in hypertensives. Weight loss begins in 2 weeks and lasts for 3 months. It should not be necessary to give drug therapy for longer, and it is likely to be ineffective anyway. Some dependence occurs and abrupt withdrawal can cause depression which is especially marked after 4 days; withdrawal should be gradual.

Adverse effects include sleepiness, depression, diarrhoea, impotence and increased dreaming. Dependence can occur; avoid abrupt withdrawal (above). Heavy overdose can cause central nervous system stimulation and cardiac dysrhythmias.

Interactions. Dexfenfluramine does not antagonise antihypertensive therapy as do the amphetamines, indeed there may be some potentiation. Hypertension may occur with MAOIs. Sedatives and antidiabetics may be potentiated. In a few patients, fenfluramine has been associated with the development of pulmonary hypertension.

Fluoxetine (Prozac) is an antidepressant that inhibits serotonin re-uptake into nerve endings; it has anorectic action; it may be effective in bulimia nervosa (see p. 344).

Biguanide antidiabetics reduce intestinal carbohydrate absorption and may induce weight loss without reducing blood glucose concentration. But their use is probably best confined to diabetics.

Bulk preparations, e.g. methylcellulose or sterculia, are used to fill the stomach with non-nutrient material and induce a feeling of satiety.[16] Their use is probably based on a wrong physiological concept (unless enormous amounts are taken). Animals eat for calories, not bulk; it is possible to feel hungry in the absence of a stomach. Patients might as well be invited to eat flavoured toilet paper.

Thyroxine (T_4) or tri-iodothyronine (T_3) has long history of misuse in obesity. It is probably beneficial only when a diet so restricted as to amount to starvation has diminished the normal conversion of T_4 to T_3, a rare situation. Otherwise administration of T_4 or T_3 suppresses normal hormone production by the familiar feedback mechanism, and should not be used in the usual weight-losing regimens.

---

[16] This approach has been carried to the extreme of inflating a balloon in the stomach.

Appetite stimulation

Cyproheptadine (Periactin) blocks serotonin and histamine H_1-receptors. It has the unusual effect of increasing appetite, probably via an action on serotonin receptors in the hypothalamus. It is sometimes used as adjuvant therapy in anorexia nervosa that is without bulimic episodes. In general, little or nothing is gained by seeking to stimulate appetite by drugs.

Cyproheptadine also reduces corticotrophin release by blocking the serotonergic path controlling corticotrophin releasing factor and growth hormone and it has been used with variable success in Cushing's syndrome and acromegaly. It may also benefit other symptoms caused by serotonin release, e.g. postgastrectomy dumping syndrome and carcinoid tumour.

Insulin increases appetite by reducing blood glucose concentration.

Cannabis may induce hunger.

METHYLXANTHINES (XANTHINES)

The three xanthines, caffeine, theophylline and theobromine, occur in plants. They are qualitatively similar but differ markedly in potency.

- *Tea* contains caffeine and theophylline.
- *Coffee* contains caffeine.
- *Cocoa and chocolate* contain caffeine and theobromine.
- The *cola nut* ('cola' drinks) contains caffeine.

Theobromine is weak and is of no clinical importance.

Mode of action. Caffeine and theophylline have complex and incompletely elucidated effects on intracellular calcium, on adenosine (vasodilator) receptors (block) and on noradrenergic function. Their capacity to inhibit phosphodiesterase, the enzyme that breaks down cyclic AMP (formation of which is stimulated by adrenoceptor agonists), occurs significantly only at concentrations higher than those reached in therapeutic use. When theophylline is used alongside salbutamol in asthma their actions add up to increased *benefit* to the bronchi, but increased *risk* to the heart.

Pharmacokinetics. Absorption of xanthines after

oral or rectal administration varies with the preparation used. It is generally extensive but erratic. Caffeine metabolism is dose-dependent (saturation kinetics) with a $t^{1/2}$ rising from 4 h to more than 10 h in heavy coffee drinkers who are prone to adverse effects (see Chronic overdose, below). Xanthines are metabolised (more than 90%) by numerous enzymes, including xanthine oxidase. (For further details on theophylline, see Asthma.)

Actions on mental performance. Caffeine is more potent than theophylline, but both drugs stimulate mental activity where it is below normal. They do not raise it above normal; thought is more rapid and fatigue is removed or its onset delayed. The effects on mental and physical performance vary according to the mental state and personality of the subject. Reaction-time is decreased. Performance that is inferior because of excessive anxiety may become worse.

Caffeine can (like amphetamine) also improve *physical performance* both in tasks requiring more physical effort than skill (athletics) and in tasks requiring more skill than physical effort (monitoring instruments and taking corrective action in an aircraft flight simulator). It is uncertain whether the improvement consists only of restoring to normal performance that is impaired by fatigue or boredom, or whether caffeine (and amphetamine) can also enable subjects to improve their normal maximum performance. The drugs may produce their effects by altering both physical capacity and mental attitude.

There is insufficient information on the effects on learning to be able to give any useful advice to students preparing for examination other than that *intellectual performance* may be assisted when it has been reduced by fatigue or boredom. Effects on *mood* vary greatly amongst individuals and according to the environment and the task in hand. In general, caffeine (and amphetamine) induce feelings of alertness and well-being, euphoria or exhilaration. Onset of boredom, fatigue, inattentiveness and sleepiness is postponed.

Overdose can cause anxiety, tension and tremors and will certainly reduce performance.

The regular, frequent use of caffeine-containing drinks is part of normal social life and mild over-dose is common. Habitual tea and coffee drinkers are seldom willing to recognise that they have a psychological drug dependence.

Other effects

Respiratory stimulation occurs with substantial doses.

Sleep. Caffeine affects sleep of older more than it does of younger people and this may be related to the fact that older people show greater catecholamine turnover in the central nervous system than do the young. Onset of sleep (sleep latency) is delayed, bodily movements are increased, total sleep time is reduced, there are increased awakenings. Tolerance to this effect does not occur, as is shown by the provision of decaffeinated coffee.[17]

Skeletal muscle. Metabolism is increased, and this may play a part in the enhanced athletic performance mentioned above. There is significant improvement of diaphragmatic function in chronic obstructive pulmonary disease.

Cardiovascular system. Both caffeine and theophylline directly stimulate the myocardium and cause increased cardiac output, tachycardia and sometimes ectopic beats and palpitations. This effect occurs almost at once after i.v. injection and lasts half an hour. Theophylline relieves acute left ventricular failure. There is peripheral (but not cerebral) vasodilatation due to a direct action of the drugs on the blood vessels, but stimulation of the vasomotor centre tends to counter this. Changes in the blood pressure are therefore somewhat unpredictable, but 250 mg caffeine (single dose) usually causes a transient rise of blood pressure of about 14/10 mmHg in occasional coffee drinkers (but no additional effect in habitual drinkers); this effect can be used advantageously in patients with *autonomic nervous system failure* who experience postprandial hypotension (2 cups of coffee with breakfast may suffice for the day). In occasional cof-

---

[17] The European Community regulations define 'decaffeinated' as coffee (bean) containing 0.3% or less of caffeine (normal content 1–2%).

fee drinkers 2 cups of coffee (about 160 mg caffeine) per day raise blood pressure by 5/4 mmHg. Increased coronary artery blood flow may occur but increased cardiac work counterbalances this in angina pectoris.

When theophyllines (aminophylline) are given i.v. slow injection is essential in order to avoid transient peak concentrations which are equivalent to administering an overdose (below).

Smooth muscle (other than vascular muscle, which is discussed above) is relaxed. The only important clinical use for this action is in reversible airways obstruction (asthma) (theophylline). Therapeutic effect is variable but can be excellent.

Kidney. Diuresis occurs in normals chiefly due to reduced tubular reabsorption of Na, similar to thiazide action, but weaker.

Miscellaneous effects. Gastric secretion is increased by caffeine given as coffee (by decaffeinated coffee too) more than by caffeine alone, and the basal metabolic rate may increase slightly (see Skeletal muscle, above).

Acute overdose, e.g. aminophylline (see p. 509) i.v., can cause convulsions, hypotension, cardiac dysrhythmia and sudden death (chronic overdose, see below).

Preparations and uses of caffeine and theophylline

Aminophylline. The most generally useful preparation is aminophylline which is a soluble, irritant salt of theophylline with ethylenediamine (see Asthma).

Attempts to make nonirritant orally reliable preparations of theophylline have resulted in choline theophyllinate and numerous variants. Sustained-release formulations are convenient for asthmatics, but they cannot be assumed to be bioequivalent and repeat prescriptions should adhere to the formulation of a particular manufacturer. Suppositories are available.

Aminophylline is used in

- *Asthma*. In severe asthma when β-adrenoceptor

agonists fail (often given i.v.); and orally to provide a background bronchodilator effect
- *Paroxysmal nocturnal dyspnoea* (i.v. for immediate effect), to terminate an attack
- *Neonatal apnoea*; caffeine is also effective
- *The dying patient*: aminophylline i.v. may cause brief and unrepeatable but socially useful recovery of consciousness and coherence
- *Caffeine* is used as an additional ingredient in analgesic tablets; about 60 mg potentiates NSAIDs. Also to *enhance oral ergotamine absorption* in migraine; in hypotension of *autonomic failure*.

Xanthine-containing drinks

(see also above)

Coffee, tea and cola drinks in excess can make people tense and anxious and exacerbate peptic ulcer. Small children are not usually given tea and coffee because they are thought to be less tolerant of the central nervous system stimulant effect, but cola drinks irrationally escape this prohibition. It is possible to make an imposing list of diseases which may be caused or made worse by caffeine-containing drinks, but there is no conclusive evidence to warrant any general prohibitions. High doses of caffeine in animals damage chromosomes and cause fetal abnormalities; but studies in man suggest that normal consumption poses no risk. Epidemiological studies are not conclusive but *suggest* either no, or only slight, increased risk ($\times$ 2–3) of coronary heart disease in heavy (including decaffeinated) coffee consumers (>4 cups/day) (see Lipids, below).

Dependence and tolerance. Slight tolerance to the effects of caffeine (on all systems) occurs. Withdrawal symptoms, attributable to psychological and perhaps mild physical dependence occur in habitual coffee drinkers (5 or more cups/day) 12–16 h after the last cup; they include headache (lasting up to 6 days), irritability, jitteriness; they may occur with transient changes in intake, e.g. high at work, lower at the weekend.

Chronic overdose. Excessive prolonged consumption of caffeine causes anxiety, restlessness, tremors, insomnia; headache, cardiac extrasystoles and confusion; diarrhoea may occur with coffee and constipation with tea. The cause can easily be overlooked if specific enquiry into habits is not made; including children regarding cola drinks. Of coffee drinkers, up to 25% who complain of anxiety may benefit from reduction of caffeine intake. A heavy *adult* user may be defined as one who takes more than 300 mg caffeine/day, i.e. 4 cups of 150 ml of brewed coffee, each containing 80 ± 20 mg caffeine per cup or 5 cups (60 ± 20) of instant coffee. The equivalent for tea would be 10 cups at approx 30 mg caffeine per cup; and of cola drinks about 2.0 l. Plainly, caffeine drinks brewed to personal taste of consumer or vendor must have an extremely variable concentration according to source of coffee or tea, amount used, method and duration of brewing. There is also great individual variation in the effect of coffee both between individuals and sometimes in the same individual at different times of life (see Sleep, above).

Decaffeinated coffee[17] contains about 3 mg per cup; cola drinks contain 8–13 mg caffeine/100 ml; cocoa as a drink, 4 mg per cup; chocolate (solid) 6–20 mg per 30 g.

In young people high caffeine intake has been linked to behaviour disorders and a limit of 125 mg/l has been proposed for cola drinks.

Blood lipids. Cessation of coffee drinking can reduce serum cholesterol concentration in hypercholesterolaemic men.

Drinking 5 cups of *boiled* coffee/day increases serum total cholesterol by up to 10%; this does not occur with coffee made by simple filtration.

Breast-fed infants may become sleepless and irritable if there is high maternal intake.

Fetal cardiac dysrhythmias have been reported with exceptionally high maternal caffeine intake, e.g. 1.5 l cola drinks/day.

Fertility. Women who drink excess of coffee may have difficulty in conceiving, but causal attribution of the association is not conclusive.

GINSENG

Ginseng is the root of 2 plants of the same family (oriental, *Panax ginseng*; Siberian, *Eleutherococcus senticosis*). It contains a range of biologically active substances (ginsenosides).

It has been used as a tonic or stimulant for thousands of years. In animal studies ginseng doubles the time that mice placed in water can swim before becoming exhausted; it appears to have antifatigue effects in various other tests in mice (climbing up a rope that is moving downwards) and it increases sexual activity. In man, ginseng has been claimed to benefit performance of (Russian) athletes and astronauts (fewer fatigue-caused errors), and to reduce absenteeism due to respiratory illness in mining and steel workers and truck drivers. Oriental soldiers at war have used ginseng.

Despite accumulating evidence and wide use by the public, the medical profession in Western countries remains sceptical of the value of this tonic. A range of adverse effects is reported, including oedema, hypertension, rashes, diarrhoea, sleeplessness and oestrogen-like effects.

GUIDE TO FURTHER READING

Anonymous 1983 A schizophrenic describes his recovery. Lancet 2: 562
Beumont P J, Russell J D, Touyz S W 1993 Treatment of anorexia nervosa. Lancet 341: 1635–1640
Black D 1991 Psychotropic drugs for problem children. British Medical Journal 302: 190
Freeman H 1993 Moclobemide. Lancet 342: 1528–1532
Garrow J S 1992 Treatment of obesity. Lancet 340: 409–413
Gelder M 1990 Psychological treatment for depressive disorder. British Medical Journal 300: 1087
Gram L 1994 Fluoxetine. New England Journal of Medicine 331: 1354–1361
Kane J M 1996 Drug therapy: schizophrenia. New England Journal of Medicine 334: 34–41
Levy M et al 1983 Caffeine metabolism and coffee-attributed sleep disturbances. Clinical Pharmacology and Therapeutics 33: 770
Paykel E S, Priest R G et al 1992 Recognition and management of depression in general practice: consensus statement. British Medical Journal 305: 1198–1202
Pickar D 1995 Prospects for pharmacotherapy of schizophrenia. Lancet 345: 557–562
Sharp D S et al 1990 Pharmacoepidemiology of the effect of caffeine on blood pressure. Clinical Pharmacology and Therapeutics 47: 57
Song F, Freemantle N et al 1993 Selective serotonin

reuptake inhibitors: meta-analysis of efficacy and acceptability. British Medical Journal 306: 683–687

Thelle D S 1991 Coffee, cholesterol and coronary heart disease. British Medical Journal 302: 804

Tonks C M 1977 Lithium intoxication induced by dieting and saunas. British Medical Journal 2: 1396

Epilepsy, parkinsonism and allied conditions

SYNOPSIS

Epilepsy, in one form or another, affects 4–10 per 1000 of general populations.

- Antiepilepsy drugs: principles of management; withdrawal of therapy; pregnancy; epilepsy in children
- Pharmacology of: carbamazepine, phenytoin, sodium valproate, lamotrigine, vigabatrin, gabapentin, clonazepam

Parkinsonism affects about 1:200 of the elderly population.

- Objectives of therapy
- Drugs used and special problems of longterm treatment

Other disorders of movement

Tetanus

Antiepilepsy drugs

Bromide (1857) was the first effective antiepilepsy drug, but is now obsolete. When phenobarbitone was introduced in 1912 it was found to control patients resistant to bromides.

The next success was the discovery in 1938 of phenytoin (a hydantoin) which is structurally relat-ed to the barbiturates. Since then many drugs have been discovered, but phenytoin still remains a drug of choice in the treatment of major epilepsy.

Epilepsy comprises sudden, excessive depolarisation of groups of cerebral neurons, which may remain localised (focal epilepsy) or which may spread to cause a generalised seizure.

Mode of action. Antiepileptic (anticonvulsant) drugs inhibit the neuronal discharge or its spread, and do so in one of three ways:

- altering cell membrane permeability to ions, e.g. Na^+, Ca^{++}
- enhancing the activity of natural inhibitory neurotransmitters such as gamma-aminobutyric acid (GABA), which induces hyperpolarisation
- inhibition of excitatory neurotransmitters, e.g. glutamate.

Principles of management
- Educate the patient about the disease, duration of treatment and need for compliance
- Treat causative factors, e.g. cerebral neoplasm
- Avoid precipitating factors, e.g. alcohol, stress
- Anticipate natural variation, e.g. fits may occur only at night or shortly after waking
- Give antiepilepsy drugs

GENERAL DRUG THERAPY

The decision whether or not to initiate drug therapy after a single major seizure remains controversial.

- Therapy should start with a single well-tried and relatively nontoxic drug. The majority of patients can be and should be controlled on *one drug* (*monotherapy*).
- Dosage should be adjusted according to known pharmacokinetic properties. Measurement of plasma (or saliva) concentrations (if practicable) is useful at the outset of therapy and where any problems of efficacy or adverse reactions arise (see below). In the absence of facilities for measurement of plasma concentration then it may be necessary to establish the *maximum tolerated dose*.
- Attention to detail, including measurement of plasma (or salivary) concentrations, allows 80% of patients, or more, to be managed on a single drug. Few patients benefit from more than 2 drugs.
- If the first drug fails to give complete control there is a choice between withdrawing it completely (*slowly*, if it has had any useful effect at all) and *substituting* concurrently a drug of a different chemical group; or else of *adding* a second drug of a different chemical group.
- *Abrupt withdrawal*. Effective therapy must never be stopped suddenly either by the doctor (carelessness) or by the patient (carelessness, intercurrent illness or ignorance), or status epilepticus may occur. But if sudden withdrawal is imposed by occurrence of toxicity, a substantial dose of another antiepileptic should be given at once.
- This trial of drug after drug should be continued until the epilepsy is controlled, or until there are no more drugs to try. Up to 3 months may be needed to try a drug thoroughly in an individual.
- In cases where fits are liable to occur at a particular time of day, dosage should be adjusted to achieve maximal drug effect at that time.
- The patient should keep a *diary* of seizures.

Dosage

Start with about one-third of the expected maintenance dose and increase it weekly to reach the maintenance dose in 3 to 4 weeks, by which time any enzyme induction will have occurred and a

steady state reached after the most recent dose increment. If plasma concentration measurements are available, a blood sample, taken at the end of the longest interval between doses, i.e. trough or minimal concentration (usually, and inconveniently, early morning), provides useful background information for further dose adjustment.

If fits continue the dose should be adjusted upwards until fits cease or adverse effects occur (maximum tolerated dose).

Frequency of administration. In general, taking into account convenience as well as pharmacokinetics, 2 equal daily doses morning and evening are recommended for routine practice. It is practicable to use once-daily administration with some drugs (having regard to the $t^{1/2}$) but there will be higher peaks and lower troughs of plasma concentration, and the consequences of a forgotten dose will be greater; sustained-release formulations for once daily use are available.

Interval between dose increments. If fits are infrequent it is obviously difficult to adjust dosage by therapeutic response. With phenytoin, a useful plan is to get the plasma concentration into the therapeutic range (measure it 1–2 weeks after instituting therapy and make appropriate adjustment) or, where this is not available, raise the dose gradually at 1–2 week intervals until an unwanted effect (nystagmus, dysarthria, ataxia) occurs and then reduce it slightly (maximum tolerated dose); but control may be achieved below this dose.

A fit or series of fits in a known epileptic often presents to a doctor who has never seen the patient before. It is important to consider the cause, whether it is noncompliance (which can be due to intercurrent disease), an inadequate drug regimen or an advance in the severity of the disease. Obviously measurement of drug plasma concentrations will help. It is important to avoid casual or impulsive alterations of regimen of drugs, which take a week or more to reach a steady state (long $t^{1/2}$), in the absence of accurate diagnosis.

PLASMA OR SALIVA MONITORING

Routine drug concentration monitoring is particularly useful with phenytoin (which shows saturation kinetics). It is seldom really useful with other drugs unless there is a specific problem to be solved. Unnecessary monitoring wastes expensive resources. *Monitoring is useful* in the following circumstances:

- 2–4 weeks after commencing therapy
- When fits occur with standard dosage: the patient may be noncompliant, or compliant and simply need more drug
- When adverse effects occur
- When sodium valproate is added to another drug (pharmacokinetic interaction)
- When another antiepilepsy drug is withdrawn in the presence of sodium valproate
- In pregnancy
- When there is hepatic or renal disease.

Note. Many patients are controlled at plasma concentrations below the lower limit of the therapeutic range, and substantial diurnal fluctuations may occur.

DRUG TREATMENT, DURATION, WITHDRAWAL

60–95% of patients with treatable epilepsies, i.e. patients with fits but who are otherwise normal, can be completely relieved within 1 year. Plainly it is undesirable in principle to continue drug therapy for the rest of the patient's life if it can be safely withdrawn for, apart from general concerns about longterm drug therapy, there is evidence suggestive of adverse effects on behaviour and cognitive function that must be a particular cause for disquiet during childhood (development and education).

After at least 2 years, and preferably 3 or 4 years, of complete freedom from attacks, withdrawal of medication should be considered. In adult epilepsy, drug withdrawal is associated with about 20% relapse during withdrawal and a further 20% relapse over the following 5 years, after which relapse is unusual.

Relapse is more likely when the epilepsy has been severe and prolonged, and with major than with minor epilepsies.

Withdrawal should be slow, over about 6 months. If a fit occurs, full therapy must be resumed again for 2–3 years. A daytime fit during or after the process results in loss of driving licence for at least a year; some patients may prefer not to risk this at all, or only after 5 years of freedom. Adverse effects of prolonged treatment can be a significant factor in the decision.

Car driving and epilepsy. The UK allows patients to drive a car (but not a truck or bus) if they have not had a daytime fit for 1 year (or for 3 years if subject to asleep fits).

PREGNANCY AND EPILEPSY

Pharmacokinetics

Pharmacokinetics are altered due to physiological changes (see p. 114). Since what is important therapeutically is the concentration of free drug, and what is measured is the concentration of the free plus bound drug (total drug), it is evident that acceptance of the total plasma concentration as a guide to therapy when protein binding has changed can be misleading. Hepatic drug metabolism may increase. Erratic fluctuations in plasma concentrations may occur. Drug concentration should be kept at the lower end of the therapeutic range.

In practice, the patient is closely watched clinically and the dose of drug increased if seizures occur more often than expected. After delivery the pharmacokinetics revert to prepregnancy state over a few days.

Antiepilepsy drugs pass into breast milk, but the total quantities ingested by the baby are small and breast feeding may be considered safe (except when taking phenobarbitone; $t^{1/2}$ 100 h). Though there is possibility of sedation of the baby the advantages of breast feeding outweigh this but if somnolence and poor suckling occur breast feeding may have to be abandoned.

Fetal abnormality

Children of mothers taking antiepilepsy drugs show an approximately $\times$ 2.5 increased rate of malformations at birth (above the background 1–2%), especially cleft palate and lip, and heart abnormalities. This is probably due to the drugs rather than to the disease. Withdrawal of effective therapy during early pregnancy cannot be recommended because seizures are dangerous to both the woman and the fetus (except perhaps in minor epilepsy, when consciousness is not lost). Women of reproductive age should be treated with the simplest possible regimen (one drug at minimum effective dose, which will be assisted by measuring plasma concentration). Folate deficiency due to altered folate metabolism also occurs with hydantoin and barbiturate antiepileptics and is a suspected cause of fetal neural tube defects (spina bifida). Sodium valproate carries a definite risk of spina bifida (even as much as 1–2%); and carbamazepine perhaps less.

A folate supplement is advisable in a woman who wishes to become, as well as who has become, pregnant.

Carbamazepine may be considered the drug of choice for women of childbearing potential. A curious multiple syndrome has been tentatively named *fetal hydantoin syndrome*.

Newborn babies of mothers taking antiepilepsy drugs sometimes have reduced clotting factors, remediable by giving vitamin K antenatally; it is attributed to the drugs, perhaps by enzyme induction.

Contraception

Because of induction of steroid metabolising enzymes by some antiepileptic drugs (carbamazepine, phenytoin, barbiturates) with possible failure of contraception, it is prudent either to prescribe the higher dose oestrogen-containing oral contraceptives (at a level that avoids breakthrough bleeding, e.g. oestrogen 50 µg,) or, perhaps better, use a different mode of contraception.

EPILEPSY IN CHILDREN

Fits in children are treated as in adults, but children may respond differently and become irritable, e.g. with sodium valproate or phenobarbitone.

It remains uncertain whether antiepilepsy drugs interfere with later development and education and it is certainly unwise to assume they do not. The sensible course is to control the epilepsy with monotherapy in minimal doses and with special attention to precipitating factors, with drug withdrawal when it is deemed safe to attempt it (see above).

When a child has *febrile convulsions* the decision to embark on continuous prophylaxis is serious for the child and depends on an assessment of risk factors, e.g. age, nature and duration of fit. Most children who have febrile convulsions do not develop epilepsy. Prolonged drug therapy, e.g. with phenytoin or phenobarbitone, has been shown to interfere with cognitive development, the effect persisting for months after the drug is withdrawn. Parents may be supplied with specially formulated rectal *solution* of diazepam (absorption from a suppository is too slow) for easy and early administration, and advised on managing fever, e.g. use paracetamol at the first hint of fever, and tepid sponging.

POST-TRAUMATIC EPILEPSY

Developed epilepsy after head injury is treated in the usual way. Prevention of epilepsy in the first week after severe head injury may be accomplished by phenytoin. No drug has been proved effective in preventing late development of epilepsy.

STATUS EPILEPTICUS

Status epilepticus is a medical emergency. Treatments of choice are shown in Table 20.1. Diazepam may cause hypotension and respiratory depression if combined with other antiepileptics or if the seizures are due to acute brain injury (when phenytoin is preferred). If i.v. injection of diazepam is impracticable, give a *solution* per rectum. Absorption from i.m. injection is slow and erratic. Duration of antiepileptic effect of diazepam is short and it should be followed at once by phenytoin i.v. (monitor ECG) to avoid relapse. Alternative drugs include clonazepam, lorazepam and chlormethiazole. Paraldehyde, which has little respiratory depressant effect, is still used where full resuscitation facilities are not available. General anaesthesia with or without neuromuscular block may even be necessary. Once the emergency is over, exploration of the reason for the episode and reinstitution of therapy, guided if possible by plasma concentrations, is immediately required. For the fits of pre-eclamptic toxaemia of pregnancy, recent studies have demonstrated the clear superiority of magnesium sulphate over phenytoin.[1,2 (see overleaf)]

Table 20.1 Drugs of choice in treatment of epileptic seizures[4]

Seizure disorder	Drugs	Usual daily dosage		Usual therapeutic serum concentrations
		Adults	Children	
PRIMARY GENERALISED TONIC-CLONIC (GRAND MAL)				
Drugs of Choice:	Valproate	1000–3000 mg	15–60 mg/kg	50–120 µg/ml
OR	Carbamazepine	800–1600 mg	10–30 mg/kg	6–12 µg/ml
OR	Phenytoin	300–400 mg	4–8 mg/kg	10–20 µg/ml
Alternatives:	Lamotrigine	100–500 mg	Not approved	Not established
	Primidone	750–1250 mg	10–20 mg/kg	6–12 µg/ml
	Phenobarbital	90–150 mg	2–5 mg/kg	15–35 µg/ml
PARTIAL, INCLUDING SECONDARILY GENERALISED				
Drugs of Choice:	Carbamazepine	800–1600 mg	10–30 mg/kg	6–12 µg/ml
OR	Phenytoin	300–400 mg	4–8 mg/kg	10–20 µg/ml
OR	Valproate	1000–3000 mg	15–60 mg/kg	50–120 µg/ml
Alternatives:	Primidone	750–1250 mg	10–20 mg/kg	6–12 µg/ml
	Phenobarbital	90–150 mg	2–5 mg/kg	15–35 µg/ml
	Lamotrigine (as adjunct)	100–500 mg	Not approved	Not established
	Gabapentin (as adjunct)	900–2400 mg	Not approved	Not established
	Vigabatrin (as adjunct)	2000–4000 mg	Not approved	Not established
ABSENCE (PETIT MAL)				
Drugs of Choice:	Ethosuximide	750–1250 mg	20–40 mg/kg	40–100 µg/ml
OR	Valproate[1]	1000–3000 mg	15–60 mg/kg	50–120 µg/ml
Alternatives:	Clonazepam	1.5–20 mg	0.05–0.2 mg/kg	20–80 ng/ml
	Lamotrigine	100–500 mg	Not approved	Not established
ATYPICAL ABSENCE, MYOCLONIC, ATONIC				
Drug of Choice:	Valproate	1000–3000 mg	15–60 mg/kg	50–120 µg/ml
Alternatives:	Clonazepam	1.5–20 mg	0.05–0.2 mg/kg	20–80 ng/ml
	Felbamate (as adjunct)	1200–3600 mg	15–60 mg/kg	Not established

STATUS EPILEPTICUS

Drugs of choice		Usual initial dose	Usual rate	Repeat doses PRN	Maximum 24 h
Diazepam, IV	Adults	5–10 mg	1–2 mg/min[3]	5–10 mg q20–30 min	100 mg
	Children	0.25–0.4 mg/kg[2]		0.25–0.4 mg/kg[2] q20–30 min	40 mg
Phenytoin, IV	Adults	15–20 mg/kg	30–50 mg/min	100–150 mg q30 min	1.5 g
	Children	15–20 mg/kg	0.5–1.5 mg/kg/min	1.5 mg/kg q30 min	20 mg/kg
Phenobarbital, IV	Adults	10–20 mg/kg	25–50 mg/min	120–240 mg q20 min	1–2 g
	Children	20 mg/kg	25–50 mg/min	6 mg/kg q20 min	40 mg/kg

[1] First choice if primary generalised tonic–clonic seizures also present.
[2] To a maximum of 5–10 mg.
[3] Slower rate of administration should be used for children.
Notes:
Doses may vary if more than one drug is used.
The term 'not approved' refers to decisions of the Food and Drug Administration (FDA) USA.
[4] The Table is based, by permission, on Tables published (1991, 1995) by the Medical Letter on Drugs and Therapeutics (USA) whom we thank.

[1] Eclampsia Trial Collaborative Group 1995 Which anticonvulsant for women with eclampsia? Evidence from the collaborative eclampsia trial. Lancet 345: 1455–1463.

[2] Lucas M J, Leveno K J, Cunningham F G 1995 A comparison of magnesium sulfate with phenytoin for the prevention of eclampsia. New England Journal of Medicine 333: 201–205.

Pharmacology of individual drugs

CARBAMAZEPINE

Carbamazepine (Tegretol) is structurally related to imipramine. Because another antiepileptic (phenytoin) is sometimes beneficial in *trigeminal* neuralgia, carbamazepine was tried in this condition, for which it is now the drug of choice. It has since become a drug of choice for generalised tonic-clonic and partial seizures. It impairs cognitive function less than does phenytoin.

Pharmacokinetics. The $t^{1/2}$ of carbamazepine falls from 35 h to 20 h over the first few weeks of therapy due to induction of hepatic enzymes that metabolise it as well as other drugs, including steroids (adrenal and contraceptive), theophylline and warfarin. Cimetidine and valproate inhibit its metabolism. There are *complex interactions* with other antiepilepsy drugs, which constitute a reason for monodrug therapy.

Standard tablets are taken twice a day.

Adverse effects include CNS symptoms (reversible blurring of vision, diplopia, dizziness) and depression of cardiac AV conduction. Also, gut symptoms, skin rashes, blood disorders and liver and kidney dysfunction. Osteomalacia by enhanced metabolism of vitamin D (enzyme induction) occurs over years; also folate deficiency.

HYDANTOINS: PHENYTOIN

Phenytoin (diphenylhydantoin, Epanutin, Dilantin) (1938) alters ionic fluxes (Na, K, Ca) across cell membranes; its effect is described as membrane stabilising, which prevents the initiation and spread of repetitive neuronal discharges. Phenytoin orally is well absorbed but there have been pharmaceutical bioavailability problems in relation to the nature of the diluent in the capsule; patients should always use the same formulation.

Phenytoin provides a major example of the importance of knowledge of pharmacokinetics for successful prescribing. The important aspects are:

- Plasma protein binding
- Saturation (zero-order) kinetics
- Hepatic enzyme induction and enzyme inhibition
- Opportunities for *clinically* important unwanted interactions are extensive.

Phenytoin is 90% bound to plasma albumin so that quite small changes in binding, e.g. a drop to 80%, will have a major effect on the concentration of free drug. Simple displacement interaction is generally not clinically important when first-order kinetics applies (metabolism increases in proportion to the rise in free drug concentration) but when there is saturation and, in addition, enzyme inhibition (see below), toxicity may result.

Phenytoin is hydroxylated in the liver and this process becomes saturated at about the doses needed for therapeutic effect. Thus phenytoin at low doses shows first-order kinetics but this changes to saturation kinetics or zero-order kinetics as the therapeutic plasma concentration is approached, i.e. smaller dose increments at longer intervals are needed to obtain the same proportional rise in plasma concentration.

A clinically meaningful single half-life can be quoted where a drug is subject only to first-order kinetics. At low doses, giving subtherapeutic plasma concentrations, the $t^{1/2}$ of phenytoin is 6–24 h. But at higher doses, giving therapeutic plasma concentrations (the enzyme system has become saturated), the $t^{1/2}$ can be up to 60 h. This has major implications for patient care, e.g. the time taken to reach a steady-state plasma concentration after a dose increment (about $5 \times t^{1/2}$) is 2–3 days at low dose and about 2 weeks at high doses. Thus dose increments should become *smaller and less frequent* as dosage increases (this is why there is a 25 mg capsule). Plainly serial plasma concentration measurement will help the prescriber.

Enzyme induction. Phenytoin is a potent inducer of hepatic metabolising enzymes affecting itself, other drugs and dietary and endogenous substances (including vitamin D and folate). The consequences of this are: a slight fall of steady state phenytoin level over the first few weeks of therapy, though this may not be noticeable if dose increments are being given; enhanced metabolism of other drugs including other antiepileptics, e.g. carbamazepine, warfarin, steroids (adrenal and gonadal), thyroxine, tricyclic antidepressants, doxycycline; naturally this can also work in reverse, and introduction of other enzyme inducers may lower phenytoin concentrations when there is capacity for increase in enzyme induction, e.g. rifampicin, ethanol.

Inhibition of phenytoin metabolism either by competition for the enzyme or by direct inhibition of enzyme activity can occur; plasma concentration of phenytoin rises. Drugs that inhibit phenytoin metabolism include: valproate, cimetidine, co-trimoxazole, isoniazid, chloramphenicol, some NSAIDs, disulfiram. There is a considerable body of mediocre and contradictory data, the lesson of which is that possible interaction should be in the mind wherever other drugs are prescribed to a patient taking phenytoin.

Adverse effects of phenytoin, many of which can be very slow to develop, include a considerable variety of central nervous system effects:

- Recognition that there is impairment of cognitive function, especially in learning situations, has led many physicians to prefer carbamazepine and valproate
- Other effects range from sedation to delirium to acute cerebellar disorder to convulsions
- Peripheral neuropathy
- Rashes (dose related)
- Gum hyperplasia (perhaps due to inhibition of collagen catabolism) more marked in children and when there is poor gum hygiene
- Coarsening of facial features
- Hirsutism
- Dupuytren's contracture, pseudolymphoma
- Megaloblastic anaemia that responds to folate (perhaps partly due to increased folate requirements, for folate is a cofactor in some hydroxylations that are increased as a result of enzyme induction by phenytoin)
- Anaemia probably only occurs when dietary folate is inadequate, but some degree of macrocytosis is common
- Osteomalacia due to increased metabolism of vitamin D occurs after years of therapy.

Overdose (cerebellar symptoms and signs, coma, apnoea) is treated according to general principles.

The patient may remain unconscious for a long time because of saturation kinetics, but will recover if respiration and circulation are sustained.

Other uses. The membrane-stabilising effect of phenytoin is used in cardiac dysrhythmias and, rarely, in resistant pain, e.g. trigeminal neuralgia.

Preparations: capsules for oral use should be taken (in 2–4 doses/day) with at least half a glass (120 ml) of water (if nausea occurs, they should be taken with food); phenytoin is also available for i.v. injection; it should not be given i.m. if this can be avoided as the pH of the solution has to be high to render it soluble: the fall in pH in the muscle leads to precipitation of the drug with slow absorption.

SODIUM VALPROATE: VALPROIC ACID

Sodium valproate (Epilim) acts by inhibiting the enzyme responsible for the breakdown of the inhibitory neurotransmitter, GABA, i.e. it inhibits GABA transaminase.

Pharmacokinetics. Valproate is about 90% bound to plasma albumin. It is metabolised in the liver and has a $t\frac{1}{2}$ of 13 h.

Valproate inhibits the metabolism of itself at *low* (but not at high) doses; and that of phenobarbitone, phenytoin and carbamazepine. It displaces phenytoin from plasma albumin but (when first-order kinetics apply) the rise in free phenytoin is accompanied by increased phenytoin elimination and so the total phenytoin plasma concentration falls; but the concentration of free phenytoin is not much changed.

Valproate does not induce drug metabolising enzymes but its metabolism is enhanced by induction due to other antiepileptics.

Adverse effects are generally minor, e.g. nausea, but can include: liver failure (risk maximal at 2–12 weeks); transient rise in liver enzymes without sinister import (but patients should be closely monitored until the biochemical measures return to normal); pancreatitis; coagulation disorder due to inhibition of platelet aggregation (coagulation should be assessed before surgery); increased alertness and appetite, with weight gain. A curious effect is change in hair colour and temporary hair loss following which regrowth may be curly:

> We thought the change might be welcomed by the patients, but one girl preferred her hair to be long and straight, and one boy was mortified by his curls and insisted on a short hair cut.[3]

Ketone metabolites may cause confusion in urine testing in diabetes.

See also Pregnancy and epilepsy (above).

BARBITURATES
(see Index)

Antiepileptic members include phenobarbitone (phenobarbital) ($t\frac{1}{2}$ 100 h), methylphenobarbitone and primidone (Mysoline), which is largely metabolised to phenobarbitone (i.e. it is a prodrug). Sedation is usual.

CLONAZEPAM

Clonazepam (Rivotril) ($t\frac{1}{2}$ 25 h) is a benzodiazepine used for routine control of a variety of epilepsies (see Table 20.1); clobazam is an alternative. Other benzodiazepines have antiepileptic action, but only at doses causing unacceptable sleepiness. For *status epilepticus* clonazepam may be given i.v. slowly (30 s); it should not be given i.m. lest absorption be as slow as diazepam i.m. when peak plasma concentration can be delayed as long as 2 h, which is useless for the urgent control needed in this medical emergency, and complicates any other therapy given in the interval. Lorazepam, i.m. is somewhat more rapidly absorbed.

Vigabatrin (Sabril) (1989) ($t\frac{1}{2}$ 6 h) is structurally related to the inhibitory CNS neurotransmitter GABA and it acts by irreversibly inhibiting GABA-transaminase so that GABA accumulates. Vigabatrin is effective in generalised tonic-clonic and partial seizures which are not adequately controlled by other drugs. GABA-transaminase is resynthesised over 6 days.

It is not metabolised and does not induce hepatic

drug metabolising enzymes. Adverse effects on the CNS are similar to those of other antiepilepsy drugs and include confusion and psychosis. Increase in weight also occurs in up to 40% of patients during the first 6 months of treatment.

Lamotrigine (1993) may be used as adjuvant or monotherapy. Its primary action is to stabilise presynaptic neuronal membranes by blockade of voltage dependent sodium channels. This blockade leads secondarily to reduced release of excitatory amino acids, such as glutamate and aspartate. Lamotrigine has similar efficacy to older agents, but is associated with slightly less frequent CNS adverse effects (the same as for carbamazepine). Withdrawal has been most commonly due to a transient maculopapular rash. The $t\frac{1}{2}$ of 24 h allows for a single daily dose. The dose needs to be higher when used in combination with carbamazepine, phenytoin or primidone, which induce its metabolism, and less frequent when combined with valproate, which inhibits metabolism of lamotrigine.

Gabapentin is an analogue of GABA but appears not to work through the GABA pathway. It is excreted unchanged and unlike other antiepileptic agents does not induce or inhibit hepatic metabolism of other agents. Like vigabatrin, its place is limited at present to combination with older agents.

Topiramate is a sulphamate-substituted monosaccharide, whose antiepileptic activity is due to blockade of voltage sensitive sodium channels, enhanced GABA activity and possibly weak blockade of a glutamate receptor. It is indicated as adjunct treatment for partial seizures. Its $t\frac{1}{2}$ of 21 hours renders it suitable for once daily dosing, and its lack of extensive metabolism reduces the interactions with other antiepileptics.

Succinimides: ethosuximide (Zarontin) ($t\frac{1}{2}$ 55 h) is used in absence seizures (petit mal). Adverse effects are gastric upset, CNS effects and allergic reactions including eosinophilia and other blood disorders, and lupus erythematosus.

Acetazolamide (Diamox) is a carbonic anhydrase inhibitor that, by producing acidosis, sometimes benefits atypical absence and other seizures in children.

---

[3] Jeavons P M et al 1977 Lancet 1: 359.

Parkinsonism

Objectives of therapy

Parkinsonism is due to degeneration of the substantia nigra[4] in the hind brain, and consequent loss of dopamine-containing neurons in the nigrostriatal pathway. Drugs do not cure but can, if properly managed, greatly improve quality of life in this progressive disease. *Two balanced systems* are important in the extrapyramidal control of motor activity at the level of the corpus striatum and substantia nigra: in one the neurotransmitter is *acetylcholine*; in the other it is *dopamine*. In Parkinson's disease there is degenerative loss of nigrostriatal dopaminergic neurons and the symptoms of the disease are due to dopamine depletion. The *symptom triad* of the disease is hypokinesia, rigidity and tremor.

RESTORING DOPAMINERGIC/CHOLINERGIC BALANCE

1. *Reduce* cholinergic activity by antimuscarinic (anticholinergic[5]) drugs; this approach is most effective in the acute treatment of rigidity (including iatrogenic, caused by dopamine receptor antagonists); or
2. *Enhance* dopaminergic activity by dopaminergic drugs which may:

   - *replenish* neuronal dopamine by supplying levodopa, which is its natural precursor; administration of dopamine itself is ineffective as it does not pass into the brain from the blood
   - *prolong* the action of dopamine through selective inhibition of its metabolism (selegiline)
   - act as *dopamine agonists* (bromocriptine, lysuride, apomorphine);

---

[4] *Substantia nigra* is (Latin): black substance. A coronal section at this point in the brain shows the distinctive black areas, visible with the naked eye in normal brain, but absent from the brains of patients with Parkinson's disease.

[5] The term *antimuscarinic* is now preferred to anticholinergic (p. 399).

- *release* dopamine from stores and inhibit re-uptake (amantadine).

This approach is most effective against hypokinesia and rigidity, and less effective in the treatment of tremor.

Both approaches are effective in therapy and may usefully be combined. It therefore comes as no surprise that drugs which prolong the action of acetylcholine (anticholinesterases) or drugs which deplete dopamine stores (reserpine) or block dopamine receptors (neuroleptics, e.g. chlorpromazine) will exacerbate the symptoms of parkinsonism or induce a Parkinson-like state.

Other parts of the brain in which dopaminergic systems are involved include the medulla (induction of vomiting), the hypothalamus (suppression of prolactin secretion) and certain paths to the cerebral cortex. Different effects of dopaminergic drugs can be explained by activation of these systems, namely emesis, suppression of lactation (mainly bromocriptine) and occasionally psychotic illness. Neuroleptics used to manage psychotic behaviour act by blockade of dopamine receptors and, as is to be expected, they are also antinauseant, may sometimes cause galactorrhoea, and can induce parkinsonism. Neuroleptic-induced parkinsonism is alleviated by antimuscarinics, but not by levodopa or amantadine, because the neuroleptics block dopamine receptors via which these drugs act. But many neuroleptics also have some antimuscarinic activity; those with greatest efficacy in this respect, e.g. thioridazine, are the least likely to cause parkinsonism.

Drugs for Parkinson's disease

DOPAMINERGIC DRUGS

Levodopa and dopa-decarboxylase inhibitors

Levodopa (dopa stands for dihydroxyphenylalanine) is a natural amino acid precursor of dopamine. The latter cannot be used because it is rapidly metabolised in the gut, blood and liver by monoamine oxidase and catechol-O-methyltransferase; even intravenously administered dopamine, or dopamine formed in peripheral tissues, is insufficiently lipid-soluble to penetrate the CNS. But levodopa is readily absorbed from the upper small intestine by active amino acid transport and has a t½ of 1.5 h. It can traverse the blood–brain barrier by a similar active transport, and within the brain it is decarboxylated (by dopa decarboxylase) to the neurotransmitter dopamine. But a major disadvantage is that levodopa is also extensively decarboxylated to dopamine in peripheral tissues so that only 1–5% of an oral dose of levodopa reaches the brain. Thus large quantities of levodopa have to be given. These inhibit gastric emptying, delivery to the absorption site is erratic and fluctuations in plasma concentration occur. The drug and its metabolites cause significant adverse effects by peripheral actions, notably nausea, but also cardiac dysrhythmia and postural hypotension. This problem has been largely circumvented by the development of *decarboxylase inhibitors*, which do not enter the central nervous system, so that they prevent only the *extracerebral* metabolism of levodopa. The inhibitors are given in combination with levodopa and there is a range of formulations comprising a decarboxylase inhibitor with levodopa in various proportions:

- *co-careldopa* (carbidopa + levodopa in proportions 12.5/50 mg, 10 /100, 25/100, 25/250) (Sinemet)
- *co-beneldopa* (benserazide + levodopa in proportions 12.5 mg/50 mg, 25/100, 50/200) (Madopar).

The combinations produce the same brain concentrations as with levodopa alone, but only 25% of the dose of levodopa is required, which smooths the action of levodopa and reduces the incidence of adverse effects, especially nausea, from about 80% to less than 15%.

Interactions. With nonselective MAOI, the monoamine dopamine formed from levodopa is protected from destruction; it accumulates and also follows the normal path of conversion to noradrenaline (norepinephrine), by dopamine β-hydroxylase; *severe hypertension results*. The interaction with the selective MAO-B inhibitor, selegiline, is therapeutic (see below). Tricyclic antidepressants are safe. Levodopa antagonises neuroleptics (dopamine

receptor blockers). Some antihypertensives enhance hypotensive effects of levodopa. Metabolites of dopamine in the urine interfere with some tests for phaeochromocytoma, and in such patients it is best to measure the plasma catecholamines directly.

Dopa-decarboxylase is a pyridoxine-dependent enzyme and concomitant use of pyridoxine (e.g. in self-medication with a multivitamin preparation) can enhance peripheral conversion of levodopa to dopamine so that less is available to enter the CNS, and benefit is lost. This effect does not occur, of course, with the now usual levodopa-decarboxylase inhibitor combinations. Dopamine receptor agonists reverse benefit.

Adverse effects: Postural hypotension occurs.

Nausea may be a limiting factor if the dose is increased too rapidly; it may be helped by cyclizine 50 mg taken 30 min before food and by domperidone (little of which enters the brain). Levodopa-induced *involuntary movements* may take the form of general restlessness or head, lip or tongue movements or choreoathetosis.
Mental changes may be seen: these include depression, which is common (best controlled with a tricyclic antidepressant), dreams and hallucinations.
Agitation and confusion occur but it may be difficult to decide whether these are due to drug or to disease.
Cardiac dysrhythmias are a rare feature.
Increased sexual activity may occur and may or may not be deemed an adverse effect. It is probably due to improved mobility and resulting enthusiasm rather than to a pharmacodynamic effect of levodopa.

Dosage. Levodopa alone and in combination (see above) are introduced gradually and titrated according to response, the dose being altered every 2–3 days. A compromise is reached between benefit and adverse effects (generally involuntary movements and mental changes).

Compliance is important. Abrupt discontinuation of therapy leads to dramatic relapse.

OTHER DRUGS

These need to mimic the effects of dopamine, the

endogenous agonist, which stimulates both the main two types of dopamine receptor, D_1 and D_2. It is the latter, coupled to adenylyl cyclase stimulation, which is the principal target in Parkinson's disease, but *chronic* D_1 stimulation appears to potentiate the response to D_2 stimulation despite acutely having an opposing inhibitory action on adenylyl cyclase. The main problems with dopamine use (i.e. the prodrug, levodopa) are its short $t^{1/2}$ and, possibly, the consequences of delivering large amounts of substrate to an oxidative pathway, MAO (see below). On the other hand, the problems of developing synthetic alternatives are:

- reproducing the 'right' balance of D_1 and D_2 stimulation (dopamine itself is slightly D_1 selective, in test systems, but its net effect in vivo is determined also by the relative amounts and locations of receptors — which differ in Parkinsonian patients from normal
- avoiding the undesired effects of peripheral, mainly gastric, D_2 receptors
- synthesising a full, not partial, agonist.

Amantadine antedates the discovery of dopamine receptor subtypes, and its own discovery as an antiparkinsonian drug was an example of serendipity. It is an antivirus drug which, given for influenza to a parkinsonian patient, was noticed to be beneficial. The two effects are probably unrelated. It appears to act by increasing synthesis and release of dopamine, and by diminishing neuronal re-uptake. It also has slight antimuscarinic effect. The drug is much less efficacious than levodopa, whose action it will slightly enhance. It is more effective than the standard antimuscarinic drugs, with which it has an additive effect. Advantages include simplicity of use (initial oral dose 100 mg, daily, increasing to twice or thrice daily, but rarely more than this) and relative freedom from adverse effects, which, however, include ankle oedema (probably a local effect on blood vessels), postural hypotension, livedo reticularis and central nervous system disturbances — insomnia, hallucinations and, rarely, fits.

Bromocriptine (Parlodel) (a derivative of ergot, p. 662) is a D_2 receptor agonist, but also weak α-adrenoreceptor antagonist. It is commonly used with levodopa. The drug is rapidly absorbed; the

$t^{1/2}$ is 5 h, so that its action is smoother than that of levodopa, which can be an advantage in patients who develop end-of-dose deterioration with levodopa. Dosing should start very low, increasing at approximately weekly intervals and according to clinical response.

Nausea and vomiting are the commonest adverse effects; these may respond to domperidone but tend to become less marked as treatment continues. Postural hypotension may cause dizziness or syncope. In high dose confusion, delusions or hallucinations may occur and, after prolonged use, pleural effusion and retroperitoneal fibrosis.

Lysuride (Revanil) ($t^{1/2}$ 2 h) and **pergolide** ($t^{1/2}$ 6 h) are similar to bromocriptine, though the latter also stimulates D_1 receptors. **Cabergoline** has a $t^{1/2}$ of more than 80 hours making it suitable for once daily dosing (or even twice weekly), but clinical experience in Parkinson's disease is still limited. **Quinagolide** is another D_2 agonist.

Apomorphine is a derivative of morphine having structural similarities to dopamine; it is a full agonist at D_1 and D_2 receptors. It can be useful in parkinsonism to treat difficulty in emptying the urinary bladder and the on–off phenomenon. Apomorphine has to be given by injection, either s.c. or by continuous infusion. It may need to be accompanied by an antiemetic, e.g. domperidone (which does not cross the blood–brain barrier as does metoclopramide), to prevent its characteristic emetic action. Overdose causes respiratory depression; it is antagonised by naloxone. Apomorphine can induce penile erection (without causing sexual excitement) and it enhances the penile response to visual erotic stimulation. The rapid onset of action after an s.c. dose (which the patient can be taught to self-administer) enables the 'off' component of the on–off phenomenon to be aborted without the patient waiting 45–60 minutes to absorb another oral dose of levodopa.

Selegiline (Eldepryl) is a selective, irreversible inhibitor of monoamine oxidase (MAO) type B; MAO enzymes have an important function in modulating the intraneuronal content of neurotransmitter. The enzymes exist in two principal forms, defined by specific substrates some of which cannot be metabolised by the other form (see Table 20.2). The therapeutic importance of recognising these two forms arises because they are to some extent present in different tissues, and the enzyme at these different locations can be selectively inhibited by the selective inhibitors: moclobemide for MAO-A (p. 345) and selegiline for MAO-B (Table 20.2).

MAO inhibitors have two therapeutic uses: in Parkinson's disease, described here, and in depression (see p. 344). The problem with nonselective MAO inhibitors is that they prevent degradation of dietary amines, especially tyramine, which is then able to act systemically as a sympathomimetic: the hypertensive 'cheese reaction'. As will be apparent from Table 20.2, selegiline does not cause the cheese reaction, because tyramine is metabolised as it traverses the liver by MAO-A, which is not inhibited. There is a further line of protection by MAO-A in the sympathetic nerve endings (tyramine is an indirect acting amine which needs to displace noradrenaline from the nerve endings). In the CNS selegiline has no effect on synaptic cleft concentrations of those amines like serotonin and noradrenaline, which are normally potentiated by the MAOI used in depression; therefore selegiline has no antidepressant action. Why then is it able to help in Parkinson's disease? The probable explanation relates to the degeneration of the nigrostriatal neurons, leaving glial cells as the main source of MAO

at the site of dopamine action (in the corpus striatum, where the nigrostriatal neurons normally terminate). Since the glial cells contain mainly MAO-B, and dopamine is itself a slightly better substrate for MAO-B than MAO-A, inhibition of MAO-B by selegiline is sufficient to potentiate the therapeutic action of dopamine in Parkinson's disease.

The principal therapeutic benefit of selegiline is to extend the availability of levodopa in those patients who experience end-of-dose akinesia rather than on–off swings. The claim that selegiline delays progress of the disease has not been supported by subsequent trials. This claim arose initially from the theory that saturation of MAO by dopamine in therapy leads to the production of damaging free oxygen radicals, and appeared to gain support from studies in experimental forms of Parkinson's disease, one case-control study of patients, and a prospective study of selegiline and a tocopherol (an antioxidant).[6]

Selegiline is given orally; as an irreversible enzyme-inhibitor, dosage cannot be accurately titrated as with a competitive receptor agonist. Its adverse effects are those of increased dopamine

[6] Lees A J 1995 Comparison of therapeutic effects and mortality data of levodopa and levodopa combined with selegiline in patients with early, mild Parkinson's disease. British Medical Journal 311: 1602–1607.

Table 20.2 Isoforms of monoamine oxidase: MAO-A and MAO-B: an explanation
The table shows the definition of the isoforms by their specific substrates, and then their selectivity (or nonselectivity) towards a number of other substrates and inhibitors. Determination of therapeutic and adverse effects is a function of selectivity of the inhibitor **and** of tissue location of the enzyme.

Enzyme	MAO-A	MAO-A and B	MAO-B
Substrate	Serotonin (see below)	Noradrenaline Adrenaline Dopamine	Phenylethylamine (see below)
Inhibitors	Moclobemide	Tyramine Tranylcypromine Phenelzine Iproniazid	Selegiline
Tissues	Liver CNS (neurons) Sympathetic neurons	See MAO-A, MAO-B	Gut CNS (glial cells)

Explanation: the specific substrate for MAO-A is serotonin, whilst for MAO-B it is the nonendogenous amine, phenylethylamine (present in many brands of chocolate). Noradrenaline, tyramine and dopamine can be metabolised by both isoforms of MAO. MAO-A is the major form in liver and in neurons (both CNS and peripheral sympathetic); MAO-B is the major form in gut, but is also present in the liver, lungs and glial cells of the CNS.

activity (see p. 365); insomnia (give in morning); interaction with pethidine (see p. 346). Selegiline will approximately halve the daily requirement for levodopa. This limit to its efficacy reflects the presence of more than one route for dopamine disposal. Drugs such as entacapone and tolcapone are being developed which inhibit catechol-O-methyltransferase; in theory such drugs are attractive since this enzyme metabolises levodopa itself as well as dopamine itself.

ANTIMUSCARINIC (ANTICHOLINERGIC) DRUGS
(see also p. 407)

Antimuscarinic drugs benefit parkinsonism by blocking acetylcholine receptors in the central nervous system, thereby partially redressing the imbalance created by decreased dopaminergic activity. Their use originated when hyoscine was given to parkinsonian patients in an attempt to reduce sialorrhoea by peripheral effect, and it then became apparent that they had other beneficial effects in this disease. Synthetic derivatives are now used orally. These include *benzhexol, orphenadrine, benztropine, procyclidine, biperiden.* There is little to choose between these. Antimuscarinics produce modest improvements in tremor, rigidity, sialorrhoea, muscular stiffness and leg cramps, but little in hypokinesia.

They are effective i.m. or i.v. in acute drug-induced dystonias.

Unwanted effects include dry mouth, blurred vision, constipation, urine retention, glaucoma, hallucinations, memory defects, toxic confusional states and psychoses (which should be distinguished from presenile dementia).

Treatment

The main features that require alleviation are *tremor*, *rigidity* and *hypokinesia*.

General measures include the encouragement of regular physical activity and specific help such as physiotherapy and speech therapy.

DRUG THERAPY

Drugs play an important role in symptom relief. No drug has yet been proved to delay progress of the disease, though the suggestion has been made for selegiline. If and when such an action is confirmed, early diagnosis of the disease will become important.

Initial treatment. Drugs should be started only when symptoms interfere with activities that are important to the patient. Antimuscarinics benefit rigidity, tremor and sialorrhoea, but have little or no effect on hypokinesia. Antimuscarinic drugs should be avoided in patients with glaucoma, difficulty in micturition, constipation and psychiatric disturbance.

Amantadine may be effective in the early stages of the disease, either alone or in combination with an antimuscarinic.

Selegiline, by preventing cerebral dopamine breakdown, can postpone the need to use levodopa (with all its complications, see below).

LONGTERM TREATMENT

But, sooner or later treatment will involve dopamine replacement with *levodopa* (combined with a decarboxylase inhibitor) to replace CNS dopamine.[7] Rigidity and hypokinesia respond best to this but the combination is less effective in relieving tremor. Levodopa initially restores normal or near-normal physical activity in more than 75% of patients. Indeed, failure to respond should prompt the physician to question whether the patient has another basal ganglia defect (multisystem atrophy, cerebrovascular disease) or whether other drugs, e.g. phenothiazines, are involved. Dosage is best increased gradually, every 3 or 4 days (3–4 doses/d) using the smallest quantity that is effective. The optimum dose varies substantially from patient to patient and within each patient with passage of time. The preparation co-careldopa contains a relatively large proportion of carbidopa to ensure that

---

[7] An alternative strategy to minimise the special problems of longterm levodopa therapy (see below) is to use low-dose levodopa plus a dopamine receptor agonist (e.g. bromocriptine) from the commencement of levodopa therapy.

there is adequate decarboxylase inhibition when only a small dose of levodopa is required. The varying amounts of levodopa in the various preparations of co-careldopa and co-beneldopa (p. 365) permit flexible dose adjustment; small alterations may be beneficial.

Eventually, after 2–5 years, the progress of the disease demands that the total dosage be increased to the level at which adverse effects become troublesome. It is then of advantage to reduce each individual dose and increase the frequency of administration. After 6 years, on average 25% of patients will still derive substantial or moderate benefit from levodopa and experience an almost normal life expectancy. About 50%, however, fail to sustain the effect or find they cannot tolerate its adverse effects.

Another major problem with longterm treatment is *fluctuation in response to levodopa*. This is often a gradual process beginning with:

- early morning akinesia, progressing to
- peak dose dyskinesia and
- end-of-dose akinesia; then the most severe form
- the 'on–off' phenomenon: this describes random fluctuations from mobility to dyskinesia or to parkinsonian immobility.

Severe dystonic muscle cramps of hand or foot may accompany the dyskinesia. In some patients, fluctuations are related to the timing of drug administration, when peak plasma concentrations coincide with the dyskinetic phase and low plasma concentrations with immobility, but other patients swing between states of mobility and akinetic mutism without apparent relation to the timing of doses. After receiving levodopa for 10 years, over 50% of patients experience such swings. It is tempting to relate the 'on–off' effect to simultaneous contrary trends, after dosing, in the levels of agonist and receptor (as a result of down-regulation); it is likely that the mechanism is more complex.

Management of these tribulations is difficult; it may involve the following:

- Gradual partial substitution of levodopa with *selegiline*, which delays CNS dopamine breakdown (if the drug has not been used at the outset). This is effective for end-of-dose

deterioration in about 40% of patients but does not alleviate severe on–off fluctuations.

- Shortening the interval between doses of levodopa to hourly or less (adding levodopa between the doses of the combination formulation). Timing of dose in relation to meals is important for these interfere with absorption of the drug, especially when the protein content is high.
- Use of a modified-release levodopa preparation: co-careldopa (Sinemet) or co-beneldopa (Madopar).
- Use of a dopamine receptor agonist, e.g. bromocriptine, apomorphine.

DRUG-INDUCED PARKINSONISM

Parkinsonism due to dopamine-receptor blocking drugs should be distinguished from idiopathic Parkinson's disease. In one series[8] of 95 new cases of parkinsonism referred to a department of geriatric medicine, 51% were associated with prescribed drugs and half of these required hospital admission. The clinical features of the drug-

---

SUMMARY — epilepsy, parkinsonism

- Antiepileptic drugs dampen CNS neuronal discharges by blocking voltage-dependent ion-channels, or by enhancing inhibitory neurotransmitter (GABA), or by blocking excitatory neurotransmitters (glutamate).
- First-line drugs for prevention of grand-mal seizures are carbamazepine and valproate.
- Alternative drugs, lamotrigine, gabapentin, vigabatrin, are used mainly as add-on therapy.
- Treatment of Parkinson's disease redresses the imbalance of dopamine and acetylcholine in the nigrostriatal system.
- The mainstay of treatment is the amino acid, levodopa, in combination with an inhibitor of peripheral dopa decarboxylase activity, allowing targeted delivery of dopamine in the CNS.
- The problems of levodopa therapy are progressive neuronal loss and swings in the response between dyskinesias (overshoot of response) and excessive hypokinesia/rigidity.
- Possible remedies are protection of dopamine from inactivation, using the selective monoamine oxidase-B inhibitor, selegiline, or substitution of long-acting synthetic dopamine agonists, pergolide or lysuride.

induced disease were very similar to those of idiopathic parkinsonism. After withdrawal of the offending drug most cases resolved completely in 7 weeks. Amongst the neuroleptic phenothiazines the commonest agent was prochlorperazine (Stemetil), usually given for vague 'postural instability' and which no longer seemed indicated in any case.

> One old lady who had received trifluoperazine (for a minor fright and anxiety) for 5 weeks, took 36 weeks to recover from the drug-induced parkinsonism but never managed to get home again.[8]

Treatment is by an antimuscarinic drug.

Other disorders of movement

Essential tremor is often, and with justice, called benign, but a few individuals may be incapacitated by it. Alcohol, through a central action, helps about 75% of patients but is plainly unsuitable for long-term use and a β-adrenoceptor blocker will benefit about 50%; diazepam or primidone are sometimes beneficial.

Drug induced dystonic reactions are seen:

- As acute reaction, often of the torsion type, and occur following administration of dopamine receptor blocking neuroleptics and antiemetics. An antimuscarinic drug, e.g. benztropine, given i.v. or i.m. and repeated as necessary, provides relief
- In some patients who are receiving levodopa for Parkinson's disease
- In patients on longterm neuroleptic treatment, who develop tardive dyskinesia (see p. 331).

Hepatolenticular degeneration (Wilson's disease) is caused by a genetic failure to eliminate copper absorbed from food so that it accumulates in the liver, brain, cornea and kidneys. A negative copper

balance is established (with some clinical improvement if treatment is started early) by chelating copper in the gut with penicillamine (p. 261) or trientine. The patients also have cirrhosis, and the best treatment for both may be orthotopic liver transplantation.

Chorea from whatever cause may be alleviated by dopamine receptor blocking neuroleptics; also tetrabenazine (Nitoman), which inhibits neuronal storage of dopamine and serotonin.

Involuntary muscle spasm: including tics, blepharospasm, hemifacial spasm and spasmodic torticollis. These may respond to a range of drugs including antimuscarinic, levodopa, dopamine agonist, neuroleptic, clonidine, benzodiazepine. *Botulinum toxin*, which irreversibly blocks release of acetylcholine from cholinergic nerve endings has been injected locally with success in facial spasm, blepharospasm, squint, torticollis and a variety of dystonias; its effect lasts about 3 months. Although not licensed universally for all these indications, the toxin is at least partially effective in up to 90% of patients with these conditions. It is, however, not without toxicity; for instance aspiration being a real risk when dysphagia occurs in ~30% of patients receiving injections into their neck and shoulder muscles for torticollis.

Spasticity results from lesions of various types and sites within the central nervous system. Drugs used include the GABA agonist baclofen and diazepam.

Myotonic states in which voluntary muscle fails to relax after contraction may be symptomatically benefited by drugs that increase muscle refractory period, e.g. procainamide, phenytoin, quinidine.

Multiple sclerosis

Until recently, there has been no treatment of proven efficacy in this relapsing and remitting condition, where the placebo effect of most drugs can appear quite powerful. Although its pathogenesis remains unknown, the evidence points to some

---

[8] Stephen P J, Williamson J 1984 Lancet 2: 1082.

form of altered immune response to injury. This has led to the testing of both old and new forms of drugs which might modify the immune response and release of cytokines.

Beta-interferon is set to test the resilience of patients, doctors, health economists and administrators. For in placebo controlled trials it is the first treatment to show a significant lengthening of the intervals between relapses, without however affecting either overall prognosis or quality of life. 372 patients with relapsing-remitting disease, able to walk 100 metres without aid or rest, were randomised to receive 8 M units or 1.6 M units of β-interferon or placebo by s.c. injection on alternate days. After 2 years there was a reduction in the relapse rate from 1.27 per year in the placebo group to 0.84 per year in the patients receiving the higher dose.[9]

The drug is not indicated in patients with progressive forms of disease, or in severely disabled patients. At £15 000 ($20 000) per annum per patient, the cost–benefit analysis has dampened initial excitement among neurologists at the drug's arrival. In the UK, beta-interferon can be prescribed only by designated neurologists, who have the unenviable task of choosing which patients should receive the drug.

Motor-neuron disease

The cause of the progressive destruction of upper and lower motor neurons is unknown. The only drug available, riluzole, may inhibit accumulation of the toxic neurotransmitter, glutamate. In 959 patients, riluzole prolonged median survival time from 13 to 16 months, with no effect on motor function.

Tetanus

Objectives

- Immediately neutralise with antitoxin any

bacterial toxin that has not yet become attached irreversibly to the central nervous system.
- Kill the tetanus bacteria by chemotherapy, thus stopping toxin production.
- Control the convulsions whilst maintaining respiratory and cardiovascular function (which latter may be disordered by the toxin, see below).
- Prevent intercurrent infection (usually pulmonary).
- Prevent electrolyte disturbances and maintain nutrition.

The acute control of the convulsive state will be considered here.

TREATMENT

Therapy for convulsions may be initiated with chlorpromazine (which has a powerful muscle relaxant effect and which neither paralyses nor causes loss of consciousness); it is given 4–8 hourly. Diazepam or a barbiturate is added as necessary. The drugs may be given orally when the convulsions are mild and there is no dysphagia, then i.m. An excess of chlorpromazine may make the convulsions worse, probably by stimulating the brainstem reticular formation. Opioids are contraindicated.

The dosage and route of administration can only be decided when confronted with the patient. A regimen which should control convulsions of almost any severity would be chlorpromazine 1–1.5 mg/kg 4–8 hourly plus diazepam 3.0 mg/kg/d or phenobarbitone 0.5 mg/kg intermittently (between the chlorpromazine doses), as required. It may be impossible to avoid abolishing consciousness at times.

An alternative, in severe cases, is to paralyse the patient with tubocurarine or gallamine (on theoretical grounds these are preferable to depolarising agents) and to provide artificial respiration and enough sedation to impair awareness and memory. This requires skill and much equipment, with facilities for measuring blood pH, electrolytes and gases as well as ability to understand the meaning of the results. Unfortunately these requirements limit its applicability, particularly in the countries where tetanus is common, so that it is especially difficult

[9] The IFNB Multiple Sclerosis Study Group and the University of British Columbia MS/MRI Analysis Group 1995. Interferon-beta-1b in the treatment of multiple sclerosis: Final outcome of the randomised controlled trial. Neurology 45: 1277–1285.

to know whether results are superior to the more conservative anticonvulsant regimens.

Paralysis and artificial respiration should be seriously considered in all cases with laryngospasm, respiratory failure, severe chest infection and spasms so severe that they can only be controlled by making the patient unconscious. The action of the toxin in the CNS may cause *overactivity of the sympathetic autonomic system* (tachycardia, hypertension), which may be sufficient to require administration of α- and β-adrenoceptor blocking drugs. Attacks of hypotension can also occur.

Anticonvulsant therapy may be needed for 2 weeks or more and so attention to nutrition and to body electrolytes is vital right from the start, as is care of the respiratory tract (to avoid pneumonia) and gentle nursing (to minimise convulsions).

GUIDE TO FURTHER READING

Brodie M J 1992 Lamotrigine. Lancet 339: 1397–1400

Calne D B 1993 Treatment of Parkinson's disease. New England Journal of Medicine 329: 1021–1027

Chadwick D 1994 Gabapentin. Lancet 343: 89–91

Chadwick D 1995 Do antiepileptics alter the natural course of epilepsy? Case for early treatment is not established. British Medical Journal 310: 177–178

Dichter M A, Brodie M J 1996 New antileptic drugs. New England Journal of Medicine 334: 1583

Reynolds E H 1995 Do antiepileptics alter the natural course of epilepsy? Treatment should be started as early as possible. British Medical Journal 310: 176–177

Clough C G 1991 Parkinson's disease: management. Lancet 337: 1324

Davis K L 1995 Tacrine. Lancet 345: 625–630

Editorial 1991 Antiepileptic drug withdrawal — hawks or doves. Lancet 337: 1193

Hughes A J et al 1990 Apomorphine test to predict dopaminergic responsiveness in parkinsonian syndrome. Lancet 336: 32

Lees A J 1995 Comparison of therapeutic effects and mortality data of levodopa and levodopa combined with selegiline in patients with early, mild Parkinson's disease. British Medical Journal 311: 1602–1607

Mardsen C D 1990 Parkinson's disease. Lancet 335: 948

O'Brien M D, Gilmour White S 1993 Epilepsy and pregnancy. British Medical Journal 307: 492–495

Quinn N 1995 Drug treatment of Parkinson's disease. British Medical Journal 310: 575–579

21

Anaesthesia and neuromuscular block

SYNOPSIS

General anaesthetics and neuromuscular blocking agents belong to the few classes of drugs whose actual administration is, by general consent, virtually confined to trained specialists.

Nevertheless, anaesthesia as well as perioperative care must sometimes be conducted by nonspecialists and their needs are particularly borne in mind in this chapter.

- General anaesthesia
- Pharmacology of anaesthetics
- Inhalation agents
- Intravenous agents
- Muscle relaxants: neuromuscular blocking drugs
- Local anaesthetics
- Obstetric analgesia and anaesthesia
- Anaesthesia in patients already taking drugs
- Anaesthesia in the diseased, the elderly and children; sedation in intensive therapy units

Acknowledgement: we are grateful to the World Health Organization for permission to quote WHO Model prescribing information: drugs used in anaesthesia (1989).

General anaesthesia

Until the mid-19th century such surgery as was possible had to be done at tremendous speed. Surgeons did their best for terrified patients with alcohol, opium, hyoscine[1] and cannabis; occasionally by concussion with a wooden bowl or partial suffocation; the great French surgeon Dupuytren (1777–1835) prepared a patient for surgery by making a brutal remark which caused the subject to faint. With the introduction of general anaesthesia surgeons could operate for the first time with careful deliberation. The problem of inducing quick, safe and easily reversible unconsciousness for any desired length of time in man only began to be solved in the 1840s when the long-known substances nitrous oxide, ether, and chloroform were introduced in rapid succession.

The details surrounding the first use of surgical anaesthesia make unedifying reading at times for there were bitter disputes on priority following an attempt to take out a patent for ether.

Sir James Simpson, who was to popularise chloroform (1847), heard of the initial trials of ether in

---

[1] A Japanese pioneer of about 1800 wished to test the anaesthetic efficacy of a herbal mixture including solanaceous plants (hyoscine-type alkaloids). His elderly mother volunteered as subject since she was anyway expected to die soon. But the pioneer administered it to his wife for, 'as all three agreed, he could find another wife, but could never get another mother' (1966 Journal of the American Medical Association 197: 10).

1846 and wrote,[2] 'It is a glorious thought, I can think of naught else'. Just before his death in 1870 he summarised the chief events of the introduction of anaesthesia in the USA.

It appears to me that we might correctly state the whole matter as follows:

1. That on the 11th December, 1844, Dr. Wells had, at Hartford, by his own desire and suggestion, one of his upper molar teeth extracted without any pain, in consequence of his having deeply breathed nitrous oxide gas for the purpose, as suggested nearly half a century before by Sir Humphrey Davy.

2. That having with others proved, in a limited series of cases, the anaesthetic powers of nitrous oxide gas, Dr. Wells proceeded to Boston to lay his discovery before the Medical School and Hospital there, but was unsuccessful in the single attempt which he made, in consequence of the gas-bag being removed too soon, and that he was hooted away by his audience, as if the whole matter were an imposition, and was totally discouraged.

3. That Dr. Wells' former pupil and partner, Dr. Morton of Boston, was present with Dr. Wells when he made his experiments there.

4. That on the 30th September, 1846, Dr. Morton extracted a tooth without any pain, whilst the patient was breathing sulphuric ether, this fact and discovery of itself making a NEW ERA in anaesthetics and in surgery.

5 & 6. That ether was soon used in general surgery[3] and midwifery.

The next important developments in anaesthesia

were in the 20th century when the appearance of new drugs both as primary general anaesthetics and as adjuvants (muscle relaxants), new apparatus, and clinical expertise in rendering prolonged anaesthesia safe, enabled surgeons to increase their range. No longer was the duration and kind of surgery determined by patients' capacity to endure pain.

STAGES OF GENERAL ANAESTHESIA

Surgical anaesthesia using a single agent is classically divided into four stages, of which the third stage is subdivided into four planes (obviously, each merges with the next). Figure 21.1 shows the procession of stages, and is provided to illustrate these from descriptions of ether anaesthesia (now obsolete) in unpremedicated patients, a slow unpleasant process.

But the attainment of balanced surgical anaesthesia (hypnosis with analgesia and muscular relaxation) with a single drug requires high doses that are liable to carry inconveniences and hazards, e.g. slow and unpleasant recovery, depression of cardiovascular and respiratory function. Modern practice employs different drugs to attain each objective so that the classic stages of anaesthesia no longer occur in visible succession.

With modern techniques of i.v. induction of anaesthesia and of inhalation induction with premedication, stages 1 and 2 may hardly be noticed by patient or anaesthetist. Nevertheless, since these stages provide a background to understanding how surgical anaesthesia is reached, an account is provided, as follows:

Stage 1: analgesia. Analgesia is partial until stage 2 is about to be reached. Consciousness and sense of touch are retained and sense of hearing is increased.

Stage 2: delirium. The patient is unconscious, but automatic movements may occur. He may shout coherently or incoherently, become violent or leap up and run about. Laryngospasm may develop. Sudden death, probably due to vagal inhibition of the heart or to sensitisation of the heart to adrenaline (endogenous or exogenous) by the anaesthetic agent, may occur in a violent second stage. Recall

---

[2] Comrie J D 1932 History of Scottish medicine, 2nd edn. Bailliére, Tindall and Cox, London, for Wellcome History of Medicine Museum.

[3] In December 1846 the first operation in England under ether (amputation of the leg of a butler from Harley Street) was conducted at University College Hospital, London. The surgeon, Robert Liston, after removing the leg in 28 s, a skill necessary to compensate for the previous lack of anaesthetics, turned to the watching students, saying, 'This Yankee dodge, Gentlemen, beats mesmerism hollow'. That night he anaesthetised his House Surgeon 'in the presence of two ladies'. Merrington W R 1976 University College Hospital and its Medical School: A history. Heinemann, London.

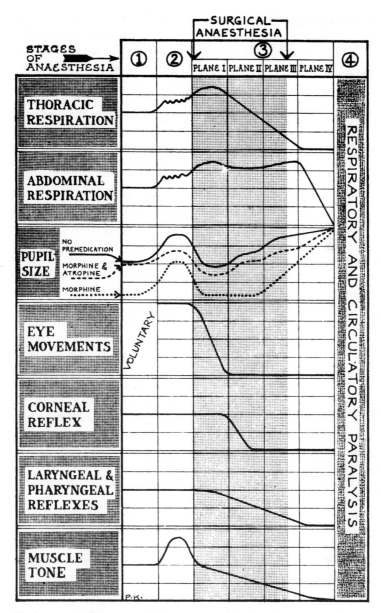

Fig. 21.1 The stages of anaesthesia

that these stages derive from descriptions of ether anaesthesia; *preventing* such unpleasant manifestations lies in a skilful, smooth and quick induction in quiet surroundings.

Stage 3: surgical anaesthesia. This is divided into four planes (see Fig. 21.1) and the required depth differs according to the kind of operation to be performed. Depth is determined by noting characteris-

tic changes in respiration, pupils, spontaneous eyeball position, reflexes and muscle tone.

Stage 4: medullary paralysis. Arrival at this stage constitutes an overdose.

DRUGS USED

The anaesthetist has 3 main areas of practice:

Before surgery, assessment of:

- the patient's physical and psychological condition
- any intercurrent illness
- the relevance of any existing drug therapy

all of which may influence the choice of anaesthetic drugs.

During surgery, the maintenance of:

- unconsciousness
- analgesia
- muscular relaxation when required
- physiological monitoring, e.g. of pulse, BP, respiration.

Whilst these can be produced by a single drug, e.g. halothane, thiopentone, to do so carries the disadvantages of toxic dosage (cardiac and respiratory depression, slow recovery); professional anaesthetists generally employ a drug for each purpose.

After surgery

- recovery, i.e. reversal of anaesthesia and neuromuscular block
- relief of pain, nausea
- other aspects of postoperative care.

These components are interdependent, and drugs play a part in each. The anaesthetist's job is complicated by the fact that patients are often already taking drugs affecting the central nervous and cardiovascular systems.

The techniques of administration of anaesthetic drugs and the physical control of respiration are of great importance, but are outside the scope of this book. Premedication is treated more fully as nonanaesthetists are more likely to find themselves concerned with it than with surgical anaesthesia.

Before surgery (premedication)

The principal aims are to provide:

Anxiolysis and amnesia. A patient who is going to have a surgical operation is naturally apprehensive, and it is kind to attempt to reduce this by explanation, reassurance and drugs. Preoperative preparation is not solely humanitarian, for the discharge of adrenaline from the suprarenal medulla and the increased metabolic rate, which are concomitants of

anxiety, render the patient both more difficult to anaesthetise and more liable to cardiac dysrhythmias with some anaesthetics. Stress-induced increase in plasma cortisol is usually suppressed by adequate premedication.

Benzodiazepines promote desirable anxiolysis and amnesia for the immediate presurgical period; temazepam, midazolam or diazepam (oral, rectal, i.v.) are appropriate. Promethazine may be used for its sedative and antiemetic actions.

Analgesia (an opioid) may be needed when there is existing pain or as a supplement to an anaesthetic agent having analgesic effect, e.g. nitrous oxide. If postoperative pain is expected, however, an analgesic may be given both before and at the end of the operation without waiting for the patient to complain of pain. This helps to avoid the postoperative restlessness that occurs if only sedatives were used preoperatively.

Inhibition of the parasympathetic autonomic system (by antimuscarinic agent) may be helpful to limit bronchial and salivary secretions which may collect in the lungs and predispose to infection, and to reduce any tendency to bronchospasm. Atropine, hyoscine or glycopyrronium may be used. Hyoscine can cause confusion in the old; glycopyrronium does not readily enter the brain but should be avoided when the patient has closed-angle glaucoma.

In general, light premedication is used and adjusted to the patients' temperaments, age, disease and medical history, the duration of surgery and whether it will be followed by severe pain, and of the anaesthetic agents that it is intended to use. Premedication is commonly given by mouth.

Timing premedication depends on the drug used, e.g. for diazepam 2 h, for temazepam 1 h before surgery.

Gastric contents. A single dose of a gastric antacid, e.g. sodium citrate, may be given before a general anaesthetic as prophylaxis against aspiration of acid gastric contents (acid aspiration pneumonitis or Mendelson's syndrome) in vulnerable (e.g. obstetric) patients; a histamine H_2-receptor blocker, e.g. ranitidine, is an alternative, to reduce gastric secretion volume as well as acidity. Metoclopramide hastens gastric emptying, usefully increases the tone of the lower oesophageal sphincter and is an antiemetic.

During surgery

The aim is to induce *unconsciousness, analgesia* and *muscular relaxation* often with separate drugs. This triad can be produced with a single drug in large doses but the consequences of the resulting deep anaesthesia are unpleasant and may be dangerous.

A typical general anaesthetic consists of:

- *Induction*: with thiopentone, etomidate (but see p. 393), methohexitone, or propofol i.v. The airway is rendered secure with a face mask or laryngeal mask; insertion of an endotracheal tube requires brief neuromuscular block with suxamethonium.
  - *Maintenance*:
    1. usually, with nitrous oxide and oxygen (or an oxygen/air mixture) plus a volatile agent, e.g. halothane or isoflurane;
    2. less often, with nitrous oxide and oxygen plus i.v. analgesic, e.g. fentanyl, morphine, pethidine, plus a competitive neuromuscular blocking agent if muscle relaxation is needed for abdominal surgery (respiration will necessarily have to be provided by the anaesthetist); where neuromuscular block is used there is risk of a paralysed patient regaining consciousness (see Awareness under anaesthesia, p. 386).

If a neuromuscular blocking drug is not used, muscle relaxation can be provided by deep anaesthesia with an inhalation agent, e.g. enflurane, though this involves high doses; or by nerve block with a local anaesthetic, or neural axis block, e.g. spinal or epidural, according to circumstances.

In addition, special techniques such as the production of hypotension or hypothermia may be required.

After surgery

The anaesthetist ensures that the effects of neuromuscular blocking agents and opioid-induced respiratory depression have either worn off or have been adequately reversed by an antagonist; the patient must never be left alone until conscious, with protective reflexes restored and a stable circulation.

Relief of pain after surgery presents many problems. Morphine and its derivatives are commonly used, usually intermittently, but sometimes by continuous (patient-controlled) i.v. infusion, or intra/extradurally. Since opioids constipate, may cause vomiting and depress cough and respiration, they are not recommended, e.g. after operations on the bowel and chest and for day-case surgery. Pethidine neither constipates nor suppresses spontaneous cough significantly, although it can also be useful, given i.v., to reduce cough from an endotracheal tube. There is a wide choice from amongst the opioids and NSAIDs. Inhalation of nitrous oxide/oxygen mixture (Entonox) is also effective (see nitrous oxide) for brief analgesia, as is epidural anaesthesia (see p. 390), e.g. for defaecation after haemorrhoidectomy.

Postoperative vomiting is largely preventable by skilled technique including avoidance of drugs that are particularly liable to cause it (thiopentone, nitrous oxide). Antiemetics can be effective, e.g. metoclopramide, ondansetron, prochlorperazine.

SOME SPECIAL TECHNIQUES

Dissociative anaesthesia, i.e. a state of analgesia and light hypnosis (the eyes may remain open) (see ketamine) is particularly useful where modern equipment and the necessary trained staff are lacking; also at scenes of major accidents and in war.

Neuroleptanalgesia, in which the patient is in a state of analgesia but is cooperative, is produced by a combination of a neuroleptic, e.g. droperidol, and a high-efficacy opioid analgesic, e.g. fentanyl or alfenatil. It is also used as a supplement to general anaesthesia, e.g. with nitrous oxide (neuroleptanaesthesia).

Sedation and amnesia without analgesia is provided by diazepam and midazolam i.v. They can be used alone for procedures causing discomfort but not pain, e.g. endoscopy, and with a local anaesthetic where pain is expected, e.g. removal of impacted wisdom teeth. Anterograde amnesia is characteristic but probably not retrograde amnesia; the patient remains cooperative. (For a general account of benzodiazepines and the competitive antagonist flumazenil, see Ch. 18.)

Respiratory depression and apnoea can occur with the above especially in the elderly with cerebral atherosclerosis and patients with respiratory insufficiency. Laryngeal reflexes are not spared and inhalation of oral secretions or dental debris can occur.

Patient-controlled analgesia, e.g. with nitrous oxide/oxygen mixtures (Entonox), is effective for brief procedures. Special apparatus allows the patient to control intravenous analgesics.

Pharmacology of anaesthetics

All successful general anaesthetics are given i.v. or by inhalation because these routes allow closest control over blood concentrations and so of effect on the brain.

Mode of action

General anaesthetics act on the brain, primarily on the midbrain reticular activating system and the cortex. A principal site of action (of both general and local anaesthetics) seems to be along the *neuronal lipid bilayer membrane*, which is disordered by the drugs so that cation (Na, K) movements through the protein pores (ion channels) which are associated with action potentials, are obstructed. The fact that increased atmospheric pressure can reverse anaesthesia is held to be compatible with this hypothesis. Other sites of action include neurotransmitter release and effects on postsynaptic membranes.

Many anaesthetics are *lipid soluble* and there is good correlation between this and anaesthetic effectiveness (the Overton–Meyer hypothesis); the more lipid soluble tend to be the more effective/powerful anaesthetics, but such a correlation is not invariable. Some anaesthetic agents are not lipid soluble and many lipid soluble substances are not anaesthetics. There are no properties common to every

agent and it is likely that there are several modes of action.

Clinical trials

Comparisons of general anaesthetics under routine clinical conditions are difficult to arrange, but they can be done.

Now that existing techniques of anaesthesia are so safe it is hard to expect a patient undergoing the anxiety of approaching surgery to consent to an experimental trial of a new drug; but to administer the drug, in however cautious a fashion, without the patient's (informed) consent is certainly immoral and assuredly illegal. The problem can be approached by paying volunteers to undergo careful administration of graduated doses in a laboratory, with extensive monitoring of cardiovascular, respiratory and central nervous functions.

Comparison of inhalational drugs for efficacy and adverse effects, e.g. cardiac depression, may be made by measuring the minimum alveolar concentration (MAC) in air or oxygen required to prevent reflex response to a surgical skin incision in 50% of subjects (MAC_{50}), or the MAC that prevents response in 95% of subjects (MAC_{95}), which is closer to real life clinical practice. A second point on the dose–response curve can be obtained for the MAC that just allows response to a spoken command. For nonvolatile i.v. anaesthetics of which a dose can be accurately administered as a bolus or infusion, the equivalent is the anaesthetic dose (AD) that prevents movement in response to the noxious stimulus (AD_{95}); or the minimum infusion dose (as for MAC).

Inhalation agents

Preferred agents

The preferred inhalation agents are those that are minimally irritant and nonflammable, and comprise nitrous oxide and the fluorinated hydrocarbons, i.e. halothane and its analogues.

Pharmacokinetics (volatile liquids, gases)

The level of anaesthesia is correlated with the

tension (partial pressure) of anaesthetic drug in the brain tissue and this is dependent on the development of a series of tension gradients from the high partial pressure delivered to the alveoli and decreasing through the blood to the brain and other tissues. These gradients are dependent on the blood/gas and tissue/gas solubility coefficients, as well as on alveolar ventilation and organ blood flow.

An anaesthetic that has *high solubility* in blood, i.e. a high blood/gas partition coefficient, will provide a *slow induction* and adjustment of the depth of anaesthesia. This is because the blood acts as a reservoir (store) for the drug so that it does not enter the brain easily until the blood reservoir has been filled. A rapid induction can be obtained by increasing the concentration of drug inhaled initially and by hyperventilating the patient.

Agents that have *low solubility* in blood, i.e. a low blood/gas partition coefficient (nitrous oxide, desflurane, sevoflurane), on the other hand, provide a *rapid induction* of anaesthesia because the blood reservoir is small and agent is available to pass into the brain sooner.

During induction of anaesthesia the blood is taking up anaesthetic agent selectively and rapidly and the resulting loss of volume in the alveoli leads to a flow of agent into the lungs that is independent of respiratory activity. When the anaesthetic is discontinued the reverse occurs and there is a flow of the agent from the blood into the alveoli. In the case of nitrous oxide, this can account for as much as 10% of the expired volume and so can significantly lower the alveolar oxygen concentration. Thus mild clinical hypoxia occurs, and it may last for as long as 10 minutes. Though harmless to most, it may be a factor in cardiac arrest in patients with reduced pulmonary and cardiac reserve, especially when administration of the gas has been at high concentration and prolonged, when the outflow is especially copious. Oxygen should therefore be given to such patients during the last few minutes of anaesthesia and the early postanaesthetic period.

This phenomenon, *diffusion hypoxia*, occurs with all gaseous anaesthetics, but is most prominent with gases that are relatively insoluble in blood, for they will diffuse out most rapidly when the drug is no longer inhaled, i.e. just as induction is faster, so is elimination. Nitrous oxide is especially powerful in this respect because it is used at concentrations of up to 70%. Highly blood-soluble agents will diffuse out more slowly, so that recovery will be slower just as induction is slower, and with them diffusion hypoxia is insignificant (and, in addition, these agents are used only in low concentration).

Nitrous oxide

Nitrous oxide (1844) is a gas with a slightly sweetish smell. It is neither flammable nor explosive. It produces light anaesthesia without demonstrably depressing the respiratory or vasomotor centre provided that normal oxygen tension is maintained.

Advantages. Nitrous oxide reduces the requirement for other more effective/powerful and intrinsically more toxic anaesthetic agents. It has a strong analgesic action. Induction is rapid and not unpleasant although transient excitement may occur, as with all agents. Recovery time rarely exceeds 4 min even after prolonged administration.

Disadvantages. Nitrous oxide is expensive to buy and to transport. It must be used in conjunction with more effective anaesthetics and muscle relaxants to produce a state of full surgical anaesthesia.

Uses. Nitrous oxide is used to maintain surgical anaesthesia in combination with other anaesthetic agents (halothane, isoflurane, thiopentone or ketamine) and muscle relaxants. In 50% concentration with oxygen (Entonox), it provides analgesia for obstetric practice, for emergency management of injuries, during postoperative physiotherapy and for refractory pain in terminal illness. It was the prolonged use (hours) of nitrous oxide in intensive therapy units that revealed its capacity to cause bone marrow depression.

Dosage and administration. For the maintenance of anaesthesia, nitrous oxide must always be mixed with at least 30% oxygen. For analgesia, a concentration of 50% nitrous oxide with 50% oxygen usually suffices.

Contraindications. Any closed air-filled space expands during administration of nitrous oxide which moves into it from the blood. It is therefore contraindicated in patients with: demonstrable collections of air in the pleural, pericardial or peritoneal spaces; intestinal obstruction; occlusion of the middle ear; arterial air embolism; decompression sickness; severe chronic obstructive airway disease; emphysema.

Precautions. Continued administration of oxygen may be necessary during recovery especially in elderly patients (see Diffusion hypoxia, above).

Adverse effects. The incidence of nausea and vomiting increases with the duration of anaesthesia. Because prolonged and repeated exposure of staff as well as of patients may be associated with bone-marrow depression and teratogenic risk, precautions should be taken to minimise ambient concentrations in operating theatres and intensive therapy units (extraction systems, closed-circuit use).

Drug interactions. Addition of 50% nitrous oxide/oxygen mixture to another inhalational anaesthetic reduces the required dosage (minimum alveolar concentration, MAC) of the latter by about 50%.

Storage. Nitrous oxide is supplied under pressure in cylinders, which for safety must be maintained below 25°C.

Cylinders containing premixed oxygen 50% and nitrous oxide 50% (Entonox) are available for analgesia. The constituents separate out at −6°C, in which case adequate mixing must be assured before use (store at > 5°C for 24 h and invert the cylinder several times before use).

Halogenated agents

Halothane was the first halogenated agent to be widely used although it is being replaced by analogues. We provide a description of halothane, and of the others mainly in so far as they differ.

Halothane is a colourless, volatile liquid with a sweet smell. In anaesthetic dosage it depresses both cerebral function and sympathetic autonomic activity and produces little, if any, preliminary excitement.

Advantages. Halothane has high therapeutic efficacy, is nonirritant and nonflammable. As its

blood/gas partition coefficient is low, induction is smooth and rapid and surgical anaesthesia can be produced in 2–5 min. It does not augment salivary or bronchial secretions. The recovery time is rapid and the incidence of postoperative nausea and vomiting is low, and diffusional hypoxia (see above) is insignificant (the MAC in oxygen is 0.8%). It does not react with soda lime and can be used in a closed-circuit (CO_2 absorption) system.

Disadvantages. Little margin exists between the doses needed to produce respiratory and vasomotor depression. Because of its cardiodepressant effect halothane is usually combined with another inhalational agent, such as nitrous oxide. Muscle relaxants are usually required to prepare the patient for abdominal surgery.

Although it suppresses endogenous sympathetic activity halothane sensitises the heart to the dysrhythmic effects of catecholamines (endogenous and exogenous) and hypercapnia.

About 20% of halothane is metabolised and it induces hepatic enzymes, including those of anaesthetists and operating theatre staff (see also hepatitis, below).

Contraindications include a history of unexplained jaundice following previous exposure to halothane (however long ago, see below), a family history of malignant hyperthermia and raised cerebrospinal fluid pressure (increased cerebral blood flow, cf. isoflurane, below).

Precautions. The patient's anaesthetic history should be carefully taken to determine previous exposure and previous reactions to halothane, e.g. unexplained fever or jaundice.

Adverse effects. *Hepatic damage* occurs in a small proportion of exposed patients. Typically fever develops 2 or 3 days after anaesthesia accompanied by anorexia, nausea and vomiting. In more severe cases this is followed by transient jaundice or, very rarely, fatal hepatic necrosis. *Severe hepatitis* is a recognised complication of repeatedly administered halothane anaesthesia (incidence 1 : 50 000). It follows immune sensitisation to an oxidative metabolite of halothane in susceptible individuals.[4]

---

[4] Kharasch E D et al 1996 Lancet 347: 1367.

Cardiac dysrhythmias may be induced, in particular atrioventricular dissociation, nodal rhythm and ventricular extrasystoles.

Drug interactions. Halothane potentiates the response to antihypertensive agents. Premedication with atropine reduces the risk of hypotension and bradycardia. Interaction occurs with adrenaline (see above).

Enflurane is more likely to cause respiratory depression such that hypercapnia is almost inevitable in patients breathing spontanously. Only 2% is metabolised, i.e. less than halothane, and so it is safer regarding the liver, and sensitisation to adrenaline. Prolonged administration or use in enzyme-induced patients results in release of sufficient free inorganic fluoride from the drug molecule to cause polyuric renal failure. Diffusional hypoxia is negligible as the MAC is 1.7%.

Isoflurane, an *isomer* of enflurane, has the most favourable risk–benefit profile of the inhalational agents in current use. Its low solubility in blood (low blood/gas partition coefficient) allows rapid induction and adjustment of the depth of anaesthesia, although its tendency to cause bronchial irritation may delay induction. Isoflurane is minimally metabolised (0.2%), has least effect in increasing cerebral blood flow (and thus intracranial pressure) and causes least depression of the myocardium. It dilates coronary arteries and there is suggestion that blood may be diverted away from areas of the myocardium supplied by stenosed vessels ('coronary steal'). As with enflurane but to a lesser extent, prolonged use releases free inorganic fluoride which may be toxic to the kidneys.

Desflurane has the lowest blood/gas partition coefficient of any inhaled anaesthetic agent and thus gives particularly rapid onset and offset of effect. As it undergoes almost no metabolism (0.03%), any release of free inorganic fluoride is minimised; this characteristic favours its use for prolonged anaesthesia. It may cause bronchoconstriction.

Sevoflurane is pleasant to inhale and provides rapid induction, having a very low blood/gas solubility. It is 3% metabolised and is thus more likely,

e.g. than isoflurane, to release renally toxic free organic fluoride.

Ether (diethyl ether) was a safe inhalational agent in untrained hands, and a reliable and potent anaesthetic that was particularly useful when elaborate apparatus was not available. Because ether is both flammable and explosive it could be used in hot dry climates only when special precautions were taken to prevent sparking and combustion; diathermy was contraindicated when ether was used with oxygen. Ether is now obsolete.

Oxygen in anaesthesia

Oxygen should be added routinely to inhalational agents, even when air is used as the carrier gas, to protect against hypoxia. This is an essential precaution whenever a volatile agent is used.

The concentration of oxygen in inspired anaesthetic gases should never be less than 21% (the concentration in air). It may be administered with the anaesthetic gases, or from a face mask or via a nasal catheter.

Combustion or sparking creates a danger of fire or explosion at high oxygen tensions. Reducing valves should not be greased, since this creates a danger of explosion.

Oxygen should not be used for longer or at a greater concentration than is necessary to prevent hypoxaemia.

After prolonged administration, concentrations greater than 80% at atmospheric pressure have a toxic effect on the lungs, which presents initially as a mild substernal irritation progressing to pulmonary congestion, exudation and atelectasis.

Use of unnecessarily high concentrations of oxygen in incubators has led to the development of retrolental fibroplasia and permanent blindness in premature infants.

Oxygen is supplied under pressure in cylinders, which must be kept below 25°C.

Cylinders containing premixed oxygen 50% and nitrous oxide 50% are available for analgesia in some countries. However, the constituents separate out at −6°C, and adequate mixing must be assured before use (see above). When the two components are supplied from separate cylinders a safety device must be installed that cuts off the flow of nitrous oxide should the oxygen pressure fall.

Atmospheric pollution of operating theatres

Pollution by inhalation anaesthetics and other volatile substances (skin cleansers) has been suspected of being harmful to theatre personnel. An anaesthetist working with halothane can accumulate in 3–4 h amounts that will not be eliminated completely by the following morning. Epidemiological studies have raised questions relating to excess of fetal malformations and miscarriages, hepatitis and cancer in operating theatre personnel. Sensible use of preventive measures probably renders the risks negligible, e.g. use of circle systems that allow low fresh gas flows, scavenging systems, improved ventilation of theatres (a minor contribution), filters that absorb volatile agents though not nitrous oxide; by using regional anaesthesia or total i.v. anaesthesia, i.e. no vapours or gases used, in preference to inhalation wherever feasible.

Precautions against atmospheric pollution, e.g. by frequent use of nitrous oxide, are also necessary in intensive therapy units.

Intravenous agents

Pharmacokinetics

While intravenous anaesthetics allow an extremely rapid induction because the blood concentration can be raised rapidly, there is no channel of elimination that can compete with the lungs for speed. The metabolic breakdown of useful agents does not occur fast enough for really quick recovery and so reliance is put on rapid distribution of the drug, e.g. thiopentone, which is satisfactory only for induction of anaesthesia. Repeated doses of thiopentone result in accumulation; attempts to use it i.v. as a sole anaesthetic agent in war casualties led to its being described as an ideal form of euthanasia.[5]

Therefore substances that are rapidly absorbed

---

[5] Halford J J 1943 A critique of intravenous anaesthesia in war surgery. Anesthesiology 4: 67.

and rapidly excreted through the lungs still offer the best prospect of precise control (with continuous administration) even in the presence of pulmonary disease, except perhaps severe emphysema. Elimination of inhaled anaesthetics can be hastened by inducing hyperventilation. There is no quick method of eliminating drugs whose action is normally terminated by metabolism or by redistribution. For the present it is usual to approach the ideal by using a combination of drugs in such a way that the disadvantages of each become less prominent.

Thiopentone (thiopental)

Thiopentone is a very short-acting barbiturate which, administered i.v. as a single dose, rapidly induces hypnosis and anaesthesia without analgesia. This rapidity of onset is ensured by extensive distribution in the highly vascular tissues of the brain and other organs and is reflected by an initial steep decline in plasma concentration ($t^1/_2$ 9 min). Next, thiopentone distributes more slowly to lean tissues ($t^1/_2$ 60 min) and recovery from its effects occurs during this phase (hence the brevity of its effect). A final slow decline in plasma concentration ($t^1/_2$ 9 h) reflects distribution to poorly perfused fat and metabolism in the liver. The action of further doses would be prolonged because of this slow elimination phase.

Advantages. Thiopentone, in a single dose, usually exerts its cerebral depressant effect within 30 s (one arm-to-brain circulation time) and it persists for about 4–7 min. Anaesthesia is induced rapidly, pleasantly and without excitement.

Disadvantages. Thiopentone has insignificant analgesic action. Any muscular relaxation that occurs is too brief to be of practical value. In contrast to ketamine (below), it cannot be used alone as an anaesthetic agent because the large and repeated doses required accumulate in fatty tissues and are subsequently only slowly released; this results in prolonged anaesthesia and delayed recovery characterised by somnolence and respiratory and circulatory depression.

Uses: to induce anaesthesia prior to administration of inhalational and other anaesthetics.

Dosage and administration. Adults and children: 3–5 mg/kg given by intravenous injection over 10–15 s and repeated, if necessary, after 20–30 s. Dosage requirements vary; they are reduced in the elderly, in hypovolaemic patients, and in patients heavily premedicated with narcotics or other cerebral depressants.

Contraindications. Thiopentone should not be used if there is doubt that a clear airway can be maintained or if there is: allergy to barbiturate; severe cardiovascular disease or hypotension; dyspnoea or obstructive respiratory disease; status asthmaticus; Addison's disease; hepatic dysfunction; myxoedema; a history of acute intermittent or variegate porphyria.

Precautions. Thiopentone should, whenever possible, be administered under the supervision of an experienced specialist anaesthetist.

Equipment for resuscitation and endotracheal intubation should be immediately available and ready for use.

The patient must always lie supine as even a small overdose can cause hypotension.

Concentrations greater than 25 mg/ml are liable to cause thrombophlebitis. Local extravasation can result in extensive necrosis and sloughing. Intra-arterial injection causes intense pain and may result in arteriospasm necessitating local use of vasodilators, supplemented, if necessary, by brachial plexus block and anticoagulation.

Adverse effects. A short period of apnoea may follow intravenous injection. Rapid injection may result in severe hypotension and hiccoughs. Coughing, sneezing or laryngeal spasm may occur during induction.

Drug interactions. Other cerebral depressants, e.g. opioids, may augment the action of thiopentone. Antihypertensives or diuretics may augment the hypotensive effect.

Overdosage. Serious overdosage results in respiratory depression necessitating assisted ventilation with oxygen, and hypotension progressing to circulatory collapse. In the latter event the head of the table must immediately be tilted down. Plasma expanders and pressor agents may be of value in patients who are unresponsive to this measure.

Methohexitone is a barbiturate similar to thiopentone.

Propofol (a phenol derivative) is notable for quick recovery (4 min) from a single dose: it is used both for induction and maintenance (by i.v. infusion) for procedures lasting up to about 1 h. The effect of a single dose is terminated by distribution; the elimination $t^1/_2$ is 45 min.

Ketamine

Ketamine is a phencyclidine (hallucinogen) derivative. In anaesthetic doses it produces a trance-like state known as *dissociative anaesthesia* (sedation, amnesia, dissociation, analgesia). It may be preferred where circumstances require anaesthesia to be undertaken by the nonprofessional.

Advantages. Anaesthesia persists for up to 15 min after a single intravenous injection and is characterised by profound analgesia. Ketamine may be used as the sole analgesic agent for diagnostic and minor surgical interventions. It is less likely than other anaesthetic agents to induce vomiting. Since it does not induce hypotension the patient does not have to remain supine and its sympathomimetic effects are of particular value in patients who are shocked, severely dehydrated or severely anaemic. Because pharyngeal and laryngeal reflexes are only slightly impaired, the airway may be less at risk than with other general anaesthetic techniques. It is of particular value in children and poor-risk patients, and also in asthmatic patients, because it rarely induces bronchospasm. (See also Dissociative anaesthesia, p. 377.)

Disadvantages. Ketamine produces no muscular relaxation. It tends to raise heart rate and intracranial and intraocular pressure. In hypertensive patients it may raise blood pressure unduly. Hallucinations can occur during recovery (emergence reaction), although rarely in children, but they are avoided if ketamine is used solely as an induction agent and followed by a conventional inhalational anaesthetic. Their incidence may also be greatly reduced by administration of diazepam both as a premedication and after the procedure.

Uses. Subanaesthetic doses of ketamine may be used to provide analgesia for painful procedures of short duration such as the dressing of burns, radiotherapeutic procedures, marrow sampling and minor orthopaedic procedures.

Ketamine may be used for induction of anaesthesia prior to administration of inhalational anaesthetics, or for both induction and maintenance of anaesthesia for short-lasting diagnostic and surgical interventions, including dental procedures, that do not require skeletal muscle relaxation. It is of particular value for children requiring frequent repeated anaesthetics.

Dosage and administration. Administration of ketamine (i.m. or i.v.) should always be preceded by premedication with atropine to reduce salivary secretions.

Premedication with diazepam reduces the subsequent requirement for ketamine and the incidence of emergence reactions but in this case there may be a need for endotracheal intubation.

Induction. Intravenous route: 1–2 mg/kg by slow intravenous injection over a period of 60 s. More rapid administration may result in respiratory depression or apnoea and an enhanced pressor response. A dose of 2 mg/kg produces surgical anaesthesia within 1–2 min which may be expected to last 5–10 min.

Intramuscular route: 5–10 mg/kg by deep intramuscular injection. This dose produces surgical anaesthesia within 3–5 min and may be expected to last up to 25 min.

Maintenance. Following induction, as above, serial doses of 50% of the original intravenous dose or 25% of the intramuscular dose are administered as required. The need for supplementary doses is established largely by movement in response to surgical stimuli.

Tonic and clonic movements resembling seizures occur in some patients. These are not indicative of a light plane of anaesthesia or of a need for additional doses of the anaesthetic.

As an analgesic. 500 microgram/kg i.m. or i.v.

followed, if necessary, by a dose of 250 microgram/kg.

Recovery. Return to consciousness is gradual. Emergence reactions with delirium may occur. Their incidence is reduced if unnecessary disturbance of the patient is avoided during recovery (although vital signs may be monitored) and they are unlikely to occur if diazepam is administered preoperatively and supplemented, if necessary, by a further 5–10 mg i.v. at the end of the procedure. Hypnotic doses of thiopentone (50–100 mg i.v.) may be required to suppress overt reactions but this will considerably prolong the recovery period.

Contraindications include: moderate to severe hypertension, congestive cardiac failure or a history of stroke; acute or chronic alcohol intoxication, cerebral trauma, intracerebral mass or haemorrhage or other causes of raised intracranial pressure; eye injury and increased intraocular pressure; psychiatric disorders such as a schizophrenia and acute psychoses.

Precautions. Ketamine should, whenever possible, be used under the supervision of an experienced specialist anaesthetist who is confident of intubating the patient should this become necessary. Pulse and blood pressure should be closely monitored.

Supplementary analgesia is often required in surgical procedures involving visceral pain pathways. Morphine may be used but the addition of nitrous oxide will often suffice.

During recovery, patients must remain undisturbed and under observation.

Use in pregnancy. Ketamine is contraindicated in pregnancy before term, since it has oxytocic activity. It is also contraindicated in patients with eclampsia or pre-eclampsia. It may be used for assisted vaginal delivery by an experienced anaesthetist. It is better suited for use during caesarean section; ketamine results in less fetal and neonatal depression than do other anaesthetics and the short exposure required has not been associated with emergence reactions when diazepam is used concomitantly.

Adverse effects: see above.

Neuroleptanalgesia/anaesthesia: see page 377.

Muscle relaxants

NEUROMUSCULAR BLOCKING DRUGS

A lot of surgery, especially of the abdomen, requires that voluntary muscle tone and reflex contraction be inhibited. This can be attained by deep general anaesthesia which carries hazard, e.g. cardiovascular depression, respiratory complications and slow recovery: also by nerve blocks, which can be difficult to do, or impracticable. Selective relaxation of voluntary muscle with neuromuscular blocking drugs allows surgery under light general anaesthesia with analgesia; it also facilitates tracheal intubation, quick induction and quick recovery. But it requires mechanical ventilation and technical skill. Neuromuscular blocking agents should be given only after induction of anaesthesia.

Neuromuscular blocking agents first attracted scientific notice because of their use as arrow poisons by the natives of South America, who used the most famous of all, curare, for killing food animals as well as enemies. In 1811 Sir Benjamin Brodie smeared 'woorara paste' on wounds of guinea-pigs and noted that death could be delayed by inflating the lungs through a tube introduced into the trachea. Though he did not continue until complete recovery, he did suggest that the drug might be of use in tetanus.

Despite attempts to use curare for a variety of diseases including epilepsy, chorea and rabies, the lack of pure and accurately standardised preparations as well as the absence of convenient routine techniques of mechanical ventilation if overdose occurred, prevented it from gaining any firm place in medical practice until 1942, when these difficulties were removed.

Drugs acting at the myoneural junction produce complete paralysis of all voluntary muscle so that movement is impossible and mechanical ventilation is needed. It is plainly important that a paralysed patient should be in a state of full analgesia and unconscious during surgery (see below).

Mechanisms

When an impulse passes down a motor nerve to voluntary muscle it causes release of acetylcholine from the nerve endings into the synaptic cleft. This activates receptors on the membrane of the motor endplate, a specialised area on the muscle fibre, opening ion channels for momentary passage of sodium which depolarises the endplate and initiates muscle contraction.

Neuromuscular blocking agents used in clinical practice interfere with this process. Natural substances that prevent the release of acetylcholine at nerve endings exist, e.g. *Clostridium botulinum* toxin (see p. 370) and some venoms.

There are two principal mechanisms by which drugs used clinically interfere with neuromuscular transmission:

1. **By competition** with acetylcholine (atracurium, cisatracurium, gallamine, mivacurium, pancuronium, rocuronium, tubocurarine, vecuronium). These drugs are competitive antagonists of acetylcholine. They do not cause depolarisation themselves but protect the endplate from depolarisation by acetylcholine. The result is a flaccid paralysis.

Reversal of this type of neuromuscular block can be achieved with anticholinesterase drugs, such as neostigmine, which prevent the destruction by cholinesterase of acetylcholine released at nerve endings, allow the concentration to build up and so reduce the competitive effect of a blocking agent.

2. **By depolarisation** of the motor endplate (suxamethonium). Such agonist drugs activate the acetylcholine receptor on the motor endplate and at their first application voluntary muscle contracts but, as they are not destroyed immediately, like acetylcholine, the depolarisation persists. It might be expected that this prolonged depolarisation would result in muscles remaining contracted but this is not so (except in chickens). With prolonged administration a depolarisation block changes to a competitive block (dual block). Because of the uncertainty of this situation a competitive blocking agent is preferred for anything other than short procedures.

COMPETITIVE ANTAGONISTS

Nondepolarising neuromuscular blocking agents: tubocurarine

The introduction of tubocurarine into surgery made

it desirable to decide once and for all whether the drug altered consciousness. Doubts were resolved in a single experiment.[6] A normal subject was slowly paralysed (curarised) after arranging a detailed and complicated system of communication. Twelve minutes after beginning the slow infusion of curare, the subject, having artificial respiration, could move only his head. He indicated that the experience was not unpleasant, that he was mentally clear and did not want an endotracheal tube inserted. After 22 min, communication was possible only by slight movement of the left eyebrow and after 35 min paralysis was complete and direct communication lost. An airway was inserted. The subject's eyelids were then lifted for him and the resulting inhibition of alpha rhythm of the electroencephalogram suggested that vision and consciousness were normal. After recovery, aided by neostigmine, the subject reported that he had been mentally 'clear as a bell' throughout, and confirmed this by recalling what he had heard and seen. The insertion of the endotracheal airway had caused only minor discomfort, perhaps because of the prevention of reflex muscle spasm. During artificial respiration he had 'felt that (he) would give anything to be able to take one deep breath' despite adequate oxygenation. In another study[7] curare was excluded from one arm by an inflated cuff so that the subject could make finger signals, and this isolated forearm technique can be used to detect wakefulness in clinical anaesthesia.

Awareness. It is essential to ensure that paralysed patients do not regain awareness unnoticed during surgery. That this is not merely a theoretical risk is shown by the occasion when an anaesthetist, visiting his patient the day after the operation, was horrified when she sympathetically remarked, 'I had no idea you doctors were so badly paid'. He had discussed the inadequacy of his salary with a colleague during the operation. The patient had felt her bowels being manipulated but no pain.

Pain can occur on such occasions, however, and both anaesthetists and patients will wish to avoid them. Awareness is most likely when nitrous oxide and oxygen are being used with neuromuscular block, and reflex signs suggestive of pain include bronchospasm, sweating and response of the pupil to light, as well as movement; but awareness can occur without these accompaniments. Patients have successfully claimed financial compensation from anaesthetists who have failed to prevent awareness.

In addition to its neuromuscular blocking effect tubocurarine blocks autonomic ganglia (acetylcholine antagonism) and causes tissue *histamine release.* Both these effects may cause an initial transient drop in blood pressure, and the latter may induce bronchospasm.

Curare is insignificantly absorbed from the alimentary tract, a fact known to the South American Indians, who use it to procure food.

Dose: after an i.v. injection of a standard dose the action is maximal in 4 min and lasts usefully for 30 min (the $t^{1/2}$ for effect is about 50 min).

Gallamine differs from tubocurarine in that it acts a little sooner (2 min) and does not release histamine, both desirable properties. It causes tachycardia by vagal block and crosses the placenta, unlike other competitive antagonists; 80% is eliminated by the kidney and 20% is metabolised.

Atracurium is unique in that it is altered spontaneously in the body to an inactive form ($t^{1/2}$ 30 min) by a passive chemical process (Hofman elimination). The duration of action (15–35 min) is thus uninfluenced by the state of the circulation, the liver or the kidneys, a real advantage in patients with hepatic or renal disease and in the aged. It is suitable for Caesarian section. Like tubocurarine it causes histamine release (locally).

Cisatracurium is a stereoisomer of atracurium; it appears less prone to cause histamine release.

Mivacurium, pancuronium, rocuronium and *vecuronium* are alternatives that differ in detail.

Antagonism of competitive neuromuscular block: neostigmine

The action of competitive acetylcholine blockers is antagonised by anticholinesterase drugs which

---

[6] Smith S M et al 1947 Anesthesiology 8: 1. Note: a randomised controlled trial is not required for this kind of investigation.

[7] Campbell E J M et al 1969 Clinical Science 36: 323.

allow accumulation of acetylcholine. Neostigmine (p. 403) is usually given i.v., preceded by atropine or glycopyrronium to prevent the parasympathetic autonomic effects of the neostigmine (especially the vagal bradycardia and salivation). It acts in 4 min and lasts for about 30 min so that the patient may relapse into paralysis again and must be carefully watched. Too much neostigmine can cause neuromuscular block by depolarisation, which will cause confusion unless there have been some signs of recovery before neostigmine is given. Progress can be monitored with a nerve stimulator.

DEPOLARISING AGENT

Suxamethonium
(succinylcholine) (Scoline)

Paralysis is usually preceded by muscular fasciculation, and this may be the cause of the muscle pain lasting 1–3 days that is a common sequence of its use and which rarely can simulate meningeal irritation. The pain can be largely prevented by preceding the suxamethonium with a small dose of a competitive blocking agent. Total paralysis with suxamethonium lasts up to 4 min with 50% recovery in about 10 min ($t^{1/2}$ for effect). It is particularly useful for brief procedures such as tracheal intubation or electroconvulsion therapy. Suxamethonium is destroyed by plasma pseudocholinesterase and so its persistence in the body is increased by neostigmine, which inactivates that enzyme, and in patients with hepatic disease or severe malnutrition whose plasma enzyme concentrations may be lower than normal. Procaine and amethocaine also are destroyed by plasma pseudocholinesterase and so, by competing with suxamethonium for the enzyme, may prolong its action and vice versa (lignocaine and prilocaine are metabolised differently). In addition there are individuals (about 1 in 2500 of the population) with hereditary defects in amount or kind of enzyme, who cannot destroy the drug as rapidly as normals.[8] Paralysis then lasts for hours; there is no practicable way of restoring the enzyme or of eliminating the drug. Treatment consists in ventilating until recovery.

---

[8] When cases are discovered the family should be investigated for low plasma cholinesterase activity and abnormal individuals warned.

Repeated injections of suxamethonium can cause bradycardia, extrasystoles, other cardiac irregularities and even ventricular arrest. These are probably due to activation of cholinoceptors in the heart and are prevented by atropine. High doses stimulate the pregnant uterus and can cause premature labour. It can be used in Caesarian section as it does not readily cross the placenta.

Suxamethonium depolarisation causes a release of potassium from muscle which can be enough to cause cardiac arrest in patients who already have raised plasma potassium (burns, muscle trauma).

Uses of neuromuscular blocking agents

These agents should be employed only by those who can intubate and ventilate.

- In surgery and in intensive therapy units they are used to provide muscular relaxation.
- In convulsions, e.g. electroconvulsion therapy, they are used to prevent injury due to the violence of the fit. In status epilepticus, tetanus or convulsant drug poisoning, neuromuscular blocking agents with mechanical ventilation are used when lesser means are insufficient.

OTHER MUSCLE RELAXANTS

Drugs that provide muscle relaxation by an action on the central nervous system or on the muscle itself are not useful for this purpose in surgery; they are insufficiently selective and full relaxation, even if achievable, is accompanied by general cerebral depression.

But there is a place for drugs that reduce spasm of the voluntary muscles without impairing voluntary movement. Such drugs can be useful in neurological spastic states, low back syndrome and rheumatism with muscle spasm.

Baclofen (Lioresal) ($t^{1/2}$ 3 h) is structurally related to gamma-aminobutyric acid (GABA), an inhibitory central nervous system transmitter; it inhibits reflex activity mainly in the spinal cord. Baclofen reduces spasticity and flexor spasms, but as it has no action on voluntary muscle power, function is commonly not improved. Ambulant patients may need their leg spasticity to provide support and reduction of spasticity may expose the weakness of the limb. It benefits some cases of trigeminal neuralgia. Baclofen is given orally.

Dantrolene (Dantrium) acts directly on muscle and prevents the release of calcium from sarcoplasm stores (see Malignant hyperthermia, p. 394).

Alternative centrally acting muscle relaxants include *orphenadrine* (Norflex), *diazepam* (Valium), *carisoprodol* (Carisoma), *chlormezanone* (Trancopal) and *methocarbamol* (Robaxin). Most are prone to cause objectionable sedation (see Quinine).

Botulinum toxin: see page 370

ALLERGIC AND PSEUDO-ALLERGIC REACTIONS

Anaphylactic type allergic and pseudo-allergic reactions occur particularly to intravenous anaesthetics and muscle relaxants, and particularly during induction. They may be fatal. Treatment is as for anaphylactic shock.

Local anaesthetics

Cocaine had been suggested as a local anaesthetic for clinical use when Sigmund Freud investigated the alkaloid in Vienna in 1884 with Carl Koller. The latter had long been interested in the problem of local anaesthesia in the eye, for general anaesthesia has disadvantages in ophthalmology. Observing that numbness of the mouth occurred after taking cocaine orally he realised that this was a local anaesthetic effect. He tried cocaine on animals' eyes and introduced it into clinical ophthalmological practice, whilst Freud was on holiday. Freud had already thought of this use and discussed it but, appreciating that sex was of greater importance than surgery, he had gone to see his fiancée. The use of cocaine spread rapidly and it was soon being used to block nerve trunks. Chemists then began to search for less toxic substitutes, with the result that procaine was introduced in 1905.

Desired properties. Innumerable compounds have local anaesthetic properties, but few are suitable for clinical use. Useful substances must be water-solu-

ble, sterilisable by heat, have a rapid onset of effect, a duration of action appropriate to the operation to be performed, be nontoxic both locally and when absorbed into the circulation, and leave no local after-effects.

Mode of action. Local anaesthetics prevent the initiation and propagation of the nerve impulse (action potential). By reducing the passage of sodium through voltage-gated Na ion channels they raise the threshold of excitability; in consequence, conduction is blocked at afferent nerve endings, and by sensory and motor nerve fibres. The fibres in nerve trunks are affected in order of size, the smallest (autonomic, sensory) first, probably because they have a proportionately greater surface area, and then the larger (motor) fibres. Paradoxically the effect in the central nervous system is stimulation (see below).

Pharmacokinetics. The *distribution rate* of a single dose of a local anaesthetic is determined by diffusion into tissues with concentrations approximately in relation to blood flow (blood $t^{1}/_{2}$ only a few minutes). By injection or infiltration local anaesthetics are usually effective within 5 min and have a useful duration of effect of 1–1.5 h, which may be doubled by adding a vasoconstrictor (below).

Most local anaesthetics are used in the form of the acid salts, as these are both soluble and stable. The acid salt (usually HCl) dissociates in the tissues to liberate the free base, which is biologically active. This dissociation is delayed in abnormally acid, e.g. inflamed, tissues; but the risk of spreading infection makes local anaesthesia undesirable in infected areas.

Absorption from mucous membranes on topical application varies according to the compound. Those that are well absorbed are used as surface anaesthetics (cocaine, lignocaine, prilocaine). Absorption of topically applied local anaesthetic can be extremely rapid and give plasma concentrations comparable to those obtained by injection. This had led to deaths from overdosage, especially via the urethra.

For topical effect on intact skin for needling procedures a eutectic[9] mixture of bases of prilocaine or

---

[9] A mixture of two solids that becomes a liquid that melts and solidifies at one temperature.

lignocaine is used (EMLA = eutectic mixture of local anaesthetics). Absorption is very slow and a cream is applied under an occlusive dressing for at least 1 h.

Ester compounds (*cocaine, procaine, amethocaine, benzocaine*) are hydrolysed by liver and plasma esterases (and their effects may be prolonged where there is genetic enzyme deficiency).

Amide compounds (*lignocaine, prilocaine, bupivacaine*) are dealkylated in the liver.

It is evident that defective liver function, whether due to primary cellular insufficiency or to low liver blood flow in cardiac failure or due to β-adrenoceptor block, may both delay elimination and allow higher peak plasma concentrations of both types of local anaesthetic. This is likely to be important only with large or repeated doses or infusions. The rate of elimination from the blood once equilibration with all body tissues has been achieved (steady state) is longer than that for distribution, e.g. lignocaine $t^{1}/_{2}$ is 1.5 h. These considerations are important in the management of cardiac dysrhythmias by i.v. infusion of lignocaine (p. 461).

PROLONGATION OF ACTION BY VASOCONSTRICTORS

The effect of a local anaesthetic is terminated by its removal from the site of application. Anything that delays its absorption into the circulation will prolong its local action and can reduce its systemic toxicity where large volumes/doses are used. Adrenaline or noradrenaline generally (1 : 200 000–1 : 400 000) are commonly used (dentists use 1 : 80 000) and they double the duration of effect, e.g. from 1 to 2 h. A vasoconstrictor should not be used for nerve block of an extremity (finger, toe, nose, penis). For obvious anatomical reasons, the whole blood supply may be cut off by intense vasoconstriction so that the organ may be damaged or even lost. In dentistry particularly it is sometimes useful to terminate local anaesthesia promptly when the operative job is done. This can be achieved by reversal of adrenaline vasoconstriction by injecting an α-adrenoceptor blocker (phentolamine) into the site.

Enough adrenaline or noradrenaline can be absorbed to affect the heart and circulation and reduce the plasma potassium. This can be dangerous in cardiovascular disease, with general anaesthetics that sensitise the heart to catecholamines (halothane) and with tricyclic antidepressants and potassium-losing diuretics. An alternative vasoconstrictor is *felypressin* (synthetic vasopressin), which, in the concentrations used, does not affect the heart rate or blood pressure and may be preferable in patients with cardiovascular disease. There is no significant added hazard to the use of catecholamines in patients taking an MAOI, except perhaps where there is cardiovascular disease, and felypressin is preferable in these patients in any case.

OTHER EFFECTS

Local anaesthetics also have the following clinically important effects in varying degree:

- Excitation of parts of the central nervous system, which may show itself by anxiety, restlessness, tremors, euphoria, agitation and even convulsions, which are followed by depression.
- Quinidine-like actions on the heart.

USES

Local anaesthesia is generally used when loss of consciousness is neither necessary nor desirable and also as an adjunct to major surgery to avoid high dose general anaesthesia. It can be used for major surgery, with sedation, though many patients prefer unconsciousness. It is invaluable when the operator must also be the anaesthetist. Local anaesthetics can also be used topically for short periods to give relief from local pain or itching (but skin allergy is common).

For any but the most trivial operation premedication with a benzodiazepine is theoretically desirable to counteract the central excitant action of local anaesthetics, especially of cocaine, but the doses given may in fact provide little or no protection.

Local anaesthetics may be used in several ways to provide:

- Surface anaesthesia, as solution, jelly, cream or lozenge. Chronic use is liable to cause allergy
- Infiltration anaesthesia, to paralyse the sensory nerve endings and small cutaneous nerves
- Regional anaesthesia.

Regional anaesthesia

Nerve block means to anaesthetise a region, which may be small or large, by injecting the drug around, not into, the appropriate nerves, usually either a peripheral nerve or a plexus. Nerve block provides its own muscular relaxation as motor fibres are blocked as well as sensory fibres, although with care differential block can be achieved. Areas of selective sensory, but not motor, nerve block are found at the edges of some regional nerve blocks. Even when motor fibres are intact, provided there is sensory block, muscular relaxation will occur if the patient's consciousness is blunted with a hypnotic drug. There are various specialised forms: brachial plexus, paravertebral, paracervical, pudendal block. Sympathetic nerve blocks may be used in vascular disease to induce vasodilatation.

Intravenous. A double cuff is applied to the arm, inflated above arterial pressure after elevating the limb to drain the venous system, and the veins filled with local anaesthetic, e.g. 0.5% prilocaine *without* adrenaline. The arm is anaesthetised in 6–8 min, and the effect lasts for up to 40 min if the cuff remains inflated. The cuff cannot be deflated safely until 20 min have passed. The technique is useful in providing anaesthesia for the treatment of injuries speedily and conveniently, and many patients can leave hospital as soon as 15 min after the cuff has been let down (during which time sensation and power return). The technique must be meticulously conducted, for if the *full* dose of local anaesthetic is accidentally suddenly released into the general circulation severe toxicity and even death may result. Even if correctly performed, drug enters the general circulation through vessels in the bone that are not obstructed by the tourniquet. If toxicity occurs, convulsions and cardiac arrest may have to be treated. Patients should be fasted and someone (in addition to the surgeon) who is fully able to resuscitate should be present.

Extradural (epidural) anaesthesia can be used in thoracic, lumbar and sacral (caudal) regions: it is widely used in obstetrics. As the term implies, the drug is injected into the extradural space where it acts on the nerve roots. This technique avoids the potentially serious hazards of putting foreign sub-

stances into the CSF; the risk of headache and hypotension is less than with spinal anaesthesia.

Subarachnoid (intrathecal) block (spinal anaesthesia). By using a solution of appropriate specific gravity and tilting the patient the drug can be kept at an appropriate level. Hypotension due to block of the sympathetic nervous system outflow occurs in younger rather than older patients. Headache due to CSF leakage can be troublesome and prolonged but is lessened by the use of atraumatic 'pencil point' needles.

Serious local neurological complications have occurred rarely, both from the formulation and from accidentally introduced bacteria.

Opioid analgesics may also be used *intrathecally* and *extradurally*. They diffuse into the spinal cord and are highly effective in skilled hands for intractable pain, including postsurgical pain. They are less effective in childbirth. Respiratory depression may occur. The effect begins in 20 min and lasts about 5 h. Morphine or other more lipid-soluble opioids may be used.

Regional anaesthesia requires considerable knowledge of anatomy and attention to detail for both success and safety.

ADVERSE REACTIONS

Excessive absorption results in paraesthesiae (face and tongue) nervousness, tremors and even *convulsions*. These latter are very dangerous and are followed by respiratory depression. Diazepam or thiopentone, or even suxamethonium, may be necessary to control the convulsions as in status epilepticus. Respiratory stimulants are useless and dangerous as the patient has already passed through a phase of overstimulation. Nausea, vomiting and abdominal pain may occur, and also sudden *cardiovascular collapse* and *respiratory failure* for which there is no specific treatment other than respiratory and cardiac resuscitation. When systemic toxicity follows injection of a local anaesthetic into an extremity, a tourniquet may be used to delay entry of what remains into the general circulation, but resuscitation is the first priority. Hypertension can occur with cocaine (below).

Allergic reactions such as rashes, asthma and anaphylactic shock rarely occur, and the subject may be allergic to more than one drug. Frequent users are wise if they take care to keep them off their own skin when filling syringes.

INDIVIDUAL LOCAL ANAESTHETICS
(Table 21.1)

Lignocaine (lidocaine; Xylocaine) (amide) ($t^{1/2}$ 1.5 h) is a first choice drug for surface use as well as for injection, combining efficacy with comparative lack of toxicity. It is also useful in cardiac dysrhythmias (see Index). Structurally, lignocaine differs from most other local anaesthetics and so is especially suitable for trial in cases of known allergy to other drugs.

Prilocaine (Citanest) (amide) ($t^{1/2}$ 1.5 h) is used similarly to lignocaine, but it is less toxic. Crystals of prilocaine and lignocaine base, when mixed, dissolve in one another to form a eutetic emulsion that penetrates skin and is used for dermal anaesthesia (EMLA, see p. 389), e.g. for premedication venepuncture in children.

Bupivacaine (Marcain) (amide) ($t^{1/2}$ 3 h) is long-acting (see Table 21.1) and is used for nerve blocks in general, including obstetric epidural anaesthesia and for postsurgical and chronic pain relief. Whilst onset of effect is comparable to the above, peak effect occurs later (30 min).

Table 21.1 Reference data (approx) on 3 widely used local anaesthetics (amide class) (Other concentrations are used, especially in dentistry)

		Solution	Dose by vol. (adult)	Duration of effect
Lignocaine	*infiltration*	0.25–0.5% + adrenaline	up to 60 ml	
	nerve block (peripheral)	1% + adrenaline	up to 50 ml	
		2% + adrenaline	up to 25 ml	1.5 h
	surface *anaesthesia*	2%	up to 20 ml	
		4%	up to 5 ml	
Bupivacaine	*infiltration*	0.25%	up to 60 ml	
	nerve block (peripheral)	0.25%	up to 60 ml	3–4 h
		0.5%	up to 30 ml	
Prilocaine	*infiltration*	0.5%	up to 80 ml	
	nerve block (peripheral)	1%	up to 40 ml	1.5–3 h
		2%	up to 20 ml	
		3% + felypressin (dental use)	up to 20 ml	

Notes:

1. Time to peak effect is about 5 min, except bupivacaine (see text).
2. Maximum doses of local anaesthetic plus vasoconstrictor are toxic in absence of the vasoconstrictor and so substantially less should be used. All doses are approximate only; larger amounts may be safe, but deaths have occurred with smaller amounts, so that the minimum dose that will suffice should be used.
3. Maximum dose of adrenaline is 500 micrograms (see below).
4. Concentrations of solutions and dose of drug: errors of calculation occur with sometimes fatal results. We provide these figures because experience of conducting examinations with medical students has taught us that they frequently lack the facility of calculating the dose of a drug in a given volume of known concentration.

1% means one gram in 100 ml = 1000 mg in 100 ml = 10 mg per ml: 2% = 20 mg per ml, and so on.

It is traditional to express adrenaline concentrations as 1 in 200 000, or 1 in 80 000, or 1 in 1000.
1 in 1000 means 1000 mg (1.0 g) in 1000 ml = 1 mg per ml.
1 in 200 000 means 1000 mg (1.0 g) in 200 000 ml = 5 micrograms per ml.

Thus the maximum dose of adrenaline, 500 micrograms (see above), is contained in 100 ml of 1 in 200 000 solution.

Adverse reactions, see above.

Cocaine (alkaloid and ester) is used medicinally solely as a surface anaesthetic (for abuse toxicity, see p. 181) usually as a 4% solution, because adverse effects are both common and dangerous when it is injected. Even as a surface anaesthetic sufficient absorption may take place to cause serious adverse effects and cases continue to be reported; it should be used only by specialists and the dose *must* be checked and restricted. Cocaine prevents the uptake of catecholamines (adrenaline, noradrenaline) into sympathetic nerve endings, thus increasing their concentration at receptor sites, so that cocaine has a built-in vasoconstrictor action, which is why it retains a (declining) place as a surface anaesthetic for surgery involving mucous membranes, e.g. nose. Other local anaesthetics do not have this action, indeed are vasodilator and added adrenaline is not so efficient.

There are numerous other local anaesthetics, e.g. *procaine, amethocaine, proxymetacaine, cinchocaine, benzocaine, oxybuprocaine, butacaine, orthocaine,* and their omission here is not meant to imply that good results are not obtainable with them.

CHOICE OF LOCAL ANAESTHETIC

The many agents available are proof that all have disadvantages and that no agent is unchallengeably the best for all occasions. This is particularly the case for *surface* anaesthesia, although a claim that lignocaine is safest and best could not easily be dismissed; prilocaine is a contender when dosage must be heavy. For *infiltration injection* by the occasional user lignocaine or prilocaine are satisfactory.

Warning. There have been many deaths due to confusion of the names, all ending in 'caine, and to the use of wrong concentrations of unfamiliar drugs.

Obstetric analgesia and anaesthesia

Although this soon ceased to be considered immoral on religious grounds, it has been a technically controversial topic since 1853 when it was announced that Queen Victoria had inhaled chloroform during the birth of her eighth child. The *Lancet* recorded 'intense astonishment … throughout the profession' at this use of chloroform, 'an agent which has unquestionably caused instantaneous death in a considerable number of cases'. But the Queen (perhaps ignorant of these risks) took a different view, writing in her private journal of 'that blessed chloroform' and adding that 'the effect was soothing, quieting and delightful beyond measure'.

Pain-free labour sometimes occurs spontaneously but most women in Western civilisations anticipate pain and demand relief. The reason for lack of general agreement on which drugs are best is that requirements are stringent, and much depends on the skill with which they are used. The *ideal drug* must relieve pain without making the patient confused or uncooperative. It must not interfere with uterine activity nor must it influence the fetus; respiratory depression is the chief disadvantage and may occur by a direct action of the drug on the fetus, by prolonging labour or by reducing uterine blood supply. It should also be suitable for use by a midwife without supervision.

Innumerable schemes have been proposed and good results can be obtained with many. Generally, strong analgesic drugs should not be started before uterine contractions are well advanced as they can arrest labour if started sooner. The following may be taken as a general guide:

- Onset of labour and up to three-quarter dilatation of cervix: noninhalational tranquillisers and analgesics, e.g. pethidine.
- From three-quarter dilatation of cervix till birth: inhalation analgesia, e.g. nitrous oxide / oxygen (below) to avoid respiratory depression of the fetus, which occurs with effective doses of narcotic analgesics.

Pethidine is widely used. It seldom causes serious respiratory depression but has been shown to reduce respiratory minute volume in the baby. The mother may experience drowsiness and nausea. Morphine depresses fetal respiration more than pethidine. Opioids may impair infant feeding for 48 h. Naloxone administered to the mother before birth or to the child after birth will reverse opioid effect. Opioids delay gastric emptying, which can carry hazard of vomiting if general anaesthesia is then needed. The effect is not antagonised by meto-clopramide.

Diazepam, as tranquilliser during labour and as anticonvulsant in pre-eclampsia and eclampsia, has a depressant effect on the newborn if the maternal dose exceeds 30 mg in the 15 h before delivery (apnoeic spells, failure to feed, hypothermia), and these effects can last several days.

In general the baby will be about as depressed as the mother at the time of birth, and respiratory depressant should be withheld if birth is imminent. The intervals between doses are judged on clinical progress.

Nitrous oxide and oxygen (50% of each: Entonox) may be administered for each pain from a machine the patient works herself or supervised by a midwife (about 10 good breaths are needed for maximal analgesia). Nitrous oxide and air mixtures are obsolete because hypoxia is unavoidable at effective concentrations of nitrous oxide.

Special techniques, e.g. extradural, caudal and pudendal nerve block, are highly effective in skilled hands.

General anaesthesia during labour presents special problems. Regurgitation and aspiration are a particular risk (see p. 376). The safety of the fetus must be considered; all anaesthetics and analgesics in general use cross the placenta in varying amounts and, apart from respiratory depression, produce no important effects except that high doses interfere with uterine retraction and may be followed by uterine haemorrhage. Neuromuscular blocking agents can be used safely, although gallamine is best avoided as it crosses the placenta; suxamethonium stimulates the uterus but is the speediest at producing the conditions for tracheal intubation (crucial for general anaesthesia for Caesarian section); none interferes with uterine retraction.

Anaesthesia in patients already taking medication

Anaesthetists are in an unenviable position. They are expected to provide safe service to patients in any condition, taking any drugs. Sometimes there is opportunity to modify drug therapy before surgery but often there is not. Anaesthetists require a particularly complete drug history of the patient.

DRUGS THAT AFFECT ANAESTHESIA

Adrenal steroids: chronic corticosteroid therapy within the previous 2 years can be associated with collapse due to the failure of the hypothalamic-pituitary-adrenal system to respond to stress (see Ch. 38). *Etomidate* depresses the *hypothalamic-pituitary* adrenal axis; for this reason it is no longer used as a continuous i.v. infusion, but single bolus injections are safe.

Antibiotics: aminoglycosides, e.g. neomycin, gentamicin, are themselves neuromuscular blocking agents in high dose and are additive with nondepolarising neuromuscular blocking drugs.

Anticholinesterases: can potentiate suxamethonium.

NSAIDs: interfere with platelet function and may cause oozing at the operation site.

Antiepileptic drugs: continued medication is essential to avoid status epilepticus. Drugs must be given parenterally until the patient can swallow. Valproate can impair coagulation.

Antihypertensives of all kinds: hypotension may complicate anaesthesia, but it is best to continue therapy. Hypertensive patients are particularly liable to excessive rise in blood pressure and heart rate during intubation, which can be dangerous if there is ischaemic heart disease. Postoperatively, parenteral therapy may be needed for a time.

Calcium channel blocking drugs: patients taking verapamil may develop heart block with halothane, and those taking nifedipine may become hypotensive if they receive isoflurane.

Digoxin: cardiac dysrhythmias are more likely with general anaesthesia, especially if there is hypokalaemia.

β-*adrenoceptor blocking drugs*: can prevent the homeostatic sympathetic cardiac response to cardiac depressant anaesthetics and to blood loss.

Diuretics: if hypokalaemia occurs, this will potentiate neuromuscular blocking agents and perhaps general anaesthetics.

Oral contraceptives containing oestrogen and post-menopausal hormone replacement therapy: predispose to thromboembolism (see p. 655).

Psychotropic drugs: neuroleptics potentiate or synergise with opioids, hypnotics and general anaesthetics. Those with antihypertensive properties, e.g. chlorpromazine, may cause severe hypotension during anaesthesia.

Antidepressants: monoamine oxidase inhibitors can cause hypertension when combined with certain amines, e.g. pethidine, and sometimes general anaesthetics as well as some indirect-acting sympathomimetics, e.g. ephedrine. Tricyclics potentiate catecholamines and some other adrenergic drugs.

Lithium: may be continued unless there is serious risk of electrolyte disturbance or renal insufficiency, when it should be stopped a week before surgery.

Anaesthesia in the diseased, the elderly and in children

The normal response to anaesthesia may be greatly modified by disease. The possibilities are vast and only some of the more important aspects will be mentioned here.

Respiratory disease and smoking predispose the patient to postanaesthetic pulmonary complications such as collapse and pneumonia. The site of operation and the occurrence of pain are also relevant when they cause defective ventilation due to pain and fear of coughing.

Cardiac disease. The aim is to avoid the circulatory stress (with increased cardiac work which can compromise the myocardial oxygen supply) caused by struggling, coughing, laryngospasm and breath holding. Drugs given i.v. should be injected slowly to avoid hypotension, which may occur with many substances if they are given too fast.

Patients with fixed cardiac output, e.g. mitral stenosis or constrictive pericarditis, are specially liable to a drop in cardiac output with drugs that depress the myocardium and vasomotor centre, for

they cannot compensate. Thiopentone induction is liable to do this and inhalation induction may be preferable. Hypoxia is obviously harmful. It will be seen that skilled technique rather than choice of drugs on pharmacological grounds is the important factor.

Hepatic and renal disease. Disease of these organs is liable to lead to increased drug effects and should be taken into account when selecting drugs and their doses. General anaesthetics can also impair hepatic function.

Malignant hyperthermia occurs in about $1:20\,000$ subjects of general anaesthesia. It is a result of an inherited muscle disorder (autosomal dominant). The condition occurs during or within several hours of anaesthesia and is precipitated by almost any drug but especially by potent inhalation agents (especially halogenated) and by suxamethonium. The patient may previously have safely experienced a general anaesthetic. The mechanism involves a sudden rise in release of bound (stored) calcium of the sarcoplasm, stimulating contraction and a hypermetabolic state.

Malignant hyperthermia is a life-threatening medical emergency. Oxygen consumption increases by up to 3 times normal, and body temperature may rise as fast as 1°C every 5 min, reaching as high as 43°C. Rigidity of voluntary muscles may not be evident at the outset or in mild cases.

Administration of dantrolene ($t^1/_2$ 9 h) i.v., 1 mg/kg, is urgently required; further doses are given if there is not a quick response (5 min); the average total effective dose is 2.5 mg/kg, but as much as 10 mg/kg may be needed. Dantrolene probably acts by preventing the release of calcium from the sarcoplasm store that ordinarily follows depolarisation of the muscle membrane.

Nonspecific treatment is needed for the hyperthermia (cooling, sodium bicarbonate i.v. infusion to correct acidosis, oxygen). Cardiac dysrhythmias occur (due to potassium release from contracted muscle).

Any *future anaesthesia* in patients who have experienced the syndrome can be achieved with minimal risk by using opioids, barbiturates, diazepam, nitrous oxide, probably propofol or ester-class local anaesthetics; pancuronium or atracurium may be safe for neuromuscular block. Dantrolene orally may be used as prophylaxis.

It is recommended that i.v. formulation of dantrolene should be available in every surgical theatre. The relation of malignant hyperthermia syndrome with neuroleptic malignant syndrome (for which dantrolene may be used as adjunctive treatment) is uncertain.

Diabetes mellitus: see page 630.
Thyroid disease: see page 640.
Porphyria: see page 128.

Muscle diseases. Patients with myasthenia gravis are very sensitive (intolerant) to competitive but not to depolarising neuromuscular blocking drugs. Those with dystrophia myotonica may recover less rapidly than normal from central respiratory depression and neuromuscular block; they may fail to relax with suxamethonium. All patients with generalised muscular weakness or disease should be treated with special attentiveness.

Sickle-cell disease: hypoxia can precipitate a crisis.

Atypical (deficient) pseudocholinesterase. There is serious delay in the metabolism of suxamethonium.

Raised intracranial pressure will be made worse by inhalation agents, e.g. halothane, nitrous oxide, by hypoxia or hypercapnia and in response to intubation; depression of the respiratory centre occurs. These patients are also liable to respiratory failure with central nervous depressants, especially opioids, and premedication may consist of atropine alone.

The elderly (see p. 113) are liable to become confused by cerebral depressants, especially by hyoscine, and atropine is usually substituted. Apart from this there are no special problems for anaesthesia, but mistakes and overdose are less easily retrieved in the old and frail than in the young and healthy. In general, elderly patients require smaller doses than the young. Hypotension should be especially avoided as it readily causes cerebral hypoxia.

Children (see p. 112). The problems with children are more technical, physiological and psychological than pharmacological. Premedication is often by sedatives, e.g. benzodiazepine, orally or by rectum, rather than by injected morphine or papaveretum with hyoscine, although children in fact tolerate these well.

Sedation in intensive therapy units. Patients who are not too sick are likely to feel anxious. Good practice requires that they be relieved by sympathetic care and, if necessary, by drugs. Benzodiazepines are an obvious choice, e.g. midazolam; also propofol, chlormethiazole, neuroleptics.

There are other reasons for sedation. Some patients will 'fight' the mechanical ventilator and may experience discomfort from the endotracheal tube. Opioids are an obvious choice, e.g. phenoperidine (where short duration of action is desired). These not only relieve pain and discomfort, but tranquillise and depress respiration so that the patient fights the ventilator less. A competitive neuromuscular blocking agent may have to be added to reduce the need for high doses of opioids, especially where there is reduced renal and hepatic function. Neuromuscular blockers do not impair consciousness and an aware and paralysed patient is in great distress and unable to communicate this to attendants. Everyone will wish to avoid this and it can be done by skilled use of sedatives and opioids.

GUIDE TO FURTHER READING

Collis R E et al 1995 Randomised comparison of combined spinal-epidural and standard epidural analgesia in labour. Lancet 345: 1413

Editorial 1989 Nausea and vomiting after general anaesthesia. Lancet 1: 651

Editorial 1992 Steroid anaesthetic agents. Lancet 340: 83

Hunter J M 1995 New neuromuscular blocking drugs. New England Journal of Medicine 332: 1691

Jacobsen B et al 1990 Opiate addiction in adult offspring through possible imprinting after obstetric treatment. British Medical Journal 301: 1067

Jones M J T et al 1990 Cognitive and functional competence after anaesthesia in patients aged over 60: controlled trial of general and regional anaesthesia for elective hip and knee replacements. British Medical Journal 300: 1683

Neil H A W et al 1987 Mortality among male anaesthetists in the United Kingdom 1957–83. British Medical Journal 295: 360

Ponte J 1995 Neuromuscular blockers during general anaesthesia. British Medical Journal 310: 1218

Rothen H U et al 1995 Prevention of atelectasis during general anaesthesia. Lancet 345: 1387

CARDIORESPIRA-TORY AND RENAL SYSTEMS

22

Cholinergic and antimuscarinic (anticholinergic) drugs

SYNOPSIS

Acetylcholine acts as a chemotransmitter at a wide variety of sites, mediating a wide variety of physiological effects.

Cholinergic drugs (acetylcholine agonists) mimic acetylcholine at all sites but with differences of emphasis.

Acetylcholine receptor (cholinoceptor) blocking drugs are selective for different physiological classes of receptor which have been selectively defined by use of the alkaloids, nicotine (from tobacco) and muscarine (from a fungus).

Acetylcholine antagonists (blockers) that oppose the nicotine-like effects (neuromuscular blockers and autonomic ganglion blockers) are described elsewhere (see Index).

Acetylcholine antagonists that block the muscarine-like effects, e.g. atropine, are often imprecisely called anticholinergics. The more precise term antimuscarinic is preferred here.

- Cholinergic drugs
  Classification
  Sites of action
  Pharmacology
  Choline esters
  Alkaloids with cholinergic effects
  Anticholinesterases
  Disorders of neuromuscular
    transmission: myasthenia gravis
- Drugs which oppose acetylcholine
  Antimuscarinic drugs

Cholinergic (cholinomimetic) drugs

These drugs act on acetylcholine receptors (cholinoceptors) at all the sites in the body where acetylcholine is the transmitter of the nerve impulse. They stimulate and later paralyse. In addition, like acetylcholine, they act on noninnervated dilator receptors on peripheral blood vessels.

USES OF CHOLINERGIC DRUGS

- For myasthenia gravis, both to diagnose (edrophonium) and to treat (neostigmine, pyridostigmine, distigmine)
- To stimulate the bladder and bowel after surgery (bethanechol, carbachol, distigmine)
- To lower intraocular pressure in chronic simple glaucoma (pilocarpine)

CLASSIFICATION

Direct-acting

- Choline esters (carbachol, bethanechol) which act at all sites like acetylcholine. Muscarinic effects are more prominent than nicotinic (see p. 401).
- Alkaloids (pilocarpine, muscarine) which act selectively on end-organs of postganglionic, cholinergic neurons.

Indirect-acting

- Cholinesterase inhibitors, or anticholinesterases (physostigmine, neostigmine, pyridostigmine, distigmine), which inactivate the enzyme that destroys acetylcholine, allowing the chemical transmitter to persist and produce intensified effects.

SITES OF ACTION

- Autonomic nervous system
  — *Parasympathetic division*
    ganglia
    postganglionic endings (all)
  — *Sympathetic division*
    ganglia
    a minority of postganglionic endings, e.g. sweat glands
- Neuromuscular junction
- Central nervous system
- Noninnervated sites: blood vessels, chiefly arterioles.

Acetylcholine is the chemotransmitter of the nerve impulse at all these sites, acting on a postsynaptic receptor, except on most blood vessels in which the action of cholinergic drugs is unrelated to cholinergic vasodilator nerves. It is also produced in tissues unrelated to nerve endings, e.g. placenta, ciliated

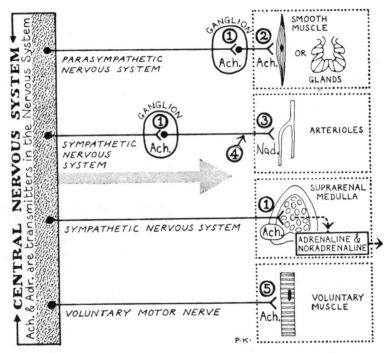

Fig. 22.1 Diagram showing sites of chemical transmitters of nerve impulse (this is the classic oversimplification that is sufficient for this account)
Ach. = acetylcholine
Nad. = noradrenaline
Site 1 is blocked by ganglion-blocking agents and stimulated by nicotine and big doses of some choline esters and anticholinesterases.
Site 2 is blocked by atropine and stimulated by some choline esters, anticholinesterases and pilocarpine.
Site 3 is blocked by adrenoceptor blocking agents and function is interfered with by drugs that deplete norepinephrine (noradrenaline) stores in nerve endings and end-organs (reserpine).
    Sympathomimetic amines stimulate here.
Site 4 is blocked by adrenergic neuron-blocking agents (guanethidine).
Site 5 is blocked by neuromuscular blocking agents and stimulated by choline esters and anticholinesterases.

epithelial cells, where it acts as a local hormone (autacoid) on local receptors.

A list of principal effects is given below. Not all occur with every drug and not all are noticeable at therapeutic doses. For example, central nervous system effects of cholinergic drugs are best seen in cases of anticholinesterase poisoning. Atropine antagonises all the effects of cholinergic drugs except those at *autonomic ganglia* and the *neuromuscular junction*, i.e. it does not act at receptors served by neurons arising in the central nervous system; it has antimuscarinic but not antinicotinic effects (see below).

PHARMACOLOGY

Autonomic nervous system

Parasympathetic division. Stimulation of cholinoceptors in autonomic ganglia and at the postganglionic endings affects chiefly the following organs:

Eye: miosis and spasm of the ciliary muscle occur so that the eye is accommodated for near vision. Intraocular pressure falls due, perhaps, to dilation of vessels at the point where intraocular fluids pass into the blood.

Exocrine glands: there is increased secretion most noticeably of the salivary, lachrymal, bronchial and sweat glands. The last are cholinergic, although anatomically part of the sympathetic system; some sweat glands, e.g. axillary, may be adrenergic.

Heart: bradycardia occurs with atrioventricular block and eventually cardiac arrest.

Bronchi: bronchoconstriction occurs, also increased secretion, which effects may be clinically serious in asthmatic or other allergic subjects, in whom cholinergic drugs should be avoided as far as possible.

Alimentary tract: there is increased motor activity and exocrine secretion and colicky pain may occur. Sphincter tone is reduced and the patient may defaecate embarrassingly. Lowering of oesophageal sphincter tone creates a risk of regurgitation and inhalation, e.g. in anaesthesia.

Bladder and ureters contract and the drugs promote micturition.

Sympathetic division. *The ganglia only are stimu-* lated, also the cholinergic nerves to the adrenal medulla. These effects are overshadowed by effects on the parasympathetic system and are commonly evident only if atropine has been given to block the latter, when tachycardia, vasoconstriction and hypertension occur.

Neuromuscular (voluntary) junction

The neuromuscular junction has a cholinergic nerve ending and so is activated, causing muscle fasciculation, followed if excess is given by a depolarisation neuromuscular block.

Central nervous system

There is usually stimulation followed by depression but variation between drugs is great, possibly due to differences in penetration into the nervous system. In overdose, mental excitement occurs, with confusion and restlessness, insomnia (with nightmares when sleep does come), tremors and dysarthria and sometimes even convulsions and coma.

Blood vessels

There is stimulation of cholinergic vasodilator nerve endings in addition to the more important dilating action on arterioles and capillaries mediated through noninnervated receptors. Anticholinesterases potentiate acetylcholine which exists in the vessel walls independently of nerves.

Nicotinic and muscarinic effects

The actions of acetylcholine and substances acting like it at autonomic ganglia and the neuromuscular junction (i.e. at the end of cholinergic nerve fibres which arise in the central nervous system) are described as *nicotinic* because they are like the stimulant effects of nicotine. The actions at postganglionic cholinergic endings (parasympathetic endings plus the cholinergic sympathetic nerves to the sweat glands) and those noninnervated receptors on blood vessels are described as *muscarinic* because they resemble those of the alkaloid, muscarine. The central nervous system actions are not included in this curious categorisation. The terms are useful because it is more concise to say that atropine blocks the muscarinic but not the nicotinic effects of neostigmine than it is to describe this antagonism in any other way, i.e. jargon is useful in the right place.

CHOLINE ESTERS

Acetylcholine

Since acetylcholine has such great importance in the body it is not surprising that attempts have been made to use it in therapeutics. But a substance with such a huge variety of effects and so rapidly destroyed in the body is unlikely to be useful when given systemically, as its history in psychiatry illustrates.

Acetylcholine was first injected intravenously as a therapeutic convulsant in 1939, in the justified expectation that the fits would be less liable to cause fractures than those following therapeutic leptazol convulsions. Recovery rates of up to 80% were claimed in various psychotic conditions. Enthusiasm began to wane however when it was shown that the fits were due to anoxia resulting from cardiac arrest and not to pharmacological effects on the brain.[1] The following description is illustrative:

> A few seconds after the injection (which was given as rapidly as possible, to avoid total destruction in the blood) the patient sat up 'with knees drawn up to the chest, the arms flexed and the head bent forward. There were repeated violent coughs, sometimes with flushing. Forced swallowing and loud peristaltic rumblings could be heard'. Respiration was laboured and irregular. 'The coughing abated as the patient sank back in the bed. Forty seconds after the injection the radial and apical pulse were zero and the patient became comatose.' The pupils dilated, and deep reflexes were hyperactive. In 45 seconds the patient went into opisthotonos with brief apnoea. Lachrymation, sweating and borborygmi were prominent. The deep reflexes became diminished. The patient then relaxed and 'lay quietly in bed –

cold moist and gray. In about 90 seconds, flushing of the face marked the return of the pulse'. The respiratory rate rose and consciousness returned in about 125 seconds. The patients sometimes micturated but did not defaecate. They 'tended to lie quietly in bed after the treatment'. 'Most of the patients were reluctant to be treated'.[2]

OTHER CHOLINE ESTERS

Carbachol is not destroyed by cholinesterase, its actions are most pronounced on the bladder and bowels, so that the drug is used to stimulate these organs, e.g. after surgery. Carbachol is stable in the alimentary tract; it is extremely dangerous if given i.v. but may be administered s.c.

Bethanechol is not destroyed by cholinesterase. It acts chiefly on the bowel and bladder and is preferable to carbachol because of this partial selectivity.

ALKALOIDS WITH CHOLINERGIC EFFECTS

Nicotine (see also p. 161) is a social drug that finds its medicinal use as an adjunct to stopping its own use as tobacco. It is available as either gum (Nicorette) or as patches (Nicotrol, Habitrol, Nicoderm). They deliver a lower dose of nicotine than cigarettes and appear to be safe in patients with ischaemic heart disease. The patches are slightly better tolerated than the gum, which needs to be chewed for 20–30 minutes of every hour, with avoidance of beverages (coffee, carbonated drinks) that reduce acidity of saliva and therefore absorption. Nicotine treatment has been reported to be 2–3 times more effective than placebo in achieving sustained withdrawal from smoking (e.g. 25% vs. 9% in one trial.[3] Treatment is much more likely to be successful if it is used as an aid to, not a substitute for, continued counselling. Some reinforcement may be provided by the high cost of treatment, likely to be several hundred US dollars for the recommended 3–4 months, and which is not reimbursable by health care providers in most

---

[2] Cohen L H et al 1944 Archives of Neurology and Psychiatry 51: 171.

[3] Sachs D P et al 1993 Archives of Internal Medicine 153: 1881.

---

[1] Harris M et al 1943 Archives of Neurology and Psychiatry 50: 304.

countries. Of course, compared to the financial, not to mention physical, costs of smoking, the investment is trivial! Subjects should, of course, not smoke when using nicotine formulations.

Pilocarpine, from an American plant (*Pilocarpus* spp.), acts directly on end-organs innervated by postganglionic nerves (parasympathetic system plus sweat glands); it also stimulates and then depresses the central nervous system. The chief clinical use of pilocarpine is to lower intraocular pressure in chronic simple glaucoma, as an adjunct to a topical β-blocker; it produces miosis, opens drainage channels in the trabecular network and improves the outflow of aqueous humour. Oral pilocarpine is available for the treatment of xerostomia (dry mouth) in Sjogren's syndrome, or following irradiation of head and neck tumours. The commonest adverse effect is sweating; adverse cardiac effects have not been reported.

Arecoline is an alkaloid in the betel nut which is chewed in the East. It produces a mild dependence for, like other parasympathomimetic drugs, it stimulates the brain.

Muscarine is of no therapeutic use but it has pharmacological interest. It is present in small amounts in the fungus *Amanita muscaria* (Fly agaric), named after its capacity to kill the domestic fly (*Musca domestica*); muscarine was so named because it was thought to be the insecticidal principle, but it is relatively nontoxic to flies (orally administered). The fungus may contain other antimuscarinic substances and GABA-receptor agonists in amounts sufficient to be psychoactive in man.

Poisoning with these fungi may present with antimuscarinic, with cholinergic or with GABA-ergic effects. All have CNS actions. Happily, poisoning by *Amanita muscaria* is seldom serious. Species of *Inocybe* contain larger amounts of muscarine (see Ch. 9).

The lengths to which man is prepared to go in taking 'chemical vacations' when life is hard, are shown by the inhabitants of Eastern Siberia who used *Amanita muscaria* recreationally, for its cerebral stimulant effects. They were apparently prepared to put up with the autonomic actions to escape briefly from reality. The fungus was scarce

in winter and the frugal devotees discovered that by drinking their own urine they could prolong the intoxication. Sometimes, in generous mood, the intoxicated person would offer his urine to others as a treat.

ANTICHOLINESTERASES

In the region of cholinergic nerve endings and in erythrocytes there is an enzyme that specifically destroys acetylcholine, true cholinesterase or acetylcholinesterase. In various tissues, especially blood plasma, there are other esterases which are not specific for acetylcholine but which also destroy other esters, e.g. suxamethonium, procaine. These are called nonspecific or *pseudocholinesterases*. Chemicals which inactivate these esterases (anticholinesterases) are used in medicine and in agriculture as pesticides. They act by allowing naturally formed acetylcholine to accumulate instead of being destroyed and their effects are almost entirely due to this accumulation in the central nervous system, at the neuromuscular junction, autonomic ganglia, postganglionic cholinergic nerve endings (which are principally in the parasympathetic nervous system) and in the walls of blood vessels, where acetylcholine is a local hormone not necessarily associated with nerve endings. Some of these effects oppose each other, e.g. the effect of anticholinesterase on the heart will be the resultant of stimulation at sympathetic ganglia and the opposing effect of stimulation at parasympathetic (vagal) ganglia and at postganglionic nerve endings.

Physostigmine (eserine) is an alkaloid, obtained from the seeds of a West African plant (Physostigma), which has long been used both as a weapon and as an ordeal poison.[4] It acts for a few hours. Physostigmine is used synergistically with pilocarpine to reduce intraocular pressure. It has been shown to have some efficacy in improving cognitive function in Alzheimer type dementia.

Neostigmine (Prostigmin) ($t^{1}\!/_2$ 2 h) is a synthetic

---

[4] To demonstrate guilt or innocence according to whether the accused died or lived after the judicial dose. The practice had the advantage that the demonstration of guilt provided simultaneous punishment.

reversible anticholinesterase whose actions are more prominent on the neuromuscular junction and the alimentary tract than on the cardiovascular system and eye. It is therefore principally used in myasthenia gravis, to stimulate the bowels and bladder after surgery, and as an antidote to competitive neuromuscular blocking agents. Neostigmine is effective orally (5–30 mg, 3 or 4 times a day), and by injection (usually s.c.) 0.5–2.0 mg. But higher doses may be used in myasthenia gravis, often combined with atropine to reduce the unwanted muscarinic effects.

Pyridostigmine (Mestinon) is similar to neostigmine but has a less powerful action that is slower in onset and slightly longer in duration, and perhaps fewer visceral effects. It is used in myasthenia gravis.

Distigmine (Ubretid) is a variant of pyridostigmine (2 linked molecules as the name implies).

Edrophonium (Tensilon) is structurally related to neostigmine but its action is brief and autonomic effects are minimal except at high doses. The drug is used to diagnose *myasthenia gravis* and to differentiate a *myasthenic* crisis (weakness due to inadequate anticholinesterase treatment or severe disease) from a *cholinergic* crisis (weakness caused by overtreatment with an anticholinesterase). Myasthenic weakness is substantially improved by edrophonium whereas cholinergic weakness is aggravated but the effect is transient; the action of 3 mg i.v. is lost in 5 minutes.

Metriphonate is used for urinary schistosomiasis (precise mode of action is uncertain).

A developing new use for anticholinesterase drugs is in the treatment of Alzheimer's disease, where both the degree of dementia and pathological count of number of amyloid plaques correlate with degree of cholinergic involvement. (See p. 335 for a discussion of the use of tacrine.)

Anticholinesterase poisoning

The anticholinesterases used in therapeutics are generally those which reversibly inactivate cholinesterase for a few hours. *Pesticides* of the carbamate type act by reversible inhibition of cholinesterase but organophosphorus compounds inhibit the enzyme almost or completely irreversibly so that recovery depends on formation of fresh enzyme. This process may take weeks although clinical recovery is usually evident in days. Cases of poisoning are usually met outside therapeutic practice, e.g. after agricultural, industrial or transport accidents. Substances of this type have also been developed and used in war, especially the 3 G agents, GA (tabun), GB (sarin) and GD (soman). Although called nerve 'gas', they are actually volatile liquids, which facilitates their use.[5] Where there is known risk of exposure prior use of pyridostigmine, which occupies cholinesterases reversibly for a few hours (the lesser evil), competitively protects them from access by the irreversible warfare agent (the greater evil); soldiers expecting attack have been provided with self-injection loaded syringes. Organophosphorus agents are absorbed through the skin, the gastrointestinal tract and by inhalation. Diagnosis depends on observing a substantial part of the list of actions below.

Typical features involve the gastrointestinal tract (salivation, vomiting, abdominal cramps, diarrhoea, involuntary defaecation), the respiratory system (bronchorrhoea, bronchoconstriction, cough, wheezing, dyspnoea), the cardiovascular system (bradycardia), the genitourinary system (involuntary micturition), the skin (sweating), the skeletal system (muscle weakness, twitching) and the nervous system (miosis, anxiety, headache, convulsions, respiratory failure). Death is due to a combination of the actions in the central nervous system, to paralysis of the respiratory muscles by peripheral depolarisation neuromuscular block, and to excessive bronchial secretions and constriction causing respiratory obstruction. At autopsy, ileal intussusceptions are commonly found.

Treatment. Since the most common circumstance of accidental poisoning is exposure to pesticide spray or spillage, contaminated clothing should be

---

[5] In recent times, there have been major instances of use against populations by both military and terrorist bodies (in the field and in an underground transport system).

removed and the skin washed. Gastric lavage is needed if any of the substance has been ingested. Attendants should take care to ensure that they themselves do not become contaminated.

- *Atropine* is the mainstay of treatment; 2 mg is given i.m. or i.v. as soon as possible and repeated every 15–60 min until dryness of the mouth and a heart rate in excess of 70 beats per minute indicate that its effect is adequate. A poisoned patient may require 100 mg or more for a single episode. Atropine antagonises the parasympathomimetic effects of the poison, i.e. due to stimulation at postganglionic nerve endings (excessive secretion) and vasodilatation, i.e. the muscarinic actions. Neuromuscular block is not relieved, for atropine does not antagonise acetylcholine at the endings of nerve fibres which arise in the central nervous system (nicotinic effects).
- *Mechanical ventilation* may therefore be needed to assist the respiratory muscles; special attention to the airway is vital because of bronchial constriction and excessive secretion.
- *Diazepam* may be needed for convulsions.
- *Atropine eyedrops* may relieve the headache caused by miosis.
- *Enzyme reactivation*. The organophosphorus pesticides inactivate cholinesterase by irreversibly phosphorylating the active centre of the enzyme. Substances that reactivate the enzyme hasten the destruction of the accumulated acetylcholine and, unlike atropine, they have both antinicotinic and antimuscarinic effects. The principal agent is *pralidoxime*, 1.0 g of which should be given 4-hourly i.m. or (diluted) by slow i.v. infusion, as indicated by the patient's condition; efficacy is best if it is administered within 12 hours of poisoning and is probably valueless after 24 hours for by then insecticide and enzyme are irreversibly bound. Muscle power may improve within 30 min.

Poisoning with *reversible* anticholinesterases is appropriately treated by atropine and the necessary general support; it lasts only hours.

In poisoning with *irreversible* agents, erythrocyte or plasma cholinesterase content should be measured if possible, both for diagnosis and to determine when a poisoned worker may return to his task in the event of his being willing to do so. This should not be allowed until the cholinesterase exceeds 70% of normal, which may take several weeks.

DISORDERS OF NEUROMUSCULAR TRANSMISSION

Myasthenia gravis

In myasthenia gravis synaptic transmission at the neuromuscular junction is impaired; most cases appear to have an autoimmune basis, for 90% of patients have a raised titre of autoantibodies to the acetylcholine receptor; but the condition is probably heterogeneous as a minority do not have antibodies.

Neostigmine was introduced in 1931 for its stimulant effects on intestinal activity. In 1934 it occurred to Dr Mary Walker that since the paralysis of myasthenia had been (erroneously) attributed to a curare-like substance in the blood, physostigmine (eserine), an anticholinesterase drug known to antagonise curare, might be beneficial. It was and she reported this important observation in a short letter.[6] Soon after this she used neostigmine by mouth with greater benefit. The sudden appearance of an effective treatment for an hitherto untreatable chronic disease must always be a dramatic event for its victims. The impact of the discovery of the action of neostigmine has been described by one patient.

> My myasthenia started in 1925, when I was 18. For several months it consisted of double vision and fatigue . . . An ophthalmic surgeon . . . prescribed glasses with a prism. However, soon more alarming symptoms began. [Her limbs became weak and she] 'was sent to an eminent neurologist. This was a horrible experience. He . . . could find no physical signs . . . declared me to be suffering from hysteria and asked me what was on my mind. When I answered truthfully, that nothing except anxiety over my symptoms, he replied 'my dear child, I am not a perfect fool . . .', and showed me out. [She became worse and at times she was unable to turn over in bed. Eating and even speaking were difficult. Eventually, her fiancé, a medical student, read about myasthenia gravis and she was correctly diagnosed in 1927.] There was at

---

[6] Walker M B 1934 Lancet 1: 1200.

that time no known treatment and therefore many things to try. [She had gold injections, thyroid, suprarenal extract, lecithin, glycine and ephedrine. The last had a slight effect.] Then in February 1935, came the day that I shall always remember. I was living alone with a nurse . . . It was one of my better days, and I was lying on the sofa after tea . . . My fiancé came in rather late saying that he had something new for me to try. My first thought was 'Oh bother! Another injection, and another false hope'. I submitted to the injection with complete indifference and within a few minutes began to feel very strange . . . when I lifted my arms, exerting the effort to which I had become accustomed, they shot into the air, every movement I attempted was grotesquely magnified until I learnt to make less effort . . . it was strange, wonderful and at first, very frightening . . . we danced twice round the carpet. That was my first meeting with neostigmine, and we have never since been separated.[7]

Pathogenesis. The clinical features of myasthenia gravis are caused by specific antibodies which either block or cause complement-mediated lysis of the acetylcholine receptor. In common with all body tissues, receptors are constantly being broken down and resynthesised. Cholinoceptors exist for about 7 days in normal individuals but for only one day in myasthenic patients. The thymus gland is in some way involved in the process and three-quarters of patients have either thymitis or a thymoma.

Diagnosis is made with the anticholinesterase drug, edrophonium, which dramatically and transiently (5 min) relieves muscular weakness. A syringe is loaded with edrophonium 10 mg; 2 mg are given i.v. and if there is no improvement in weakness in 30 s the remaining 8 mg are injected. A syringe loaded with atropine should be at hand to block severe cholinergic autonomic (muscarinic) effects, e.g. bradycardia, should they occur. Acetylcholine receptor antibodies should also be measured in the plasma for an elevated titre confirms the diagnosis.

Treatment involves immunosuppression, thymec-

tomy (unless contraindicated) and symptom relief with drugs.

● *Immunosuppressive* treatment is directed at eliminating the acetylcholine receptor antibody. *Prednisolone* induces improvement or remission in 80% of cases. The dose should be increased slowly using an alternate day regimen until the minimum effective amount is attained; an immunosuppressive improvement may take several weeks. *Azathioprine* may be used as a steroid-sparing agent. Prednisolone is effective for ocular myasthenia, which is fortunate, for this variant of the disease responds poorly to thymectomy or anticholinesterase drugs. Some acute and severe cases respond poorly to prednisolone with azathioprine and, for these, intermittent plasmapheresis (to remove circulating antibody) can provide dramatic short-term relief.

● *Thymectomy* should be offered once the clinical state allows and unless there are powerful contraindications to surgery, for most cases benefit and about 25% can discontinue drug treatment. Thymectomy should also be undertaken in all myasthenic patients who have a thymoma, but the main reason is to prevent local infiltration for the procedure is less likely to relieve the myasthenia.

● *Symptomatic* drug treatment is decreasingly used. Its aim is to increase the concentration of acetylcholine at the neuromuscular junction with anticholinesterase drugs. The mainstay is usually *pyridostigmine*, starting with 60 mg by mouth 6-hourly. It is preferred because its action is smoother than that of neostigmine, but the latter is more rapid in onset and can with advantage be given in the mornings to get the patient mobile. Either drug can be given parenterally if bulbar paralysis makes swallowing difficult. An antimuscarinic drug, e.g. propantheline, should be added if muscarinic effects are troublesome.

Too high a dose of anticholinesterase drugs may make the weakness worse by causing excess build-up of acetylcholine (*cholinergic crisis*) and it is important to distinguish this from an exacerbation of the disease (*myasthenic crisis*). A dose of edrophonium will make the diagnosis; a myasthenic crisis gets better and cholinergic crisis gets worse — dangerously so if the vital bulbar and respiratory muscles are involved; this test is best left to those with

---

[7] Disabilities and how to live with them. Lancet Publications (1952), London.

special experience, and mechanical ventilation facilities should be at hand.

A cholinergic crisis should be treated by withdrawing all anticholinesterase medication, mechanical respiration if required, and atropine i.v. for muscarinic effects of the overdosage. The neuromuscular block is a nicotinic effect and will be unchanged by atropine. A resistant myasthenic crisis may be treated by withdrawal of drugs and artificial respiration for a few days. Plasmapheresis may be beneficial by removing antibodies.

Lambert-Eaton syndrome

Separate from myasthenia gravis is the Lambert-Eaton syndrome, where similar symptoms to those in myasthenia gravis occur in association with a carcinoma; in 60% of patients this is a small-cell lung cancer. In this syndrome, there is a deficiency of acetylcholine release, not response, due to an antibody directed against voltage-gated calcium channels.

Patients with the Lambert-Eaton syndrome do not usually respond well to anticholinesterases. 3,4-Diaminopyridine (3,4-DAP) increases neurotransmitter release and also the action potential (by blocking potassium conductance); these actions lead to a nonspecific excitatory effect on the cholinergic system. It needs to be taken, orally, 4–5 times daily; adverse effects due to CNS excitation (insomnia, seizures) can occur. 3,4-DAP is an example of an orphan drug without product licence, available for 'named patient' use in the UK from the pharmacy at the Radcliffe Infirmary, Oxford.

Drug-induced disorders of neuromuscular transmission

Quite apart from the neuromuscular blocking agents used in anaesthesia, a number of drugs possess actions that impair neuromuscular transmission and, in appropriate circumstances, give rise to:

- postoperative respiratory depression in people whose neuromuscular transmission is otherwise normal
- aggravation or unmasking of myasthenia gravis
- a drug-induced myasthenic syndrome.

These drugs include:

Antibiotics: Aminoglycosides (neomycin, streptomycin, gentamicin), polypeptides (colistin, polymyxin B) and perhaps the 4-quinolones (e.g. ciprofloxacin) may cause postoperative breathing difficulty if they are instilled into the peritoneal or pleural cavities. It appears that the antibiotics both interfere with the release of acetylcholine and also have a competitive curare-like effect on the acetylcholine receptor.

Cardiovascular drugs: Those that possess local anaesthetic properties (quinidine, procainamide, lignocaine) and certain β-blockers (propranolol, oxprenolol) act by interfering with acetylcholine release and may aggravate or reveal myasthenia gravis.

Other drugs: *Penicillamine* causes some patients, especially those with rheumatoid arthritis, to form antibodies to the acetylcholine receptor and a syndrome indistinguishable from myasthenia gravis results. Spontaneous recovery occurs in about two-thirds of cases when penicillamine is withdrawn. *Phenytoin* may rarely induce or aggravate myasthenia gravis, or induce a myasthenic syndrome, possibly by depressing acetylcholine release. *Lithium* may impair presynaptic neurotransmission by substituting for sodium ions in the nerve terminal.

Drugs which oppose acetylcholine

These may be divided into:

Antimuscarinic drugs which act principally at postganglionic cholinergic (parasympathetic) nerve endings, i.e. atropine-related drugs (see Fig. 22.1, site 2). Muscarinic receptors can be subdivided into M_1, M_2 and M_3 whose principal sites are, respectively, in the brain, heart and smooth muscle cells. As with many receptors, the molecular basis of the subtypes has been defined together with two further subtypes (M_4 and M_5) for which no functional counterpart has yet been described.

Antinicotinic drugs

Ganglion-blocking drugs (Fig. 22.1, site 1) (see Ch. 24)

Neuromuscular blocking drugs (Fig. 22.1, site 5) (see Ch. 21).

ANTIMUSCARINIC DRUGS

The principal effect of atropine and related drugs is to block competitively the binding of acetylcholine to receptors at the postganglionic cholinergic (parasympathetic) endings (Fig. 22.1, site 2) and at the noninnervated receptors on blood vessels; hence their description as antimuscarinic drugs. They also block effects of acetylcholine in the central nervous system; some have a blocking effect at autonomic ganglia also, but none blocks the neuromuscular junction at clinical doses.

The actions of atropine will first be described; other drugs will be dealt with chiefly in so far as they differ. Many antimuscarinic drugs have a variety of other actions, e.g. antihistamine, but find a place in therapeutics as antimuscarinic agents.

Atropine

Atropine ($t\frac{1}{2}$ 2 h) is an alkaloid from the plant *Atropa belladonna.*[8] In general, the effects of atropine are inhibitory but in large doses it stimulates the CNS (see poisoning, below). Atropine also blocks the muscarinic effects of injected cholinergic drugs both peripherally and on the central nervous system. The clinically important actions of atropine at parasympathetic postganglionic nerve endings are listed below; they are mostly the opposite of the activating effects on the parasympathetic system produced by cholinergic drugs.

Exocrine glands. All secretions except milk are diminished. Dry mouth and dry eye are common.

---

[8] The first name commemorates its success as a homicidal poison, for it is derived from the senior of three legendary Fates, Atropos, who cuts with shears the web of life spun and woven by her sisters Clotho and Lachesis (there is a minor synthetic atropine-like drug called lachesine). The term belladonna (Italian: beautiful woman) refers to the once fashionable female practice of using an extract of the plant to dilate the pupils (incidentally blocking ocular accommodation) as part of the process of making herself attractive.

USES OF ANTIMUSCARINIC DRUGS

- **For their actions in the central nervous system** some (benzhexol, orphenadrine) are used against the rigidity and tremor of *parkinsonism*, in which disease doses higher than the usual therapeutic amounts are often needed and tolerated.

    They are used as *antiemetics* (principally hyoscine, promethazine). Their *sedative* action is used in anaesthetic premedication (hyoscine).

- **For their peripheral actions**, atropine, homatropine and cyclopentolate are used in *ophthalmology* to dilate the pupil and to paralyse ocular accommodation. Patients should be warned of a transient, but unpleasant stinging sensation, and that they cannot read or drive (at least without dark glasses) for at least 3–4 hours. Tropicamide is the shortest acting of the mydriatics. If it is desired to dilate the pupil and to spare accommodation, a sympathomimetic, e.g. phenylephrine, is useful.

    In *anaesthesia*, atropine, glycopyrronium and hyoscine block the vagus and reduce secretion.

    In the *respiratory tract* ipratropium is an effective bronchodilator.

- **For their actions on the alimentary tract** against muscle spasm and hypermotility, e.g. against colic (pain due to spasm of smooth muscle) and to reduce morphine-induced smooth muscle spasm when the analgesic is used against acute colic.

- **In the urinary tract**, flavoxate, propantheline and oxybutynin are used to relieve muscle spasm accompanying infection in cystitis, and for detrusor instability.

- In disorders of the **cardiovascular system** atropine is useful in bradycardia following myocardial infarction.

- In **cholinergic poisoning**, atropine is an important antagonist of both central nervous, parasympathomimetic and vasodilator effects though it has no effect at the neuromuscular junction and will not prevent voluntary muscle paralysis. It is also used to block muscarinic effects when cholinergic drugs, such as neostigmine, are used for their effect on the neuromuscular junction in myasthenia gravis.

Disadvantages of the antimuscarinics include glaucoma, and urinary retention where there is prostatic hypertrophy.

Gastric acid secretion is reduced but so also is the total volume of gastric secretion so that H$^+$ concentration (pH) may be little altered. *Sweating* (sympathetic nerve supply, but largely cholinergic) is inhibited. *Bronchial* secretions are reduced and may become viscid, which can be a disadvantage, as removal of secretion by cough and ciliary action is rendered less effective.

Smooth muscle is relaxed. In the gastrointestinal tract there is reduction of tone and peristalsis. Muscle spasm of the intestinal tract induced by morphine is reduced, but such spasm in the biliary tract is not significantly affected. Atropine relaxes bronchial muscle, an effect which is useful in some asthmatics. Micturition is slowed and urinary retention may be induced especially when there is pre-existing prostatic enlargement.

Ocular effects. Mydriasis occurs with a rise in intraocular pressure in an eye predisposed to narrow-angle glaucoma (but only rarely in chronic open-angle glaucoma). This is due to the dilated iris blocking drainage of the intraocular fluids from the angle of the anterior chamber. An attack of glaucoma may be induced. There is no significant effect on pressure in normal eyes. The ciliary muscle is paralysed and so the eye is accommodated for distant vision. After atropinisation, normal pupillary reflexes may not be regained for 2 weeks. Atropine is a cause of unequal sized and unresponsive pupils.

Cardiovascular system. Atropine reduces vagal tone thus increasing the heart rate, and enhancing conduction in the bundle of His, effects which are less marked in the elderly in whom vagal tone is low. Full atropinisation may increase rate by 30 beats/min in the young, but has little effect in the old. Transient vagal stimulation, probably in the CNS, may cause bradycardia, e.g. if atropine is given i.v. with neostigmine and the effects of the two drugs summate.

Atropine has no significant effect on peripheral blood vessels in therapeutic doses but, in poisoning, there is marked vasodilatation.

Atropine is effective against both tremor and rigidity of *parkinsonism*. It prevents or abates *motion sickness*.

Antagonism to cholinergic drugs. Atropine opposes the effects of all cholinergic drugs on the CNS, at postganglionic cholinergic nerve endings and on the peripheral blood vessels. It does not oppose cholinergic effects at the neuromuscular junction or significantly at the autonomic ganglia, i.e. atropine opposes the muscarine-like but not the nicotine-like effects of acetylcholine.

Pharmacokinetics. Atropine is readily absorbed from the alimentary tract and may also be injected by the usual routes. The occasional cases of atropine poisoning following use of eye drops are due to the solution running down the lacrimal ducts into the nose and being swallowed. Atropine is in part destroyed in the liver and in part excreted unchanged by the kidney (t½ 2 h).

Dose. 0.25–2.0 mg by mouth or 0.4–1.0 mg i.v.; for chronic use it has largely been replaced by other antimuscarinic drugs.

Poisoning with atropine (and other antimuscarinic drugs) presents with the more obvious peripheral effects: dry mouth (with dysphagia), mydriasis, blurred vision, hot, flushed, dry skin, and, in addition, hyperthermia (CNS action plus absence of sweating), restlessness, anxiety, excitement, hallucinations, delirium, mania. The cerebral excitation is followed by depression and coma or, as it has been described with characteristic American verbal felicity, 'hot as a hare, blind as a bat, dry as a bone, red as a beet and mad as a hen.[9] It may occur in children who have eaten berries of solanaceous plants, e.g. deadly nightshade and henbane. When the diagnosis is doubtful, it is said to be worth putting a drop of the patient's urine in one eye of a cat. Mydriasis, if it results, confirms the diagnosis, but absence of effect proves nothing.

Treatment of atropine poisoning involves giving activated charcoal to adsorb the drug, and diazepam for excitement.

Other antimuscarinic drugs

In the following accounts of drugs, the principal peripheral atropine-like effects of the drugs may be assumed; differences from atropine are described.

Hyoscyamine is less active in the central nervous system. Atropine is racemic hyoscyamine;

---

[9] Cohen et al 1944 Archives of Neurology and Psychiatry 51: 171.

'hyoscyamine' is the laevo form; the dextro form is only feebly active. Atropine is more stable chemically and so is preferred.

Hyoscine (scopolamine) is structurally related to atropine. It differs chiefly in being a central nervous system depressant, although it may sometimes cause excitement. The old are often confused by hyoscine and so it is avoided in their anaesthetic premedication. Mydriasis is briefer than with atropine.

Hyoscine butylbromide (Buscopan) also blocks autonomic ganglia. If injected, it is an effective relaxant of smooth muscle, including the cardia in achalasia, the pyloric antral region and the colon, which properties are utilised by radiologists and endoscopists. It may sometimes be useful for colic.

Homatropine is used for its ocular effects (1% and 2% solutions as eye drops). Its action is shorter than atropine and therefore less likely to cause serious rise of intraocular pressure; the effect wears off in a day or two. Complete cycloplegia cannot always be obtained unless repeated instillations are made every 15 min for 1–2 h. It is especially unreliable in children, in whom cyclopentolate or atropine is preferred. The pupillary dilation may be reversed by physostigmine eyedrops.

Tropicamide (Mydriacyl) and *cyclopentolate* (Mydrilate) are useful (as 0.5 or 1% solutions) for mydriasis and cycloplegia. They are quicker and shorter acting than is homatropine. The differences between the two are trivial. Mydriasis occurs in 10–20 min and cycloplegia shortly after. The duration of action is 4–12 h.

Ipratropium (Atrovent) is used by inhalation as a bronchodilator, and can be useful when cough is a pronounced symptom in an asthmatic patient.

Flavoxate (Urispas) is used for urinary frequency, tenesmus and urgency incontinence because it increases bladder capacity and reduces unstable detrusor contractions (see Ch. 27).

Oxybutynin is also used for detrusor instability, but antimuscarinic adverse effects may limit its value.

Glycopyrronium is used in anaesthetic premedication to reduce salivary secretion; given i.v. it causes less tachycardia than does atropine.

Propantheline (Pro-Banthine) also has ganglion-blocking properties. It may be used as a smooth muscle relaxant, e.g. for irritable bowel syndrome and diagnostic procedures.

Dicyclomine (Merbentyl) is an alternative.

Benzhexol and orphenadrine: see parkinsonism.

Promethazine: see page 506.

Oral antimuscarinics have occasional use in the treatment of *hyperhidrosis*, and of peptic ulcer in patients intolerant of more modern therapies, e.g. pirenzepine (p. 570).

SUMMARY

- Acetylcholine is the most important receptor agonist neurotransmitter in both the brain and peripheral nervous system.
- It acts on neurons in the CNS and at autonomic ganglia, on skeletal muscle at the neuromuscular junction, and at a variety of other effector cell types, mainly glandular or smooth muscle.
- The effector response is rapidly terminated through enzymatic destruction by acetylcholinesterase.
- Outside the CNS, acetylcholine has 2 main classes of receptor: those on autonomic ganglia and skeletal muscle responding to stimulation by nicotine and the rest that respond to stimulation by muscarine.
- Drugs which mimic or oppose acetylcholine have a wide variety of uses. For instance, the muscarinic agonists (e.g. pilocarpine) and antagonists (e.g. atropine) stimulate or inhibit glandular secretions, and reverse vagal slowing of the heart (atropine).
- The main use of drugs at the neuromuscular junction is to relax muscle in anaesthesia, or to inhibit acetylcholinesterase in diseases where nicotinic receptor activation is reduced, e.g. myasthenia gravis.

GUIDE TO FURTHER READING

Cohen H L et al 1944 Acetylcholine treatment of schizophrenia. Archives of Neurology and Psychiatry 51: 171

Davis K L 1995 Tacrine. Lancet 345: 625–630

Drachman D B 1994 Myasthenia gravis. New England Journal of Medicine 330: 1797–1810

Goyal R K 1989 Muscarinic receptor subtypes. New England Journal of Medicine 321: 1022

Hawkins J R et al 1956 Intravenous acetylcholine therapy in neurosis. A controlled trial (p. 43); Carbon dioxide inhalation therapy in neurosis. A controlled clinical trial (p. 52); The placebo response (p. 60). Journal of Mental Science 102: 43

HMSO 1987 Medical manual of defence against chemical agents. (No. 0117725692) JSP: 312

Lambert D 1981 (personal paper) Myasthenia gravis. Lancet 1: 937

Morita H et al 1996 Sarin poisoning in Matsumoto, Japan. Lancet 346: 290–293

Morton H G et al 1939 Atropine intoxication. Journal of Pediatrics 14: 755

Adrenergic mechanisms (sympathomimetics, shock, hypotension)

SYNOPSIS

Anyone who administers drugs acting on cardiovascular adrenergic mechanisms requires an understanding of how they act in order to use them to the best advantage and with safety.

- Adrenergic mechanisms
- Classification of sympathomimetics: by mode of action and selectivity for adrenoceptors
- Individual sympathomimetics
- Mucosal decongestants
- Shock
- Chronic orthostatic hypotension

Adrenergic mechanisms

The discovery in 1895 of the hypertensive effect of adrenaline (epinephrine) was initiated by Dr Oliver, a physician in practice, who conducted a series of experiments on his young son into whom he injected an extract of bovine suprarenal. The effect was confirmed in animals and led eventually to the isolation and synthesis of adrenaline in the early 1900s. Many related compounds were examined and, in 1910, Barger and Dale invented the word *sympathomimetic*[1] and also pointed out that noradrenaline mimicked the action of the sympa-

thetic nervous system more closely than did adrenaline.

Adrenaline, noradrenaline and dopamine are formed in the body and are used in therapeutics. The natural synthetic path is:

tyrosine → dopa → **dopamine** → **noradrenaline** → **adrenaline**.

Classification of sympathomimetics

BY MODE OF ACTION

Noradrenaline is synthesised and stored in adrenergic nerve terminals and can be released from these stores by stimulating the nerve or by drugs (ephedrine, amphetamine). These noradrenaline stores may be replenished by i.v. infusion of noradrenaline, and abolished by reserpine or by cutting the sympathetic neuron.

Sympathomimetics may be classified as those that act:

---

[1] 'Compounds which ... simulate the effects of sympathetic nerves not only with varying intensity but with varying precision ... a term ... seems needed to indicate the types of action common to these bases. We propose to call it "sympathomimetic". A term which indicates the relation of the action to innervation by the sympathetic system, without involving any theoretical preconception as to the meaning of that relation or the precise mechanism of the action.' Barger G, Dale H H 1910 Journal of Physiology XLI: 19–50.

1. **directly**, i.e. *adrenoceptor agonists* (adrenaline, noradrenaline, isoprenaline (isoproterenol), methoxamine, xylometazoline, oxymetazoline, metaraminol, entirely; and dopamine and phenylephrine mainly)
2. **indirectly**, by causing a release of noradrenaline from stores at nerve endings (amphetamines, tyramine; and ephedrine, largely)
3. **by both mechanisms** (1) and (2), though often with a preponderance of one or other: other synthetic agents.

It is evident that *tachyphylaxis* (diminishing response to frequent or continuous administration) is particularly to be expected with drugs in group 2, and that they are less suitable for use in maintaining blood pressure than drugs of group 1. Tachyphylaxis to group 1 may be due to receptor changes.

Interactions of sympathomimetics with other drugs affecting the vascular system are complex. Some drugs prevent the uptake of noradrenaline from the circulation into stores (this may account for the potentiation of the pressor effect of administered noradrenaline by tricyclic antidepressants) and some drugs deplete or destroy the stores (reserpine) and thus block the action of sympathomimetics that act by releasing noradrenaline from stores. Some drugs will act differently after acute and after chronic administration, according to whether the noradrenaline stores are depleted or not, and receptors may change in number and activity; and there are subclasses of receptors.

Many sympathomimetics are racemic compounds and one form is commonly much more active: for instance levo-noradrenaline is at least 50 times as active as the dextro form.

History. Up to 1958 it was known that the peripheral motor (vasoconstriction) effects of adrenaline were preventable and that the peripheral inhibitory (vasodilatation) and the cardiac stimulant actions were not preventable by the then available antagonists (ergot alkaloids, phenoxybenzamine).

In 1948, Ahlquist introduced a hypothesis to account for this. He proposed two different sorts of adrenoceptors (α and β). For a further 10 years, only antagonists of α-receptor effects (α-adrenoceptor block) were known, but in 1958 the first substance selectively and competitively to prevent β-receptor effects (β-adrenoceptor block), dichloroisoprenaline, was synthesised. However, it was unsuitable for clinical use (it also had strong agonist activity, i.e. it was a partial agonist or agonist/antagonist), and it was not until 1962 that the first reasonably satisfactory β-adrenoceptor blocker (pronethalol) was introduced to medicine. Unfortunately it had a low therapeutic index and was carcinogenic in mice, and was soon replaced by propranolol (Inderal).

It is evident that the site of action has an important role in selectivity, e.g. drugs that act on end-organ receptors *directly* and stereospecifically may be highly selective, whereas drugs that act *indirectly* by discharging noradrenaline indiscriminately from nerve endings, e.g. amphetamine, will have a wider range of effects.

Subclassification of adrenoceptors is shown in Table 23.1.

Consequences of activating the adrenoceptor

Catecholamines (adrenaline, noradrenaline, dopamine) act at β-adrenoceptors as *first messenger* transmitters, combining with receptors on the outside of the cell membrane of the end-organ, thus activating the enzyme adenylyl cyclase on the inside of the cell membrane, which causes an increase in intracellular cyclic AMP, the *second messenger* (destroyed by intracellular phosphodiesterase[2]). This second messenger initiates a sequence (cascade) of changes that differ among tissues. They include contraction of cardiac muscle, relaxation of vascular and bronchial smooth muscles, and release of glucose or potassium from liver cells. Many hormones act via cyclic AMP. Specificity is provided by the receptor, not by the messengers. Mechanisms of action at α_1- and α_2-adrenoceptors differ in detail.

Complexity of adrenergic mechanisms

Drugs may mimic or impair adrenergic mechanisms:

---

[2] Aminophylline (in high does only) inhibits phosphodiesterase and so enhances cyclic AMP concentrations. In the treatment of asthma with a β-receptor agonist plus aminophylline there is thus a desired interaction on the bronchi, but an undesired interaction on the heart.

Table 23.1 Clinically relevant aspects of adrenoceptor functions and actions of agonists and antagonists

α_1-adrenoceptor effects[1]	β-adrenoceptor effects
Eye:[2] mydriasis	**Heart (β_1, β_2)**[3] increased *rate* (SA node) increased *automaticity* (AV node and muscle) increased *velocity* in conducting tissue increased *contractility* of myocardium increased O_2 consumption decreased *refractory period* of all tissues
Arterioles: constriction (only slight in coronary and cerebral)	**Arterioles:** dilatation (β_2) **Bronchi** (β_2): relaxation **Anti-inflammatory effect:** inhibition of release of autacoids (histamine, leukotrienes) from mast cells, e.g. asthma in type I allergy
Uterus: contraction (pregnant)	**Uterus** (β_2): relaxation (pregnant)
	Skeletal muscle: tremor (β_2)
Skin: sweat, pilomotor	
Male ejaculation	**Blood platelet**: aggregation
Metabolic effect: hyperkalaemia	**Metabolic effects:** hypokalaemia (β_2) hepatic glycogenolysis (β_2) lipolysis (β_1, β_2)
Bladder sphincter: contraction	**Bladder detrusor**: relaxation

Intestinal smooth muscle relaxation is mediated by α- and β-adrenoceptors.

α_2-**adrenoceptor effects**:[1] α_2-receptors on the nerve ending, i.e. presynaptic autoreceptors mediate negative feedback which inhibits noradrenaline release.

---

[1] For the role of subtypes (α_1 and α_2) see prazosin.

[2] Effects on intraocular pressure involve both α- and ß-adrenoceptors as well as cholinoceptors.

[3] Cardiac β_1-receptors mediate effects of sympathetic nerve stimulation. Cardiac β_2-receptors mediate effects of circulating adrenaline, when this is secreted at a sufficient rate, e.g. following a myocardial infarction or in heart failure. Both receptors are coupled to the same intracellular signalling pathway (cyclic AMP production) and mediate the same biological effects.

The use of the term *cardioselective* to mean β_1-receptor selective only, especially in the case of β-receptor blocking drugs, is no longer appropriate. Although in most species the β_1-receptor is the only cardiac β-receptor, this is not the case in humans. What is not generally appreciated is that the endogenous sympathetic neurotransmitter, noradrenaline, has about a 20-fold selectivity for the β_1-receptor — similar to that of the antagonist, atenolol — with the consequence that under most circumstances, in most tissues, there is little or no β_2-receptor stimulation to be affected by a nonselective β-blocker. Why asthmatics should be so sensitive to β-blockade is paradoxical: all the bronchial β-receptors are β_2, and the bronchi themselves are not innervated by adrenergic fibres; the circulating adrenaline levels are, if anything, low in asthma.

- *directly,* binding on adrenoceptors: agonist (adrenaline) or antagonist (propranolol)
- *indirectly,* by discharging noradrenaline stored in nerve endings[3] (amphetamine)
- by preventing re-uptake into the adrenergic nerve ending of released noradrenaline (and dopamine) in the nerve ending (cocaine, tricyclic antidepressants)
- by preventing the destruction of noradrenaline (and dopamine) in the nerve ending (monamine oxidase inhibitors)
- by depleting the stores of noradrenaline in nerve endings (reserpine)

---

[3] Fatal hypertension can occur when this class of agent is taken by a patient treated with monoamine oxidase inhibitor.

- by preventing the release of noradrenaline from nerve endings in response to a nerve impulse (guanethidine)
- by causing the nerve ending to synthesise a false transmitter instead of noradrenaline (methyldopa)
- by blocking sympathetic autonomic ganglia (pentolinium, trimetaphan).

All the above mechanisms operate in both the *central* and *peripheral* nervous systems. This discussion is chiefly concerned with agents that influence peripheral adrenergic mechanisms.

SELECTIVITY FOR ADRENOCEPTORS

The following classification of sympathomimetics and antagonists is based on selectivity for receptors and on use. But selectivity is relative, not absolute; some agents act on both α- and β-receptors, some are partial agonists and, if enough is administered, many will extend their range; the same applies to selective antagonists (receptor blockers); e.g. a β_1-selective adrenoceptor blocker can cause severe exacerbation of asthma (β_2) even at low dose. It is important to remember this because patients have died in the hands of doctors who have forgotten or been ignorant of it.[4]

Adrenoceptor agonists (Table 23.1)

$\alpha + \beta$ **effects, nonselective: adrenaline (epinephrine)** is now used as vasoconstrictor (α) with local anaesthetics, as a mydriatic and in the emergency treatment of anaphylactic shock, for which condition it has the right mix of effects (bronchodilator, positive cardiac inotropic, vasoconstriction at high dose); it has been superseded for asthma by more selective (β_2) agents.

α_1 **effects: noradrenaline** (with slight β effect on heart) is best left to its essential role in physiology;

---

[4] While it is simplest to regard the selectivity of a drug as relative, being lost at higher doses, it is more strictly correct to point out that it is the *benefits* of the receptor selectivity of an agonist or antagonist which are dose-dependent. A 10-fold selectivity of an agonist at the β_1-receptor, for instance, is a property of the agonist independent of its dose, and means simply that 10 times less of the agonist is required to activate this receptor compared to the β_2-subtype.

it is selectively released where it is wanted. As a therapeutic agent it has been almost entirely superseded for hypotensive states by dopamine and dobutamine; also having predominantly α_1 effects are methoxamine and imidazolines (xylometazoline, oxymetazoline), metaraminol, phenylephrine, phenylpropanolamine, ephedrine, pseudoephedrine: some are used solely for topical vasoconstriction (nasal decongestants).

α_2 **effects in the central nervous system:** clonidine.

β **effects, nonselective** (i.e. $\beta_1 + \beta_2$): **isoprenaline (isoproterenol).** Its uses as bronchodilator (β_2), for positive cardiac inotropic effect and to enhance conduction in heart block (β_1, β_2) have been largely superseded by agents with a more appropriately selective profile of effects. Other agents with nonselective β effects: ephedrine, orciprenaline are also obsolescent for asthma.

β_1 **effects, with some α effects:** dopamine, used in vascular shock.

β_1 **effects:** dobutamine, used for cardiac inotropic effect.

β_2 **effects,** used in *asthma*, or to relax the *uterus*, include: salbutamol, terbutaline, fenoterol, pirbuterol, reproterol, rimiterol, isoxsuprine, orciprenaline, ritodrine.

Adrenoceptor antagonists (blockers)
See page 435

Effects of a sympathomimetic

The *overall effect* of a sympathomimetic depends on the *site* of action (receptor agonist or indirect action), on *receptor specificity* and on *dose*; for instance adrenaline ordinarily dilates muscle blood vessels (β_2; mainly arterioles, but veins also) but in very large doses constricts them (α). The end results are often complex and unpredictable, partly because of the variability of homeostatic reflex responses and partly because what is observed, e.g. a change in blood pressure, is the result of many factors, e.g. vasodilatation [β] in some areas, vasoconstriction [α] in others, and cardiac stimulation [β].

To block all the effects of adrenaline and noradrenaline, antagonists for both α- and β-receptors must be used. This can be a matter of practical importance, e.g. in phaeochromocytoma.

Adverse effects may be deduced from their actions (Table 23.1, Fig. 23.1). Tissue necrosis due to intense vasoconstriction (α) around injection sites occurs as a result of leakage from i.v. infusions. The effects on the heart (β₁) include tachycardia, palpitations, cardiac dysrhythmias including ventricular tachycardia and fibrillation, and muscle tremor (β₂). Sympathomimetic drugs should be used with great caution in patients with heart disease.

Sympathomimetics are particularly likely to cause cardiac dysrhythmias (β₁) in patients under halothane anaesthesia. The effect of the sympathomimetic drugs on the pregnant uterus is variable and difficult to predict, but serious fetal distress can occur, due to reduced placental blood flow as a result both of contraction of the uterine muscle (α) and arterial constriction (α). β₂-agonists are used to relax the uterus in premature labour, but unwanted cardiovascular actions can be troublesome.

Sympathomimetics and plasma potassium. Adrenergic mechanisms have a role in the physiological control of plasma potassium concentration. The biochemical pump that shifts K into cells is activated by β₂-adrenoceptor agonists (adrenaline, salbutamol, isoxsuprine) and can cause hypo-kalaemia. The effect is blocked by β₂-adrenoceptor antagonists.

The hypokalaemia effects of administered (β₂) sympathomimetics may be clinically important, particularly in patients having pre-existing hypokalaemia, e.g. due to intense adrenergic activity such as occurs in myocardial infarction,[5] in fright

---

[5] Normal subjects, infused i.v. with adrenaline in amounts that approximate to those found in the plasma after severe myocardial infarction, show a fall in plasma K of about 0.8 mmol/l (Brown M J 1983 New England Journal of Medicine 309: 1414).

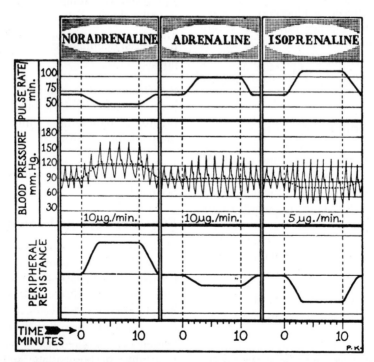

Fig. 23.1 Cardiovascular effects of noradrenaline (norepinephrine), adrenaline (epinephrine) and isoprenaline (isoproterenol): pulse rate/min, blood pressure in mmHg (dotted line is mean pressure), peripheral resistance in arbitrary units.

The differences are due to the differential α and β agonist selectivities of these agents (see text).

(By permission, after Ginsburg J, Cobbold A F 1960 In: Vane J R et al (eds) Adrenergic mechanism. Churchill, London)

(admission to hospital is accompanied by transient hypokalaemia), or with previous diuretic therapy, and taking digoxin. In such subjects use of a sympathomimetic infusion or of an adrenaline-containing local anaesthetic may precipitate cardiac dysrhythmia. Hypokalaemia may occur during treatment of severe asthma, particularly where the β_2-receptor agonist is combined with theophylline.

β-adrenoceptor blockers, as expected, enhance the hyperkalaemia of muscular exercise; and one of their benefits in preventing cardiac dysrhythmias after myocardial infarction may be due to block of β_2-receptor-induced hypokalaemia.

Pharmacokinetics

Catecholamines (adrenaline, noradrenaline dopamine, dobutamine, isoprenaline) (plasma $t^{1/2}$ approx. 2 min) are metabolised by two enzymes, monoamine oxidase (MAO) and catechol-O-methyltransferase (COMT). These enzymes are present in large amounts in the liver and kidney and account for most of the metabolism of injected catecholamines. MAO is also present in the intestinal mucosa (and in nerve endings, peripheral and central). Because of these enzymes catecholamines are ineffective when swallowed (though isoprenaline in enormous dose can be used by this route to treat heart block: Saventrine); noncatecholamines, e.g. salbutamol, amphetamine, are effective orally.

Physiological note

The termination of action of noradrenaline released at nerve endings is by

- re-uptake into nerve endings where it is stored and also subject to MAO degradation
- diffusion away from the area of the nerve ending and the receptor (junctional cleft)
- metabolism (by extraneuronal MAO and COMT).

These processes are slower than the extraordinarily swift destruction of acetylcholine at the neuromuscular junction by acetylcholinesterase situated outside the cells alongside the receptors. The difference reflects a different physiological requirement; the almost instantaneous (millisecond) responses required of voluntary muscle are not required (indeed might be disastrous) of arteriolar muscle.

Synthetic noncatecholamines in clinical use have $t^{1/2}$ of hours, e.g. salbutamol (albuterol) 4 h, because they are more resistant to enzymatic degradation and conjugation. They may be given orally. They penetrate the central nervous system and may have prominent effects, e.g. amphetamine. Substantial amounts appear in the urine.

Overdose of sympathomimetics

Overdose is treated according to rational consideration of mode and site of action (see Adrenaline, below).

Individual sympathomimetics

The actions are summarised in Table 23.1. The classic, mainly endogenous substances will be described first despite their limited role in therapeutics, and then the more selective analogues that have largely replaced them.

CATECHOLAMINES[6]

For Pharmacokinetics, see above.

Adrenaline (epinephrine)

Adrenaline (epinephrine) (α- and β-adrenoceptor effects) is used

- as a vasoconstrictor with local anaesthetics (1:80 000 or weaker) to prolong their effects (about × 2)
- as a topical mydriatic (sparing accommodation; it also lowers intraocular pressure)
- for allergic reactions, s.c., i.m. (or i.v.).

---

[6] Traditionally catecholamines have had a dual nomenclature (as a consequence of a company patenting the name Adrenalin), broadly European and N. American. The latter has been chosen by the World Health Organization as International Nonproprietary Names (INN) (see Ch. 6), and the European Union has directed member states to use INN. Because uniformity has not yet been achieved and because of the scientific literature we state both classes of name.

The route must be chosen with care. Given s.c. there is intense vasoconstriction, which slows absorption and so prolongs and smooths effects. If there is circulatory collapse (as in anaphylactic shock) absorption will be too much delayed and the i.m. route is preferred; i.v. use requires dilution of the standard solution (1:1000, i.e. 1 mg/ml) and careful, frequent monitoring of heart rate and blood pressure. Intracardiac (or intra-airway) injection is used in cardiac arrest; even though ventricular fibrillation may be provoked, normal rhythm can be restored by electric cardioversion.

In anaphylactic shock adrenaline is used (i.m.) because its mix of actions, cardiovascular and bronchial, provide the best compromise for speed and simplicity of use in an emergency; it may also stabilise mast cell membranes and reduce release of vasoactive autacoids; see page 505.

Adrenaline (topical) decreases intraocular pressure in chronic open-angle glaucoma, as does dipivefrine, an adrenaline ester prodrug. They are contraindicated in closed-angle glaucoma because they are mydriatics. Hyperthyroid patients are intolerant of adrenaline.

Accidental overdose with adrenaline occurs occasionally. It is rationally treated by propranolol to block the cardiac β effects (cardiac dysrhythmia) and phentolamine or chlorpromazine to control the α effects on the peripheral circulation that will be prominent when the β effects are abolished; labetalol would be an alternative. β-adrenoceptor block alone is hazardous as the then unopposed α-receptor vasoconstriction causes (severe) hypertension (see Phaeochromocytoma). Antihypertensives of most other kinds are irrational and some may also potentiate the adrenaline.

Noradrenaline (norepinephrine) (chiefly α and β_1 effects)

The main effect of administered noradrenaline is to raise the blood pressure by constricting the arterioles and so raising the total peripheral resistance, with *reduced bloodflow* (except in coronary arteries which have few α_1-receptors). Though it does have slight cardiac stimulant (β_1) effect, the tachycardia of this is masked by the profound reflex bradycar-

dia caused by the hypertension. Noradrenaline is given by i.v. infusion to obtain a gradual sustained response; the effect of a single i.v. injection would last only a minute or so. It is obsolete except where strong peripheral vasoconstriction is specifically desired, which is very rare. It can cause peripheral gangrene and local necrosis; tachyphylaxis occurs; withdrawal must be gradual. Despite this noradrenaline is still used in a last resort to raise the blood pressure in severely shocked patients. A better alternative in such patients is angiotensin II (Hypertensin).

Isoprenaline (isoproterenol)

Isoprenaline (isopropylnoradrenaline) is a nonselective β-receptor agonist, i.e. it activates both β_1- and β_2-receptors. It relaxes smooth muscle, including that of the blood vessels, has negligible metabolic or vasoconstrictor effects, but a vigorous stimulant effect on the heart. This latter is its main disadvantage in the treatment of bronchial asthma. Its principal uses are in complete heart block and occasionally in cardiogenic shock (hypotension). It can be given by infusion, or as tablets: either to be dissolved under the tongue or as a sustained-release preparation (Saventrine) to be swallowed. In asthma it has been superseded by selective β_2-agonists. (See Pharmacokinetics, above.)

Dopamine

Dopamine is an agonist for specific *dopamine (D_1) receptors* in the CNS and the renal and other vascular beds (dilator); it also activates presynaptic autoreceptors (D_2) which suppress release of noradrenaline. In addition it is an agonist at β_1-adrenoceptors in the heart and at high doses activates β_1-adrenoceptors (vasoconstrictor) and also releases noradrenaline from nerve endings. It is given by continuous i.v. infusion because, like all catecholamines, its $t\frac{1}{2}$ is 2 min. An i.v. infusion (2–5 micrograms/kg/min) causes increased renal blood flow. As the dose rises the heart is stimulated, with tachycardia and increased cardiac output. On the peripheral circulation the combination of effects usually causes overall slight reduction in total peripheral resistance.

This combination of effects renders dopamine a

drug of choice in management of shock (**provided** any intravascular volume deficit has been corrected). But at rates exceeding 5 micrograms/kg/h vasoconstriction and hypertension may occur. An i.v. infusion should start at about 2 micrograms/kg/min and may be increased (by 5–10 micrograms/kg/min) at intervals of 15–30 min until the desired effect or adverse effects occur, e.g. excessive tachycardia or dysrhythmia. Increasingly close monitoring (blood pressure, urine output, etc.) should be conducted as the rate exceeds 5 micrograms/kg/min; it should rarely be taken above 20 micrograms/kg/min. The infusion should be withdrawn gradually over hours to avoid hypotension.

Dopamine is stable for about 24 h in sodium chloride or dextrose; it is inactivated by alkaline solutions, e.g. sodium bicarbonate. Subcutaneous leakage causes vasoconstriction and necrosis and should be treated by local injection of an α-adrenoceptor blocking agent (phentolamine 5 mg, diluted).

It may be mixed with dobutamine.

For CNS aspects of dopamine, agonists and antagonists: see Neuroleptics, Parkinsonism.

Dobutamine is primarily a β_1-adrenoceptor agonist with greater inotropic than chronotropic effects on the heart; it has some α-agonist effect, but less than dopamine. It may be useful in shock (with dopamine) and in low output heart failure (in the absence of severe hypertension).

Dopexamine is a synthetic catecholamine whose principal action is as an agonist for cardiac β_2-adrenoceptors (positive inotropic effect). It is also a weak dopamine agonist (causing renal vasodilatation) and inhibitor of noradrenaline uptake (enhancing noradrenaline's stimulation of cardiac β_1-receptors. It is used for short-term treatment of low cardiac output states, e.g. after cardiac surgery.

NONCATECHOLAMINES

Salbutamol, fenoterol, rimiterol, reproterol, pirbuterol, salmeterol, ritodrine and terbutaline are β-adrenoceptor agonists that are relatively *selective for β_2-receptors*, so that cardiac (chiefly β_1-receptor) effects are less prominent. Tachycardia still occurs because of atrial (sinus node) β_2-receptor stimulation; the β_2-adrenoceptors are less numerous in the ventricle and there is probably less risk of serious ventricular dysrhythmias than with the use of nonselective catecholamines. The synthetic agonists are also longer acting than isoprenaline because they are not substrates for catechol-O-methyltransferase, which methylates catecholamines in the liver. They are used principally in asthma, and to reduce uterine contractions in premature labour.

Salbutamol (see also Asthma)

Salbutamol (Ventolin) ($t^{1/2}$ 4 h) is taken orally, 2–4 mg up to 4 times/d; it also acts quickly by inhalation and the effect can last as long as 4 h, which makes it suitable for both prevention and treatment of asthma. Of an inhaled dose about 20% is absorbed and can cause cardiovascular effects. It can also be given by injection, e.g. in asthma, premature labour (β_2-receptor) and for cardiac inotropic (β_1) effect in heart failure (where the β_2 vasodilator action is also useful). Clinically important hypokalaemia can occur (shift of K into cells). The other drugs above are similar.

Salmeterol (Serevent) is a variant of salbutamol that has additional binding property to a site adjacent to the β_2-adrenoceptor, which results in slow onset and long duration of action (about 12 h) (see p. 509).

Clenbuterol is similar to salbutamol. It has found an unorthodox use as a growth promoter in cattle, and an illicit use for a similar indication in athletes. Liver from treated cattle eaten by humans has caused illness compatible with its pharmacology.[7]

Ephedrine

Ephedrine ($t^{1/2}$ approx. 4 h) is a plant alkaloid with actions similar to adrenaline though it acts indirectly; but it has a relatively greater stimulant effect on the central nervous system in adults, producing alertness, anxiety, insomnia, tremor and nausea. Children may be sleepy when taking it. In practice central effects limit its use as a sympathomimetic in asthma.

Ephedrine is well absorbed when given by

---

[7] Deaths have been reported in farmers who inhaled clenbuterol powder when (illicitly) adding it to cattle food.

mouth and unlike most other sympathomimetics is not much destroyed by the liver: it is largely excreted unchanged by the kidney. It is usually given by mouth but can be injected. It differs from adrenaline principally in that its effects come on more slowly and last longer. Tachyphylaxis occurs, probably because it acts by discharging noradrenaline from stores, which it exhausts.

Ephedrine can be used as a bronchodilator, in heart block, as a mydriatic and as a mucosal vasoconstrictor, but it is being displaced by newer drugs, which are often better for these purposes. It is sometimes useful in myasthenia gravis (adrenergic agents enhance cholinergic neuromuscular transmission). Pseudoephedrine is similar.

Phenylpropanolamine (norephedrine) is similar but with less CNS effect.

Amphetamine (Benzedrine) and dexamphetamine (Dexedrine) act indirectly. They are seldom used for their peripheral effects, which are similar to those of ephedrine, but usually for their effects on the central nervous system (narcolepsy, attention deficit in children). (For a general account of amphetamine, see p. 349.)

Phenylephrine has actions qualitatively similar to noradrenaline but a longer duration of action, up to an hour or so. It can be used as a nasal decongestant (0.25–0.5% solution), but sometimes irritates. In the doses usually given, the central nervous effects are minimal, as are the direct effects on the heart. It is also used as a mydriatic and briefly lowers intraocular pressure.

Xamoterol

Xamoterol (Corwin) is a partial agonist at β_1-adrenoceptors; it acts as agonist or antagonist according to circumstances, particularly the level of sympathetic autonomic activity present. At low levels of sympathetic activity it increases heart rate and contractility (inotropic) by its agonist effect, and at high rates it reduces them by its antagonist action. It has little action on bronchial (β_2) receptors. Xamoterol may benefit mild chronic heart failure only; it is likely to worsen moderate and severe failure because sympathetic activity increases with worsening heart failure.[8] It has benefited some cases of hypotension caused by autonomic neuropathy.

Mucosal decongestants

Nasal and bronchial decongestants (vasoconstrictors) are widely used in allergic rhinitis, colds, coughs and sinusitis, and to prevent otitic barotrauma, as nasal drops or as sprays to be sniffed; sprays reach a greater area of the mucous membrane. All the sympathomimetic vasoconstrictors, i.e. with α effects, have been used for the purpose, with or without an antihistamine (H_1-receptor), and there is little to choose between them. If used more often than 3-hourly and for above 3 weeks the mucous membrane is likely to be damaged. The occurrence of rebound congestion or of allergic reaction is liable to lead to overuse. The least objectionable drugs are ephedrine 0.5% and phenylephrine 0.5%. Xylometazoline 0.1% (Otrivine) should be used, if at all, for only a few days since longer application reduces the ciliary activity and leads to rebound congestion. Naphazoline and adrenaline should not be used, and nor should blunderbuss mixtures of vasoconstrictor antihistamine, adrenal steroid and antibiotics. Oily drops and sprays, used frequently and longterm, may enter the lungs and eventually cause lipoid pneumonia.

It may sometimes be better to give the drugs orally rather than up the nose. They interact with antihypertensives and can be a cause of unexplained failure of therapy unless enquiry into patient self-medication is made. Deaths (hypertension) have occurred when such preparations have been taken by patients treated for depression with a monoamine oxidase inhibitor.

Shock

Definition: Shock is a state of inadequate capillary perfusion (oxygen deficiency) of vital tissues to an extent that adversely affects cellular metabolism

---

[8] However, recent studies of β-receptor antagonists (metoprolol, bisoprolol and carvedilol) have shown that these can be introduced in some patients with more severe heart failure, if the dose is carefully titrated from a very low starting point (see p. 476).

(capillary endothelium and organs) causing malfunction, including release of enzymes and vasoactive substances,[9] i.e. it is a *low flow* or *hypoperfusion* state.

The cardiac output and blood pressure are low in fully developed cases. But a maldistribution of blood (due to constriction, dilatation, shunting) can be sufficient to produce tissue injury even in the presence of high cardiac output and arterial blood pressure (warm shock), e.g. some cases of septic shock.

The essential element, hypoperfusion of vital organs, is present whatever the cause, whether pump failure (myocardial infarction), maldistribution of blood (septic shock) or loss of total intravascular volume (bleeding or increased permeability of vessels damaged by bacterial cell products, by burns or by anoxia). Function of vital organs, brain (consciousness, respiration) and kidney (urine formation) are clinical indicators of adequacy of perfusion of these organs.

Treatment may be summarised:

- *Treatment of the cause*: pain, wounds, bleeding, infections, adrenocortical deficiency
- *Replacement of any fluid* lost from the circulation; but extra fluid is dangerous when the primary fault is in the heart or pulmonary circulation
- *Maintenance* of the diastolic blood pressure and *perfusion of vital organs* (brain, heart, kidneys).

Blood flow (oxygen delivery) rather than blood pressure is of the greatest immediate importance for the function of vital organs. But a reasonable blood pressure is needed to ensure organ perfusion, e.g. brain and myocardium, and pressure for formation of urine. Hypotension due to low peripheral resistance is of little importance if the patient is horizontal or tilted head down, for venous return to the heart, and so the cardiac output, is then maintained; blood flow to brain, myocardium and kidneys remains adequate until the diastolic pressure falls below about 40 mmHg. But *low cardiac output* is always serious even though compensatory vaso-

constriction maintains the arterial pressure, for blood flow is reduced.

The decision how to treat shock depends on assessment of the pathophysiology:

- whether cardiac output, and so peripheral blood flow, is inadequate (low pulse volume, cold-constricted periphery)
- whether cardiac output is normal and peripheral blood flow is adequate (good pulse volume and warm dilated periphery), but there is maldistribution of blood
- whether the patient is hypovolaemic or not, or needs a cardiac inotropic agent, a vasoconstrictor or a vasodilator.

In poisoning by a cerebral depressant the principal cause of hypotension is low peripheral resistance due to sympathetic block. The cardiac output can be restored by tilting the patient head-down and by increasing the venous filling pressure by cautiously raising the blood volume with a plasma expander. Use of vascular drugs is unnecessary and may be harmful.

In central circulatory failure (cardiogenic shock, e.g. myocardial infarction) the cardiac output and blood pressure are low due to loss of pumping power; myocardial perfusion is dependent on aortic pressure. Venous return (central venous pressure) is normal or high. The low blood pressure may trigger the sympathoadrenal mechanisms of peripheral circulatory failure summarised below.

Not surprisingly, the use of drugs in low output failure due to acute myocardial damage is disappointing. Vasoconstriction (by an α-adrenoceptor agonist), by increasing peripheral resistance, may raise the blood pressure by increasing afterload, but this additional burden on the damaged heart can further reduce cardiac output. Cardiac stimulation with a β1-adrenoceptor agonist may fail; it increases myocardial oxygen consumption and may cause a dysrhythmia. Dobutamine, dopexamine or dopamine offer a reasonable choice if a drug is judged necessary.

If there is bradycardia (as there sometimes is in myocardial infarction), minute output can be increased by vagal block with atropine.

Vasodilators may be needed to treat *severe cardiac failure*.

---

[9] In fact, a medley of substances (autacoids), kinins, prostaglandins, leukotrienes, histamine, endorphins, serotonin, vasopresssin, have been implicated. In endotoxic shock, the toxin also induces synthesis of nitric oxide, the endogenous vasodilator, in several types of cells other than the endothelial cells which are normally its main source.

Septic shock is caused by endotoxins from Gram-negative organisms and other cell products from Gram-positive organisms; they injure tissues and cause release of cytokines, e.g. interleukin-1, that are responsible for many of the adverse manifestations of shock. First there is a peripheral vasodilatation with eventual fall in arterial pressure. This initiates a vigorous sympathetic discharge that causes constriction of arterioles and venules; the cardiac output may be high or low according to the balance of these influences. There is a progressive peripheral anoxia of vital organs and acidosis. The veins (venules) dilate and venous pooling occurs so that blood is sequestered in the periphery and effective circulatory volume falls because of this and of fluid loss into the extravascular space.

The immediate aim of treatment is to restore cardiac output and vital organ perfusion by increasing venous return to the heart and to reverse the maldistribution of blood. This can be done by increasing intravascular volume (plasma or plasma substitute transfusion), keeping a close watch on central venous pressure to avoid overloading the heart, and by tilting the patient head-down. Oxygen is useful as there is often uneven pulmonary perfusion.

In addition a drug with a mix of cardiac inotropic and peripheral vascular actions may restore essential blood flow to vital organs. Dopamine provides such actions, is least likely to do harm and may even do good. Dobutamine may be added for extra cardiac inotropic effect.

Drugs that increase peripheral resistance (sympathomimetics with α effects and no β_1 effect, e.g. methoxamine) are likely only to make matters worse by further reducing blood flow to vital organs, in the event of the resistance vessels (arterioles) retaining their reactivity and responding to them, which they may not do. Noradrenaline does have some cardiac inotropic (β_1) effect and may be used if substantial vasoconstriction is judged to be the principal requirement. Administration of a vasodilator drug to a patient with low blood volume is, of course, disastrous.

Hypotension in patients with atherosclerosis (occlusive vascular disease) is more serious than in others, for they are specially dependent on pressure to provide the necessary blood flow in vital organs

because the vessels are less able to dilate. Dopamine may be considered.

CHOICE OF DRUG IN SHOCK

On present knowledge the best drug would be one that stimulates the myocardium as well as selectively modifying peripheral resistance to increase flow to vital organs.

> *Dopamine* comes closest to meeting these requirements. Where high doses are used and vasoconstriction predominates it may sometimes be useful to add a vasodilator, e.g. an α-adrenoceptor blocking drug (e.g. phentolamine).
> *Dobutamine* is used when cardiac inotropic effect is the primary requirement.
> *Dopexamine* combines some of the properties of dopamine and dobutamine.
> *Noradrenaline* is used when vasoconstriction is the first priority, plus some slight cardiac inotropic effect.
> *Angiotensin II* is available in some countries, generally on a named patient basis. It may be especially useful when tachyphylaxis to noradrenaline has occurred.

As well as reducing peripheral blood flow, prolonged vasoconstriction reduces blood volume due to passage of fluid into the extravascular space; this contributes to the drop in cardiac output that occurs with abrupt withdrawal.

Monitoring drug use

Modern monitoring by both invasive and noninvasive techniques has reached such heights of complexity that it can give more information than some doctors know how to put to good use, even if it is indeed the right information. We are liable

> to measure everything at once, losing ourselves in a sea of numbers many of which are derived by arithmetical exercises from other numbers.[10]

At least the heart rate and rhythm, blood pressure and urine flow should be closely watched. No

---

[10] Thompson W L 1977 Proceedings of the Royal Society of Medicine 70: 25.

attempt should be made to raise the pressure to normal; about 80–90 mmHg systolic pressure is enough, for the drugs are not restoring normal physiology. Prognostic indices tell us

> whether the patient will live or die, but such studies do not reveal by which parameters we should 'fly' the patient, and so we end up flying the patient by the seat of our pants instead of our other end.[10]

These words of an expert may give some comfort when the complexities of rational management seem overwhelming.

Warning. The use of drugs in shock is secondary to accurate assessment of cardiovascular state (especially of peripheral flow) and to other essential management, treatment of infection and maintenance of intravascular volume.

Restoration of intravascular volume

Ideally the transfusion should be similar to that which has been lost: blood for haemorrhage, plasma for burns, saline for gastrointestinal loss.

In an emergency, speed of replacement is more important than its nature. Isotonic saline and saline/lactate (crystalloid) solutions are immediately effective and are cheap, but they leave the circulation quickly. Macromolecules (colloids) remain in the circulation longer. The two classes (crystalloids and colloids) may be used together. Isotonic solutions of human plasma proteins and human albumin are available (concentrated solution of albumin is used in severe hypovolaemia with oedema to move fluid into the circulation).

Colloidal isotonic solutions of macromolecules include: dextrans (glucose polymer), gelatin (hydrolysed collagen) and hetastarch (hydroxyethyl starch).

Dextran 70 (i.e. mol. wt. 70 000) has a plasma $t^{1/2}$ of 12 h. Dextran 40 is used to decrease blood sludging and so to improve peripheral blood flow, e.g. prophylaxis of postsurgical thrombosis.

Gelatin products (Haemaccel, Gelofusine) have a plasma $t^{1/2}$ of 5 h.

Etherified starch (Hetastarch, Pentastarch) has a plasma $t^{1/2}$ of 17 d.

Adverse effects include anaphylactoid reactions; dextran and hetastarch can impair haemostatic mechanisms; dextran interferes with blood group cross matching and clinical biochemical measurements.

Chronic orthostatic hypotension

Chronic orthostatic hypotension occurs most commonly with age, in primary progressive autonomic failure and secondary to parkinsonism and diabetes. The clinical features can be mimicked by saline depletion. The two conditions are clearly separated by measurement of plasma levels of noradrenaline (supine and erect) and renin. These are elevated in saline depletion, but depressed in most causes of hypotension due to autonomic failure.

Since blood pressure can be considered as a product of 'volume' and 'vasoconstriction' the logical initial treatment of orthostatic hypotension is by expansion of blood volume using a sodium-retaining adrenocortical steroid (fludrocortisone[11]) or desmopressin (p. 645) — plus elastic support stocking to reduce venous pooling of blood when erect.

It is more difficult to reproduce the actions of the endogenous vasoconstrictors, and especially their selective release on standing, in order to achieve erect normotension without supine hypertension. Drugs which may be tried often have a mix of receptor actions: β_1-adrenoceptor agonist, β_2-adrenoceptor block, α-adrenoceptor agonist (on veins) and dopamine receptor block; they include pindolol, xamoterol, dihydroergotamine, metoclopramide and domperidone. Because of the risk of hypertension when the patient is supine, only a modest increase in erect blood pressure should be sought; fortunately a systolic blood pressure of 85–90 mmHg is usually adequate to maintain cerebral perfusion in these patients.

Postprandial fall in blood pressure (probably due to redistribution of blood to the splanchnic area) is characteristic of this condition; it especially occurs

---

[11] Effective doses may not affect blood volume and may work by sensitising vascular adrenoceptors.

after breakfast (blood volume is lower in the morning). Substantial doses of caffeine (2 large cups of coffee) can mitigate this, but they need to be taken before or early in the meal. The action may be due to block of splanchnic vasodilator adenosine receptors. Administration of the somatostatin analogue, octreotide, prevents postprandial hypotension, but the requirement for twice daily subcutaneous injections makes the drug an unlikely candidate for regular use in this group of patients.

Some of the variability in reported results of drug therapy may be due to differences in adrenergic function dependent on whether the degeneration is central, peripheral, preganglionic, postganglionic or due to age-related changes in the adrenoceptors on end-organs. In central autonomic degeneration, 'multisystem atrophy', noradrenaline is still present in peripheral sympathetic nerve endings. In these patients, an indirect amine may be successful, and one patient has been described who titrated the amount of Bovril (a tyramine-rich meat extract drink) she required in order to stand up.[12]

Erythropoietin has been used with success (increases blood volume).

SUMMARY

- The adrenergic arm of the autonomic system uses noradrenaline (norepinephrine) as its neurotransmitter.
- Adrenaline (epinephrine), unlike noradrenaline, is a circulating hormone.
- These two catecholamines act on the same adrenoceptors: α_1 and α_2 which are blocked by phenoxybenzamine but not by propranolol, and β_1 and β_2 which are blocked by propranolol but not phenoxybenzamine. However, noradrenaline is a 20-fold weaker agonist at β_2-receptors than is adrenaline.
- Distinction between receptor classes is made initially by defining differing ability of two agonists (or antagonists) to mimic (or block) two effects of catecholamines.
- Often these differences correlate with a difference in receptor type on two different tissues: e.g. stimulation of cardiac contractility by β_1-receptors and bronchodilatation by β_2-receptors.
- The distinction between α_1- and α_2-receptors corresponds to their principal location on blood vessels (causing vasoconstriction) and neurons.
- Catecholamines themselves can be used in therapy when rapid onset and offset is useful. Selective mimetics at each of the 4 main receptor subtypes are used for individual locations, e.g: α_1 for nasal decongestion, α_2 for systemic hypotension, β_1 for heart failure or shock, β_2 for bronchoconstriction.
- α- and β-blockade are both used in hypertension, and β-blockade also in angina.

GUIDE TO FURTHER READING

Ahlquist R P 1948 A study of adrenotropic receptors. American Journal of Physiology 153: 586

Bond R A et al 1995 Physiological effects of inverse agonists in transgenic mice with myocardial overexpression of the beta 2-adrenoceptor. Nature 374: 272–276

Brown M J 1995 To β block or better block? British Medical Journal 311: 701–702

Brown M J et al 1981 Increased sensitivity and accuracy of phaeochromocytoma diagnosis achieved by plasma adrenaline estimations and a pentolinium suppression test. Lancet II: 174–177

Califf R M, Bengtson J R 1994 Cardiogenic shock. New England Journal of Medicine 330: 1724–1730

Cryer P E 1980 Physiology and pathophysiology of the human sympathoadrenal neuroendocrine system. New England Journal of Medicine 303: 436

Editorial 1968 Gas gangrene from adrenaline. British Medical Journal 1: 721

Edwards J D 1993 Management of septic shock. British Medical Journal 306: 1661–1664

Fowler M B et al 1982 Comparison of haemodynamic responses to dobutamine and salbutamol in cardiogenic shock after acute myocardial infarction. British Medical Journal 284: 73

Jack D 1991 A way of looking at agonism and antagonism: lessons from salbutamol, salmeterol and other β-adrenoceptor agonists. British Journal of Clinical Pharmacology 31: 501

Motulsky H J et al 1982 Adrenergic receptors in man: direct identification, physiologic regulation and clinical alterations. New England Journal of Medicine 307: 18

---

[12] Karet F E et al 1994 Bovril and moclobemide: a novel therapeutic strategy for central autonomic failure. Lancet 344: 1263–1265.

Arterial hypertension, angina pectoris, myocardial infarction

SYNOPSIS

Hypertension and angina are common diseases of great importance. Hypertension affects above 20% of the total population of the USA with its major impact on those over age 50. Management requires attention to detail, both clinical and pharmacological.

The way drugs act in these diseases is outlined and the drugs are described according to class.

- Hypertension and angina pectoris: how drugs act
- Drugs used in both hypertension and angina
    Diuretics
    Vasodilators
        organic nitrates, calcium channel blockers, ACE inhibitors, angiotensin receptor antagonists
    Adrenoceptor blocking drugs, α and β
    Peripheral sympathetic nerve terminal
    Autonomic ganglion-blocking drugs
    Central nervous system
    Treatment of angina pectoris
- Myocardial infarction
- Treatment of arterial hypertension
- Sexual function and cardiovascular drugs
- Phaeochromocytoma

Hypertension: how drugs act

- Dilatation of arteriolar *resistance vessels*; the heart pumps against lower resistance (afterload), with more rapid run-off of pressure
- Dilatation of venous *capacitance vessels*; reduced venous return to the heart (preload) leads to reduced cardiac output, especially in the upright position
- Reduction of *cardiac contractility and rate* leads to reduced output at lower pressure, especially in response to stress, e.g. upright posture, exercise
- Depletion of *body sodium* reduces plasma volume (transiently), and reduces arteriolar response to noradrenaline (norepinephrine)
- Inhibition of *angiotensin II formation or action* leads to vasodilatation (above).

Modern antihypertensive drugs lower blood pressure with minimal interference with homeostatic control, i.e. posture, exercise. Postural and exercise hypotension was particularly limiting with antihypertensives that block the sympathetic neuron (they are more effective at high rates of impulse transmission, i.e. standing, than at low rates, i.e. lying) and can still be a problem with α-adrenoceptor blockers, and with drugs that dilate capacitance vessels (venules).

Drugs that reduce sympathetic autonomic activity may act in the central nervous system or on peripheral nerves.

Angina pectoris: how drugs act

Drugs used in angina pectoris are those that reduce *cardiac work* and *myocardial oxygen need* by:

- unloading the heart
- dilating capacitance and resistance vessels
- dilating coronary arteries
- blocking β-adrenoceptors.

Some drugs benefit both hypertension and angina pectoris and the following account embraces drugs used in both conditions.

Drugs used in both hypertension and angina

Diuretics (see also Ch. 27)

Diuretics, particularly the thiazides, are useful antihypertensives. They cause sodium loss with reduced volume of blood and extracellular fluid (up to 10% with chronic treatment though this may not be maintained beyond 3 months). The main blood pressure lowering effect is probably due to reduced responsiveness of resistance vessels to endogenous vasoconstrictors, principally noradrenaline. While this hyposensitivity may be a consequence of the sodium depletion, thiazides are generally more effective antihypertensive agents than are the loop diuretics, despite causing less salt loss, and evidence suggests an independent action of thiazides on an unidentified ion-channel on vascular smooth muscle cell membranes. Maximum effect on blood pressure is delayed for several weeks and other drugs are best added after this time. Adverse metabolic effects of thiazides on K^+, blood lipids, glucose tolerance, and uric acid metabolism led to suggestions that they should be replaced by newer agents not having these effects. However it is now recognised that unnecessarily high doses of thiazides have been used in the past

and that with low doses, e.g. bendrofluazide 1.25–2.5 mg/d or less (or cyclopenthiazide 125 micrograms), thiazides are both effective and well-tolerated. Moreover, they are not only by far the cheapest antihypertensive agents available worldwide but have proved to be the most effective in several outcome trials in preventing the major complications of hypertension, myocardial infarction and stroke. The characteristic *reduction in renal calcium excretion* induced by thiazides may, in longterm therapy, reduce the occurrence of hip fractures in older patients and benefit women with postmenopausal osteoporosis.

Vasodilators

Organic nitrates

Organic nitrates (and nitrite) were introduced into medicine in the 19th century. Denitration in the smooth muscle cell releases nitric oxide (NO), which is the main physiological vasodilator, normally produced by endothelial cells. Both nitrates and NO activate the soluble guanylate cyclase in vascular smooth muscle cells and cause an increase in intracellular cyclic GMP (guanosine monophosphate) levels. This is the second messenger that alters calcium fluxes in the cell and induces relaxation. The result is a *generalised dilatation of venules* (capacitance vessels) and to a less extent of arterioles (resistance vessels), causing a fall of blood pressure that is postural at first; the larger coronary arteries especially dilate. Whereas some vasodilators can 'steal' blood away from atheromatous arteries, with their fixed stenoses, to other, healthier arteries, nitrates probably have the reverse effect as a result of their supplementing the endogenous NO. There is increasing evidence that atheroma is associated with impaired endothelial function, resulting in reduced release of the endogenous vasodilator and, possibly, its accelerated destruction by the oxidised LDL in atheroma (see p. 482, and Ch. 26).

The venous dilatation causes a reduction in venous return, a fall in left ventricular filling pressure with reduced stroke volume, but cardiac output (per min) is sustained by the reflex tachycardia induced by the fall in blood pressure.

Uses. Nitrates are chiefly used to relieve angina pectoris and sometimes left ventricular failure. An excessive drop in blood pressure will reduce coronary flow as well as cause fainting due to reduced cerebral blood flow, and so it is important to ensure that an overdose is not taken. Patients with angina should be instructed on the signs of overdose — palpitations, dizziness, blurred vision, headache and flushing followed by pallor — and what to do about it (below). The optimum dose is probably just below that which causes slight tachycardia and a feeling of fullness in the heart.

Transient relief of pain due to spasm of other smooth muscle (colic), can sometimes be obtained, so that relief of chest pain by nitrates does not prove the diagnosis of angina pectoris.

Pharmacokinetics. The nitrates are generally well absorbed through oral and intestinal mucosal and the skin and are used by these routes. They are subject to extensive and rapid metabolism in the liver at first-pass after absorption from the gut, as is shown by the substantially larger doses required by that route over sublingual (this is why it is acceptable to swallow a sublingual tablet of glyceryl trinitrate to terminate excess effect should it be socially embarrassing to spit it out). They are first denitrated to mononitrates (and to glycerol) and then conjugated with glucuronic acid. The $t^1/2$ periods vary, (see below). The *systemic* bioavailability of swallowed formulations and $t^1/2$ increase when there is hepatic insufficiency.

Tolerance to the characteristic vasodilator headache comes and goes quickly (hours). Explosives factory workers exposed to a nitrate-contaminated environment lost it over a weekend and some chose to maintain their intake by using nitrate impregnated headbands (transdermal absorption) rather than have to accept the headaches and reacquire tolerance so frequently. In therapeutics tolerance is prevented by ensuring that *steady-state plasma concentration* is avoided. This is easy with occasional use of glyceryl trinitrate, but with nitrates having longer $t^1/2$ (see below) and sustained release formulations it is necessary to plan the dosing to allow low plasma concentration for 4–8 h, e.g. at night; transdermal patches may be removed for a few hours if tolerance is suspected.

Adverse effects. Collapse due to fall in blood pressure resulting from overdose or allergy may occur. The patient should remain supine, and the legs should be raised above the head to restore venous return to the heart.

These drugs are contraindicated as the sole treatment for myocardial infarction. However, the discovery that coronary artery occlusion by thrombosis is itself 'stuttering' — developing gradually over hours — and associated with vasospasm in other parts of the coronary tree has made the use of nitrates a logical, and often effective, form of analgesia when used on the coronary care unit. They are contraindicated in angina due to anaemia.

Nitrate headache, which may be severe, is probably due to the stretching of pain-sensitive tissues around the meningeal arteries resulting from the increased pulsation that accompanies the local vasodilatation. If headache is severe the dose should be halved.

Methaemoglobinaemia occurs with heavy dosage.

Glyceryl trinitrate (see also above)

Glyceryl trinitrate (1879) (trinitrin, nitroglycerin) ($t^1/2$ 3 min) is an oily, nonflammable liquid that explodes on concussion with a force greater than that of gunpowder. However, physicians meet it mixed with inert substances and made into a tablet, in which form it is both innocuous and fairly stable. Tablets more than 8 weeks old or exposed to heat or air will have lost potency by evaporation and should be discarded.

Glyceryl trinitrate is the drug of choice in the treatment of an attack of angina pectoris. The tablets should be chewed and dissolved under the tongue, or placed in the buccal sulcus, where absorption is rapid and reliable. Time spent ensuring that patients understand the way to take the tablets and that the feeling of fullness in the head is harmless is time well spent. The action begins in 2 min and lasts up to 30 min. The initial dose of the standard tablet is 300, 500 or 600 micrograms, but the amount required for each patient must be found by trial, up to 6 mg a day total. It is taken at the onset of pain, when stopping exercise to find and take the tablet no doubt contributes to the relief, and as a prophylactic immediately before any exertion that experience has taught usually brings on the pain.

Sustained release buccal tablets are available (Suscard), 1–5 mg. Absorption from the intestine is good, but there is such extensive hepatic first-pass metabolism that the sublingual or buccal route is ordinarily preferred; an oral metered aerosol (spray under the tongue and close the mouth) (Nitrolingual Spray) is an alternative.

For prophylaxis, glyceryl trinitrate can be given as an oral (buccal, or to swallow, Sustac) sustained-release formulation or via the skin as a patch (or ointment); these formulations can be useful for victims of nocturnal angina.[1]

Venepuncture: the ointment can assist difficult venepuncture and a transdermal patch adjacent to an i.v. infusion site can prevent extravasation and phlebitis and prolong infusion survival.

An i.v. formulation (Isoket) is available for use in *left ventricular failure* and unstable angina.

Isosorbide dinitrate (Cedocard) ($t^{1}/_{2}$ 20 min) is used for prophylaxis of angina pectoris and for congestive heart failure (tabs sublingual, and to swallow).

Isosorbide mononitrate (Elantan) ($t^{1}/_{2}$ 4 h) is used for prophylaxis of angina (tabs to swallow). Hepatic first-pass metabolism is much less than for the dinitrate so that systemic bioavailability is more reliable.

Pentaerythritol tetranitrate (Peritrate) ($t^{1}/_{2}$ 8 h) is less efficacious than its metabolite pentaerythritol trinitrate ($t^{1}/_{2}$ 11 h).

Amyl nitrite (1867) is a flammable volatile liquid. It is inhaled through the open mouth. The social disadvantage of having to break (pop) a glass capsule and the distinctive smell, with no compensatory advantage, has rendered it obsolete for angina pectoris; but as 'poppers' amyl nitrite has acquired a spurious reputation as an aphrodisiac[2] and indeed may seem so to those individuals who cannot dis-

tinguish between genital vasodilatation and true sexual pleasure. No sympathy need be expended on individuals who suffer severe hypotension by such misuse nor on its use to relax the anal sphincter to accommodate sexual procedures; also *isobutyl nitrite*.

Calcium channel blockers

Calcium is involved in the initiation of smooth muscle and cardiac cell contraction and in the propagation of the cardiac impulse. *Actions on cardiac pacemaker cells and conducting tissue* are described in Chapter 25.

Vascular smooth muscle cells. Contraction of these cells requires an influx of calcium across the cell membrane. This occurs through ion channels that are largely specific for calcium and are called 'slow calcium channels' to distinguish them from 'fast' channels that allow the rapid influx and efflux of sodium.

Activation of calcium channels by an action potential allows calcium to enter the cells. There follows a sequence of events which results in activation of the contractile proteins, myosin and actin, with shortening of the myofibril and contraction of smooth muscle. During relaxation calcium is released from the myofibril and, as it cannot be stored in the cell, it passes out through the channel.

The calcium channel blockers inhibit the passage of calcium through the voltage gated L- (for 'large') type membrane channels of smooth and cardiac muscle, reduce available intracellular calcium and cause the muscle to relax. There are 3 structurally different classes of calcium blocker:

- Dihydropyridines (the most numerous)
- Phenylalkylamines (principally verapamil)
- Benzothiazepine, diltiazem.

The slight differences between their clinical

---

[1] Useful, but not always safe. Defibrillator paddles and nitrate patches make an explosive combination, and it is not always in the patient's interest to have the patch as unobtrusive as possible (Canadian Medical Association Journal (1993) 148: 790).

[2] From *Aphrodite*, the Greek name for Venus, the goddess of beauty, the mother of love, the queen of laughter ... and the patroness of courtesans (Lemprière). An aphrodisiac would be a drug that provided a reliable, selective, dose-related increase in sexual desire and performance, lasting ideally, we suppose, a few hours; there should be a competitive antagonist. Perhaps fortunately there is no such drug. If there were, its social disadvantages might well be found to outweigh any benefits to an occasional individual.

effects can be explained in part by their binding to different parts of the L-type calcium channel. All members of the group are vasodilators, and some have weakly *negative* cardiac inotropic action and negative chronotropic effect via pacemaker cells and depress conducting tissue. Blockade of a T-type ('T' = transient, because the channel is open only briefly during the cardiac cycle) channel on conducting tissue and neuronal cells may enhance the antihypertensive efficacy of calcium blockade by reducing heart rate and reflex sympathetic activation. A phenylalkylamine which blocks T-channels, mibefradil, is under development.

The therapeutic benefit of the calcium blockers, in hypertension and angina, is due mainly to their action as vasodilators. Their action on the heart gives some of them an additional role as class 4 antidysrhythmics, but the dihydropyridines (except amlodipine) should not generally be used for this indication because of their negative inotropism.

Indications for use

- *Hypertension*: amlodipine, isradipine, nicardipine, nifedipine, verapamil
- *Angina*: amlodipine, diltiazem, nicardipine, nifedipine, verapamil
- *Raynaud's disease*: nifedipine
- Prevention of *ischaemic neurological damage following subarachnoid haemorrhage*: nimodipine
- *Cardiac dysrhythmia*: verapamil (see p. 460).

Pharmacokinetics. Calcium channel blockers in general are well absorbed from the gut. The first generation drugs undergo first-pass elimination in the liver and their action is terminated by hepatic metabolism. Dose adjustments for patients with impaired renal function are therefore either minor or unnecessary.

Adverse effects. Headache, flushing, dizziness, palpitations and hypotension may occur during the first few hours after dosing, as the plasma concentration is increasing, particularly if the initial dose is too high or increased too rapidly. Ankle oedema may also develop. This is due to a rise in intracapillary pressure as a result of the selective vasodilatation by calcium blockers of the precapillary

arterioles. The oedema is not a sign of sodium retention. It is not therefore relieved by diuretics but disappears after lying flat (e.g. overnight). In theory the oedema should also be attenuated by combining the calcium blocker with another vasodilator which is more effective (than calcium blockers) at relaxing the postcapillary *venules* (e.g. nitrates or ACE inhibitors). Bradycardia and dysrhythmia may occur. Gastrointestinal effects include constipation, nausea and vomiting; palpitation and lethargy may be felt.

Interactions. As many of the drugs in this group in general are extensively metabolised, there is risk of decreased effect with enzyme inducers, e.g. rifampicin, and increased effect with enzyme inhibitors, e.g. cimetidine. Beta-adrenoceptor blockers may aggravate atrioventricular (AV) block and cardiac failure. Diltiazem, nicardipine and verapamil raise plasma cyclosporin concentration.

Individual calcium blockers

Nifedipine ($t^1/2$ 2 h) is the prototype dihydropyridine. It selectively dilates arteries with little effect on veins; its negative myocardial inotropic and chronotropic effects are less than those of verapamil. There are sustained-release formulations of nifedipine that permit once daily dosing with minimal peaks and troughs in plasma concentration so that adverse effects due to rapid fluctuation of concentrations are also minimised. Various methods have been used to prolong, and smooth, drug delivery, and bioequivalence between these formulations cannot be assumed; prescribers should specify the brand to be dispensed. The adverse effects of calcium blockers with a short duration of action may include the hazards of activating the sympathetic system, each time a dose is taken. The dose range for nifedipine is 30–90 mg daily. In addition to the adverse effects listed above, gum hypertrophy may occur. Nifedipine can be taken sublingually, by crushing a capsule and squeezing the contents under the tongue. The vagaries and risks of this route of administration outweigh the largely illusory idea of delivering the drug rapidly into the systemic circulation in a hypertensive emergency (see p. 453).

Amlodipine is the prototype second generation dihydropyridine, and probably still the only one with a $t^1/2$ sufficient to permit the same benefits as the longest acting formulations of nifedipine without requiring a special formulation. The $t^1/2$ of 40 h is indeed so long that the initial effects are cumulative over several days, and therefore amlodipine is not suitable for emergency reduction of blood pressure. On the other hand a missed dose is of little consequence. Amlodipine differs from all other dihydropyridines listed in this chapter in being safe to use in patients with cardiac failure (the PRAISE[3] Study).

Diltiazem ($t^1/2$ 5 h) is given $\times$ 3/d, or $\times$ 2/d if a slow release formulation is prescribed. It causes less myocardial depression and prolongation of AV conduction than does verapamil but should not be used where there is bradycardia, second or third degree heart block or sick sinus syndrome.

Isradipine ($t^1/2$ 8 h) is given $\times$ 1–2/d (it is similar to nifedipine).

Nicardipine ($t^1/2$ 4 h) is given $\times$ 3/d.

Nimodipine has a moderate cerebral vasodilating action. Cerebral ischaemia after subarachnoid haemorrhage may be partly due to vasospasm; clinical trial evidence[4] indicates that nimodipine given after subarachnoid haemorrhage reduces cerebral infarction (incidence and extent). Although the benefit is small, the absence of any more effective alternatives has led to the routine administration of nimodipine (60 mg $\times$ 4/d) to all patients for the first few days following subarachnoid haemorrhage. No benefit has been found in similar trials following other forms of stroke.

Verapamil ($t^1/2$ 4 h) is an arterial vasodilator with some venodilator effect; it also has marked negative myocardial inotropic and chronotropic actions. It is given $\times$ 3/d as a conventional tablet or $\times$ 1/d as a sustained-release formulation. Because of its negative effects on myocardial conducting and contracting cells it should not be given to patients with

bradycardia, second or third degree heart block, or patients with Wolff–Parkinson–White syndrome who have atrial flutter or fibrillation. Amiodarone and digoxin increase the AV block. Verapamil increases plasma quinidine concentration and this interaction may cause dangerous hypotension.

Other members include: felodipine, nisoldipine, nitrendipine, lacidipine, isradipine.

There has been some concern that the shorter acting Ca^{++}-blockers may adversely affect the risk of myocardial infarction and cardiac death. The evidence is based on case-control studies which cannot escape the possibility that sicker patients (i.e. worse hypertension or angina) received Ca^{++}-blockade. The safety and efficacy of the class will be resolved by current prospective comparisons with other antihypertensives.

Angiotensin converting enzyme (ACE) inhibitors and angiotensin (AT) receptor antagonists

Renin is an enzyme produced by the kidney in response to a number of factors including adrenergic activity (β_1-receptor) and sodium depletion. Renin converts a circulating glycoprotein (angiotensinogen) into the biologically inert angiotensin I, which is then changed by *angiotensin converting enzyme* (ACE or kininase II) into the highly potent *vasoconstrictor* angiotensin II (ACE is located on the luminal surface of capillary endothelial cells, particularly in the lungs; and there are also renin-angiotensin systems in many organs, e.g. brain, heart, the relevance of which is uncertain). Angiotensin II acts on two G-protein coupled receptors, of which the angiotensin 'AT_1' subtype accounts for all the classic actions of angiotensin. As well as vasoconstriction these include also stimulation of aldosterone (sodium-retaining hormone) production by the adrenal cortex. It is evident that angiotensin II can have an important effect on blood pressure. In addition, it stimulates cardiac and vascular smooth muscle cell growth, contributing probably to the progressive amplification of hypertension once the process is initiated. Limited studies to date have shown that the AT_2 receptor subtype is coupled to inhibition of muscle growth or proliferation. Bradykinin (an endogenous

---

[3] PRAISE = Prospective Randomised Amlodipine Survival Evaluation (see Packer M et al 1996 The effect of amlodipine on morbidity and mortality in severe chronic heart failure. New England Journal of Medicine 335: 1107–1114).

[4] Packard J D et al 1989 British Medical Journal 289: 636.

vasodilator occurring in blood vessel walls) is also a substrate for ACE; it is probably a minor contributor to the vasodilator action of ACE inhibitors, except in patients without kidneys or other low-renin causes of hypertension. However either bradykinin or one of the neurokinin substrates of ACE (such as substance P) may cause cough (below). The AT_1 blockers have no effect on bradykinin, and are likely to be even less effective than ACE inhibitors in the absence of renin secretion.

Uses. The antihypertensive effect of ACE inhibitors and AT_1 receptor blockers results primarily from vasodilatation (reduction of peripheral resistance) with little change in cardiac output or rate; renal blood flow may increase (desirable): a fall in aldosterone production may also contribute. ACE inhibitors may reverse the vascular remodelling and cardiac hypertrophy of hypertension, and postpone diabetic nephropathy, and there is increasing (if not yet definitive) evidence that these effects of ACE inhibitors are greater than to be expected from blood pressure reduction alone.[5]

Both these classes are particularly efficacious when the raised blood pressure results from excess renin production (renovascular hypertension). The effect is immediate and there may be an initial brisk, even serious, drop in blood pressure (*first dose effect*) so that therapy is best initiated at bedtime and the patient warned. Patients already taking a diuretic should omit this for a few days before the first dose. The antihypertensive effect increases progressively over weeks with continued administration (as with other antihypertensives) and the dose may be increased at intervals of 2 weeks.

ACE inhibitors have a useful vasodilator and diuretic-sparing (but not diuretic-substitute) action in all grades of *heart failure*. Their reduction of mortality in this condition, due possibly to their being the only vasodilator which does not reflexly activate the sympathetic system, has made the ACE inhibitors more critical to the treatment of heart failure than of hypertension, where they are not usually an essential part of management. The AT_1 blockers have not yet been introduced for the treatment of cardiac failure; this is likely to be a matter of time, although the introduction of new drugs in cardiac failure can be faced with the problem of demonstrating efficacy against a background of ACE inhibitor therapy, with a placebo control no longer being ethically acceptable.

Dose. The elderly and patients on concomitant antihypertensive therapy should be started on half the standard dose.

Captopril (Capoten) has a $t^1/2$ of 2 h and is partly metabolised and partly excreted unchanged; in renal failure elimination is reduced and adverse effects are more common; it is given × 2/d. Captopril is the shortest acting of the ACE inhibitors, one of the few where the oral drug is itself active, not requiring de-esterification after absorption.

Enalapril (Innovace) is a prodrug ($t^1/2$ 35 h) that is converted to the active enalaprilat ($t^1/2$ 10 h). Some enzyme inhibition is still present at 24 h and enalapril may usually be given once a day.

Other members include lisinopril, perindopril, ramipril, cilazapril, moexipril, trandolapril and quinapril. Fosinopril is cleared by both liver and kidney, but this is rarely of clinical importance. Trandolapril is one of the few ACE inhibitors with a sufficiently long $t^1/2$ to guarantee high trough/peak plasma ratios on once daily dosing, but once again the clinical significance of this is insufficient to recommend any claim of superiority over other drugs in the class.

Adverse effects include persistent dry cough, angioneurotic oedema which may be severe, other rashes, loss of taste (which may recover though therapy is continued), stomatosis (like aphthous ulcers), abdominal pain, neutropenia, liver injury, raised plasma K (see effect on aldosterone above), deterioration of renal function, proteinuria and blood disorders.

---

[5] It will be fascinating to see whether longterm differences in regression of cardiac hypertrophy or of hypertension itself are confirmed, and whether there are practical consequences of the pharmacological differences between ACE inhibitors and the AT_1 receptor blockers. Thus the former may inhibit cellular growth through their potentiation of bradykinin, which stimulates NO production, whilst the AT_1 blockers cause a reflex increase in circulating angiotensin concentration that can act on the unblocked antiproliferative AT_2 receptor.

Losartan (Cozaar) is the first AT_1 receptor antagonist. It is a competitive blocker with a noncompetitive active metabolite. The drug is only one-third absorbed after oral dosing ($t^1/2$ 2 h). That of the metabolite is much longer, permitting adequate once daily doses. No significant drug-related adverse effects have been reported, other than those due to excessive hypotension in salt-depleted subjects, and it is certain that losartan does not cause a dry cough. Until further experience of the drug is gained, its main use is in patients responding to an ACE inhibitor who develop the cough.

Other vasodilators

Diazoxide (Eudemine) ($t^1/2$ 36 h) is a thiazide but without diuretic effect; indeed it causes salt and water retention. It is a potent antihypertensive by reducing arteriolar peripheral resistance through activation of the ATP-dependent K+ channel, with little effect on veins.

It is chiefly used to obtain immediate control of *severe hypertension* and heart failure: 1–3 mg/kg (max 150 mg) is given i.v. *rapidly* (< 30 s) (repeat after 5–15 min); the patient must be lying down. The reason for speed was thought to be that diazoxide was so extensively bound to plasma protein that a sufficiently high free plasma concentration may not be attained if the dose was given slowly; but this is probably not so. The maximum effect occurs within 5 min and lasts for at least 4 h. It is strongly alkaline and extravasation should be avoided. The dose may be repeated according to response; i.v. use will rarely need to be prolonged beyond 24 h. Alternative therapy suitable for longterm use should be instituted at the same time.

Diazoxide causes sodium retention, and concurrent use of a nonthiazide diuretic will be needed; blood glucose and potassium should be monitored. It also relaxes the *uterus* and may stop labour, which may be restarted with oxytocin.

Diazoxide causes hyperglycaemia by inhibiting release of stored (but not of newly synthesised) insulin from β-islet cells; the hyperglycaemia can be antagonised by a sulphonylurea. This action (reversible on withdrawal) renders it unsuitable for longterm oral use in hypertension. But it can be used orally in treatment of insulinoma.

Hydralazine ($t^1/2$ 1 h) has little place now in the routine oral therapy of hypertension, but might be used as a vasodilator together with nitrates in congestive cardiac failure. It reduces peripheral resistance by directly relaxing *arterioles*, but has negligible effect on veins. For this reason postural hypotension is not generally a problem in treatment of hypertension. The compensatory baroreceptor-mediated sympathetic discharge induced by the hypotension causes tachycardia and increased cardiac output, even causing angina pectoris in predisposed subjects. This can be eliminated by a β-adrenoceptor blocker. The usual compensatory increases in blood volume that occur with all drugs that increase the intravascular capacity lead to loss of effect (tolerance); a diuretic can eliminate this. Therefore combination therapy is usual practice. Some of the adverse effects of hydralazine can be accounted for by the hyperkinetic circulatory changes: headache, flushing, nasal and conjunctival congestion, lacrimation, palpitations and vomiting. With prolonged use of doses above 100 mg total/day (the safe maximum oral dose) a reversible syndrome of myalgia and arthralgia proceeding to disseminated lupus erythematosus is liable to occur.

Hydralazine is metabolised by acetylation with the same genetic bimodal distribution as isoniazid. But the difference is more evident in presystemic metabolism and so affects systemic bioavailability rather than postsystemic elimination. Twice-daily dosing is usual.

In most hypertensive emergencies except for dissecting aneurysm hydralazine 5–20 mg i.v. may be given over 20 min; the maximum effect will be seen in 10–80 min; it can be repeated according to need and the patient transferred to oral therapy within 1–2 days.

Minoxidil (Loniten) is a vasodilator selective for *arterioles* rather than for veins, similar to diazoxide and hydralazine. Like the former, it is now realised to be an ATP-dependent K+ channel opener. It is highly effective in severe hypertension, but causes increased cardiac output, tachycardia, fluid retention and hypertrichosis (see alopecia). Minoxidil is also available indeed as a topical solution for the treatment of baldness, although it is effective only in the minority of such patients.

Sodium nitroprusside (Nipride) is a highly effective antihypertensive agent when given i.v. Its effect is almost immediate and lasts for 1–5 min. Therefore it must be given by a precisely controllable infusion. It dilates both *arterioles and veins*, which would be disastrous if the patient stood up. But no patient who needs this drug is likely to want to stand up. There is a compensatory sympathetic discharge with tachycardia and tachyphylaxis to the drug. Nitroprusside action is terminated by metabolism. It penetrates erythrocytes where electron transfer from haemoglobin iron to nitroprusside yields methaemoglobin and an unstable nitroprusside radical. This breaks down, liberating cyanide radicals. Most of the cyanide remains in the erythrocytes and is firmly bound; it is the free cyanide that passes into the plasma that is toxic, diffusing throughout the body and inhibiting cellular respiration (cytochrome oxidase). The cyanide is converted to thiocyanate and so accumulates over days as the infusion is prolonged (a few hours should not normally be exceeded).

Measurement of plasma thiocyanate may be useful in determining whether the patient is suffering from toxicity from prolonged (days) infusion. Poisoning can cause delirium and psychotic symptoms. Metabolic acidosis may occur as a result of cell metabolism becoming anaerobic. Animals and man poisoned by nitroprusside are reputed to manifest the characteristic cyanide smell.

Clearly nitroprusside infusion should not be undertaken without meticulous regard for the manufacturer's recommendations and precautions; outside specialist units it may be safer overall to choose another more familiar drug.

Sodium nitroprusside is used in *hypertensive emergencies*, *refractory heart failure* and for *controlled hypotension in surgery*. An infusion[6] may be begun at 0.3–1.0 micrograms/kg/min and control of blood pressure is likely to be established at 0.5–6.0 micrograms/kg/min; close monitoring of blood pressure is mandatory; rate changes of infusion may be made every 5–10 min.

Nicorandil (Ikorel) is a newer, orally effective vasodilator with mixed nitrate and ATP-dependent K+ channel opening actions (i.e. it is a *potassium channel activator*). It is indicated for use in angina, where it has similar efficacy to β-blockade, nitrates or Ca++-blockade. It is an alternative to nitrates when tolerance to these is a problem, or to the other classes when contraindicated by asthma or cardiac failure. Adverse effects to nicorandil are similar to nitrate adverse effects, with headache reported in 35% of patients.

Papaverine is an alkaloid present in opium, but is structurally unrelated to morphine. It inhibits phosphodiesterase and its principal effect is relaxation of smooth muscle throughout the body, especially in the vascular system. It is occasionally injected into an area where local vasodilatation is desired, especially into and around arteries and veins to relieve spasm during vascular surgery and when setting up i.v. infusions. It is also used to treat *male sexual impotence* by self-injection into the corpora cavernosa of the penis shortly before intercourse (sometimes with phentolamine).[7] (Papaveretum has occasionally been supplied in error, to the surprise, distress and hazard of the subject.) A physician who prescribes papaverine for this purpose must be ready to treat the occasional case of priapism (defined as erection lasting more than 4 h) (aspirate the corpora cavernosa and inject an α-adrenoceptor agonist, e.g. metaraminol).

Alprostadil (Caverject) is prostaglandin E_1. It is effective in both psychogenic and neuropathic penile erectile dysfunction. A double-blind crossover trial in men with the former found that 5 or 10 micrograms produced an erection sufficient for sexual intercourse in 32 of 42 attempts, while placebo injections were ineffective.[8] It acts by increasing arterial inflow and reducing venous outflow by contracting the corporal smooth muscle that occludes draining venules. The site of injection is

---

[6] Light causes sodium nitroprusside in solution to decompose; when made, a solution should be immediately protected by an opaque cover, e.g. metal foil, and used fresh; the fresh solution has a faint brown colour; if the colour is strong it should be discarded.

[7] Brindley G S 1986 Pilot experiments on the actions of drugs injected into the human corpus cavernosum penis. British Journal of Pharmacology 87: 495 — an account of self-experimentation with 17 drugs.

[8] Schramek P, Waldhauser M 1989 British Journal of Clinical Pharmacology 28: 567.

along the dorsolateral aspect of the proximal third of the penis, alternating sides and sites for each injection. The patient package insert from the manufacturer provides some helpful drawings. The dose is arrived at by titration initially in the doctor's office, aiming for an erection lasting not more than one hour. Adverse effects are as for papaverine. Prostaglandin E_1 is also used i.v. to maintain patency of the ductus arteriosus in the newborn with congenital heart disease.

Vasodilators in heart failure (see p. 475)

Vasodilators in peripheral vascular disease

The aim has been to produce peripheral arteriolar vasodilatation without a concurrent significant drop in blood pressure, so that an increased blood flow in the limbs will result. Drugs are naturally more useful in patients in whom the decreased flow of blood is due to *spasm* of the vessels (Raynaud's phenomenon) than where it is due to *organic obstructive* changes that may make dilatation in response to drugs impossible (arteriosclerosis, intermittent claudication, Buerger's disease).

Vasodilators such as naftidrofuryl (Praxilene) and oxpentifylline (Trental) increase blood flow to skin rather than muscle; they have also been successfully used in the treatment of *venous leg ulcers* (varicose and traumatic).

Intermittent claudication. Patients should 'stop smoking and keep walking' — i.e. take *frequent exercise* within their capacity. Other risk factors should be treated vigorously, especially hyperlipidaemia, and patients should also receive aspirin 75–150 mg daily as an antiplatelet agent. Most patients with intermittent claudication succumb to ischaemic or cerebrovascular disease, and therefore a major objective of treatment should be prevention of such outcomes. Naftidrofuryl or oxpentifylline may be tried but should be withdrawn if there is no benefit in a few weeks. Naftidrofuryl has several actions. It is classed as a metabolic enhancer since it activates the enzyme succinic dehydrogenase, increasing the supply of ATP and reducing lactate levels in muscle. Oxpentifylline is thought to improve oxygen supply to ischaemic tissue by improving erythrocyte deformability and reducing *blood viscosity*, in

part by reducing plasma fibrinogen. Neither of these drugs is a direct vasodilator, as is the third drug used for intermittent claudication, inositol nicotinate. However the evidence in favour of any benefit is stronger for the first two, with ~50% increase in walking distance. There have been few adequate placebo-controlled studies of any of these agents. Most vasodilators act selectively on healthy blood vessels, causing a steal from atheromatous vessels. *Night cramps* occur in the disease and *quinine* has a somewhat controversial reputation in their prevention. However, meta-analysis of 6 double-blind trials of nocturnal cramps (not necessarily associated with peripheral vascular disease) shows that the number, but not severity or duration of episodes, is reduced by a night-time dose. The benefit may not be seen for 4 weeks. (see *ticlopidine*).

Raynaud's phenomenon may be helped by nifedipine, reserpine, an α-adrenoceptor blocker (in subhypotensive dose) and also by topical glyceryl trinitrate; indeed any vasodilator is worth trying in resistant cases; enalapril (ACE inhibitor) seems to lack efficacy. In severe cases, especially patients with ulceration, intermittent infusions over several hours of the endogenous vasodilators, prostacyclin (epoprostenol) or calcitonin-gene-related-peptide achieve long-lasting improvements in symptoms, possibly by desludging capillaries.

β-adrenoceptor blockers exacerbate peripheral vascular disease and Raynaud's phenomenon by reducing perfusion of a circulation that is already compromised. There is no benefit in using β_1-selective blockers, since the adverse effect is due to reduced cardiac output rather than leaving α-receptor vasoconstriction unopposed.

Dextran 40 reduces blood viscosity briefly.

Adrenoceptor blocking drugs

Adrenoceptor blocking drugs occupy the adrenoceptor in competition with adrenaline (epinephrine) and noradrenaline (and other sympathomimetic amines) whether released in the body or injected; circulating adrenaline and noradrenaline are antagonised more readily than are the effects of adrenergic nerve stimulation.

Some adrenoceptor blocking drugs have to be altered in the body before they become effective, i.e. they are prodrugs, and this explains the slow onset of action of phenoxybenzamine.

There are two principal classes of adrenoceptor, α and β: for details of *receptor effects* see Table 23.1.

α-ADRENOCEPTOR BLOCKING DRUGS

There are two main subtypes of α-adrenoceptor, defined by their relative affinity for the drugs which occupy them:

- Classic α_1-adrenoceptors, on the effector organ (postsynaptic), mediate vasoconstriction
- α_2-adrenoceptors are present both on some effector tissues (postsynaptic), and on the nerve ending (presynaptic). The presynaptic receptors (or *autoreceptors*) mediate a reduction of release of chemotransmitter (noradrenaline), i.e. they provide a negative feedback control of transmitter release. CNS α-adrenoceptors also belong to the α_2 subtype.

The first generation of α-adrenoceptor blockers were nonselective, blocking both α_1- and α_2-receptors. When subjects taking such a drug rise from supine to erect posture or take exercise, the sympathetic system is physiologically activated (via baroreceptors). The normal vasoconstrictive (α_1) effect (to maintain blood pressure) is blocked by the drug and the failure of this response causes the sympathetic system to be further activated and to release more and more transmitter. This increase in transmitter would normally be reduced by negative feedback via the α_2-autoreceptors; but these are blocked too.

The β-adrenoceptors however are not blocked and the excess transmitter released at adrenergic endings is free to act on them, causing a tachycardia that may be unpleasant. It is for this reason that nonselective α-adrenoceptor blockers are not used alone in hypertension.

An α_1-adrenoceptor blocker that spares the α_2-receptor so that negative feedback inhibition of noradrenaline release is maintained, is more useful in hypertension (less tachycardia and postural and exercise hypotension); prazosin is such a drug (below).

Adverse effects of α-adrenoceptor block are postural hypotension, nasal stuffiness, red sclerae and, in the male, failure of ejaculation. Effects peculiar to each drug are mentioned below.

Prazosin (Hypovase) ($t^{1/2}$ 3 h) acts as just described, i.e. it blocks postsynaptic α_1-receptors but not presynaptic α_2-autoreceptors. It has a curious transient disadvantage, the 'first-dose effect'; within 2 h of the first (rarely after another) dose there may be a brisk hypotension sufficient to cause loss of consciousness. It is prudent to initiate treatment with a low dose, with food, at home and on going to bed, since to experience this effect would not be a reassuring introduction to what is likely to be life-long therapy. Lower doses of prazosin may be used if it is combined with a diuretic or β-adrenoceptor blocker. For use in prostatic hypertrophy, see page 498. The converse of the benefit in the treatment of prostatism is an adverse effect of micturition incontinence in women.

Doxazosin (Cardura) ($t^{1/2}$ 8 h) is suitable for once daily prescribing. The first dose effect is less marked, although it is still advisable to start patients at a lower dose than intended for maintenance. It is convenient, for instance, to prescribe 1 mg daily, increasing after 1 week to twice this dose without repeating the blood pressure measurement at this stage.

Alfuzosin and *terazosin* are similar.

Indoramin (Baratol) is an older α_1-blocker, which is a less useful antihypertensive, but (perhaps because of this) still popular for prostatic symptoms.[9] It is taken × 2–3/day.

Phentolamine (Rogitine) is a nonselective α-adrenoceptor blocker. It is given i.v. for brief effect in adrenergic hypertensive crises, e.g. phaeochromocytoma or MAOI-sympathomimetic interaction. It can be used to terminate dental anaesthesia when adrenaline has been used to provide vasoconstriction (for

---

[9] It can be the reflex sympathetic activation, as much as hypotension itself, which causes problems. More than one cardiologist have had their efforts at controlling angina in elderly patients sabotaged when the patient visits a urologist for his prostatic symptoms, and is treated with one of the newer, more powerful α_1-blockers.

convenience or to reduce self-injury by cheek and tongue chewing as is liable to occur in mentally retarded subjects). In addition to α-receptor block it has direct vasodilator and cardiac inotropic actions. Dose for hypertensive crisis is 5–10 mg i.v. or i.m. repeated as necessary (minutes to hours). The use of phentolamine as a diagnostic test for phaeochromocytoma is only appropriate when biochemical measurements are impracticable, since it is less reliable.

Phenoxybenzamine (Dibenyline) is a powerful nonselective α-adrenoceptor blocking drug whose effects may last 2 days or longer. Accumulation may therefore occur at the beginning of treatment and the dose must be increased slowly. It is impossible to reverse the circulatory effects of an overdose by noradrenaline or other sympathomimetic drugs, because, although the amount of receptor binding at the outset is competitive, once the drug is on the receptor it binds irreversibly and is not displaced by administering increased amounts of agonist. Its effects are thus insurmountable, which make it the preferred α-blocker for treating phaeochromocytoma.

It is wise to observe the effects of a single test dose closely before starting regular administration.

Indigestion and nausea can occur with oral therapy, which is best given with food.

Thymoxamine (Opilon) is a nonselective α-blocker.

Labetalol has both α- and β-receptor blocking activities (see under β-adrenoceptor block, below). The different actions are due to different isomers.

Ergot alkaloids (see Index). The naturally occurring alkaloids with effective α-adrenoceptor blocking actions are also powerful α-adrenoceptor agonists (i.e. they are partial agonists); the latter action obscures the vasodilatation that is characteristic of α-adrenoceptor blocking drugs.

Chlorpromazine has many actions of which α-adrenoceptor block is a minor one, but sufficient to cause hypotension, and to be clinically useful in amphetamine overdose.

Yohimbine is an alkaloid from a West African tree. It is a weak α_2-adrenoceptor (autoreceptor) block-

ing agent, i.e. it blocks the negative feedback receptor so that adrenergic activity is enhanced. It also stimulates the central nervous system, causing a release of antidiuretic hormone. When given with a barbiturate it causes seminal ejaculation in mice, but despite this it neither affects penile diameter in healthy volunteers, nor enhances the response to visual erotic stimuli. A number of more selective α_2-adrenoceptor blockers have been developed, but none has found a secure clinical indication.

USES OF α-ADRENOCEPTOR BLOCKING DRUGS

- Hypertension
  — essential: doxazosin, prazosin
  — phaeochromocytoma: phenoxybenzamine; phentolamine (for crises)
- Peripheral vascular disease
- Miscellaneous
  — in benign prostatic hypertrophy (to relax capsular smooth muscle that may contribute to urinary obstruction), e.g. prazosin
  — in chilblains, with dubious benefit
  — in causalgia, the mechanism of relief, if any, is obscure but anything (also i.v. regional guanethidine block) is worth trying in this diabolical condition.

β-ADRENOCEPTOR BLOCKING DRUGS

Pharmacodynamics. These drugs selectively block the β-receptor effects of noradrenaline and adrenaline. They may be pure antagonists or may have some agonist activity in addition (when they are described as partial agonists).

The *cardiovascular* effects of β-adrenoceptor block depend on the amount of sympathetic tone present. The chief *cardiac* effects result from reduction of sympathetic drive:

- Reduced automaticity (heart rate)
- Reduced myocardial contractility (rate of rise of pressure in the ventricle).

With reduced rate the cardiac output/min is reduced and the overall cardiac oxygen consumption falls. These effects are more evident on the response to exercise than at rest.

With acute administration of a pure β-adrenoceptor blocker, i.e. one without any agonist effect, *peripheral vascular resistance* tends to rise — probably chiefly a reflex response to the reduced cardiac output, but also because the α-adrenoceptor (vasoconstrictor) effects are no longer partially opposed by β-adrenoceptor (dilator) effects; peripheral flow is reduced. With chronic use peripheral resistance returns to about pretreatment levels or a little below, varying according to presence or absence of partial agonist activity. But peripheral blood flow remains reduced. *Hepatic blood flow* may be reduced by as much as 30% and this is enough to prolong the $t\frac{1}{2}$ of the lipid-soluble members whose metabolism is much dependent on hepatic flow, i.e. those with extensive hepatic first-pass metabolism, including propranolol itself; also lignocaine, which is liable to be used concomitantly for cardiac dysrhythmias. The cold extremities that are characteristic of chronic therapy are probably due chiefly to reduced cardiac output with reduced peripheral blood flow, rather than to the blocking of peripheral (β_2) dilator receptors, for the effect occurs also with the β_1 selective agents.

Effects. At first sight the *cardiac effects* might seem likely to be disadvantageous rather than advantageous, and indeed maximum exercise capacity is reduced, but the heart has substantial functional reserves so that use may be made of the desired properties in the diseases listed below, without inducing heart failure. But heart failure due to the drug does occur in patients with seriously diminished cardiac reserve.

With longterm use the *resting blood pressure* falls because cardiac output falls and the normal physiological reflex response (increased peripheral resistance) passes off; indeed there may be a fall in peripheral resistance (the mechanism is obscure). But in some patients the normal compensatory reflex persists, and these nonresponders must be treated with other drugs.

Most of the blood pressure effect occurs quickly (hours, days) but there is often a modest further decrease over several weeks.

A substantial advantage of β-blockade in hypertension is that physiological stresses such as *exercise, upright posture* and *high environmental temperature* are not accompanied by hypotension, as they are with agents that interfere with α-adrenoceptor-mediated homeostatic mechanisms. With β-blockade these necessary adaptive α-receptor constrictor mechanisms remain intact.

Effect on *plasma potassium concentration*, see page 416.

β-adrenoceptor selectivity

Some β-adrenoceptor blockers have higher affinity for cardiac β_1-receptors than for cardiac and peripheral β_2-receptors (see Table 24.1). The *ratio* of the amount of drug required to block two receptor subtypes is often described as the *selectivity* of the drug. (See note to Table 23.1 regarding use of the terms β_1 *selective* and *cardioselective*.) The question is whether the differences between selective and nonselective β-blockers constitute clinical advantages. In theory there is less likelihood of causing bronchoconstriction, but in practice none of the available β_1-blockers is sufficiently selective to be safely used in asthma. The main practical use of β_1-selective blockade is in diabetics where β_2-receptors mediate both the symptoms of hypoglycaemia and the counter-regulatory metabolic responses that reverse the hypoglycaemia.

Some β-blockers (antagonists) also have agonist action, i.e. they are *partial agonists*. This is sometimes described as having *intrinsic sympathomimetic activity* (ISA). These agents cause less fall in resting heart rate than do the pure antagonists and may be less effective in severe angina pectoris in which reduction of heart rate is particularly important. There is also less fall in cardiac output and possibly fewer patients experience unpleasantly cold extremities, though intermittent claudication may be worsened by β-block whether or not there is partial agonist effect. Both classes of drug can precipitate heart failure and indeed no important difference is to be expected since patients with heart failure already have high sympathetic drive.

Abrupt withdrawal may be less likely to lead to a rebound effect if there is some partial agonist action, since up-regulation of receptors, such as occurs with prolonged receptor block, may not have occurred.

Some β-blockers have *membrane stabilising* (quinidine-like or local anaesthetic) effect, but this, with currently available drugs, is probably clinically insignificant except that agents having this effect will anaesthetise the eye (undesirable) if applied topically for glaucoma (timolol is used in the eye and does not have this action).

The *ankle jerk relaxation time* is prolonged by β_2-adrenoceptor block, which may be misleading if the reflex is being relied on in diagnosis and management of hypothyroidism.

Intrinsic heart rate

If the sympathetic (β) and the parasympathetic (vagus) drives to the heart are simultaneously adequately blocked by a β-adrenoceptor blocker plus atropine, the heart will be its own master and will beat at its 'intrinsic' rate. The intrinsic rate at rest is usually about 100/min, i.e. normally there is parasympathetic vagal dominance, which decreases with age.

Pharmacokinetics

First-order kinetics applies to elimination from plasma, but receptor block follows a *zero-order* decline. The reasons for this are complex but the practical application is important, e.g. within 4 h of 20 mg propranolol i.v. the plasma concentration falls by 50%, but the receptor block (as measured by exercise tachycardia) falls by only 35%.

Most β-adrenoceptor blockers can be given orally once daily in either ordinary or sustained-release formulations because the $t^1/2$ of pharmacodynamic effect exceeds the elimination $t^1/2$ of the substance in the blood.

Solubility of β-blockers relevant to their use.

Lipid-soluble agents are extensively metabolised (hydroxylated, conjugated) to water-soluble substances (some of which are active) that can be eliminated by the kidney. They are subject to hepatic first-pass metabolism after oral administration, especially propranolol (up to 80% metabolised). Plasma concentrations of drugs subject to extensive hepatic first-pass metabolism vary greatly between subjects (up to $\times$ 20) because the process is so much affected by two highly variable factors, speed of absorption and hepatic blood flow, which latter is the rate-limiting factor.

Lipid-soluble agents readily cross cell membranes into and inside the body and so have a high apparent volume of distribution; they readily enter the central nervous system, e.g. propranolol reaches concentrations in the brain $\times$ 20 those of the water-soluble atenolol. Propranolol has a shorter $t^1/2$ (about 4 h) than atenolol (7 h). For some of the lipid-soluble β-blockers, especially timolol, plasma $t^1/2$ may not reflect the duration of β-blockade since the drug remains bound to the tissues near the receptor long after therapeutic concentrations of drug have disappeared from the bloodstream.

Water-soluble agents show more predictable plasma concentrations because they are less subject to liver metabolism, being excreted unchanged by the kidney; thus their half-lives are much prolonged in renal failure, e.g. atenolol $t^1/2$ is increased from 7 to 24 h. Patients with renal disease are best not given drugs (of any kind) having a long $t^1/2$ and an action terminated by renal elimination. Water-soluble agents are less widely distributed and may have a lower incidence of effects attributed to penetration of the central nervous system, e.g. nightmares.

- *The most lipid-soluble agents* are propranolol, metoprolol, oxprenolol, labetalol
- *The least lipid-soluble (water-soluble)* agents are atenolol, sotalol, nadolol
- *Others* are intermediate.

Considerations of pharmacokinetics are of importance not only because β-adrenoceptor blockers are widely used but also because a high proportion of patients is elderly. Although propranolol is the oldest and still most widely used and tested member of the class, it is probably the most difficult to use well and in some patients the most poorly tolerated.

Classification of β-adrenoceptor blocking drugs

- *Pharmacokinetic*: lipid-soluble, water-soluble, see above.
- *Pharmacodynamic* (Table 24.1). The associated properties (partial agonist action and membrane stabilising action) have only minor clinical importance with current drugs at doses ordinarily used and may be insignificant in most

cases. But it is desirable that they be known, for they can sometimes matter and they may foreshadow future developments.

β-adrenoceptor blockers[10] not listed in Table 24.1 include:

nonselective: bunolol, carteolol, bufuralol, bunitrolol

$β_1$-*receptor selective:* betaxolol, bevantolol, pafenolol, tolamolol, esmolol (ultra-short acting: minutes)

β *and* α-*receptor block:* bucindolol, carvedilol
Partial agonists (i.e. both agonist and antagonist actions): celiprolol, xamoterol. Depending on the degree of intrinsic activity (defined as the ratio of maximal agonist activity to that of a full agonist like isoprenaline), these drugs may have a role in treatment of heart failure. However they need to be introduced at much lower than normal doses, and under careful observation (see xamoterol).

Agents with other combinations of actions are to be expected.

USES OF β-ADRENOCEPTOR BLOCKING DRUGS

Any condition where reduction of adrenergic activity involving β-adrenoceptors can be beneficial:

- peripheral sympathetic autonomic
- adrenal medullary secretion
- CNS adrenergic activity
- Such conditions are various.

Cardiovascular uses

Angina pectoris (β-blockade reduces cardiac work and oxygen consumption).

Hypertension (β-blockade reduces cardiac output and rate): there is little interference with homeostatic reflexes. Some concurrent prevention of sudden cardiovascular deaths may occur with metoprolol.

Cardiac tachydysrhythmias: β-blockade reduces

---

[10] More than 40 are available worldwide.

drive to cardiac pacemakers: subsidiary properties (see Table 24.1) may also be relevant.

Myocardial infarction and β-adrenoceptor blockers. There are two modes of use that reduce acute mortality and prevent recurrence: the so-called 'cardioprotective' effect.

— *Early use* within 6 hours (or at most 12 h) of onset (i.v. for 24 h then oral for 3–4 weeks). Benefit has been demonstrated only for atenolol. Cardiac work is reduced, resulting in a reduction in infarct size by up to 25% and protection against cardiac rupture. Surprisingly, tachydysrhythmias are not less frequent — perhaps because the cardiac $β_2$-receptor is not blocked by atenolol. Maximum benefit is in the first 24–36 h but mortality remains lower for up to one year.
Contraindications to early use include bradycardia (<55/min), hypotension (systolic <90 mm Hg) and left ventricular failure.
A patient already taking a β-blocker may be given additional doses.
— *Late use* for secondary prevention of another myocardial infarction. The drug is started between 4 days and 4 weeks after the onset of the infarct and is continued for at least 2 years.
— *Choice of drug.* The agent should be a pure antagonist, i.e. without agonist action.

Aortic dissection and *after subarachnoid haemorrhage*: by reducing force and speed of systolic ejection (contractility) and blood pressure.

Obstruction of ventricular outflow where sympathetic activity occurs in the presence of anatomical abnormalities, e.g. Fallot's tetralogy (cyanotic attacks): hypertrophic subaortic stenosis (angina); some cases of mitral valve disease.

Hepatic portal hypertension and oesophageal variceal bleeding: reduction of portal pressure.

Cardiac failure. At present, specialist use in some cases of dilated cardiomyopathy and hypertrophic obstructive cardiomyopathy to reduce disadvantageous catecholamine effects (mild congestive failure, see xamoterol). Recent prospective studies of carvedilol in over 1000 patients, in which the drug improved survival by 40%, suggest that use of some β-blockers may become more widespread. Their introduction will always need to be cautious, and at

Table 24.1 β-adrenoceptor blocking drugs: properties at therapeutic doses

	Drug	Partial agonist effect (intrinsic sympathomimetic effect)	Membrane stabilising effect (quinidine-like effect)
Division I: nonselective ($\beta_1 + \beta_2$) blockade			
Group I	oxprenolol	+	+
Group II	propranolol	−	+
Group III	pindolol	+	−
Group IV	sotalol		
	timolol	−	−
	nadolol		
Division II: β_1-('cardio')[1]-selective blockade[2]			
Group I	acebutolol	+	+
Group IV	atenolol		
	bisoprolol		
	metoprolol	−	−
	betaxolol		
Division III: nonselective β-blockade + α-blockade			
Group II	labetalol	+	−

[1] See Table 23.1, page 414 regarding use of the term *cardioselective*. Note: Hybrid agents having ß-receptor block plus vasodilatation unrelated to adrenoceptor have been developed, e.g. carvedilol.

[2] β_1-selective drugs are considered to be up to 50 times as effective against β_1-receptors than β_2-receptors. However, what selectivity really means is that 50 times more of the blocker is required to achieve the *same* blockade of the β_2-receptor as of the β_1-receptor. Therefore as the dose (concentration at receptors) rises the benefit of selectivity is gradually lost.

very low doses, to avoid initial exacerbation of cardiac failure.

Endocrine uses

Hyperthyroidism: β-blockade reduces unpleasant symptoms of sympathetic overactivity; there may also be an effect on metabolism of thyroxine.

Phaeochromocytoma: blockade of β-agonist effects of circulating catecholamines always in combination with α-adrenoceptor block. Only small doses of a β-blocker are required.

● Central nervous system

Anxiety with somatic symptoms (see anxiety). *Migraine* prophylaxis (nonselective β-blockade may be more effective than β_1-selective). *Essential tremor*, some cases. *Alcohol and opioid* acute *withdrawal* symptoms.

● Eyes

Glaucoma: (timolol or carteolol eye drops) act by altering production and outflow of aqueous humour.

Adverse reactions due to β-adrenoceptor block

Bronchoconstriction (β_2-receptor) occurs as expected, especially in *asthmatics* (in whom even eye drops can be **fatal**).[11] In elderly chronic bronchitics there may be gradually increasing bronchoconstriction over weeks (even with eye drops). Plainly risk is

---

[11] A 36-year-old asthmatic collected from a pharmacy, chlorpheniramine for herself and oxprenolol for a friend. She took a tablet of oxprenolol by mistake. Wheezing began in one hour and worsened rapidly; she experienced a convulsion, respiratory arrest and ventricular fibrillation. She was treated with positive-pressure ventilation (for 11 h) and i.v. salbutamol, aminophylline and hydrocortisone. She survived (Williams I P et al 1980 Thorax 35: 160). There is a logical — or rather *pharmaco*logical — link between the use of timolol as eye drops and the risk of asthma. For local administration, a drug needs high potency, meaning that half the maximal response is achieved with a physically small (and therefore locally administrable) amount of drug. The principal determinant of potency of a receptor antagonist is its affinity for the receptor, which in turn reflects how long each molecule remains bound to the receptor — technically, the dissociation rate constant. This is why one drop of timolol down the lacrimal duct can kill!

greater with nonselective agents, but β_1-receptor selective members are not totally selective and may precipitate asthma.

Cardiac failure. Patients near to cardiac failure need sympathetic drive to provide adequate cardiac output/min: a drop in rate may be enough to induce cardiac failure.

Heart block may be made dangerously worse.

Incapacity for vigorous exercise due to failure of the cardiovascular system to respond to sympathetic drive.

Hypotension when the drug is given after myocardial infarction.

Hypertension may occur whenever block of β-receptors allows pre-existing α-effects to be unopposed, e.g. phaeochromocytoma.

Reduced peripheral blood flow, especially with nonselective members, leading to cold extremities which, rarely, can be severe enough to cause necrosis; intermittent claudication may be worsened.

Reduced blood flow to liver and kidneys, reducing metabolism and biliary elimination of drugs, is liable to be important if there is hepatic or renal disease.

Hypoglycaemia, especially with nonselective members, which block β_2-receptors, and especially in diabetes and after substantial exercise, due to impairment of the normal sympathetic-mediated homeostatic mechanism for maintaining the blood glucose, i.e. recovery from iatrogenic hypoglycaemia is delayed. But since α-adrenoceptors are not blocked, hypertension (which may be severe) can occur as the sympathetic system discharges in an 'attempt' to reverse the hypoglycaemia. In addition, the symptoms of hypoglycaemia, in so far as they are mediated by the sympathetic (anxiety, palpitations), will not occur (though cholinergic sweating will) and the patient may miss the warning symptoms of hypoglycaemia and slip into coma. β_1-selective drugs are preferred in diabetes.

Plasma lipoproteins, high density and low density, are altered in a direction adverse for coronary heart disease (decrease of HDL/LDL ratio). The effect is small, and mainly on HDL. Since many patients with hyperlipidaemia also have an indication for β-blocker therapy, the hyperlipidaemia should not generally be regarded as a contraindication.

Sexual function: interference is unusual.

Abrupt withdrawal of therapy can be dangerous in angina pectoris and after myocardial infarction and withdrawal should be gradual, e.g. reduce to a low dose and continue this for a few days. The existence and cause of a β-blocker withdrawal phenomenon is debated, but probably occurs due to upregulation of β_2-receptors. It is particularly inadvisable to initiate an α-blocker at the same time as withdrawing a β-blocker in patients with ischaemic heart disease, since the α-blocker causes reflex activation of the sympathetic system. The β-blocker withdrawal phenomenon appears to be least common with partial agonists and most common with β_1-selective antagonists. Rebound hypertension is insignificant.

Adverse reactions not certainly due to β-adrenoceptor blockade

Effects include loss of general well-being, tired legs, fatigue, depression, sleep disturbances including insomnia, dreaming, feelings of weakness, gut upsets, rashes.

Oculomucocutaneous syndrome occurred with chronic use of practolol (now obsolete) and even occasionally after cessation of use.[12] Other members

---

[12] *Practolol* was developed to the highest current scientific standards; it was marketed (1970) as the first cardioselective β-blocker and only after independent review by the UK drug regulatory body. All seemed to go well for about 4 years (though skin rashes were observed) by which time there had accumulated about 200 000 patient years of experience with the drug, and then, wrote the then Research Director of the industrial developer, 'came a bolt from the blue and we learnt that it could produce in a small proportion of patients a most bizarre syndrome, which could embrace the skin, eyes, inner ear, and the peritoneal cavity' and also the lung (oculomucocutaneous syndrome). The cause is likely to be an immunological process to which a small minority of patients are prone, 'with present knowledge we cannot say it will not happen again with another drug'. That the drug caused this peculiar syndrome was recognised by an alert ophthalmologist who ran a special clinic for external eye diseases. In 1974 he suddenly became aware that he was seeing patients complaining of dry eyes but with unusual features. Instead of the damage (blood vessel changes with metaplasia and keratinisation of the conjunctive) being on the front of the eye exposed by the open lids, it was initially in the areas behind and protected by the lids. He noted that these patients were all taking practolol. Quite soon the whole system was defined, as above. Some patients became blind and some required surgery for the peritoneal disorder and a few died as a consequence.

either do not cause it, or so rarely do so that they are under suspicion only and, properly prescribed, the benefits of their use far outweigh such a very low risk. The mechanism of the syndrome is uncertain.

Overdose, including self-poisoning, causes bradycardia, heart block, hypotension and low output cardiac failure that can proceed to cardiogenic shock; death is more likely with agents having membrane stabilising action (see Table 24.1). Bronchoconstriction can be severe, even fatal, in patients subject to any bronchospastic disease; loss of consciousness may occur with lipid-soluble agents that penetrate the central nervous system. Receptor blockade will outlast the persistence of the drug in the plasma.

Rational treatment includes:

- *Atropine* (1–2 mg i.v. as 1 or 2 bolus doses) to eliminate the unopposed vagal activity that contributes to bradycardia
- *Glucagon*, which has cardiac inotropic and chronotropic actions independent of the β-adrenoceptor (dose 5–10 mg i.v. followed by infusion of 1–10 mg/h) to be used at the outset in severe cases.
- If there is no response, i.v. injection or infusion of a β-adrenoceptor agonist is used, e.g. isoprenaline (4 microgram/min, increasing at 1–3 min intervals until the heart rate is 50–70 beats/min).
- In severe poisoning the dose may need to be high and prolonged to surmount the competitive block.[13]
- Other sympathomimetics may be used as judgement counsels, according to the desired receptor agonist actions (β$_1$, β$_2$, α) required by

the clinical condition, e.g. dobutamine, dopamine, dopexamine, noradrenaline, adrenaline.

- For bronchoconstriction salbutamol may be used; aminophylline has nonadrenergic cardiac inotropic and bronchodilator actions and should be given i.v. very slowly to avoid precipitating hypotension.

Treatment may be needed for days. With prompt treatment death is unusual.

Interactions

Pharmacokinetic. Agents metabolised in the liver provide higher plasma concentrations when another drug that inhibits hepatic metabolism, e.g. cimetidine, is added. Enzyme inducers enhance the metabolism of this class of β-blockers. β-adrenoceptor blockers themselves reduce hepatic blood flow (fall in cardiac output) and reduce the metabolism of other β-blockers, of lignocaine and of chlorpromazine.

Pharmacodynamic. The effect on the blood pressure of sympathomimetics having both α- and β-receptor agonist actions is increased by block of β-receptors leaving the α-receptor vasoconstriction unopposed (adrenaline added to local anaesthetics may cause hypertension); the pressor effect of abrupt clonidine withdrawal is enhanced, probably by this action. Other cardiac antidysrhythmic drugs are potentiated (hypotension, bradycardia, heart block, etc). Combination with verapamil (i.v.) is hazardous in the presence of atrioventricular nodal or left ventricular dysfunction because the latter has stronger negative inotropic and chronotropic effects than do other calcium channel blockers.

Most NSAIDs attenuate the antihypertensive effect of β-blockers (but not perhaps of atenolol), presumably due to inhibition of formation of renal vasodilator prostaglandins.

β-adrenoceptor blockers potentiate the effect of other antihypertensives particularly when an increase in heart rate is part of the homeostatic response (Ca^{++}-blockers and α-adrenoceptor blockers).

Nonselective β-receptor blockers potentiate hypoglycaemia of insulin and sulphonylureas.

The drug was first restricted to brief use by injection in emergency control of disorders of heart rhythm, but is now obsolete even for that.

The developer acknowledged moral (though not legal) liability for the harm done and paid compensation to affected patients. He was not *negligent* because current science did not provide a possibility of predicting the effect, i.e. 'state of the art defence' applied. The law did not provide for strict liability or no-fault compensation (see p. 10).

[13] The present published record seems to be 115 mg isoprenaline i.v. over 65 h held by Lagerfelt J et al 1976 Acta Medica Scandinavica 199: 517.

Pregnancy

β-adrenoceptor blocking agents are used in hypertension of pregnancy, including pre-eclampsia. Both lipid- and water-soluble members enter the fetus and may cause neonatal bradycardia and hypoglycaemia. In early pregnancy they appear not to be teratogenic.

Individual β-adrenoceptor blockers

(For General pharmacokinetics, see p. 83)

Propranolol (Inderal) is available in standard (× 2–3/d) and sustained-release (once daily) formulations. When given i.v. (1 mg/min over 1 min, repeated every 2 min up to 10 mg) for *cardiac dysrhythmia* or *thyrotoxicosis* it should be preceded by atropine (1–2 mg i.v.) to prevent excessive bradycardia; hypotension may occur.

Atenolol (Tenormin) is used for angina pectoris and hypertension, 25–100 mg orally once a day. The tendency in the past has been to use higher than necessary doses. When introduced, atenolol was considered not to need dose-ranging, unlike propranolol, but this was in part because the initial dose was already at the top of the dose-response curve.

Bisoprolol (Monocor, Emcor) is the most β$_1$-selective blocker available since the withdrawal of practolol. Although a relatively lipid-soluble agent, its t$^1/_2$ is one of the longest (11 h), and there is not the wide range of dose-requirement seen with propranolol. As with atenolol, it is worth starting at a low dose, to avoid causing unnecessary tiredness, and especially when trying to obtain the maximum benefit of its selectivity. There is no need to alter doses when renal or hepatic function is reduced.

Oxprenolol is used similarly.

β- + α-adrenoceptor blocking drug

Labetalol (Trandate) is a racemic mixture, one isomer is a β-adrenoceptor blocker (nonselective), another blocks α-adrenoceptors; its dual effect on blood vessels minimises the vasoconstriction characteristic of nonselective β-block so that for practical purposes the outcome is similar to using a β$_1$-selective β-blocker (see Table 24.1).

The β-blockade is 4–10 times greater than the α-blockade, varying with dose and route of administration. Labetalol can be useful as a parenterally administered drug in the rare patient who requires emergency blood pressure reduction. Ordinary β-blockers lower blood pressure slowly, in part because reflex stimulation of unblocked α-receptors opposes the fall in blood pressure. In most patients, even those with severe hypertension, a gradual reduction in blood pressure is desirable to avoid the risk of cerebral or renal hypoperfusion, but in the presence of a great vessel dissection or of fits a more rapid effect is required (below).

Chronic use of labetalol is accompanied by normal cardiac output with reduced peripheral resistance and about normal peripheral blood flow; whereas chronic pure β-receptor blockade is accompanied by low cardiac output, about normal peripheral resistance and reduced peripheral blood flow.

Postural hypotension (characteristic of α-receptor blockade) is liable to occur at the outset of therapy and if the dose is increased too rapidly. But with chronic therapy when the β-receptor component is largely responsible for the antihypertensive effect it is not a problem.

Labetalol (but not propranolol) reduces the hypertensive response to orgasm in women.

The t$^1/_2$ is 4 h; it is extensively metabolised in the hepatic first-pass. The drug needs to be taken × 2–3/d.

For emergency control of severe hypertension 50 mg i.v. may be given over 1 min with the patient supine, and repeated at 5 min intervals up to a maximum of 200 mg; atropine reverses or prevents severe bradycardia. After i.v. labetalol patients are highly responsive to posture for about 3 h.

Serotonin (5-HT) receptor + α-adrenoceptor blocking drugs

Ketanserin appears to act principally to block serotonin vasoconstrictor (subtype 5-HT$_2$) receptors and also has some α-adrenoceptor blocking effect (its affinity ratio of serotonin block to adrenoceptor block is 1 : 5). It is of interest as an example of an 'hybrid' drug, but has been of limited use in hypertension. It is unavailable in many countries.

Serotonin (5-hydroxytryptamine, 5-HT) is synthesised in enterochromaffin cells, largely in the gut, and also extensively taken up into blood platelets from which it is released to have vascular effect. It has complex effects on the cardiovascular system, varying with the vascular bed and its physiological state; it generally constricts arterioles and veins and induces blood platelet aggregation; it stimulates intestinal and bronchial smooth muscle. Because platelets store and release serotonin, and because serotonin itself activates platelets, the longterm efficacy of ketanserin in preventing the complications of atheroma has been investigated. Carcinoid tumours secrete serotonin and symptoms may be benefited by serotonin antagonists, e.g. cyproheptadine, methysergide and sometimes by octreotide (see Index). It is a neurotransmitter in the brain.

Peripheral sympathetic nerve terminal

Adrenergic neuron blocking drugs

Adrenergic neuron blocking drugs are selectively taken up into adrenergic nerve endings by the active, energy-requiring, saturable amine (noradrenaline) pump mechanism. They accumulate in the noradrenaline storage vesicles from which they are released in response to nerve impulses, diminishing the release of noradrenaline and so all sympathetic function. They do not adequately control supine blood pressure and are prone to interactions with other drugs affecting adrenergic function, e.g. tricyclic antidepressants and topical nasal decongestants. They are virtually obsolete in hypertension.

Guanethidine has been used to reduce intraocular pressure in open angle glaucoma and to reduce thyrotoxic eyelid retraction for cosmetic effect. Other members of the group are debrisoquine and bethanidine. Metaiodobenzylguanidine is used diagnostically, with a radioiodine label, to locate chromaffin tumours (mainly phaeochromocytoma) which accumulate drugs in this class (p. 455).

Depletion of stored transmitter

(noradrenaline)

Reserpine (Serpasil) is an alkaloid from plants of the genus *Rauwolfia*, used in medicine since ancient times in southern Asia, particularly for insanity; reserpine was extensively used in psychiatry but is now obsolete, though it retains a minor place in combination therapy (with a diuretic) of hypertension.

Reserpine depletes adrenergic nerves of noradrenaline primarily by blocking or destroying the storage mechanism within the nerve ending, so that there is less transmitter available for release. It does not block the amine pump by which extraneuronal noradrenaline is taken up into nerve endings. Its antihypertensive action is due chiefly to peripheral action, but it enters the CNS, where it can cause severe depression which persists after withdrawal; suicide has occurred. The lowest possible dose must be used, and a history of depression contraindicates the drug.

Older domestic male turkeys are liable to fatal hypertensive dissecting aneurysm of the aorta. This can cause serious economic loss. The addition of reserpine to their drinking water reduces their blood pressure and preserves their lives without noticeably moderating their natural rage,[14] as may β-adrenoceptor blockers.

Inhibition of synthesis of transmitter

Metirosine (α-methyltyrosine) is a competitive inhibitor of the enzyme tyrosine hydroxylase, which converts tyrosine to dopa; lack of dopa means lack of dopamine and therefore of noradren-

---

[14] Conference on use of tranquillising agent Serpasil in animal and poultry production 1959 College of Agriculture, Rutgers State University, USA. Wild turkeys have a blood pressure of 120/60 mmHg, but domestic turkeys are hypertensive (204/144 mmHg). Digoxin increases the incidence of aneurysm. It seems that it is the *rate* of rise of pressure in the aorta that is important in this disease (probably in man also) and that reserpine and β-adrenoceptor blockers benefit by attenuating this.

aline and adrenaline, which are made from it by further enzyme processes. It acts also in the adrenal medulla and is used to treat phaeochromocytomas that cannot be removed surgically. Catecholamine synthesis is reduced by up to 80% over 3 days. Because the drug readily penetrates the CNS and depletes brain noradrenaline, it tends to cause severe depression. In patients whose life expectancy is threatened more by tumour invasion than by mild or moderate hypertension, the need for the drug should be weighed carefully.

Autonomic ganglion-blocking drugs

Because they are not selective and block sympathetic and parasympathetic systems alike, the ganglion-blockers are obsolete in routine therapy of hypertension; they cause severe postural hypotension.

Trimetaphan (Arfonad), a short-acting agent (given by i.v. infusion), also has direct vasodilator effect; it is used for producing hypotension to provide a blood-free field during surgery, and can be used for emergency control of hypertension; pressure may be adjusted by tilting the body; it provides 'minute-to-minute' control, when the lack of selectivity is important.

Pentolinium is used in a diagnostic test for phaeochromocytoma; patients with the tumour do not demonstrate the normal rapid reduction in plasma noradrenaline and adrenaline concentrations after a bolus i.v. injection (p. 456).

Central nervous system

α_2-ADRENOCEPTOR AGONIST

Clonidine (Catapres) is an imidazoline which is an agonist to α_2-adrenoceptors (postsynaptic) in the brain, suppressing sympathetic outflow and reducing blood pressure. At high doses it also activates peripheral α_2-adrenoceptors (*presynaptic* autorecep-

tors) on the adrenergic nerve ending; ate negative feedback suppression of line release. (In overdose clonidine can stimulate peripheral α_1-adrenoceptors (*postsynaptic*) and thus cause hypertension by vasoconstriction), i.e. there is a therapeutic window. Clonidine was discovered to be hypotensive, not by the pharmacologists who tested it in the laboratory but by a physician who used it on himself as nose drops for a common cold.[15]

Clonidine reduces blood pressure with little postural or exercise drop and would be a drug of first choice were it not for a *serious handicap*. Abrupt or even gradual withdrawal, e.g. forgetfulness, intercurrent illness, need for surgery, causes a rebound hypertension (in up to 50% of cases) (with high plasma catecholamine concentration) akin to the hypertensive attacks of phaeochromocytoma. The onset may be rapid (a few hours) or delayed for as long as 2 days; it subsides over 2–3 days. Treatment is either to reinstitute clonidine, i.m. if necessary ($t^1/2$ 6 h), or to treat as for phaeochromocytoma. Although it does not occur invariably on withdrawal the disadvantage is potentially serious and therefore clonidine cannot be regarded as a drug of first choice. It should never be used with a β-adrenoceptor blocker which exacerbates withdrawal hypertension (see phaeochromocytoma). Patients taking clonidine will need to be assessed for reliability of compliance as well as given careful instructions. Common adverse effects include sedation and dry mouth. Tricyclic antidepressants antagonise the antihypertensive action and increase the rebound hypertension of abrupt withdrawal. It also has a minor role, in low doses (Dixarit) in migraine prophylaxis, and perhaps menopausal flushing and choreas.

Rebound hypertension is a less important problem with longer acting imidazolines, since omission of a single dose will not trigger the rebound. Such drugs include *moxonidine*, *rilmenidine* and *guanfacine*. No drug has yet certainly succeeded in separating the sedative and hypotensive effects; although there is good evidence for the existence of an imidazoline receptor in the CNS distinct from the α_2-receptor, it is not certain that desired and undesired effects of a drug will be mediated through different receptors.

---

[15] Page L H 1981 New England Journal of Medicine 304: 1371.

FALSE TRANSMITTER

Chemotransmitters and receptors in the CNS and in the periphery are similar, and the drug in this section also has peripheral actions, as is to be expected.

Methyldopa (Aldomet) ($t^{1}/2$ 1.5 h) probably acts primarily in the brain stem vasomotor centres. It is a substrate for other enzymes that synthesise noradrenaline. α-Methylnoradrenaline synthesis results in tonic stimulation of CNS α_2-receptors since after its release α-methylnoradrenaline cannot be metabolised by monoamine oxidase, and selectively stimulates the α_2-adrenoceptor. Stimulation of this receptor in the hindbrain nuclei concerned with blood pressure control results in a fall in blood pressure, i.e. methyldopa acts in the same way as clonidine. α-Methylnoradrenaline is also produced at peripheral adrenergic endings, but to a lesser extent and peripheral action is clinically insignificant.

Methyldopa is reliably absorbed from the gut and readily enters the CNS.

Adverse effects are largely those expected of its mode of action; they include: sedation (frequent), headache, nightmares, depression, involuntary movements, nausea, flatulence, constipation, sore or black tongue, positive Coombs test with, occasionally, haemolytic anaemia, leucopenia, thrombocytopenia, hepatitis.

Gynaecomastia and lactation occur due to interference with dopaminergic suppression of prolactin secretion. Any failure of male sexual function is probably secondary to sedation. Because of its adverse effects methyldopa is no longer a drug of first choice in routine longterm management of hypertension, but remains popular with obstetricians.

Treatment of angina pectoris[16]

Cause: an attack of angina pectoris[17] occurs when the need of the myocardium for oxygen exceeds the amount delivered to it by the coronary circulation.

The principal forms relevant to choice of drug therapy are angina of exercise (more common) and its worsening form, unstable (preinfarction,

crescendo) angina, which occurs at rest. Variant (Prinzmetal) angina (less common) results from spasm of a large coronary artery.

Treatment objective is to unload the heart or to prevent/relax spasm of the coronary arteries so that oxygen need is adequately met.

Myocardial oxygen consumption is chiefly determined by:

- *Preload*, i.e. the venous filling and stretching of the heart and its muscle fibres, which evokes the contractility (extent and velocity of fibre-shortening during systole)
- *Afterload*, i.e. the peripheral arteriolar resistance against which the heart must eject blood, and including the peak systolic pressure that must be reached
- *Heart rate*, which determines the duration of diastole during which intramyocardial pressure is low enough to allow myocardial perfusion to occur via the coronary arteries.

All these determinants of oxygen consumption are influenced by the activity of *the sympathetic nervous system* and it is no surprise that continuous use of a β-adrenoceptor blocking drug benefits angina pectoris, reducing the frequency of attacks whether induced by exercise, anxiety or excitement.

The heart can be unloaded, i.e. its oxygen needs diminished, by:

- halting the provocative exercise (physical or emotional)
- reducing the preload (venous return)
- reducing the afterload (arteriolar resistance)
- reducing the rate
- dilating the coronary arteries (even though diseased, the larger arteries may double their diameter).

Antianginal drugs act as follows:

- Organic nitrates reduce preload and afterload

---

[16] For a personal account by a physician of his experiences of angina pectoris, coronary bypass surgery, ventricular fibrillation and recovery, see Swyer G I M 1986 British Medical Journal 292: 337. Compelling and essential reading.

[17] Angina pectoris: *angina*, a strangling; *pectoris*, of the chest.

and dilate the main coronary arteries (rather than the arterioles).

- β-adrenoceptor blocking drugs reduce myocardial contractility and slow the heart rate. They may increase coronary artery spasm in variant angina.
- Calcium channel blocking drugs reduce cardiac contractility, dilate the coronary arteries (where there is evidence of spasm) and reduce afterload (dilate peripheral arterioles).

These classes of drug complement each other and can be used together. The combined nitrate and K+ channel activator, *nicorandil*, is an alternative when any of the other drugs is contraindicated.

Summary of treatment

- Any contributory cause is treated when possible, e.g. anaemia, dysrhythmia.
- Life style is changed so as to reduce the number of attacks. Weight reduction can be very helpful; stop smoking.
- For immediate pre-exertional prophylaxis: glyceryl trinitrate sublingually or nifedipine (bite capsule and hold liquid in mouth or swallow it).
- For an acute attack: glyceryl trinitrate (sublingual): nifedipine (bite capsule, as above).

For longterm prophylaxis:

1. *β-adrenoceptor block*, e.g. propranolol (nonselective) or a $β_1$-selective member: given continuously (not merely when an attack is expected). Dosage is adjusted by response. Some put an arbitrary upper limit to dose, but others recommend that if complete relief is not obtained the dose should be raised to the maximum tolerated, provided the resting heart rate is not reduced below 55/min; or raise the dose to a level at which an increase causes no further inhibition of exercise tachycardia. In severe angina a pure antagonist, i.e. an agent lacking partial agonist activity, is preferred, since the latter may not slow the heart sufficiently. Warn the patient of the risk of abrupt withdrawal.
2. *Calcium channel blocking drug*, e.g. nifedipine or diltiazem, an alternative to a β-adrenoceptor blocker: use especially if coronary spasm is suspected or if the patient has myocardial insufficiency or any bronchospastic disease. It can also be used with a β-blocker, or
3. *A long-acting nitrate*, isosorbide dinitrate or mononitrate: use so as to avoid tolerance (p. 82).
4. *Nicorandil*, a long-acting K+ channel activator: this does not cause tolerance like the nitrates.

- Drug therapy may be adapted to the time of attacks, e.g. nocturnal (transdermal glyceryl trinitrate, or isosorbide mononitrate orally at night).
- Antiplatelet therapy (aspirin) reduces the incidence of fatal and of nonfatal myocardial infarction in patients with unstable angina, used alone or with low dose heparin.
- Surgery in selected cases.

As well as the objective of reducing symptoms in angina, it is important to remember the objective of preventing complications, particularly myocardial infarction and sudden death. This requires vigorous treatment of all risk factors — hypertension, hyperlipidaemia, diabetes mellitus — and, of course, no smoking. There is little evidence that the symptomatic treatments, medical or surgical, themselves affect outcome except in patients with stenosis of the main stem of the left coronary, who require surgical intervention. Although aspirin has not specifically been studied in patients with stable angina, it is now reasonable to extrapolate from the studies of aspirin in other patient groups. There is now evidence that high doses of vitamin E (α-tocopheryl acetate) can usefully reduce the risk of myocardial infarction in patients with severe (angiographically proven) coronary disease. Confirmatory studies are in progress.

Myocardial infarction (MI) (also Ch. 29)

The immediate objectives are relief of pain and initiation of treatment demonstrated to reduce mortality. Subsequent management is concerned with treatment of complications, *dysrhythmias, heart failure* and *emboli*, and then secondary prevention of further myocardial infarctions.

The initial treatment can appropriately be administered by a general practitioner or paramedic before a definite diagnosis is established or the patient reaches hospital:

- morphine or diamorphine (2.5 or 5 mg *intravenously*, because of the certainty of haematoma formation when intramuscular injections are followed by thrombolytic therapy)
- aspirin 150 or 300 mg orally
- 60% oxygen.

In certain areas, GPs or paramedics may be trained to administer an appropriate thrombolytic drug, anistreplase, where the journey to hospital is likely to take more than an hour. This agent has a $t^{1/2}$ of almost 2 hours, which enables administration as a slow bolus, rather than as a controlled infusion. Following arrival at hospital, preferably directly to the coronary care unit to avoid further delays, thrombolytic therapy should be initiated in any patient with ischaemic chest pain who has ST elevation on the ECG and in whom there are no contraindications to thrombolysis (see below). Patients with a typical history but without ST elevation may still be eligible, especially those with left bundle branch block. However several trials have shown that patients without ECG changes (or with ST depression), and patients with unstable angina, benefit slightly if at all from thrombolytic therapy.

The choice of thrombolytic is in most places dictated by (1) a wealth of comparative outcome data from well designed trials and (2) relative costs. For a first infarct, patients should receive streptokinase 1 500 000 units infused over 1 hour, unless they are in cardiogenic shock. For subsequent infarcts within 1–2 years, the presence of antistreptokinase antibodies dictates the use of recombinant tissue plasminogen activator alteplase. This drug was one of the first naturally occurring human proteins to be manufactured in bulk by recombinant DNA technology. Both alteplase and streptokinase bind plasminogen and convert it to plasmin, which lyses fibrin. Alteplase has a much higher affinity for plasminogen bound to fibrin than in the circulation. This selectivity does not, however, confer any therapeutic advantage as originally anticipated, since severe haemorrhage following thrombolysis is

Table 24.2 Drugs for myocardial infarction

Drug	t½	Recommended usage
Streptokinase	80 min	1 500 000 units over 1 hour
Alteplase (rt-PA)	30 min	10 mg bolus, 50 mg over 1st hour, 40 mg over subsequent 2 hours
		Also heparin 5000 U bolus, then 1000 U/hour
Anistreplase	105 min	30 units over 5 min (suitable for use outside hospital)

almost always due to lysis of an appropriate clot at previous sites of bleeding or trauma. Indeed, the tendency for some lysis of circulating fibrinogen as well as fibrin by streptokinase gives this drug some anticoagulant activity which is lacking from alteplase, so that administration of alteplase needs to be accompanied and followed by administration of heparin.

> **Principal contraindications to thrombolysis**
> 1. Haemorrhagic diathesis
> 2. Recent symptoms of peptic ulcer, or GI bleeding
> 3. Recent stroke
> 4. Recent surgery, especially neurosurgery
> 5. Prolonged cardiopulmonary resuscitation (during current presentation)
> 6. Severe, uncontrolled hypertension

In addition to thrombolysis and aspirin, a third treatment has been shown to reduce mortality, namely intravenous β-blockade. In the ISIS-1 study,[18] atenolol 50 mg was given intravenously followed by the same dose orally. The reduction in mortality is due mainly to prevention of cardiac rupture, which appears interestingly to remain the only complication of MI which is not reduced by thrombolysis. The usual contraindications to β-blockade apply, but most patients with a first MI should be able to receive this treatment.

SECONDARY PREVENTION (also Ch. 29)

The best predictor of risk of a myocardial infarction

[18] ISIS = International Studies of Infarct Survival.

is myocardial infarction. After the first few hours, the principal objective of treatment therefore becomes prevention of future infarcts. Most patients should enter a formal rehabilitation programme after discharge from hospital, in which they are encouraged to exercise and diet, and advice about these should be given before discharge. All patients need to reduce saturated fat intake, and there is increasing evidence to support increased intake of fish and olive oil.

DRUGS FOR SECONDARY PREVENTION (also Ch. 29)

All patients should receive aspirin and β-blockade for at least two years, unless contraindicated. The commonest contraindication to β-blockade post-MI is heart failure, although this should now be uncommon after a first MI. In such patients, β-blockade should be replaced by an ACE inhibitor. All three of these drug groups have been shown to reduce the incidence of reinfarction by 20–25%, although additivity has not been demonstrated. In the 'SAVE' study, captopril 50 mg × 3/d or placebo was started 3–16 days after a myocardial infarction in 2231 patients without overt cardiac failure but with a left ventricular ejection fraction of <40%. The captopril group had a lower incidence of recurrent myocardial infarction (133) and deaths (228) than the placebo group (170 and 275). Similar results have been achieved in several other trials, except for the CONSENSUS-II study which found no benefit from enalapril started within 24 hours of myocardial infarction. Whereas most studies have used echo or isotope scanning to assess cardiac function, the AIRE study showed a reduction in deaths (170 vs. 222) in the active group, receiving ramipril 5 mg × 2/d, started 3–10 days after a myocardial infarction in 2006 patients with *clinical* evidence only of cardiac failure.[19]

In addition to these drugs, many patients should receive a cholesterol lowering drug, usually a statin, which will reduce mortality by a similar further percentage in patients whose cholesterol remains >5.2 mmol/L after dietary therapy.

There is no place for *routine* antidysrhythmic prophylaxis, and longterm anticoagulation is similarly out of place, except when indicated by arrhythmias or poor left ventricular function.

SUMMARY

- The treatment of both hypertension and angina drugs which reduce the work of the heart either directly or via reduction of peripheral vascular resistance.
- β-blockade, which acts mainly through reduced cardiac output, and Ca^{++}-channel blockade (selective arterial dilatation) may be used in either condition.
- Other vasodilators are suited preferentially to hypertension (ACE inhibitors, angiotensin AT_1 receptor antagonists and α-adrenoceptor blockade) or to angina (nitrates).
- The treatment of myocardial infarction requires thrombolysis, aspirin and β-adrenoceptor blockade acutely, with the latter two continued for at least two years as secondary prevention of a further myocardial infarction.
- Other important steps in secondary prevention include ACE inhibitors and statins in selected patients with cardiac failure and hypercholesterolaemia, respectively.

Treatment of arterial hypertension

Clinical evaluation of antihypertensives falls into two classes:

1. Whether longterm reduction of blood pressure benefits the patient by preventing complications and prolonging life; these studies take years, require enormous numbers of patients and cost millions (£ or $).[20]

---

[19] SAVE = Survival and Ventricular Enlargement Trial; AIRE = Acute Infarction Ramipril Efficacy study; CONSENSUS = Cooperative New Scandinavian Enalapril Survival Study. References: Rutherford J D et al 1994 Effects of captopril on ischemic events after myocardial infarction. Results of the Survival and Ventricular Enlargement trial. SAVE Investigators. Circulation 90: 1731–1738. AIRE Study Investigators 1993 Effect of ramipril on mortality and morbidity of survivors of acute myocardial infarction with clinical evidence of heart failure. Lancet 342: 821–828. Swedberg K P et al 1992 Effects of the early administration of enalapril on mortality in patients with acute myocardial infarction. New England Journal of Medicine 327: 678–684.

[20] The biggest trial ever done in hypertension was single blind for logistic, not scientific, reasons. It was deemed to be

2. Whether a drug is capable of effective, safe and comfortable control of blood pressure for about one year. Such studies are deemed sufficient to allow the introduction of a new drug. There is sufficient evidence that reduction of blood pressure is beneficial that trials of the first kind are not demanded for all new drugs by regulatory authorities. However it is recognised that the shorter trials may not reveal the longterm consequences of some metabolic effects, e.g. on blood lipids, which may adversely affect the risk of coronary heart disease. Placebo effects are prominent in these shorter trials and must be carefully controlled in trial design.

AIM OF TREATMENT

The principal longterm aim in most patients is prevention of stroke with prevention of myocardial infarction, requiring attention to other risk factors such as plasma lipids. The more immediate aim of treatment is to reduce the blood pressure as near to normal as possible in the erect posture, and to keep it there whether the patient is lying, standing or exercising and whether the environment is hot or cold. This is expecting a lot, but it often can be achieved though there may be a price to pay in well-being (quality of life).

When this aim is achieved in *severe cases* there is great symptomatic improvement: retinopathy clears and vision improves; headaches are abolished. However, a variable amount of irreversible damage has often been done by the high blood pressure before treatment is started; renal failure may progress despite treatment; arterial damage leads to cardiac or cerebral catastrophes.

It is obviously desirable to start treatment before irreversible changes occur and in *mild and moderately severe cases* this often means advising treatment to symptom-free people discovered by screening.

impracticable to manage a study involving treatment adjustments in 17 354 patients and lasting 5.5 years if the double blind technique was used. The study cost £4.5 million (US$5.85 million at then current values) (Medical Research Council Working Party 1985 British Medical Journal 291: 97). The time from commencement to publication was 8 years. The choice of drugs as well as the dose is liable to become outdated in such trials. Calcium agonists were introduced into medicine during the course of this study.

Which patient to treat

Effective treatment reduces the risk of strokes, renal failure and heart failure though, in many trials, not the risk of myocardial infarction. An exception is in the elderly. Treatment will almost always be life-long. However, in the younger patients treated in the decade before complications are likely to occur, there is a case for a trial of discontinuation after a year or two of very good control and provided there is attentive follow-up monitoring.

The *relative* risks of hypertension and benefits of treating hypertension in the elderly are less than in the under 65s, but it is very clear now that the *absolute* risks and benefits are greater. Given the large choice of treatments available, doctors cannot cite improved quality of life as an excuse for not treating hypertension in the elderly. However, starting doses should often be halved and, pending further evidence, it may be permissible to seek less aggressive targets for blood pressure reduction.

It is obvious that adverse effects of therapy are important in that *very large* numbers of patients must be treated in order that *very small* numbers may gain; this is a salient feature of the use of drugs to prevent disease.

PRINCIPLES OF ANTIHYPERTENSIVE THERAPY

General measures may be sufficient to control mild cases as follows:

- Obesity: reduce it
- Alcohol: minimise intake
- Smoking: stop it
- Diet: *no added salt*; avoid highly salted foods. *Add potassium and oily fish.* Dietary supplementation with potassium reduces blood pressure; as does a high intake of fish oil, a source of eicosapentaenoic and related acids, the high intake of which in the diet of Inuit (Eskimos) may be responsible for the rarity amongst them of severe hypertension. There is not yet a consensus on the role of these items in routine antihypertension therapy beyond ensuring adequate dietary intake (in the healthy as well as in hypertensives) and avoiding diuretic-induced potassium depletion

- Relaxation therapy: worth considering for highly motivated borderline patients.

DRUG THERAPY

Blood pressure may be reduced by any one or more of the actions listed at the beginning of this chapter. It is difficult to predict the best drug for individual patients, though younger patients are more likely to respond to a β-blocker or ACE inhibitor, and older patients to a diuretic or Ca^{++}-blocker. By systematic trial and error, a target of 140/90 mmHg can be reached in about 40% of patients.

Since each drug acts on only one or two of the blood pressure control mechanisms, the factors that are uninfluenced by monotherapy are liable to adapt (homeostatic mechanism), to oppose the useful effect and to restore the previous state. There are two principal mechanisms of such adaptation or tolerance:

1. *Increase in blood volume* occurs with any drug that reduces peripheral resistance (increases intravascular volume) or cardiac output (reduces glomerular flow) due to activation of the renin-angiotensin-aldosterone system. The result is that cardiac output and blood pressure rise. This compensatory effect can be prevented by using a diuretic in combination with the other drug.

2. *Baroreceptor reflexes.* A fall in blood pressure evokes reflex activity of the sympathetic system, causing increased peripheral resistance and cardiac activity (rate and contractility).

Therefore, whenever high blood pressure is proving difficult to control and whenever a number of hypotensive drugs are used in combination, the drugs chosen should between them act on *all three main determinants of blood pressure:*

blood volume, peripheral resistance and the heart.
Such combinations will achieve three objectives:

- maximise antihypertensive efficacy by adding actions exerted at 3 different points in the cardiovascular system;
- minimise the opposing homeostatic effects by blocking the compensatory changes in blood volume, vascular tone and cardiac function;
- minimise side-effects by permitting smaller

doses of each drug each acting at a different site and having different side-effects.[21]

First-dose hypotension is now uncommon and occurs mainly with drugs having an action on veins (α-adrenoceptor blockers, ACE inhibitors) when baroreflex activation is impaired, e.g. old age; or intravascular volume is depleted, e.g. by diuretics.

TREATING HYPERTENSION

A graded well-tried and conventional regimen is as follows:

1. Start with a single morning dose of either a *β-adrenoceptor blocker*, e.g. atenolol, or a *diuretic*, e.g. bendrofluazide. Efficacy will begin to be seen within 2–3 d and most of it will have developed within 14 d (dose of β-blocker can be monitored by heart rate response to standard exercise).

2. If the pressure is not controlled in 2–3 weeks, either change to a single drug of a different group (monodrug therapy is preferred where it is possible) or add the second drug, above. The dose of diuretic will be fixed, but that of the β-adrenoceptor blocker will be in the small-to-moderate range.[22]

3. If blood pressure control is still inadequate, the patient should be given a trial of either an ACE inhibitor (in younger patients) or Ca^{++}-blocker (in older patients). Initial severity and response to the β-blocker and diuretic will determine whether these drugs are simultaneously withdrawn. If one of these drugs is continued, the logical combinations are of either:

- β-blocker plus Ca^{++}-blocker (since the former blocks part of the baroreflex response to the latter), or
- ACE inhibitor plus diuretic (since the latter stimulates the renin-angiotensin system and

---

[21] Chalmers J P 1977 Australian Prescriber 2: 6.

[22] Drugs having a *short steep dose-response curve* for efficacy (that quickly reach a plateau) are given in fixed dose (e.g. to increase the diuretic does not add to efficacy though it does add to toxicity). Drugs having *long sloping dose-response curves* can be titrated for efficacy as well as being used as fixed-dose components of multidrug regimens.

turns nonrenin dependent hypertension into renin-dependent hypertension).

The choice between these will be influenced by which of the β-blocker or diuretic appeared to cause the greater initial fall in blood pressure but, as with monotherapy, trial and error are often required.

4. Most patients still uncontrolled at this stage will have had a contraindication or adverse response to one of the drugs. In these patients the combination of the two newer drug classes, Ca^{++}-channel blocker (nifedipine or amlodipine) plus ACE inhibitor (enalapril or lisinopril), is effective. If an ACE inhibitor has been precluded by the dry cough which occurs in around 20% of patients, an effective alternative now is an angiotensin-receptor antagonist (losartan).

5. If additional therapy is required, α-blockade (e.g. doxazosin) is particularly effective at this stage by blocking the vasoconstrictor component of the baroreflex response to some of the other drugs. A very small number of patients may need reversion to an older class of drug such as minoxidil (provided that diuretics and β-blockers can also be given) or methyldopa.

Treatment and severity

Mild hypertension will commonly be adequately treated by a single drug, stage 1 above.

Moderate and severe hypertension may be treated from the start as in stage 2 above (2-drug regimen). However, optimal blood pressure control is rarely an emergency (see below) and it is preferable in most patients to follow the systematic route to this goal so that the efficacy and tolerability of individual drugs can be assessed in each patient.

In a few patients with severe hypertension, lowering the blood pressure may make the patient worse, e.g. if there is severe renal impairment (blood urea above 17 mmol/l), or advanced cerebral or coronary atherosclerosis. In these cases blood flow to vital organs may depend upon a high perfusion pressure; but when such patients have severe hypertensive symptoms a very cautious trial of antihypertensive drugs is worthwhile.

Monitoring

The blood pressure must be monitored by a doctor (particularly important in the old) and also sometimes by the patient. 24-hour ambulatory blood pressure monitoring (ABPM) is possible with an increasing number of user-friendly, semi-automatic devices, but they are still an expensive ideal for which data on their influence on outcome is not yet available.

Diuretics and potassium. The potassium-losing (kaliuretic) diuretics used in hypertension deplete body potassium by 10–15%. Routine potassium chloride supplements are not required, but hypokalaemia will occasionally occur. Uncomplicated patients may not need monitoring if the lowest possible doses are used, but vulnerable patients, e.g. the elderly, should be monitored for K loss at 3 months and thereafter every 6–12 months. In general a potassium-retaining diuretic (amiloride) in a fixed-dose combination with a thiazide, e.g. Dyazide, is preferred over the use of potassium supplements. With such use, a potassium supplement then becomes dangerous.

Control of K balance is particularly important if the patient is also taking digoxin. It is also important in patients receiving combinations of diuretic and ACE inhibitors, though here it is the risk of an elevated K^+ (and low Na^+), due to reduced aldosterone secretion, that is the danger.

Fixed-dose diuretic/potassium formulations contain only a little K and provide only marginal protection.

Compliance. It is obvious that multidrug therapy will pose a substantial problem of compliance. Since treatment will be life-long it is well worthwhile taking trouble to find the most convenient regimen for each individual. A single daily dose would be ideal and to achieve this sustained release formulations and fixed-dose combinations are used. Examples include: Tenoretic (atenolol + chlorthalidone), Tenif (atenolol and nifedipine) and Zestoretic (lisinopril and hydrochlorothiazide).

Treatment of hypertension emergencies

It is important to distinguish three circumstances

which may exist separately or together, as illustrated in Figure 24.1, the Venn diagram.[23] The diagram emphasises that

- *Severe* hypertension is not on its own an indication for *urgent* (or large) reductions in blood pressure
- Blood pressure (BP) can occasionally require urgent reduction even when the hypertension is not severe
- *Accelerated phase* (malignant) *hypertension* rarely requires urgent reduction, and specifically the blood pressure must be lowered *slowly* during the first few days.

The indications for *emergency* reduction of blood pressure are rare. They are

- Hypertensive encephalopathy (including eclampsia)
- Acute left ventricular failure (due to hypertension)
- Dissecting aneurysm.

In these conditions, blood pressure should be

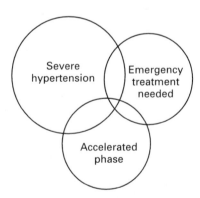

Fig. 24.1 Venn diagram, illustrating intersections among three overlapping clinical states which are defined above

---

[23] J Venn (1834–1923) English logician who 'adopted the diagrammatic method of illustrating propositions by inclusive and exclusive circles' (Dictionary of National Biography). A medical pilgrimage to Cambridge, where Venn worked, should take in Caius College (named after its founder and early president of the London College of Physicians in the 16th century); as well as stained glass windows celebrating Venn's circles, the visitor may see a portrait of the most famous medical Caian, William Harvey.

reduced over the course of an hour. In patients with a dissecting aneurysm, where the BP may have been *completely normal* prior to dissection, the target is a low BP of 110/70 mmHg. Otherwise only small reductions are necessary to remove the emergency.

Accelerated phase hypertension (previously called malignant hypertension when the lack of treatment heralded death within a year of diagnosis) is characterised pathologically by fibrinoid necrosis of the small arteries. This has the important consequence that autoregulation of the cerebral and renal circulations is lost, meaning that reduction of blood pressure causes a proportional reduction in perfusion. It is therefore vital not to reduce diastolic BP by more than 20 mmHg on the first day of treatment. The consequences of ignoring this can frequently include cerebral infarction.

Unless contraindicated, the best treatment for all circles in the Venn diagram is β-blockade, given as atenolol 25 or 50 mg orally. In emergencies, an intravenous vasodilator should be used in addition.

A useful alternative is methyldopa 250 mg orally. Both these treatments are gradual in onset and unlikely to cause excessive hypotension. A theoretically preferable, but often impractical alternative is i.v. infusion of the vasodilator, nitroprusside (see p. 433). In patients with dissecting aneurysm, vasodilators should not be used unless patients are first β-blocked since any increase in the rate of rise of the pulse stroke is undesirable. Labetalol provides a convenient method of treating all patients within the three circles (except asthmatics), using either oral or parenteral therapy as appropriate. However it is not the most effective, and should be changed if blood pressure does not fall at the desired rate.

Alternatives for parenteral use are diazoxide, and the trimetaphan; when using the latter, the position of the patient can be used to facilitate (head-up, feet-down) or counter the effects of the drug, depending on response (or over-response).

Lower-than-usual doses of all drugs should be used if antihypertensive drugs have recently been taken or if renal function is impaired.

Oral maintenance treatment for severe hypertension should be started at once if possible; parenteral therapy is seldom necessary for more than 48 h.

Pregnancy hypertension

Effective treatment of pregnancy-induced hypertension improves fetal and perinatal survival. Controlled trials are difficult to do and present considerable ethical problems. Methyldopa has long been a favoured agent for oral therapy,[24] and parenteral hydralazine for emergency reduction of blood pressure (but not in early pregnancy: risk of teratogenesis). Because of possible consequence to the fetus choice of drug is conservative. But β-adrenoceptor blockers (labetalol, atenolol) are increasingly regarded as effective and safe for both mother and fetus. Severe hypotension in the mother jeopardises the fetus. But where patients enter pregnancy with mild essential hypertension, drug therapy may not benefit, and atenolol (but probably not methyldopa) may retard fetal growth.[24]

A diuretic should not be used in prevention or treatment of pre-eclampsia as there is no evidence of efficacy and metabolic effects may increase risk to both mother and fetus.

If a woman entering labour is still hypertensive, she has a 1% chance of a fit. The most effective *prophylaxis* is magnesium sulphate (4 g over 5 min i.v. or i.m. followed by 1 g/hour for 24 hours). This regimen prevented any fits in 1049 women with a BP >140/90 mmHg randomised to magnesium, compared to 10 fits in 1089 women given phenytoin. However this trial does not mean that either of the drugs is necessary in such women. By contrast, if a woman has one fit (treat with diazepam), then the magnesium regimen is superior to diazepam or phenytoin in preventing further fits.[25]

Aspirin, in low dose, was reported in early studies to reduce the incidence of pre-eclampsia in at-risk patients, but a more recent meta-analysis has contradicted these reports.

---

[24] Methyldopa: follow-up studies show no intellectual impairment in children up to age 7.5 years (for atenolol, see: Butters L 1990 British Medical Journal 301: 587).

[25] Lucas M J, Leveno K J, Cunningham F G 1995 A comparison of magnesium sulfate with phenytoin for the prevention of eclampsia. New England Journal of Medicine 333: 201–205.

The Eclampsia Trial Collaborative Group 1995 Which anticonvulsant for women with eclampsia? Evidence from the Collaborative Eclampsia Trial. Lancet 345: 1455–1463.

Unwanted interactions with antihypertensive drugs
(see also individual drugs)

Alcohol is the commonest contributing factor, or even cause of hypertension, and should always be considered as a cause of erratic or failed responses to treatment.

Sympathomimetics including appetite suppressants (but excluding dexfenfluramine) and tricyclic antidepressants can, even in small doses, reverse the effects of the rarely used adrenergic neuron blockers, but are otherwise unlikely to interfere with treatment.

Phenothiazine and butyrophenone *neuroleptics* interact unpredictably.

Methyldopa plus an MAO inhibitor may cause excitement and hallucinations.

Nonsteroidal anti-inflammatory drugs (NSAIDs), e.g. indomethacin, attenuate the antihypertensive effect of β-adrenoceptor blockers and of diuretics, perhaps by inhibiting the synthesis of vasodilator prostaglandins. This effect can also be important when a diuretic is used for severe *left ventricular failure*.

Cimetidine inhibits hepatic metabolism of lipid-soluble β-adrenoceptor blockers, increasing their effect.

Surgical anaesthesia may lead to a brisk fall in blood pressure in patients taking antihypertensives. Antihypertensive therapy should not ordinarily be altered before surgery, although it obviously can complicate care both during and after the operation. Anaesthetists **must** be informed.

Sexual function and cardiovascular drugs

All drugs that interfere with sympathetic autonomic activity, including diuretics, can interfere with sexual function. In men they cause failure of ejaculation and difficulty with erection. Substitution of a drug having a different site of action (e.g. ACE inhibitor or calcium antagonist; or even changing the drug within a group) may solve this problem, in which pharmacological effects may be potentiated by psychology. Centrally acting drugs (methyldopa, clonidine) cause sedation as well as reducing sympathetic drive, and this is an additive factor. Also, hypertensive patients are commonly of an age when nondrug causes of decline in sexual activity are increasingly common and patients may be influenced by fear of ill-health and of the consequences for their disease in general and the likelihood that sexual activity may be hazardous, as indeed it sometimes may be.

Sexual intercourse and the cardiovascular system

Normal sexual intercourse with orgasm is accompanied by transient but brisk physiological changes, e.g. tachycardia of up to 180 beats/min, with increases of 100 beats/min over less than one min, can occur. Systolic blood pressure may rise by 120 mmHg and diastolic by 50 mmHg. Orgasm may be accompanied by transient pressure of 230/130 mmHg in normotensive individuals. Electrocardiographic abnormalities may occur in healthy men and women. Respiratory rate may rise to 60/min.

Such changes in the healthy may reasonably be thought to bode ill for the unhealthy (hypertension, angina pectoris, post-myocardial infarction):

sudden deaths do occur during or shortly after sexual intercourse [ventricular fibrillation or subarachnoid haemorrhage], usually in clandestine circumstances such as the bordello or the mistress's boudoir, or when the relationship is between an older man and a younger woman — or are these the ones that make the news? In one series, 0.6% of all sudden deaths were [reportedly] attributable to sexual intercourse and in about half of these cardiac disease was present. Clearly it is undesirable that the patient with coronary heart disease should achieve the haemodynamic heights attainable in youth . . . [26]

There appears to be no record of sudden cardiovascular death in a woman.

If there is substantial concern about cardiovascular stress (hypertension, dysrhythmia) during sexual intercourse in either sex, a dose of labetalol about

2 hours before the event may well be justified (taking account of other therapy already in use). But patients taking a β-blocker long term for angina prophylaxis have shown reductions in peak heart rate during coitus from 122 to 82 beats/min. Excessive doses of these drugs may attenuate performance and satisfaction.

Patients suffering from angina pectoris will use glyceryl trinitrate or isosorbide dinitrate as usual for pre-exertional prophylaxis 10 min before intercourse.

Phaeochromocytoma

This tumour of the adrenal medulla secretes principally noradrenaline, but also variable amounts of adrenaline. Symptoms are related to this. Hypertension may be sustained or intermittent.

Diagnostic tests include measurement of catecholamine metabolites in urine followed by catecholamine concentrations in blood when the urine results are equivocal or high. With modern techniques interference by drugs and diet is less troublesome than formerly.

Antihypertensive drugs may alter catecholamine concentrations (particularly those that induce a reflex increase in sympathetic activity, e.g. vasodilators). False-positive results in tests can then occur and in the past patients have undergone unnecessary operations.[27]

A variety of *pharmacological tests* is now available,

---

[26] Editorial 1976 British Medical Journal 1: 414.

[27] On the other hand, a positive test must not be ignored. In 1954, a hospital clinical chemistry laboratory was asked to set up a biological assay for catecholamines in the urine. The head of the laboratory tested urine from the lab staff to obtain a reference range for the assay. All were negative except his own which was strongly positive. He felt well and regarded the result as showing insufficient specificity of the test. Two years later a fluorometric assay became available. The urines of the lab staff were tested again with the same result. The head of the laboratory still felt well, but this time he decided to consult a physician colleague. A few days later, before the consultation, he was quietly reading a newspaper at home in the evening when he had a fatal cerebral infarction. Autopsy revealed a phaeochromocytoma. (Robinson R 1980 Tumours that secrete catecholamines. Wiley, Chichester.

though best performed in specialist units to avoid erroneous results, e.g. pentolinium suppression test. Provocation tests are dangerous.

A phaeochromocytoma may also be stimulated to secrete and cause a hypertensive attack by metoclopramide and by any drug that releases histamine (opioids, curare, trimetaphan).

Establishment of the diagnosis ('does the patient have a phaeochromocytoma?') should always precede the radiological search for a tumour. The accurate measurement of adrenaline in plasma is itself invaluable in determining whether the tumour is likely to be adrenal or extra-adrenal for only adrenal tumours can synthesise adrenaline.

Control of blood pressure and **heart rate** preoperatively or when the tumour cannot be removed is achieved best by a combination α- and β-adrenoceptor blockade.

The α-blockade controls the blood pressure chiefly by abolishing peripheral vasoconstriction, and the β-blockade controls the tachycardia. A **β-receptor blocker should not be given alone**, since abolition of the peripheral vasodilator effects of adrenaline leaves the powerful α effects unopposed. The combined β- and α-receptor blocker (labetalol) can be used successfully, but the preferred treatment is the irreversible α-blocker, phenoxybenzamine, whose blockade cannot be overcome by a catecholamine surge. Treatment should be for several weeks, if possible, prior to surgery, to allow the intravascular volume depletion which is always present in phaeochromocytoma patients to be reversed.

During surgical removal, phentolamine (or sodium nitroprusside) should be at hand to control rises in blood pressure when the tumour is handled. When the adrenal veins have been clamped, volume expansion is often required to maintain blood pressure even after adequate preoperative α-blockade. A pressor infusion may also be needed, with isoprenaline or angiotensin (Hypertensin) being more use than the usual α-agonists, to which the patient will be insensitive, due to existing α-receptor blockade.

Metirosine (α-methyltyrosine) has been used with some success to block catecholamine synthesis in malignant phaeochromocytomas (see p. 444).

Metaiodobenzylguanidine (m^{131}IBG, an analogue of guanethidine) is actively taken up by adrenergic tissue and is concentrated in phaeochromocytomas. Radioactive forms allow localisation of tumours and detection of metastases; also selective therapeutic irradiation of functioning metastases or other tumours of chromaffin tissue, e.g. carcinoid.

GUIDE TO FURTHER READING

Antiplatelet Trialists' Collaboration 1994 Collaborative overview of randomised trials of antiplatelet therapy. I: Prevention of death, myocardial infarction, and stroke by prolonged antiplatelet therapy in various categories of patients. British Medical Journal 308: 81–107

Baver K et al 1991 Assessment of systemic effects of different ophthalmic β-blockers in healthy volunteers. Clinical Pharmacology and Therapeutics 49: 658

Beard K et al 1992 Management of elderly patients with sustained hypertension. British Medical Journal 304: 412–416

Braunwald E 1996 Acute myocardial infarction — the value of being prepared. New England Journal of Medicine 334: 51–53

Brown M J 1995 Phaeochromocytoma. In: Weatherall D, Ledingham J, Warrell D (eds) Oxford textbook of medicine. Oxford University Press, Oxford, pp. 2553–2557

Bulpitt C J et al 1990 The measurement of quality of life in hypertensive patients: a practical approach. British Journal of Clinical Pharmacology 30: 353; Palmer A et al p. 365; (editorial) Callender J S p. 351

Cairns J A 1995 Medical management of unstable angina. Lancet 346: 1644–1645

Calhoun D A et al 1990 Treatment of hypertensive crisis. New England Journal of Medicine 323: 1177 and subsequent correspondence

Cameron H A et al 1988 Drug treatment of intermittent claudication: a critical analysis of the methods and findings of published clinical trials. British Journal of Clinical Pharmacology 26: 569

Cooke E D et al 1990 Raynaud's syndrome. British Medical Journal 300: 553

Cunningham F G, Lindheimer M D 1992 Hypertension in pregnancy. New England Journal of Medicine 326: 927–932

Dickerson J E C, Brown M J 1995 Influence of age on general practitioners' definition and treatment of hypertension. British Medical Journal 310: 574

Flapan A D 1994 Management of patients after their first myocardial infarction. British Medical Journal 309: 1129–1134

Fletcher A E, Bulpitt C J 1992 How far should blood pressure be lowered? New England Journal of Medicine 326: 251–254

Goodfriend T L, Elliott M E, Catt K J 1996 Angiotensin receptors and their antagonists. New England Journal of Medicine 334: 1649–1654

Krane R J et al 1989 Impotence. New England Journal of Medicine 321: 1148

Johnston C I 1995 Angiotensin receptor antagonists: focus on losartan. Lancet 346: 1403–1407

Lau J et al 1992 Cumulative meta-analysis of therapeutic trials for myocardial infarction. New England Journal of Medicine 327: 248–254

McMurray J, Rankin A 1994 Cardiology — I: Treatment of myocardial infarction, unstable angina, and angina pectoris. British Medical Journal 309: 1343–1350

Norwegian Multicentre Study Group 1981 Timolol-induced reduction in mortality and reinfarction in patients surviving acute myocardial infarction. New England Journal of Medicine 304: 803 — a classic

Orme M 1990 Thiazides in the 1990s: the risk:benefit ratio still favours the drug. British Medical Journal 300: 1668

Redman C W G, Roberts J M 1995 Management of pre-eclampsia. Lancet 341: 1451–1454

Roberts J M 1995 Magnesium for preeclampsia and eclampsia. New England Journal of Medicine 333: 250–251

Scandinavian Simvastatin Survival Study Group 1994 Randomised trial of cholesterol lowering in 4444 patients with coronary heart disease: the Scandinavian Simvastatin Survival Study (4S). Lancet 344: 1383–1389

Shawket S et al 1989 Selective suprasensitivity to CGRP, the potent endogenous vasodilator, in the hands of patients with Raynaud's phenomenon. Lancet ii: 1354–1357

Sibai B M et al 1993 Prevention of preeclampsia with low-dose aspirin in healthy, nulliparous pregnant women. The National Institute of Child Health and Human Development Network of Maternal-Fetal Medicine Units. New England Journal of Medicine 329: 1213–1218

Swales J D 1994 Pharmacological treatment of hypertension. Lancet 344: 380–385

25

Cardiac dysrhythmia and failure

SYNOPSIS

The pathophysiology of cardiac dysrhythmias is complex and the actions of drugs that are useful in stopping or controlling them may seem equally so. Nevertheless many patients with dysrhythmias respond well to therapy with drugs and a working knowledge of their effects and indications pays dividends, for irregularity of the heart-beat is at least inconvenient and at worst fatal.

- Drugs for cardiac dysrhythmias
- Principal drugs by class
- Specific treatments, including that for cardiac arrest
- Drugs for cardiac failure

Drugs for cardiac dysrhythmias

OBJECTIVES OF TREATMENT

In almost no other condition is it as important to remember the dual objectives:

- To reduce morbidity
- To reduce mortality.

Dysrhythmias are frequently asymptomatic and only rarely fatal. The same cannot be said of most anti-dysrhythmics, which should therefore be avoided in the absence of clear indications. All anti-dysrhythmics are also pro-dysrhythmic. Except for digoxin and amiodarone, they are to a variable degree negatively inotropic.

A second reason for an empirical approach to anti-dysrhythmic treatment is the gulf between the theoretical classification of their mechanism of action and the lack of understanding this offers for their different clinical uses. On the side of normal physiology, we can see the spontaneous generation and propagation of the cardiac impulse requiring a combination of specialised conducting tissue and intermyocyte conduction. The heart also has backstops in case of problems such as the variety of pacemakers. By contrast, the available drugs may be considered still to be at an early stage of evolution, and useful anti-dysrhythmic actions — such as that of adenosine — continue to be discovered as much by chance as by design.

Doctors and drugs interfere with cardiac electronics at their peril. In emergencies, action often needs to be taken by the most junior doctor in the team, and some *rote* recommendations are then necessary. However, the diagnosis and elective treatment of chronic, or episodic dysrhythmias require greater skill to ensure that the risk–benefit equation receives the correct solution. As will become clear, anti-dysrhythmic drugs have a hard time proving superior safety or efficacy over use of the defibrillator and pacing wire.

SOME PHYSIOLOGY AND PATHOPHYSIOLOGY

There are broadly two types of cardiac tissue.

- *The first type* is ordinary myocardial (atrial and ventricular) muscle, responsible for the pumping action of the heart.
- *The second type* is specialised *conducting* tissue that initiates the cardiac electrical impulse and determines the order in which the muscle cells contract. The important property of being able to form impulses spontaneously is called *automaticity* and is a feature of certain parts of the conducting tissue, i.e. the sinoatrial (SA) and atrioventricular (AV) nodes. The SA node has the highest frequency of spontaneous discharge, 70 times per minute, and thus controls the contraction rate of the heart, making the cells more distal in the system fire more rapidly than they would do spontaneously, i.e. it is the pacemaker. If the SA node fails to function, the next fastest part takes over. This is often the AV node (45 discharges per min) or a site in the His-Purkinje system (25 discharges per min).

Altered rate of automatic discharge, or abnormality of the mechanism by which an impulse is generated from a centre in the nodes or conducting tissue, is one cause of cardiac dysrhythmia, e.g. atrial fibrillation, flutter or tachycardia.

Ionic movements into and out of cardiac cells

Nearly all cells in the body exhibit a difference in electrical voltage between their interior and exterior, the membrane potential. Some cells, including the conducting and contracting cells of the heart, are excitable; an appropriate stimulus alters the properties of the cell membrane, ions flow across it and elicit an action potential. This spreads to adjacent cells, i.e. is conducted as an electrical impulse and, when it reaches a muscle cell, causes it to contract, i.e. excitation–contraction coupling.

In the resting state the interior of the cell (conducting and contracting types) is electrically *negative* with respect to the exterior due to the disposition of ions (mainly sodium, potassium and

calcium) across its membrane, i.e. it is polarised. The ionic changes of the action potential first result in a rapid redistribution of ions such that the potential alters to *positive* within the cell (depolarisation); subsequent and slower flows of ions restore the resting potential (repolarisation). These ionic movements may be separated into *phases* which are briefly described here and in Figure 25.1, for they help to explain the actions of antidysrhythmic drugs.

VAUGHAN-WILLIAMS CLASSIFICATION OF ANTI-DYSRHYTHMICS[1]

This is based on the phases of the cardiac cycle depicted in Figure 25.1.

Phase 0 is a rapid depolarisation of the cell membrane that is associated with a fast inflow of sodium ions through channels that are selectively permeable to these ions.

Phase 1 is a short initial period of rapid repolari-

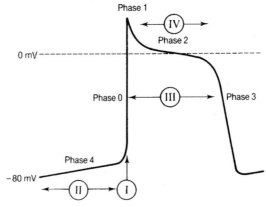

Fig. 25.1 The action potential of a cardiac cell that is capable of spontaneous depolarisation (SA or AV nodal, or His-Purkinje) indicating phases 0–4; the figure illustrates the gradual increase in transmembrane potential (mV) during phase 4; cells that are not capable of spontaneous depolarisation do not exhibit increase in voltage during this phase (see text). The modes of action of antidysrhythmic drugs of classes I, II, III and IV are indicated in relation to these phases

---

[1] Vaughan Williams E M 1984 Journal of Clinical Pharmacology 24: 129.

sation brought about mainly by an outflow of *potassium ions*.

Phase 2 is a period when there is a delay in repolarisation caused mainly by a slow movement of *calcium ions* from the exterior into the cell through channels that are selectively permeable to these ions.

Phase 3 is a second period of rapid repolarisation during which potassium ions move out of the cell.

Phase 4 is the fully repolarised state during which potassium ions move back into and sodium and calcium ions move out of the cell. During this phase, the interior of cells that discharge automatically becomes gradually less negative until a potential is reached (threshold) which allows rapid depolarisation (phase 0) to occur, and the cycle is repeated. Cells that do not discharge spontaneously rely on the arrival of an action potential from another cell to initiate depolarisation.

In phases 1 and 2 the cell is in an *absolutely refractory* state and is incapable of responding further to any stimulus but during phase 3, the *relative refractory* period, the cell will depolarise again if a stimulus is unusually strong. The orderly transmission of an electrical impulse (action potential) throughout the conducting system may be retarded in an area of disease, e.g. ischaemia. Thus an impulse travelling down a normal Purkinje fibre may spread to an adjacent fibre which has transiently failed to transmit, and pass up it in reverse direction. If this retrograde impulse should in turn re-excite the cells which provided the original impulse, a repetitively-firing *re-entrant circuit* is established and may cause a dysrhythmia, e.g. paroxysmal supraventricular tachycardia.

In summary most cardiac dysrhythmias are probably due either to:

- *altered rate of spontaneous discharge* in conducting tissue, or
- *impaired conduction* in part of the system leading to the formation of re-entry circuits.

CLASSIFICATION OF DRUGS

Class I: sodium channel blockade. These drugs restrict the rapid inflow of sodium during phase 0 and thus slow the maximum rate of depolarisation.

Another term for this property is *membrane stabilising activity*; it may contribute to stopping dysrhythmias by limiting the *responsiveness to excitation* of cardiac cells. The drugs may be subclassified as follows:

A. Drugs that lengthen action potential duration and refractoriness, e.g. quinidine, disopyramide, procainamide
B. Drugs that shorten action potential duration and refractoriness, e.g. lignocaine, mexiletine, tocainide, phenytoin
C. Drugs that have negligible effect on action potential duration and refractoriness, e.g. flecainide, propafenone.

The value of the classification is that drugs in class 1B are ineffective for supraventricular dysrhythmias, whereas they all have some action in ventricular dysrhythmias. However, the classification is not useful in explaining *why* the classes differ anatomically in their efficacy.

Class II: catecholamine blockade. Propranolol and other β-adrenoceptor antagonists reduce background sympathetic tone in the heart, reduce automatic discharge (phase 4) and protect against adrenergically stimulated ectopic pacemakers.

Class III: lengthening of refractoriness (without effect on sodium inflow in phase 0). Prolongation of cellular refractoriness (phases 1,2,3,) beyond a critical point may prevent a re-entry circuit being completed and may thereby abolish a re-entrant tachycardia (see above), e.g. amiodarone, bretylium, also sotalol.

Class IV: calcium channel blockade. These drugs depress the slow inward calcium current (phase 2) and prolong conduction and refractoriness particularly in the SA and AV nodes, which may explain their effectiveness in terminating paroxysmal supraventricular tachycardia, e.g. verapamil.

Although the antidysrhythmics have been entered into this classification according to a characteristic major action, most have other effects as well. For example, quinidine (class I) has class III effects; propranolol (class II) has class I effects, bretylium (class III) has class II effects and sotalol (class II) has class III effects.

Principal drugs by class

(For further data see Table 25.1)

CLASS IA (sodium channel blockade with lengthened refractoriness)

Disopyramide

Disopyramide ($t^{1/2}$ 6 h) is now the most commonly used drug in this class. It also has significant antimuscarinic activity. The drug is effective in both ventricular dysrhythmias, especially after myocardial infarction, and in supraventricular dysrhythmias. It may also be used for paroxysmal supraventricular tachycardias of the Wolff–Parkinson–White (WPW) syndrome.

Adverse reactions. The antimuscarinic activity is a significant problem and may lead to dry mouth, blurred vision, glaucoma and micturition hesitancy and retention. Gastrointestinal symptoms, rash and agranulocytosis occur. Effects on the cardiovascular system include hypotension and cardiac failure (negative inotropic effect), and tachydysrhythmia, e.g. torsade de pointes. This last may be preceded by widening of the QT interval (ECG) and is unusual if disopyramide is not combined with other class IA or class III drugs.

Pharmacokinetics. Disopyramide is used both orally and intravenously (see Table 25.1) and is well absorbed. It is both excreted unchanged and metabolised. The drug is variably protein bound.

Quinidine

Quinidine is considered the prototype class I drug, although not now the most frequently used.[2] Its residual use is in the chronic treatment of difficult supraventricular tachycardias. In addition to class IA, quinidine depresses the contractility of the myocardium (negative inotropic effect), and reduces vagus nerve activity on the heart (antimuscarinic effect). At therapeutic doses there is lengthening of ventricular systole and atrioventricular conduction block.

Pharmacokinetics. Absorption of quinidine from the gut is rapid, 75% of the drug is metabolised and the remainder is eliminated unchanged in the urine. Active metabolites may accumulate when renal function is impaired.

Adverse reactions. Quinidine must never be used alone to treat atrial fibrillation or flutter as its antimuscarinic action enhances AV conduction and the heart rate may accelerate. Other cardiac effects include serious ventricular tachydysrhythmias associated with electrocardiographic QT prolongation, e.g. torsade de pointes, the probable cause of 'quinidine syncope'. The negative inotropic action of quinidine may result in hypotension and cardiac failure. Plasma digoxin concentration is raised by quinidine (displacement from tissue binding and impairment of renal excretion) and the dose of digoxin should be decreased when the drugs are used together.

Noncardiac effects, called *cinchonism*, include diarrhoea and other gastrointestinal symptoms, rashes, thrombocytopenia and fever.

CLASS IB (sodium channel blockade with shortened refractoriness)

Lignocaine

Lignocaine (lidocaine) is used principally for ventricular dysrhythmias, especially those complicating myocardial infarction. Its kinetics make it unsuitable for oral administration and therefore restrict its application to the treatment of acute dysrhythmias.

Adverse reactions are uncommon unless infusion

---

[2] In 1912 K F Wenckebach, a Dutch physician (who described 'Wenckebach block') was visited by a merchant who wished to get rid of an attack of atrial fibrillation (he had recurrent attacks which, although they did not unduly inconvenience him, offended his notions of good order in life's affairs). On receiving a guarded prognosis, the merchant enquired why there were heart specialists if they could not accomplish what he himself had already achieved. In the face of Wenckebach's incredulity he promised to return the next day with a regular pulse, which he did, at the same time revealing that he had done it with quinine (an optical isomer of quinidine). Examination of quinine derivatives led to the introduction of quinidine in 1918 (Wenckebach K F 1923 Journal of the American Medical Association 81: 472).

Table 25.1 Drugs for cardiac dysrhythmia

Drug		Usual doses* and interval	Effect on ECG	Usually effective plasma concentration
IA:	Quinidine	p.o.: 200 mg test dose, then 200–400 mg × 6–8 h	Prolongs QRS QT and (±) PR	2–5 mg/l
	Procainamide	p.o.: mg/kg/d in divided doses × 3–4 h or × 6 h (sust. release). i.v.: see specialist literature	Prolongs QRS QT and (±) PR	4–10 mg/l (NAPA: active metabolite, 10–20 mg/l)
	Disopyramide	p.o.: 300–800 mg/d in divided doses. i.v.: see specialist literature	Prolongs QRS QT and (±) PR	2–5 mg/l
IB:	Lignocaine (lidocaine)	i.v. loading: 100 mg as a bolus over a few min; i.v. maintenance: 1–4 mg/min	No significant change	1.5–6 mg/l
	Mexiletine	p.o.: initial dose 400 mg, then after 2 h 200–250 mg × 6–8 h. i.v.: see specialist literature	No significant change	0.5–2 mg/l
	Tocainide	p.o.: 1.2 g/d in divided doses to 2.4 g/d max.; i.v.: see specialist literature	No significant change	3–10 mg/l
	Phenytoin	i.v.: 3.5–5 mg/kg by caval catheter not exceeding 50 mg/kg with ECG and BP monitoring	No significant change	5–20 mg/l
IC:	Flecainide	p.o.: 100–200 mg × 12 h; and i.v.: see specialist literature	Prolongs PR and QRS	0.2–1 mg/l
	Propafenone	p.o.: see specialist literature	Prolongs PR and QRS	Active metabolite precludes establishment
II:	Propranolol	p.o.: 10–80 mg × 6 h i.v.: 1mg over 1 min intervals to 10 mg max. (5 mg in anaesthesia)	Prolongs PR (±). No change in QRS. Shortens QT Bradycardia	Not established
	Esmolol	i.v.: 40 mg over 1 min + 4 mg/min: see specialist literature	As for propranolol	0.15–2 mg/l
III:	Amiodarone	p.o.: loading: 200 mg × 8 h for 1 week, then 200 mg × 12 h for1 week; maintenance 200 mg/d	Prolongs PR, QRS and QT Sinus bradycardia	Not established
	Bretylium	i.v.: see specialist literature	No change. Sinus bradycardia	Not established
IV:	Verapamil	p.o.: 40–120 mg × 8–12 h i.v.: see specialist literature	Prolongs PR	Probably 100–300 μg/l
Other:	Digoxin	p.o.: (tablets): 0.5–0.75 mg initially; additional 0.25–0.5 mg × 6–8 h maintenance: 0.125–0.5 mg/d	Prolongs PR Depresses ST segment Flattens T wave	1–2 μg/l

*Doses based on British National Formulary recommendations. Patients with decreased hepatic or renal function may require lower doses (see text).
This table is adapted from that published in the Medical Letter on Drugs and Therapeutics (USA) 1991. We are grateful to the Chairman of the Editorial Board for allowing us to use this material.

is rapid or there is significant cardiac failure; they include hypotension, dizziness, blurred sight, sleepiness, slurred speech, numbness, sweating, confusion and convulsions.

Pharmacokinetics. Lignocaine is used by the i.v, or occasionally the i.m. route; dosing by mouth is unsatisfactory because the t½ (90 min) is too short to maintain a constant plasma concentration by repeated administration and because the drug undergoes extensive presystemic (first-pass) elimination in the liver.

Mexiletine is similar to lignocaine but is effective by the oral route ($t^{1/2}$ 10 h). It is used for ventricular dysrhythmias especially those complicating myocardial infarction, and those induced by cardiac glycosides. *Adverse reactions* are dose related and include nausea, vomiting, hiccough, tremor, drowsiness, confusion, dysarthria, diplopia, ataxia, cardiac dysrhythmia and hypotension.

CLASS IC (sodium channel blockade with minimal effect on refractoriness)

Flecainide

Flecainide slows conduction in all cardiac cells including the anomalous pathways responsible for the Wolff–Parkinson–White (WPW) syndrome. Together with encainide and moricizine, it underwent clinical trials to establish if suppression of asymptomatic premature beats with antidysrhythmic drugs would reduce the risk of death from dysrhythmia after myocardial infarction.[3] The study was terminated after preliminary analysis of 1727 patients revealed that mortality in the groups treated with flecainide or encainide was 7.7% compared with 3.0% in controls. The most likely explanation for the result was the *induction* of lethal ventricular dysrhythmias by flecainide and encainide, i.e. a *prodysrhythmic* effect. In the light of these findings the *indications for use* of flecainide are restricted to treatment of AV nodal tachycardia in patients with WPW syndrome or similar conditions with anomalous pathways, symptomatic sustained ventricular tachycardia and premature ventricular contractions and/or nonsustained ventricular tachycardia causing disabling symptoms where other drugs are ineffective or cannot be tolerated. Flecainide may also be useful as a prelude to DC conversion in patients with atrial fibrillation (AF) who have previously reverted to AF.

Pharmacokinetics. Its action is terminated by metabolism in the liver and by elimination unchanged in the urine. The $t^{1/2}$ is 14 h in healthy adults but may be over 20 h in patients with cardiac disease, in the elderly and in those with poor renal function.

Adverse reactions. Flecainide is *contraindicated* in patients with sick sinus syndrome, with cardiac failure, and in those with a history of myocardial infarction who have asymptomatic ventricular ectopic beats or asymptomatic nonsustained ventricular tachycardia. Minor adverse effects include nausea, dizziness, blurred vision, tremor, abnormal taste sensations and paraesthesiae.

Propafenone

In addition to the properties of this class, propafenone also has β-adrenoceptor blocking activity equivalent to low doses of propranolol. It may be used to suppress nonsustained ventricular dysrhythmias in patients whose left ventricular function is well preserved.

Pharmacokinetics. It is metabolised by the liver and 7% of patients are poor metabolisers (see p. 110) who thus for equivalent doses have higher plasma concentrations than the remainder of the population who are extensive metabolisers.

Adverse reactions are similar to those caused by flecainide and are commoner in poor oxidisers. In addition, conduction block may occur, cardiac failure may worsen and ventricular dysrhythmias may be exacerbated, especially in patients with sustained ventricular tachycardia and poor left ventricular function.

CLASS II (catecholamine blockade)

Beta-adrenoceptor antagonists
(see also Ch. 24)

Beta-adrenoceptor blockers are effective probably because they counteract the dysrhythmogenic effect of catecholamines. The following actions appear to be relevant:

- The rate of automatic firing of the SA node is accelerated by β-adrenoceptor activation and

---

[3] Cardiac arrhythmia suppression trial investigators 1989 New England Journal of Medicine 321: 406.

this effect is abolished by β-blockers. Some ectopic pacemakers appear to be dependent on adrenergic drive.

- β-blockers prolong the refractoriness of the AV node which may prevent re-entrant tachycardia at this site.
- Many β-blocking drugs (propranolol, oxprenolol, alprenolol, acebutolol, labetalol) also possess membrane stabilising (class I) properties; sotalol prolongs cardiac refractoriness (class III) but has no class I effects; it is often preferred when a β-blocker is indicated. Esmolol is a short-acting $β_1$-selective agent, whose sole use is in the treatment of dysrhythmias. Its short duration and $β_1$-selectivity mean that it could be considered in some patients with contraindications to other β-blocking drugs.
- Beta-adrenoceptor antagonists are effective for a range of supraventricular dysrhythmias, in particular those associated with exercise, emotion or hyperthyroidism. They may be used in Wolff–Parkinson–White syndrome and in digoxin-induced dysrhythmias. Sotalol may be used to suppress ventricular ectopic beats and ventricular tachycardia.

Pharmacokinetics. For longterm use, any of the oral preparations of β-blocker is suitable. In emergencies, propranolol or esmolol may be given i.v. (see Table 25.1). Esmolol has a $t^1/2$ of 9 min, which allows infusion of the drug and rapid increments in dose, titrated against response. The range is 4–12 mg/min after an initial bolus of 40 mg over 1 minute.

Adverse reactions. Adverse cardiac effects from overdosage include heart block or even cardiac arrest. Heart failure may be precipitated when a patient is dependent on sympathetic drive to maintain output (see Ch. 24 for an account of other adverse effects).

Interactions: concomitant i.v. administration of calcium channel blockers that affect conduction (verapamil, diltiazem) increases the risk of bradycardia and AV block. In patients with depressed myocardial contractility, the combination of oral or i.v. β-blockade and Ca^{++}-channel blockade (nifedipine, verapamil) may cause hypotension or cardiac failure.

CLASS III (lengthening of refractoriness without sodium channel blockade)

Amiodarone

Amiodarone is now the most powerful anti-arrhythmic available for the treatment and prevention of both atrial and ventricular dysrhythmias. Even short-term use, however, can cause serious toxicity, and its use should always follow consideration or trial of alternatives. Amiodarone prolongs the effective refractory period of myocardial cells, the AV node and of anomalous pathways. It also blocks β-adrenoceptors noncompetitively.

Amiodarone is used in chronic ventricular dysrhythmias; in atrial fibrillation it slows the ventricular response and may restore sinus rhythm; it may be used to maintain sinus rhythm after cardioversion for atrial fibrillation or flutter. Amiodarone is also effective for the management of resistant re-entry supraventricular tachycardias associated with the Wolff–Parkinson–White syndrome. Despite one trial showing benefit from routine administration of amiodarone to patients with congestive cardiac failure, such treatment has not entered everyday practice, and further trials will be required.[4]

Pharmacokinetics. Amiodarone is effective given orally; its enormous apparent distribution volume (70 l/kg) indicates that little remains in the blood. It is stored in fat and many other tissues and the $t^1/2$ of 54 days after multiple dosing signifies slow release from these sites (and slow accumulation to steady state means that a loading dose is necessary, see Table 25.1). The drug is metabolised in the liver and eliminated via the biliary and intestinal tracts.

Adverse reactions. Adverse cardiovascular effects include bradycardia, heart block and induction of ventricular dysrhythmia. Other effects are the development of corneal microdeposits which cause visual haloes and photophobia. These are dose-related, resolve when the drug is discontinued and are not a longterm threat to vision. Amiodarone

---

[4] Singh S N et al 1995 Amiodarone in patients with congestive heart failure and asymptomatic ventricular arrhythmia. New England Journal of Medicine 333: 77–82; Doval H C et al 1994 Randomised trial of low-dose amiodarone in severe congestive heart failure. Lancet 344: 493–498.

contains iodine and both hyperthyroidism and hypothyroidism are reported; thyroid function should be monitored before and during therapy. Photosensitivity reactions are common and amiodarone may cause a bluish discolouration on exposed areas of the skin. Less commonly, pulmonary fibrosis and hepatitis occur, sometimes rapidly during short-term use of the drug.

Interaction with digoxin (by displacement from tissue binding sites and interference with its elimination) and with warfarin (by inhibiting its metabolism) increases the effect of both these drugs. Beta-blockers and calcium channel antagonists augment the depressant effect of amiodarone on SA and AV node function.

Bretylium ($t^{1}/2$ 9 h) prevents the release of noradrenaline (norepinephrine) from sympathetic nerves. It prolongs the cardiac refractory period. It may be used for resistant ventricular tachyrhythmias, especially those complicating myocardial infarction or cardiac surgery. The main adverse effects are nausea, vomiting, hypotension and bradycardia.

CLASS IV (calcium channel blockade)

Calcium is involved in the contraction of cardiac and vascular smooth muscle cells, and in the automaticity of cardiac pacemaker cells. Actions of *calcium channel blockers* on vascular smooth muscle cells are described with the main account of these drugs in Chapter 24. Although the three classes have similar effects on vascular smooth muscle in the arterial tree, their cardiac actions differ. The phenylalkylamine, verapamil, depresses myocardial contraction more than the others, and both verapamil and the benzothiazepine, diltiazem, slow conduction in the sino-atrial and atrio-ventricular nodes.

Calcium and cardiac cells

Cardiac muscle cells are normally depolarised by the fast inward flow of sodium ions, following which there is a slow inward flow of calcium ions through the L-channel (L=large) (phase 2, in Fig. 25.1); the consequent rise in free intracellular calcium ions activates the contractile mechanism.

Pacemaker cells in the SA and AV nodes rely heavily on the slow inward flow of calcium ions (phase

4) for their capacity to discharge spontaneously, i.e. for their automaticity.

Calcium channel blockers inhibit the passage of calcium through the membrane channels; the result in myocardial cells is to depress contractility, and in pacemaker cells to suppress their automatic activity. Members of the group therefore may have negative cardiac inotropic and chronotropic actions. These actions can be separated; nifedipine, at therapeutic concentrations, acts almost exclusively on noncardiac ion channels and has no clinically useful antidysrhythmic activity whilst verapamil is a useful antidysrhythmic.

Verapamil (see also p. 430) prolongs conduction and refractoriness in the AV node and depresses the rate of discharge of the SA node. If adenosine is not available, verapamil should be used to terminate paroxysmal supraventricular tachycardia. Adverse effects include nausea, constipation, headache, fatigue, hypotension, bradycardia and heart block. Chemically related drugs acting on a different Ca^{++}-channel (the 'T-channel') in conducting tissue are under development, e.g. mibefradil; they may find a role.

OTHER ANTIDYSRHYTHMICS

Digoxin and other cardiac glycosides[5]

Crude digitalis is a preparation of the dried leaf of the foxglove plant *Digitalis purpurea*. Digitalis (purpurea or lanata) contains a number of active glyco-

---

[5] In 1775 Dr William Withering was making a routine journey from Birmingham (England), his home, to see patients at the Stafford Infirmary. Whilst the carriage horses were being changed half way, he was asked to see an old dropsical woman. He thought she would die and so some weeks later, when he heard of her recovery, was interested enough to enquire into the cause. Recovery was attributed to a herb tea containing some 20 ingredients, amongst which Withering, already the author of a botanical textbook, found it 'not very difficult . . . to perceive that the active herb could be no other than the foxglove'. He began to investigate its properties, trying it on the poor of Birmingham, whom he used to see without fee each day. The results were inconclusive and his interest flagged until one day he heard that the principal of an Oxford College had been cured by foxglove after 'some of the first physicians of the age had declared that they could do no more for him'. This put a new complexion on the matter and, pursuing his investigation,

sides (digoxin, digitoxin, lanatosides) whose actions are qualitatively similar, differing principally in rapidity of onset and duration; the pure individual glycosides are used. The following account refers to all the cardiac glycosides but *digoxin* is principally used.

Mode of action. Cardiac glycosides affect the heart both directly and indirectly in complex interactions, some of which oppose each other. The *direct* effect is to inhibit the membrane-bound adenosinetriphosphatase (ATPase) enzyme that, by hydrolysing ATP, supplies energy for the system that pumps sodium out of and transports potassium into conducting and contracting cells. The resulting rise in intracellular sodium and fall in intracellular potassium is accompanied by an influx of calcium ions. The *indirect* effect is to enhance vagal activity by complex peripheral and central mechanisms.

The clinically important consequences are:

- *On the contracting cells*: increased contractility and excitability
- *On SA and AV nodes and conducting tissue*: decreased generation and propagation.

Uses of cardiac glycosides:

- Atrial fibrillation, benefiting chiefly by the vagal effect on the AV node, reducing conduction through it and thus slowing the ventricular rate
- Paroxysmal supraventricular tachycardia, benefiting chiefly by the vagal effect on the SA node, slowing its rate of discharge, and on the AV node, as above
- Atrial flutter. Cardioversion is preferred, but digoxin may be effective, chiefly by the vagus nerve action of shortening the refractory period of the atrial muscle, to convert flutter to fibrillation, in which the ventricular rate is more readily controlled
- Cardiac failure, benefiting the patient chiefly by the direct action to increase myocardial contractility. Digoxin is used in left ventricular or congestive cardiac failure due to ischaemic, hypertensive or valvular heart disease, especially in the short term.

Withering found that foxglove extract caused diuresis in some oedematous patients. He defined the type of patient who might benefit from it and, equally important, he standardised his foxglove leaf preparations and was able to lay down accurate dosage schedules. His advice, with little amplification, would serve today (Withering W 1785 An account of the foxglove. Robinson, London).

Pharmacokinetics. Digoxin may be administered by mouth or i.v. It is eliminated 85% unchanged by the kidney and the remainder is metabolised by the liver. The $t^{1/2}$ is 36 h. By contrast digitoxin is extensively metabolised and the $t^{1/2}$ is 150 h.

Dose and therapeutic plasma concentration: see Table 25.1.

Reduced dose of digoxin is called for in: renal impairment (see above); the elderly (probably from decline in renal clearance with age); electrolyte disturbances (hypokalaemia accentuates the effects of digoxin, as does hypomagnesaemia); hypothyroid patients (they are intolerant of digoxin).

Adverse effects. *Abnormal cardiac rhythms* usually take the form of ectopic dysrhythmias (ventricular ectopic beats, ventricular tachydysrhythmias, paroxysmal supraventricular tachycardia) and heart block. *Gastrointestinal effects* include anorexia which usually precedes vomiting and is a warning that dosage is excessive. Diarrhoea may also occur. *Visual effects* include disturbances of colour vision, e.g. yellow (xanthopsia) but also red or green vision, photophobia and blurring. *Gynaecomastia* may occur in men and breast enlargement in women with longterm use (cardiac glycosides have structural resemblance to oestrogen). *Mental effects* include confusion, restlessness, agitation, nightmares and acute psychoses.

Acute digoxin poisoning causes initial nausea and vomiting and hyperkalaemia because inhibition of the sodium-potassium ATPase pump prevents intracellular accumulation of potassium. The ECG changes (see Table 25.1) of prolonged use of digoxin may be absent. There may be exaggerated sinus dysrhythmia, bradycardia and ectopic rhythms with or without heart block.

Treatment of overdose. Phenytoin 100 mg i.v. is useful in the management of digoxin-induced ventricular dysrhythmias. Atropine is effective for bradycardia. Electrical pacing may be needed, but direct current shock may lead to ventricular fibrillation. For severe digoxin poisoning infusion of the *digoxin-specific binding (Fab) fragment* (Digibind) of the antibody to digoxin, neutralises digoxin in the plasma and is an effective treatment. Because it lacks the Fc segment, this fragment is nonimmunogenic and it is sufficiently small to be eliminated as the digoxin-antibody complex in the urine.

Interactions. Cardiac dysrhythmias may develop due to depletion of body *potassium* from therapy with *diuretics* or with adrenal steroids. Verapamil, nifedipine, quinidine and amiodarone raise steady-state plasma digoxin concentrations (see above) and the digoxin dose should be lowered when any of these is added. AV block caused by digoxin is increased by verapamil and by β-adrenoceptor blockers.

Adenosine

Adenosine is an endogenous purine nucleotide which slows atrioventricular conduction and dilates coronary and peripheral arteries. It is rapidly metabolised by circulating adenosine deaminase. It enters cells; hence its residence in plasma is brief ($t^{1}/_2$ several seconds) and it must be given i.v. Administered as a bolus injection, adenosine is useful for distinguishing the origin of (ECG) 'broad QRS complex' tachycardias, i.e. whether ventricular, or supraventricular with aberrant conduction. If the latter is the case AV block with adenosine allows the P waves to be seen and the diagnosis to be made; adenosine thus has the same effect as carotid massage (see below). Evidence also indicates that adenosine is effective for terminating paroxysmal supraventricular (re-entrant) tachycardias, including episodes in patients with Wolff–Parkinson–White syndrome. The initial dose in adults is 3 mg over 2 seconds with continuous ECG monitoring, with doubling increments every 1–2 minutes. The average total dose is 125 micrograms/kg, which is superior to verapamil and also safer if used mistakenly in a ventricular tachycardia (because adenosine is not negatively inotropic). Adverse effects are not serious because of the brevity of its action but dyspnoea, facial flushing, chest pain and transient dysrhythmias, e.g. bradycardia, may occur. Adenosine should not be given to asthmatics or to patients with second or third degree AV block or sick sinus syndrome (unless a pacemaker is in place).

The autonomic system

Some drugs used for dysrhythmias exert their actions through the *autonomic nervous system* by mimicking or antagonising the effects of the sympathetic or parasympathetic nerves that supply the heart. The neurotransmitters in these two branches of the autonomic system, noradrenaline and acetylcholine, are functionally antagonistic by having opposing actions on cyclic AMP production within the cardiomyocyte. Their receptors are coupled to the two trimeric GTP-binding proteins, Gs and Gi, which stimulate and inhibit adenylyl cyclase, respectively.

The sympathetic division (adrenergic component of the autonomic nervous system), when stimulated, has the following *effects on the heart* (receptor effects):

- Tachycardia due to increased rate of discharge of the SA node
- Increased automaticity in the AV node and His-Purkinje system
- Increase in conductivity in the His-Purkinje system
- Increased force of contraction
- Shortening of the refractory period.

Isoprenaline, a β-adrenoceptor agonist, may be used to accelerate the heart and to raise cardiac output when there is extreme bradycardia due to heart block, prior to the insertion of an electrical pacemaker. The dose is: i.v. 0.5–10 mg per minute; by mouth 30 mg every 8 h to a maximum of 840 mg per day. Adverse effects are those expected of β-adrenoceptor agonists and include tremor, flushing, sweating, palpitation, headache and diarrhoea.

The vagus nerve (cholinergic, parasympathetic), when stimulated, has the following effects on the heart:

- Bradycardia due to depression of the SA node
- Slowing of conduction through and increased refractoriness of the AV node
- Shortening of the refractory period of atrial muscle cells
- Decreased myocardial excitability.

These effects are used in the therapy of dysrhythmias.

There is also reduced force of contraction of atrial and ventricular muscle cells.

The vagus nerve may be stimulated reflexly by various physical manoeuvres. Vagal stimulation may slow or terminate supraventricular dysrhythmias and should if possible be carried out under ECG control.

Carotid sinus massage activates stretch receptors: external pressure is applied gently to one side at a time but never to both sides at once. Some individuals are very sensitive to the procedure and develop severe bradycardia and hypotension.

Other methods include the *Valsalva manoeuvre* (deep inspiration followed by expiration against a closed glottis, which both stimulates stretch receptors in the lung and reduces venous return to the heart); the Muller procedure (deep expiration followed by inspiration against a closed glottis); production of nausea and retching by inviting patients to put their own fingers down their throat.

The effects of vagus nerve activity are blocked by *atropine* (antimuscarinic action), an action that is used to accelerate the heart during episodes of sinus bradycardia as may occur after myocardial infarction. The dose is 0.6 mg i.v. and repeated as necessary to a maximum of 3 mg per day. Adverse effects are those of muscarinic blockade, namely dry mouth, blurred vision, urinary retention, confusion and hallucination.

Other antidysrhythmia drugs that have a vagal antimuscarinic action include quinidine, procainamide and disopyramide.

PRODYSRHYTHMIC EFFECTS

Antidysrhythmic drugs can also *cause* dysrhythmia. Such prodysrhythmic effects are most commonly seen with drugs that prolong the QT interval or QRS complex of the ECG; hypokalaemia aggravates the danger. Quinidine may cause tachydysrhythmia in an estimated 1–4% of patients. A prodysrhythmic effect of flecainide resulting in a doubling of mortality was revealed by the Cardiac Arrhythmia Suppression Trial (CAST) (see p. 463).

Digoxin can induce a variety of brady- and tachydysrhythmias (see above).

CHOICE BETWEEN DRUGS AND ELECTROCONVERSION

Direct current (DC) electric shock applied externally is often the best way to convert cardiac dysrhythmias to sinus rhythm. Many atrial or ventricular dysrhythmias start as a result of transiently operating factors but, once they have begun, the abnormal mechanisms are self-sustaining. When an electric shock is given, the heart is depolarised, the ectopic focus is extinguished and the SA node, the part of the heart with the highest automaticity, resumes as the dominant pacemaker.

Electrical conversion has the advantage that it is immediate, unlike drugs, which may take days or longer to act; also, the effective doses and adverse effects of drugs are largely unpredictable, and can be serious.[6]

Uses of electrical conversion: in supraventricular and ventricular tachycardia, ventricular fibrillation and atrial fibrillation and flutter. Drugs can be useful to prevent a relapse, e.g. sotalol, amiodarone.

SPECIFIC TREATMENTS[7]

Sinus bradycardia

Sinus bradycardia requires treatment if there is hypotension or escape rhythms; extreme bradycardia may allow a ventricular focus to take over and lead to ventricular tachycardia. The foot of the bed should be raised to assist venous return and atropine should be given i.v.

Atrial ectopic beats

Reduction in the use of tea, coffee and other

---

[6] To the layman, 'shock' treatment could be interpreted as frights (which stimulate the vagus, as described above), or as the electrical sort. Dr James Le Fanu describes a Belfast doctor who reported a farmer with a solution that covered both possibilities. He had suffered from episodes of palpitations and dizziness for 30 years. When he first got them, he would jump from a barrel and thump his feet hard on the ground at landing. This became less effective with time. His next 'cure' was to remove his clothes, climb a ladder and jump from a considerable height into a cold water tank on the farm. Later, he discovered the best and simplest treatment was to grab hold of his 6-volt electrified cattle fence — although if he was wearing wellington boots he found he had to earth the shock, so besides grabbing the fence with one hand he simultaneously shoved a finger of the other hand into the ground.

[7] See also European Resuscitation Council guidelines (Fig. 25.2).

methylxanthine-containing drinks, and of tobacco, may suffice for ectopic beats not due to organic heart disease. When action is needed, a small dose of a β-adrenoceptor blocker may be effective.

Paroxysmal supraventricular (AV re-entrant) tachycardia

If vagal stimulation (by carotid massage, or swallowing ice-cream) is unsuccessful, *adenosine* has the dual advantage of being effective in most such tachycardias, while having no effect on a ventricular tachycardia. The response to adenosine is therefore of diagnostic value. If, however, the patient is in circulatory shock as a result of the tachycardia, or drug treatment fails, a DC shock should be administered, for immediate effect. A β-adrenoceptor blocker, e.g. sotalol, may be effective at preventing attacks.

Atrial fibrillation (AF)

The treatment decision tree is:

- Treatment vs no treatment
- Conversion vs rate control
- Immediate vs delayed conversion
- Drugs or DC conversion.

The information required is:

- Apical (ventricular) rate ('normal' or high)
- Haemodynamic state ('normal' or compromised)
- Atrial size ('normal' or enlarged).

In the majority of patients, AF is an incidental finding on the background of some existing cardiovascular disease, and with a large atrium. Most such patients require chronic digitalisation, unless the radial pulse rate is usually less than 80 bpm, which can be introduced over several days without a loading dose. Where the atrium is small, or there has been a recent onset of heart failure or shock, conversion should be attempted. DC conversion is favoured where treatment is either urgent or likely to be successful in holding the patient in sinus rhythm. Pharmacological conversion can often be achieved over hours to days by amiodarone, and this is useful in patients who revert rapidly to AF after DC conversion.

When conversion is not urgent, it should be delayed for a month to permit institution of anticoagulation by warfarin, and this should be continued for a month subsequently. In patients who have reverted to AF after previous conversions, flecainide has been used with some anecdotal success to prevent reversion.

Additional treatments in chronic atrial fibrillation. Longterm treatment with warfarin is almost mandatory to reduce embolic complications. The efficacy of aspirin as an anti-embolic agent is probably less in this group, but has been shown to be of value in patients where warfarin is considered inappropriate.[8]

Where digoxin is ineffective alone in controlling the ventricular rate, it may be combined with either a Ca^{++}-channel blocker, such as verapamil, or a β-blocker.

Atrial flutter

It is doubtful whether this differs in its origins or sequelae from atrial fibrillation. However the ventricular rate is usually faster (typically, half an atrial rate of 300, where 2:1 block is present), which is too fast to be left without treatment for a month. Since, similarly, the patient is unlikely to have been in this rhythm for a prolonged period, there is less likelihood that atrial thrombus has accumulated and it is therefore safe to attempt conversion without prior anticoagulation. Patients should not be left in chronic atrial flutter, and DC conversion will usually restore either sinus rhythm or atrial fibrillation. The latter is treated as above. Patients who fail to convert, or who revert repeatedly to atrial flutter, may be treated with either flecainide or a class III antidysrhythmic (sotalol or amiodarone).

---

[8] Next to hypertension, AF is the most preventable cause of stroke, and yet implementation of trial findings has been slow. Perhaps the estimate that warfarin carries a net benefit, except where a patient is considered to have a 6-fold increased risk of bleeding (e.g. due to a bleeding diathesis, or active peptic ulcer) will help to convince the wavering practitoners (Caro J J et al 1993 Atrial fibrillation and anticoagulation: from randomised trials to practice. Lancet 341: 1381–1384).

EMERGENCY TREATMENT

PERI-ARREST ARRHYTHMIAS

If not already done, give oxygen and establish IV access

Doses based on adult of average body weight

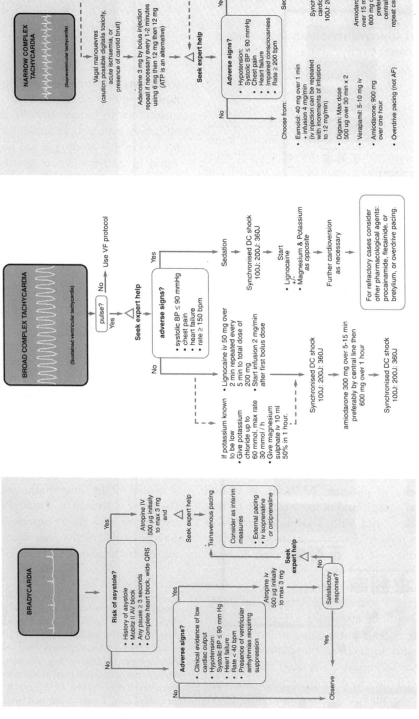

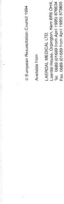

Fig. 25.2 Protocol for the treatment of pericardiac arrest arrhythmias (dysrhythmias) in hospitals. With permission, European Resuscitation Council

ADVANCED CARDIAC LIFE SUPPORT

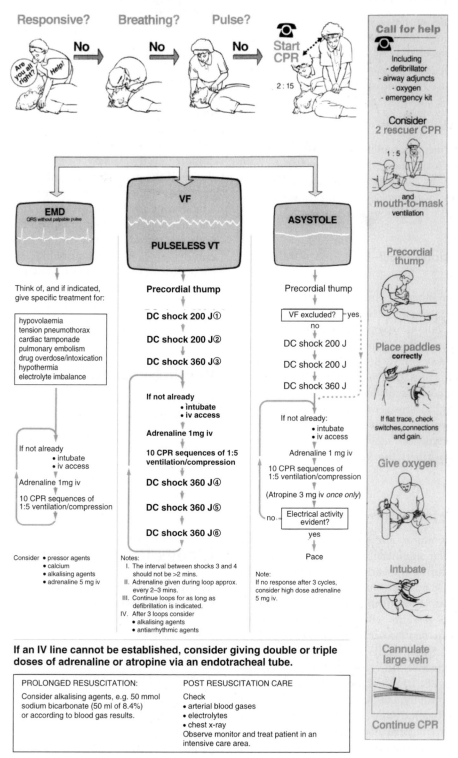

Responsive? No → **Breathing?** No → **Pulse?** No → Start CPR 2:15

Call for help
Including
- defibrillator
- airway adjuncts
- oxygen
- emergency kit

Consider 2 rescuer CPR
1:5
and **mouth-to-mask** ventilation

Precordial thump

Place paddles correctly

If flat trace, check switches, connections and gain.

Give oxygen

Intubate

Cannulate large vein

Continue CPR

EMD
QRS without palpable pulse

Think of, and if indicated, give specific treatment for:

hypovolaemia
tension pneumothorax
cardiac tamponade
pulmonary embolism
drug overdose/intoxication
hypothermia
electrolyte imbalance

If not already
- intubate
- iv access

Adrenaline 1mg iv

10 CPR sequences of 1:5 ventilation/compression

Consider
- pressor agents
- calcium
- alkalising agents
- adrenaline 5 mg iv

VF
PULSELESS VT

Precordial thump

DC shock 200 J①

DC shock 200 J②

DC shock 360 J③

If not already
- intubate
- iv access

Adrenaline 1mg iv

10 CPR sequences of 1:5 ventilation/compression

DC shock 360 J④

DC shock 360 J⑤

DC shock 360 J⑥

Notes:
I. The interval between shocks 3 and 4 should not be >2 mins.
II. Adrenaline given during loop approx. every 2–3 mins.
III. Continue loops for as long as defibrillation is indicated.
IV. After 3 loops consider
  - alkalising agents
  - antiarrhythmic agents

ASYSTOLE

Precordial thump

VF excluded? — yes
no

DC shock 200 J

DC shock 200 J

DC shock 360 J

If not already:
- intubate
- iv access

Adrenaline 1 mg iv

10 CPR sequences of 1:5 ventilation/compression

(Atropine 3 mg iv *once only*)

no — Electrical activity evident?
yes

Pace

Note:
If no response after 3 cycles, consider high dose adrenaline 5 mg iv.

If an IV line cannot be established, consider giving double or triple doses of adrenaline or atropine via an endotracheal tube.

PROLONGED RESUSCITATION:	POST RESUSCITATION CARE
Consider alkalising agents, e.g. 50 mmol sodium bicarbonate (50 ml of 8.4%) or according to blood gas results.	Check - arterial blood gases - electrolytes - chest x-ray Observe monitor and treat patient in an intensive care area.

Fig. 25.3 Advanced cardiac life support. With permission, European Resuscitation Council

Atrial tachycardia with variable AV block

The atrial rate is 120–250/min, and commonly there is AV block. If the patient is taking digoxin, it should be suspected as the cause of the dysrhythmia, and stopped. If the patient is not taking digoxin, it may be used to control the ventricular rate.

Heart block

The use of artificial pacemakers is beyond the scope of this book. In an emergency, AV conduction may be improved by atropine (antimuscarinic vagal block) (0.6 mg i.v.) or by isoprenaline (β-adrenoceptor agonist) (0.5–10 micrograms/min, i.v.).

Pre-excitation (Wolff–Parkinson–White) syndrome

This occurs in otherwise healthy people, who possess an anomalous (accessory) atrioventricular pathway; they often experience attacks of paroxysmal AV re-entrant tachycardia or atrial fibrillation. Drugs that delay conduction through the AV node are used to prevent it, i.e. a β-adrenoceptor blocker (sotalol), amiodarone or flecainide. Verapamil and digoxin may increase conduction through the anomalous pathway and should not be used. Electrical conversion may be needed to restore sinus rhythm when the ventricular rate is very rapid.

Ventricular premature beats

These are common after myocardial infarction. Their particular significance is that an ectopic beat developing during the early or peak phases of the T-wave (ECG) may precipitate ventricular tachycardia or fibrillation (the R-on-T phenomenon). About 80% of patients with myocardial infarction who proceed to ventricular fibrillation have preceding ventricular premature beats. Lignocaine (lidocaine) is effective in suppression of ectopic ventricular beats. In the absence of clear evidence that routine prophylaxis reduces mortality, many specialists in coronary care give lignocaine: if there are more than 6 ventricular ectopics per minute; if they occur near to the peak of the T-wave; if there are runs of 2 or more in succession or if they are multifocal. Propafenone, mexiletine, disopyramide or sotalol are alternatives.

Ventricular tachycardia

Ventricular tachycardia demands urgent treatment since it frequently leads to ventricular fibrillation and circulatory arrest. A powerful thump of the fist on the mid-sternum or precordium may stop a tachycardia. If there is rapid haemodynamic deterioration, electrical conversion is the treatment of choice. If the patient is in good condition i.v. treatment may begin with lignocaine or, should that fail, amiodarone i.v. For recurrent ventricular tachycardia amiodarone is often preferred but the choice is wide and includes: mexiletine, tocainamide, disopyramide, procainamide, quinidine, propafenone or sotalol by mouth. The selection of a particular drug may be influenced by anticipated adverse effects, e.g. disopyramide and quinidine have antimuscarinic effects that would be undesirable in a patient with glaucoma or prostatism.

Ventricular fibrillation and cardiac arrest

Ventricular fibrillation is usually caused by myocardial infarction or ischaemia, or serious organic heart disease and is one of the reasons for cardiac arrest. Guidelines for the management of cardiac arrest are issued by the Resuscitation Council of the United Kingdom.[9] A protocol depicting these appears on page 471.

Drugs for cardiac failure

SOME PHYSIOLOGY AND PATHOPHYSIOLOGY

Cardiac output (CO) depends on the heart rate (HR) and the volume of blood that is ejected with each beat, i.e. the stroke volume (SV). Their relation is expressed by the equation:

$$CO = HR \times SV$$

---

[9] British Medical Journal (1989) 209: 446. We are grateful to the Resuscitation Council (UK) and to (Laerda) Medical for permission to publish this information.

There are three factors that regulate the stroke volume, namely preload, afterload and contractility.

● *Preload* is the load on the heart created by the volume of blood injected into the left ventricle by the left atrium (at the end of ventricular diastole) and that it must eject with each contraction. It can also be viewed as the amount of stretch to which the left ventricle is subject. As the preload rises so also does the degree of stretch and the length of cardiac muscle fibres. Preload is thus a *volume* load and can be excessive, e.g., when there is valvular incompetence.

● *Afterload* refers to the load on the contracting ventricle created by the resistance to the blood injected by the ventricle into the arterial system, i.e. the total peripheral resistance. Afterload is thus a *pressure* load and is excessive, e.g., in arterial hypertension.

● *Contractility* refers to the capacity of the myocardium to generate the force necessary to respond to preload and to overcome afterload.

DEFINITION OF CARDIAC FAILURE

Cardiac failure is present when the heart cannot provide all organs with the blood supply appropriate to demand. This definition emphasises two features of cardiac failure: that cardiac output may be normal at rest; and that, when demand is increased, perfusion of the vital organs (brain and kidneys) is maintained at the expense of other tissues, especially skeletal muscle. Overall systemic arterial pressure is also maintained until a late stage.

The therapeutic importance of recognising this pathophysiology is that many of the neuroendocrine abnormalities of cardiac failure — particularly, the elevated renin and sympathetic activity — are caused more by the treatments than the disease. Renal perfusion is not altered early in heart failure, whereas diuretics and vasodilators stimulate renin and noradrenaline production through actions at the juxtaglomerular apparatus in the kidney and on the arterial baroreflex, respectively. In recent years we have learned that the earliest endocrine abnormality in almost all types of cardiac disease is increased release of the heart's own hormones, the natriuretic peptides ANP and BNP (A for atrial, B for brain, where it was first discovered). These peptides normally *suppress* renin and aldosterone pro-

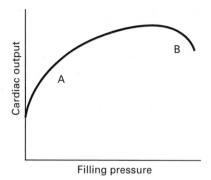

Fig. 25.4 Starling curve of relationship between cardiac filling pressure and cardiac output
In phase A, reduction in blood volume (by diuretics) reduces filling pressure and cardiac output
In phase B, reduction in blood volume reduces filling pressure and increases cardiac output

duction, but this suppression appears to be overridden in cardiac failure.

THE STARLING CURVE AND CARDIAC FAILURE

The Starling relationship (Fig. 25.4) describes the increased contractility of cardiac muscle fibres in response to increased stretch, and can be extrapolated to the whole ventricle to explain the normal relationship between filling pressure and ejection fraction. Contrary to popular belief, most patients with heart failure have not entered the decompensation phase ('B' in Fig. 25.4) of the relationship, which does not occur until the ventricle is grossly dilated. While diuretics, therefore, improve the congestive symptoms of cardiac failure which are due to the increased filling pressure (*preload*), they actually reduce cardiac output in most patients. Whether patients feel better or worse as a result depends on whether their predominant symptom was dyspnoea (due to pulmonary venous congestion) or fatigue. It is likely that a principal benefit of using ACE inhibitors in cardiac failure is their diuretic sparing effect.

NATURAL HISTORY OF CARDIAC FAILURE

The severity of cardiac failure can be classified at the bedside according to how much the patient is able to do without becoming dyspnoeic, and this so-called New York Heart Association (NYHA) classification offers also an approximate prognosis, with that of the worst grade (NYHA Class 4) being as bad as most cancers.[10] Most patients with cardiac failure die from a dysrhythmia, rather than from terminal decompensation, and prognosis is improved most by drugs which do not increase further the heart's exposure to elevated catecholamine concentrations (some vasodilators, but see below).

OBJECTIVES OF TREATMENT

As for cardiac dysrhythmias, these are

- To reduce morbidity
- To reduce mortality.

However, in this case, most patients are symptomatic, and are likely to die from their disease. There is some tension between the two objectives of reducing morbidity and mortality. Few of the longer established treatments have been shown to improve outcome, and it is clear that some drugs which temporarily improve symptoms can reduce survival. There is a further tension between the needs of treating the features of *forwards* failure, or low output, and *backwards* failure, or the congestive features. The principal symptom of a low cardiac output, tiredness, is difficult to quantify, and patients have tended to have their treatment tailored more to the consequences of venous congestion.

Haemodynamic aims of drug therapy

Cardiac output can be increased by strengthening the heart (by a direct inotropic action) or by reducing the resistance against which it has to work (*afterload*). Despite numerous attempts over recent years, digoxin remains the only inotropic drug available for chronic oral use. Afterload reduction by *vasodilators* includes more options, and the ACE inhibitors are the most widely used. The nitrates also act partly by reducing afterload, but also

improve coronary blood flow, as discussed in Chapter 24.

The heart may fail from disease of the myocardium itself, mainly ischaemic, or from an excessive afterload imposed on it by arterial hypertension, valvular disease or an arteriovenous shunt. The management of cardiac failure requires both the relief of any treatable underlying or aggravating cause, e.g. hypertension, and therapy directed at the failure itself.

The distinction between the capacity of the myocardium to pump blood and the load against which the heart must work is useful in therapy. The failing myocardium is so strongly stimulated to contract by increased sympathetic drive that therapeutic efforts to induce it to function yet more vigorously are in themselves alone unlikely to be of benefit. Drugs can be used however to alleviate the load imposed on the failing heart by the physiological adjustments to cardiac failure; agents that reduce preload or afterload are very effective, especially where the left ventricular volume is raised (less predictably so for failure of the right ventricle). The main hazard of their use is a drastic fall in cardiac output in those occasional patients whose output is dependent on a high left ventricular filling pressure, e.g. those who are volume depleted by diuretic use or those with severe mitral stenosis.

CLASSIFICATION OF DRUGS

Drugs used may therefore be classified as producing:

Reduction of preload

Diuretics increase salt and water loss, reduce blood volume and lower excessive venous filling pressure (see Ch. 27). The congestive features of oedema, in the lungs and periphery, are alleviated; when the heart is grossly enlarged, cardiac output will also increase (see discussion of Starling curve, above).

Nitrates (see also Ch. 24) dilate the smooth muscle in venous capacitance vessels, increase the volume of the venous vascular bed (which normally may comprise 80% of the whole vascular system), reduce ventricular filling pressure, thus decreasing heart wall stretch, and reduce myocardial O_2

---

[10] NYHA Class 1 = minimal dyspnoea (except after moderate exercise)
  Class 2 = dyspnoea while walking on the flat
  Class 3 = dyspnoea on getting in/out of bed
  Class 4 = dyspnoea lying in bed.

requirements. Their arteriolar dilating action is relatively slight. Glyceryl trinitrate may be given sublingually 0.3–1 mg for acute left ventricular failure and repeated as often as necessary or by i.v. infusion, 10–200 micrograms/min. For chronic left ventricular failure isosorbide dinitrate 40–160 mg/d or isosorbide mononitrate 40–80 mg/d may be given by mouth in divided doses. Exercise capacity is improved but tolerance to nitrates may develop with chronic use. Headache, which tends to limit the dose of nitrate used for angina, is less of a problem in cardiac failure perhaps because the patients are more vasoconstricted.

Reduction of afterload

Hydralazine (see also Ch. 24) relaxes arterial smooth muscle and reduces peripheral vascular resistance. Reflex tachycardia, however, limits its usefulness and lupus erythematosus may be induced when the dose exceeds 100 mg per day.

Reduction of preload and afterload

Angiotensin converting enzyme (ACE) inhibitors (see also Ch. 24) act by:

- reduction of afterload, by preventing the conversion of angiotensin I to the active form, angiotensin II, which is a powerful arterioconstrictor and is present in the plasma in high concentration in cardiac failure
- reduction of preload, because the formation of aldosterone, and thus retention of salt and water (increased blood volume), is prevented by the reduction of angiotensin II.

ACE inhibitors are the only drugs which reduce peripheral resistance (afterload) without causing a reflex activation of the sympathetic system.

Captopril or **enalapril** are effective. A test dose should always be given to patients who are in cardiac failure (or who are already taking a diuretic for other reasons, e.g. hypertension); maintenance of blood pressure in such individuals may depend greatly on the activated renin-angiotensin-aldosterone system and a standard dose of an ACE

inhibitor can cause a catastrophic fall in blood pressure. Except for captopril, most ACE inhibitors (including enalapril) are prodrugs, which are inactive for several hours after dosing. This has favoured the use of captopril for the initial dose(s) given under medical supervision; captopril also has the shortest $t^{1/2}$ so that hypotension will be reversed the most quickly. Although there has been less experience with the many ACE inhibitors developed after captopril and enalapril (see p. 430), some of these have a sufficiently long $t^{1/2}$ to suggest that the initial doses would have a cumulative effect on blood pressure over several days; such long-acting ACE inhibitors might avoid the risk of sudden falls in blood pressure or renal function (glomerular filtration) after the first dose. More information is required in order to facilitate the wider use of these drugs outside a hospital environment.

Phentolamine or sodium nitroprusside (see Ch. 24) may rarely be used (by i.v. infusion) when *acute* cardiac failure is accompanied by a high blood pressure.

Stimulation of the myocardium

Digoxin improves myocardial contractility (positive inotropic effect) most effectively in the dilated, failing heart and in the longer term once an episode of cardiac failure has been brought under control. This effect occurs in patients in sinus rhythm and is separate from its (negative chronotropic) action of reducing ventricular rate and thus improving ventricular filling in atrial fibrillation. Over 200 years after the first use of digitalis for dropsy, the DIG trial has brought some relief for doctors wishing evidence of longterm benefit.[11] This trial was a prospective randomised comparison of digoxin with placebo in 7788 patients in Class II to III heart failure and sinus rhythm, of whom, most also received an ACE inhibitor and a diuretic. Unlike all other positive isotropes digoxen caused no increase in overall mortality or dysrhythmias, and slightly reduced the number of deaths from worsening heart failure.

The phosphodiesterase inhibitors, *enoximone* and

---

[11] Yusuf S et al 1996 Need for a large randomised trial to evaluate the effects of digitalis on morbidity and mortality in congestive heart failure. American Journal of Cardiology 69: 64G-70G.

milrinone have positive inotropic effect due to selective myocardial enzyme inhibition and may be used for short-term treatment of severe congestive cardiac failure.

Dopamine, dobutamine, dopexamine, xamoterol: see Chapter 23.

DRUG MANAGEMENT OF CARDIAC FAILURE

Mild cardiac failure should be treated with a thiazide diuretic, if renal function is normal. If not, or if oedema persists on a thiazide, the next step is a loop diuretic in low daily dose, e.g. frusemide 40 mg, to which amiloride 5 mg may be added to help conserve potassium; if necessary the frusemide may be increased. The addition of a thiazide, usually metolazone, to a loop diuretic is usually effective in stimulating a diuresis (if necessary, with the drugs given i.v. for the first few days) in patients who have accumulated many litres of oedema fluid despite more routine diuretic management. The converse risk of such a regime is a slide (rapid or insidious) into intravascular volume depletion and severe hyponatraemia; it is always wise to restrict total fluid intake during such aggressive diuretic therapy, in order to limit dilutional hyponatraemia, and to monitor patients closely in a hospital environment. It is not yet clear whether the endogenous natriuretic peptides, ANP and BNP (see p. 473) can be harnessed to therapeutic use, with a drug such as candoxatril which inhibits their destruction and overcomes partially the resistance to their effects in cardiac failure.

All patients requiring chronic diuretic treatment for heart failure should also now receive an ACE inhibitor, in view of the several longterm studies showing improved survival even in mild failure. For instance, in the SOLVD studies where enalapril was compared with placebo in patients with either clinical features of heart failure, or reduced left ventricular function in the absence of symptoms, treatment reduced serious events (myocardial infarction and unstable angina) by ~20% and hospital admissions with progressive heart failure by up to 40%.[12] In the more severe patients, the ACE inhibitors have a diuretic sparing effect, which improves the patients' symptoms by maintaining peripheral per-

fusion, and reducing the neurohumoral response to excessive diuresis. An alternative to ACE inhibition as a vasodilator is isosorbide mononitrate with which hydralazine may later be combined. Cough appears to be a less common adverse effect of ACE inhibition in cardiac failure than in hypertension, perhaps because of confusion with other causes of cough. It seems likely that the angiotensin receptor antagonists (e.g. losartan) may prove to be a satisfactory alternative.

Digoxin should be added if failure persists, and the diuretic regimen may be intensified, e.g. by increasing the amount of loop diuretic and by replacing amiloride with spironolactone.

None of the available phosphodiesterase inhibitors has become established in routine therapy, because the short-term benefit of the increased contractility has been offset by an increased mortality (presumably due to dysrhythmias) on chronic dosing. A similar fate befell flosequinan, which was a positive inotrope which acted through the phosphatidylinositol system. In contrast to these inotropes, a longterm role has been suggested for β-blockers, particularly carvedilol, which has vasodilating action not related to β-blockade. This may reduce mortality, protecting against the increased sympathetic nervous stimulation of the heart in cardiac failure.[13] If used at all, it will be important (as in the trials) to introduce β-blockers at about one quarter of their usual starting dose in hypertension or angina.

Acute left ventricular failure

This common medical emergency (less common perhaps since the advent of thrombolysis for myocardial infarction) is treated by reassuring the intensely anxious patient, who should sit upright with the legs dependent to reduce systemic venous return. A loop diuretic, e.g. frusemide 40–80 mg

---

[12] SOLVD = Studies of Left Ventricular Dysfunction. The SOLVD Investigators 1991 Effect of enalapril on survival in patients with reduced left ventricular ejection fractions and congestive heart failure. New England Journal of Medicine 325: 293–302.

[13] Packer M et al 1996. Effect of carvedilol on morbidity and mortality in patients with chronic heart failure. New England Journal of Medicine 334: 1349–1355.

i.v., is the mainstay of therapy and provides benefit both by a rapid and powerful venodilator effect reducing preload, and by the subsequent diuresis. Oxygen should be given, if the patient can tolerate a face mask, and diamorphine or morphine i.v. which in addition to relieving anxiety and pain, have a valuable vasodilator effect.

While there can be a case for short-term use of inotropic drugs (see Ch. 23) for cardiac failure where low output is a predominant feature, it is important to remember that most such drugs substantially increase the risk of dysrhythmias when the heart is hypoxic. Digoxin's pharmacokinetics do not lend themselves to emergency use. Aminophylline (5 mg/kg over 20 min) can be administered i.v., following even more carefully than in status asthmaticus the precautions regarding dose and monitoring (see p. 514). By this stage, the possibility of the patient's requiring assisted ventilation should be considered: where pulmonary oedema is the main problem, ventilation is likely to be both safer and more effective than inotropic drugs.

CARDIAC TRANSPLANTATION

While this lies outside the scope of clinical pharmacology, an important element in meeting the objectives of treatment (p. 474) is to recognise when further drug treatment is likely to be counter-productive in improving symptoms or prognosis. It is the physician who must first consider the possibility of a surgical intervention (which increasingly may involve procedures short of transplantation itself); on occasion, it can help the patient to be made aware that failure of both the heart and the drugs is not necessarily the end of the road.

GUIDE TO FURTHER READING

Braunwald E 1991 ACE inhibitors — a cornerstone of the treatment of heart failure. New England Journal of Medicine 325: 351

Camm A J and Garratt C J 1991 Adenosine and supraventricular tachycardia. New England Journal of Medicine 325: 1621–1629

Cohn J N 1989 Inotropic therapy for heart failure. New England Journal of Medicine 320: 729

Dargie H J, McMurray J J 1994 Diagnosis and management of heart failure. British Medical Journal 308: 321–328

de Bono D 1994 Digoxin in eurhythmic heart failure: PROVED or 'not proven'? Lancet 343: 128–129

Garratt C et al 1989 Lessons from the cardiac dysrhythmia suppression trial (CAST). British Medical Journal 299: 805

Lip G Y H, Watson R D S, Singh S P 1994 ABC of atrial fibrillation: drugs for a trial. British Medical Journal 309: 1631–1635

Onunain S, Ruskin J 1993 Cardiac arrest. Lancet 341: 1641–1647

Packer M et al 1993 Withdrawal of digoxin from patients with chronic heart failure treated with angiotensin converting enzyme inhibitors. New England Journal of Medicine 329: 1–7

Roden D M 1994 Risks and benefits of antiarrhythmic therapy. New England Journal of Medicine 331: 785–791

Ruskin J N 1989 The cardiac dysrhythmia suppression trial (CAST). New England Journal of Medicine 321: 386

The SOLVD Investigators 1991 Effect of enalapril on survival in patients with reduced left ventricular ejection fractions and congestive heart failure. New England Journal of Medicine 325: 293–302

SUMMARY

- The treatment of dysrhythmias can be directly physical, electrical, pharmacological or surgical.
- The choice among drugs is influenced partly by theoretical predictions from their action on the cardiac cycle but largely by short and longterm observations of their efficacy and safety.
- All antidysrhythmics can be dangerous, and should not be used unless patients are symptomatic or haemodynamically compromised.
- Adenosine is the treatment of choice for diagnosis and reversal of supraventricular dysrhythmias.
- Amiodarone is the most effective drug at reversing atrial fibrillation, and in prevention of ventricular dysrhythmias, but has several adverse effects.
- Digoxin retains a unique role as a positively inotropic antidysrhythmic, being most useful in slowing atrioventricular conduction in atrial fibrillation.
- The treatment of heart failure requires both diuretics and ACE inhibitors.
- Treatments which improve symptoms in heart failure do not necessarily improve prognosis — and vice versa.

Hyperlipidaemias

SYNOPSIS

Correction of blood lipid abnormalities offers scope for a major impact on cardiovascular disease. Dietary adjustment plays an important primary role in the management of hyperlipidaemias while drugs help in selected cases, and agents with a variety of modes of action are available.

- Classification
- Management
- Drugs used in treatment: anion-exchange resins; nicotinic acid and derivatives; fibric acid derivatives; statins

SOME PHYSIOLOGY

Dietary triglyceride is carried in the blood stream on chylomicrons which become progressively smaller as lipolysis takes place. This is accomplished by the enzyme lipoprotein lipase attached to the capillary endothelium of certain tissues including adipose tissue and skeletal and cardiac muscle. Fatty acids released during lipolysis are taken up by the tissues and the chylomicron remnants are cleared by the liver.

Endogenous triglyceride, synthesised by the liver and carried bound to very low density lipoproteins (VLDL) is progressively removed from the circulation by the same lipolytic mechanism as above. The low density lipoproteins (LDL), which include cholesterol, are formed as a result of this process and constitute the major system for delivering cholesterol to the tissues in man. LDL are small enough to pass through the vascular endothelium, bind to specific high-affinity LDL receptors on cell membranes and enter cells by active uptake. Cholesterol within the cell is needed for membrane growth and repair, and in the liver to form bile acids.

High density lipoproteins (HDL), the other cholesterol-rich particles in the blood, appear to act as reverse transport mediators, accepting cholesterol from peripheral cells, e.g. in arterial walls, and taking it to the liver; they are thus protective against ischaemic heart disease (IHD).

There appears to be no homeostatic regulation of circulating LDL levels, perhaps because there is no survival value in preventing the onset of LDL-induced diseases after the reproductive age. What is tightly regulated is the intracellular level of cholesterol in the hepatocyte. The three possible sources — diet, de novo synthesis, and circulating LDL (via the LDL receptor) — are reciprocally regulated; thus any fall in intracellular cholesterol following diet or drugs leads to increased expression of LDL receptors. These actively transport LDL out of the plasma, with a resulting fall in the circulating concentration.

Classification

Hyperlipidaemias have been classified[1] thus:

Type I is very rare, characterised by high concentrations in the blood of chylomicrons and triglycerides due to genetic deficiency of lipoprotein lipase, and is associated with abdominal pain, pancreatitis and eruptive xanthomata.

Type IIa is common, characterised by high concentrations of LDL and cholesterol in the blood, and is associated with IHD in 50% of males by 50 years and females by 60 years of age. A proportion of these patients (0.2% of the general population) have heterozygous monogenic familial hypercholesterolaemia (FH) which is associated with severe premature heart disease and tendon xanthomata.

Type IIb is common, characterised by high concentrations of LDL and VLDL, cholesterol and triglycerides in the blood, and is associated with IHD.

Type III is uncommon, characterised by high concentrations of 'broad-beta' lipoprotein, cholesterol and triglyceride in the blood due to an inherited abnormal apolipoprotein, and is associated with palmar xanthomata and ischaemic heart and peripheral vascular disease.

Type IV is common, characterised by high concentrations of VLDL and triglyceride in the blood, may be associated with obesity, diabetes and high alcohol intake and gives rise to ischaemic heart and peripheral vascular disease.

Type V is uncommon, characterised by high concentrations of plasma triglyceride on chylomicrons and VLDL, in some patients in part due to excessive alcohol intake or diabetes. These patients are liable to develop pancreatitis.

Management

The management of hyperlipidaemias should be viewed against the background of the following observations.

● Hyperlipidaemias are common; 66% of the adult UK population have a plasma cholesterol concentration in excess of 5.2 mmol/l (the lowest concentration associated with cardiovascular risk).

● Investigation of hyperlipidaemia must be directed initially at excluding contributory causes which include: liver and biliary disease, obesity, hypothyroidism, diabetes, diet, alcohol excess and drugs (β-adrenoceptor blockers, thiazide diuretics, oral contraceptive steroids, etretinate). However, none of these should be assumed to be the sole cause, even if present. Longterm decisions on management should not be initiated on the basis of a single blood lipid estimate.

● The vast majority of cases of hyperlipidaemia seen in general medical practice and perhaps half those who attend special lipid clinics can be managed by *diet* alone; all patients and their spouses, if appropriate, should have effective dietary counselling. Much of the work of lipid clinics is taken up with attending to patients' other risk factors including hypertension, diabetes, thyroid disease and smoking, as well as to the lipid abnormality.

● Lipid lowering drugs should not usually be considered until other measures have failed. The decision to use them is made on the basis of the overall IHD risk, e.g. evidence of existing IHD, hypertension, diabetes mellitus, positive family history. The justification is easiest in two groups: as primary prevention in the relatively small number of asymptomatic patients who have major abnormalities of their lipid profiles, and as secondary prevention in patients who have recently sustained a myocardial infarction. The Scandinavian '4S' Study[2] found in 4444 patients with a total cholesterol

[1] Beaumont J L et al 1970 Bulletin of the World Health Organization 43: 891.

[2] Scandinavian Simvastatin Survival Study Group 1994 Randomised trial of cholesterol lowering in 4444 patients

> 5.2 mmol after a myocardial infarction who were randomised to simvastatin (see below) or placebo that treatment reduced total mortality by 30%, deaths from coronary heart disease by 42% and recurrent myocardial infarction risk by 35%.[2] The authors estimated that addition of simvastatin to the treatment regimens of 100 patients with coronary heart disease would, over 6 years, preserve the lives of 4 out of 9 patients who would otherwise die and prevent a nonfatal myocardial infarction in 7 of an expected 21 cases.

More controversial is the extent to which primary prevention (treatment of clinically unaffected) patients with moderate elevation of cholesterol levels) should include drugs, and whether secondary prevention could ever start with drugs rather than diet. Dietary treatment can lower cholesterol levels in committed subjects, and are obviously less costly than drug treatment. Unfortunately numerous studies have shown that over any substantial period of time (e.g. one year) diet has no clinically significant influence on cholesterol; and the wait for diet to have an effect often results in patients being lost from hospital follow-up after their initial myocardial infarction. Concerns that primary prevention could have a net adverse outcome (that cholesterol reduction increased the risk of cancer or violent deaths) have been largely laid to rest by the first primary prevention trial with a statin. In the WOSCOPS study[3] where pravastatin and placebo were compared in 6590 men age 50–70 with LDL 4–6 mmol/l, pravastatin reduced coronary heart disease (fatal and nonfatal events) by 31% with a nonsignificant reduction in overall mortality.[3] The authors estimated that treatment of 1000 such subjects each year would prevent 20 heart attacks. Increasingly, the implications from such trials for practising doctors and public health officials will depend on such calculations of absolute risk for each patient of coronary events and the cost–benefit equations of prevention versus treatment of such events.

with coronary heart disease: the Scandinavian Simvastatin Survival Study (4S). Lancet 344: 1383–1389.

[3] WOSCOPS = West of Scotland Pravastatin Study. Shepherd J et al 1995 Prevention of coronary heart disease with pravastatin in men with hypercholesterolemia. New England Journal of Medicine 333: 1301–1307.

Management may proceed as follows:

1. *Any medical disorder* that may be causing hyperlipidaemia, e.g. diabetes, hypothyroidism, should be treated first.
2. *Dietary adjustment*. The following applies to all patients:

   - Those who are overweight should reduce their total caloric intake until they have returned to the weight that is appropriate for their height (i.e. body mass index); this automatically assumes reduced intake of alcohol and total (especially animal) fat. Elevated triglyceride concentrations may respond particularly well to alcohol withdrawal.
   - Those who fail to achieve adequate weight reduction or who are already at their ideal weight should reduce their total fat intake; poly- and mono-unsaturated fats or oils may be taken partially to substitute for the reduction in animal fats. Reduction in dietary cholesterol is a much less important element of the diet, but excess egg yolks should be avoided.

3. Specific types of hyperlipidaemia are treated thus:

   - *Type I and some type V*. Reduce dietary fat to 10% of total caloric intake; this may be assisted by partial substitution of fat by medium chain triglycerides which are not carried to the systemic circulation on chylomicrons but enter the liver directly by the portal circulation.
   - *Mild/moderate (common) hypercholesterolaemia (type IIa)* usually responds to diet but those with familial hypercholesterolaemia almost always need an ion exchange resin (cholestyramine or colestipol) and/or another agent, usually a statin. In older patients, the latter is the more effective and better tolerated and should now be the preferred starting treatment. For patients in their 20s and 30s it may be preferable to use the nonabsorbed resin for which there are no concerns about longterm systemic effects.
   - *Type IIb and IV* patients usually have symptoms related to overweight, to diabetes,

food and alcohol, and respond to the measure indicated in (2) above; fibrates are often more effective than statins, and the resins should be avoided.

- *Type III* patients are usually diet-sensitive, failing which, fibrates are the drugs of choice and are normally very effective.
- Poorly responsive patients with familial hypercholesterolaemia (type IIa) and those with severe (types III, IV and V) hyperlipidaemia should preferably be advised by a specialist.

Drugs used in treatment

STATINS

Simvastatin (Zocor) inhibits the rate-limiting enzyme in endogenous cholesterol synthesis, hydroxy-methyl-glutaryl coenzyme A (HMG CoA) reductase. This results in increased synthesis of LDL receptors (up-regulation) in the liver and clearing of LDL from the circulation; plasma total cholesterol and LDL-cholesterol undergo a dose-related reduction (LDL-cholesterol falls by about 30% at a dose of 20 mg/d).

It is well tolerated orally, the commonest adverse effect being transient, and usually minor, abnormality of liver function tests. Elevation of muscle enzymes (creatine phosphokinase) and myositis occur rarely, most reports being in transplant patients receiving cyclosporin.

Other statins are pravastatin, lovastatin, fluvastatin and atorvastatin. There are no clear differences among them, except that the newest, atorvastatin, is the only one to cause substantial reductions in triglyceride as well as cholesterol levels.

FIBRIC ACID DERIVATIVES (fibrates)

These drugs inhibit hepatic lipid synthesis, causing plasma cholesterol to **decline** by 10–15% and triglyceride by 20–30%; associated with this is a rise in the 'protective' HDL-cholesterol which may have contributed to the reduction in nonfatal myocardial infarction with gemfibrozil in the Helsinki Heart Study.[4] Fibric acid derivatives are well absorbed from the gastrointestinal tract, extensively bound to plasma proteins and excreted mainly by the kidney. They are the drugs of choice for mixed hyperlipidaemia (elevated cholesterol plus triglycerides) but may be used in hypercholesterolaemia, alone or with anion exchange resins. They are contraindicated where hepatic or renal function is severely impaired (but gemfibrozil has been used in uraemic and nephrotic patients without aggravating deterioration in kidney function); all may induce a myositis-like syndrome, particularly in patients with poor renal function. Interactions may occur with oral anticoagulants and oral antidiabetic agents due to displacement of these drugs from plasma proteins, enhancing their effect.

The group includes: bezafibrate, fenofibrate, ciprofibrate, gemfibrozil and clofibrate (the latter increases the risk of gallstones and should be used only in patients who have had a cholecystectomy). There is some evidence of varying efficacy among these both in cholesterol-lowering and in additional beneficial effects, such as reduction in blood fibrinogen and urate concentration. Unless compared in outcome trials, it will be difficult to know how clinically important these differences are.

ANION-EXCHANGE RESINS
(bile acid sequestrants)

Cholestyramine is an oral anion-exchange resin[5] which binds bile acids in the intestine. Bile acids are formed from cholesterol in the liver, pass into the gut in the bile and are reabsorbed at the terminal ileum. The total bile acid pool is only 3–5 g but, because such enterohepatic recycling takes place 5–10 times a day, on average 20–30 g of bile acid are delivered into the intestine every 24 hours. Bile acids bound to cholestyramine are lost in the faeces and the depletion of the bile acid pool stimulates conversion of cholesterol to bile acid: the result is a fall in intracellular cholesterol in hepatocytes, and

---

[4] Frick M H et al 1987 New England Journal of Medicine 317: 1237.

[5] The resins consist of aggregations of large molecules carrying a fixed positive charge which therefore bind negatively charged ions (anions).

an increase (up-regulation) in both LDL receptors and cholesterol synthesis. The former has the predominant influence on plasma LDL cholesterol, which falls by 20–25%. In many patients there is some compensatory increase in hepatic triglyceride output. Anion exchange resins therefore may be used first line for hypercholesterolaemia but not for hypertriglyceridaemia, which may be aggravated in such patients.

About half the patients who take cholestyramine experience constipation and some complain of anorexia, abdominal fullness and occasionally of diarrhoea; these effects may limit or prevent its use. Because the drug binds anions, drugs such as warfarin, digoxin, thiazide diuretics, phenobarbitone and thyroid hormones should be taken 1 h before or 6 h after cholestyramine to avoid impairment of their absorption.

Colestipol is similar to cholestyramine.

NICOTINIC ACID AND DERIVATIVES

Nicotinic acid (t½ 1 h) lowers plasma triglyceride and cholesterol concentrations. It acts as an antilipolytic agent in adipose tissue, reducing the supply of nonesterified free fatty acids and hence the availability of substrate for hepatic triglyceride synthesis. Treatment of hyperlipidaemias by nicotinamide requires about × 100 the normal human nutritional needs. Flushing of the skin (preventable by low dose aspirin) and gastrointestinal upset commonly occur; the unpleasantness may be diminished by gradually building up the oral dose over 6 weeks and in time tolerance develops. Rarely there is major disturbance of liver function.

Acipimox is better tolerated than nicotinic acid and has a longer duration of action. However, unlike nicotinic acid, it does not reduce circulating levels of the prothrombotic protein, lipoprotein-(a), better known as Lp(a). The reduction achieved by nicotinic acid may contribute to overall protection against the complications of atheroma, although the pathogenetic significance of lipoprotein-(a) is still unclear.

OTHER DRUGS

Omega-3 marine triglycerides (Maxepa) contain the triglyceride precursors of two polyunsaturated fatty acids (eicosapentaenoic acid and docosahexaenoic acid) derived from sea fish. They have no place in treating hypercholesterolaemia. Some patients with moderate to severe hypertriglyceridaemia may respond to oral use, although LDL-cholesterol may rise. There is an associated 90 calorie per day energy load.

Probucol (Lurselle) increases the excretion of bile acids and reduces cholesterol biosynthesis; the resulting fall in plasma lipid concentration affects both LDL and the 'protective' HDL. The drug is well tolerated orally but some patients experience gastrointestinal upset and abdominal pain.

Alpha-tocopherol acetate (vitamin E) has no effect on lipid levels but is a powerful anti-oxidant. Considerable evidence points to oxidation of LDL as an essential step in the development of atheroma, and therefore interest has centred on the role of either endogenous or therapeutic vitamin E in prevention of atheroma. Average levels of vitamin E in both blood and fat (vitamin E is a fat soluble vitamin) are reduced in both the inhabitants of coun-

---

SUMMARY

- The commonest and most important hyperlipidaemia is hypercholesterolaemia, which is one of the major risk factors for ischaemic heart disease.
- Most treatment works by reducing the intracellular concentration of cholesterol in hepatocytes, leading to compensatory overexpression of low density lipoprotein (LDL) receptors on their surface, and increased uptake of cholesterol-rich LDL particles from the bloodstream.
- The most effective drugs are the statins, which inhibit the rate limiting step in cholesterol synthesis.
- These drugs reduce blood cholesterol levels by 25–35% and cause a 35–45% reduction in risk of ischaemic heart disease.
- The main indications for their use are in patients with even slight elevations of cholesterol after a myocardial infarction, and in patients with gross excess of cholesterol and a family history of ischaemic heart disease.

tries with a high prevalence of ischaemic heart disease, and (within these countries) in patients who develop ischaemic heart disease. A high dose reduced by half the risk of myocardial infarction in 2000 patients with angina and positive coronary angiogram. A number of other, prospective studies of either vitamin E, or vitamin E combined with other anti-oxidants (vitamin C, β-carotene) which are in progress will establish in which patients one or other of these may have a role.

GUIDE TO FURTHER READING

Betteridge D J 1989 High density lipoprotein and coronary heart disease. British Medical Journal 298: 974

Brunzell J D, Austin M A 1989 Plasma triglyceride levels and coronary disease. New England Journal of Medicine 320: 1273

Editorial 1989 Low cholesterol and increased risk. Lancet 1: 1423

Gordon D J, Rifkind B M 1989 High density lipoprotein — the clinical implications of recent studies. New England Journal of Medicine 321: 1311

Grundy S M 1988 HMG-CoA reductase inhibitors for treatment of hypercholesterolaemia. New England Journal of Medicine 319: 24

Haq I U et al 1995 Sheffield risk and treatment table for cholesterol lowering for primary prevention of coronary heart disease. Lancet 346: 1467–1471

Law M R et al 1994 By how much and how quickly does reduction in serum cholesterol concentration lower risk of ischaemic heart disease. British Medical Journal 308: 367–372

Mansell P, Reckless J P D 1991 Garlic. British Medical Journal 303: 379

Oliver M et al 1995 Lower patient's cholesterol now. British Medical Journal 310: 1280–1281

Ramsay L E et al 1991 Dietary reduction of serum cholesterol concentration: time to think again. British Medical Journal 303: 953–957

Sacks F M, Pfeffer M A, Moye L A et al 1996 The effect of pravastatia on coronary events after myocardial infarction in patients with average cholesterol levels. New England Journal of Medicine 335: 1001–1009

Scandinavian Simvastatin Survival Study Group 1994 Randomised trial of cholesterol lowering in 4444 patients with coronary heart disease: the Scandinavian Simvastatin Survival Study (4S). Lancet 344: 1383–1389

Shepherd J et al 1995 Prevention of coronary heart disease with pravastatin in men with hypercholesterolemia. New England Journal of Medicine 333: 1301–1307

Steinberg D 1993 Antioxidant vitamins and coronary heart disease. New England Journal of Medicine 328: 1487–1489

Stephens N G et al 1996 Randomised controlled trial of vitamin E in patients with coronary disease: Cambridge heart antioxidant study. Lancet 347: 781–786

Kidney and urinary tract

SYNOPSIS

- Diuretic drugs: their sites and modes of action, classification, adverse effects and uses in cardiac, hepatic, renal and other conditions
- Carbonic anhydrase inhibitors
- Cation-exchange resins and their uses
- Alteration of urine pH

Drugs and the kidney

- Adverse effects
- Drug-induced renal disease: by direct and indirect biochemical effects and by immunological effects
- Prescribing for renal disease: adjusting the dose according to the characteristics of the drug and to the degree of renal impairment
- Nephrolithiasis and its management
- Pharmacological aspects of micturition
- Benign prostatic hyperplasia

Diuretic drugs

(See also Ch. 24)

Definition: a diuretic is any substance which increases urine and solute excretion. This wide definition, however, includes substances not commonly thought of as diuretics, e.g. water. To be therapeutically useful a diuretic should increase the output of sodium as well as of water, for diuretics are normally required to remove oedema fluid which is composed of water and solutes, of which sodium is the most important.

Each day the body produces 180 l of glomerular filtrate which is modified in its passage down the renal tubules to appear as 1.5 l of urine. Thus a 1% reduction in reabsorption of tubular fluid will more than double urine output. Clearly, drugs that act on the tubule have considerable scope to alter body fluid and electrolyte balance. Most clinically useful diuretics are organic anions and are transported from the blood, through the tubular cells and into tubular fluid. The following brief account of tubular function with particular reference to sodium transport will help to explain where and how diuretic drugs act; it should be read with reference to Figure 27.1.

SITES AND MODES OF ACTION[1]

As a result of active reabsorption of sodium chloride and sodium bicarbonate from the renal tubular lumen and passive reabsorption of accompanying water, 65% of the glomerular filtrate is reabsorbed iso-osmotically from the proximal tubule. The epithelium of the proximal tubule is described as 'leaky' because of its free permeability to water and a number of solutes.

---

[1] Beavers occupying a watery habitat have nephrons with short loops, while those of the desert rat have long loops.

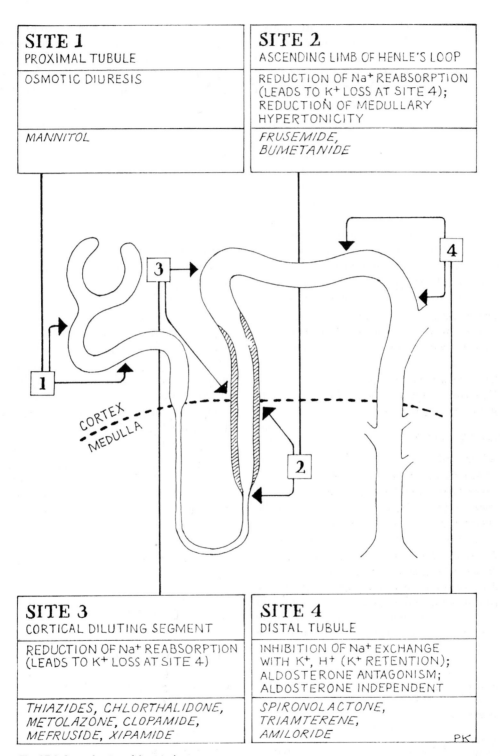

SITE 1 PROXIMAL TUBULE	SITE 2 ASCENDING LIMB OF HENLE'S LOOP
OSMOTIC DIURESIS	REDUCTION OF Na^+ REABSORPTION (LEADS TO K^+ LOSS AT SITE 4); REDUCTION OF MEDULLARY HYPERTONICITY
MANNITOL	FRUSEMIDE, BUMETANIDE

CORTEX

MEDULLA

SITE 3 CORTICAL DILUTING SEGMENT	SITE 4 DISTAL TUBULE
REDUCTION OF Na^+ REABSORPTION (LEADS TO K^+ LOSS AT SITE 4)	INHIBITION OF Na^+ EXCHANGE WITH K^+, H^+ (K^+ RETENTION); ALDOSTERONE ANTAGONISM; ALDOSTERONE INDEPENDENT
THIAZIDES, CHLORTHALIDONE, METOLAZONE, CLOPAMIDE, MEFRUSIDE, XIPAMIDE	SPIRONOLACTONE, TRIAMTERENE, AMILORIDE

PK

Fig. 27.1 Sites of action of diuretic drugs

Osmotic diuretics such as mannitol are solutes which are not reabsorbed in the proximal tubule (site 1, Fig. 27.1) and therefore carry into the urine equivalent volumes of fluid.

The tubular fluid now passes into the loop of Henle where 25% of the filtered sodium is reabsorbed. There are two populations of nephron: those that have short loops and are confined to the cortex; and the juxtamedullary nephrons whose long loops penetrate into the inner parts of the medulla and are principally concerned with water conservation; the following discussion refers to the latter. The physiological changes are best understood by considering first the ascending limb. In the thick segment (site 2, Fig. 27.1), chloride ion is transported actively from the tubular fluid into the interstitial fluid, taking with it sodium ion but not water, to which this part of the tubule is impermeable. In consequence, the tubular fluid becomes dilute, the interstitium becomes hypertonic and fluid in the descending limb, which is permeable to water, becomes more concentrated as it approaches the tip of the loop, because the hypertonic interstitial fluid sucks water out of the tubule. The 'hairpin' structure of the loop thus confers on it the property of a *countercurrent multiplier* which by active transport of ions converts a small change in osmolality into a steep osmotic gradient; the high osmotic pressure in the medullary interstitium is sustained by the vasa rectae which lie close to the loops of Henle and act as *countercurrent exchangers*, for the incoming blood receives sodium from the outgoing blood.[2] Frusemide, bumetanide, piretanide, torasemide and ethacrynic acid act principally at site 2 by inhibiting active chloride ion transport, which thus prevents sodium ion reabsorption and lowers the osmotic gradient between cortex and medulla; the result is that large volumes of dilute urine are formed. These drugs are called the *loop diuretics*.

---

[2] The most easily comprehended countercurrent exchange mechanism (in this case for heat) is that in wading birds in cold climates whereby the veins carrying cold blood from the feet pass closely alongside the arteries carrying warm blood from the body and heat exchange takes place. The result is that the feet receive blood below body temperature (which does not matter) and the blood from the feet which is often very cold, is warmed before it enters the body so that the internal temperature is more easily maintained. The principle is the same for maintaining renal medullary hypertonicity.

As the ascending limb of the loop re-enters the renal cortex, sodium and chloride continue to be actively passed into the interstitial tissue (site 3) but are rapidly removed because cortical blood flow is high and there are no vasa rectae present; consequently the urine becomes more dilute. *Thiazides* act principally at the cortical diluting segment of the ascending limb, preventing sodium reabsorption.

In the distal tubule (site 4), sodium ions are exchanged for potassium ions and hydrogen ions. In part the mechanism of this exchange is aldosterone-dependent and may be inhibited by the competitive mineralocorticoid receptor antagonist, spironolactone; an aldosterone-independent mechanism(s) also operates and is inhibited by triamterene and amiloride. Only 5% of filtered sodium is reabsorbed by the distal tubule, but by reducing sodium/potassium exchange these diuretics cause potassium retention. Diuretics that act proximal to this point bring about potassium *loss* because they allow more sodium to be delivered to the site at which sodium may be exchanged for potassium.

The collecting tubule then travels back down into the medulla to reach the papilla; in doing so it passes through a gradient of increasing osmotic pressure which tends to draw water out of tubular fluid. This final concentration of urine is under the influence of antidiuretic hormone (ADH) whose action is to make the collecting ducts permeable to water, and in its absence water remains in the collecting tubule; ethanol causes diuresis by inhibiting the release of ADH from the posterior pituitary gland.

Diuresis may also be achieved by extrarenal mechanisms, by raising the cardiac output and increasing renal blood flow, e.g. with dobutamine and dopamine.

CLASSIFICATION

The maximum efficacy in removing salt and water that any drug can achieve is related to its site of action, and it is clinically appropriate to rank diuretics according to their natriuretic capacity, as follows:

The percentages quoted in this rank order refer to the highest fractional excretion of filtered sodium under carefully controlled conditions and should not be taken to represent the average fractional sodium loss during clinical use.

High efficacy

Frusemide, bumetanide, piretanide, torasemide and ethacrynic acid (loop diuretics) can cause 5–25% of filtered sodium to be excreted. Their action impairs the powerful urine-concentrating mechanism of the loop of Henle and confers higher efficacy compared to drugs that act in the relatively hypotonic cortex (see below). Progressive increase in dose is matched by increasing diuresis, i.e. they have a high 'ceiling' of effect. Indeed, they are so efficacious that overtreatment can readily dehydrate the patient. Loop diuretics remain effective at glomerular filtration rates below 10 ml/min (normal 120 ml/min).

Moderate efficacy

The *thiazide* family, bendrofluazide and the related chlorthalidone, clopamide, indapamide, mefruside, metolazone, xipamide, etc. cause 5–10% of filtered sodium load to be excreted. Increasing the dose beyond a small range produces no added diuresis, i.e. they have a low 'ceiling' of effect. Such drugs tend to be ineffective once the glomerular filtration rate has fallen below 20 ml/min (except metolazone).

Low efficacy

Potassium sparing triamterene, amiloride, spironolactone, cause 5% of filtered sodium to be excreted. They are usefully combined with more efficacious diuretics to prevent the potassium loss which other diuretics cause.

Osmotic diuretics, e.g. mannitol, and methylxanthines, e.g. aminophylline, also fall into this category.

Individual diuretics

HIGH EFFICACY LOOP DIURETICS
(frusemide)

Frusemide (furosemide, Lasix) acts on the thick portion of the ascending limb of the loop of Henle

(site 2) to produce the effects described above. Because more sodium is delivered to site 4, exchange with potassium leads to urinary potassium loss and hypokalaemia. Magnesium and calcium loss are increased by frusemide to about the same extent as sodium; the effect on calcium is utilised in the emergency management of hypercalcaemia (see Index).

Pharmacokinetics. Frusemide is well absorbed from the gastrointestinal tract and is highly bound to plasma proteins. The $t^{1/2}$ is 2 h, but this rises to over 10 h in renal failure.

Uses. Frusemide is highly successful for the relief of oedema. Progressive increase of dose of frusemide is matched by increase in urine production. Taken orally it acts within an hour and diuresis lasts about 6 hours. Enormous urine volumes can result and overtreatment may lead to hypovolaemia and circulatory collapse. Given i.v. it acts within 30 minutes and can relieve acute pulmonary oedema, partly by a vasodilator action which precedes the diuresis. An important feature of frusemide is its efficacy when the glomerular filtration rate is 10 ml/min or less.

The dose is 20–120 mg by mouth per day; i.m. or i.v.; 20–50 mg is given initially. For use in renal failure, special high dose tablets (500 mg) are available, and a solution of 250 mg in 25 ml which should be infused i.v. at a rate not greater than 4 mg/min.

Adverse effects are uncommon, apart from excess of therapeutic effect (electrolyte disturbance, hypotension due to low plasma volume) and those mentioned in the general account for diuretics (below). They include nausea, pancreatitis and, rarely, deafness which is usually transient and associated with rapid i.v. injection in renal failure. NSAIDs, notably indomethacin, reduce frusemide-induced diuresis probably by inhibiting the formation of vasodilator prostaglandins in the kidney.

Bumetanide (Burinex), piretanide (Arelix) and ethacrynic acid are similar to frusemide. Torasemide (Torsemide) is also similar, but has also been demonstrated to be an effective anti-hypertensive agent at lower, non-natriuretic doses

(2.5–5 mg/d) than those used in oedema states (5–40 mg). Ethacrynic acid is less widely used as it is more prone to cause adverse effects, especially nausea and deafness.

MODERATE EFFICACY DIURETICS
(thiazide and related diuretics)

(See also Hypertension, Ch. 24)
Thiazides depress sodium reabsorption at site 3 which is just proximal to the region of sodium–potassium exchange. These drugs thus raise potassium excretion to an important extent. Thiazides lower blood pressure, chiefly due to reduction in intravascular volume but probably also to reduction of peripheral vascular resistance. In chronic use they diminish the responsiveness of vascular smooth muscle to noradrenaline (norepinephrine); but they may also have a direct action on vascular smooth muscle membranes, acting on an as yet unidentified ion channel.

Thiazides are generally well absorbed from the gut and most begin to act within an hour. There are numerous derivatives and their differences lie principally in duration of action. The relatively *water soluble*, e.g. cyclopenthiazide, chlorothiazide, hydrochlorothiazide, are most rapidly eliminated, their peak effect occurring within 4–6 h and passing off by 10–12 h. They are excreted unchanged in the urine and active secretion by the proximal renal tubule contributes to their high renal clearance and t$\frac{1}{2}$ of < 4 h. The relatively *lipid soluble* members of the group, e.g. polythiazide, hydroflumethiazide, distribute more widely into body tissues and act for over 24 h, which can be objectionable if the drug is used for diuresis, though useful for hypertension. Thiazides are not effective when renal function is severely impaired.

Adverse effects in general are discussed below. Rashes (sometimes photosensitive), thrombocytopenia and agranulocytosis occur. Treatment with thiazide-type drugs causes an increase in total serum cholesterol, but on longterm usage even of high doses this is less than 5%. The questions about the appropriateness of use of these drugs for mild hypertension, of which ischaemic heart disease is a common complication, have been laid to rest by their proven success in randomised outcome comparisons.

Bendrofluazide is a satisfactory member for routine use.

- *Used primarily for a diuresis* oral dose is 5–10 mg which usually lasts less than 12 h so that it should be given in the morning. It may be given daily for the first few days then, say, 3 days a week.
- *As an antihypertensive* bendrofluazide 2.5 mg is given daily; in the absence of a diuresis clinically important potassium depletion is uncommon, but plasma potassium concentration should be checked in potentially vulnerable groups such as the elderly (see Ch. 25).

Cyclopenthiazide is a satisfactory alternative.
Other members of the group include: benzthiazide, chlorothiazide, hydrochlorothiazide, hydroflumethiazide, methyclothiazide, polythiazide.

Diuretics related to the thiazides. Several compounds, although strictly not thiazides, share structural similarities with them and probably act at the same site on the nephron; they therefore exhibit moderate therapeutic efficacy. Overall, these substances have a greater duration of action, are used for oedema and hypertension and their profile of adverse effects is similar to that of the thiazides. They are listed below.

Chlorthalidone acts for 48–72 h after a single oral dose.

Xipamide is structurally related to chlorthalidone and to frusemide. It induces a diuresis for about 12 h that is brisker than with thiazides, which may trouble the elderly.

Clopamide also acts for about 24 h.

Metolazone is effective when renal function is impaired. It potentiates the diuresis produced by frusemide and the combination can be effective in resistant oedema, provided the patient's fluid and electrolyte loss are carefully monitored.

Mefruside has its peak effect 6–12 h after administration and its duration may be 24 h.

Indapamide is structurally related to chlorthalidone but lowers blood pressure at subdiuretic doses, perhaps by altering calcium flux in vascular smooth muscle. It has little apparent effect on potassium, glucose or uric acid excretion (see below).

LOW EFFICACY DIURETICS
(potassium-sparing diuretics)

Spironolactone

Spironolactone (Aldactone) is structurally similar to aldosterone and competitively inhibits its action (sodium reabsorption and potassium loss in the distal tubule); excessive secretion of aldosterone contributes to fluid retention in hepatic cirrhosis, nephrotic syndrome and congestive cardiac failure, in which conditions as well as in primary hypersecretion (Conn's syndrome) it is most useful.

After oral administration, spironolactone is largely converted in the gut and liver to the active metabolite *canrenone*, which has a plasma $t^{1}/2$ of 9 h. Most of the diuretic effect of spironolactone is probably due to this metabolite which is available as a drug in its own right, *potassium canrenoate*. Canrenone has been shown to improve myocardial contraction, an additional action which may prove beneficial in cardiac failure.

Spironolactone is relatively ineffective when used alone, causing less than 5% of the filtered sodium load to be excreted. It may, however, be more effective when combined with a drug that reduces sodium reabsorption proximally in the tubule, e.g. a loop diuretic. Spironolactone (and amiloride and triamterene, see below) also reduces the potassium loss that occurs with loop diuretics, but its combination with another potassium-sparing diuretic leads to hyperkalaemia. Dangerous potassium retention may also develop if spironolactone is given to patients with impaired renal function. Spironolactone is given orally in one or more doses. The maximum diuresis is delayed for up to 4 days but if after 5 days the response is inadequate, the dose may be increased to 200 mg/d.

Adverse effects are uncommon but include gynaecomastia, which is often painful but reverses when the drug is withdrawn; unfortunately, unnecessary mastectomies have been performed in ignorance of the iatrogenic nature of the problem. Other adverse effects are mental confusion, drowsiness, rashes, abdominal pain and menstrual irregularities including amenorrhoea. It causes negligible urate retention. Possible human metabolites are carcinogenic in rodents. Spironolactone induces hepatic microsomal enzymes.

Amiloride (Midamor) increases sodium loss and *reduces* potassium loss by a direct action on ion transport in the distal tubule, i.e. it does not antagonise the action of aldosterone and, in contrast to spironolactone, it is effective when there is no aldosterone excess. Its action is therefore complementary to that of the thiazides and, used with them, it increases sodium loss and reduces potassium loss. One such combination, co-amilozide, (Moduretic) (amiloride 5 mg plus hydrochlorothiazide 50 mg), is used for moderate hypertension or oedema. The maximum effect of amiloride occurs about 6 h after an oral dose and the action may last 24 h. The oral dose is 5–20 mg daily.

Triamterene (Dytac) is a potassium-sparing diuretic which has an action and use similar to that of amiloride. The diuretic effect extends over 10 h. Gastrointestinal upsets occur. Reversible, non-oliguric renal failure may occur when triamterene is used with indomethacin (and presumably other NSAIDs).

ADVERSE EFFECTS CHARACTERISTIC OF DIURETICS

Potassium depletion. Diuretics, which act at sites 1, 2 and 3 (Fig. 27.1), cause more sodium to reach the sodium–potassium exchange site in the distal tubule (site 4) and so increase potassium excretion. This subject warrants discussion since hypokalaemia may cause cardiac dysrhythmia.

The safe lower limit for serum potassium concentration is normally quoted as 3.5 mmol/l. Whether or not diuretic therapy causes significant lowering of serum potassium depends both on the drug and on the circumstances in which it is used.

● *The loop diuretics* cause a smaller fall in serum potassium than do the thiazides, for equivalent diuretic effect, but have a greater capacity for diuresis, i.e. higher efficacy especially in large dose, and so are associated with greater decline in potassium. If diuresis is brisk and continuous, clinically important potassium depletion is likely to occur.

• *Low dietary intake* of potassium predisposes to hypokalaemia; the risk is particularly notable in the elderly, many of whom ingest less than 50 mmol per day (the dietary normal is 80 mmol).

• Hypokalaemia during diuretic therapy is also more likely in *hyperaldosteronism*, whether primary or more commonly secondary to severe liver disease, congestive cardiac failure or nephrotic syndrome.

• Potassium loss occurs with *diarrhoea, vomiting or small bowel fistula,* and may be aggravated by diuretic therapy.

• When a thiazide diuretic is used for *hypertension*, there is probably no case for routine prescription of a potassium supplement if no predisposing factors are present (see Ch. 24).

Potassium depletion can be minimised or corrected by:

• Maintaining a good dietary potassium intake
• Combining a potassium-depleting with a potassium-sparing drug
• Intermittent use of potassium-losing drugs, i.e. drug holidays
• Potassium supplements: potassium chloride is preferred because chloride is the principal anion excreted along with sodium when high efficacy diuretics are used, i.e. they cause hypochloraemic alkalosis. Potassium supplements are a less effective alternative than combination with potassium-sparing diuretic since the thiazide or loop diuretic increases clearance of the supplements. Satisfactory formulations include: potassium chloride sustained-release tabs (Slow-K tabs) containing 8 mmol each of K and Cl; potassium chloride effervescent tabs (Sando-K tabs) containing 12 mmol of K and 8 mmol of Cl. All forms of potassium are irritant to the gastrointestinal tract. If, for example, the tablet is held up in the oesophagus, ulceration may result. The elderly, in particular, should be warned never to take such tablets dry but always with a large cupful of liquid and sitting upright or standing.

Hyperkalaemia may occur especially if a potassium-sparing diuretic is given to a patient with impaired renal function. Angiotensin-converting enzyme (ACE) inhibitors cause modest elevation of plasma potassium which may aggravate hyperkalaemia if they are also being taken.

Treatment of hyperkalaemia depends on the severity and the following measures are appropriate:

• The potassium-sparing diuretic should be discontinued.
• A cation exchange resin, e.g. polystyrene sulphonate resin (Resonium A, Calcium Resonium, see later) can be used orally (more effective than rectally) to remove body potassium via the gut.
• Potassium may be moved rapidly from plasma into cells by giving

(1) sodium bicarbonate
   — i.v. (40–160 mmol) and repeating this in a few minutes if the characteristic ECG changes persist;
(2) glucose 20%, 300–500 ml plus insulin 1 unit/3 g glucose by i.v. infusion.
   — If ECG changes are marked, calcium gluconate 10% solution, 10 ml i.v. and repeated if necessary in a few minutes, may be given to oppose the myocardial effect of potassium. Calcium may potentiate digoxin and should be used cautiously, if at all, in a patient taking this drug. Sodium bicarbonate and calcium salt must not be mixed in a syringe or reservoir because calcium precipitates.

• Dialysis is, of course, highly effective.

Hypovolaemia can result from overtreatment. Acute loss of excessive fluid leads to postural hypotension and dizziness. A more insidious state of chronic hypovolaemia can develop especially in the elderly. After initial benefit, the patient becomes sleepy and lethargic. Blood urea concentration rises but sodium and chloride concentrations are usually normal. Renal failure may result.

Urinary retention. Sudden vigorous diuresis can cause acute retention of urine in the presence of bladder neck obstruction, e.g. due to prostatic enlargement.

Hyponatraemia may result if sodium loss occurs in patients who drink a large quantity of water. Other mechanisms are probably involved, including enhancement of antidiuretic hormone release. Such patients have reduced total body sodium and extracellular fluid and are oedema-free. Discontinuation of the diuretic and water restriction usually suffice to correct the state. The condition should be distinguished from hyponatraemia with oedema which develops in some patients with congestive cardiac failure, cirrhosis or nephrotic syndrome. Here salt and water intake should be restricted because extracellular fluid volume is expanded.

The combination of a potassium-sparing diuretic and ACE inhibitor can also cause severe *hypo*natraemia.

Urate retention with hyperuricaemia and sometimes clinical gout occurs with the high and moderate efficacy diuretics, but the effect is unimportant or negligible with the low efficacy diuretics.

Two mechanisms appear to be responsible. First, diuretics cause volume depletion, reduction in glomerular filtration and increased absorption of almost all solutes in the proximal tubule including urate. Second, diuretics and uric acid are organic acids and compete for the transport mechanism which carries such substances from the blood into the urine. Diuretic-induced hyperuricaemia can be prevented by allopurinol or probenecid.

Magnesium deficiency. Loop and thiazide diuretics, and in particular chlorthalidone, cause significant urinary loss of magnesium; potassium-sparing diuretics probably also cause magnesium retention. Magnesium deficiency brought about by diuretics seems rarely to be severe enough to induce the classic picture of neuromuscular irritability and tetany but cardiac dysrhythmias, mainly of ventricular origin, do occur and respond to repletion of magnesium (magnesium chloride 35–50 mmol may be added to 1 litre of glucose 5% and infused over 12–24 h).

Carbohydrate intolerance is caused by those diuretics which produce prolonged hypokalaemia, i.e. the loop and thiazide type. It appears that intracellular potassium is necessary for the formation of insulin, and glucose intolerance is probably due to insulin deficiency. Insulin requirements thus increase in established diabetics and the disease may become manifest in latent diabetics. The effect is generally reversible over several months.

Calcium homeostasis. Renal calcium loss is increased by the loop diuretics; in the short term this is not a serious disadvantage and indeed frusemide may be used in the management of hypercalcaemia after rehydration has been achieved. In the long term hypocalcaemia may be harmful especially in elderly patients who tend in any case to be in negative calcium balance. Thiazides, by contrast, decrease renal excretion of calcium and this property may influence the choice of diuretic in a potentially calcium deficient or osteoporotic individual, for thiazide use is associated with reduced risk of hip fracture in the elderly. The hypocalciuric effect of the thiazides has also been used effectively in patients with idiopathic hypercalciuria, the commonest metabolic cause of renal stones.

Interactions

Loop diuretics potentiate ototoxicity of aminoglycosides and nephrotoxicity of some cephalosporins. NSAIDs tend to cause sodium retention which counteracts the effect of diuretics; the mechanism may involve inhibition of renal prostaglandin formation. Diuretic treatment of a patient taking lithium can precipitate toxicity from this drug (see Index).

Abuse of diuretics

Psychological abnormality sometimes takes the form of abuse of diuretics and/or purgatives. The subject usually desires to slim to become attractive or healthy or may have anorexia nervosa. There can be severe depletion of sodium and potassium, with renal tubular damage due to chronic hypokalaemia.

OSMOTIC DIURETICS

Osmotic diuretics are small molecular weight substances that are filtered by the glomerulus but are not reabsorbed by the renal tubule, and thus increase the osmolarity of the tubular fluid. Their principal site of action is the proximal tubule and probably also the loop of Henle, where they prevent the reabsorption of water and also, by more complex mechanisms, of sodium. The result is that urine volume increases according to the load of osmotic diuretic.

Mannitol, a polyhydric alcohol (mol. wt. 452), is most commonly used; it is given i.v. In addition to its effect on the kidney, mannitol encourages the movement of water from inside cells to the extracellular fluid, which is thus transiently expanded. These properties define its uses, which are for rapid reduction of *intracranial* or *intraocular pressure,* and to maintain urine flow to prevent *renal tubular necrosis.* Mannitol is contraindicated in congestive cardiac failure and pulmonary oedema; where it is uncertain that the drug will be excreted the dose (normal 50–200 g) should be reduced.

METHYLXANTHINES

The general properties of the methylxanthines (theophylline, caffeine) are discussed elsewhere (see p. 509). Their mild diuretic action probably depends in part on smooth muscle relaxation in the afferent arteriolar bed increasing renal blood flow, and in part on a direct inhibitory effect on salt reabsorption in the proximal tubule. Their uses in medicine depend on their other properties.

INDICATIONS FOR DIURETICS

● *Oedematous states* associated with sodium overload, e.g. cardiac, renal or hepatic disease, and also without sodium overload, e.g. acute pulmonary oedema following myocardial infarction. Note that oedema may also be localised, e.g. angioedema, or due to low plasma albumin, or immobility in the elderly, in which circumstances a diuretic is not indicated.

● *Hypertension,* by reducing intravascular volume and probably by other mechanisms too, e.g. reduction of sensitivity to noradrenergic vasoconstriction.

● *Hypercalcaemia.* Frusemide reduces calcium reabsorption in the ascending limb of the loop of Henle and this action may be utilised in the emergency reduction of elevated plasma calcium in addition to rehydration and other measures (see Index).

● *Idiopathic hypercalciuria,* a common cause of renal stone disease, may be reduced by thiazide diuretics; reduction of intravascular volume favours proximal renal tubular reabsorption of calcium.

● *The syndrome of inappropriate secretion of antidiuretic hormone secretion* (SIADH) may be treated with frusemide if there is a dangerous degree of volume overload. Other measures will also be required; these include: withdrawal of a drug if it is the cause (e.g. chlorpropamide), water restriction, demeclocycline (see Index) and salt replacement.

● *Nephrogenic diabetes insipidus,* paradoxically, may respond to diuretics which, by contracting vascular volume, increase salt and water reabsorption in the proximal tubule, and thus reduce urine volume.

THERAPY

Congestive cardiac failure

The main account appears in Chapter 25. It is sufficient here to note that because diuretics by mouth are easily given repeatedly, lack of supervision can result in insidious overtreatment. Relief at disappearance of the congestive features can mask exacerbation of the low output symptoms of heart failure, such as *tiredness* and *postural dizziness* due to reduced blood volume. A *rising blood urea* is usually evidence of reduced glomerular blood flow consequent on a fall in cardiac output, but does not distinguish whether the cause of the reduced output is overdiuresis or deterioration of the heart failure itself. The simplest guide to the success or failure of diuretic regimens is to monitor *body weight.* Fluid intake and output charts are more demanding of nursing time, and often less accurate.

Acute pulmonary oedema: left ventricular failure (See Ch. 25, p. 476)

Renal oedema

The chief therapeutic aims are to reduce dietary sodium intake and to prevent excessive sodium retention using diuretic drugs. Reduction of sodium reabsorption in the renal tubule by diuretics is most effective where glomerular filtration has not been seriously reduced by disease. Frusemide and bumetanide are effective even when the filtration rate is very low; frusemide may usefully be combined with metolazone but the resulting profound diuresis requires careful monitoring.

Secondary hyperaldosteronism complicates the

nephrotic syndrome because albumin loss causes plasma colloid pressure to fall, and the resulting diversion of intravascular volume to the interstitium activates the renin-angiotensin-aldosterone system; then spironolactone may be added usefully to potentiate a loop diuretic and to conserve potassium, loss of which can be severe.

Hepatic ascites. Ascites and oedema are due to portal venous hypertension together with decreased plasma colloid osmotic pressure causing hyperaldosteronism as with nephrotic oedema (above). Furthermore, diversion of renal blood flow from the cortex to the medulla favours sodium retention. In addition to dietary sodium restriction, a loop diuretic plus spironolactone are used to produce a *gradual* diuresis; too vigorous depletion of sodium with added potassium loss and hypochloraemic alkalosis may cause hepatic coma. Abdominal paracentesis, usually undertaken for the sake of speed, aggravates hypoproteinaemia, and should be avoided if at all possible.

Carbonic anhydrase inhibitors

Carbonic anhydrase facilitates the reaction between carbon dioxide and water to form carbonic acid:

$$CO_2 + H_2O \rightleftharpoons \overset{\text{carbonic}}{\underset{}{\text{anhydrase}}} H_2CO_3 \rightleftharpoons H^+ + HCO_3^-$$

The rate is slow in the absence of the enzyme. By making available hydrogen and bicarbonate ions, this reaction is fundamental to the production of either acid or alkaline secretions and high concentrations of carbonic anhydrase are present in the gastric mucosa, pancreas, eye and kidney. Inhibitors of carbonic anhydrase are obsolete as diuretics, but they still have uses in medicine.

Reduction of intraocular pressure. This action is due not to diuresis (thiazides actually raise intraocular pressure slightly). The formation of aqueous humour is an active process requiring a supply of bicarbonate ions, which depends on carbonic anhy-

drase. Inhibition of carbonic anhydrase reduces the formation of aqueous humour and lowers intraocular pressure. This is a local action and is not affected by the development of acid-base changes elsewhere in the body, i.e. tolerance does not develop. *Acetazolamide* is the most widely used carbonic anhydrase inhibitor. In patients with glaucoma, acetazolamide can be taken either orally, or locally as eye-drops.

Prevention of high altitude (mountain) sickness. This condition may affect unacclimatised people at altitudes in excess of 3000 metres especially if ascent has been rapid and exertion great; symptoms range from nausea, lassitude and headache to pulmonary and cerebral oedema. The initiating cause is hypoxia: at high altitude, the normal hyperventilatory response to falling oxygen tension is inhibited because alkalosis is also induced. A carbonic anhydrase inhibitor induces metabolic acidosis, increases respiratory drive, notably at night when apnoeic attacks may occur, and thus helps to maintain arterial oxygen tension; it should be started on the day before the ascent and continued for 2 days after reaching the intended altitude.

High doses of acetazolamide may cause drowsiness and fever, rashes and paraesthesiae may occur, and blood disorders have been reported. Renal calculi may occur, perhaps because the urine calcium is in less soluble form owing to low citrate content of the urine.

The drug has two other uses. In *periodic paralysis*, where sudden falls in plasma K^+ occur due to its exchange with Na^+ ions in cells, the rise in plasma H^+ caused by acetazolamide provides an alternative cation to K^+ for exchange with Na^+. In *petit-mal seizures*, acetazolamide is a second-line drug after carbamazepine (see p. 360).

Dichlorphenamide is similar.

Cation-exchange resins

Cation-exchange resins may be used to remove potassium from the intestinal contents, as a means of treating *hyperkalaemia* when urine formation is poor or has ceased, or in potential dialysis patients. The resins consist of aggregations of big insoluble molecules carrying fixed negative charges, which therefore loosely bind positively charged ions (cations); these latter readily exchange with cations in the fluid environment to an extent that depends on their affinity for the resin and their concentration. Resins loaded with sodium or calcium exchange these cations preferentially with potassium cations in the intestine (about 1 mmol of potassium per gram of resin); the freed cations are absorbed and the resin with the bound potassium is passed in the faeces. The resin does not merely prevent absorption of ingested potassium, but it also takes up the potassium normally secreted into the intestine and ordinarily reabsorbed.

In hyperkalaemia, oral administration or retention enemas of a *polystyrene sulphonate resin* may be used. A sodium phase resin (Resonium A) should obviously not be used in patients with renal or cardiac failure as sodium overload may result. A calcium phase resin (Calcium Resonium) may cause hypercalcaemia and should be avoided in predisposed patients, e.g. with multiple myeloma, metastatic carcinoma, hyperparathyroidism and sarcoidosis. Enemas should be retained for as long as possible, although patients rarely manage for as long as necessary (at least 9 h) to exchange K^+ at all available sites on the resin.

Alteration of urine pH

Alteration of urine pH by drugs is sometimes desirable. The most common reason is in the treatment of poisoning (a fuller account appears on p. 142). A summary of the main indications appears below.

Alkalinisation of urine

- increases the elimination of salicylate, phenobarbitone and chlorophenoxy herbicides, e.g. 2,4-D, MCPA
- reduces irritation of an inflamed urinary tract
- discourages the growth of certain organisms, e.g. *Escherichia coli.*

The urine can be made alkaline by sodium bicarbonate i.v., or by potassium citrate by mouth. Sodium overload may exacerbate cardiac failure, and sodium or potassium excess are dangerous when renal function is impaired.

Acidification of urine

- is used as a test for renal tubular acidosis
- increases elimination of amphetamine, dexfenfluramine, quinine and phencyclidine, although it is very rarely needed.

The urine is made acid by ammonium chloride by mouth, taken with food to avoid vomiting. It should not be given to patients with impaired renal or hepatic function. Other means include arginine HCl, ascorbic acid and $CaCl_2$ by mouth.

Drugs and the kidney

ADVERSE EFFECTS

The kidneys comprise only 0.5% of body weight, yet they receive 25% of the cardiac output. Thus, it is hardly surprising that drugs can *damage* the kidney and that disease of the kidney affects *responses* to drugs.

DRUG-INDUCED RENAL DISEASE

Drugs and other chemicals damage the kidney by:

1. **Direct biochemical effect**
Substances that cause direct toxicity include:

- Heavy metals, e.g. mercury, gold, iron, lead
- Antimicrobials, e.g. aminoglycosides, amphotericin, sulphonamides, cephalosporins
- X-ray contrast media, e.g. agents for visualising the biliary tract
- Analgesics, e.g. NSAID combinations
- Solvents, e.g. carbon tetrachloride, ethylene glycol.

2. **Indirect biochemical effect**

- Cytotoxic drugs and uricosurics may cause urate to be precipitated in the tubule.
- Calciferol may cause renal calcification by causing hypercalcaemia.
- Diuretic and laxative abuse can cause tubule

damage secondary to potassium and sodium depletion.

- Anticoagulants may cause haemorrhage into the kidney.

3. Immunological effect

A wide range of drugs produces a wide range of injuries.

- *Drugs* include: phenytoin, gold, penicillins, sulphonamides (especially the long-acting and extensively protein bound), hydralazine, isoniazid, rifampicin, procainamide, penicillamine, probenecid.
- *Injuries* include: arteritis, glomerulitis, interstitial nephritis, systemic lupus erythematosus.

A drug may cause damage by more than one of the above three mechanisms, e.g. sulphonamides.

The sites and pathological types of injury are as follows:

Glomerular damage. The large surface area of the glomerular capillaries renders them susceptible to damage from circulating immune complexes; glomerulonephritis, proteinuria and nephrotic syndrome may result, e.g. following treatment with penicillamine when the patient has made an immune response to the drug. The degree of renal impairment is best reflected in the *creatinine clearance* which measures the glomerular filtration rate because creatinine is eliminated entirely by this process.

Tubule damage. By concentrating 180 l of glomerular filtrate into 1.5 l of urine each day, renal tubule cells are exposed to much greater amounts of solutes and environmental toxins than are other cells in the body. The proximal tubule, through which most water is reabsorbed, experiences the greatest concentration and so suffers most drug-induced injury. Specialised transport processes concentrate acids, e.g. salicylate (aspirin), cephalosporins, and bases, e.g. aminoglycosides, in renal tubular cells. Heavy metals and radiographic contrast media also cause damage at this site. Proximal tubular toxicity is manifested by leakage of *glucose, phosphate, bicarbonate and aminoacids* into the urine.

The counter current multiplier and exchange systems of urine concentration (see p. 486) cause some drugs to accumulate in the renal medulla. Analgesic nephropathy is often first evident at this site partly because of high tissue concentration and partly, it is believed, because of ischaemia through inhibition of locally produced vasodilator prostaglandins by NSAIDs. The distal tubule is the site of lithium-induced nephrotoxicity; damage to the medulla and distal nephron is manifested by failure to *concentrate* the urine after fluid deprivation and by failure to *acidify* urine after ingestion of ammonium chloride.

Tubule obstruction. Given certain physicochemical conditions, crystals can deposit within the tubular lumen. Methotrexate is relatively insoluble at low pH and can precipitate in the distal nephron when the urine is acid.

Successful treatment of a leukaemia may be followed by the development of fatal urate nephropathy if breakdown of nucleic acids, released by destruction of leukaemic cells, delivers large amounts of insoluble urate to tubular fluid. This outcome can be prevented by starting the patient on allopurinol before the leukaemia is treated, for allopurinol inhibits xanthine oxidase, and the more soluble precursor, hypoxanthine, is excreted.

Other drug-induced lesions of the kidney include:

- Vasculitis, caused by sulphonamides, allopurinol, isoniazid
- Allergic interstitial nephritis, caused by penicillins (especially), sulphonamides, thiazides, allopurinol, phenytoin
- Systemic lupus erythematosus, caused by hydralazine, procainamide.

Drugs may thus induce any of the common clinical syndromes of renal injury, namely:

Acute renal failure, e.g. aminoglycosides, cisplatin

Nephrotic syndrome, e.g. penicillamine, gold, captopril (only at higher doses than now recommended)

Chronic renal failure, e.g. NSAIDs

Functional impairment, i.e. reduced ability to dilute and concentrate urine (lithium), potassium loss in urine (loop diuretics), acid base imbalance (acetazolamide).

PRESCRIBING FOR RENAL DISEASE

Drugs may:

- exacerbate renal disease
- be potentiated by accumulation due to failure of renal excretion
- be ineffective, e.g. thiazide diuretics in moderate or severe renal failure; uricosurics.

Problems of safety arise especially in patients with impaired renal function who must be treated with drugs that are potentially toxic and that are wholly or largely eliminated by the kidney.

A knowledge of, or at least access to, sources of pharmacokinetic data is essential for safe therapy for such patients.[3] The profound influence of impaired renal function on the elimination of some drugs is illustrated in Table 27.1.

The $t^{1/2}$ of other drugs, whose activity is terminated by metabolism, is unaltered by renal impairment. Many such drugs, however, produce *pharmacologically active metabolites* which tend to be more water-soluble than the parent drug, are dependent on the kidney for their elimination, and accumulate in renal failure, e.g. acebutolol, diazepam, warfarin.

The majority of drugs fall into an intermediate class and are partly metabolised and partly eliminated unchanged by the kidney.

Administering the correct dose to a patient with renal disease must therefore take into account both the extent to which the drug normally relies on renal elimination, and the degree of renal impairment; the most convenient and useful guide to the

Table 27.1 Drug t½ (h) with normal and with severely impaired renal function

	Normal	Severe renal impairment*
captopril	2	25
amoxycillin	2	14
gentamicin	2.5	5
atenolol	6	100
digoxin	36	90

* glomerular filtration rate < 5 ml/min (normal is 120 ml/min)
These are examples of drugs that are excreted almost unchanged; the prolongation of their t½ indicates that special care must be exercised if they are used in patients with impaired renal function.

latter is the *creatinine clearance*. These issues are now discussed.

DOSE ADJUSTMENT FOR PATIENTS WITH RENAL IMPAIRMENT

Adjustment of the *initial dose* (or where necessary the priming or loading dose, see p. 105) is generally unnecessary, for the volume into which the drug has to distribute should be the same in the uraemic as in the healthy subject.

Adjustment of the *maintenance dose* involves either reducing each dose given or lengthening the time between doses.

Special caution is needed when the patient is hypoproteinaemic and the drug is usually extensively plasma protein bound, or in advanced renal disease when accumulated metabolic products may compete for protein binding sites; particular care is required in the early stages of dosing until response to the drug can be gauged.

General rules

1. Drugs that are wholly or largely excreted by the kidney or drugs that produce active, renally-eliminated metabolites: give a normal or, if there is special cause for caution (above), a slightly reduced initial dose, and lower the maintenance dose or lengthen the dose interval in proportion to the reduction in creatinine clearance.

2. Drugs that are wholly or largely metabolised to inactive products: give normal doses. When the special note of caution (above) applies, a modest reduction of initial dose and the maintenance dose rate are justified while drug effects are assessed.

3. Drugs that are partly eliminated by the kidney and partly metabolised: give a normal initial dose and modify the maintenance dose or dose interval in the light of what is known about the patient's renal function and the drug, its dependence on renal elimination and its inherent toxicity.

Recall that the *time to reach steady-state blood concen-*

---

[3] e.g. manufacturers' data, formularies and other books and specialist journals.

tration (p. 85) is dependent only on drug $t\frac{1}{2}$ and a drug reaches 97% of its ultimate steady-state concentration in $5 \times t\frac{1}{2}$. Thus if $t\frac{1}{2}$ is prolonged by renal impairment, so also will be the time to reach steady state.

Schemes for modifying drug dosage for patients with renal disease do not altogether remove their increased risk of adverse effects; such patients should be observed particularly carefully throughout a course of drug therapy. Ideally, dosing should be monitored by drug plasma concentration measurements, but this service is not available to most of the world population.

Nephrolithiasis

Calcareous stones result from hypercalciuria, hyperoxaluria and hypocitraturia. Hypercalciuria and hyperoxaluria render urine supersaturated in respect of calcium salts; citrate makes calcium oxalate more soluble and inhibits its precipitation from solution.

Noncalcareous stones occur most commonly in the presence of urea-splitting organisms which create conditions in which magnesium ammonium phosphate (struvite) stones form. Urate stones form when urine is unusually acid (pH <5.5).

Management. Recurrent stone-formers should maintain a urine output exceeding 2.5 l/d. Some benefit from restricting dietary calcium or reducing the intake of oxalate-rich foods (rhubarb, spinach, tea, chocolate, peanuts).

- Thiazide diuretics reduce the excretion of calcium and oxalate in the urine and reduce the rate of stone formation.
- Sodium cellulose phosphate (Calcisorb) binds calcium in the gut, reduces urinary calcium excretion and may benefit calcium stoneformers.
- Allopurinol is effective in those who have high excretion of uric acid in the urine.
- Potassium citrate, which alkalinises the urine, should be given to prevent formation of pure uric acid stones.

Pharmacological aspects of micturition

SOME PHYSIOLOGY

The *detrusor*, whose smooth muscle fibres comprise the body of the bladder, is innervated mainly by parasympathetic nerves which are excitatory and cause the muscle to contract. The *internal sphincter*, a concentration of smooth muscle at the bladder neck, is well developed only in the male and its principal function is to prevent retrograde flow of semen during ejaculation. It is rich in α_1-adrenoceptors, activation of which causes contraction. There is an abundant supply of oestrogen receptors in the distal two-thirds of the female urethral epithelium which degenerates after the menopause causing loss of urinary control.

When the detrusor relaxes and the sphincters close, urine is stored; this is achieved by central inhibition of parasympathetic tone accompanied by a reflex increase in α-adrenergic activity. Voiding requires contraction of the detrusor, accompanied by relaxation of the sphincters. These acts are coordinated by a micturition centre probably in the pons.

FUNCTIONAL ABNORMALITIES

The main abnormalities that require treatment are:

- *Unstable bladder* or detrusor instability, characterised by uninhibited, unstable contractions of the detrusor which may be of unknown aetiology or secondary to an upper motor neuron lesion or bladder neck obstruction.
- *Decreased bladder activity* or hypotonicity due to a lower motor neuron lesion or overdistension of the bladder or to both.
- *Urethral sphincter dysfunction* which is due to various causes including weakness of the muscles and ligaments around the bladder neck, descent of the urethrovesical junction and periurethral fibrosis; the result is stress incontinence.
- *Atrophic change* affects the distal urethra in females.

Drugs may be used to alleviate abnormal micturition.

Antimuscarinics block the parasympathetic supply to the bladder and are effective for incontinence due to detrusor instability. Oxybutynin or propantheline give considerable benefit to some sufferers but often at the cost of the adverse effects that accompany muscarinic blockade.

Tricyclic antidepressants. Imipramine, amitriptyline and nortriptyline are effective, especially for nocturnal but also for daytime incontinence. Their parasympathetic blocking (antimuscarinic) action is probably in part responsible but imipramine may also benefit by altering the patient's sleep profile.

Smooth muscle relaxants may benefit urinary frequency and incontinence, e.g. flavoxate which has a papaverine-like action.

Oestrogens either applied locally to the vagina or taken by mouth may benefit urinary incontinence due to atrophy of the urethral epithelium in menopausal women.

Parasympathomimetic drugs, e.g. bethanechol, carbachol and distigmine, may be used to stimulate the detrusor when the bladder is hypotonic, e.g. due to an upper motor neuron lesion. Distigmine is preferred but, as its effect is not sustained, intermittent catheterisation is also needed when the hypotonia is chronic.

BENIGN PROSTATIC HYPERPLASIA (BPH)

One of the commonest problems in men older than 50, BPH was for a long time helped only by surgical interventions, which themselves were an outstanding example of the different (usually absent) rules that apply in the assessment of surgical compared to pharmacological treatments. Many are the men who would have opted for continuing micturition frequency in preference to the impotence, incontinence or pulmonary emboli that awaited them after transurethral resection; few are the drugs which would survive such complications, whatever the

benefits. Now there is a limited choice between medical and surgical approaches, although these have never been formally compared, and the drugs are not a substitute for surgery if urinary retention has occurred. The prostate is a mixture of capsular and stromal tissue, rich in α_1-adrenoceptors, and glandular tissue under the influence of androgens. Both these, the α-receptors and androgens, are targets for drug therapy. Because the bladder itself has few α-receptors, it is possible to use selective α_1-blockade without affecting bladder contraction.

Alpha-adrenoceptor antagonists. Prazosin, afluzosin, indoramin, terazosin and doxazosin are α-adrenoceptor blockers, with selectivity for the α_1-subtype. They cause significant increases (compared to placebo) in objective measures such as maximal urine flow rate, and drugs also improve semi-objective symptoms scores. In normotensive men, they cause generally negligible falls in blood pressure; in hypertensive patients, the fall in pressure can be regarded as an added bonus (provided concurrent treatment is adjusted accordingly). These drugs can cause dizziness and asthenia even in the absence of marked changes in blood pressure.

Finasteride. An alternative drug for prostatic symptoms is the type II 5α-reductase inhibitor, finasteride (Proscar), which inhibits conversion of testosterone to its more potent metabolite, dihydrotestosterone. It reduces prostatic volume by ~20% and increases urinary flow rates by a similar degree. These changes translate into only modest clinical benefits. Finasteride has a $t^1/2$ of 6 h, and is taken as a single 5 mg tablet orally each day. The clinical benefit appears over 6 months (as the prostate shrinks in size) and in 5–10% of patients may be at the cost of some loss of libido. The serum concentration of prostate-specific antigen is approximately halved. While this may reflect a real reduction in risk of prostatic cancer, it is safer to regard as abnormal concentrations of the antigen in the upper half of the usual range, in patients receiving finasteride. Other anti-androgens, such as the gonadorelin agonists, are used in the treatment of prostatic cancer, but the need for parenteral administration makes them less suitable for BPH.

SUMMARY

- The actions of drugs on the kidney are of an importance disproportionate to the low prevalence of kidney disorders.
- The kidney is the main site of loss, or potential loss, of all body substances. It is among the functions of drugs to help reduce losses of desirable substances and increase losses of undesired substances.
- The kidney is also at increased risk of toxicity from foreign substances because of the high concentrations these can achieve in the renal medulla.
- Diuretics are among the most commonly used drugs, perhaps because the evolutionary advantages of sodium retention have left an ageing population without salt-losing mechanisms of matching efficiency.
- Loop diuretics, acting on the ascending loop of Henle, are the most effective, and are used mainly to treat the oedema states. K^+ is lost as well as Na^+.
- Thiazides, acting on the early distal tubule, have lower natriuretic efficacy, but slightly greater antihypertensive efficacy than loop diuretics. K^+ loss is rarely a problem with thiazides, and thiazides reduce loss of Ca^{++}.
- K^+ retention with even hyperkalaemia can occur with the third group of K^+-sparing diuretics, which block Na^+ transport in the last part of the distal tubule, either directly (e.g. amiloride) or by blocking aldosterone receptors (spironolactone).
- Drugs have little ability to alter the filtering function of the kidney, when this is reduced by nephron loss. The filtration of many substances, especially drugs, is reduced according to their extent of protein-binding.
- The main disease of the lower urinary tract requiring drugs to postpone, or avoid, surgery is prostatic enlargement. The symptoms of benign prostatic hyperplasia are partially relieved either by α_1- adrenoceptor blockade or by inhibiting synthesis of dihydrotestosterone in the prostate.

GUIDE TO FURTHER READING

Editorial 1987 Acetazolamide in acute mountain sickness. British Medical Journal 295: 1161

Johnson T S, Rock P B 1988 Acute mountain sickness. New England Journal of Medicine 319: 841

LaCroix A Z et al 1990 Thiazide diuretic agents and the incidence of hip fractures. New England Journal of Medicine 322: 286

Lepon H, Williford W O, Barry M J et al 1996 The efficacy of terazosin, finasteride, or both in benign prostatic hyperplasia. New England Journal of Medicine 335: 533–539

Mason P D, Pusey C D 1994 Glomerulonephritis: diagnosis and treatment. British Medical Journal 309: 1557–1563

Oesterling J E 1995 Benign prostatic hyperplasia. New England Journal of Medicine 332: 99–107

Orme M L E (editorial) 1990 Thiazides in the 1990s. The risk:benefit ratio still favours the drug. British Medical Journal 300: 1668

Resnick N M, Subbaro V Y 1985 Management of urinary incontinence in the elderly. New England Journal of Medicine 313: 800

Rittmaster R S 1994 Drug therapy: finasteride. New England Journal of Medicine 330: 120–125

Robertson G L (editorial) 1989 Syndrome of inappropriate antidiuresis. New England Journal of Medicine 321: 538

Wickham J E 1993 Treatment of urinary tract stones. British Medical Journal 307: 1414–1417

Respiratory system

- Cough: modes of action and uses of antitussives
- Respiratory stimulants: their place in therapy
- Pulmonary surfactant
- Oxygen therapy: its uses and dangers
- Histamine, antihistamines and allergies
- Bronchial asthma: types, modes of prevention, agents used for treatment and their use in asthma of varying degrees of severity
- Infections, see Ch. 13

Cough

There are two sorts of cough: the useful and the useless. Cough is useful when it effectively expels secretions, exudates, transudates or extraneous material from respiratory tracts, i.e. when it is *productive*; it is useless when it is *unproductive*. Useful cough should be allowed to serve its purpose and suppressed only when it is exhausting the patient or is dangerous, e.g. after eye surgery. Useless cough should be stopped, or, if it is due to thick secretions that cannot be expelled, made useful if possible.

Clinical assessment of the frequency and intensity of cough of disease by objective recording via a microphone, allows assessment of antitussives despite the great spontaneous fluctuations. Such recording has shown patients' own reports of their cough to be too unreliable to provide valid drug comparisons. Placebo effects in cough are great.

SITES OF ACTION FOR TREATMENT

Peripheral sites

On *the afferent side* of the cough reflex: by reducing input of stimuli from throat, larynx, trachea, e.g. a warm moist atmosphere, demulcents[1] in the pharynx.

On the *efferent side* of the cough reflex: measures to render secretions more easily removable (mucolytics, postural drainage) will reduce the amount of coughing needed, by increasing its efficiency.

The *best antitussive* is removal of the cause of the cough by, e.g. chemotherapy or surgery. In patients with hypertension or cardiac failure, a common cause of a dry cough is treatment by an ACE inhibitor.

Central nervous system

Agents may act on

- the medullary paths of the cough reflex (opioids)
- the cerebral cortex

---

[1]Latin: *demulcere*, to caress soothingly.

- the subcortical paths (opioids and sedatives in general).

Cough is also under substantial voluntary control, as witness the increase during the louder passages of a winter orchestral concert. A good spouse with a cough may sleep better alone and free from fear of depriving an exhausted companion of sleep, whilst a child may cough less if in reassuring company in the parents' room. A cough can be induced by psychogenic factors (such as anxiety not to cough when it is socially disadvantageous to do so, e.g. during the quiet parts of a musical concert) and reduced by a placebo. Considerations such as these are relevant to practical therapeutics.

COUGH SUPPRESSION

Antitussives that act peripherally

The patient should stop smoking.

When the cough arises *above the larynx*, syrups and lozenges that glutinously and soothingly coat the pharynx (*demulcents*) may be used, e.g. Simple linctus (mainly syrup; sugar). Small children are prone to swallow lozenges and so a confection on a stick may be preferred.

Linctuses are demulcent preparations that can be used alone and as vehicles of other antitussives. That their exact constitution is not critical was known and taught to medical students in 1896.

> Many of you know that this (simple) linctus used to be very much thicker than it is now, and very likely the thicker linctus was more efficacious. The reason why it was made thinner was this. It was discovered that a large number of children came to the surgery complaining of cough, and they were given the linctus, but instead of their using it as a medicine, they took it to an old woman out in Smithfield, who gave them each a penny, took their linctus, and made jam tarts with it.[2]

When cough arises *below the larynx* water aerosol inhalations and a warm environment often give relief. If it is wished to make the inhalation smell therapeutic (aromatic inhalation), compound benzoin tincture[3] may be added to the hot water. Benzoin inhalation may also promote secretion of dilute mucus and so help to give a protective coating to the inflamed mucous membrane. Menthol and eucalyptus provide similar therapeutic smell.

Intractable cough can be a severe problem in patients with bronchial carcinoma. Lignocaine administered by a nebuliser appears to control it effectively and may delay the need to use sedative opioids such as diamorphine.

Antitussives that act on the CNS

In general, when it is desired to suppress cough, drugs that act on the pathways of the cough reflex in the medulla are used. Where these drugs are opioids then part of the effect may result from their actions on higher nervous centres as tranquillisers. The morphine-related antitussives are relatively nonaddicting and have little depressant effect on the respiratory centre, though they may dry the mucosa and thicken the sputum. They include codeine and pholcodine.

It appears that as good results can be obtained with these as with more addicting opioids, e.g. morphine, diamorphine and methadone which are powerful respiratory depressants. Linctuses of codeine, pholcodine and methadone are often used. Codeine needs to be given in high dose, say 60 mg, and a tablet is equally satisfactory. In bronchogenic carcinoma a strong pholcodeine linctus or even diamorphine linctus may be required to control cough. Dextromethorphan does not possess the CNS pharmacology of the opioids (though structurally related) and binds with high affinity and selectivity to medullary sites; it is widely used in over-the-counter antitussive preparations; overdose is antagonised by naloxone.

Sedation reduces cough. Antihistamines (H_1-receptor) having also sedative and antimuscarinic actions, e.g. diphenhydramine, can suppress cough by these (but not by antihistamine) actions; they may need to be given in doses which also cause drowsiness and thus they are usually combined with other drugs.

---

[2]Brunton L 1897 Lectures on the action of medicines. Macmillan, London.

[3]Friar's Balsam.

MUCOLYTICS AND EXPECTORANTS

Normally about 100 ml of fluid is produced from the respiratory tract each day and most of it is swallowed. Respiratory mucus consists largely of water and its slimy character is due to glycoproteins linked together by disulphide bonds to form polymers. In pathological states much more mucus may be produced; an exudate of plasma proteins which bond with glycoproteins and form larger polymers results in the mucus becoming more viscous. Patients with chest disease can have difficulty in clearing their chest of viscous sputum by cough because the bronchial cilia are rendered ineffective. They can be assisted by drugs that liquefy mucus.

Mucolytics

Acetylcysteine, carbocisteine and methyl cysteine have free sulphydryl groups that open disulphide bonds in mucus and reduce its viscosity. They are given by inhalation (or instillation) and may be useful chiefly where particularly viscous secretion is a problem (cystic fibrosis, care of tracheostomies). Acetylcysteine may also be taken by mouth (swallowed) and achieves high concentration in the lung. Mucolytics may cause gastrointestinal irritation and allergic reaction.

Iodide stimulates the production of thin bronchial secretion by a direct action on secretory cells. It must generally be given to the limits of tolerance and so is not popular. Iodide has an unpleasant metallic taste and may cause painful swelling of the salivary and lachrymal glands after a few doses. With longterm treatment gastric intolerance or hypothyroidism may occur but these are largely avoided if treatment is intermittent. *Water inhalation* as an aerosol (breathing over a hot basin), though cheap, is not to be despised. Simply hydrating a dehydrated patient can have a beneficial effect in lowering sputum viscosity.

Dornase alfa is a deoxyribonuclease which can be inhaled. It is of modest value only in patients with cystic fibrosis, whose genetic defect in chloride transport causes particularly viscous sputum. The blocked airways, as well as the sputum itself, are a trap for pathogens.

CHOICE OF DRUG THERAPY FOR COUGH

As always, it is necessary to have a clear idea of the underlying problem before starting to use drugs. For example, the approach to cough due to invasion of a bronchus by a neoplasm differs from that due to post-nasal drip from chronic sinusitis or to that due to chronic bronchitis. The following are general recommendations.

● **Simple suppression of useless cough.**
Codeine, pholcodine, dextromethorphan and methadone linctuses may be used in large, infrequent doses. In children, cough is nearly always useful and sedation at night is more effective to give rest than is codeine. A sedative antihistamine is convenient (e.g. promethazine), although sputum thickening may be a disadvantage. In pertussis infection (whooping cough), codeine and atropine methonitrate may be tried.

● **To increase bronchial secretion slightly and to liquefy what is there.** Water aerosol with or without menthol and benzoin inhalation, or menthol and eucalyptus inhalation may provide comfort harmlessly.
Acetylcysteine or another mucolytic orally may be useful.
Preparations containing any drug having antimuscarinic action are undesirable as muscarinic receptor blockade thickens bronchial secretion. Oxygen inhalation dries secretions, so rendering them even more viscous; oxygen must be bubbled through water and patients having oxygen may need measures to liquefy sputum.

● **Cough originating in the pharyngeal region.**
Glutinous sweets or lozenges (demulcents), incorporating a cough suppressant or not, as appropriate, are used.

Expectorants

These are held to encourage productive cough by increasing the volume of bronchial secretion but may have no more than placebo value. The group includes iodide, chlorides, bicarbonates, acetates, squill, guaiphenesin, ipecacuanha, creosotes and volatile oils.

Cough mixtures

Every formulary is replete with combinations of antitussives, expectorants, mucolytics, bronchodilators and sedatives. Although choice is not critical, a knowledge of the active ingredients is useful, for some contain sedative antimuscarinic antihistamines or ephedrine (which may antagonise antihypertensives).

Respiratory stimulants

(Analeptics)

The drugs used are central nervous system stimulants and the therapeutic dose is close to that which causes convulsions. Their use must therefore be carefully monitored.

Nikethamide is obsolescent. It causes an increase in the rate and depth of respiration by stimulating the medullary respiratory centres both directly and reflexly through the carotid body. It is less safe than doxapram.

Doxapram acts like nikethamide but has a larger margin between therapeutic and toxic doses. A continuous i.v. infusion of 1.5–4.0 mg/min is given according to the patient's response. Coughing and laryngospasm that develop after its use may represent a return of normal protective responses. The adverse effects include restlessness, twitching, itching, vomiting, flushing and cardiac dysrhythmias, and in addition it causes patients to experience a feeling of perineal warmth; in high doses the blood pressure is elevated.

Ethamivan is similar to nikethamide.

Aminophylline is a respiratory stimulant and may be infused slowly i.v. (500 mg in 6 h).

Acetazolamide (see also p. 493) promotes bicarbonate diuresis and metabolic acidosis which may be a useful stimulus to respiration during exacerbations of chronic obstructive lung disease or weaning from mechanical ventilation.

USES

Respiratory stimulants have a place in some cases of acute ventilatory failure due to:

- Acute exacerbations of chronic lung disease with hypercapnia, drowsiness and inability to cough or to tolerate low (24%) concentrations of inspired oxygen (air is 21% O_2). A respiratory stimulant can arouse the patient enough to allow effective physiotherapy and, by stimulating respiration, can improve ventilation–perfusion matching. As a short-term measure, this may obviate tracheal intubation and mechanical ventilation and 'buy time' for chemotherapy to control infection.
- Apnoea in premature infants; aminophylline and caffeine may benefit some cases.

Avoid respiratory stimulants if possible in patients with epilepsy (risk of convulsions).

Contraindications include ischaemic heart disease, status asthmaticus, severe hypertension and thyrotoxicosis.

Irritant vapours, to be inhaled, have an analeptic effect in fainting, especially if it is psychogenic, e.g. aromatic solution of ammonia (Sal Volatile). No doubt they sometimes 'recall the exorbitant and deserting spirits to their proper stations'.[4]

Pulmonary surfactant

The endogenous surfactant system produces stable low surface tension in the alveoli, preventing their collapse. Failure of production of natural surfactant occurs in respiratory distress syndrome (RDS), including that in the neonate. A number of synthetic phospholipids is now available for instillation down the intratracheal tube to act as surfactants: e.g. ALEC (named after the inventor of liposomes, or synthetic membrane vesicles, Dr Alec Banham), colfosceril palmitate, poractant alfa, beractant, pumactant. These need to be stored chilled, and the manufacturer's instructions followed carefully since on reaching body temperature their physicochemical properties rapidly change. Their function is to coat the surface of the alveoli and maintain their patency, and their administration to premature neonates with RDS is now an important and successful part of reducing mortality.

---

[4]Thomas Sydenham, 1624–89.

Oxygen therapy

Oxygen used in therapy should be prescribed with the same care as any drug; there should be a well defined purpose and its effects should be monitored objectively.

The absolute indication to supplement inspired air is inadequate tissue oxygenation. As clinical signs may be imprecise, arterial blood gases should be measured whenever suspicion arises. Tissue hypoxia can be assumed when the PaO_2 falls below 6.7 kPa (50 mmHg) in a previously normal acutely ill patient, e.g. with myocardial infarction, acute pulmonary disorder, drug overdose, musculoskeletal or head trauma. Chronically hypoxic patients may maintain adequate tissue with a PaO_2 below 6.7 kPa by compensating through raised red cell mass. Oxygen therapy is used as follows:

High concentration oxygen therapy is reserved for where a low PaO_2 is associated with a normal or low $PaCO_2$, as in: pulmonary embolism, pneumonia, pulmonary oedema, myocardial infarction, and young patients with status asthmaticus. Concentrations of O_2 up to 60% may be used for short periods, for there is little risk of inducing hypoventilation and CO_2 retention.

Low concentration oxygen therapy is reserved for patients with low PaO_2 and raised $PaCO_2$, notably those with chronic obstructive lung disease during an infective exacerbation. The normal stimulus to respiration is elevation of the $PaCO_2$ but this control is blunted in chronically hypercapnic patients whose respiratory drive comes from hypoxia. Elevating the PaO_2 in such patients by giving them high concentrations of oxygen removes their stimulus to ventilate, exaggerates CO_2 retention and may cause fatal respiratory acidosis. The objective of therapy in such patients is to provide just enough oxygen to alleviate hypoxia without exaggerating the hypercapnia and respiratory acidosis; normally the inspired oxygen concentration should not exceed 28% and in some 24% may be sufficient.

Continuous longterm domiciliary oxygen therapy is given to patients with severe persistent hypoxaemia and cor pulmonale due to chronic bronchitis and emphysema. Either oxygen cylinders are delivered to the patients' homes or they are provided with an oxygen concentrator. Clinical trial evidence indicates that taking oxygen for more than 15 h per day improves survival.

Histamine, antihistamines and allergies

Histamine is a naturally-occurring amine that has long fascinated pharmacologists and physicians. It is found in most body tissue in an inactive bound form, often in mast cells, and pharmacologically active free histamine is released from cells in response to stimuli such as physical trauma or antigen–antibody reactions. Various chemicals can also cause release of histamine. The more powerful of these (proteolytic enzymes and snake venoms) have no place in therapeutics, but a number of useful drugs, such as tubocurarine, morphine and even some antihistamines, cause histamine release, although not usually enough to do more than transiently lower blood pressure or cause a local reaction; but significant bronchospasm may occur in asthmatics.

The physiological functions of histamine are suggested by its distribution in the body.

- In body epithelia (the alimentary canal, the respiratory tract and in the skin) it is released in response to invasion by foreign substances.
- In glands (gastric, intestinal, lachrymal, salivary) it mediates part of the normal secretory process.
- In most cells near blood vessels it plays a role in regulating the microcirculation.

Histamine acts as a local hormone (autacoid) similarly to serotonin or prostaglandins, i.e. it is a local chemical transmitter between the cell from which it is released and cells in the immediate vicinity. In the context of gastric secretion, for example, stimulation of receptors on the histamine-containing cell causes release of histamine which in turn acts on receptors on parietal cells which then secrete hydrogen ions (see Gastric secretion, Ch. 32). The clinical (diagnostic) uses of histamine, in equivocal cases of phaeochromocytoma or to stimulate gastric acid secretion, have been superseded by more accurate and better tolerated procedures.

Actions. The actions of histamine which are clinically important are those on:

Smooth muscle. In general, histamine causes smooth muscle to contract (excepting arterioles, but including the larger arteries). Stimulation of the pregnant human uterus is insignificant. A brisk attack of bronchospasm may be induced in subjects who have any allergy, particularly asthma, when it may occur even in the presence of an antihistamine.

Arterioles are dilated, with a consequent fall in blood pressure. The characteristic throbbing headache that occurs after histamine injections is due to stretching pain-sensitive structures in the dura mater by fluctuations in pressure in blood vessels and cerebrospinal fluid.

Capillaries dilate and their permeability to plasma increases, which responses comprise two parts (the flush and the wheal) of the triple response described by Thomas Lewis.[5] The third part, the flare, is arteriolar dilatation due to an axon reflex.

Skin. Histamine release in the skin can cause itch.

Gastric secretion. Histamine increases the acid and pepsin content of gastric juices.

As may be anticipated from the above actions, anaphylactic shock, which is largely due to histamine release, is characterised by circulatory collapse and bronchoconstriction. The most rapidly effective antidote is adrenaline (epinephrine) (see below), and an antihistamine (H_1-receptor) may be given as well.

Metabolism. Histamine is formed from the amino acid histidine and is inactivated by metabolism, largely by deamination and by methylation. In common with other local hormones, this process is extremely rapid.

HISTAMINE H_1- AND H_2-RECEPTOR ANTAGONISTS

The effects of histamine can be *opposed* in three ways:

● By using a drug with opposite effects, e.g.

histamine constricts bronchi, causes vasodilatation and increases capillary permeability. Adrenaline opposes these effects by a mechanism unrelated to histamine. This is *physiological antagonism.*

● By preventing histamine from reaching its site of action (receptors), e.g. *by competition*, the H_1- and H_2-receptor antagonists.

● By preventing the release of histamine from cells in which it is stored; adrenal steroids and sodium cromoglycate can suppress the effects on cells of antigen–antibody reactions.

Drugs that competitively block H_1-histamine receptors were the first to be introduced and are conventionally called the 'antihistamines'. They effectively inhibit the increased capillary permeability, flare and itch skin responses of histamine; they also partially prevent the vascular smooth muscle (blood pressure lowering) action but they have *no effect* on histamine-induced gastric secretion. Indeed, the standard method of testing a patient's capacity to secrete gastric acid used to be to inject histamine after first giving a large dose of a conventional (H_1-receptor) antihistamine to block the other (undesired) effects of the injection. Thus, if a group of drugs could block some actions of histamine but not others, it was reasoned that there must be more than one kind of histamine receptor. This was the basis for the search for drugs that block histamine-induced gastric secretion (see Ch. 32) and its success established that there are at least two types of *histamine receptor*:

● H_1-receptor: mediates the oedema and vascular effects of histamine (see above)

● H_2-receptor: mediates the effect on gastric secretion.

Thus, histamine antagonists are classified as:

● Histamine H_1-receptor antagonists (see account below)

● Histamine H_2-receptor antagonists: cimetidine, famotidine, nizatidine, ranitidine (see Ch. 32).

HISTAMINE H_1-RECEPTOR ANTAGONISTS

The term antihistamine is unsatisfactory, for the drugs have numerous other actions. This partly

---

[5]Lewis T et al 1924 Heart 11: 209.

derives from the fact that there is a considerable similarity of structure amongst such local hormones as histamine, adrenaline, serotonin and acetylcholine. A compound which may block the action of one substance may also be capable of blocking the action of another. Thus, the H_1-antihistamines may also have antimuscarinic, sedative or sometimes α-adrenoceptor antagonist effects, and antimuscarinic drugs may exhibit some antihistaminic actions. Thus H_1-antihistamines are used as hypnotics, antitussives, expectorants, in motion sickness and in parkinsonism, all actions which are not evidently related to antihistaminic effect. These features are a disadvantage when H_1-antihistamines are used specifically to antagonise the effects of histamine, e.g. for allergies, but the introduction of drugs that are more selective H_1-antagonists and are largely free of antimuscarinic and sedative effects (see below) has been a useful advance. They can be discussed together.

Actions. H_1-receptor antihistamines oppose, to varying degrees, the effects of liberated histamine, i.e. the oedema-producing and vascular effects. They are of negligible use in asthma, in which numerous mediators other than histamine are involved. Conventional H_1-antihistamines are competitive, surmountable inhibitors of the action of histamine except for astemizole (at therapeutic doses) and terfenadine (at very high doses) which dissociate very slowly from the receptor and exhibit insurmountable antagonism (see p. 80). H_1-antihistamines are more effective if used *before* histamine has been liberated. Reversal of effects of histamine after it has been released is more readily achieved by *physiological* antagonism by adrenaline which should be used first in life-threatening allergic reactions.

The older H_1-antihistamines cause drowsiness and there is need to warn patients, e.g. about driving or operating machinery, and about additive effects with alcohol. Paradoxically, CNS stimulation may occur and absence epilepsy (petit mal) made worse. The newer H_1-antihistamines which penetrate the blood–brain barrier poorly are largely devoid of these effects. Antimuscarinic effects benefit parkinsonism and motion sickness.

Pharmacokinetics. H_1-antihistamines taken orally are readily absorbed. They are mainly metabolised in the liver. Enough may be excreted in the milk to cause sedation in infants. They are generally administered orally and can also be given i.m. or i.v.

Uses. The H_1-antihistamines are used for symptomatic relief of allergies such as hay fever and urticaria (see below). They are of broadly similar therapeutic efficacy.

INDIVIDUAL H_1-RECEPTOR ANTIHISTAMINES

Non- (or less) sedative

These newer drugs are relatively selective for H_1-receptors and enter the brain less readily than do the earlier antihistamines. Differences lie principally in their duration of action.

Cetirizine ($t^1/_2$ 7 h), *loratadine* ($t^1/_2$ 15 h) and *terfenadine* ($t^1/_2$ 20 h) are effective taken once daily and are suitable for general use. The choice may lie between cetirizine which is possibly more effective but may sedate some patients, and terfenadine which may be less effective.

Acrivastine ($t^1/_2$ 2 h) must be given × 3/d and is best reserved for intermittent therapy, e.g. when breakthrough symptoms occur in a patient using topical therapy for hay fever.

Astemizole has a slow onset of effect. Because of its long $t^1/_2$ (5 days; 10 days for an active metabolite) it takes a longer time to reach steady state, and dose titration is more difficult than with short $t^1/_2$ drugs.

Sedative

Mequitazine is less sedative than most members of this group.

Chlorpheniramine ($t^1/_2$ 20h) is effective when urticaria is prominent, and its sedative effect is then useful.

Diphenhydramine ($t^1/_2$ 32 h) is strongly sedative and has antimuscarinic effects; it is also used in parkinsonism and motion sickness.

Promethazine ($t^1/_2$ 12 h) is so strongly sedative that it is used as an hypnotic in adults and children. It may sedate the next day.

Azatadine, brompheniramine, buclizine, clemastine, cyproheptadine, dimethindene, diphenhydramine, diphenylpyraline, hydroxyzine, mebhydrolin, oxatomide, phenindamine, pheniramine, trimeprazine and *triprolidine* are similar.

Adverse effects. Apart from sedation, these include: dizziness, fatigue, insomnia, nervousness, tremors, and antimuscarinic effects, e.g. dry mouth, blurred vision and gastrointestinal disturbance. Dermatitis and agranulocytosis can occur. Severe poisoning due to overdose results in coma and sometimes in convulsions.

DRUG MANAGEMENT OF SOME ALLERGIC STATES

Histamine is released in many allergic states, but it is not the sole cause of symptoms, other chemical mediators, e.g., leukotrienes and prostaglandins, also being involved. Hence the usefulness of H_1-receptor antihistamines in allergic states is variable, depending on the extent to which histamine, rather than other mediators, is the cause of the clinical manifestations.

Hay fever. If symptoms are limited to rhinitis, a *corticosteroid* (beclomethasone, betamethasone, budesonide or flunisolide), *ipratropium* or *sodium cromoglycate* applied topically as a spray or insufflation is often all that is required. Ocular symptoms alone respond well to sodium cromoglycate drops. When both nasal and ocular symptoms occur, or there is itching of the palate and ears as well, a systemic nonsedative H_1-antihistamine is indicated. *Sympathomimetic vasoconstrictors*, e.g. ephedrine, are immediately effective if applied topically, but rebound swelling of the nasal mucous membrane occurs when medication is stopped. Rarely, a *systemic corticosteroid*, e.g. prednisolone, is justified for a severely affected patient to provide relief for a short period, e.g. during academic examinations.

Urticaria, see page 281.
Anaphylactic shock, see page 127.

Bronchial asthma

Asthma affects 2–5% of the UK population; this incidence is increasing.

SOME USEFUL PATHOPHYSIOLOGY

The bronchi become hyperreactive as a result of a persistent inflammatory process in response to a number of stimuli which include biological agents, e.g. allergens, viruses and environmental chemicals, e.g. ozone. Inflammatory mediators are liberated from mast cells, eosinophils, neutrophils, monocytes and macrophages. Some mediators such as histamine are preformed and their release causes an immediate bronchial reaction. Others are formed after activation of cells and produce more sustained bronchoconstriction; these include metabolites of arachidonic acid from both the cyclo-oxygenase, e.g. prostaglandin D_2, and lipoxygenase, i.e. leukotrienes, pathways. In addition platelet activating factor (PAF) is being increasingly recognised as an important mediator.

The relative importance of many of the mediators is not precisely defined but they interact to produce mucosal oedema, secretion of mucus which is hard to dislodge and damage to the ciliated epithelium. Breaching of the protective epithelial barrier allows hyperreactivity to be maintained by bronchoconstrictor substances or by local axon reflexes through exposed nerve fibres. Wheezing and breathlessness result. The bronchial changes also obstruct access of inhaled drug to the periphery, which is why they can fail to give full relief.

Asthma, like many of the common chronic disorders (hypertension, diabetes mellitus), is a polygenic disorder and already genetic loci for either increased production of IgE or bronchial hyperreactivity have been found in some families with an increased incidence of asthma.

Early in an attack there is hyperventilation so that PaO_2 is maintained and $PaCO_2$ is lowered but with increasing airways obstruction the PaO_2 declines and $PaCO_2$ rises, signifying a serious asthmatic episode.

The mechanisms underlying late-onset and exercise-induced asthma are poorly understood.

TYPES OF ASTHMA

The following are recognised:

Asthma associated with specific allergic reactions

This *extrinsic* type is the commonest and occurs in

patients who develop allergy to antigenic substances in the inspired air. In some (atopic) individuals, who have a special liability to develop allergy, the resulting reaction is of the immediate (type 1) type involving IgE antibodies; in other (nonatopic) people the reaction is delayed for some hours (type 3) and is associated with the production of precipitating antibodies. Avoidance of exposure to allergens is particularly relevant to managing this type of asthma.

Asthma not associated with known allergy

Some patients exhibit wheeze and breathlessness that is not attributable to any allergic reaction. They are considered to have *intrinsic* asthma and it follows that attempting to avoid an allergen has no place.

Exercise-induced asthma

Some patients develop wheeze that regularly follows within a few minutes of exercise; they should take a β-adrenoceptor agonist or sodium cromoglycate (see below) prior to the activity.

Asthma associated with chronic obstructive lung disease

A number of patients who have persistent airflow obstruction also exhibit considerable variation in airways resistance and are benefited by drugs used for asthma. It is important to recognise the association and to test their responses to bronchodilators or corticosteroids.

APPROACHES TO TREATMENT

With the foregoing discussion in mind, the following approaches to treatment are logical:

- Prevention of exposure to antigen(s)
- Reduction of the bronchial inflammation and hyperreactivity
- Dilatation of narrowed bronchi.

These objectives may be achieved as follows:

Prevention of exposure to antigen(s)

This approach is appropriate for extrinsic asthmatics. Identifying an antigen may be aided by the patient's history (wheezing in response to contact with grasses, pollens, animals), by skin prick or by intradermal injection of selected antigens or by demonstrating antibodies in the patient's serum. Avoiding an allergen may be practicable when it is related to some special situation, e.g. occupation, but is not feasible if it is widespread, as with house-dust mite. Hyposensitisation is an option for insect venoms and grass pollens but should be undertaken only where facilities for cardiopulmonary resuscitation are immediately available.

Reduction of the bronchial inflammation and hyperreactivity

As persistent inflammation is central to bronchial hyperreactivity, the use of anti-inflammatory drugs is sensible.

Corticosteroids bring about a gradual reduction in bronchial hyperreactivity. The exact mechanisms of this action are disputed but they probably include: inhibition of the influx of inflammatory cells into the lung that follows exposure to an allergen; inhibition of the release of mediators from macrophages and eosinophils and reduction of the microvascular leakage which these mediators cause. Some of the actions of corticosteroids may be mediated by their induction of the formation of lipocortin, a protein which inhibits phospholipase-A, the enzyme that is responsible for generating arachidonic acid and which in turn gives rise to prostaglandins, leukotrienes and platelet activating factor. Corticosteroids used in asthma include prednisolone, beclomethasone, betamethasone and budesonide (see Ch. 35).

Sodium cromoglycate[6] (cromolyn, Intal) impairs

---

[6]Cromoglycate was introduced in 1968 as the culmination of work carried out by the asthmatic research director of the company (REC Altounyan) on himself. We can admire Dr Altounyan without recommending this as the best way of screening new chemical entities.

the immediate response to allergen and was formerly thought to act by inhibiting the release of mediators from mast cells. Evidence now suggests that the late allergic response and bronchial hyperreactivity are also inhibited, and points to effects of cromoglycate on other inflammatory cells and also on local axon reflexes.

Cromoglycate is poorly absorbed from the gastrointestinal tract but is well absorbed from the lung, which is fortunate, so that it can be given by inhalation; it is eliminated unchanged in the urine and bile.

Since it does not antagonise the bronchoconstrictor effect of the active substances after they have been released, cromoglycate is *not* effective at terminating an existing attack, i.e. it *prevents bronchoconstriction* as opposed to inducing bronchodilatation.

Sodium cromoglycate is chiefly of value in extrinsic (allergic) asthma including asthma in children, and in exercise-induced asthma. The benefit may be delayed by several weeks. It may reduce the need to use oral adrenocortical steroid in some patients and allows a lower dose to be used (steroid-sparing effect).

The drug may be inhaled as an aerosol, as a powder (using a special insufflator) or as a nebulised solution. Special formulations are used for *allergic rhinitis* (Rynacrom) and *allergic conjunctivitis* (Opticrom). Sodium cromoglycate may also be used (as Nalcrom) by mouth for food allergy, in association with avoidance of known allergens.

It is remarkably nontoxic. Apart from cough and bronchospasm induced by the powder it may rarely cause allergic reactions. Application to the eye may produce a local stinging sensation and the oral form may cause nausea.

Nedocromil sodium (Tilade) is structurally unrelated to cromoglycate but has a similar profile of actions. Its use is by metered aerosol in patients with reversible airways obstruction. There is little experience of nedocromil administration to children.

Other drugs. Ketotifen is a histamine H_1-receptor blocker which may also have some antiasthma effects but its benefit has not been conclusively demonstrated. In common with other antihistamines it causes drowsiness.

Dilatation of narrowed bronchi

This is achieved by physiological antagonism of bronchial muscle contraction.

β_2-**adrenoceptor agonists.** These are drugs of choice because the adrenoceptors in bronchi are mainly β_2 type and their stimulation causes bronchial muscle to relax. They include: *salbutamol, terbutaline, fenoterol, pirbuterol, reproterol, eformoterol* and *rimiterol*, and are discussed in Chapter 23. *Salmeterol* is longer acting because its lipophilic side chain anchors the drug in the membrane, slowing washout from the receptor. The drug may have some action in reducing release of mediators from inflammatory cells, which themselves have a β_2-receptor on their surface.

Less selective adrenoceptor agonists such as adrenaline (epinephrine), *ephedrine, isoetharine, isoprenaline* and *orciprenaline* are less safe, being more likely to cause cardiac dysrhythmias. Alpha-adrenoceptor activity contributes to bronchoconstriction but α-adrenoceptor antagonists have not proved effective.

Methylxanthines include theophylline, aminophylline and choline theophyllinate. An account of theophylline will suffice.

Theophylline relaxes bronchial muscle. Its mode of action is not understood with certainty but probably involves competitive inhibition of adenosine receptors, for theophylline is structurally similar to adenosine and blocks many of its biological actions at concentrations within the therapeutic range. Adenosine can cause bronchoconstriction in asthmatics. Theophylline also inhibits phosphodiesterase (PDE), the enzyme that metabolises cyclic AMP. Although this effect is negligible at therapeutic concentrations, there does appear to be a better correlation between the efficacy of xanthines as bronchodilators and their rank order as PDE inhibitors than with their rank order as adenosine antagonists. The explanation of this paradox may prove to lie in the large number of subtypes of both the PDE enzyme and of the adenosine receptor. An advantage of old, nonselective drugs can be that their targets are more likely to include the 'correct' enzyme or receptor subtype, if an atypical subtype proves to be responsible for most of the therapeutic benefit. However, an alternative explanation (of how methylxanthines inhibit bronchoconstriction) is that plasma concentrations of a lipophilic drug like theophylline may markedly underrepresent the concentration of drug at an intracellular site of action, like the enzyme PDE. Xanthines have also been found to improve diaphragmatic contraction, which may be relevant to their role in respiratory disease.

Other actions of theophylline are to increase the rate and force of cardiac contraction, and to raise the rate of urine production (diuresis).

Absorption of theophylline from the gastrointestinal tract is usually rapid and complete. It is widely distributed and 90% is metabolised by the liver. There is evidence that the process is saturable at therapeutic doses. The $t^{1/2}$ is 8 h, with substantial variation, and it is prolonged in patients with severe cardiopulmonary disease and cirrhosis. Obesity and prematurity are associated with reduced rates of elimination, whereas smoking tobacco or cannabis enhances theophylline clearance by inducing hepatic enzymes. Attention to these factors may explain lack of responsiveness or adverse reactions to theophylline. Best therapeutic results are obtained when the plasma concentration is 10–20 mg/l (55–110 μmol/l). Theophylline is relatively insoluble and commercial formulations increase its solubility or duration of action. *Aminophylline* is a mixture of theophylline with ethylenediamine which is sufficiently soluble for i.v. use; there are numerous sustained-release oral forms. Theophylline is used for both chronic asthma (by mouth, choline theophyllinate) and status asthmaticus (i.v. aminophylline); a suppository at night may be effective for those whose asthma is especially worse in the early morning ('morning dippers'). It is also used in the emergency treatment of left ventricular failure (see p. 476).

At high therapeutic doses some patients experience nausea and diarrhoea and when the plasma concentration exceeds the recommended range there is danger of cardiac dysrhythmia and epileptic seizures. The latter are prone to occur with rapid intravenous injection, which exposes the heart and brain to high concentrations before distribution is complete. It follows that i.v. injection must be slow (5 mg/kg over 20 min) and reduced i.v. dose must be given to any patient who is already taking a xan-

thine preparation (*always enquire* about this before injecting). Enzyme inhibition by erythromycin, ciprofloxacin, allopurinol or oral contraceptives increases the plasma concentration of theophylline; enzyme inducers such as carbamazepine, phenobarbitone and phenytoin reduce the concentration.

Overdose with theophylline has assumed greater importance with the advent of sustained-release preparations which prolong toxic effects, with peak plasma concentrations being reached 12–24 h after ingestion. Vomiting may be severe but the chief dangers are cardiac dysrhythmia, hypotension, hypokalaemia and seizures. After gastric lavage, activated charcoal should be given every 2–4 h until the plasma concentration is below 20 mg/l. Potassium replacement is important to prevent dysrhythmias. Diazepam is used to control convulsions.

Antimuscarinic bronchodilators competitively inhibit the postsynaptic receptor action of acetylcholine at vagal nerve endings that constrict bronchial smooth muscle. Atropine has been used thus but has largely been replaced for asthma by ipratropium.

Ipratropium and *oxitropium* are synthetic analogues of atropine but, unlike the latter, are negligibly absorbed after inhalation. They act nonselectively on the various subtypes of muscarinic receptor in the lung to inhibit cholinergic activation of airway smooth muscle and thereby cause bronchodilation. Tolerance does not appear to develop. Ipratropium is a less effective bronchodilator than are the β-adrenoceptor agonists in asthma. This is mainly because it antagonises only one of the endogenous bronchoconstrictors, whereas physiological antagonists oppose all of them. Additionally, it is theoretically possible that nonselective muscarinic blockade increases release of acetylcholine (and possibly other mediators) by blocking the presynaptic M_2 autoreceptor that provides negative feedback to acetylcholine release. Currently there are no selective postsynaptic M_3 muscarinic antagonists available. Ipratropium is a useful adjunct to β_2-agonists and particularly benefits some, notably older, patients with intrinsic asthma and chronic bronchitis. It is administered by aerosol and by nebuliser.

Zileuton (Leutrol) is the first antileukotriene

antagonist to become available for chronic treatment of asthmatics, who are not controlled by conventional therapy. The drug inhibits 5-lipoxygenase, thus preventing formation of all the leukotrienes, including LTB4 (which stimulates cellular infiltration, chemotaxis aggregation and degranulation) and LTC4, LTD4 and LTE4, which cause airway constriction, vasopermeability, mucous hypersecretion, mucosal oedema and reduced mucociliary clearance. At the recommended dose of 600 mg 4 times daily, the drug increases FEV_1 by 12–15%, reduced β-agonist use by 25%, and in one study reduced the need for steroids from 22% of placebo treated controls to 8% in patients receiving zileuton.

INHALATION OF DRUGS

The inhalational route has been developed to advantage because the undesirable effects of systemic administration are reduced by the smaller doses that are needed. Drugs intended to be inhaled must first be converted into particulate form and the optimum particle size to reach and be deposited in the small bronchi is 2 μm. An *aerosol* consists of particles dispersed in a gas and may be produced as follows:

Pressurised aerosol. Drug is dissolved in a low boiling point liquid in a canister under pressure; when the valve is opened, a metered dose of liquid is ejected into the atmosphere, the carrier liquid evaporates instantly leaving an aerosol of the drug and is inhaled. Until recently the vehicle has been one or more of the CFCs (chlorofluorocarbons), but these are slowly being replaced by hydrofluoroalkanes (HFAs) which do not damage the atmospheric ozone.

Coordinating the act of opening the valve with that of inhalation can be difficult, especially for the young and the elderly; the problem can be overcome by interposing between the aerosol source and the patient's mouth, an extension tube (*spacer*) which prevents dispersion of the aerosol before the patient inhales.

Nebulisers convert a solution or suspension of drug into an aerosol. *Jet* nebulisers require a driving gas, usually air from a compressor unit for home use, or oxygen in hospital; the solution in the nebulising chamber is broken into droplets by the jet and the larger droplets are filtered off leaving the smaller ones to be inhaled. *Ultrasonic* nebulisers convert a solution into particles of uniform size by vibrations created by a piezo electric crystal.[7] With either method the nebulised solution is delivered to the patient by a mouthpiece or facemask, so no coordination is called for, and the dose can be altered by changing the strength of the solution.

Much larger doses can be administered by nebuliser than by pressurised aerosol.

Dry powder inhalers. The drug is formulated as a micronised powder and placed in a device, e.g. a Spinhaler, from which it is inhaled. Some patients can use these when they fail with metered dose aerosols. Inhalation of powder can cause transient bronchoconstriction.

DRUG TREATMENT

This varies with the severity and type of asthma. It is a general rule that the effectiveness of changes in drug and dose should be monitored by serial measurements of the simpler respiratory function tests such as peak expiratory flow rate (PEFR) or forced expiratory volume (FEV_1). Neither the patients' feelings nor ordinary physical examination are alone sufficient to determine whether there is still room for improvement. When an asthmatic attack is severe, arterial blood gases should be monitored. The British Thoracic Society guidelines recommend a 5-step approach, summarised below.

Constant and intermittent asthma

A β-adrenoceptor agonist should be given by metered dose aerosol and dosing adjusted to the patients' symptoms. Salbutamol is suitable, and the other $β_2$-adrenoceptor agonists referred to above; their effect is immediate. The usual dose is 1–2 puffs 4–8 hourly. *The patient should be carefully instructed how to use the inhaler* when treatment is begun, since failure to benefit is often due to improper use; time spent on this is never wasted. Patients should be *observed* to ensure their skill. An

---

[7]Converts electricity into mechanical vibration.

5-STEP TREATMENT OF ASTHMA

Step 1	Intermittent use of inhaled bronchodilator (β-agonist)
Step 2	+ Regular use of inhaled anti-inflammatory agent (cromoglycate or glucocorticoid)
Step 3	+ Regular use of high dose of glucocorticoid (or alternative)

If the above does not achieve

- **Minimal symptoms and exacerbations**
- **Infrequent need for bronchodilators and good exercise tolerance**
- **Peak expiratory flow rate (PEFR) 80% of predicted with < 20% diurnal variation**

then proceed to

Step 4	High dose inhaled adrenal steroids and regular bronchodilators
	+ Sequential trial of other inhaled treatments or oral methylxanthine
Step 5	Best of above + Oral prednisolone

oral β-adrenoceptor agonist can be used, e.g. salbutamol 4 mg, 3–4 times daily, but this route is more likely to give rise to tremor and headache. Salmeterol is slow in onset and acts for about 12 h. It is thus unsuitable for relief of acute attacks of asthma and its principal advantage over other $β_2$-agonists lies in its prevention of nocturnal asthma. It is not an alternative to corticosteroids.

If attacks recur, *sodium cromoglycate* or *nedocromil sodium* should be added and continued for about 4 weeks properly to assess benefit. They are most likely to prevent attacks in extrinsic asthmatics, especially children.

Ipratropium by metered dose aerosol, 1–2 puffs 3–4 times daily, may benefit some asthmatics, especially elderly intrinsic asthmatics who may also have chronic bronchitis.

For the patient who fails to improve on sodium cromoglycate an inhaled *corticosteroid* by metered dose aerosol may control symptoms. Since the drug is delivered directly to the site of action only a fraction of the oral dose is used (50–250 micrograms per puff). Furthermore 90% of the inhaled dose is either exhaled or is swallowed and then both poorly absorbed from the gut and rapidly metabolised in the hepatic first pass. Although reduced hypothalamic-pituitary-adrenal responsiveness has been demonstrated with inhaled corticosteroid, it is not ordinarily a clinical problem. Dysphonia and candidiasis of the mouth and throat can develop in a minority of cases; the latter is readily treated with nystatin mouthwashes or amphotericin lozenges without interrupting asthma therapy. Washing out the mouth with water after each inhalation reduces the chance of recurrence. Beclomethasone, betamethasone, budesonide or fluticasone are used 2–4 times a day, and adjusted to the minimum effective dose. They are about as effective as prednisolone 5–10 mg by mouth. Fluticasone has the highest first-pass metabolism of any inhaled steroid, > 99%. However, the lack of adrenal suppression by the other inhaled corticosteroids has made it difficult to demonstrate any practical advantage from using fluticasone.

To abort exacerbations, a β-receptor agonist aerosol, e.g. salbutamol, may be sufficient.

For more severe relapses, short courses of oral corticosteroid may be used, thus:

days 1 and 2: prednisolone 20 mg a day
days 3 and 4: 15 mg a day
days 5 and 6: 10 mg a day
day 7: 5 mg.

Such use does not cause withdrawal problems (Ch. 35).

Chest infections will increase reversible airways resistance and should be treated vigorously. The requirement of $β_2$-receptor agonist may increase.

Severe chronic asthma

Additions to therapy should be made sequentially with objective assessment, e.g. by peak expiratory flow rate, so that only treatments that are beneficial are continued. These are likely to include a check of the inhaler technique, a trial of sodium cromoglycate, of ipratropium and of theophylline. It is likely that higher doses of a β_2-adrenoceptor agonist will be required, possibly given by nebuliser at home.

Longterm oral therapy with *adrenal corticosteroid* is used only when all else has failed in patients who relapse repeatedly into status asthmaticus or who are too disabled to lead a reasonably normal working life. This is more often the case with intrinsic asthma. Therapy may begin with prednisolone, say 40 mg/d total, reducing it as soon as feasible to a maintenance dose of 10 mg/d, which is generally well tolerated. If relapses occur, as they may, the dose may be increased to 30 mg for one day, after which it is reduced by 5 mg/d until the maintenance dose is re-established. Adrenal suppression may be minimised by giving the corticosteroid as a single dose in the early morning when endogenous cortisol is at its peak and there is less negative feedback effect on the hypothalamic-pituitary-adrenal system. Although the $t^{1/2}$ of prednisolone is 3 h, once daily administration is reasonable as the *biological* effect $t^{1/2}$ is 18–36 h.

Patients taking longterm systemic (oral) adrenal steroid therapy should also use an inhaled steroid. The reason for this is that the inhaled steroid may allow the dose of oral (systemic) steroid to be lower than it otherwise would be, and so contribute to reducing the incidence of adverse effects of longterm systemic adrenal steroid therapy.

If systemic adrenal corticosteroid therapy has lasted more than 6 months, great caution is required during withdrawal, because of a risk of catastrophic relapse.

STATUS ASTHMATICUS

This a medical emergency requiring early vigorous treatment, for the bronchi may become refractory to β-receptor agonists (refractory to one means refractory to all) after about 36 h, perhaps the result of respiratory acidosis. In addition, drugs given by metered dose aerosol may fail to reach bronchi narrowed and blocked by mucus plugs. These are the

pathological hallmark of the condition, which render essential the early and adequate use of adrenal corticosteroids. No other treatment affects mucus production. The following lists, with some explanation, the recommendations of the British Thoracic Society.[8]

Immediate treatment

- *Oxygen* should be given to relieve the distress of dyspnoea (*humidified*, to help liquefy mucus). CO_2 narcosis is rare in asthma and 60% can be used if the diagnosis is not in doubt. In older patients, or when there is any concern about chronic CO_2 retention, it is safer to start with O_2 28% and to check that the $PaCO_2$ has not risen before delivering O_2 35%.
- *Salbutamol* should be given by nebuliser in a dose of 2.5–5 mg over about 3 min, repeated in 15 min. *Terbutaline* 5–10 mg is an alternative.
- *Prednisolone* 30–60 mg by mouth must be given at the outset, or *hydrocortisone* 200 mg i.v. to very sick patients.
- *No sedation of any kind.*
- Chest X-ray to exclude pneumothorax.

If life-threatening features are present:

- *Ipratropium* 0.5 mg should be added to the nebulised β-agonist.
- *Aminophylline* 5 mg/kg over 20 minutes or *salbutamol* 250 micrograms over 10 minutes may be given i.v. Aminophylline should not be given to patients already taking oral theophyllines.

Subsequent management
If patient is improving, continue:

- 40–60% oxygen
- Prednisolone 30–60 mg daily or hydrocortisone 200 mg 6-hourly
- Nebulised salbutamol or terbutaline 4-hourly.

If patient is **not** improving after 15–30 minutes:

- Continue oxygen and adrenal corticosteroids
- Give nebulised β-agonist more frequently, up to every 15–30 minutes
- Add ipratropium 0.5 mg to nebuliser and repeat 6-hourly until patient is improving.
  Antimuscarinics reduce, but thicken,

---

[8]British Thoracic Society and others 1993 Guidelines on the management of asthma. Thorax 48: S12.

secretion; this may be helped by keeping the patient well hydrated, if necessary by i.v. fluid.

If patient is still not improving give:

- Aminophylline infusion (small patient 750 mg/24 hours, large patient 1500 mg/24 hours); monitor blood concentrations if continued for > 24 hours
- Infusion of a β-agonist (as above) as an **alternative**.

Monitoring treatment

- By Peak Expiratory Flow Rate (PEFR) every 15–30 minutes
- Oxygen saturation: maintain > 92%
- Repeat blood gas measurements 2 hours after starting treatment if
  - initial paO_2 < 8 kPa (60 mmHg)
  - initial $paCO_2$ normal or raised (the tachypnoea is expected to *reduce* $paCO_2$ in most patients)
  - patient deteriorates.

Treatment in intensive care unit

Transfer (accompanied by doctor with facilities for intubation) is required if

- any of the above deteriorates, despite maximal treatment
- the patient becomes exhausted, drowsy, or confused
- coma or respiratory arrest occurs.

Treatment at discharge from hospital

Patients should:

- Continue inhaled adrenal corticosteroid and a reducing dose of oral prednisolone
- Be instructed to monitor their own PEFR and abort reduction in dose if the PEFR falls, or there is a recurrence of early morning dipping in the reading (patients should not generally be discharged until there is < 25% diurnal variation in PEFR readings).

Warnings

Asthma may be *precipitated* by β-adrenoceptor block and the use of β-adrenoceptor antagonists should be avoided altogether in patients with a history of asthma; *fatal asthma has been precipitated by β-blocker eye-drops.*

Overuse of β-adrenergic agonists is dangerous. In the mid-1960s, there was an epidemic of sudden deaths in young asthmatics outside hospital. It was associated with the introduction of a high dose, metered aerosol of isoprenaline (β_1 + β_2-agonist); it did not occur in countries where the high concentration was not marketed.[9] The epidemic declined in Britain when the profession was warned, and the aerosols were restricted to prescription only. Though the relationship between the use of β-receptor agonists and death is presumed to be causal, the actual mechanism of death is uncertain; overdose causing cardiac dysrhythmia is not the sole factor. The subsequent development of selective β_2-receptor agonists was a contribution to safety but a review in New Zealand during the 1980s found that the use of fenoterol (β_2-selective) by metered dose inhalation was associated with increased risk of death in severe asthma[10] and the matter remains controversial.

Any sedation that will ensure sleep in a severe asthmatic may adversely affect the respiratory drive and useful cough. If the patient tires before there is a marked improvement in the PEFR, then the appropriate treatment may be ventilation. The least dangerous sedatives and hypnotics are probably diazepam, chloral derivatives, chlorpromazine and promethazine, and an experienced physician may decide to prescribe one of these once recovery is assured.

CHRONIC OBSTRUCTIVE PULMONARY DISEASE (COPD)

Whereas asthma is characterised by reversible airways obstruction and bronchial hyperreactivity, COPD is characterised by incompletely reversible airways obstruction and mucus hypersecretion. In older years, the clinical overlap may make diagnosis uncertain. Arbitrarily, COPD is said to show less than 15% reversibility. In practice, even though —

---

[9]Stolley P D 1972 American Review of Respiratory Diseases 105: 8: 33.

[10]Crane J et al 1989 Lancet 1: 917.

indeed precisely because — most of the airways obstruction is fixed, it is important to maximise the reversible component. The assessment of this is performed by giving prednisolone 30 mg daily for 3 weeks, with measurement of Forced Expiratory Volumes or PEFR before and at the end of this period.

Drugs used to treat COPD are exactly as for asthma, except that the role of chronic adrenal corticosteroid treatment is unresolved. At present steroids should be reserved for those showing the greatest response during the 3-week therapeutic trial, and given by the inhaled route to avoid systemic effects.

Domiciliary oxygen is indicated for patients:

- whose paO_2 is < 7.5 kPa (56 mmHg) when stabilised on medical treatment
- whose $paCO_2$ is > 5.0 kPa (38 mmHg)
- who have had an episode of right-sided cardiac failure (cor pulmonale)
- whose FEV_1 is < 1.5 l and FVC > 2 l.

SUMMARY

- Asthma is characterised by hypersensitivity to the endogenous bronchoconstrictors, acetylcholine and histamine, and by reversible obstruction of the airways.
- However, drugs which block the actions of acetylcholine and histamine are weak or ineffective in the treatment of asthma.
- Most treatment is therefore aimed either at reducing release of inflammatory cytokines (glucocorticoids and sodium cromoglycate) or at direct bronchodilatation by stimulation of the bronchial β_2-receptors.
- Early use of glucocorticoids (adrenocortical steroids) is the keystone to prevention of fatalities.
- Antihistamines conventionally refer to antagonists of the H_1-receptor, and have wide applications in the treatment of allergic disorders, most importantly in anaphylaxis.
- The principal adverse effect of older antihistamines, sedation, is avoided by use of newer drugs which do not enter the CNS.
- Respiratory distress of the newborn is usually a treatable condition, using synthetic lung surfactant administration, and can often be avoided by treatment of the mother with glucocorticoids.

GUIDE TO FURTHER READING

Avery M E, Merritt T A 1991 Surfactant-replacement therapy. New England Journal of Medicine 324: 910

Ayres J G 1990 Late onset asthma. British Medical Journal 300: 1602

Barnes P J 1995 Inhaled glucocorticoids for asthma. New England Journal of Medicine 332: 868-875

Barnes P J, Fan Chung K 1989 Difficult asthma. British Medical Journal 299: 695

British Thoracic Society and others 1993 Guidelines on the management of asthma. Thorax 48: S12

du Bois R M 1995 Respiratory medicine. British Medical Journal 310: 1594–1597

Fuller R W 1994 Use of beta 2 agonists in asthma: much ado about nothing? Adverse effects are not proved. British Medical Journal 309: 795–796

Gross N J 1988 Ipratropium bromide. New England Journal of Medicine 319: 486

McFadden E R, Hejal R 1995 Asthma. Lancet 345: 1215–1220

Nelson H S 1995 β-adrenergic bronchodilators. New England Journal of Medicine 333: 499

Rees J, Price J 1995 ABC of asthma. Chronic asthma — general management. British Medical Journal 310: 1400–1401

Rees J, Price J 1995 ABC of asthma. Treatment of chronic asthma. British Medical Journal 310: 1459–1463

Shiner R J, Geddes D M 1989 Treating patients with asthma who are dependent on systemic steroids. British Medical Journal 299: 216

Stead R J, Cooke N J 1989 Adverse effects of inhaled corticosteroids. British Medical Journal 298: 403

Tattersfield A E 1994 Use of beta 2 agonists in asthma: much ado about nothing? Still cause for concern. British Medical Journal 309: 794–795

BLOOD AND NEOPLASTIC DISEASE

29

Drugs and haemostasis

SYNOPSIS

Occlusive vascular disease is a major cause of morbidity and mortality. There is now a better understanding of the mechanisms by which the haemostatic system permits blood to remain fluid within vessels, yet to form a solid plug when a vessel is breached, and of the ways in which haemostasis may be altered by drugs to prevent or reverse (lyse) pathological thrombosis.

- Coagulation system: the mode of action of drugs that promote coagulation and that prevent it (anticoagulants) and their uses
- Fibrinolytic system: the mode of action of drugs that promote fibrinolysis (fibrinolytics) and their uses to lyse arterial and venous thrombi (thrombolysis)
- Platelets: the ways that drugs that inhibit platelet activity are used to treat arterial disease

The haemostatic system is complex but can be separated into the following major components:

- Formation of fibrin (coagulation), which stabilises the platelet plug
- Degradation of fibrin (fibrinolysis)
- Platelets, which form the haemostatic plug
- Blood vessels.

Drugs that interfere with the haemostatic system (anticoagulants, thrombolytics) are valuable in the management of pathological thrombus formation within blood vessels, or of pathological bleeding. They are classified according to which component of the system they affect.

Coagulation system

The blood coagulation system is shown in simplified form in Figure 29.1.

The prothrombin time (expressed as the International Normalised Ratio, INR) primarily monitors the extrinsic system.

The kaolin–cephalin clotting time (KCCT), also known as the activated partial thromboplastin time (APTT), primarily monitors the intrinsic system. Each is affected by the final common pathway, the end-point of which is tested by the thrombin time.

SUBSTANCE THAT PROMOTES COAGULATION: VITAMIN K

Vitamin K (Koagulation vitamin) occurs naturally in two forms. K_1 is widely distributed in plants and K_2 is synthesised in the alimentary tract by bacteria, e.g. *Escherichia coli*. Bile is required for the absorption of the natural vitamins K, which are fat-soluble. A syn-

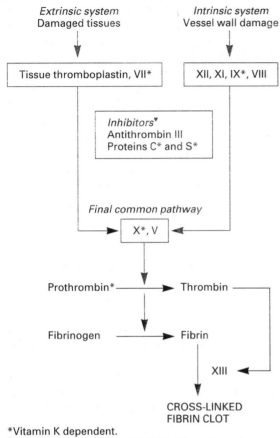

Extrinsic system
Damaged tissues

Intrinsic system
Vessel wall damage

Tissue thromboplastin, VII*

XII, XI, IX*, VIII

Inhibitors▾
Antithrombin III
Proteins C* and S*

Final common pathway

X*, V

Prothrombin* ⟶ Thrombin

Fibrinogen ⟶ Fibrin

XIII

CROSS-LINKED
FIBRIN CLOT

*Vitamin K dependent.
▾Antithrombin III inhibits IX, X, XI, XII and thrombin.
Proteins C and S inhibit V and VIII.

Fig. 29.1 Blood coagulation system (simplified)

thetic analogue (K_3) (below) of the natural vitamins also has biological activity in vivo; it is water-soluble.

Vitamin K is necessary for the final stages of the synthesis of the coagulation proteins in the liver by gamma-carboxylation of the molecule which mediates calcium binding to negatively charged phospholipid surfaces. The proteins are factors II (prothrombin), VII, IX and X, and also the anticoagulant proteins C and S. During their formation vitamin K is converted to an epoxide, an oxidation product, which is subsequently reduced again enzymatically to the active vitamin K, i.e. there exists an interconversion cycle between vitamin K epoxide and reduced and active vitamin K (KH_2). When the vitamin is deficient or where its action is inhibited, functionally impaired proteins result.

Deficiency may arise from:

- bile failing to enter the intestine, e.g. obstructive jaundice or biliary fistula
- certain malabsorption syndromes, e.g. coeliac disease, or after extensive small intestinal resection
- reduced alimentary tract flora, e.g. in newborn infants and rarely after broad-spectrum antimicrobials.

The following preparations of vitamin K are available:

Phytomenadione (phytonadione, Konakion), the naturally occurring fat-soluble vitamin K_1, acts within about 12 h. The i.v. formulation is used in emergency and must be administered slowly as an anaphylactoid reaction with facial flushing; sweating, fever, chest tightness, cyanosis and peripheral vascular collapse may occur. Patients with chronic liver disease and those using histamine H_2-receptor antagonists seem to be specially likely to react. Otherwise phytomenadione may be given i.m., s.c. or orally.

Menadiol sodium phosphate (vitamin K_3, Synkavit), the synthetic analogue of vitamin K, being water-soluble, is preferred in malabsorption or in states in which bile flow is deficient. The main disadvantage is that it takes 24 h to act, but its effect lasts for several days. The dose is 5–40 mg daily, orally, i.v. or i.m.

Menadiol sodium phosphate in moderate doses causes haemolytic anaemia and for this reason it should not be given to neonates, especially those that are deficient in glucose-6-phosphate dehydrogenase; their immature livers are unable to cope with the heavy bilirubin load and there is danger of kernicterus.

Fat-soluble analogues of vitamin K which are available in some countries include *acetomenaphthone* and *menaphthone*.

Indications for vitamin K or its analogues

- Haemorrhage or threatened bleeding due to the coumarin or indandione anticoagulants. Phytomenadione is preferred for its more rapid action; dosage regimens vary according to the degree of urgency, as described on page 523.
- Haemorrhagic disease of the newborn (and also late haemorrhagic disease which presents at

6–7 months). Prophylaxis is recommended[1] with vitamin K (phytomenadione, as Konakion) 500 microgram on the day of birth followed by 50 microgram/day (or 200 microgram/week or 500 microgram at 7–10 days and again at 4–6 weeks) during the period of vulnerability, i.e. 26 weeks in breast-fed infants. Formula-fed infants do not need a supplement. Fears that i.m. vitamin K might cause childhood cancer have been allayed.

• Hypoprothrombinaemia due to intestinal malabsorption syndromes. Menadiol sodium phosphate should be used as it is water-soluble.

DRUGS THAT PREVENT COAGULATION: ANTICOAGULANTS

There are two types of anticoagulant:

Indirect-acting: coumarin[2] and indandione drugs take about 72 h to become fully effective, act for several days, are given orally or by injection and can be antagonised (see below) by vitamin K.

Direct-acting: heparin and ancrod are rapidly effective, act for only a few hours and must be given parenterally.

Indirect-acting anticoagulants

Coumarins include warfarin and nicoumalone.

Indandione anticoagulants are practically obsolete because of allergic adverse reactions unrelated to coagulation but *phenindione* ($t\frac{1}{2}$ 5 h) is still available.

Warfarin

Mode of action. During the gamma-carboxylation of the coagulant factors II (prothrombin), VII, IX

---

[1] Report 1992 Vitamin K in infancy. British Paediatric Society, London.

[2] Coumarins are present in many plants and are important in the perfume industry; the smell of new mown hay and grass is due to coumarins. Their discovery as anticoagulants dates from investigation of an unexplained haemorrhagic disease of cattle that had eaten mouldy sweet clover. Subsequent research culminated in the isolation of the causative agent, dicoumarol.

and X (and also the anticoagulant regulatory proteins C and S) in the liver, active vitamin K (KH_2) is oxidised to an epoxide and must be reduced by the enzyme vitamin K epoxide reductase to become active again. Coumarins are structurally similar to vitamin K and competitively inhibit epoxide reductase, so limiting availability of the active form of the vitamin to form coagulant (and anticoagulant) proteins. The overall result is a shift in haemostatic balance in favour of anticoagulation because of the accumulation of clotting proteins with absent or decreased gamma-carboxylation sites. Proteins C and S, however, have a shorter $t\frac{1}{2}$ than the procoagulant proteins and their more rapid decline in concentration in advance of these proteins creates a *transient hypercoagulable state*. This can be serious in those who have inherited protein S and C deficiency and justifies initiating anticoagulation with heparin until the effect of warfarin is well established.

The great advantage over heparin is that warfarin can be given orally. Its chief disadvantage is the time lag before it exerts its effect, which is due to its indirect mode of action, i.e. although synthesis of the native proteins is quickly prevented, anticoagulation is delayed until the functioning clotting factors already present in the circulation have been used up; this process occurs at different rates for individual factors and the net result is that anticoagulant protection is not effective until about 72 h after the first dose. A similar time lag is found when warfarin dose is altered or discontinued as the $t\frac{1}{2}$ of the nonfunctioning proteins is approximately that of functioning proteins.

Pharmacokinetics. Warfarin is readily absorbed from the gastrointestinal tract and like all the oral anticoagulants it is more than 90% bound to plasma proteins. Its action is terminated by metabolism in the liver. Warfarin ($t\frac{1}{2}$ 36 h) is a racemic mixture of approximately equal amounts of two isomers S ($t\frac{1}{2}$ 35 h) and R ($t\frac{1}{2}$ 50 h) warfarin, i.e. it is in effect two drugs. S warfarin is 4 times more potent than R warfarin. Drugs which interact with warfarin affect these isomers differently.

Uses. Warfarin is the oral anticoagulant of choice, for it is reliably effective and has the lowest incidence of adverse effects. Monitoring of therapy is by the prothrombin time. Usually the test is carried out with a standardised thromboplastin and the result is expressed as the International Normalised Ratio (INR), which is the ratio of the prothrombin time in the patient to that in a normal (un-anticoagulated) person — taking account of the sensitivity of the thromboplastin used.

Oral anticoagulation is commonly undertaken in patients who are already receiving heparin. The INR reliably reflects the degree of prothrombin activity provided that the kaolin–cephalin clotting time (KCCT, the best measure of the anticoagulant effect of heparin, see below), is within the therapeutic range (1.5–2.5 × control).

Dose. There is much inter-individual variation in dose requirements. The usual dose to initiate therapy is 10 mg daily for 2 days, with the maintenance dose then adjusted according to the INR; a more detailed regimen has been suggested.[3]

The level of anticoagulation should be adjusted to match the perceived level of danger of thrombosis, by the following guidelines:[4]

- **INR 2.0–2.5** Prophylaxis of deep vein thrombosis including surgery on high-risk patients (2.0–3.0 for hip surgery and fractured femur operations).
- **INR 2.0–3.0** Treatment of deep vein thrombosis; pulmonary embolism; systemic embolism; prevention of venous thromboembolism in myocardial infarction; mitral stenosis with embolism; transient ischaemic attacks; atrial fibrillation.
- **INR 3.0–4.5** Recurrent deep vein thrombosis and pulmonary embolism; arterial disease including myocardial infarction; mechanical prosthetic heart valves.

Adverse effects. Bleeding is the commonest. The incidence of major haemorrhage is 4–8%[5] and an identifiable risk factor is often present, e.g. thrombocytopenia, liver disease or vitamin K deficiency, an endogenous disturbance of coagulation, cancer or recent surgery. Naturally, poor anticoagulant control or drug interaction with warfarin increase the risk. Haemorrhage is most likely to occur in the alimentary and renal tracts, and in the brain in those with cerebrovascular disease.

Cutaneous reactions, apart from purpura and ecchymoses in those who are excessively anticoagulated, include pruritic lesions. Skin necrosis due to a mixture of haemorrhage and thrombosis occurs rarely where induction of warfarin therapy is over-abrupt and/or the patient has a genetically determined or acquired deficiency of the anticoagulant protein C or its cofactor protein S; it can be very serious.

Warfarin used in early pregnancy may injure the fetus (other than by bleeding). It causes skeletal disorder (5%) (bossed forehead, sunken nose, foci of calcification in the epiphyses) and absence of the spleen. Women on longterm warfarin should be advised not to become pregnant while taking the drug. Heparin should be substituted prior to conception and continued through the first trimester, after which warfarin should replace heparin, as continued exposure to heparin may cause osteoporosis. Warfarin should be discontinued near term as it exacerbates neonatal hypoprothrombinaemia and its control is too imprecise to be safe in labour; heparin may be substituted at this stage for it can be discontinued just before labour and its anticoagulant effect passes off in about 6 h.

CNS abnormalities (microcephaly, cranial nerve palsies) are reported with warfarin used at any stage of pregnancy and are presumed to be due to intracranial haemorrhage.

Management of bleeding or over-anticoagulation is guided by the clinical state and the INR:[6]

- Haemorrhage threatening life or major organs. In addition to blood replacement, rapid reversal of anticoagulation is achieved with prothrombin complex concentrate (containing factors II, IX and X, and given i.v. as 50 units per kg of factor

---

[3] Fennerty A et al 1988 British Medical Journal 297: 1285–8.

[4] British Society for Haematology 1990 Guidelines on oral anticoagulants, 2nd edn. Journal of Clinical Pathology 43: 177–183 (Reproduced with permission).

[5] A study of 261 patients who received warfarin for 221 patient-years reported major haemorrhage in 5.3% after 1 year and 10.6% after 2 years. Mayo Clinic Proceedings (1995) 70: 725.

[6] Based on recommendations of the British Society for Haematology.

IX) or fresh frozen plasma. If full reversal of anticoagulation is judged necessary, phytomenadione 5 mg is then given by slow i.v. injection. This renders the patient refractory to oral anticoagulant (but not to heparin) for about 2 weeks. The thrombotic risk so created must be assessed for each patient and may be judged unacceptable in some, e.g. those with prosthetic heart valves. For lesser bleeding, warfarin should be withheld and phytomenadione 0.5–2 mg may be given by slow i.v. injection.

- *INR > 7 but without bleeding.* Correct by withholding warfarin, and giving phytomenadione 0.5 mg by slow i.v. injection if judged appropriate.
- *INR 4.5–7.0.* Manage by withholding warfarin for 1–2 days and then reviewing the INR.
- *INR 2.0–4.5 (the therapeutic range).* Bleeding, e.g. from the alimentary or renal tracts, should be fully investigated as a local cause frequently exists.

Withdrawal of oral anticoagulant. The balance of evidence is that abrupt, as opposed to gradual withdrawal of therapy does not, of itself, add to the risk of thromboembolism, for resynthesis of clotting factors takes several days.

Interactions. Oral anticoagulant control requires to be precise both for safety and efficacy. If a drug which alters the action of warfarin must be used, the INR should be monitored frequently and the dose of warfarin adjusted during the period of institution until the new stable dose of warfarin is identified; careful monitoring is also needed on withdrawal of the interacting drug.

The following list, although not comprehensive, identifies medicines which should be avoided and those which may safely be used with warfarin.

- Analgesics. Avoid if possible, all NSAIDs including aspirin because of their irritant effect on gastric mucosa and action on platelets. Paracetamol is acceptable but doses over 1.5 g/d may raise the INR. Dextropropoxyphene inhibits warfarin metabolism and compounds that contain it, e.g. co-proxamol, should be avoided. Codeine, dihydrocodeine and combinations with paracetamol, e.g. co-dydramol, are preferred.
- Antimicrobials. Aztreonam, cephamandole, chloramphenicol, ciprofloxacin, co-trimoxazole, erythromycin, fluconazole, itraconazole, ketoconazole, metronidazole, miconazole, ofloxacin and sulphonamides (including co-trimoxazole)

increase anticoagulant effect by mechanisms that include interference with warfarin or vitamin K metabolism. Rifampicin and griseofulvin accelerate warfarin metabolism (enzyme induction) and reduce its effect. Broad spectrum antimicrobials, e.g. amoxycillin, may increase sensitivity to warfarin by reducing the intestinal flora that produce vitamin K.
- Anticonvulsants. Carbamazepine, phenobarbitone and primidone accelerate warfarin metabolism (enzyme induction); the effect of phenytoin is variable. Clonazepam and sodium valproate are safe.
- Cardiac antidysrhythmics. Amiodarone, propafenone and possibly quinidine potentiate the effect of warfarin and dose adjustment is required, but atropine, disopyramide and lignocaine do not interfere.
- Antidepressants. Serotonin re-uptake inhibitors may enhance the effect of warfarin but tricyclics may be used.
- Gastrointestinal drugs. Avoid cimetidine and omeprazole which inhibit the clearance of R warfarin, and sucralfate which may impair its absorption. Ranitidine may be used but INR should be checked if the dose is high. Most antacids are safe.
- Lipid-lowering drugs. Clofibrate and the other drugs of this group, and possibly also simvastatin, enhance anticoagulant effect. Cholestyramine is best avoided for it may impair the absorption of both warfarin and vitamin K.
- Sex hormones and hormone antagonists. Oestrogens increase the synthesis of some vitamin K dependent clotting factors and progestogen-only contraceptives are preferred. The hormone antagonists danazol, flutamide and tamoxifen enhance the effect of warfarin.
- Sedatives and anxiolytics. Benzodiazepines may be used.

Nicoumalone (t$\frac{1}{2}$ 24 h) is similar to warfarin; it is eliminated in the urine mainly in the unchanged form.

Direct-acting anticoagulants: heparin

Heparin was discovered by a medical student, J McLean, working at Johns Hopkins Medical School in 1916. Seeking to devote one year to physiological research he was set to study 'the thromboplastic (clotting) substance in the body'. He found that extracts of brain, heart and liver accelerated clotting but that activity deteriorated during storage. To his surprise, the extract of liver which he had kept longest not only failed to accelerate but actually retarded clotting. His personal account proceeds:

After more tests and the preparation of other batches of heparophosphatide, I went one morning to the door of Dr. Howell's office, and standing there (he was seated at his desk), I said 'Dr. Howell, I have discovered antithrombin'. He was most skeptical. So I had the Deiner, John

Schweinhant, bleed a cat. Into a small beaker full of its blood, I stirred all of a proven batch of heparophosphatides, and I placed this on Dr. Howell's laboratory table and asked him to call me when it clotted. It never did clot. [It was heparin.][7]

Heparin is a mucopolysaccharide, occurs in mast cells and is prepared commercially from a variety of animal tisues to give preparations that vary in mol. wt. from 3000 to 30 000 (average 15 000). It is the strongest organic acid in the body and in solution carries an electronegative charge.

Mode of action. Heparin depends for its action on the presence in plasma of a protein, *antithrombin* III, which is a naturally occurring inhibitor of thrombin and of activated factor X (Xa). In the presence of heparin antithrombin becomes vastly more active. The importance of inhibition of factor Xa is that this factor is involved in both the intrinsic and extrinsic coagulation systems and heparin is effective in small quantities. This provides the rationale for giving low dose subcutaneous heparin to prevent thrombus formation. At a molecular level the capacity of heparin to inhibit factor Xa has been found to depend on a specific pentasaccharide sequence which can be isolated in fragments of average mol. wt. 5000 (low mol. wt. heparins). These fragments are too short to inhibit thrombin which is the principal action of conventional heparin (average mol. wt. 15 000). Fibrin formed in the circulation binds to thrombin and protects it from inactivation by the heparin-antithrombin III complex, which may provide a further explanation for the higher doses of heparin needed to stop extension of a thrombus than to prevent its formation. Heparin also inhibits platelet aggregation.

Apart from its anticoagulant properties, heparin inhibits the proliferation of vascular smooth muscle cells and is involved in angiogenesis. Heparin also inhibits certain aspects of the inflammatory response; this is evident in the rapid resolution of inflammation that accompanies deep vein thrombosis, when heparin is given.

---

[7] McLean gives a fascinating account of his struggles to pay his way through medical school, as well as his discovery of heparin in: McLean J 1959 Circulation XIX: 75.

Pharmacokinetics. Heparin is poorly absorbed from the gastrointestinal tract and is given i.v. or s.c.; once in the blood its effect is immediate. Heparin binds to several plasma proteins and to sites on endothelial cells; it is also taken up by cells of the reticuloendothelial system and some is cleared by the kidney. Elimination of heparin from the plasma appears to involve a combination of zero-order and first-order processes, the effect of which is that the plasma biological effect $t\frac{1}{2}$ alters disproportionately with dose, being 60 min after 75 units per kg and 150 min after 400 units per kg.

Control of heparin therapy is by the kaolin–cephalin clotting time (KCCT), the optimum therapeutic range being 1.5–2.5 times the control (which is preferably the patient's own pretreatment KCCT).

Dose

Treatment of established thrombosis. The usual intravenous regimen is a bolus i.v. injection of 5000 units (or 10 000 units in severe pulmonary embolism) followed by a constant rate i.v. infusion of 1000–2000 units per hour. Alternatively 15 000 units may be given s.c. every 12 h but control is less even. The KCCT should be measured 6 h after starting therapy and the administration rate adjusted to keep it in the optimum therapeutic ratio of 1.5–2.5; this usually requires daily measurements of KCCT preferably between 0900 h and 1200 h (noon) as the anticoagulant effect of heparin exhibits circadian changes.

Prevention of thrombosis. Postoperatively or after myocardial infarction 5000 units should be given s.c. every 8 or 12 h without monitoring (this dose does not prolong the KCCT), or in pregnancy 5000–10 000 units s.c. every 12 h with monitoring (except for pregnant women with prosthetic heart valves for whom specialist monitoring is needed).

Low mol. wt. heparins (dalteparin, enoxaparin, tinzaparin) are as effective and safe as conventional (unfractionated) heparin at preventing venous thrombosis (see above), and may be preferred for orthopaedic practice. Once daily s.c. administration will suffice as their duration of action is longer than that of conventional heparin. Low mol. wt. heparin also proved as effective as standard i.v. therapy for patients with thrombosis of popliteal or more proximal veins;[8] this simplified therapy may allow patients with uncomplicated deep-vein thrombosis to be treated without admission to hospital.

Adverse effects. Bleeding is the serious acute complication of heparin therapy. It is uncommon, but patients with impaired hepatic or renal function, with carcinoma, and those over 60 years appear to be most at risk. A KCCT ratio > 3 is associated with an 8-fold increased chance of bleeding. A further serious complication is the syndrome of thrombocytopenia with arterial thromboemboli and haemorrhage which occurs in about 2–3% of patients who receive heparin for a week or more. It occurs most commonly with heparin derived from bovine lung and least with that of intestinal origin, has an immunological pathogenesis, and recurs on rechallenge. Up to 30% of patients may require amputation or may die. Warfarin should be substituted if the platelet count falls when a patient receives heparin. Osteoporosis may occur; it is dose related and may be expected with 15 000–30 000 units/day for about 6 months. Hypersensitivity reactions and skin necrosis occur but are rare. Transient alopecia has been ascribed to heparin but in fact may be due to the severity of the thromboembolic disease for which the drug was given. Skin necrosis similar to that seen with warfarin (see above) occurs rarely.

Heparin antagonism. Heparin effects wear off so rapidly that an antagonist is seldom required except after extracorporeal perfusion for heart surgery. When antagonism is needed:

Protamine, a protein obtained from fish sperm, reverses the anticoagulant action of heparin. It is as strongly basic as heparin is acidic, which explains its immediate antagonism. Protamine sulphate is given by slow i.v. injection and 1 mg neutralises about 100 units of heparin derived from mucosa (mucous) or 80 units of heparin from lung; but if the heparin was given more than 15 min previously, the dose must be scaled down. Protamine itself has some anticoagulant effect and overdosage must be avoided. The maximum dose must not exceed 50 mg.

---

[8] Hull R D et al 1992 New England Journal of Medicine 326: 975.

The antithrombotic properties of direct inhibitors of thrombus-bound thrombin, e.g. *hirudin* (from the medicinal leech), *hirulog* and *hirugen* are being assessed.

USES OF ANTICOAGULANTS

Venous disease

Established venous thromboembolism. An anticoagulant is used to prevent extension of an existing thrombus while its size is reduced by natural thrombolytic activity. Effective anticoagulation prevents formation of fresh thrombus, which is more likely to detach and embolise, particularly if it is in large proximal veins; it also helps to recanalise veins and to clear vein valves of thrombus and should thus prevent longterm consequences such as swelling of the leg and stasis ulceration.

The site and extent of thrombosis should be established by venous ultrasound or venography. Small distal thrombi require only elevation of the limb and no anticoagulant. For a thrombus less than 10 cm long in a tibial vein heparin 15 000 units s.c. × 2/d is sufficient until the patient is fully mobile. Full anticoagulation may be required for more extensive thrombosis; heparin should be used initially because of its rapid onset of effect and continued until the signs of thrombosis (heat, swelling of the limb) have settled, which may take 5–7 days. Oral anticoagulant is usually started on the third to the fifth day in the knowledge that at least 2 days must elapse before the INR is in the therapeutic range. The patient should wear a well-fitting compression stocking to increase flow in deep veins, should exercise the leg and should be encouraged to mobilise as soon as the discomfort has settled.

Thrombolytic therapy with intravenous streptokinase or urokinase may be used when thrombosis is thought to be life-threatening, and thrombectomy is recommended where the viability of the limb is threatened.

The risk of recurrence reduces with passage of time after the initial event. In cases of deep vein thrombosis uncomplicated by pulmonary embolus, 3 months of anticoagulant therapy appears adequate. Where there is evidence of pulmonary embolus it is common practice to continue therapy for 6 months.

Anticoagulant therapy may be life-saving in thromboembolic pulmonary hypertension.

Prevention of venous thrombosis. Oral anticoagulant reduces the risk of thromboembolism in conditions in which there is special hazard, e.g. after surgery. Partly because of the danger of bleeding and partly because of the effort of maintaining control, oral anticoagulants have not been widely adopted. Numerous trials, however, have shown the protective effect of low doses of heparin (5000 units every 8–12 h s.c.) against deep leg vein thrombosis. The significant fact is that it takes a lot less heparin to prevent thrombosis than it does to treat established thrombosis, because heparin acts in low concentration at an early stage in the cascade of coagulation factors which leads to fibrin formation (see above).

Apart from its use after surgery, low-dose heparin can be used to prevent venous thromboembolism in other high-risk patients, e.g. those confined to bed and immobilised with strokes, cardiac failure or malignant disease. Spontaneous bleeding has not been a problem with this form of anticoagulant treatment.

Low mol. wt. dextrans can reduce postoperative thromboembolism if infused i.v. at the time of operation. Dextran 70 (mol. wt. 70 000) is used; it may act by reducing platelet adhesiveness.

Cardiovascular disease

Acute myocardial infarction. Anticoagulation with heparin is used to reduce the risk of venous thromboembolism, and the risk and size of emboli from mural thrombi following acute myocardial infarction.

Longterm anticoagulation with warfarin to prevent arterial thromboembolism should be considered for any patient who has a large left atrium or a low cardiac output or paroxysmal or established atrial fibrillation (with or without cardiac valvular disease). Where warfarin is considered unsuitable, aspirin may be substituted for it has also been shown to prevent stroke in patients with atrial fibrillation, though less effectively. Heparin is given for 2 h to patients after undergoing angioplasty.

Heparin, aspirin or both are used to prevent myocardial infarction in the acute phase of *unstable angina*.

Peripheral arterial occlusion. Heparin may prevent extension of a thrombus and hasten its recanalisation; it is commonly used in the acute phase following thrombosis or embolism. There is no case for treating ischaemic peripheral vascular disease with an oral anticoagulant (for prevention, see Antiplatelet drugs).

Longterm anticoagulant prophylaxis

The decision to use warfarin longterm must take into account nondrug factors. The patient should be told of the risks of haemorrhage, including those introduced by taking other drugs, and of the signs of bleeding into the alimentary or urinary tracts. All patients should carry a card stating that they are receiving an oral anticoagulant. Such therapy should be withheld from a patient who is considered to be unlikely or unable to comply with the requirements of regular medication and blood testing. The incidence of haemorrhagic complications is directly related to the level of anticoagulation; safety and good results can only be obtained by close attention to detail.

Surgery in patients receiving anticoagulant therapy

For elective surgery warfarin may be withdrawn about 5 days before the operation and resumed about 3 days after if conditions seem appropriate; low-dose heparin may be used in the intervening period. In patients with mechanical prosthetic valves, heparin is substituted at full dosage 4 days before surgery, and restarted 12–24 h after the operation. Warfarin is restarted when the patient resumes oral intake. Emergency surgery: proceed as for bleeding (p. 522). For dental extractions: omission of warfarin for 1–2 days to adjust the INR to the lower limit of the therapeutic range is adequate (INR should be tested just prior to the procedure). The usual dose of warfarin can be resumed the day after extraction.

Aspirin, taken prophylactically for thromboembolic disorders (see below), is commonly discontinued 2 weeks before elective procedures and restarted when oral intake permits.

Contraindications to anticoagulant therapy

Contraindications relate mostly to conditions in which there is a tendency to bleed, and are relative rather than absolute, the dangers being balanced against the possible benefits. They include:

- Behavioural: inability or unwillingness to cooperate, dependency on alcohol
- Neurological: stroke within 3 weeks, or surgery to the brain or eye
- Alimentary: active peptic ulcer, active inflammatory bowel disease, oesophageal varices, uncompensated hepatic cirrhosis
- Cardiovascular: severe uncontrolled hypertension
- Renal: if function is severely impaired
- Pregnancy: in early pregnancy the fetal warfarin syndrome is a hazard and bleeding may cause fetal death in late pregnancy
- Haematological: pre-existing bleeding disorder.

Fibrinolytic system

The preservation of an intact vascular system requires not only that blood be capable of coagulating but also that there should be a mechanism for removing the products of coagulation when they have served their purpose of stopping a vascular leak. This is the function of the fibrinolytic system, the essential features of which are shown in Figure 29.2.

The system depends on the formation of the fibrinolytic enzyme plasmin from its precursor protein, plasminogen, in the blood. During clotting, plasminogen binds to specific sites on fibrin. Simultaneously the natural activators of plasminogen, i.e. tissue plasminogen activator (tPA) and urokinase, are released from endothelial and other tissue cells and act on plasminogen to form plasmin. The result is that plasmin formation takes place on the fibrin surface but not generally within the circulation.

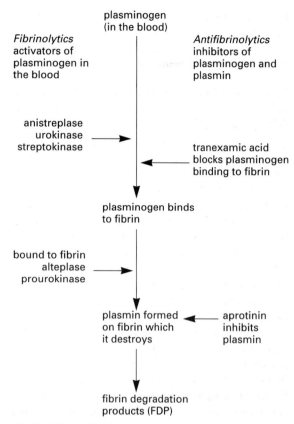

Fig. 29.2 Blood fibrinolytic system

Since fibrin is the framework of a thrombus, its dissolution clears the clot away.

Fibrinolytics (thrombolytics) can remove formed thrombi and emboli. Inhibitors of the fibrinolytic system (*antifibrinolytics*) can be of value in certain bleeding states characterised by excessive fibrinolysis.

DRUGS THAT PROMOTE FIBRINOLYSIS

An important application of fibrinolytic drugs has been to dissolve thrombi in acutely occluded coronary arteries, thereby to restore blood supply to ischaemic myocardium, to limit necrosis and to improve prognosis. The approach is to give a plasminogen activator intravenously by infusion or by bolus injection in order to increase the formation of the fibrinolytic enzyme plasmin. Those currently available include:

Streptokinase ($t\frac{1}{2}$ 80 min) is a protein derived from β-haemolytic streptococci: it forms a complex with plasminogen (bound loosely to fibrin) where it converts plasminogen to plasmin. Too rapid administration causes abrupt fall in blood pressure.

Anistreplase (anisoylated plasminogen streptokinase activator complex, APSAC) ($t^{1}/_{2}$ 90 min), is the plasminogen-streptokinase complex (above) in which the enzyme centre that converts plasminogen to plasmin is protected from deactivation, so prolonging its action.

Urokinase ($t^{1}/_{2}$ 16 min) made from human fetal kidney cells in tissue culture, is a direct activator of plasminogen.

Streptokinase, anistreplase and urokinase are not well absorbed by fibrin thrombi and are called nonfibrin-selective. They convert plasminogen to plasmin in the circulation, which depletes plasma fibrinogen and induces a general hypocoagulable coagulant state. This does not reduce their local thrombolytic potential but increases the risk of bleeding.

Recombinant prourokinase ($t^{1}/_{2}$ 7 min), as the name suggests, is produced by recombinant DNA technology; on binding to fibrin it converts to urokinase.

Alteplase (rt-PA) ($t^{1}/_{2}$ 30 min) is tissue type plasminogen activator produced by recombinant DNA technology.

Recombinant prourokinase and alteplase are termed fibrin-selective, for they bind strongly to fibrin, and are capable of dissolving ageing or lysis-resistant thrombi better than nonfibrin-selective agents. These drugs are less likely to produce a coagulation disturbance in the plasma, i.e. they are selective for thrombi.

USES OF FIBRINOLYTIC DRUGS

Coronary artery thrombolysis (See Ch. 24)

Timing of administration. The earlier thrombolysis is given the better the outcome. Treatment commencing within the first 3 h of onset is a realistic aim but thrombolysis up to 12 h is yet worth while.

Anistreplase can be given i.v. over 4–5 min (and so more easily out of hospital); its effect persists for 6–9 h. Other agents are normally infused i.v. over 1–3 h with most of the dose being given early in that period.

Reduction in mortality (see also Myocardial infarction, p. 447). There is now compelling evidence that streptokinase, anistreplase and alteplase reduce mortality with an acceptable frequency of adverse effects.[9] Comparisons between these drugs show no apparent advantage of one over the others in respect of survival.[10,11] Those under 75 years appeared to gain most from thrombus dispersal but 'physiological' age is more important than chronological age.

Stroke may complicate myocardial infarction and is considered usually to be embolic, for its incidence correlates with the extent of myocardial infarction. Evidence[12] indicates, however, that the combination of thrombolysis plus aspirin lowers the overall risk of stroke, possibly by limiting the size of the infarct, or by reducing thromboembolic episodes, or by both.

Thrombolysis may also be valuable in persistent unstable angina and especially where arteriography demonstrates substantial thrombus in coronary arteries.

Adverse effects. Bleeding is the most important complication and usually occurs at a vascular lesion, e.g. the site of injection, for fibrinolytic therapy does not distinguish between an undesired thrombus and a useful haemostatic plug. If the contraindications (below) are followed, the incidence of bleeding severe enough to require transfusion is <1%.

Nausea and vomiting may occur.

Multiple microemboli from disintegration of pre-existing thrombus anywhere in the vascular system may endanger life; these commonly originate in an enlarged left atrium, or a ventricular or aortic aneurysm.

Cardiac dysrhythmias result from reperfusion of ischaemic tissue. These vary in type and are often transient, a factor which may influence the decision whether or not to treat.

[9] Carins J A et al 1992 Chest 102 (Suppl): 482S–507S.

[10] The International Study Group 1990 Lancet 336: 71.

[11] ISIS-3 Collaborative Group 1992 Lancet 339: 753.

[12] ISIS-2 Collaborative Group 1988 Lancet 2: 349.

Allergy. Streptokinase and anistreplase are antigenic and anaphylactic reactions with rash, urticaria and hypotension may occur for most people have circulating antibodies to streptococci. Antibodies persist after exposure to these drugs and their *re-use should be avoided* between 5 days and 12 months as the recommended dose may not overcome immune resistance to plasminogen activation.

Contraindications to fibrinolytic drug use (see Myocardial infarction, p. 448).

Non-coronary thrombolysis

Pulmonary embolism. Thrombolysis is superior to heparin at relieving obstructed veins demonstrated radiologically. While a reduction in mortality is thus implied, the numbers of cases reported in clinical trials of thrombolytics have been insufficient to provide conclusive statistical proof. There is, nevertheless, a strong impression that thrombolysis is beneficial where pulmonary embolism is accompanied by signs of haemodynamic decompensation (raised jugular venous pressure, pulse rate >100 beats/min, systolic pressure <100 mm of mercury, arterial oxygen desaturation). Alteplase 100 mg may be infused over 2 h, followed by an i.v. infusion of heparin.

Deep venous thrombosis. Thrombolysis may be justified where the affected vesssels are proximal and the risk of pulmonary embolism is high.

Systemic or local thrombolysis may be considered for arterial occlusions distal to the popliteal artery, (thrombectomy being the usual therapeutic approach for occlusion of <24 h duration proximal to this site). Intravenous streptokinase will lyse 80% of occlusions if infusion begins within 12 h, and 60% if it is delayed for up to 3 days.

Thrombolysis may also be considered for ocular thrombosis (urokinase) and for thrombosed arteriovenous shunts (streptokinase).

DRUGS THAT PREVENT FIBRINOLYSIS

Antifibrinolytics are useful in a number of bleeding disorders.

Tranexamic acid occupies the sites on fibrin at which plasminogen is bound and converted to plasmin (causing dissolution of fibrin); fibrinolysis is thus retarded. The $t^{1/2}$ is 1.5 h after an i.v. bolus injection and it is excreted largely unchanged in the urine.

The principal indication for tranexamic acid is to prevent the hyperplasminaemic bleeding state that results from damage to certain tissues rich in plasminogen activator, e.g. after prostatic surgery, tonsillectomy, uterine cervical conisation, and menorrhagia, whether primary or induced by an intrauterine contraceptive device. Tranexamic acid may also reduce bleeding after ocular trauma and in haemophiliacs after dental extraction where it is normally used in combination with desmopressin. The drug benefits some patients with hereditary angioedema presumably by preventing the plasmin-induced uncontrolled activation of the complement system which characterises that condition. Tranexamic acid may be of value in thrombocytopenia (idiopathic or following cytotoxic chemotherapy) to reduce the risk of haemorrhage by inhibiting natural fibrinolytic destabilisation of small platelet plugs; the requirement for platelet transfusion is thereby reduced. It may also be used for overdose with thrombolytic agents.

Adverse effects are rare but include nausea, diarrhoea and sometimes orthostatic hypotension.

Aprotinin is a naturally occurring inhibitor of plasmin and other proteolytic enzymes which has been used to limit bleeding following open heart surgery with extracorporeal circulation, and for the treatment of life-threatening haemorrhage due to hyperplasminaemia complicating surgery of malignant tumours or thrombolytic therapy.

Platelets

SOME PHYSIOLOGY

Platelets do not stick to healthy endothelium but if a vessel wall is breached they react at the site by:

- Adhesion to the exposed tissues, especially to collagen, and release of substances including adenosine diphosphate (ADP) and the prostaglandin thromboxane-A_2, in response to which,

- Aggregation of platelets on the original deposition releases further ADP and thromboxane-A_2, whereupon,
- Transformation of platelets takes place into a solid plug and simultaneously they release their granule contents, including proteins, enzymes, enzyme inhibitors, vasoactive and other peptides and agents that participate in the coagulation process, and translocate negatively charged phospholipids to the outer surface of the plasma membrane, so providing a binding site for coagulation proteins (an activity known as platelet factor 3).

The system that enables platelets to distinguish between healthy and damaged endothelium is shown in simplified form in Figure 29.3. It is a continuation of, and should be studied in conjunction with, the general diagram for eicosanoids on page 250.

Platelet activity

1. Cyclic AMP plays a key role. High concentrations of intraplatelet cyclic AMP inhibit platelet

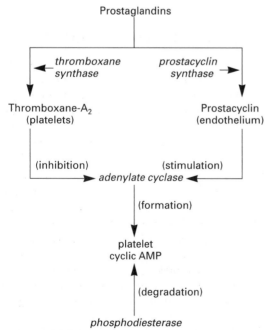

adhesion, aggregation and the release of active substances (see above), and low concentrations of cyclic AMP have the opposite effect.

2. The quantity of cyclic AMP within platelets is under enzymatic control, for it is formed by the action of adenylate cyclase and degraded by phosphodiesterase.

3. Platelet adenylate cyclase formation in turn is stimulated by prostacyclin (from the endothelium) and inhibited by thromboxane-A_2 (from within platelets). Hence the action of thromboxane-A_2 lowers cyclic AMP concentration and promotes platelet adhesion; prostacyclin raises cyclic AMP concentration and prevents platelet adhesion.

4. Prostacyclin and thromboxane-A_2 are derived from arachidonic acid which is a constituent of cell walls, both platelet and endothelial. Cyclo-oxygenase (now called prostaglandin G/H synthase), an enzyme present in cells at both sites, converts arachidonic acid to cyclic endoperoxides which are further metabolised by prostacyclin synthase to prostacyclin in the endothelium and by thromboxane synthase to thromboxane-A_2 in platelets. Thus prostacyclin is principally formed in the endothelium whereas thromboxane-A_2 is formed mainly in platelets.

5. These differences in the prostaglandins synthesised in endothelium and platelets are important. Intact vascular endothelium does not attract platelets because of the high concentration of prostacyclin in the intima. Subintimal tissues contain little prostacyclin and platelets, under the influence of thromboxane-A_2, immediately adhere and aggregate at any breach in the intima. Atheromatous plaques do not generate prostacyclin — which explains platelet adhesion and thrombosis at these sites.

Inhibitors or activators of platelet aggregation act directly or indirectly by altering the rate of formation or degradation of platelet cyclic AMP. Local concentrations of these substances determine whether the platelet adhesion/aggregation process will occur.

DRUGS THAT INHIBIT PLATELET ACTIVITY (ANTIPLATELET DRUGS)
(See also Ch. 24)

Aspirin (acetylsalicylic acid) acetylates and thus

Fig. 29.3 Prostacyclin, thromboxane and the formation of platelet cyclic AMP

inactivates prostaglandin G/H synthase (cyclo-oxygenase), the enzyme responsible for the first step in the formation of prostaglandins, the conversion of arachidonic acid to prostaglandin H_2. It follows from the diagram on page 250 (Fig. 15.1) that aspirin can prevent formation of both thromboxane-A_2 and prostacyclin. Acylation of prostaglandin G/H synthase is irreversible and, as the platelet is unable to synthesise new enzyme, prostaglandin G/H synthase activity is irreversibly lost for its lifetime (8–10 d). Therapeutic interest in the antithrombotic effect of aspirin has centred on separating its actions on thromboxane-A_2 and prostacyclin formation, and this can be achieved by using low dose. Thus 75–100 mg/d by mouth is sufficient to abolish synthesis of thromboxane-A_2 without significant impairment of prostacyclin formation, i.e. amounts substantially below the 2.4 g/d used to control pain and inflammation. Even low dose aspirin is not without risk: some 13% of episodes of peptic ulcer bleeds in people over 60 years can be attributed to prophylactic asprin (use in the community about 8%).[13]

Dipyridamole reversibly inhibits platelet phosphodiesterase (see Fig. 29.3) and in consequence cyclic AMP concentration is increased and platelet (thrombotic) reactivity reduced; evidence also suggests that its antithrombotic effect may derive from release of prostaglandin precursors by vascular endothelium. Dipyridamole is extensively bound to plasma proteins and has a $t^{1/2}$ of 12 h.

Dextrans, particularly of mol. wt. 70 000 (dextran 70), alter platelet function and prolong the bleeding time. Dextrans differ from the other antiplatelet drugs which tend to be used for arterial thrombosis; dextran 70 reduces the incidence of postoperative venous thromboembolism if it is given during or just after surgery. The dose should not exceed 10% of the estimated blood volume.

Ticlopidine inhibits the binding of fibrinogen to platelets and also interferes with a variety of platelet activities which sugggests an effect on some basic platelet function. It appears to be converted to its active form by presystemic metabolism and the $t^{1/2}$ of the parent drug varies between 30 and 50 h. Ticolopidine may be used to prevent stroke in patients who are intolerant of aspirin, providing a similar degree of protection. Clinical trials indicate that it reduces the risk of coronary and other vascular events after acute myocardial infarction and in unstable angina, and that it increases walking distance and speed in patients with peripheral arterial disease. Neutropenia is the most serious adverse effect (risk 2.4%) and is greatest in the first 12 weeks of therapy; leucocyte counts every 2 weeks are recommended during this period. Diarrhoea and other gastrointestinal symptoms may be induced in a third of patients.

Epoprostenol (prostacyclin) ($t^{1/2}$ 3 min) may be given to prevent platelet loss during renal dialysis, with or without heparin; it is infused i.v. and s.c. It is a potent vasodilator.

Abciximab is a monoclonal antibody which blocks the platelet glycoprotein IIb/IIIa receptor that is necessary for platelet binding to fibrinogen, and *dazoxiben*, an inhibitor of thromboxane-A_2 but not of prostacyclin synthesis, are being evaluated in cardiovascular disease.

USES OF ANTIPLATELET DRUGS

Antiplatelet therapy protects 'at risk' patients against stroke, myocardial infarction or death. A meta-analysis of 145 clinical trials of prolonged antiplatelet therapy versus control and 29 trials between antiplatelet regimens found that the chance of nonfatal myocardial infarction and nonfatal stroke were reduced by one third, and that there was a one sixth reduction in the risk of death from any vascular cause.[14] Expressed in another way, in the first month after an acute myocardial infarction (a vulnerable period) aspirin prevents death, stroke or a further heart attack in about 4 patients for every 100 treated. Aspirin is by far the most commonly used antiplatelet agent. The optimum dose is not known but one not exceeding aspirin 325 mg is acceptable, and 75–150 mg/d may be as effective

[13] Weil J et al 1995 Prophylactic aspirin and risk of peptic ulcer bleeding. British Medical Journal 310: 827.

[14] Antiplatelet Trialists' Collaboration 1994 British Medical Journal 308: 81.

and preferred where there is gastric intolerance. Aspirin alone (mainly) or aspirin plus dipyridamole greatly reduced the risk of occlusion where vascular grafts or arterial patency was studied systematically.[15]

Many patients who take aspirin for vascular disease may also require an NSAID for, e.g. joint disease, and it may be argued that the NSAID renders aspirin unnecessary as both act by inhibition of prostaglandin G/H synthase. As inhibition by aspirin is irreversible and that by NSAIDs may not be, continued use of aspirin in such circumstances seems prudent, especially if NSAID use is intermittent.

SUMMARY

- *Myocardial infarction.* Aspirin should be given indefinitely to patients who have survived myocardial infarction. There is as yet no case for using aspirin to prevent myocardial infarction in those without important risk factors for the disease.
- *Transient ischaemic attacks* (TIAs) or minor ischaemic stroke. There is grave risk of progression to completed stroke and patients should receive aspirin indefinitely. Before starting treatment it is important to exclude intracerebral haemorrhage (by computed tomography) and other conditions that mimic TIAs, e.g. cardiac dysrhythmia, migraine, focal epilepsy and hypoglycaemia.
- *Unstable angina.* The chance of myocardial infarction is high and aspirin should be used with other drugs , i.e. a β-adrenoceptor antagonist, a nitrite, a calcium channel blocker and possibly heparin i.v. as is judged appropriate.
- *Arterial grafts,* peripheral vascular disease. Aspirin (possibly combined with dipyridamole for grafts) should be given to prevent occlusion. These drugs may also be used to protect against thrombotic occlusion following percutaneous transluminal coronary angioplasty.

Haemostatics

Ethamsylate (Dicynene) is given systemically to reduce capillary bleeding, e.g. in menorrhagia.

---

[15] Antiplatelet Trialists' Collaboration 1994 British Medical Journal 308: 159.

Adrenaline (epinephrine) may be useful in epistaxis, stopping haemorrhage by local vasoconstriction when applied by packing the nostril with ribbon gauze soaked in adrenaline solution.

Fibrin glue consists of fibrinogen and thrombin contained in two syringes, the tips of which form a common port. The two components are thus delivered in equal volumes to a bleeding point where fibrinogen is converted to fibrin at a rate determined by the concentration of thrombin. Fibrin glue can be used to secure surgical haemostasis, e.g. on a large raw surface, and to prevent external oozing of blood in patients with haemophilia (see also below).

Sclerosing agents. Chemicals may be used to cause inflammation and thrombosis in veins so as to induce permanent obliteration, e.g. ethanolamine oleate injection, sodium tetradecyl sulphate (given i.v. for varicose veins) and oily phenol injection (given submucously for haemorrhoids). Local reactions, tissue necrosis and embolus can occur.

Haemophilia

Management of the haemophilias (genetic deficiencies of the factor VIII or IX) is a matter for those with special expertise but the following points are of general interest.

- Bleeding can sometimes be stopped by pressure; edges of superficial wounds should be strapped, not stitched.
- In haemophilia A antihaemophilic globulin (factor VIII) concentrate ($t^1/_2$ 12 h) should be used for bleeding that is more than minor.
- Factor IX ($t^1/_2$ 18 h) likewise for haemophilia B (Christmas disease).
- Tranexamic acid helps stabilise thrombi in both diseases.

Desmopressin (DDAVP) 0.3 microgram/kg body weight i.v. increases factor VIII and IX activity by 3–5 times baseline in mild to moderate haemophilia; its use may render unnecessary transfusion after minor procedures such as dental extraction. It is also effective in von Willebrand's disease for which DDAVP opens the prospect of nontransfusional treatment. Patients with severe deficiencies do not respond to DDAVP. Plasma-derived clotting factors which carry the risk of disease transmission are being replaced by recombinant-DNA derived factors. The cloning of the factor VIII gene and development of retroviral-vector delivery systems have raised the possibility that the defect in haemophilia A may be corrected by gene therapy. In a sense this is already a reality; patients with haemophilia A who underwent liver transplantation for progressive hepatic disease were found to be producing haemostatic concentrations of factor VIII.

GUIDE TO FURTHER READING

Atrah H I 1994 Fibrin glue. British Medical Journal 308: 933

Cobbe S M 1994 Thrombolysis in myocardial infarction. The earlier the better, but how late is late? British Medical Journal 308: 216

Collen D 1993 Towards improved thrombolytic therapy. Lancet 342: 34

Furie B, Furie B C 1992 Molecular and cellular biology of blood coagulation. New England Journal of Medicine 326: 800

Herbert P 1994 Suspected myocardial infarction and the GP. Give aspirin. British Medical Journal 388: 734

Hirsh J 1995 The optimal duration of anticoagulant therapy for venous thrombosis. New England Journal of Medicine 332: 1710

Hoyer L W 1994 Hemophilia. New England Journal of Medicine 330: 38

Khamashta M A, Hughes G R V 1993 Antiphospholipid syndrome. British Medical Journal 307: 883

Lefkovits J et al 1995 Platelet glycoprotein IIb/IIIa receptors in cardiovascular medicine. New England Journal of Medicine 332: 1553

Lip G Y H et al 1996 Antithrombotic treatment for atrial fibrillation. British Medical Journal 312: 45

Patrono C 1994 Aspirin as an antiplatelet drug. New England Journal of Medicine 330: 1287

Schafer A I 1994 Hypercoagulable states: molecular genetics to clinical practice. Lancet 344: 1739

Schafer A I 1966 Low–molecular–weight heparin — an opportunity for home treatment of venous thrombosis. New England Journal of Medicine 334: 724

Shearer M J 1995 Vitamin K. Lancet 345: 229

ten Cate J W 1993 Thrombolytic treatment of pulmonary embolism. Lancet 341: 1315

Underwood M J, More R S 1994 The aspirin papers. British Medical Journal 308: 71 (Refers to British Medical Journal 308: 81, 195, 235)

Ware J A, Heistad D D 1993 Platelet-endothelium interaction. New England Journal of Medicine 328: 628

Weinmann E E, Saltzman E W 1994 Deep-vein thrombosis. New England Journal of Medicine 331: 1630

World Health Organization Collaborative Study of cardiovascular disease and steroid hormone contraception 1995 Venous thromboembolic disease and combined oral contraceptives: results of international multi-centre case-control study. Lancet 346: 1575

Cellular disorders and anaemias

SYNOPSIS

- Iron: therapy, acute overdose
- Vitamin B$_{12}$ (cobalamins)
- Folic acid
- Haemopoietic growth factors
- Polycythaemia rubra vera
- Aplastic anaemia

Drug-induced cellular blood disorders: granulocytopenia, thrombocytopenia, aplastic anaemia, haemolysis.
Leukaemias and lymphomas.

Some facts and figures

- Total body iron is 3–5 g (male > female).
- Haemoglobin contains about two-thirds of total iron.
- Stores comprise about one-third (ferritin, a water-soluble protein–iron complex, and an insoluble aggregate, haemosiderin) in liver, marrow, spleen and muscle.
- Diet (average Western) contains 10–15 mg iron/day.
- Normal human absorbs 5–10% dietary iron, i.e. 0.5–1.0 mg/d, which is adequate for an adult male or postmenopausal female but the menstruating or pregnant woman requires 1–3 mg/d.
- Iron deficient or pregnant woman absorbs about 30% of dietary iron.
- Iron is lost from the body mainly in desquamated skin and gut cells.
- Menstrual loss is about 30 mg/period; menstruating women may therefore be in negative iron balance.

Iron

Iron, which was the metal symbolising strength in magical systems, used to be given to people suffering from weakness, and no doubt many were benefited, some psychologically (placebo reactors) and others because they had anaemia. The rational use of iron could not begin until both the presence of iron in the 'colouring matter' of the blood and the 'defective nature of the colouring matter' in anaemia were recognised.

IRON KINETICS

Iron absorption takes place chiefly in the duodenum where the acid environment enhances solubility, but also throughout the gut, allowing sustained-release preparations to be used. Most iron in food is present as ferric hydroxide, ferric-protein complexes or haem-protein complexes. Ferrous (Fe^{++}) iron is more readily absorbed than ferric (Fe^{+++}) and a reducing agent, such as ascorbic acid, increases the amount of the ferrous form; ascorbic acid 50 mg increases iron absorption from a meal by 2–3 times. Food reduces iron absorption.

The process of absorption regulates the amount of iron entering the body according to need, i.e. the state of the iron stores. Dietary and administered iron is actively transported into the gut mucosal cell. Iron that is not needed by the body is bound to a protein (apoferritin) as *ferritin* and this is lost into the gut lumen when the mucosal cell is shed (2–3 days); it is eliminated at near constant rate in the faeces in healthy people. Iron that is needed forms a labile pool within the cell; if this pool is excessive it stimulates production of more apoferritin to bind and lose more iron as ferritin. Labile pool iron in the Fe^{+++} form enters the blood bound to a transport globulin, *transferrin*, which delivers it to the sites of physiological need, principally erythrocyte precursors (80%) (where it forms haem), the rest to muscles (myoglobin), and to form iron-containing enzymes, e.g. cytochromes, in all body cells. There is a small amount of ferritin in the blood in balance with the iron stores.

Iron is stored as ferritin and its aggregate, *haemosiderin*, in the cells of the liver, bone marrow and spleen. A measure of the state of iron stores is provided by the amount of ferritin in the blood (normally 20–300 μmol/l) and by the relationship of serum iron concentration (normally 10–30 μmol/l; low in iron deficiency) to the binding capacity of transferrin (normally 45–70 μmol/l; high in iron deficiency). Ferritin is an acute-phase reactant and may be an inaccurate measure of iron stores in inflammatory states, e.g. rheumatoid arthritis.

Prolonged heavy excess of iron intake overwhelms the mechanism described and results in haemosiderosis, as there is no physiological mechanism to increase iron excretion in the face of increased absorption. Iron-deficient subjects absorb up to 20 times as much administered iron as those not in need. Abnormalities of the small intestine may interfere with either the absorption of iron, as in coeliac disease and other malabsorption syndromes, or possibly with the conversion of iron into a soluble and reduced form, e.g. partial gastrectomy.

The formation of insoluble iron salts (such as phosphate and phytate) in the alkaline environment of most of the small intestine explains why much of the iron taken by mouth is not absorbed, even in severe iron deficiency.

Interactions. Iron chelates in the gut with tetracy-clines, penicillamine, methyldopa, levodopa, carbidopa, ciprofloxacin, norfloxacin and ofloxacin; it also forms stable complexes with thyroxine, captopril and biphosphonates. These interactions can be clinically important. Doses should be separated by 3 h.

Ascorbic acid increases absorption (above) but its use (200 mg/day) is not clinically important in routine therapy; *desferrioxamine* binds iron and reduces absorption (see Poisoning, below); *tea* (tannins) and *bran* reduce absorption.

IRON THERAPY

Iron therapy is indicated only for the prevention or cure of iron deficiency. In general terms, making 25 mg of iron per day available to the bone marrow will allow an iron deficiency anaemia to respond with a rise of 1% of haemoglobin (0.15 g Hb/100 ml) per day (beginning after 7 days' therapy); a reticulocyte response occurs between 4 and 12 days.

Oral iron therapy. When oral therapy is used it is reasonable to assume that about 30% of the iron will be absorbed and to give 180 mg of elemental iron daily for 1–3 months according to the degree of anaemia. Iron stores are less easily replenished by oral therapy than by injection, and oral therapy (at lower dose) should be continued for 3 months after the haemoglobin concentration has returned to normal (or as long as blood loss continues).

Contraindications. It is illogical to give iron in the anaemia of *chronic infection* where utilisation of iron stores is impaired; but such patients may also have true iron deficiency which may be difficult to diagnose without direct visualisation of stores in a bone marrow aspirate. Iron should not be given in *haemolytic anaemias* unless there is also haemoglobinuria, for the iron from the lysed cells remains in the body, and adding to the iron load may cause haemosiderosis.

Iron therapy is needed in:

- Iron deficiency due to dietary lack or to chronic blood loss
- Pregnancy. The extra iron required by mother and fetus totals 1000 mg, chiefly in the latter half of pregnancy. The fetus takes iron from the

mother even if she is iron deficient. Dietary iron is seldom adequate and iron and folic acid (50–100 mg elemental iron plus folic acid 200–500 micrograms/d) should be given to pregnant women from the fourth month. Opinions differ on whether all women should receive prophylaxis or only those who can be identified as needing it. There are numerous formulations. Parents should be particularly warned *not to let children get at the tablets*

- Abnormalities of the gastrointestinal tract in which the proportion of dietary iron absorbed may be reduced, i.e. in malabsorption syndromes
- Premature babies, since they are born with low iron stores, and in babies weaned late. There is very little iron in human milk and even less in cow's milk
- Early treatment of severe pernicious anaemia with hydroxocobalamin, as the iron stores occasionally become exhausted by the surge in red cell formation.

Oral iron preparations. There is an enormous variety of official and proprietary iron preparations. For each milligram of elemental iron taken by mouth, ferrous sulphate is as effective as more expensive preparations.'It is particularly important to avoid initial overdosage with iron as the resulting symptoms may cause the patient to abandon therapy. A small dose is given at first and increased after a few days. The objective is to give 100–200 mg of elemental iron per day. Iron given on a full stomach causes less gastrointestinal upset but less is absorbed than if given between meals; however, use with food is commonly preferred to improve compliance. Commonly used preparations, given in divided doses, include:

Ferrous Sulphate Tabs, 200–600 mg/d (providing 67–195 mg/d of elemental iron)
Ferrous Gluconate Tabs, 300–1200 mg daily (providing 35–140 mg/d of elemental iron)
Ferrous Furmarate Tabs, 200–600 mg daily (providing 130–195 mg/d of elemental iron)
Ferrous succinate and *ferrous glycine sulphate* are alternatives.

Choice of oral iron preparation. Oral iron is used both for therapy and for prophylaxis (pregnancy) of anaemia in people who are often feeling little if any ill-health. Because of this, the occurrence of gastrointestinal upset is particularly important as it is liable to cause the patient to give up taking iron. The evidence as to which preparation provides best iron absorption with least adverse effects is conflicting. Gastrointestinal upset is minimal if the daily dose does not exceed 180 mg elemental iron and if iron is given with food.

A suggested course. Start a patient on ferrous sulphate taken on a full stomach once, then twice, then thrice a day. If gut intolerance occurs, stop the iron and reintroduce it with one week for each step. If this seems to cause gastrointestinal upset, try ferrous gluconate, succinate or fumarate. If simple preparations (above) are unsuccessful, and this is unlikely, then the pharmaceutically sophisticated and expensive *sustained-release* preparations may be tried; they release iron slowly and only after passing the pylorus, from resins, chelates (sodium iron edetate) or plastic matrices, e.g. Slow-Fe, Ferrograd, Feospan, so that iron is released in the lower rather than the upper small intestine. Patients who cannot tolerate standard forms even when taken with food may get as much iron with fewer unpleasant symptoms if they use a sustained-release formulation.

Liquid formulations are available for adults who prefer them and for small children, e.g. Ferrous Sulphate Oral Solution, Paediatric: 5 ml contains 12 mg of elemental iron: but they stain the teeth. Polysaccharide-iron complex (Niferex): 5 ml contains 100 mg of elemental iron. There are numerous other iron preparations which can give satisfactory results.

Sustained-release and *chelated* forms of iron (see above) have the advantage that poisoning is less serious if a mother's supply is consumed by young children, a real hazard.

Iron therapy blackens the faeces but does not generally interfere with tests for occult blood (commonly needed in investigation of anaemia), though it may give a false positive with some occult blood tests, e.g. guaiac test.

Failure of oral iron therapy is most commonly due to poor patient compliance, persistent bleeding and, as with all drug therapy, wrong diagnosis.

Adverse effects. The gastrointestinal effects of oral iron include nausea, abdominal pain, and either constipation or diarrhoea.

Intramuscular iron therapy

Intramuscular iron may be required if:

- Iron cannot be absorbed from the intestine
- The patient cannot be relied on to take it or experiences intolerable gut symptoms
- A sure response is essential in a severe iron deficiency anaemia, as in late pregnancy (though here a blood transfusion may be preferred).

Speed of haemopoietic response is not quicker than that with full doses of oral iron reliably taken and normally absorbed, for both provide as much iron as an active marrow can use, but a course of injected iron is stored and utilised over months. The ionised salts of iron given orally are unsuitable as parenteral preparations as they are powerful protein precipitants and an un-ionised iron complex is used.

Iron sorbitol inj. (Jectofer; 50 mg of iron/ml) is an iron-sorbitol-citric-acid complex of mol. wt. < 5000 that is rapidly absorbed into the blood from the site of i.m. injection.

Iron sorbitol is bound to plasma globulin, transferrin, and is stored in the marrow and liver. It is not substantially taken up in the reticuloendothelial system. Excess unbound iron is excreted in the urine (about 30% of the dose) which may turn black transiently at the time of peak iron excretion or only on standing for some hours (probably due to formation of iron sulphide by bacterial action).

Oral iron therapy should be stopped 24 h before injections begin; not only is continuation unnecessary, but it may promote adverse reactions by saturating the plasma protein (transferrin) binding capacity so that the injected iron gives a higher unbound plasma iron concentration than is safe.

Dose: 1.5 mg/kg/d (up to a maximum of 100 mg/injection) until the total amount of iron required has been given. The approximate *total requirement* is ascertained from manufacturers' dosage schedules which relate the number of injections to the haemoglobin deficit. Iron sorbitol is normally given daily or on alternate days where tolerance is low. It is given by deep i.m. injection, which can be painful. It stains the skin (for up to 2 years) but this can be minimised by inserting the needle through the skin and then moving the skin and subcutaneous tissue laterally before entering the muscle so that the needle track becomes angulated when the needle is withdrawn.

The injections are usually painful and general reactions (headache, dizziness, nausea, vomiting, disorientation, pressure sensations in the chest) occur and sometimes a metallic taste, up to 2 h after injection. Iron sorbitol has been found to increase the urinary leucocyte excretion rate in patients with urinary tract infections or noninfective renal disease (which can mislead diagnosis).

Iron dextran inj. may be given as a single total dose i.v. infusion. It is stored in the reticuloendothelial system whence utilisable iron is released over months.

Folic acid deficiency may be unmasked by effective iron therapy. Where there is a deficiency of both iron and folic acid, the deficiency of the latter may not be obvious because haemopoiesis is held back by lack of iron. If iron is supplied there will be an increased formation of red cells and the folic acid deficiency will be disclosed. This is liable to happen in pregnancy and so folic acid is commonly given to all pregnant patients with anaemia (see below); it also occurs in malabsorption syndromes.

Acute overdose: poisoning

High doses of iron salts by mouth can cause severe gastrointestinal irritation and even necrosis of the mucous membrane. Autopsy shows severe damage to brain and liver. Iron poisoning is particularly dangerous in children. Sustained-release forms are safer in homes where heedless parents live with small children. Ferrous sulphate is the most toxic.

Typically acute oral iron poisoning has the following phases:

- First, 0.5–1 h after ingestion there is abdominal pain, grey/black vomit, diarrhoea, leucocytosis and hyperglycaemia. Severe cases are indicated by acidosis and cardiovascular collapse which may proceed to coma and death.

- Second, there follows a period of improvement lasting 6–12 h, which may be sustained or which may deteriorate to the next stage.
- Third, jaundice, hypoglycaemia, bleeding, encephalopathy, metabolic acidosis and convulsions are followed by cardiovascular collapse, coma and sometimes death 48–60 h after ingestion.
- Fourth, 1–2 months later, upper gastrointestinal obstruction may result from scarring and stricture.

Treatment of acute iron poisoning is urgent and immediate efforts must be made to chelate iron in the blood and in the stomach and intestine. Raw egg and milk help to bind iron until a chelating agent is available.

The first step should be to give *desferrioxamine* 1–2 g i.m.; the dose is the same in adults and children. Only after this should gastric aspiration or emesis be performed. If lavage is used, the water should contain desferrioxamine 2 g/l. After emptying the stomach, desferrioxamine 10 g in 50–100 ml water should be left in the stomach; it is not absorbed.

Subsequently, desferrioxamine should be administered by i.v. infusion not exceeding 15 mg/kg/h (maximum 80 mg/kg/24 h) or further i.m. injections (2 g in sterile water 10 ml) should be given 12-hourly. Poisoning is severe if the plasma iron concentration exceeds the total iron binding capacity (upper limit 75 μmol/l) or the plasma becomes pink due to the large formation of ferrioxamine (see below); i.v. rather than i.m. administration of desferrioxamine is then indicated.

Desferrioxamine (deferoxamine) (Desferal) (t ½ 6 h) is an iron-chelating agent (see Chelating agents). During a systematic investigation of actinomycete metabolites, iron-containing substances (sideramines) were discovered. One of these substances was ferrioxamine. The iron in this can be removed chemically, leaving desferrioxamine.

When desferrioxamine comes into contact with ferric iron, its straight-chain molecule twines around it and forms a nontoxic complex of great stability (ferrioxamine), which is excreted in the

urine giving it a red/orange colour, and in the bile. It is not absorbed from the gut and must be injected for systemic effect. In acute poisoning, as opposed to chronic overload, desferrioxamine 5 g chelates the iron contained in about 10 tablets of ferrous sulphate or gluconate. It has a negligible affinity for other metals in the presence of iron excess.

Desferrioxamine has been shown to be effective in the therapy of acute iron poisoning and in the treatment and perhaps in the diagnosis of diseases associated with chronic iron accumulation. A topical formulation is available for ocular siderosis.

Serious adverse effects are uncommon but include rashes and anaphylactic reactions; with chronic use cataract, retinal damage and deafness can occur. Hypotension occurs if desferrioxamine is infused too rapidly and there is danger of (potentially fatal) adult respiratory distress syndrome if infusion proceeds beyond 24 h.[1]

Chronic iron overload

The body is unable to excrete any excess of iron so that, if there is uncontrolled iron intake, it accumulates. Grossly excessive parenteral iron therapy or a hundred or more blood transfusions (as in treatment of thalassaemia[2]) can lead to haemosiderosis. Oral iron therapy over many years has also been reported to cause it.

Treatment of chronic iron overload, e.g. haemochromatosis, haemolytic anaemias and thalassaemia with transfusional iron overload: iron may be removed by repeated venesection when there is not anaemia (haemochromatosis) or by chelation (transfusional overload).

A single venesection of 450 ml of blood, *in the absence of anaemia*, removes 200 mg of iron and can be repeated weekly. Chelation can be effectively carried out by 12 h nocturnal s.c. infusion of desferrioxamine (on 5 nights per week). Oral ascorbic

---

[1] Tenenbein M et al 1992 Lancet 339: 699.

[2] A 26-year-old subject with beta-thalassaemia major had been transfused 404 units of blood over his lifetime. His iron stores were so high (estimated at above 100 g) that he triggered a metal detector at an airport security checkpoint (Jim R T S 1979 Lancet 2: 1028).

acid increases the availability of free iron for chelation. This regimen can put a patient living a life dependent on red-cell transfusions into the desired negative iron balance. The expense of doing this over a long period is currently enormous and raises serious ethical problems in economically poor countries where most of these patients live. *Deferiprone*, which is taken by mouth, may provide an alternative but the risk of agranulocytosis restricts its use.

Vitamin B$_{12}$

PERNICIOUS ANAEMIA

In 1925, it was demonstrated that 2 factors were required to cure pernicious anaemia: one in the food (extrinsic factor) and one in gastric juice (intrinsic factor).

- The *extrinsic factor, cyanocobalamin (vitamin B$_{12}$)*, was isolated in 1948.
- The *intrinsic factor* (a glycoprotein secreted by the gastric acid-forming cells) acts solely as a vehicle for carrying the important extrinsic factor into the body via receptors in the ileum. Some cyanocobalamin may be absorbed by diffusion, i.e. independently of intrinsic factor, though less reliably and only with large doses.

THE COBALAMINS

The active cellular coenzymes (vitamin B$_{12}$) are necessary for demethylation of tetrahydrofolate and thus for DNA synthesis. They are formed in the body from administered *hydroxocobalamin* and cyanocobalamin. Hydroxocobalamin is preferred for clinical use.

Deficiency of vitamin B$_{12}$ in the body leads to:

- Megaloblastic anaemia
- Degeneration of the brain, spinal cord (subacute combined degeneration) and peripheral nerves; symptoms may be psychiatric and physical
- Abnormalities of epithelial tissue, particularly of the alimentary tract, e.g. sore tongue and malabsorption.

Requirements of cobalamins are about 3.0 micrograms/d. Absorption takes place mainly in the terminal ileum, and they are carried in plasma bound to proteins (transcobalamins). They are not significantly metabolised and pass into the bile (there is enterohepatic circulation which can be interrupted by intestinal disease and hastens the onset of clinical deficiency), and are excreted via the kidney. Body stores amount to about 5 mg (mainly in the liver) and are sufficient for 2–4 years if absorption ceases. Most animals cannot synthesise cobalamin and so are directly or indirectly dependent upon microorganisms for it. Humans get most of their cobalamins from meat; bacteria in the human colon synthesise it but it is not absorbed from this part of the intestine. Rabbits in the wild would suffer from B$_{12}$ deficiency if they did not eat their own faeces.

Dietary deficiency is virtually confined to people who have not enough money to buy meat, and to Vegans, a sect of particularly uncompromising vegetarians.

INDICATIONS FOR VITAMIN B$_{12}$

Indications for administration are the prevention and cure of conditions due to its deficiency.

Pernicious (Addisonian) anaemia. The atrophic gastric mucosa is unable to produce intrinsic factor (and acid); there is failure to absorb vitamin B$_{12}$ so that deficiency results. Despite its name (given when no treatment was known), the prognosis of a patient with uncomplicated pernicious anaemia, properly treated with hydroxocobalamin, is little different from that of the rest of the population. The neurological complications, particularly spasticity, develop only after prolonged severe deficiency but may be permanent. Total removal of the stomach or atrophy of the mucous membrane in a postgastrectomy remnant may, after several years, lead to a similar anaemia.

Malabsorption syndromes. In stagnant loop syndrome (which can be remedied by a broad-spectrum antimicrobial), ileal resection, Crohn's disease and chronic tropical sprue, vitamin B$_{12}$ and folic acid deficiency are common although megaloblastic anaemia occurs only relatively late.

Tobacco amblyopia has been attributed to cyanide intoxication from strong tobacco which interferes with the coenzyme function of vitamin B_{12}; hydroxocobalamin (**not** cyanocobalamin) may be given.

DIAGNOSIS OF B_{12} DEFICIENCY

The serum concentration of vitamin B_{12} is low (normal 170–925 ng/l). In addition, absorption of radioactive vitamin B_{12} (*Schilling test*) helps to distinguish between gastric and intestinal causes.

First: the patient is given a small dose of radioactive vitamin B_{12} *orally*, with a simultaneous large dose of nonradioactive vitamin B_{12} *intramuscularly*. The large injected dose saturates binding sites so that any of the oral radioactive dose that is absorbed cannot bind and will be eliminated in the urine where it can easily be measured (normally >10% of the administered dose appears in urine collected for 24 h, if renal function is normal). In pernicious anaemia gut absorption, and therefore radioactivity in the plasma (measured 8–12 h later), and urine are negligible.

Second: the test is repeated with intrinsic factor added to the oral dose. The radioactive vitamin B_{12} is now absorbed in pernicious anaemia (but not in intestinal malabsorption) and is detected in plasma and urine. Both stages of the test are needed to maximise reliability of diagnosis of pernicious anaemia.

CONTRAINDICATIONS TO VITAMIN B_{12}

Inadequately diagnosed anaemia is an important contraindication. Therapy of pernicious anaemia must be both adequate and life-long, so that accurate diagnosis is essential. Even a single dose of vitamin B_{12} interferes with the haematological picture for weeks, although the Schilling test remains diagnostic.

PREPARATIONS AND USE

Hydroxocobalamin is bound to plasma protein to a greater extent than is cyanocobalamin, with the result that there is less free to be excreted in the urine after an injection and rather lower doses at longer intervals are adequate. This is why it is preferred to cyanocobalamin, though the latter can give satisfactory results.

The initial dose in cobalamin deficiency anaemias, including uncomplicated pernicious anaemia, is hydroxocobalamin 1 mg i.m. every 2–3 days for 5 doses to induce remission and to replenish stores. Maintenance may be 1 mg every 3 months; higher doses will not find binding sites and will be eliminated in the urine. But higher doses should probably be used in renal and hepatic disease (due to defects in conversion to the active coenzyme and excretion).

After initiation of therapy, patients feel better in 2 days, reticulocytes peak at 7 days and haemoglobin concentration rises by 0.1 g/dl/d.

Failure to respond implies wrong or incomplete diagnosis. The initial stimulation of haemoglobin synthesis often depletes the *iron* and *folate* stores and supplements of these may be needed.

Hypokalaemia may occur at the height of the erythrocyte response in severe cases. It is attributed to uptake of potassium by the rapidly increasing erythrocyte mass. Oral potassium should be given.

Inadequate response should be treated by increased frequency of injections as well as increased amount (because of urinary loss with high plasma concentrations).

Haemoglobin estimations are necessary at least every 6 months to check adequacy of therapy and for early detection of iron deficiency anaemia due to carcinoma of the stomach, which occurs in about 5% of patients with pernicious anaemia.

When injections are refused or are impracticable (rare allergy, bleeding disorder), administration as snuff or aerosol has been effective, but these routes are potentially less reliable. Large daily oral doses (1000 micrograms) are probably preferable; monitoring of the blood must be more frequent. *Cyanocobalamin* remains available.

Adverse effects virtually do not occur, but use of vitamin B_{12} as a 'tonic' is an abuse of a powerful remedy for it may obscure the diagnosis of pernicious anaemia, which is a matter of great importance in a disease requiring life-long therapy and prone to serious neurological complications.

In pernicious anaemia, folic acid should not be used alone. Although the anaemia improves (because vitamin B_{12} plays a role in folate metabolism), it allows progression of subacute combined degeneration of the nervous system.

Folic acid (pteroylglutamic acid)

Folic acid[3] was so named because it was discovered as a bacterial growth factor present in spinach leaves. It is one of the B group of vitamins and was soon shown to be the same substance as that present in yeast and liver which cured a nutritional macrocytic anaemia in Indian women.

Functions

Folic acid is itself inactive; it is converted into the biologically active coenzyme, tetrahydrofolic acid, which is important in the biosynthesis of amino acids and DNA and therefore in cell division. The formyl derivative of tetrahydrofolic acid is *folinic acid* and this can be used to bypass the block when the body fails to effect the conversion of folic acid (see Folic acid antagonists).

Ascorbic acid protects the active tetrahydrofolic acid from oxidation; the anaemia of scurvy, although usually normoblastic, may be megaloblastic due to deficiency of tetrahydrofolic acid.

Deficiency of folic acid leads to a megaloblastic anaemia probably because it is necessary for the production of the purines and pyrimidines, which are essential precursors of deoxyribonucleic acid (DNA). The megaloblastic marrow of cobalamin deficiency is due to interference with folic acid utilisation and the morphological changes of such deficiency can be reversed by folic acid. It is, however, vital to realise that folic acid **does not** provide adequate treatment for pernicious anaemia. Nor does vitamin B_{12} provide adequate treatment for the megaloblastic anaemia of folic acid deficiency although a partial response may occur.

Occurrence and requirements

Folic acid is widely distributed, especially in green

vegetables, yeast and liver. Daily requirement of folic acid is some 50–100 micrograms and a diet containing 400 micrograms of polyglutamates will provide this. Body stores last several months.

Indications

Folic acid is used to prevent or cure deficiency of folate.

Pregnancy. Folic acid requirement is increased to 300–400 microgram a day. This cannot be met from the diet by one-third of women in Western societies and the problem is greater in less economically developed countries where nutritional deficiency may be aggravated by high red cell turnover due to haemoglobinopathies and endemic malaria. For this reason folic acid is added to iron for prophylaxis of anaemia. The dose needed is about 300 micrograms folic acid a day, which is insufficient to alter the blood picture of pernicious anaemia and so there is no risk of masking that disease, which is also very rare in women of reproductive age and is probably incompatible with a successful pregnancy. A large number of preparations of iron with folic acid is available (see also Iron therapy, p. 535). They are suitable only for prevention. Larger doses may be used in therapy of anaemia during pregnancy (see below); it will remit spontaneously some weeks after delivery. Vigorous iron therapy in pregnancy may unmask a folate deficiency.

Prevention of fetal neural tube defect (spina bifida). Folic acid supplement taken before conception and during the early weeks of pregnancy has been shown in an 8-year trial to prevent the condition in pregnancies subsequent to an affected birth.[4] Women hoping to conceive and who have had an affected child are advised to take folic acid 5 mg/d; to prevent a first occurrence 0.4 mg/d should be taken both before conception, or as soon as possible after diagnosis, and for the first 12 weeks of pregnancy.

Premature infants. Supplementation is needed because these infants miss the build-up of folate stores which normally occurs in the last few weeks of pregnancy.

---

[3] Latin: *folium*, a leaf.

[4] MRC Vitamin Study research group 1991 Lancet 338: 131.

Malabsorption syndromes. Particularly in gluten-sensitive enteropathy and tropical sprue, poor absorption of folic acid from the small intestine often leads to a megaloblastic anaemia.

Drugs. Antiepileptics, particularly phenytoin, primidone and phenobarbitone, occasionally cause a macrocytic anaemia that responds to folic acid. This may be due to enzyme induction by the antiepileptics increasing the need for folic acid to perform hydroxylations (see Epilepsy) but other factors may be involved. Some antimalarials, e.g. pyrimethamine, may interfere with conversion of folates to the active tetrahydrofolic acid, causing macrocytic anaemia. Methotrexate, another folate antagonist, may cause a megaloblastic anaemia especially when used longterm for leukaemia or psoriasis.

Miscellaneous causes of excess utilisation or loss. In chronic haemolytic states, where erythropoiesis is accelerated, and in myelofibrosis, where haemopoiesis is inefficient, folate requirement is increased. Extensive shedding of skin cells in exfoliative dermatitis, inflammatory states, e.g. rheumatoid arthritis, and malignant disease, e.g. lymphoma, can similarly lead to folate deficiency. Folate loss during chronic haemodialysis may be sufficient to require replacement.

Contraindications

Imprecisely diagnosed megaloblastic anaemia is the principal contraindication. Some cancers are folate dependent and folic acid should be used in malignant disease only where there is a confirmed folate deficiency anaemia.

Preparations and dosage

Synthetic folic acid is taken orally; for therapy 5 mg daily is usually given for 4 months, or indefinitely if the cause of deficiency cannot be removed; 15 mg/d may be needed in malabsorption states. There is no advantage in giving folinic acid instead of folic acid, except in the treatment of the toxic effects of folic acid antagonists (folinic acid 'rescue', see p. 547).

- For prophylaxis, with iron, in pregnancy, see page 536
- For prophylaxis in haemolytic diseases and in renal dialysis: 5 mg per day or per week depending on need.

Adverse reactions: allergy occurs rarely, and status epilepticus may be precipitated.

Haemopoietic growth factors

Once a cell growth factor has been identified, the cloning of the relevant gene and recombinant DNA technology allow the production of amounts sufficient for clinical use. Growth factors are now available to stimulate both erythroid and myeloid cell lines. These factors are potentially useful whenever there is deficiency of blood cell function, whether due to disease or to cytotoxic chemotherapy.

Epoetin (recombinant derived human erythropoietin) Erythropoietin is a glycoprotein hormone made in the kidney (90%; the remainder in the liver and other sites) in response to hypoxia. The anaemia of chronic renal failure is largely due to failure of the diseased kidney to make enough erythropoietin. The principal action of the hormone is to stimulate the proliferation and differentiation of erythrocyte precursors.

The manufacture of enough epoetin for clinical use became possible when the human gene for erythropoietin was successfully inserted into cultured hamster ovary cells.

Epoetin must be given s.c. (which may be more effective) or i.v.; the $t^1/2$ is 4 h and appears not to be affected by dialysis. Maximum reticulocyte response occurs in 4 days. Self-administration at home 3 times a week is practicable; the dose is adjusted by response. Iron reserves must be adequate for optimum erythropoiesis, i.e. serum ferritin should exceed 100 micrograms/l. Epoetin is available as two preparations, epoetin alpha and epoetin beta, which are interchangeable.

Epoetin is effective in the anaemia of chronic renal failure to an extent that it significantly enhances the patients' quality of life. Patients become independent of blood transfusion, with great benefit to blood transfusion services as well as to themselves.

The hormone has also been used in anaemia of rheumatoid arthritis, prematurity, following cancer chemotherapy and zidovudine-treated AIDS, and to improve the quality of presurgical autologous blood collection. It is misused by sports people seeking advantage.

Adverse effects. A dose-dependent increase in arterial blood pressure follows the rise in red cell mass and encephalopathy may occur in some previously hypertensive patients. Arteriovenous shunts, especially those that are compromised, may thrombose as a result of increased blood viscosity.

Iron deficiency may occur, as increased haematopoiesis outstrips available iron stores, and this can be a cause of inadequate response to the hormone; parenteral iron therapy may be needed.

Transient influenza-like symptoms may accompany the first i.v. injections.

COLONY-STIMULATING FACTORS

A number of cytokines (see p. 250) are known to stimulate the growth, differentiation and functional activity of colonies of myeloid cells. As the name implies the function of these polypeptides was defined in in vitro colonies assays of bone marrow progenitors. They have effects on all myeloid cells including the multipotential stem cells (but probably not the more immature pluripotential cells), intermediate progenitors and circulating mature cells. Some of those that have been developed for clinical use are described below.

Filgrastim (recombinant human granulocyte colony stimulating factor: G-CSF) speeds the maturation and proliferation of neutrophil precursors and activates their functional activity; a single dose will cause the neutrophil count to rise $\times$ 4–5 within hours and the increased count persists up to 72 h.

The drug is rapidly cleared after i.v. injection ($t^1/2$ 2 h) and administration by i.v. infusion or s.c. is necessary to prolong plasma concentration. High concentrations are found in plasma, bone marrow and kidneys. It is degraded to its component amino acids.

The principal use of filgrastim is for patients suffering neutropenia from cytotoxic chemotherapy (except myeloid malignancies). It may also be used to raise the neutrophil count and reduce the risk of infection after bone marrow transplantation, in aplastic anaemia, AIDS, and congenital, cyclical and idiopathic neutropenia.

Adverse effects. Medullary bone pain occurs with high i.v. doses. Musculoskeletal pain, dysuria, splenomegaly, allergic reactions and abnormality of liver enzymes also occur.

Lenograstim is similar.

Molgramostim (recombinant human granulocyte macrophage-colony stimulating factor: GM-CSF) ($t^1/2$ 3 h) has a broader spectrum of activity than filgrastim, stimulating both monocyte and granulocyte production with functional effects on the mature cells of both cell lines. Administration by i.v. infusion or s.c. is needed to maintain plasma concentration.

Molgramostim is used to reduce cytotoxic-induced neutropenia and in bone marrow transplantation, aplastic anaemia and for neutropenia caused by ganciclovir and for AIDS-related cytomegalovirus retinitis.

Adverse effects. Molgramostim causes medullary bone pain, skin rashes, lethargy and myalgia in 10–20% of patients. It may also cause fever, the interpretation of which presents a clinical dilemma in neutropenic patients who are subject to sepsis. Pleural and pericardial effusions occur after high doses.

Sargramostim is similar.

Polycythaemia rubra vera

The principles of treatment are:

All patients: reduce packed cell volume to normal by venesection (300–500 ml) every 2 days.

Attempt to maintain normal status by occasional venesection. Iron deficiency may occur and need treatment although this may result in a need for more frequent venesection.

If frequent venesection is required to maintain a normal haematocrit or if the platelet count continues high (added risk of thrombosis) then:

Younger patients: use cytotoxic chemotherapy with continuous hydroxyurea or intermittent busulphan (see Ch. 31) to maintain a normal haematocrit.

Older patients: radiophosphorus may provide prolonged control of erythroid hyperproliferation.

Radiophosphorus (^{32}P, sodium radiophosphate) is given i.v. Phosphorus is concentrated in bone and in cells that are dividing rapidly, so that the erythrocyte precursors in the bone marrow receive most of the β-irradiation. The effects are similar to those of whole-body irradiation, and in polycythaemia rubra vera ^{32}P is now a treatment of choice for those >65 years (accumulation in the gonads precludes its use in younger patients). The maximum effect on the blood count is delayed 1–2 months after the dose; a single dose usually provides control for 1–2 years. Excessive depression of the bone marrow including leucocytes and platelets is the main adverse effect, but is seldom serious.

Secondary leukaemia occurs with both classes of therapy.

Pruritus is troublesome and difficult to relieve; it may be helped by H$_1$- and H$_2$-histamine receptor blockers alone or together.

Hyperuricaemia, due to cell destruction, is prevented by allopurinol; and *iron* and *folate deficiency* by replacement doses.

Low dose aspirin (for antiplatelet action) may be used if the platelet count continues high or thrombosis occurs despite the above treatment.

Aplastic anaemia

Treatment will be chosen according to the severity of the cytopenia, the age of the patient, the availability of a suitable bone marrow donor and, less commonly, the cause (if known). Choices include bone marrow transplantation and immunosuppression, e.g. with antilymphocytic globulin, corticosteroid and perhaps cyclosporin; and haemopoietic growth factors (see above).

GUIDE TO FURTHER READING

Armitage J O 1994 Bone marrow transplantation. New England Journal of Medicine 330: 827

Bates C J et al 1989 Vitamins, iron, and physical work. Lancet 2: 313

Campbell N R C et al 1991 Iron supplements: a common cause of drug interactions. British Journal of Clinical Pharmacology 31: 251

Canadian Orthopedic Perioperative Erythropoietin Study Group 1993 Effectiveness of perioperative recombinant human erythropoietin in elective hip replacement. Lancet 341: 1227

Castle W B 1966 Treatment of pernicious anaemia: historical aspects. Clinical Pharmacology and Therapeutics 7: 347

Chanarin I 1992 Pernicious anaemia. British Medical Journal 304: 1584

Charache S et al 1995 Effect of hydroxyurea on the frequency of painful crises in sickle cell anaemia. New England Journal of Medicine 332: 1317

Ferner R E et al 1989 Drugs in donated blood. Lancet 2: 93

George J N et al 1994 Chronic idiopathic thrombocytopenic purpura. New England Journal of Medicine 331: 1207

Hoeldtke R D et al 1993 Treatment of orthostatic hypotension with erythropoietin. New England Journal of Medicine 329: 611

Lieschke G J et al 1992 Granulocyte colony-stimulating factor and granulocyte-macrophage colony-stimulating factor. New England Journal of Medicine 327: 28 (first part), 99 (second part)

MRC Vitamin study research group 1991 Prevention of neural tube defects: results of the Medical Research Council vitamin study. Lancet 338: 131, also 153 (Editorial) 379 (subsequent correspondence)

Oliveri N F et al 1995 Iron-chelating therapy with deferiprone in patients with thalassaemia major. New England Journal of Medicine 332: 918

Steward W P 1993 Granulocyte and granulocyte-macrophage colony-stimulating factors. Lancet 342: 153

Neoplastic disease and immunosuppression

SYNOPSIS

Neoplastic disease

About 75% of cancers are due to environmental factors, some of which are within the control of the individual, e.g. tobacco smoking, exposure to sunlight. When cancer has developed patients are naturally not interested in being told that they might have avoided it by personal action over past decades. Here we discuss treatment, cure and palliation of cancer with emphasis on drugs and hormones.

- Prevention and cure
- Cytotoxic drugs
- Cytotoxic chemotherapy
- Adverse effects
- Endocrine therapy
- Immunotherapy and biological control of cancer
- Chemoprophylaxis of cancer

Immunosuppression

- Uses
- Hazards

Neoplastic disease

Prevention and cure

Malignant disease is of immense variety.

Prevention, by drugs, of the change that converts a normal cell to an invasive malignant cell has only now begun to be attained (p. 561). Some cancers can be prevented, wholly or in part, by protecting people or inviting them to protect themselves from exposure to known carcinogens (industrial cancers, bronchial cancer).

Attempts to cure or palliate cancer employ five principal modes:

1. surgery
2. radiotherapy
3. chemotherapy[1]
4. endocrine therapy
5. immunotherapy, including cytokines.

Details of the exploitation of all of these techniques, whether alone, sequentially or concurrently

---

[1] Although not in strict accord with the definition of Chapter 11, the word chemotherapy is in general use in this connection and it would be pedantic to avoid it. It arose because some malignant cells can be cultured and the disease transmitted by inoculation, as with bacteria. Some prefer to call it anticytotic or cytotoxic therapy.

is beyond the scope of a book on clinical pharmacology. This account will be substantially confined to drugs.

ENDOCRINE INFLUENCE ON CANCER

The possibility of interfering with cancer other than by surgery, e.g. by endocrine manipulation, was first tested in 1895 when a Scottish surgeon faced with a woman aged 33 years with advanced breast cancer

> put it to her husband and herself as to whether she should have performed the operation of removal of the [fallopian] tubes and ovaries. Its nature was fully explained to them both, and also that it was a purely experimental one ... She readily consented ... as she knew and felt her case was hopeless. [Eight months after operation] all vestiges of her previous cancerous disease had disappeared. [The surgeon concluded, after treating two further cases, that there may be ovarian influences in breast cancer and added that] whether [this is] accepted or not, I am sure I shall be acquitted of having acted thoughtlessly or recklessly.[2]

The treatment had indeed been based on reason. The author, 20 years previously, had agreed to take charge of a Scottish landowner 'whose mind was affected'. His duties 'were at times exciting, but never onerous', and, having the time and the interest to observe the weaning of lambs on a local farm, he observed a similarity 'up to a point' between the proliferation of epithelial cells of the milk ducts in lactation and in cancer; he learned that some farmers practised oophorectomy to prolong lactation in cows; and he had the idea that cancer of the breast might be due to an abnormal ovarian stimulus and that removal of the ovaries might have a therapeutic effect on cancer of the genital tract.

In 1941[3] it was shown that prostatic cancer with metastases was made worse by androgen and made better by oestrogen (stilboestrol). Activity of this cancer is particularly readily observable since the plasma prostate-specific antigen concentration provides a reliable marker. Indeed the availability of some means of reliably measuring effect is crucial to the use of drugs in cancer.

Cytotoxic drugs

Cytotoxic chemotherapy began with sulphur mustards (oily vesicant liquids) which had been developed and used as chemical weapons in World War I (1914–18). Amongst their actions depression of haemopoiesis and of lymphoid tissues were observed.

Preparations for World War II (1939–45) included research to increase the potency and toxicity ('efficacy') of these odious substances. It was found that substitution of a nitrogen atom for the sulphur atom, i.e. making nitrogen mustards, had the desired result. The disappearance of lymphocytes and granulocytes from the blood of rabbits was a useful marker of toxicity and gave rise to the idea of possible efficacy in lymphoid cancer.

> The problem was fundamental and simple: could one destroy a tumour with this group of cytotoxic agents before destroying the host?[4]

Nitrogen mustards, as anticancer agents, were first tested on experimental lymphoma in mice and the results were sufficiently encouraging to warrant a therapeutic trial in man. 'The response of the first patient was as dramatic as that of the first mouse', following 10 days treatment. But severe bone marrow depression occurred and, disappointingly, as the bone marrow recovered so did the tumour; in addition, with further courses, it rapidly became resistant.

> Twenty years later (1963) we can appreciate how accurately this first patient reflected the future trials and tribulations of therapy with alkylating agents.[4]

The development of other classes of agents, e.g. antimetabolites, soon followed.

Chemotherapy depends on developing drugs that *kill* malignant cells or modify their growth and

---

[2] Beatson G T 1896 Lancet 2: 104, 162.

[3] Huggins C et al 1941 Cancer Research 1: 293.

[4] Gilman A 1963 American Journal of Surgery 105: 574.

leave those of the host unharmed or at least recoverable.

The comparative success of antimicrobial chemotherapy is due to the fact that the metabolism of the parasite differs qualitatively from that of host cells. But cancer cells are host cells that differ from normal cells quantitatively rather than qualitatively, and to attain *adequate selectivity* it is necessary to take into account and exploit every possible factor that may improve the therapeutic index:

- the sensitivity of the malignant cell to drugs
- the endocrine environment
- the number of cells dividing at any one time
- the total number of cells (size of the tumour)
- the kinetics of the drugs
- the sensitivity of normal tissue and its rate of recovery from the unavoidable toxic effects of the drugs (most important).

Apoptosis[5] or 'programmed' or 'physiological' cell death is a process by which single cells are removed from the midst of living tissue without disturbing its architecture or function, or eliciting an inflammatory response. The instructions for the response are built into the cell's genetic material. Dysregulated apoptosis is involved in the pathogenesis of various forms of neoplastic disease; understanding its mechanisms and the defective processes offers scope for novel approaches to the treatment of cancer.[6]

Infection with microorganisms normally causes an *immune response* and antibacterial drugs that are merely cytostatic can be used, for the host defence mechanisms of the body eliminate the pathogens whose replication has been arrested. But there is less immune response to cancer (attempts are being made to strengthen it) and cure has to be achieved only by killing or otherwise removing cancer cells.

Drug therapy cannot be conducted rationally without some understanding of the disease as well as of the drugs. Since cancer is not one disease but many, although they share certain characteristics (see below), the following notes must be confined to what is usually true.

Classes of cytotoxic agents

A list of drugs used appears in Table 31.1. Table 31.2 provides detail of toxicity of individual agents. The following is an overview of the mode of action and toxicity of the principal groups of drugs.

ALKYLATING AGENTS

Alkylating agents (nitrogen mustards and ethyleneimines) act by transferring alkyl groups to DNA in the N–7 position of guanine during cell division. There follows either DNA strand breakage or cross-linking of the two strands so that normal synthesis is prevented.

Examples include: busulphan, carmustine, chlorambucil, cyclophosphamide, estramustine (a combination of oestrogen and mustine), ifosfamide, lomustine, melphalan, mustine (mechlorethamine), thiotepa, treosulfan; platinum drugs (cisplatin, carboplatin).

Alkylating agents particularly cause nausea and vomiting, and bone marrow depression (delayed with carmustine and lomustine) and cystitis[7] (cyclophosphamide, ifosfamide) and pulmonary fibrosis (especially busulphan). Male infertility and premature menopause may occur.

ANTIMETABOLITES

Antimetabolites are synthetic analogues of normal metabolites and act by competition, i.e. they 'deceive' or 'defraud' bodily processes.

Methotrexate, for example, a *folic acid antagonist*, competitively inhibits dihydrofolate reductase, preventing the synthesis of tetrahydrofolic acid (the coenzyme important in synthesis of amino and nucleic acids). This drug also provides a cogent illustration of the need to exploit every possible means of enhancing selectivity. Where it

---

[5] Greek: *apo*, off; *ptosis*, a falling

[6] Bellamy C O et al 1995 Cell death in health and disease: the biology and regulation of apoptosis. Seminars in Cancer Biology 6 (1): 3–16.

[7] A metabolite, acrolein, of cyclophosphamide and ifosfamide causes haemorrhagic cystitis. A high urine volume plus use of mesna (sodium 2-mercaptoethanesulphonate), which provides free thiol groups that bind acrolein, are used to prevent this serious complication.

Table 31.1 Reference data: Drugs commonly used for different types of cancer

Cancer type	Drugs of choice
Adrenocortical carcinoma[**]	Mitotane; cisplatin
Bladder (urinary)[*]	*Local*: instillation of doxorubicin or BCG (bacille Calmette-Guérin)
	Systemic: methotrexate + vinblastine + doxorubicin (Adriamycin) + cisplatin (MVAC)
Brain	
anaplastic astrocytoma[*]	Procarbazine + lomustine + vincristine
glioblastoma[**]	Carmustine or lomustine
Breast (see also text)	*Adjuvant*: cyclophosphamide + methotrexate + fluorouracil (CMF); cyclophosphamide + doxorubicin (Adriamycin) ± fluorouracil (AC or CAF); tamoxifen
	Metastatic: cyclophosphamide + methotrexate + fluorouracil (CMF) or cyclophosphamide + doxorubicin ± fluorouracil (AC or CAF) for receptor-negative and/or hormone-refractory; tamoxifen for receptor-positive and/or hormone-sensitive
Cervix uteri[**]	Cisplatin + cyclophosphamide; ifosfamide with mesna; bleomycin + ifosfamide with mesna + cisplatin
Choriocarcinoma	Methotrexate ± folinic acid; dactinomycin (cactinomycin)
Colorectal[*]	*Adjuvant*:
	fluorouracil + levamisole;
	fluorouracil + folinic acid
	Metastatic: fluorouracil + folinic acid
Endometrial[**]	Megestrol or another progestin;
	doxorubicin + cisplatin ± cyclophosphamide
Ewing's sarcoma[∞]	Cyclophosphamide (or ifosfamide with mesna) + doxorubicin (Adriamycin) + vincristine (CAV) ± dactinomycin (cactinomycin)
Gastric[**]	Fluorouracil ± folinic acid
Head and neck, squamous cell[*]	Cisplatin + fluorouracil; methotrexate
Islet cell (pancreas)[**]	Streptozotocin + doxorubicin
Kaposi's sarcoma[*] (AIDS-related)	Etoposide or interferon alfa or vinblastine;
	Doxorubicin (Adriamycin) + bleomycin + vincristine or vinblastine (ABV)
Leukaemias	
Acute lymphocytic leukaemia (ALL)	*Induction*: vincristine + prednisolone + crisantaspase (asparaginase) ± doxorubicin
	CNS prophylaxis: intrathecal methotrexate ± systemic high-dose methotrexate with folinic acid rescue ± intrathecal cytarabine ± intrathecal hydrocortisone
	Maintenance: methotrexate + mercaptopurine; bone marrow transplant
Acute myelogenous leukaemia (AML)	*Induction*: cytarabine + either daunorubicin or idarubicin
	Post-induction: high-dose cytarabine ± other drugs such as etoposide; bone marrow transplant
Chronic lymphocytic leukaemia (CLL)	Chlorambucil ± prednisolone;
	fludarabine
Chronic myelogenous leukaemia (CML)	
Chronic phase	Hydroxyurea;
	bone marrow transplant Interferon alfa
Accelerated	Bone marrow transplant
Hairy cell leukaemia	Pentostatin or cladribine or interferon alfa
Liver[**]	Doxorubicin; fluorouracil
Lung, small cell (oat cell)	Cyclophosphamide + doxorubicin (Adriamycin) + vincristine (CAV); cisplatin + etoposide (PE); PE alternated with CAV
Lung (non-small cell)[**]	Cisplatin + etoposide;
	cisplatin + vinblastin ± mitomycin
Lymphomas	
Hodgkin's disease	Mustine (mechlorethamine) + vincristine (Oncovin) + procarbazine ± prednisolone (MOPP);
	doxorubicin + bleomycin + vinblastine + dacarbazine (ABVD);
	ABVD alternated with MOPP
Non-Hodgkin's lymphoma Burkitt's lymphoma	Cyclophosphamide + vincristine + methotrexate
Diffuse large-cell lymphoma	Cyclophosphamide + doxorubicin + vincristine (Oncovin) + prednisolone (CHOP[1])

Table 31.1 (cont'd)

Cancer type	Drugs of choice
Follicular lymphoma	Cyclophosphamide or chlorambucil + prednisolone
Melanoma[**]	Interferon alfa; dacarbazine
Mycosis fungoides[*]	PUVA (psoralen + untraviolet A);
	mustine (mechlorethamine) (topical);
	interferon alfa; electron beam radiotherapy; methotrexate
Myeloma[*]	Melphalan (or cyclophosphamide) + prednisolone;
	melphalan + carmustine + cyclophosphamide + prednisolone + vincristine
Oesophageal[*]	Cisplatin + fluorouracil
Osteogenic sarcoma[∞]	Doxorubicin + cisplatin ± etoposide + ifosfamide
Ovary	Cisplatin (or carboplatin) + cyclophosphamide (CP) ± doxorubicin
	(Adriamycin) (CAP); paclitaxel
Pancreatic[**]	Fluorouracil ± folinic acid
Prostate	Leuprorelin (or goserelin) ± flutamide; estramustine
Renal[**]	Aldesleukin
	interferon alfa
Sarcomas, soft tissue, adult[*]	Doxorubicin + dacarbazine ± cyclophosphamide ± ifosfamide with mesna
Testicular	Cisplatin (Paraplatin) + etoposide (or vinblastine) + bleomycin (PEB), (PVB)
Wilms' tumour[∞]	Dactinomycin (cactinomycin) + vincristine ± doxorubicin ± cyclophosphamide
(nephroblastoma)	

[*]Chemotherapy has only moderate activity.
[**]Chemotherapy has only minor activity.
[∞]Drugs have major activity only when combined with surgical resection, radiotherapy or both.
Reproduced by courtesy of the Medical Letter on Drugs and Therapeutics (1995) New York (abbreviated; numerous alternative regimens omitted).
[|] The original use of hydroxydoxorubicin gave rise to this acronym.

is desired to maximise the effect of methotrexate a potentially fatal dose is given and is followed 24 h later by a dose of tetrahydrofolic (folinic) acid as Ca folinate (Ca Leucovorin), to bypass and terminate its action. This is called folinic acid 'rescue', since if it is not given the patient will die. The therapeutic justification for this manoeuvre is that high concentrations of methotrexate are obtained and that the bone marrow cells recover better than the tumour cells and some degree of useful selectivity is achieved (also effective with fluorouracil).

Purine antagonists (azathioprine, mercaptopurine, thioguanine) and *pyrimidine antagonists* (cytarabine, fludarabine, fluorouracil) similarly deprive cells of essential metabolites.

Antimetabolites cause gastrointestinal upsets including ulceration and bone marrow depression; renal impairment potentiates their toxicity, especially methotrexate. Active excretion of methotrexate by the renal tubule is blocked by salicylate, which also displaces it from plasma protein, increasing the risk of toxicity.

CYTOTOXIC ANTIBIOTICS

These antibiotics interfere with DNA/RNA synthesis. They include: aclarubicin, bleomycin, dactinomycin (cactinomycin), daunorubicin, doxorubicin (and amsacrine which is similar), epirubicin (and the related mitozantrone), idarubicin, plicamycin (mithramycin), mitomycin and streptozotocin (for islet-cell pancreatic tumour). Antibiotics depress the bone marrow, cause gastrointestinal upsets and stomatitis, alopecia, cardiomyopathy (daunorubicin and doxorubicin) and pulmonary fibrosis and skin rashes (bleomycin). The effects of some are radiomimetic, and use of radiation causes additive toxicity.

SPINDLE POISONS

The plant alkaloids (vincristine, vinblastine, vindesine and vinorelbine) and taxoids (paclitaxel, docetaxel) inhibit microtubule assembly and cause cell cycle arrest in mitosis. They particularly cause bone marrow depression, peripheral neuropathy (vincristine) and alopecia. Etoposide blocks the cell cycle before mitosis.

BIOLOGICAL AGENTS

Interferons and interleukins are described on page 250, and in Table 31.2. They are used in hairy cell leukaemia and Kaposi's sarcoma.

MISCELLANEOUS AGENTS

Crisantaspase, crisantaspase (asparaginase), starves tumour cells dependent upon a supply of the amino acid, asparagine (except those able to synthesise it for themselves); its use is almost confined to acute lymphoblastic leukaemia. Other agents include procarbazine, dacarbazine, hydroxyurea, and razoxane.

REFERENCE TABLE

Tables 31.1 and 31.2 provide reference data that would otherwise complicate the main text. We offer this authoritative source as useful background, presented in tabular form for ease of access.

Cytotoxic chemotherapy

TUMOUR CHARACTERISTICS[8]

Cancers, despite their variability, share some common characteristics:

- Growth that is not subject to normal restrictions for that tissue, and in which a high proportion of cells are dividing, i.e. there is a high 'growth fraction'
- Local invasiveness
- Tendency to spread to other parts of the body (metastasis)
- Less differentiated cell morphology
- Tendency to retain some characteristics of the tissue of origin.

---

[8] WHO 1977 Chemotherapy of solid tumours. Technical Report, 605, Geneva.

Survival. In experimental leukaemia:

- survival time is inversely related to the initial number of leukaemia cells, or to the number remaining after treatment
- a single leukaemia cell is capable of multiplying and eventually killing the host.

Cell kinetics and mode of action of drugs. Cytotoxic drugs act against all cells that are multiplying. Bone marrow, mucosal surfaces (gut), hair follicles, reticuloendothelial system, germ cells, are all dividing more rapidly than many cancers and so are also targets for cytotoxic drugs, as is shown by the occurrence of adverse effects on these tissues during chemotherapy. Most solid tumours in man divide slowly and recovery from cytotoxic agents is slow but normal marrow and gut recover rapidly. This rapid recovery of normal tissues is exploited in devising intermittent courses of chemotherapy.

In cancer, the normal feedback mechanisms that mediate cell growth are defective, perhaps from faulty cell contact signalling processes (transduction defects). Cell multiplication, when it has reached its optimum, does not stop. These signalling processes offer multiple targets for developers of new anticancer drugs. Cancer cells continue to multiply, at first exponentially, as the numbers increase, until later there is a slowing down and the volume-doubling time becomes prolonged due to several factors, most of which conspire to render the ageing cancer *less susceptible* to drugs:

- Increased cell cycle (division) time
- Decrease in the number of cells actively dividing, with more in the resting state (decrease in 'growth fraction')
- Increased cell death within the tumour as it ages
- Overcrowding of cells leading to defective nutrition (poor vascular supply) with defective access of drugs.

All cells, normal and malignant, engaged in division (cycling) go through a series of phases of synthesis of DNA, RNA, mitosis and rest. Cytotoxic drugs interfere with cell division at various points, e.g. synthesis of nucleotides from purines and pyrimidines, of DNA and RNA, and interference with mitosis. They are also mutagenic.

In general drugs are most active against *actively*

cycling cells (normal and malignant) and least active against *resting cells*. These latter are particularly sinister in that, although inactive, they retain the capacity to proliferate and may start cycling again after a completed course of chemotherapy. In order to eliminate them it is necessary to develop drugs that are active against the resting phase, to prolong chemotherapy to catch them when they become active, or to induce synchronous activity so that they may all be simultaneously vulnerable to cycle or phase-specific drugs. There are also *circadian rhythms* in cell metabolism and proliferation and those of leukaemic cells differ from those of normal leucocytes. Evidence is increasing that the time of day at which therapy is administered does influence the outcome; for example, maintenance chemotherapy of some leukaemias is more effective if given in the evening (chronopharmacology).

Plainly all this has important implications for the practice of chemotherapy.

Principles of chemotherapy

- Determine that there is no better (more effective and safe) treatment available.
- Decide whether expected benefit (cure, palliation and the expected quality of life) justifies the risk.
- Determine the marker(s) (symptom, sign, laboratory measure) that will allow progress to be assessed.
- Ensure that the patient is fit to accept chemotherapy (infection treated, anaemia corrected).
- Treat sensitive tumours early in the course of the disease to increase likelihood of total cell kill.
- Choose drugs that are cycle-nonspecific or cycle-specific, as appropriate; or that have been shown empirically to be effective.
- Use combinations of drugs.
- Repeat courses of high dose chemotherapy with intervals for recovery of normal tissues; this is ordinarily more effective than continuous low dose therapy.
- Use adjuvant therapy to eliminate micrometastases.
- Recognise that contraindications include very advanced disease and existing bone marrow depression.

Objectives. When there is realistic expectation of cure or major life prolongation of quality acceptable to the patient, then it is appropriate to risk severe drug toxicity.

Where expectation is confined to palliation or modest life prolongation of indifferent quality, then less toxic drug regimens should be devised.

Plainly patients should understand the issues with the aid of appropriate counselling.

Whilst **selectivity** of drugs for the cancer cell is generally low compared with selectivity of drugs against bacteria, in some tumours it can be substantial, as in lymphoma, in which the tumour cell kill with some drugs is 10 000 times as great as that of marrow cells. Techniques for targeting drugs to cancer cells are greatly needed.

Cell destruction by drugs follows first-order kinetics, i.e. a given dose of drug kills a constant *fraction* of cells (not a constant *number*) regardless of the number of cells present, i.e. a treatment reducing a cell population from 1 000 000 to 10 000 will reduce a cell population of 100 to one. Therefore, where there are many cells (late presentation, macroscopic disease) it is necessary to use several drugs, and to repeat administration to the limit of patient tolerance.[9] With some cancers final complete cell kill can be unattainable without unacceptable risk; therefore adjuvant chemotherapy is used (see below).

But cells remaining after initial doses are likely to be more resistant to drugs since cell sensitivity is not homogeneous at the outset due to random mutations as the tumour grows.

Drug action. Drugs that kill cancer cells may be:

- *Cycle-nonspecific*: these kill cells whether resting or actively cycling (as in low growth fraction cancer such as solid tumours, e.g. alkylating agents, doxorubicin and allied anthracyclines)
- *Cycle-specific*: these kill only cells that are actively cycling (often because their site of action is confined to one part of the cell cycle, e.g. antimetabolite drugs).

These considerations are relevant to the choice of drugs in combination chemotherapy, and to the desirability of attaining synchronisation of cell cycling to achieve maximum cell kill.

---

[9] And even beyond, e.g. methotrexate with folinic acid 'rescue' (p. 547), and bone marrow transplant following remission induced by aggressive chemotherapy in leukaemia.

> However well-chosen the drug, it will be ineffective if it does not reach the malignant cells at a high enough concentration for a long enough time at the right stage of the cell cycle.

Considerations of pharmacokinetics in relation to cell kinetics are of the first importance, as drug treatment alters the activity of both malignant and normal cells. Large solid tumours are better removed by surgery (the proportion of cells multiplying is often small), even if this is incomplete, and what remains treated by cytotoxic drugs.

Cell resistance to single drugs is both frequently present at the outset (primary resistance), and develops readily with repeated exposure (acquired resistance). Increased dosage is limited by toxicity, e.g. to bone marrow, which does not become tolerant. Therefore combination therapy is the routine. But *multiple drug resistance* is now a major problem. It appears to be due to activation of an ATP-dependent membrane efflux pump acting via a protein called P-glycoprotein (developed as a protective mechanism against environmental toxins). The genetic expression of P-glycoprotein is being unravelled and the possibility exists of interfering with it pharmacologically. Cytotoxic drugs vary in their capacity to stimulate P-glycoprotein and some, e.g. cisplatin, do not induce this type of resistance.

Well-designed treatment at the outset lessens this problem. In those tumours where cures can be achieved by chemotherapy (acute lymphoblastic leukaemia in childhood, Hodgkin's lymphoma, choriocarcinoma) *adequate initial chemotherapy* is of the first importance. If inadequate therapy is used, drug-resistant cells emerge and subsequent cure with intensive chemotherapy becomes difficult or even impossible.

Intermittent combination chemotherapy. Combinations of drugs are commonly used to obtain maximum cell kill; these are selected and repeated (scheduling, or pulsed courses) according to considerations of:

- Choosing drugs that act at different biochemical sites in the cell
- Using drugs that attack cells at different phases of the growth cycle
- Synchronising the active cell cycles
- Giving drugs that do not suppress bone marrow in between courses of those that do
- Using clinical experience of successful regimens, i.e. empirically.

The logical basis of the first two considerations (above) is obvious. But synchronisation (3 above) represents a refinement. For example, cells are killed or are arrested in mitosis by vincristine, which is then withdrawn. Cells then enter a new reproductive cycle more or less synchronously and when the majority are judged to be in a phase sensitive to a particular phase-specific drug, e.g methotrexate or cytarabine, it is given.

In spite of the important kinetic considerations discussed above it remains true that the majority of chemotherapy regimens have been devised by using a commonsense empiricism, and do not rely on detailed knowledge of tumour kinetics (which is at best meagre).

The drugs have been chosen because:

- They are known to be effective as single agents
- The toxicities do not overlap greatly
- In empirical (trial and error) use, the margins of safety of the combination have been determined, and it is reasonably hoped that by mixing differing classes of agents with differing effects in the cell cycle a spectrum of activity against both dividing and nondividing cells can be achieved, e.g. cycle-nonspecific agents first to reduce tumour cell mass and cycle-specific drugs second.

After an attempt to get maximum malignant cell kill using drugs to the limit of normal host tolerance, including exploitation of special routes of administration (intrathecal, arterial organ perfusion), an interval must be left for sufficient recovery of the normal cells, including the recovery of immunological mechanisms that have been suppressed. An interval between courses of 2–4 weeks is usually enough.

The aggressive pursuit of cure by total cell kill is conducted with repeated courses of combinations of drugs known by their abbreviations (usually the initial letter of the nonproprietary or proprietary name) (see Table 31.1). But *single drug therapy* is adequate in some cancers (cervix uteri, choriocarcinoma, although two or more drugs are often used, see Table 31.1).

Adjuvant chemotherapy is therapy given after the initial surgery or radiation in order to eliminate any persisting micrometastases; it is chiefly used for tumours known for their propensity to such spread, e.g. breast cancer. It may be cytotoxic or endocrine. The objective is to remove tumour cells that may be present but undetectable at the early stage of growth when the cells of a tumour are more rapidly dividing and more sensitive to drugs. Over-liberal use of adjuvant therapy carries the risk of treating patients who in fact have been cured by the initial therapy and so exposing them needlessly to the risk of a second, drug-induced, tumour.

Adverse effects

Principal adverse effects (see Table 31.2) are manifest as, or follow damage to, the following:

- Nausea and vomiting
- Bone marrow and lymphoreticular system: pancytopenia and immunosuppression (depression of both antibody and cell-mediated immunity), leading to opportunistic microbial infection
- Gut epithelium and other mucosal surfaces: diarrhoea, mouth ulcers
- Hair: alopecia due to effect on hair bulb (recovers 2–6 months after ceasing treatment); prevention by scalp hypothermia helps with certain drugs, e.g. vindesine
- Delayed wound healing
- Local toxicity if extravasation occurs
- Various organ damages (see Table 31.2)
- Germ cells and reproduction: sterility, teratogenesis, mutagenicity
- Second cancers (see below).

The first six occur immediately or in the short term and are liable to be troublesome with any vigorously pursued regimen.

Nausea and vomiting. This is common, can be extremely severe and prolonged and cause patients to refuse treatment. Management is of the first importance (see also pp 298, 574).

Vomiting commonly begins in 1–5 h and lasts from 6–48 h, depending on the agent. Drugs most likely to cause nausea and vomiting, and the severity are shown in Table 31.2.

Since emesis is largely predictable, preventive action can be taken. The most effective drugs are competitive antagonists at serotonin (5-HT$_3$) receptors (ondansetron) and at the dopamine D$_2$-receptor (metoclopramide). They are used in combination with a benzodiazepine (anxiety is a major factor in promoting emesis when the patient knows that it will occur, as with cisplatin), and dexamethasone which benefits by an unknown mechanism. Other effective agents include prochlorperazine, domperidone and nabilone.

Combinations, e.g. benzodiazepine plus dexamethasone, plus a 5-HT$_3$ or dopamine D$_2$-receptor blocker (ondansetron or metoclopramide) are more effective than a single drug.

Routes of administration are chosen as commonsense counsels, e.g. prophylaxis may be oral, but when vomiting occurs injections and suppositories are available.

Bone marrow suppression is the single most important dose-limiting factor. Repeated blood counts are essential and transfusion of all formed elements of the blood may be needed, e.g. platelet transfusion for thrombocytopenic bleeding or where the platelet count falls below $25\,000 \times 10^9/1$. Cell growth factors, e.g. the natural granulocyte colony stimulating factor (filgrastim), are effective in neutropenia.

Septicaemia is often an opportunistic infection by Gram-negative bacteria from the patient's own flora, e.g. from the gut, which has been injured by the drugs. Vigorous antimicrobial prophylaxis and therapy, often in combination, are used. Infections with virus (herpes zoster), fungus (candida) and protozoa (pneumocystis) are also prominent. Fever in a patient under this treatment requires collection of samples for microbiological studies and urgent treatment.

Immune responses. Vigorous and prolonged

chemotherapy can impair the immune responsiveness of patients for as long as 3 years after ceasing therapy.

Gonadal cells and reproduction. *Sterility* may occur. The *mutagenic* effects of anticancer drugs mean that reproduction should be avoided during and for several months after therapy (but both men and women have reproduced normally whilst undergoing chemotherapy). When treatment may cause permanent sterility, men are offered the facility for prior storage of sperm. Most cytotoxic drugs are *teratogenic* and should not be used during pregnancy. Contraceptive advice should be given before cancer chemotherapy begins.

Urate nephropathy. Too-rapid destruction of malignant cells releases purines and pyrimidines, which are converted to uric acid and may crystallise in and block the renal tubule (urate nephropathy). In practice this occurs only when there is a large cell mass and the tumour is very sensitive to drugs, e.g. acute lymphocytic leukaemia and lymphomas. High fluid intake, alkalinisation of the urine and use of allopurinol during the early stages of chemotherapy averts this outcome.

Carcinogenicity (second tumours). Many cytotoxic drugs are carcinogenic, and a patient may be cured of the primary disease only to succumb to a second, treatment-induced cancer 5–20 years later. Whether this is due to a mutagenic effect, to immunosuppression, or both, remains undecided. Alkylating agents are particularly incriminated and also some antimetabolites (mercaptopurine) and antibiotics (doxorubicin). The risk can be as high as 10–20 times that of unexposed people and the cancers include leukaemia, lymphoma and squamous carcinoma.

In Hodgkin's lymphoma life is greatly prolonged by chemotherapy, but in ovarian cancer it is not; these aspects are plainly relevant to acceptance of risk of second tumours. Use of radiation concurrently does not increase risk of leukaemia.

Quality of life. Over-enthusiastic and aggressive use of cytotoxic drug therapy may destroy the quality of the brief time remaining to a patient. When cure is not feasible, but there is prospect of prolonging survival, then the quality of the life that is gained is of paramount importance.

Hazards to staff handling cytotoxic agents. The urine of some nurses and of pharmacists who prepare infusions and injections of anticancer drugs was found to contain drugs even to the extent of being sometimes mutagenic to bacteria. When they stopped handling the drugs the contamination ceased. It can be assumed that absorption of even small amounts of these drugs is harmful (mutagenesis, carcinogenesis), especially when it occurs repeatedly over long periods.

Contamination occurs from spilt drugs and carelessly handled syringes (there should be a swab on the tip of the needle when expelling air); even opening an ampoule can create an aerosol. Used ampoules, syringes and absorbent swabs constitute a hazard, as may body wastes of treated patients.

Precautions appropriate to different drugs range from simply avoiding spillage, through gloves, surgical masks, goggles and aprons, to the use of laminar flow cabinets. Special training of nominated drug handlers is essential. Pregnant staff should not handle these drugs.

INTERACTIONS OF CYTOTOXICS WITH OTHER DRUGS

Many examples of *therapeutic* interactions (drug combinations) are shown in Table 31.1. *Non-therapeutic* interactions can be serious. Inhibition of metabolism of cytotoxic drugs can cause toxicity, e.g. cimetidine increases the toxicity of fluorouracil and allopurinol increases toxicity of mercaptopurine and cyclophosphamide.

REFERENCE TABLE

The table below displays reference data on the toxic effects of cytotoxic chemotherapeutic agents indicating, by emphasis, the effects that limit therapeutic dose. This authoritative source is offered as useful background in tabular form for ease of access. It should be read in conjunction with the above text.

Table 31.2 Reference data: Toxicity of some anticancer drugs and hormones
Reproduced (abbreviated and adapted) by courtesy of the Medical Letter on Drugs and Therapeutics (1995) New York.

	Dose-limiting effects are in bold type	
Drug	**Acute toxicity**	**Delayed toxicity***[*]
Aldesleukin (interleukin-2)	**Fever; fluid retention; hypotension; respiratory distress;** rash, anaemia, thrombocytopenia; nausea and vomiting; diarrhoea, capillary leak syndrome, nephrotoxicity; myocardial toxicity, hepatotoxicity; erythema nodosum; neutrophil chemotactic defects	Neuropsychiatric disorders; hypothyroidism; nephrotic syndrome; possibly acute leucoencephalopathy; brachial plexopathy; bowel perforation
Altretamine (hexamethyl-melamine)	Nausea and vomiting	**Bone marrow depression**; CNS depression; peripheral neuropathy; visual hallucinations; ataxia; tremors; alopecia; rash
Aminoglutethimide	Drowsiness; nausea; dizziness; rash	Hypothyroidism (rare); bone marrow depression; fever; hypotension; masculinisation
Amsacrine	Nausea and vomiting; diarrhoea; pain or phlebitis on infusion; anaphylaxis	**Bone marrow depression**; hepatic injury; convulsions; stomatitis; ventricular fibrillation; alopecia; congestive heart failure; renal dysfunction
BCG (bacille Calmette-Guérin)	Bladder irritation; nausea and vomiting; fever; sepsis	Granulomatous pyelonephritis; hepatitis; urethral obstruction; epididymitis; renal abscess
Bleomycin	Nausea and vomiting; fever; anaphylaxis and other allergic reactions; phlebitis at injection site	**Pneumonitis and pulmonary fibrosis**; rash and hyperpigmentation; stomatitis; alopecia; Raynaud's phenomenon; cavitating granulomas; haemorrhagic cystitis
Busulfan	Nausea and vomiting; rare diarrhoea	Bone marrow depression; pulmonary infiltrates and fibrosis; alopecia; gynaecomastia; ovarian failure; hyperpigmentation; azoospermia; leukaemia; chromosome aberrations; cataracts; hepatitis; seizures and veno-occlusive disease with high doses
Carboplatin	Nausea and vomiting	**Bone marrow depression**; peripheral neuropathy (uncommon); hearing loss; transient cortical blindness; haemolytic anaemia
Carmustine	Nausea and vomiting; local phlebitis	**Delayed leukopenia and thrombocytopenia** (may be prolonged); pulmonary fibrosis (may be irreversible); delayed renal damage; reversible liver damage; leukaemia; myocardial ischaemia
Chlorambucil	Nausea and vomiting; seizures	**Bone marrow depression**; pulmonary infiltrates and fibrosis; leukaemia; hepatic toxicity; sterility
Cisplatin	Nausea and vomiting; diarrhoea; anaphylactic reactions	**Renal damage**; ototoxicity; bone marrow depression; haemolysis; hypomagnesaemia; peripheral neuropathy; hypocalcaemia; hypokalaemia; Raynaud's disease; sterility; teratogenesis; hypophosphataemia; hyperuricaemia
Cladribine	Fever	**Bone marrow depression**; peripheral neuropathy at high doses
Crisantaspase, (asparaginase)	Nausea and vomiting; fever, chills; headache; hypersensitivity, anaphylaxis;	CNS depression or hyperexcitability; acute haemorrhagic pancreatitis; (Cont'd)

Table 31.2 *(cont'd)*

	Dose-limiting effects are in bold type	
Drug	**Acute toxicity**	**Delayed toxicity**[*]
Crisantaspase, (asparaginase) *(cont'd)*	abdominal pain; hyperglycaemia leading to coma	coagulation defects; thrombosis; renal damage; hepatic damage
Cyclophosphamide	Nausea and vomiting; Type I (anaphlactoid) hypersensitivity; facial burning with i.v. administration; visual blurring	**Bone marrow depression**; alopecia; haemorrhagic cystitis; sterility (may be temporary); pulmonary infiltrates and fibrosis; hyponatremia; leukaemia; bladder cancer, inappropriate antidiuretic hormone secretion; cardiac toxicity
Cytarabine	Nausea and vomiting; diarrhoea; anaphylaxis; sudden respiratory distress with high doses	**Bone marrow depression**; conjunctivitis; megaloblastosis; oral ulceration; hepatic damage; fever; pulmonary oedema and central and peripheral neurotoxicity with high doses; rhabdomyolysis; pancreatitis when used with crisantaspase (asparaginase); rash
Dacarbazine	Nausea and vomiting; diarrhoea; anaphylaxis, pain on administration	**Bone marrow depression**; alopecia; flu-like syndrome; renal impairment; hepatic necrosis; facial flushing; paraesthesiae; photosensitivity; urticarial rash
Dactinomycin (cactinomycin)	Nausea and vomiting; hepatic toxicity with ascites; diarrhoea; severe local tissue damage and necrosis on extravasation; anaphylactic reaction	**Stomatitis; oral ulceration; bone marrow depression**; alopecia; folliculitis; dermatitis in previously irradiated areas
Daunorubicin	Nausea and vomiting; diarrhoea; red urine (not haematuria); severe local tissue damage and necrosis on extravasation; transient ECG changes; anaphylactoid reaction	**Bone marrow depression; cardiotoxicity** (may be delayed for years); alopecia; stomatitis; anorexia; diarrhoea; fever and chills; dermatitis in previously irradiated areas; skin and nail pigmentation; photosensitivity
Diethylstilbestrol	Nausea and vomiting; abdominal cramps; headaches	Gynaecomastia in males; breast tenderness; loss of libido; thrombophlebitis and thromboembolism; hepatic injury; sodium retention with oedema; hypertension; change in menstrual flow; peptic ulcer
Doxorubicin	Nausea and vomiting; red urine (not haematuria); severe local tissue damage and necrosis on extravasation; diarrhoea; fever, transient ECG changes; ventricular arrhythmia; anaphylactoid reaction	**Bone marrow depression; cardiotoxicity** (may be delayed for years); alopecia; stomatitis; anorexia; conjunctivitis; acral (extremities) pigmentation; dermatitis in previously irradiated areas; hyperuricaemia
Estramustine	Nausea and vomiting; diarrhoea	Mild gynaecomastia; increased frequency of vascular accidents; myelosuppression (uncommon); oedema; dyspnoea; pulmonary infiltrates and fibrosis; decreased glucose tolerance; thrombosis; hypertension
Etoposide	Nausea and vomiting; diarrhoea; fever; hypotension; anaphylactoid reactions; phlebitis at infusion site	**Bone marrow depression**; rashes; alopecia; peripheral neuropathy; mucositis and hepatic damage with high doses; leukaemia
Etretinate		Dryness of mucous membranes; chapped lips; hair loss; bone and joint pain; eye irritation; peeling skin; pseudotumour cerebri; premature epiphyseal closure; hepatic injury; major teratogenic effects *(Cont'd)*

Table 31.2 (cont'd)

Drug	Acute toxicity	Delayed toxicity*
	Dose-limiting effects are in bold type	
Finasteride		Impotence; decreased libido; teratogenic
Floxuridine	Nausea and vomiting; diarrhoea	**Oral and gastrointestinal ulceration; bone marrow depression;** alopecia; dermatitis; hepatic dysfunction with hepatic infusion
Fludarabine	Nausea and vomiting	**Bone marrow depression;** CNS effects; visual disturbances; renal damage with higher doses; pulmonary infiltrates; tumour lysis syndrome
Fluorouracil (5-FU)	Nausea and vomiting; diarrhoea; hypersensitivity reaction (rare)	**Oral and GI ulcers; bone marrow depression;** diarrhoea (especially with fluorouracil-folinic acid); neurological defects, usually cerebellar; cardiac arrhythmias; angina pectoris; alopecia; hyperpigmentation; palmar-plantar erythrodysaesthesia; conjunctivitis; heart failure; seizures
Flutamide (anti-androgen)	Nausea; diarrhoea	Gynaecomastia; hepatotoxicity
Goserelin	Transient increase in bone pain (see p. 559) and urethral obstruction in patients with metastatic prostatic cancer; hot flushes	Impotence; testicular atrophy; gynaecomastia
Hydroxyurea	Nausea and vomiting; allergic reactions to tartrazine dye (e.g. in medicinal formulations)	**Bone marrow depression;** stomatitis; dysuria; alopecia; rare neurological disturbances; pulmonary infiltrates
Idarubicin	Nausea and vomiting; tissue damage on extravasation	**Bone marrow depression;** alopecia; stomatitis; myocardial toxicity; diarrhoea
Ifosfamide	Nausea and vomiting; confusion; coma; nephrotoxicity; metabolic acidosis and renal Fanconi's syndrome; cardiac toxicity with high doses	**Bone marrow depression; haemorrhagic cystitis** (prevented by concurrent mesna); alopecia; inappropriate ADH secretion; neurotoxicity (somnolence, hallucinations, blurring of vision, coma)
Interferon alfa-2a, alfa-2b, alfa-n3, alfa-2b	Fever; chills; myalgias; fatigue; headache; arthralgias; hypotension	Bone marrow depression; anorexia; neutropenia; anaemia; confusion; depression; renal toxicity; possible hepatic injury; facial and peripheral oedema; cardiac arrhythmias
Isotretinoin	Fatigue; headache; nausea and vomiting; pruritis	**Teratogenicity; cheilitis;** xerostomia; rash; conjunctivitis and eye irritation; anorexia; hyper-triglyceridaemia; pseudotumour cerebri
Leuprolein (LHRH analogue)	Transient increase in bone pain and ureteral obstruction in patients with metastatic prostatic cancer; hot flushes	Impotence; testicular atrophy; gynaecomastia; peripheral oedema
Levamisole	Nausea and vomiting; diarrhoea; flu-like symptoms; metallic taste	Agranulocytosis; arthralgias; rash; encephalopathy; hyperlipidaemia; pancreatitis; fatigue; peripheral neuropathy
Lomustine	Nausea and vomiting	**Delayed (4–6 weeks) leukopenia and thrombocytopenia** (may be prolonged); transient elevation of transaminase activity; neurological reactions; pulmonary fibrosis; renal damage; leukaemia
Medroxyprogesterone acetate	Nausea; urticaria; headache; fatigue	Menstrual changes; gynaecomastia; hot flushes; weight gain; hirsutism; insomnia; fatigue; depression; oedema; (Cont'd)

Table 31.2 *(cont'd)*

	Dose-limiting effects are in bold type	
Drug	**Acute toxicity**	**Delayed toxicity**[*]
Medroxyprogesterone acetate *(cont'd)*		thrombophlebitis and thromboembolism; sterile abscess
Megestrol acetate	Nausea and vomiting; headache	Menstrual changes; hot flushes; thrombophlebitis and thromboembolism; fluid retention; oedema; weight gain
Melphalan	Mild nausea; hypersensitivity reactions	**Bone marrow depression** (especially platelets); pulmonary infiltrates and fibrosis; amenorrhoea; sterility; leukaemia
Mercaptopurine	Nausea and vomiting; diarrhoea	**Bone marrow depression**; cholestasis and rarely hepatic necrosis; oral and intestinal ulcers; pancreatitis
Mesna	Nausea and vomiting; diarrhoea; allergic reactions	
Methotrexate	Nausea and vomiting; diarrhoea; fever; anaphylaxis; hepatic necrosis	**Oral and gastrointestinal ulceration,** perforation may occur; **bone marrow depression**; hepatic toxicity including cirrhosis; renal toxicity; **pulmonary infiltrates and fibrosis**; osteoporosis; conjunctivitis; alopecia; depigmentation; menstrual dysfunction; encephalopathy; infertility; lymphoma; teratogenesis
Mitomycin	Nausea and vomiting; tissue necrosis; fever	**Bone marrow depression** (cumulative); stomatitis; alopecia; acute pulmonary toxicity; pulmonary fibrosis; hepatotoxicity; renal toxicity; amenorrhoea; haemolytic-uraemic syndrome; bladder calcification (with intravesical administration)
Mitotane	Nausea and vomiting; diarrhoea	**CNS depresssion**; rash; visual disturbance; adrenal insufficiency; haematuria; haemorrhagic cystitis; albuminuria; hypertension; orthostatic hypotension; cataracts; prolonged bleeding time
Mitozantrone	Blue-green pigment in urine; blue-green sclerae; nausea and vomiting; stomatitis; fever; phlebitis	**Bone marrow depression**; cardiotoxicity; alopecia; white hair; skin lesions; hepatic damage; renal failure; extravasation necrosis
Mustine (mechlorethamine)	Nausea and vomiting; local reaction and phlebitis	**Bone marrow depression;** alopecia; diarrhoea; oral ulcers; leukaemia; amenorrhoea; sterility; hyperuricaemia; teratogenesis
Octreotide	Nausea and vomiting; diarrhoea	Steatorrhoea; gallstones
Paclitaxel	Anaphylaxis, dyspnoea, hypotension, angioedema, urticaria (probably due to vehicle)	**Bone marrow depression**; peripheral neuropathy; alopecia; arthralgias; myalgias; cardiac toxicity; mild GI disturbances; mucositis
Pentostatin	Nausea and vomiting; rash	Nephrotoxicity; rash; **bone marrow depression**; respiratory failure; hepatic toxicity; arthralgia; myalgia; photophobia; conjunctivitis
Plicamycin	Nausea and vomiting	**Haemorrhagic diathesis;** thrombocytopenia; coagulation abnormalities; hepatic damage; hypocalcaemia and hypokalaemia; stomatitis; renal damage *(Cont'd)*

Table 31.2 (cont'd)

| Drug | Dose-limiting effects are in bold type | |
	Acute toxicity	Delayed toxicity*
Procarbazine	Nausea and vomiting; CNS depression; disulfiram-like effect with alcohol; adverse reactions typical of a MAO inhibitor	**Bone marrow depression**; stomatitis; peripheral neuropathy; pneumonitis; leukaemia
Stilboestrol, see Diethylstilbestrol		
Streptozotocin	Nausea and vomiting; local pain	**Renal damage**; hypoglycaemia; hyperglycaemia; liver damage; diarrhoea; bone marrow depression (uncommon); fever; eosinophilia; nephrogenic diabetes insipidus
Tamoxifen	Hot flushes; nausea and vomiting; transiently increased bone or tumour pain; hypercalcaemia; hyperglycaemia	Vaginal bleeding and discharge; rash; thrombocytopenia; peripheral oedema; depression; dizziness; headache; decreased visual acuity; corneal changes; retinopathy; purpuric vasculitis; thromboembolism; endometrial cancer
Teniposide	Nausea and vomiting; diarrhoea; phlebitis; anaphylactoid symptoms	**Bone marrow depression**; alopecia; peripheral neuropathy; leukaemia
Thioguanine	Occasional nausea and vomiting; diarrhoea	**Bone marrow depression**; hepatic damage; stomatitis
Thiotepa	Nausea and vomiting; rare hypersensitivity reaction	**Bone marrow depression**; menstrual dysfunction; interference with spermatogenesis; leukaemia; mucositis with high doses
Trimetrexate	Fever; chills; nausea and vomiting; diarrhoea	**Bone marrow depression**; mucositis; peripheral neuropathy; rash; pruritis; hyperpigmentation; nephrotoxicity; hepatic injury
Vinblastine	Nausea and vomiting; local reaction and phlebitis with extravasation	**Bone marrow depression**; alopecia; stomatitis; loss of deep tendon reflexes; jaw pain; muscle pain; paralytic ileus
Vincristine	Tissue damage with extravasation	**Peripheral neuropathy**; alopecia; mild bone marrow depression; constipation; paralytic ileus; jaw pain; inappropriate ADH secretion; optic atrophy

*Cutaneous reactions** (sometimes severe), hyperpigmentation, and ocular toxicity have been reported with virtually all nonhormonal anticancer drugs.

Endocrine therapy

HORMONES AND ANTIHORMONES

The growth of some cancers is inhibited by surgical removal of gonads, adrenals and pituitary, i.e. these neoplasms are hormone-dependent. The same effect is increasingly achievable, at less cost to the patient, by administering hormones, or antihormones, of oestrogens, androgens or progestogens (see Ch. 38) and inhibitors of hormone synthesis.

Prostatic cancer is androgen-dependent and metastatic disease can be helped by orchidectomy, or by a *gonadorelin analogue*, e.g. *buserelin, goserelin, leuprorelin* or *triptorelin*. These cause a transient stimulation of luteinising hormone and thus testosterone release, before inhibition occurs; some patients may experience exacerbation of tumour effects, e.g. bone pain, spinal cord compression. Where this can be anticipated, prior orchidectomy or anti-androgen treatment, e.g. with cyproterone or flutamide, is necessary.

Anti-androgen, e.g. *bicalutamide, buserelin* or *cypro-terone*: see also pages 557, 647. Benign prostatic hyper-trophy is also androgen-dependent and drug therapy includes use of *finasteride*, an inhibitor of the enzyme (5α-reductase) that activates testosterone.

Breast cancer cells may have receptors for oestro-gen, progesterone and androgen and hormonal manipulation benefits some 30% of patients with metastatic disease; when a patient's tumour is oestrogen-receptor positive the response is about 60%, and when negative it is only 10%.

After treatment of the primary cancer, endocrine therapy with *tamoxifen*, 20 mg/d, is the adjuvant therapy of choice for postmenopausal women who have disease in the lymph nodes; both the interval before the development of metastases and overall survival are increased. Adjuvant therapy with cyto-toxic drugs and/or tamoxifen is recommended for node-negative patients with large tumours or other adverse prognostic factors.

Cytotoxic chemotherapy is more useful in younger women (see Table 31.1), with tamoxifen, increasing-ly, as adjuvant therapy. The optimum duration of dosing with tamoxifen is not yet established.

For those who do not respond to tamoxifen, sec-ond-line therapy includes *progestogens*, e.g. *megestrol* or *medroxyprogesterone*. Should fluid retention prove a problem with these, *formestane* may be substituted in postmenopausal women (it inhibits aromatase, an enzyme involved in the convertion of androgens to oestrogens). *Aminoglutethimide* and *trilostane*, which inhibit the conversion of androgens to oestrogens (and have largely replaced adrenalectomy for breast cancer) are also used for postmenopausal women; concurrent glucocorticoid replacement therapy is, however, essential.

Adrenocortical steroids are used for their action on the cancer itself and also to treat some of the complications of cancer (hypercalcaemia, raised intracranial pressure, see Index).

Their principal use is in cancer of the lymphoid tissues and blood. In leukaemias they may also reduce the incidence of complications such as haemolytic anaemia and thrombocytopenia. A glu-cocorticoid is preferred, e.g. prednisolone, as high doses are used and mineralocorticoid actions are not needed and cause fluid retention.

In general, endocrine therapy carries less serious consequences for normal tissues than do the cyto-toxic agents.

Immunotherapy and biological therapy

Immunotherapy derives from an observation in the 19th century that cancer sometimes regressed after acute bacterial infections, i.e. there may be nonspecific immunostimulant effect.

Cytotoxic drugs are notable as being immuno-suppressive and so are likely to diminish what little natural immune resistance to a tumour that there may be.

Exploration of immunotherapy has involved:

- Nonspecific stimulation of active immunity with vaccines, e.g. *BCG* (bacille Calmette-Guérin) instilled into the urinary bladder for bladder cancer.
- Nonspecific stimulation of active immunity with drugs, e.g. *levamisole* (an anthelminthic), which appears to enhance function of phagocytes and T-lymphocytes when this is subnormal. It has also been used in immune deficiency states and autoimmune disease, e.g. rheumatoid arthritis.

BIOLOGICAL THERAPY OF CANCER

Natural substances that regulate cell function are increasingly used to treat cancer. They include:

- *Cytokines*, produced in response to a variety of stimuli, such as antigens, e.g. virus, cancer (see p. 250). They regulate cell growth and activity, and immune responses; they can be synthesised by recombinant DNA technology and include:
- *Interleukins* which stimulate proliferation of T-lymphocytes and activate natural killer cells. *Aldesleukin* (interleukin-2) is used in metastatic renal cell carcinoma.
- *Interferons* (see p. 250). Interferon alfa is used for hairy cell leukaemia and Kaposi's sarcoma.
- *Haemopoietic growth factors* (p. 542) or cell colony-stimulating factors are used for leukopenic patients, e.g. filgrastim (recombinant human granulocyte colony stimulating factor,

G-CSF) and molgramostim (recombinant human granulocyte macrophage-colony stimulating factor, GM-CSF).

Chemoprophylaxis of cancer

Some vitamins and derivatives and dietary micro-nutrients may inhibit the development of cancers, e.g. beta-carotene, isotretinoin, folic acid, ascorbic acid, alphatocopherol. Large scale trials of these substances and derivatives are in progress. Isotretinoin prevents second primary squamous cell tumours of the head and neck. Tamoxifen (anti-oestrogen) is being studied in women at high risk of developing breast cancer.

CANCER 'CURES': UNPROVEN REMEDIES

> So long as conventional medicine cannot cure all patients with cancer some will be willing to try anything that they think might help.[10]

This is perfectly understandable and many patients use unproven methods, including medicines (see complementary medicine). Innumerable methods are and have been offered for cancer. A recent prominent remedy was *laetrile*, a preparation of apricot seeds (pits, pips), which contains amygdalin (a β-glucoside) which incorporates cyanide. It was claimed to relieve pain, prolong survival and even to induce complete remission of cancer. Benefit was reputed to result from release of cyanide in the body which was claimed to kill cancer cells but not normal cells.

As has so often been the case in the past, and no doubt will continue to be in the future, the calm evaluation of such claims is obstructed by a mixture of emotionalism and exploitation. Scientific clinical investigation shows no benefit.

Although it was claimed that laetrile had no toxic effects, an 11-month-old girl died after swallowing tablets (1–5) being used by her father. The toxicity was due to metabolic formation of hydrocyanic acid in the intestine. Deaths have also been reported

---

[10] Editorial. British Medical Journal (1977) 1: 3.

from eating material intended for injection. There is no serious evidence that laetrile is effective.

Interestingly, despite criticism of overpermissive laxity of the drug regulatory authority (FDA) in the USA, the public is unwilling to accept the opinion of the FDA when it advises against the use of drugs such as laetrile.

There is a long and generally dishonourable history of the promotion of cancer 'cures', but as each new one appears the medical profession must yet again be willing to look dispassionately at the possibility that this time there really may be something in it, whilst avoiding the tragic raising of hopes that will not be realised — a sad and difficult task.

Immunosuppression

Suppression of immune responses mediated via mononuclear cells (lymphocytes, plasma cells) is used in therapy of:

- Autoimmune and collagen and connective tissue disease (see below)
- Organ transplantation; to prevent immune rejection.

Cytotoxic cancer chemotherapeutic agents are immunosuppressive because they interfere with mononuclear cell multiplication and function. But they are generally too toxic for the above purposes and the following are principally used for intended immunosuppression:

- Adrenocortical steroids
- Azathioprine (see below)
- Cyclosporin, tacrolimus (see below)
- Some alkylating agents: cyclophosphamide and chlorambucil (see Table 31.1)
- Antilymphocyte immunoglobulin (see below).

With the exception of *cyclosporin* and *tacrolimus*, all the above cause nonspecific immunosuppression so that the general defences of the body against infection are impaired.

Adrenal steroids destroy lymphocytes, reduce inflammation and impair phagocytosis (see Ch. 35).

Cytotoxic agents destroy immunologically competent cells. *Azathioprine*, a prodrug for the purine antagonist mercaptopurine, is used in autoimmune disease because it provides enhanced immunosuppressive activity. Cyclophosphamide is a second choice. Bone marrow is depressed as is to be expected.

Cyclosporin

Cyclosporin is a polypeptide obtained from a soil fungus. It acts selectively and reversibly by preventing the transcription of interleukin-2 and other lymphokine genes, thus inhibiting the production of lymphokines by T-lymphocytes (that mediate specific recognition of alien molecules). Cyclosporin spares nonspecific functions, e.g. of granulocytes, that are responsible for phagocytosis and metabolism of foreign substances. It does not depress haemopoiesis.

Pharmacokinetics. Cyclosporin is about 40% absorbed from the gastrointestinal tract and is metabolised in the liver; the $t^{1}/2$ is 27 h.

Uses. Cyclosporin is used to prevent and treat rejection of organ transplants (kidney, liver, heart–lung) and bone marrow transplants. It may be given orally or i.v. In the context of transplantation, administration continues indefinitely and must be carefully monitored, including measurement of plasma concentration and renal function.

Cyclosporin may also be used for severe, resistant psoriasis in hospitalised patients.

Adverse reactions. Cyclosporin is nephrotoxic; acute or chronic renal impairment may develop if the trough plasma concentration consistently exceeds 250 μg/l. In the main, renal changes resolve if the drug is withdrawn. Hypertension develops in about 50% of patients, more commonly when a corticosteroid is co-administered but possibly due in part to mineralocorticosteroid action of cyclosporin. The blood pressure can be controlled by standard antihypertensive therapy without need to discontinue cyclosporin. Other adverse effects include gastrointestinal reactions, hepatotoxicity, hyperkalaemia, hypertrichosis, gingival hypertrophy and convulsions.

Interactions. Careful attention to co-administered drugs is essential as many may interact. The plasma concentration of cyclosporin, and risk of toxicity, is increased by drugs that include ketoconazole, erythromycin, chloroquine, cimetidine, oral contraceptives, anabolic steroids and calcium channel antagonists. Curiously, grapefruit juice also elevates plasma cyclosporin concentrations; flavonoids in the juice may inhibit the cytochrome that metabolises cyclosporin. Drugs that reduce the plasma concentration of cyclosporin, risking loss of effect, include enzyme-inducing antiepileptics (e.g. phenytoin, carbamazepine, phenobarbitone) and rifampicin. Inherently nephrotoxic drugs add to the risk of renal damage with cyclosporin, e.g. aminoglycoside antibiotics, amphotericin, NSAIDs, (diclofenac). Potassium-sparing diuretics add to the risk of hyperkalaemia.

Tacrolimus is a macrolide immunosuppressant agent that is isolated from a bacterium. It acts like cyclosporin and is used to protect and treat liver and kidney grafts where conventional immunosuppresants fail. Such rescue treatment may be graft- or life-saving. Tacrolimus may cause nephrotoxicity, neurotoxicity, disturbance of glucose metabolism, hyperkalaemia and hypertrophic cardiomyopathy.

Antilymphocyte immunoglobin is used in organ graft rejection, a process in which lymphocytes are involved; it is made by preparing antisera to human lymphocytes in animals (horses); allergic reactions are common. It largely spares the patient's response to infection.

Mycophenolate selectively blocks the proliferation of T and B lymphocytes and acts like azathioprine; it is being evaluated in combination immunosuppressive regimens for organ transplantation.

USES

Diseases in which immunosuppression may be useful include: tissue transplantation, inflammatory bowel disease, rheumatoid arthritis, chronic active hepatitis, systemic lupus erythematosus, glomerulonephritis, nephrotic syndrome, some haemolytic anaemias and thrombocytopenias, uveitis, myasthenia gravis, polyarteritis, polymyositis, systemic sclerosis, Behçet's syndrome.

HAZARDS OF LIFE ON IMMUNOSUPPRESSIVE DRUGS

Impaired immune responses render the subject more liable to *bacterial* and *viral* infections. Treat all infection early and vigorously (using bactericidal drugs where practicable); use human gamma globulin to protect if there is exposure to virus infections, e.g. measles, varicella. For example, patients who have not had chickenpox and are receiving therapeutic (as opposed to replacement) doses of corticosteroid are at risk of *severe chickenpox*; they should receive varicella-zoster immunoglobulin if there has been contact with the disease within the previous 3 months.

Carcinogenicity is also a hazard, generally after 4–7 years of therapy. The cancers most likely to occur are those thought to have viral origin (leukaemia, lymphoma, skin). Where cytotoxics are used there is the additional hazard of mutagenicity, which may induce cancer.

Hazards also include those of longterm corticosteroid therapy, and of cytotoxics in general (bone marrow depression, infertility and teratogenesis).

Whilst the hazards may be acceptable to the patient who has grave life-endangering disease, they give more cause for concern when immunosuppressive regimens are proposed in younger patients with less serious disease, e.g. rheumatoid arthritis, ulcerative colitis.

ACTIVE IMMUNISATION DURING IMMUNOSUPPRESSIVE THERAPY

Response to nonliving antigens (tetanus, typhoid, poliomyelitis) is diminished and giving 1 or 2 extra doses may be wise. With living vaccines (some polio) there is a risk of serious generalised disease; boosters are safer than primary vaccination. If vaccination *must* be performed (an unlikely event) reduce or stop the immunosuppressive therapy and vaccinate lightly (6 months later); if a severe reaction occurs use an appropriate antiviral agent or a specific immunoglobulin if available (see also Adrenocorticosteroids).

IMMUNOSTIMULATION:

See Immunotherapy, page 560.

GUIDE TO FURTHER READING

Alexanian R, Dimopoulos M 1994 The treatment of multiple myeloma. New England Journal of Medicine 330: 484

Armitage J O 1994 Bone marrow transplantation. New England Journal of Medicine 330: 827

Catalona W J 1994 Management of cancer of the prostate. New England Journal of Medicine 331: 996

Cline M J 1994 The molecular basis of leukaemia. New England Journal of Medicine 330: 328

DeVita V T, Hubbard S M 1993 Hodgkin's disease. New England Journal of Medicine 328: 560

Hulka B S, Stark A T 1995 Breast cancer: cause and prevention. Lancet 346: 883

London N J et al 1995 Risk of neoplasia in renal transplant patients. Lancet 346: 403

Moertel C G 1994 Chemotherapy for colorectal cancer. New England Journal of Medicine 330: 1136

Moertel G G et al 1982 A clinical trial of amygdalin (laetrile) in the treatment of human cancer. New England Journal of Medicine 306: 201 (also Relman A S Editorial p. 236)

Morris J H H et al 1995 Viral infection and cancer. Lancet 346: 754

Mullan F 1985 Seasons of survival: reflections of a (32-year-old) physician with cancer. New England Journal of Medicine 313: 270

Naber S P 1994 Molecular pathology: detection of neoplasia. New England Journal of Medicine 331: 1508

Nevin P et al 1994 Tamoxifen and the uterus. British Medical Journal 309: 1313

Niedobitek G, Young L S 1994 Epstein-Barr virus persistence and virus-associated tumours. Lancet 343: 333

Pui C-H 1995 Childhood leukaemias. New England Journal of Medicine 332: 1618

Rosen F S et al 1995 The primary immunodeficiencies. New England Journal of Medicine 333: 431

SECTION 7

GASTRO-INTESTINAL SYSTEM

32

Stomach and oesophagus

SYNOPSIS

Drugs for peptic ulcer

- Reduction of acid secretion
- Neutralisation of secreted acid
- Enhancing mucosal resistance
- Overall management

Vomiting

- Antiemetic and prokinetic drugs
- Treatment for various forms
- Gastro-oesophageal reflux

Drugs for peptic ulcer

Peptic ulcer kills few patients but troubles many. Ulcers may be transient, recurrent or chronic, and drug therapy is valuable for the relief of symptoms, to aid healing and to prevent relapse.

SOME PATHOPHYSIOLOGY

The concept of a balance between the aggressive capacities of acid plus pepsin and the defensive mechanisms of the mucosa is useful. An ulcer is thought to develop when the equilibrium is disturbed either by enhanced aggressiveness or by lessened mucosal resistance.

On average, patients with duodenal ulcer pro-duce about twice as much HCl as normal subjects, but there is much overlap, and about half the patients with duodenal ulcer have acid outputs in the normal range. Patients with gastric ulcer produce normal or reduced amounts of acid.

The factors that protect the mucosa comprise its:

- impermeability to H^+ ion (the mucosal 'barrier' to H^+)
- ability to secrete mucus and bicarbonate ion
- blood flow and its capacity rapidly to replace damaged epithelial cells.

Endogenous prostaglandins are probably involved in all these mechanisms.

Use of nonsteroidal anti-inflammatory drugs, cigarette smoking, the presence of *Helicobacter pylori* in the stomach and heredity (male sex, blood group O) influence that equilibrium unfavourably and are associated with increased incidence of peptic ulcer.

Drugs can alter the balance towards healing and prevention of recurrence of **ulcer** in the following ways:

- Reduction of acid secretion by:
  - histamine H_2-receptor antagonists, e.g. ranitidine, cimetidine, famotidine, nizatidine
  - proton pump inhibitors, e.g. omeprazole
  - antimuscarinic drugs, e.g. pirenzepine
- Neutralisation of secreted acid by antacids, e.g. magnesium trisilicate, aluminium hydroxide
- Enhancement of mucosal resistance by various mechanisms, e.g. bismuth compounds, sucralfate, prostaglandins.

The use of drugs should be seen against the background that many ulcers heal spontaneously, especially by cessation of smoking. Medicines are justified partly because they accelerate healing with reduced risk of complications and quicker relief of symptoms, and partly because they heal some ulcers which otherwise would not heal. They may also prevent recurrence.

Reduction of acid secretion

HISTAMINE H$_2$-RECEPTOR ANTAGONISTS

A general account of the pharmacology of histamine appears in Chapter 28. Clinically, the most important histamine H$_2$-receptors are those on the gastric parietal (acid-secreting) cells. Numerous factors influence acid secretion by the stomach, including food, psychological conditioning and drugs. Their effects are mediated at the parietal cells by the transmitter substances histamine, gastrin and acetylcholine which, through a common path involving cyclic AMP and calcium ions, interact with the gastric proton pump (see p. 569) that is ultimately responsible for secreting acid into the lumen of the stomach. Histamine, however, appears to be necessary for the action of gastrin and acetylcholine, and histamine H$_2$-receptor antagonists inhibit acid secretion induced by these agents also; it is no surprise that histamine H$_2$-receptor blockade has become clinically important.

Cimetidine

Cimetidine, the first clinically important histamine H$_2$-receptor antagonist, is described fully and the others in so far as they differ. Cimetidine provides dose-related inhibition of gastric secretion stimulated by injected histamine, by insulin, caffeine, protein-rich meals and (cholinergic) muscarinic drugs. All phases of gastric secretion are reduced namely, fasting and nocturnal (completely), and food-stimulated (by about 70%) by a therapeutic daily dose. Both the volume and the hydrogen ion concentration of gastric juice are reduced. Although the concentration of pepsin is not reduced, the total

amount secreted falls because the volume of gastric juice is less. Parietal cells secrete intrinsic factor as well as hydrogen ions but in normal doses cimetidine does not have a sufficient effect on vitamin B$_{12}$ turnover to cause haematological or neurological complications. Cimetidine does not affect gastric emptying, unlike antimuscarinic drugs which delay it.

Pharmacokinetics. Cimetidine is readily absorbed from the upper small gut. The t$^1/_2$ is 2 h and 60% of an oral dose is recovered as unchanged drug in the urine, the remainder appearing as metabolites. Total absorption of cimetidine is unimpaired if it is taken with food although peak blood concentrations are lower.

Uses. Cimetidine is used for conditions in which reduction of gastric acid secretion is beneficial. These are in the main: duodenal ulcer, benign gastric ulcer, stomal ulcer and reflux oesophagitis.

When treating a gastric ulcer, it is desirable to confirm that it is benign by endoscopy and biopsy every 6–8 weeks until it is healed, for the symptoms of gastric carcinoma can be relieved by cimetidine, so that apparently successful treatment may fatally delay the correct diagnosis.

Cimetidine is also used for prophylaxis of *gastrointestinal bleeding* due to gastric erosions complicating the stress of such serious conditions as burns, fulminant hepatic failure, renal failure or trauma. This success contrasts with acute bleeding in patients with peptic ulcer, oesophagitis or Mallory–Weiss syndrome (prolonged vomiting causing laceration at the oesophagogastric junction) in which there may be erosion or trauma to larger blood vessels, and in which clinical trials have failed consistently to show benefit.

Other uses. Cimetidine is given before *anaesthesia* for emergency surgery and before *labour* to lessen the risk of pulmonary aspiration of gastric acid; it is also used to prevent peptic ulcer induced by NSAIDs in high-risk patients, e.g. elderly women and those with a previous history of ulceration, although conclusive evidence of benefit is lacking. In chronic *pancreatic insufficiency* oral enzyme supplements may fail to reach the duodenum in sufficient amount since they are destroyed by acid in the stomach; steatorrhoea and weight loss may be prevented if cimetidine is taken at the same time as the enzyme formulation.

Dose. Cimetidine 400 mg $\times$ 2/day, with breakfast and at bedtime is usually satisfactory for peptic ulcer. Alternatively, patients with duodenal ulcer who normally have a high nocturnal acid secretion, may receive 800 mg as a single daily dose at bedtime. Most patients become symptom-free in about 8 days but treatment should continue for 6–8 weeks, after which 85–90% of duodenal and 60% of gastric ulcers can be expected to heal; this is about *double the spontaneous healing rate*. Maintenance preventive dose for recurrent cases: 400 mg at night. The dose should be reduced when renal or hepatic function are significantly impaired.

Adverse effects and interactions are few in short-term use. Minor complaints include headache, dizziness, constipation, diarrhoea, tiredness and muscular pain. Bradycardia and cardiac conduction defects may also occur. Cimetidine is a weak antiandrogen, and may cause gynaecomastia and sexual dysfunction in males. In the elderly particularly, it may cause CNS disturbances including lethargy, confusion and hallucinations. Cimetidine is an inhibitor of hepatic drug-oxidising enzymes; raised plasma concentrations with enhanced activity of warfarin, phenytoin, lignocaine, propranolol and theophylline result when these drugs are administered with it. Indeed when cimetidine is given there is a potential for increased effect with any drug with a low therapeutic index that is inactivated by oxidation in the liver.

Ranitidine, famotidine, nizatidine

These histamine H_2-receptor antagonists have actions, uses and therapeutic efficacy that are essentially those of cimetidine. Differences from cimetidine lie chiefly in dose and profile of unwanted effects.

Pharmacokinetics. Ranitidine ($t^{1}/_{2}$ 2 h) is 50%, famotidine ($t^{1}/_{2}$ 3 h) is 25% and nizatidine ($t^{1}/_{2}$ 1 h) is 10% metabolised, in each case the remainder being excreted unchanged by the kidney.

Dose. Ranitidine 150 mg $\times$ 2/d taken in the morning and in the evening will usually suffice; a single dose of 300 mg at night may be used as an alternative for duodenal ulcer. A course should last at least 4 weeks and ulcers that have not healed at this stage are normally healed by a further 4 weeks of therapy. Those with a history of recurrent ulcer may benefit from a maintenance dose of 150 mg nightly.

Adverse effects. The drugs are well tolerated but headache, dizziness, reversible confusion, constipation and diarrhoea may occur. In addition, urticaria, sweating and somnolence are reported with nizatidine. The drugs *do not inhibit* hepatic microsomal enzymes and drug interactions reported with cimetidine are not to be anticipated. Ranitidine and famotidine do not block androgen receptors and do not cause gynaecomastia and impotence, like cimetidine.

PROTON PUMP INHIBITORS

Drugs of this class reduce gastric acid secretion not by blocking histamine-H_2 or muscarinic receptors, but by inhibiting the action of H^+,K^+-ATPase, an enzyme that occurs almost exclusively in the gastric parietal cell. The enzyme catalyses the exchange of protons (hydrogen ions, H^+) for potassium ions at the cell membrane, i.e. the final step in the acid secretory process, sometimes called the proton pump. Therefore they antagonise all stimulants of gastric secretion.

Omeprazole

Omeprazole ($t^{1}/_{2}$ 1 h) produces a profound, long-lasting and probably irreversible[1] enzyme inhibition of both basic and stimulated acid secretion, a single 20 mg dose decreasing acidity by 90% over 24 h. Omeprazole must be given in enteric-coated granules for it is degraded at low pH; it is absorbed in the small intestine. The drug is rapidly metabolised. Systemic availability increases with dose, probably because of saturation of first-pass effect.

Uses. Omeprazole is highly effective for ulcerative reflux oesophagitis and is the drug of choice for

---

[1] Reversible proton pump inhibitors, also called acid pump antagonists (APA) are becoming available.

Zollinger–Ellison syndrome (gastrin-producing tumour of the pancreas, causing hypersecretion of gastric acid and severe peptic ulceration). Omeprazole heals peptic ulcers at least as well as histamine H_2-receptor antagonists but the latter are generally drugs of first choice because of persisting uncertainty about the safety of profound and longterm suppression of acid secretion (see below). Omeprazole, however, should be considered for resistant ulcers including those related to therapy with NSAIDs.

Adverse effects. Nausea, headache, diarrhoea, constipation and rash occur but are uncommon. Omeprazole inhibits the oxidative metabolism of warfarin and phenytoin, enhancing the action of these drugs (but inhibition is less than with cimetidine).

Concern has arisen that longterm use of highly effective antisecretory drugs may increase the risk of gastric neoplasia. Differing mechanisms have been proposed. When acid secretion is suppressed, gastrin is released as a normal homeostatic response. Gastrin stimulates the growth of the gastric epithelium, including the enterochromaffin cells which transform into carcinoid tumours; some rats developed these tumours after prolonged and high dose exposure to omeprazole. Alternatively, prolonged hypochlorhydria favours the colonisation of the stomach by bacteria which have the potential to convert ingested nitrates into carcinogenic nitrosamines.

Surveillance studies to date have not provided evidence that this is a real hazard, and it is certainly unlikely with short-term use, e.g. up to 8 weeks.

Lansoprazole is similar.

ANTIMUSCARINIC DRUGS

A general account appears in Chapter 22. Despite expectations, based on theoretical considerations of the importance of the parasympathetic autonomic system in gastric secretion, drugs with general antimuscarinic activity have not proved successful in the therapy of peptic ulcer, because of the unwanted effects of general antimuscarinic blockade, i.e. atropine-like effects.

Pirenzepine has some selectivity, i.e. it inhibits gastric secretion at doses lower than those that affect

gastrointestinal motility, ocular, salivary, urinary and central nervous function. It owes this relative selectivity to its high affinity for and blockade of M_1-muscarinic receptors in autonomic ganglia; it has low affinity for the M_2-receptors of the smooth muscle of the ileum and urinary bladder. In the stomach pirenzepine appears to inhibit transmission in parasympathetic enteric ganglia.

Pirenzepine is poorly absorbed from the gastrointestinal tract and it is excreted mainly unchanged in the urine and bile. The $t^{1/2}$ is 11 h. It is used for duodenal and gastric ulcer.

Neutralisation of secreted acid

Antacids are basic substances that reduce gastric acidity by neutralising HCl. The *hydroxide* is the most common base but trisilicate, carbonate and bicarbonate ions are also used. The therapeutic efficacy and adverse effects depend also on the metallic ion with which the base is combined, and this is usually *aluminium*, *magnesium* or *sodium*. Calcium and bismuth have largely been abandoned for this purpose because this caused systemic toxicity.

The benefit of antacids depends on protecting the gastric mucosa from acid (by neutralisation) and from pepsin (which is inactive above pH 5, and which in addition is inactivated by aluminium and magnesium). Continuous elevation of pH by intermittent administration is limited by gastric emptying. The significant fact is that however large or small the gastric contents, if they are liquid, half will have left in about 30 minutes.

Antacids, therefore, are generally used to relieve symptoms of ulcer and nonulcer dyspepsia and they are taken when symptoms occur, i.e. intermittently. Histamine H_2-receptor antagonists are normally preferred as ulcer-healing agents but an antacid may be taken for occasional symptomatic relief, especially during the first few days of a course of treatment with an H_2-receptor blocker.

INDIVIDUAL ANTACIDS

Magnesium oxide and **hydroxide** react quickly,

but cause diarrhoea, as do all magnesium salts, which are also used as purgatives.

Magnesium carbonate is rather less effective.

Magnesium trisilicate reacts slowly, to form magnesium chloride which reacts with intestinal secretions to form the carbonate, the chloride being released and reabsorbed. Systemic acid–base balance is thus not significantly altered.

Aluminium hydroxide reacts with HCl to form aluminium chloride which reacts with intestinal secretions to produce insoluble salts, especially phosphate, the chloride being released and reabsorbed; thus it does not alter systemic acid–base balance. It tends to constipate. Sufficient aluminium may be absorbed from the intestine to create a risk of encephalopathy in patients with chronic renal failure. Hypophosphataemia and hypophosphaturia may result from binding phosphate so that it is not absorbed from the gut.

Sodium bicarbonate reacts with acid and relieves pain within minutes. It is absorbed and causes alkalosis which in short-term use may not cause symptoms but can be a serious matter in patients with renal insufficiency. Sodium bicarbonate can release enough CO_2 in the stomach to cause discomfort and belching, which may have a psychotherapeutic effect or not, according to the circumstances. Excess sodium intake may cause oedema and heart failure in patients with cardiac or renal disease.

Calcium- and *bismuth-containing antacids* are available but should be avoided. Those that contain calcium may cause rebound acid hypersecretion and, with prolonged use, hypercalcaemia and alkalosis which may rarely be associated with renal failure (the milk–alkali syndrome). Bismuth may be absorbed and cause encephalopathy and arthropathy.

Alginic acid may be combined with an antacid to encourage adherence of the mixture to the mucosa, e.g. for reflux oesophagitis.

Dimethicone is sometimes included in antacid mixtures as an antifoaming agent to reduce flatulence. It is a silicone polymer that lowers surface tension and allows the small bubbles of froth to coalesce into large bubbles that can more easily be passed up from the stomach or down from the colon. It helps distended mountaineers to belch usefully at high altitudes.

Adverse effects of antacid mixtures

Those that apply to individual antacids are described above but the following general points are also relevant.

Some antacid mixtures contain *sodium* which may not be readily apparent from the name and for this reason may be dangerous for patients with cardiac or renal disease. For example, a 10 ml dose of magnesium carbonate mixture or of magnesium trisilicate mixture contains about 6 mmol of sodium (normal daily dietary intake is approx. 120 mmol of sodium).

Aluminium- and magnesium-containing antacids may interfere with the absorption of other drugs by binding with them or by altering gastrointestinal pH or transit time. Reduced biological availability of iron, digoxin, warfarin and some NSAIDs has been ascribed to this type of interaction. It is probably advisable not to co-administer antacids with drugs that are intended for systemic effect by the oral route.

Choice and use of antacids

No single antacid is satisfactory for all circumstances and mixtures are often used. They may contain sodium bicarbonate for quickest effect, supplemented by magnesium hydroxide or carbonate. Sometimes magnesium trisilicate or aluminium hydroxide is added, but these are often used alone, though they are relatively slow-acting.

Disturbed bowel habit can be corrected by altering the proportions of magnesium salts that tend to cause diarrhoea, and aluminium salts that tend to constipate, sometimes severely.

Tablets are more convenient for the patient at work but they act more slowly unless they are sucked or chewed; a liquid may be more acceptable for frequent use. Patients will find their own optimal pattern of use.

Enhancing mucosal resistance

Drugs can increase mucosal resistance by

- protecting the base of a peptic ulcer (bismuth chelate, sucralfate)
- eradicating *Helicobacter pylori* (antimicrobials)
- 'cytoprotection' (misoprostol).

Bismuth chelate (tripotassium dicitratobismuthate, bismuth subcitrate, De-Nol).

This substance was thought to act primarily by selectively chelating with protein material in the ulcer base, so forming a coating that protects it from the adverse influences of acid, pepsin and bile. Subsequently, bismuth chelate was found to be active against *Helicobacter pylori*, especially when combined with an antimicrobial (see below).

Bismuth chelate is used for benign gastric and duodenal ulcer and has a therapeutic efficacy approximately equivalent to histamine H_2-receptor antagonists. Ulcer healing appears to persist longer after bismuth chelate than after the histamine H_2-receptor antagonists, and this may relate to the ability of the former but not of the latter to eradicate *Helicobacter pylori*.

Bismuth chelate, particularly as a liquid formulation, darkens the tongue, teeth and stool; the tablet is less likely to do so and is thus more acceptable. Systemic absorption of bismuth from the chelated preparation appears to be well below the levels at which encephalopathy occurs but bismuth is eliminated by the kidney and it is prudent to avoid giving the drug to patients with impaired renal function. Elimination in the urine continues for months after bismuth is discontinued.

Sucralfate

This is a complex salt of sucrose sulphate and aluminium hydroxide. In the acid environment of the stomach, the aluminium moiety is released so that the compound develops a strong negative charge and binds electrostatically to positively charged protein molecules that transude from damaged mucosa. The result is a viscous paste that adheres selectively and protectively to the ulcer base. Its action appears to derive also from binding to and inactivating pepsin and bile acids which are ulcerogenic; it has negligible acid neutralising capacity but may prevent damaging back-diffusion of H^+ from the lumen to the mucosa.

Sucralfate is used for benign gastric and duode-

nal ulcer and for chronic gastritis; its therapeutic efficacy is approximately equal to that of the histamine H_2-receptor antagonists but may be better at prolonging remission after healing has occurred. Maintenance treatment is effective at preventing relapse.

Sucralfate may cause constipation but is otherwise well tolerated. It is partly absorbed from the gastrointestinal tract; the concentration of aluminium in the plasma may be elevated but appears to be a problem only with longterm use by uraemic patients, especially those undergoing dialysis. As the drug is effective only in acid conditions, an antacid should not be taken 30 min before or after a dose of sucralfate. Sucralfate interferes with absorption of co-administered drugs, e.g. ciprofloxacin, theophylline, digoxin, phenytoin and amitriptyline, possibly by binding due to its strong negative charge.

Antimicrobials: eradication of *Helicobacter pylori*

The bacterium *Helicobacter pylori* is specifically adapted to living in the mucus that overlies gastric epithelial cells and in areas of ectopic gastric mucosa in the duodenum.

Duodenal ulcer is often associated with an active chronic inflammation of the duodenum and of the gastric antrum.

Gastric ulcer is associated with a more severe inflammation that involves the antrum and body of the stomach.

A causal role for *Helicobacter pylori* in gastroduodenal disease has become accepted because:

- The organism is found in about 90% of cases of duodenal ulcer or chronic antral gastritis and about 70% of cases of gastric ulcer
- Experimental infection of healthy volunteers with the organism produces gastritis
- Eradication of the bacterium protects against relapse of *duodenal* ulcer (its value in gastric ulcer is less certain).

Infection may be confirmed by mucosal histology, a radio-labelled breath test or by the detection of IgG antibodies to *Helicobacter pylori,* and should be suspected in any patient with duodenal ulcer.

Helicobacter pylori is sensitive to metronidazole, amoxycillin, clarithromycin, tetracycline and bismuth salts. Numerous regimens have been proposed to eradicate the organism and heal ulcers. It appears likely that the most efficacious will comprise one or two weeks of antimicrobial therapy (to include metronidazole, and either amoxycillin or clarithromycin or both) combined with suppression of acid secretion (with omeprazole). The position is complicated by the appearance of metronidazole-resistant strains of *Helicobacter pylori.*

Bismuth-based therapies are also effective but are more complicated and less well tolerated. Eradication of the infection usually results in longterm remission of the ulcer.

Misoprostol

Endogenous prostaglandins contribute importantly to the integrity of the gastrointestinal mucosa by a number of related mechanisms:

- Stimulation of mucus and bicarbonate secretion
- Maintenance of blood flow; an adequate flow not only ensures a supply of oxygen and nutrients but also helps to remove H^+ which readily diffuses from the lumen into damaged or ischaemic tissues
- Prevention of luminal H^+ from diffusing into the mucosa, e.g. in response to aspirin, ethanol and bile salts
- Enhancement of the rate of cell replication in the mucosa, to hasten the repair of damaged epithelium
- Reduction of gastric acid secretion.

Gastric and duodenal mucosal damage and chronic peptic ulcer associated with the use of NSAIDs may derive from interference with the above actions (sometimes collectively called 'cytoprotective') of prostaglandins, for NSAIDs inhibit the formation of prostaglandins.

Misoprostol is a synthetic analogue of prostaglandin E_1 which prevents the formation of gastric ulcers in patients who are taking NSAIDs, presumably by these mechanisms. The drug also heals chronic gastric and duodenal ulcers to an extent predictable from its inhibition of gastric acid secretion, i.e. not dependent on the cytoprotective action.

Adverse effects. Diarrhoea and abdominal pain, transient and dose-related, are the commonest. Women may experience gynaecological disturbances such as spotting and dysmenorrhoea; the drug is contraindicated in pregnancy or for women planning to become pregnant, for the products of conception may be aborted (and indeed women have resorted to using misoprostol (illicitly) as an abortifacient in parts of the world where provision of contraceptive services is poor).[2]

Liquorice derivatives, carbenoxolone and deglycyrrhizinised liquorice, formerly used for peptic ulcer, are now obsolete.

Overall management

Several therapeutic strategies are now recognised as being effective for peptic ulcer and their place in the overall management of the disease may be summarised:

- *General advice* should be to stop smoking, to avoid NSAID use and alcohol. Both smoking and NSAIDs retard ulcer healing with histamine H_2-receptor antagonists.
- *Healing* of peptic ulcer can be accelerated by a number of types of drug.

  — **A histamine H_2-receptor antagonist** is generally preferred because of safety and ease of administration. Those currently available have approximately equal therapeutic efficacy and the choice in the individual case may be determined by considerations such as cost, concurrent use of drugs such as warfarin, theophylline or phenytoin with which cimetidine will interact, and experience of adverse effects.

---

[2] A combination of methotrexate and misoprostol has been advocated as a safe and effective alternative to invasive methods to terminate early pregnancy (Hausknecht R U 1995 New England Journal of Medicine 333: 337–340).

— **Bismuth chelate** and sucralfate are alternatives that are approximately as effective as histamine H_2-receptor antagonists but the need for multiple dosing (up to $\times 4/d$) may limit compliance.

— **Antacids** as sole treatment can accelerate ulcer healing but must be taken frequently and in high dose to achieve this; their use is now limited to providing supplementary symptomatic relief, e.g. in the first few days of a course of a histamine H_2-blocker and for intermittent use subsequently.

● *Eradication of Helicobacter pylori.* Opinions differ as to whether this should be primary therapy for all ulcers.

● *Ulcers that are difficult to heal* may respond to double the normal dose of a histamine H_2-blocker or to omeprazole. For duodenal ulcers, evidence of infection with *Helicobacter pylori* should be sought and, if found, one of the regimens to eradicate the organism should be used.

● *Most ulcers induced by NSAIDs* occur in the stomach and duodenum. The first step should be to review the necessity for using the NSAID. Misoprostol may prevent peptic ulceration in those at high risk, e.g. the elderly, and those who have previously had an ulcer. Misoprostol may also be used to treat an NSAID-induced ulcer. A duodenal ulcer induced by NSAIDs may respond to a histamine H_2-blocker.

● *Prevention of relapse*, in those individuals who are prone to it, may be achieved with a histamine H_2-blocker taken as a single dose at night, on a longterm basis, for such drugs have a well-established safety record. Post-ulcer patients may reasonably be advised periodically to take a histamine H_2-blocker for a few days for indigestion.

● *Surgery* may be required for patients whose ulcers recur despite all other measures.

Vomiting

If the cause of vomiting cannot be promptly removed, it may be desirable to attempt to prevent or suppress it by drugs.

The pharmacology of vomiting was little studied until the world war of 1939–45, when motion sickness attained military importance as a possible handicap for sea landings made in the face of resistance. The British military authorities and the Medical Research Council therefore organised an investigation. Whenever there was a prospect of sufficiently rough weather, about 70 soldiers were sent to sea in small ships, again and again, after being dosed with a drug or a dummy tablet and having had their mouths inspected to detect non-compliance. The ships returned to land when up to 40% of the soldiers vomited. 'On the whole the men enjoyed their trips;' some of them, however, being soldiers, thought the tablets were given in order to make them vomit and some 'believed firmly in the efficacy of the dummy tablets'. It was concluded that, of the remedies tested, hyoscine (0.6 mg or 1.2 mg) was the most effective.[3]

SOME PHYSIOLOGY

Useful vomiting occurs as a protective mechanism for eliminating irritant or harmful substances from the upper gastrointestinal tract. The act of emesis is controlled by the vomiting centre in the medulla and close to it lie other visceral centres, e.g. for respiration, salivation and vascular control which give rise to the prodromal sensations of vomiting. These centres are not anatomically discrete but comprise interconnected networks within the nucleus tractus solitarii. The *vomiting centre* does not initiate, but rather it coordinates the act of emesis on receiving stimuli from various sources, namely,

1. The chemoreceptor trigger zone (CTZ), a nearby area that is extremely sensitive to the action of drugs and other chemicals
2. The vestibular system
3. The periphery, e.g. distension or irritation of the gut, myocardial infarction, biliary or renal stone
4. Cortical centres.

The vomiting centre and the nucleus tractus solitarii contain many muscarinic cholinergic and histamine H_1-receptors, and the CTZ is rich in dopamine D_2-receptors; drugs that block these receptors are effective antiemetics. The precise role and location of 5-HT_3-receptors (see Ondansetron, below) in

---

[3] Holling H E et al 1944 Lancet 1: 127.

relation to emesis remains to be defined but both central and peripheral mechanisms may be involved.

Antiemetic and prokinetic drugs

These may be classified as shown in Table 32.1.

Antiemetics acting on the vomiting centre have *antimuscarinic* (their principal mode) and antihistaminic action, e.g. hyoscine, promethazine; they alleviate vomiting from any cause. But drugs acting on the CTZ (haloperidol, ondansetron) are effective only for vomiting mediated by the chemoreceptors (morphine, digoxin, cytotoxics, uraemia). The most efficacious drugs act at more than one site (see Table 32.1).

Antimuscarinic drugs (including those classed primarily as histamine H_1-receptor antagonists) are described elsewhere. Drugs with antimuscarinic activity probably act both centrally and in the gastrointestinal tract. Phenothiazines and butyrophe-

Table 32.1 Classification of antiemetic drugs

Drug	Site of action
Dopamine D_2-receptor antagonists	
domperidone	CTZ and gut
metoclopramide	CTZ and gut
haloperidol	CTZ
phenothiazines, e.g.	Vomiting centre
chlorpromazine,	and CTZ
prochlorperazine,	
thiethylperazine	
5-HT$_3$-receptor antagonists	
ondansetron	CTZ and gut
granisetron	
tropisetron	
Antimuscarinics	
hyoscine and some drugs also	Vomiting centre
classed as histamine H_1-receptor	and gut
antagonists, e.g. cyclizine,	
dimenhydrinate, promethazine	
Other agents	
cisapride	Gut
corticosteroids (dexamethasone,	
methylprednisolone)	Vomiting due to
cannabinoids (nabilone)	cytotoxics
benzodiazepines (lorazepam)	

nones owe their antiemetic efficacy to blockade of dopamine D_2-receptors but they readily penetrate the brain and may produce unwanted extrapyramidal effects by blocking D_2-receptors in the basal ganglia; many also have antimuscarinic effects.

Metoclopramide

Metoclopramide (Maxolon) acts centrally by blocking dopamine D_2-receptors in the CTZ, and peripherally by enhancing the action of acetylcholine at muscarinic nerve endings in the gut. It raises the tone of the lower oesophageal sphincter, relaxes the pyloric antrum and duodenal cap and increases peristalsis and emptying of the upper gut. The peripheral actions are utilised to empty the stomach before emergency anaesthesia and in labour (the term *prokinetic* is used for this action). If an opioid has been given, metoclopramide may fail to overcome the opioid-induced inhibition of gastric emptying and thus the risk of vomiting and inhaling gastric contents remains. The direct effects on the gut are antagonised by antimuscarinic drugs. The action of metoclopramide is terminated by metabolism in the liver; the $t^{1/2}$ is 4 h.

Uses. Metoclopramide is used for nausea and vomiting associated with gastrointestinal disorders, with postsurgical conditions, and with cytotoxic drugs and radiotherapy. It is also an effective antiemetic in migraine and is used as a prokinetic agent (above).

Adverse reactions are characteristic of dopamine receptor antagonists and include extrapyramidal dystonia (torticollis, facial spasms, trismus, oculogyric crises) which occurs more commonly in children and young adults, and in those who are concurrently receiving other dopamine receptor antagonists, e.g. phenothiazine drugs. The reaction is rapidly abolished by the antimuscarinic drug, benztropine, given i.v. Longterm use of metoclopramide may cause tardive dyskinesia in the elderly. Metoclopramide stimulates prolactin release and may cause gynaecomastia and lactation. Motor restlessness and diarrhoea also occur.

Cisapride (Prepulsid) is structurally related to metoclopramide but does not block dopamine receptors; rather, it appears to enhance acetylcholine release in the myenteric plexus of the gut; it increases motility throughout the gastrointestinal tract. The $t^{1/2}$ is 10 h; its action is terminated by metabolism and there is evidence of considerable first-pass inactivation by the oral route.

Cisapride is used to relieve symptoms of gastro-oesophageal reflux, for reflux oesophagitis and where gastric motility is impaired, e.g. in diabetes and systemic sclerosis.

The drug may cause abdominal cramping and diarrhoea, which are indeed extensions of its pharmacological action. It appears to have no central sedative effects. Co-administration by mouth of cisapride with fluconazole, itraconazole, ketaconazole, miconazole, erythromycin or clarithromycin is contraindicated as serious cardiac dysrhythmias may result.

Domperidone ($t^{1/2}$ 7 h) blocks dopamine D_2-receptors in the CTZ, and peripherally in the upper gut where it increases the tone in the lower oesophageal sphincter, enhances contractions of the gastric antrum and relaxes the pyloric sphincter. It crosses the blood–brain barrier poorly; this does not limit its therapeutic efficacy, for the CTZ is functionally outwith the barrier, but there is less risk of adverse effects in the central nervous system. Domperidone is used for nausea or vomiting associated with gastrointestinal disorders and with cytotoxic and other drug treatment. Dystonic reactions with domperidone are much fewer than with metoclopramide. It may cause gynaecomastia and galactorrhoea.

Ondansetron ($t^{1/2}$ 5 h) is a selective 5-HT$_3$-receptor antagonist. Drugs with this activity appear to be highly effective against nausea and vomiting induced by cytotoxic agents and radiotherapy. Evidence suggests that such anticancer treatment releases serotonin (5-HT) from enterochromaffin cells in the gut mucosa (where resides > 80% of the serotonin in the body) which activates specific receptors in the gut and central nervous system to cause emesis.[4] The action of ondansetron is thus partly central and partly peripheral. Ondansetron may be given by i.v. injection or infusion immediately prior to cancer chemotherapy (notably with cisplatin), followed by oral administration for up to 5 days. The drug appears to be well tolerated but constipation, headache and a feeling of flushing in the head and epigastrium may occur. *Granisetron* and *tropisetron* are similar.

Nabilone is a synthetic cannabinoid and has properties similar to tetrahydrocannabinol (the active constituent of marijuana) which has an antiemetic action. It is used to relieve nausea or vomiting caused by cytotoxic drugs. Adverse effects include: somnolence, dry mouth, decreased appetite, dizziness, euphoria, dysphoria, postural hypotension, confusion and psychosis. These may be reduced if prochlorperazine is given concomitantly.

Treatment for various forms

MOTION SICKNESS

Motion sickness is more easily prevented than cured. It is due chiefly to overstimulation of the vestibular apparatus (and does not occur if the labyrinth is destroyed). Other factors also contribute. Visually, a moving horizon can be most disturbing, as can the sensations induced by the gravitational inertia of a full stomach when the body is in vertical movement. That the environment, whether close and smelly or open and vivifying, is important, is a matter of common experience amongst all who have been on a rough sea. Psychological factors, including observation of the fate of one's companions, are also important. Tolerance to the motion occurs, generally over a period of days.

Drugs that are used for motion sickness include: *cinnarizine, cyclizine, dimenhydrinate, hyoscine* and *promethazine*, all antimuscarinic.

For prophylaxis an antiemetic is best taken 1 h before exposure to the motion. About 70% protection may be expected by the right dose given at the right time. Once motion sickness has started, oral administration of drugs may fail, and the i.m., s.c. or rectal routes are required; alternatively, hyoscine may be administered as a dermal patch, so avoiding the enteral route. Prevention of symptoms may

---

[4] Cubeddu L X et al 1990 New England Journal of Medicine 322: 810.

therefore be possible only at the expense of troublesome unwanted effects: sleepiness, dry mouth, blurred vision.

DRUG-INDUCED VOMITING

If reducing the dose or withdrawing the offending drug are not options then an attempt, often unsatisfactory, may be made to oppose it by another drug. In general, *chlorpromazine* or another phenothiazine or *metoclopramide* are best. Opioid-induced vomiting responds to one of the drugs used for motion sickness (see above); cyclizine and morphine are combined as Cyclimorph.

VOMITING DUE TO CYTOTOXIC DRUGS

Prevention and alleviation of this distressing and often very severe symptom of some forms of cancer treatment may allow an optimal chemotherapeutic regimen to be used, and avoid admitting the patient to hospital. Cisplatin is notably emetic. Recognition that serotonin release probably plays a key role in cytotoxic-induced vomiting led to the introduction of *ondansetron* which proved highly effective. *Dexamethasone* is also efficacious although its mode of action is unclear. *Lorazepam*, despite dose-limiting sedation and dysphoria is a useful adjunct and provides amnesia which may limit the development of anticipatory vomiting.

Ondansetron plus dexamethasone with or without lorazepam (all given i.v.) is the most effective combination for severe vomiting due to cytotoxics and is well tolerated. Metoclopramide may be substituted for ondansetron where a less emetic regimen is used, especially in older patients who are less susceptible to its extrapyramidal reactions.

VOMITING AFTER GENERAL ANAESTHESIA

Postoperative vomiting is related to the duration of anaesthesia and the causation is multifactorial. *Metoclopramide*, a 5-HT$_3$-receptor antagonist, e.g. *ondansetron* or a butyrophenone, e.g. *haloperidol* or droperidol, may be used. The condition affects some 30% of patients and routine prophylaxis seems warranted only where the risk is high, e.g. those with a history of postoperative vomiting or of motion sickness, or where vomiting carries special hazard, e.g. eye surgery.

VOMITING IN PREGNANCY

This reaches a peak at 10–11 weeks and usually resolves by 13–14 weeks of gestation. Nausea alone does not require treatment. Much can be achieved by reassurance that the problem is transient and a discussion of diet, e.g. taking food before getting up in the morning. Rarely, a decision is taken to use a drug, and then a histamine H$_1$-receptor antagonist or a phenothiazine, e.g. promethazine (see above) is preferred. Although pyridoxine deficiency has not been shown to complicate simple pregnancy vomiting, it may occur in hyperemesis gravidarum which requires i.v. fluids and multivitamin supplement.

VERTIGO

A great range of drugs has been recommended to treat vertigo and labyrinthine disorders but antimuscarinics and phenothiazines are generally preferred. Cyclizine or prochlorperazine may be used to relieve an acute attack. *Betahistine* (a histamine analogue) is used in the hope of improving the blood circulation to the inner ear in Menière's syndrome; also cinnarizine.

Gastro-oesophageal reflux

Recurrent reflux of gastric contents into the oesophagus produces symptoms of 'heartburn' and/or oesophageal injury. This common condition may be managed as follows.

General measures include advice to avoid:

- Meals late at night, or lying down after meals
- Heavy lifting, tight clothing, bending
- Being overweight
- Smoking, because nicotine relaxes the lower oesophageal sphincter
- Substances known to aggravate the condition, e.g. hot foods or alcohol

- Drugs which encourage reflux, i.e. those with antimuscarinic activity (e.g. tricyclic antidepressants); smooth muscle relaxants (e.g. nitrates and calcium channel blockers); theophylline compounds
- Elevating the head of the patient's bed by 15–20 cm will discourage nocturnal reflux.

Drugs. An antacid, either alone or combined with alginic acid, e.g. Gaviscon, Gastrocote, provides relief for milder degrees of oesophagitis. The addition of alginic acid is supposed to produce a floating viscous gel that blocks reflux and protectively coats the oesophagus. More severe oesophagitis requires *acid suppression* with a proton pump inhibitor, e.g. omeprazole, or with a histamine H_2-receptor antagonist in a dose that is higher than that for gastric or duodenal ulcer and given for a prolonged period. Metoclopramide or cisapride may be used intermittently, especially for those patients who also complain of abdominal fullness or bloating.

Miscellaneous

Therapeutic emesis: see Drug overdose.

Diffuse oesophageal spasm may be helped by isosorbide dinitrate 5 mg sublingually or 10 mg by mouth, or by nifedipine 10 μg sublingually or swallowed.

Achalasia, in which there is failure of relaxation of the lower oesophageal sphincter, may be relieved by balloon dilatation or by surgery.

Bitters are substances taken before meals to improve appetite. They have not been scientifically investigated. They include gentian, nux vomica and quinine. Preparations can be found in formularies and at wine merchants (Dubonnet, Campari).

Carminatives are substances which are used to assist in expelling gas from the stomach and intestines. Examples are: dimethicone, peppermint, dill, anise and other herbs which are commonly included in liqueurs and (in nonalcoholic solutions) for babies, and may be useful in irritable bowel syndrome. The problem is not new: the Roman Emperor Claudius (AD 10–54)

planned an edict to legitimise the breaking of wind at table, either silently or noisily, after hearing about a man who was so modest that he endangered his health by an attempt to restrain himself (Suetonius (trans) R Graves).

GUIDE TO FURTHER READING

Andersen M, Schou J S 1994 Are H_2-receptor antagonists safe over the counter drugs? British Medical Journal 309: 494

Cohen S, Parkman H P 1995 Treatment of achalasia — from whalebone to botulinum toxin. New England Journal of Medicine 332: 815

Costa S H, Vessey M P 1993 Misoprostol and illegal abortion in Rio de Janeiro, Brazil. Lancet 341: 1258

Goodwin C S 1993 Gastric cancer and *Helicobacter pylori*: the whispering killer? Lancet 342: 507

Graham J R 1995 *Helicobacter pylori*: human pathogen or simply opportunist? Lancet 345: 1095

Grunberg S M, Hesketh P J 1994 Control of chemotherapy-induced emesis. New England Journal of Medicine 329: 1790

Lane L, Peterson W L 1994 Bleeding peptic ulcer. New England Journal of Medicine 331: 717

Maton P N 1991 Omeprazole. New England Journal of Medicine 324: 965

Patel P et al 1995 Prospective screening of dyspeptic patients by *Helicobacter pylori* serology. Lancet 346: 1315

Peterson W L 1991 *Helicobacter pylori* and peptic ulcer disease. New England Journal of Medicine 324: 1043

Pope C E 1994 Acid reflux disorders. New England Journal of Medicine 331: 656

Soll A H 1990 Pathogenesis of peptic ulcer and implications for therapy. New England Journal of Medicine 322: 909

Walsh J H, Peterson 1995 The treatment of *Helicobacter pylori* infection in the management of peptic ulcer disease. New England Journal of Medicine 333: 984

Wolfe M M, Soll A H 1988 The physiology of gastric secretion. New England Journal of Medicine 319: 1707

Vigneri S et al 1995 A comparison of five maintenance therapies for reflux esophagitis. New England Journal of Medicine 333: 1106

33

Intestines

SYNOPSIS

- Constipation: mode of action and use of drugs
- Misuse of laxatives
- Diarrhoea (importance of fluid/electrolyte replacement)
- Abnormal gut motility
- Inflammatory bowel disease

Constipation

The terms purgative, cathartic, laxative, aperient and evacuant may be considered synonymous; they are medicines that promote defaecation largely by reducing the viscosity of the contents of the lower colon.

Purgatives may be classified as:

- bulk
- osmotic
- faecal softeners
- stimulant.

Their properties confer some variation in the indications for use. The times that purgatives take to act are listed in the text, for these determine whether they should be given in the morning or evening.

BULK PURGATIVES

These comprise indigestible vegetable fibre and hydrophilic colloids. Bulk purgatives act by increasing the volume and lowering the viscosity of intestinal contents to promote a large, soft, solid stool. The substances thus encourage normal *reflex bowel activity*, rendering it more effective and generally acting within 1–3 h. They are also helpful for anal fissure, haemorrhoids, diverticular disease and irritable bowel syndrome. All bulk purgatives must be taken with 2 l/day of fluid. If taken repeatedly with too little fluid they can cause intestinal obstruction, especially if there is any organic obstruction or if peristalsis is weak.

Dietary fibre is essentially the cell walls and supporting structures of vegetables and fruits. The term 'fibre' is retained although it is imprecise because it covers a range of substances that cannot be easily measured. Increasingly reference is made to *non-starch polysacccharide* (NSP)[1] which refers to carbohydrates that are not digestible by human enzymes and which can be assayed; NSP comprises most of the fibre in our diet. Fibre may be soluble (pectins, guar, ispaghula) or insoluble (cellulose, hemicelluloses, lignin). Soluble fibre forms viscous solutions that delay gastric emptying and the absorption of nutrients from the small bowel; they have small but useful (5–10%) plasma cholesterol-lowering and appetite-suppressing effects, and are used to improve glycaemic control in diabetes mellitus, as well as treatment for constipation. Insoluble fibre has less effect on the viscosity of gut contents but is a stronger laxative: first, because it resists digestion

---

[1]The term 'unavailable complex carbohydrate' (UCC) is also used and refers to NSP plus undigested ('resistant') starch.

579

in the small gut and so enters the colon intact; second, because it has a vast capacity for retaining water, e.g. one gram of carrot fibre can hold 23 grams of water.[2] It has been proposed that as humans have refined the carbohydrates in their diet over the centuries, so they have deprived themselves of fibre, particularly from cereal, and that the resultant under-filling of the colon is an important cause of constipation, irritable bowel syndrome, haemorrhoids and diverticular disease. Adding fibre to the diet is thus a safe and natural way of treating constipation in individuals with low-fibre diets. *Bran* is the residue left when flour is made from cereals; it contains between 25 and 50% of fibre. The fibre content of normal diet can be increased by eating wholemeal bread and bran cereals but over-zealous supplementation may cause heartburn and aggravate the constipation (see above). While underfilling of the bowel causes constipation in otherwise normal individuals, it seems that some patients are constipated because their bowels are less responsive to insoluble fibre, and indeed to other stimulants. Viscous (soluble) fibres, e.g. ispaghula, are effective and more palatable than bran.

Ispaghula husk contains mucilage and hemicelluloses which swell rapidly in water.

Methylcellulose takes up water to swell to a colloid about 25 times its original volume. It is also used as a suspending agent in pharmacy, in lubricating jellies, in contact-lens wetting solutions and in artificial tears.

Sterculia,[3] similarly, swells when mixed with water.

OSMOTIC LAXATIVES

These are but little absorbed and increase the bulk and reduce viscosity of intestinal contents to promote a fluid stool.

Some inorganic salts retain water in the intestinal lumen or, if given as hypertonic solution, with-

draw it from the body. When constipation is mild, magnesium hydroxide will suffice but magnesium sulphate (Epsom[4] salt) is used when a more powerful effect is needed. Both magnesium salts act in 2–4 h. The small amount of magnesium absorbed when the sulphate is frequently used can be enough to cause magnesium poisoning in patients with renal impairment, the central nervous effects of which somewhat resemble those of uraemia. *Magnesium sulphate* 50% (hypertonic) is available as a single dose retention enema to reduce cerebrospinal fluid pressure in neurosurgery. Solutions of phosphates or sodium citrate may be used as enemas for constipation or when the bowel has to be cleared for a diagnostic procedure or surgery.

Lactulose is a synthetic disaccharide. Taken orally, it is unaffected by small intestinal disaccharidase, is not absorbed and thus acts as an osmotic laxative. Lactulose is also used in treatment of hepatic encephalopathy, which condition is aggravated by ammonia produced in the colon gaining access to the systemic circulation. In the colon lactulose is fermented to lactic and acetic acids which inhibit the growth of colonic ammonia-producing organisms and, by lowering pH, reduce non-ionic diffusion of ammonia from the colon into the blood. It takes 48 h to act. Tolerance may develop. Apart from hepatic disease, it is useful for patients with distal ulcerative colitis who tend to have faecal stasis in the proximal colon.

FAECAL SOFTENERS (emollients)

The softening properties of these agents are useful in the management of anal fissure and haemorrhoids.

Docusate sodium (dioctyl sodium sulphosuccinate) softens faeces by lowering the surface tension of fluids in the bowel which allows more water to remain in the faeces. It appears also to have bowel stimulant properties. Docusate sodium acts in 1–2 days but is relatively weak. *Poloxamers*, e.g. poloxalkol (poloxamer 188), act similarly and are used in combination with other agents.

---

[2] McConnell A A et al 1974 J Sci Food Agric 25: 1427.

[3] Named after Sterculinus, a god of ancient Rome, who presided over manuring of agricultural land.

[4] Epsom, a town near London, known for its defunct mineral spring water, and for horse racing.

Liquid paraffin is a chemically inert mineral oil and is not digested. It appears to reduce water absorption in the small intestine and it may be this effect as well as the softening powers of the oil (in the colon) that promotes the passage of softer faeces. It is often presented in emulsions with magnesium hydroxide. Some paraffin is absorbed from the intestine and collects in the mesenteric lymph nodes where paraffinomas may eventually form. Large doses may leak out of the anus causing both physical and social discomfort. Paraffin taken orally over long periods, especially at night, may be aspirated and cause chronic lipoid pneumonia. An unusual case resulted from successful attempts by a patient to lubricate his larynx with liquid paraffin. Because of these disadvantages its use is declining and it should never be used longterm as a laxative.

Arachis oil is included in enemas to soften impacted faeces.

STIMULANT PURGATIVES
(contact laxatives)

These increase intestinal motility by various mechanisms; they may cause abdominal cramps and should not be used where there is intestinal obstruction.

Bisacodyl stimulates sensory endings in the colon by direct action from the lumen. It is effective orally in 6–10 h and, as a suppository, acts in 1 h. In geriatric patients, bisacodyl suppositories reduce the need for regular enemas. There are no important unwanted effects.

Sodium picosulphate is similar and is also used to evacuate the bowel for investigative procedures and surgery.

Oxyphenisatin is administered as an enema to clear the colon for diagnostic procedures and surgery. It is not suitable for repeated use as this causes hepatitis.

Glycerol has a mild stimulant effect on the rectum when administered as a suppository.

The anthraquinone group of purgatives includes senna, danthron, cascara, rhubarb[5] and aloes. In the small intestine soluble anthraquinone derivates are liberated and absorbed. These are excreted into the colon and act there, along with those that have escaped absorption, probably after being chemically changed by bacterial action.

Patients taking some anthraquinones may notice their urine coloured brown (if acid) or red (if alkaline). Prolonged use can cause melanosis of the colon which cognoscenti can recognise through an endoscope. Anthraquinone preparations made from crude plant extracts are to be avoided as their lack of standardisation leads to erratic results.

Danthron is available as a standardised preparation in combination with the faecal softeners poloxamer 188 (as co-danthramer) and docusate sodium (as co-danthrusate). It acts in 6–12 h. As evidence from rodent studies indicates a possible carcinogenic risk, longterm exposure to danthron should be avoided but it is acceptable for use in the elderly or the terminally ill.

Senna, available as a biologically standardised preparation, is widely used to relieve constipation and to empty the bowel for investigative procedures and surgery. It acts in 8–12 h.

Drastic purgatives (castor oil, jalap,[6] colocynth, phenolphthalein and podophyllum) are obsolete.

Suppositories (bisacodyl, glycerin) may be used to obtain a bowel action in about 1 hour.

For anal and rectal disease, suppositories which are astringent (hamamelis), or anti-inflammatory (adrenal steroid) or local anaesthetic (lignocaine) are used as seems necessary.

Enemas produce defaecation by softening faeces

---

[5] In the late 18th century Britain made approaches to trade with China which were met with indifference; it seems that the mandarins held the belief that the British feared death from constipation if deprived of rhubarb (Rheum palmatum), one of China's exports.

[6] In the 19th century 'young men proceeding to Africa' were advised to take pills named Livingstone's Rousers, consisting of rhubarb, jalap, calomel and quinine. British Medical Journal (1964) 2: 1583.

and distending the bowel. They are used in preparation for surgery, radiological examination and endoscopy.[7] Preparations with sodium phosphate, which is poorly absorbed and so retains water in the gut, are generally used.

Enemas to be *retained* may be used to provide topical therapy for ulcerative colitis or Crohn's disease of the colon.

MANAGEMENT OF CONSTIPATION

Constipation may arise in the following settings:

• *Habitual constipation*, which is best corrected by adjusting the diet to contain more fibre, e.g. by including unpeeled fruit and vegetables, wholemeal bread, bran-based cereals, muesli[8] or simply by adding unprocessed bran. The latter may be sprinkled on the morning cereal or made up as a separate drink, the disagreeable nature of which is only partially disguised by mixing with fruit juice or milk. A faecal softener may be necessary and, if a stimulant is required, senna is perhaps the least objectionable.

Psychological factors are important. An explanation that normal bowel habit may vary between 3 motions per day and 2 per week, may be of more value to the patient than the prescription of a laxative.

• *Painful anal lesions* frequently lead to constipation because, when defaecation occurs, it is postponed for as long as possible, with the result that more water is absorbed and the faeces become harder and so hurt even more when they are eventually passed. This vicious cycle is best broken by the cure of the anal lesion but a bulk laxative or a faecal softener, and a local anaesthetic suppository, may give relief temporarily.

• *Pregnancy.* Constipation is best treated by ensuring that there is adequate fibre in the diet; if, despite this, the bowel sluggishness persists, one of the milder stimulant laxatives, e.g. senna, should be used, as vigorous purgation can cause abortion, though this is less reliable than some women hope.

• *Acute illness* may lead to sluggish bowel habit, especially if it involves confinement to bed and is accompanied by loss of appetite. Dependence on others for assistance to the toilet or, worse, to bring a bedpan, is also a factor. If severe enough to warrant attention, this kind of constipation can usually be dealt with by a bulk laxative, a faecal softener, senna or suppositories of glycerine or bisacodyl.

• *Elderly* patients may become constipated because their abdominal and perineal muscles lack tone and their diets are inadequate. The initial approach should be to use bran or other bulking agent, combined with improving mobility, fluid intake and establishing a regular bowel habit. Senna or bisacodyl may be used intermittently if further assistance is necessary but longterm use of a stimulant laxative may damage the myoenteric pathways. Resistant constipation may be best managed by twice-weekly phosphate enemas.

• *Drugs* may cause constipation. Opioid analgesics decrease propulsion in the gut. Drugs with *antimuscarinic* action reduce intestinal motility by blocking the muscarinic action of acetylcholine on gut smooth muscle; these include antispasmodics (hyoscine), antiparkinsonian drugs (orphenadrine), and tricyclic antidepressants (amitriptyline). *Aluminium-containing antacids*, *iron*, *calcium-channel blockers* and *benzodiazepines* all may constipate to varying degrees. Impaired propulsion enhances water absorption from the gut contents which become more viscous. When withdrawal of the causative drug is not feasible, e.g. treating intractable pain with an opioid, constipation should

---

[7] Enemas may arouse complex psychosocial/sexual impulses ranging from frequent use for imagined self-cleansing (colonic lavage) to the extraordinary case of the 'Illinois enema bandit' (USA, 1966–75), a man who broke into women students' accommodation and forcibly administered enemas. His exploits were immortalised in song by Frank Zappa (© 1978 Zappa Family Trust. Reprinted by permission):

'The Illinois Enema Bandit
I heard he's on the loose
I heard he's on the loose
Lord, the pitiful screams
Of all them college-educated women …
Boy, he'd just be tyin' 'em up
(They'd be all bound down!)
Just be pumpin' every one of 'em up with all the bag fulla
The Illinois Enema Bandit Juice …'

[8] A Swiss invention, being a delicious mixture of chopped cereals, nuts, dried fruits and honey.

be anticipated and a laxative prescribed with the analgesic.

Misuse of laxatives

Dependence (abuse) may arise following laxative use during an illness or in pregnancy, or the individual may have the mistaken notion that a daily bowel motion is essential for health, or that the bowels are only incompletely opened by nature, and so indulge in regular purgation. This effectively prevents the easy return of normal habits because the more powerful stimulant purges empty the whole colon, whereas normal defaecation empties only the descending colon. Cessation of use after a few weeks is thus inevitably followed by a few days' constipation whilst sufficient material collects to restore the normal state, which delay may convince the patient of the continued necessity for purgatives.

To prevent purgative dependence is easier than to cure it; patients feel they understand their own bowels far better than anyone else possibly could, an opinion they seldom extend to other organs, except perhaps the liver. In Britain, there is a belief that nurses have an intuitive understanding of the bowels that is denied to doctors.

Laxative dependence, which may be solely emotional at first, may be followed by *physical dependence*, i.e. the bowels will not open without a purgative. Excessive use of stimulant purgatives[9] may, especially in the old, lead to severe water and electrolyte depletion, even to hypokalaemic paralysis, malabsorption and protein-losing enteropathy. An atonic colon due to damage to gut nerves may result from prolonged abuse. Purgatives are dangerous if given to patients with undiagnosed abdominal pain, inflammatory intestinal disease or obstruction. Nor should they be used to get rid of hardened masses of faeces in the rectum, for they will fail and cause pain. Digital removal, generally

---

[9] The Roman Emperor Nero (AD 37–68) murdered his severely constipated aunt by ordering the doctors to give her 'a laxative of fatal strength'. He 'seized her property before she was quite dead and tore up the will so that nothing could escape him.' (Suetonius (trans) R Graves).

ordered by a senior and performed by a junior doctor, is required. A faecal softener helps to prevent recurrence.

Diarrhoea

Diarrhoea ranges from a mild and socially inconvenient illness to a major cause of death and malnutrition among children in less developed countries; acute diarrhoea causes 4–5 million deaths throughout the world annually. Drugs have a place in its management but the first priority of therapy is to *preserve fluid and electrolyte balance*. The condition is often assumed to be microbial (infection or toxins in food), but it may be caused by anxiety, food, drugs or other toxins. Diarrhoea is measured by volume and frequency of stools.

SOME PHYSIOLOGY

Absorption and secretion of *water* and *electrolytes* occur throughout the intestine, probably as separate processes, for absorption is a function of the cells of the intestinal villi and the surface cells of the colon, while cells in the crypts between villi are responsible for active secretion of water. Water follows the osmotic gradients which result from shifts of electrolytes across the intestinal epithelium, and sodium and chloride transport mechanisms are central to the causation and management of diarrhoea, especially that caused by bacteria and viruses.

Absorption of *sodium* into the epithelium is effected by:

Sodium-glucose-coupled entry. Glucose stimulates the absorption of sodium and the resulting water flow also sweeps additional sodium and chloride along with it (solvent drag). This important mechanism remains active in diarrhoea of various aetiologies and improvement of sodium and water absorption by glucose (and amino acids) is the basis of oral rehydration regimens (see below).

Sodium-ion-coupled entry. Na^+ and Cl^- enter the epithelial cell, either as a pair or, as seems more likely, there is a double exchange: Na^+ (extracellular) with H^+ (intracellular) and Cl^- (extracellular) with ^-OH or $^-HCO_3$ (intracellular). Oral rehydration solutions (see below) contain sodium, chloride and bicarbonate.

Secretion is the opposite process to that of absorption. In response to various stimuli, crypt cells actively transport chloride into the gut lumen and sodium and water follow. This stimulus-secretion coupling is modulated by cyclic AMP and GMP, calcium, prostaglandins and leukotrienes.

Diarrhoea has numerous causes, from infections with enteric organisms (which may stimulate secretion or damage absorption), to nutrient malabsorption due to disease. Rarely it is due to secretory tumours of the alimentary tract, e.g. carcinoid tumour, vipoma (a tumour which secretes VIP, vasoactive intestinal protein).

Motility patterns in the bowel. Segmental contractions of the smooth muscle mix the intestinal contents. Patients with diarrhoea commonly have less spontaneous activity of the sigmoid colon than do people with normal bowel habit, and patients with constipation have more. An important factor in diarrhoea may be loss of the normal segmenting contractions that delay passage of contents, so that an occasional peristaltic wave may have greater propulsive effect. Antidiarrhoeal drugs act by increasing segmentation and inhibiting peristalsis (antimotility drugs).

Therapy for diarrhoea involves, first, the correction of fluid and electrolyte imbalance and second, the use of drugs (in some cases).

FLUID AND ELECTROLYTE TREATMENT

Oral rehydration therapy (ORT) with glucose-electrolyte solution is sufficient to treat the vast majority of episodes of watery diarrhoea. As a simple, effective, cheap and readily administered therapy for a potentially lethal condition, ORT must rank as a major advance in therapy. It is effective because glucose-coupled sodium transport continues during diarrhoea and so enhances replacement of water and electrolyte losses in the stool.

Oral rehydration salts (ORS)	
The WHO/UNICEF[10] recommended formulation is:	
Sodium chloride	3.5 g/l
Potassium chloride	1.5 g/l
Sodium citrate	2.9 g/l
Anhydrous glucose	20.0 g/l
This provides Na^+ 90 mmol, K^+ 20 mmol, Cl^- 80 mmol, citrate 10 mmol, glucose 111 mmol.	

Several other formulations exist, some with less sodium, see national formularies.[11]

Rehydration therapy with commercial soft drinks alone will fail because their sodium content is too low (usually less than 4 mmol/l). The glucose may be replaced by another substrate, e.g. glycine ORS, rice powder ORS. Indeed cereal-based ORS, relying on starch (to produce glucose) from many sources, e.g. rice, wheat, corn, potato, may yet prove to be a further advance. Thus almost every household in the world can find the essential components of an effective oral rehydration mixture: cereals and salt.

Most cases can be adequately treated by assiduous attention to oral intake, but fluid and electrolyte depletion are especially dangerous in children for whom hospitalisation and intravenous replacement may be needed. Antimotility drugs are inappropriate for severe diarrhoea in young children; any marginal efficacy they may have is liable to be counterbalanced by hazard (see below).

DRUG TREATMENT

There are two types of drug which are often used in combination. Both types increase viscosity of faeces.

1. Antimotility drugs. These act on bowel muscle to delay the passage of gut contents so allowing time for more water to be absorbed.

---

[10] World Health Organization/United Nations Children's Fund (originally the words 'international' and 'emergency' were included).

[11] The higher sodium content of the WHO/UNICEF formulation is based on sodium concentrations in diarrhoeal stools, but low-sodium, high-glucose formulations may be preferred for infants, for their faecal losses of sodium are less.

Codeine (t^{1}/2 3 h) activates opioid receptors on the smooth muscle of the bowel which reduce peristalsis and increase segmentation contractions so that passage of contents is delayed and more water is absorbed. Tolerance may develop if use is prolonged, as may dependence (rarely). It should be avoided in patients with diverticular disease as it increases intraluminal pressure.

Diphenoxylate (t^{1}/2 3 h) is structurally related to pethidine and affects the bowel like morphine. The drug is offered mixed with a trivial dose of atropine (to discourage abuse) as co-phenotrope (Lomotil). Nausea, vomiting, abdominal pain and depression of the central nervous system may be caused. In overdose with Lomotil, respiratory depression may be serious and can occur up to 16 h after ingestion because gastric emptying is slowed. It is used to control colostomies.

Loperamide (t^{1}/2 10 h) is structurally similar to diphenoxylate. Its precise mode of action remains obscure but it impairs propulsion of gut contents by effects on intestinal circular and longitudinal muscle that are at least partly due to an action on opioid receptors. Loperamide may cause nausea, vomiting and abdominal cramps. Its potential for abuse appears to be low.

The actions of codeine, diphenoxylate and loperamide are antagonised by naloxone.

Warning: antimotility drugs should not be used for acute diarrhoea in children, especially babies, for there is danger of causing paralytic ileus or respiratory depression: oral rehydration salts are the treatment.

2. Drugs that increase the viscosity of gut contents directly.

Kaolin and chalk are adsorbent powders. Their therapeutic efficacy is marginal as is shown by the fact that they are often combined with an opioid. Bulk-forming agents such as *ispaghula, methylcellulose* and *sterculia* (see above) are useful for diarrhoea in diverticular disease, and for reducing the fluidity of faeces in patients with ileostomy and colostomy.

TRAVELLERS' DIARRHOEA

So familiar is diarrhoea to travellers that it has acquired regional popular names: the Aztec 2-step, Montezuma's Revenge, Delhi Belly, Rangoon Runs, Tokyo Trots, Gyppy Tummy, Hong-Kong Dog, Estomac Anglais and Casablanca Crud, all indicate some of the areas deemed dangerous by visitors. The Mexican name *turista* indicates the principal sufferers.

It is now clear that most cases are infective, and up to half of the diarrhoea that afflicts visitors to tropical and subtropical countries is associated with enterotoxigenic strains of *Escherichia coli*; other bacteria, e.g. *Shigella* and *Salmonella* spp, viruses, e.g. of the Norwalk family and parasites, e.g. *Giardia lamblia* have also been implicated. Recognition that transmission is almost invariably by ingestion of contaminated food and water points to the most effective way of reducing the risk, i.e. avoiding raw, unpeeled fruit and vegetables, and unboiled water.

Acute watery diarrhoea *in adults* can ordinarily be controlled by oral rehydration salts and one of the antimotility drugs, e.g. loperamide, codeine phosphate, although in mild cases the abdominal bloating produced by the latter may be less acceptable than the loose stools. While diarrhoea is usually limited to 2–3 days, this is socially too long. Thus if symptomatic remedies fail, an aminoquinolone, e.g. ciprofloxacin 500 mg × 2/d will be effective. The use of antimicrobials for travellers' diarrhoea continues to evoke controversy (see below) but most sufferers will appreciate the relief that even one or two tablets can bring.

Prophylactic antimicrobial therapy has been shown to reduce the incidence of attacks of diarrhoea but its routine use carries the risk of hindering the diagnosis of serious infection. A wider issue is the possible development and spread of antibiotic-resistant organisms. Thus any benefits to the individual must be weighed against the risk to *the community* in the future. In most instances prophylactic antimicrobials should not be used but ciprofloxacin 500 mg × 1/d may be justified for individuals who must remain well while travelling for short periods to high risk areas.

SPECIFIC INFECTIVE DIARRHOEAS

Chemotherapy is available for certain specific organisms, e.g. amoebae, giardiasis, typhoid fever (see Index).

DRUG-INDUCED DIARRHOEA

Antimicrobials are the commonest drugs that cause diarrhoea, probably due to alteration of bowel flora. It may range from a mild inconvenience to life-threatening enterocolitis. Magnesium-containing antacids may also produce diarrhoea, as may NSAIDs (indomethacin, mefenamic acid, flurbiprofen) and lithium.

SECRETORY DIARRHOEAS

Octreotide, a synthetic peptide which shares amino acid homology with somatostatin (see p. 643), inhibits the release of peptides that mediate certain alimentary secretions, and may be used to relieve diarrhoea due to carcinoid tumours and vipomas.

Abnormal gut motility

Abnormal activity of the gut (see Irritable bowel syndrome, below) may cause accelerated, retarded or retrograde (reflux) movement of its contents, with attendant symptomatology. Depending on the type of movement, patients may complain of diarrhoea, constipation, colic and a variety of symptoms, e.g. nausea, abdominal distension and pain, generally classed as *nonulcer dyspepsia*.[12] The symptomatic management of vomiting, constipation and diarrhoea have been discussed earlier in this and the previous chapter. In addition, certain drugs with smooth muscle relaxant properties may benefit some of these often rather intractable symptoms. They include:

Antimuscarinic drugs

These drugs block cholinergic transmission at parasympathetic postganglionic nerve endings, including those that innervate smooth muscle, causing it to relax. They include *atropine* and *hyoscine*, and the synthetic antimuscarinics *dicyclomine*, *poldine* and *propantheline*. They may be used to benefit some of the spectrum of symptoms, notably those perceived to be due to smooth muscle spasm, e.g. colic and

pain. Their therapeutic efficacy is limited by the other antimuscarinic effects which include dry mouth, paralysis of visual accommodation, urinary hesitancy and constipation. Antimuscarinics should be avoided in patients with gastro-oesophageal reflux and with paralytic ileus.

Other smooth muscle relaxants

Mebeverine is a reserpine derivative which has a direct effect on colonic muscle activity, especially, it appears, on colonic hypermotility. It may be used to relieve spasm of intestinal muscle, e.g. associated with organic disease of the gut, and in irritable bowel syndrome. Not being an antimuscarinic, it does not demonstrate the troublesome side-effects of that group of drugs.

Alverine and peppermint oil also have direct smooth muscle relaxing activity.

IRRITABLE BOWEL SYNDROME

This common condition is characterised by abnormal bowel activity (causing abdominal pain, constipation or diarrhoea), without obvious organic cause. Stress, psyche, lack of dietary fibre and food allergy contribute variably to its pathogenesis. An explanation of the functional nature of the disease and avoidance of foods that obviously precipitate symptoms are important initial measures. The condition is not regularly improved by drugs but benefit may be derived by increasing viscous (soluble) dietary fibre, e.g. with ispaghula, when constipation dominates and by antimotility drugs (loperamide, diphenoxylate) for diarrhoea (note that *insoluble* fibre such as wheat bran may actually aggravate diarrhoea and cause heartburn). Depending on the spectrum of symptoms presented, alleviation may be obtained by metoclopramide or cisapride for nausea and abdominal distension, by antimuscarinics or smooth muscle relaxants (see above) for abdominal pain, by anxiolysis with a benzodiazepine, or occasionally, by an antidepressant.

Inflammatory bowel disease

In *ulcerative colitis* and *Crohn's disease*, measures to

---

[12] Working Party 1988 Lancet 1: 576.

correct anaemia, fluid and electrolyte losses and to improve the general nutritional state are important. Drugs are useful both in the termination of an acute attack and in the maintenance of remission. The following are used:

Anti-inflammatory drugs

Corticosteroid (see Ch. 35). Prednisolone is effective principally for acute attacks of ulcerative colitis; it may also be used during remission in those patients who cannot be maintained on mesalazine alone. Prednisolone is also effective for Crohn's disease. The objective is to reduce the inflammatory process whilst avoiding the unwanted effects of the steroid. Thus prednisolone 21-phosphate, a water-soluble salt of prednisolone, is preferred for topical use within the bowel (as suppositories or enemas), for it is less absorbed than prednisolone itself, and this preparation is also suitable for i.v. administration; prednisolone itself is used orally where systemic therapy is required. *Azathioprine* is valuable when the disease, especially Crohn's disease, is severe and as a corticosteroid-sparing agent for patients who need to be maintained on prednisolone.

5-aminosalicylic acid compounds

Sulphasalazine (salicylazosulfapyridine) consists of two compounds, sulphapyridine and 5-aminosalicylic acid, joined by an azo-bond. Sulphasalazine is poorly absorbed from the small intestine and bacteria in the colon split the azo-bond to release the component parts. The therapeutically active moiety is now known to be 5-aminosalicylic acid (see below). Sulphapyridine is well absorbed, is acetylated in the liver and excreted in the urine; it has no therapeutic action in colitis but contributes to a mechanism for delivering 5-aminosalicylic acid to the colon; sulphonamide toxicity may occur.

Sulphasalazine maintains remission in patients with ulcerative colitis (relapses are reduced by a factor of 3), and may also be used with a corticosteroid for treatment of the acute attack. It is also used as a disease-modifying agent in rheumatoid arthritis (see Index), the condition for which it was originally introduced in the 1930s. It is available as an oral tablet, retention enema or suppository.

Adverse effects include headache, malaise, anorexia, nausea and vomiting; these are dose-related and commoner in slow acetylators (of the sulphonamide). Allergic reactions include rash, fever and lymphadenitis; rarely leucopenia and agranulocytosis occur. Males may become infertile due to oligospermia and reduced sperm motility; this reverses if sulphasalazine is replaced with mesalazine. Several of these adverse effects are caused by the sulphapyridine moiety.

Mesalazine is a 5-aminosalicylic acid (see above); its several actions include inhibition of prostaglandin G/H synthase and lipoxygenase but the precise explanation for its beneficial effect in inflammatory bowel disease remains obscure. Mesalazine is presented in formulations that are designed to delay its release until they reach the colon. Mesalazine that enters the blood is rapidly cleared by acetylation in the liver and renal excretion. The drug is used to maintain remission in ulcerative colitis and to treat mild to moderate exacerbations of the disease. It may be given as an oral tablet, retention enema or suppository. Patients who are intolerant of sulphasalazine usually tolerate mesalazine. The profile of adverse effects includes nausea, abdominal pain, watery diarrhoea and interstitial nephritis.

Olsalazine is 2 molecules of 5-aminosalicylic acid linked by an azo-bond which is split by colonic bacteria. It is used to maintain remission in ulcerative colitis and to treat mild to moderate attacks of the disease. Watery diarrhoea is its main adverse effect and appears to occur more often than with mesalazine. These drugs are used as follows.

Ulcerative colitis

Mild attacks can be managed outside hospital, with a regimen of prednisolone by retention enema at night and one of the preparations that contain 5-aminosalicylic acid. Alternatively, mesalazine by retention enema at night is acceptable. An antimotility drug may be used judiciously, e.g. for social purposes.

Moderately severe attacks should generally be managed initially in hospital with prednisolone 10 mg × 4/d and 5-aminosalicylic acid by mouth, and prednisolone by retention enema night and morning. The regimen should be maintained for two weeks, when the corticosteroid should be tailed off but the 5-aminosalicylic acid should continue. A course of iron by mouth may be needed for anaemia.

Severe attacks must be treated in hospital, for management involves: correcting dehydration and electrolyte upset by i.v. fluids, parenteral nutrition, blood, if necessary, and hydrocortisone 200–400 mg/d i.v. As the patient's condition improves, the intravenous corticosteroid may be replaced with oral prednisolone 40 mg/d in divided doses. 5-aminosalicylic acid should be reintroduced once improvement has been maintained, and an oral iron supplement will usually be required. Failure to respond to this intensive regimen means that colectomy will be required.

Faecal loading (visualised on abdominal radiograph) can be a cause of spurious diarrhoea and a factor that can decrease the therapeutic efficacy of prednisolone and mesalazine; the treatment is a laxative, not codeine.

Proctitis: prednisolone or 5-aminosalicylic acid by enema is appropriate.

Crohn's disease

Prednisolone is best to induce remission in acutely ill patients and give some benefit from continued corticosteroid therapy. Azathioprine may be useful as a steroid-sparing agent, and also in some patients who have fistula or who are resistant to corticosteroid. Metronidazole may be effective for disease of the perianal region. 5-aminosalicylic acid helps patients with mild or moderate disease of the colon, but is less effective than prednisolone.

GUIDE TO FURTHER READING

Almroth S, Latham M C 1995 Rational home management of diarrhoea. Lancet 345: 709

Christensen J 1992 Pathophysiology of the irritable bowel syndrome. Lancet 340: 1444

Donowitz M et al 1995 Evaluation of patients with chronic diarrhoea. New England Journal of Medicine 332: 725

Eastwood M 1995 The dilemma of laxative abuse. Lancet 346: 1115

Farthing M J G 1993 Travellers' diarrhoea. British Medical Journal 306: 1425

Goyal R K, Hirano I 1996 The enteric nervous system. New England Journal of Medicine 334: 1106

Hanauer S B 1996 Inflammatory bowel disease. New England Journal of Medicine 334: 841

Lynn R B, Friedman L S 1993 Irritable bowel syndrome. New England Journal of Medicine 329: 1940

Podolsky D K 1991 Inflammatory bowel disease. New England Journal of Medicine 325: 928, 1008

Sazawal S et al 1995 Zinc supplementation in young children with acute diarrhoea in India. New England Journal of Medicine 333: 839

Shanahan F 1993 Pathogenesis of ulcerative colitis. Lancet 342: 407

Thompson W G 1993 Irritable bowel syndrome: pathogenesis and management. Lancet 341: 1569

Liver, biliary tract, pancreas

Drugs and the liver

The liver is the most important organ in which drugs are structurally altered. Some of the resulting metabolites may be biologically inactive, some active, some toxic. Furthermore, the liver is exposed to drugs at higher concentrations than are most organs, for the following reason. Most drugs are administered orally, are absorbed from the gastrointestinal tract and thus the whole dose must pass through the liver to reach the systemic circulation; subsequently, 20% of the cardiac output also passes through the liver. It is hardly surprising therefore that:

- Drugs can cause direct cellular injury to the liver or otherwise interfere with its function.

- Pharmacokinetic and pharmacodynamic changes are caused by liver disease.

These issues are now considered.

DRUG-INDUCED LIVER INJURY

Toxic effects of drugs on the liver or its function may mimic almost every naturally occurring hepatic disease. Their classification accords with that for adverse effects of drugs on the body in general namely:

Type A (Augmented)

Liver injury occurs as the dose of some drugs is increased, causing:

- *Centrizonal necrosis*, with *paracetamol* in overdose and also *carbon tetrachloride* (dry-cleaner) (due to formation of active metabolite) and other nonmedicinal chemicals.
- *Hepatocellular necrosis* with *salicylates*, particularly in patients with collagen diseases, when >2 g/d are taken.
- *Fatty change* in liver cells and *hepatic failure* with tetracyclines with high doses; this is avoided if <2 g/day is given orally and <1 g/day i.v.
- *Hepatitis* with alcohol, especially following very heavy consumption over a short period. Alcohol hepatitis-like changes may be induced by *amiodarone*, due either to the drug or its main metabolite; the dose should be kept below 600 mg/d.

- *Interference with bilirubin metabolism and excretion* with some drugs. Jaundice is induced selectively with minimal disturbance of other liver function tests; recovery ordinarily occurs on stopping the drug. Examples are:

C–17α-substituted hormones impair bilirubin excretion into the hepatic canaliculi; the block is biochemical not mechanical. These include some androgens and anabolic steroids and oestrogens and progestogens used as oral contraceptives; but jaundice is rare with the low dose formulations now preferred.

Rifampicin impairs hepatic uptake and excretion of bilirubin; plasma unconjugated and conjugated bilirubin may be elevated during the first 2–3 weeks of dosing.

Fusidic acid interferes with hepatic bilirubin excretion to cause conjugated hyperbilirubinaemia.

Cholecystographic media compete with bilirubin for uptake into the hepatic cell, and serum bilirubin may be transiently raised after an oral cholecystogram.

Type B (Bizarre)

Many drugs can cause hepatic damage at therapeutic doses, although the incidence with any single agent is low (if it were not the drug would not be used). The injury is due to unusual properties of the patient interacting with the drug and is unrelated to dose. The reaction may or may not be associated with features of generalised allergy (fever, arthralgia, skin rash, eosinophilia, lymphadenopathy). Patterns include:

- *Acute hepatocellular necrosis.* This reaction varies from a transient disturbance of liver function tests to acute hepatitis. It can be induced by several drugs including general anaesthetics (halothane), antiepileptics (carbamazepine, phenytoin, sodium valproate, phenobarbitone), antidepressants (MAO inhibitors), anti-inflammatory drugs (indomethacin, ibuprofen), antimicrobials (isoniazid, sulphonamides, nitrofurantoin) and cardiovascular drugs (methyldopa, hydralazine).
- *Cholestatic hepatitis.* The picture is of obstructive

jaundice though the block is biochemical rather than mechanical. This type is particularly associated with the *phenothiazine neuroleptics*, especially chlorpromazine. The jaundice generally occurs within the first month of therapy, its onset may be insidious or acute with abdominal pain, and can be accompanied by features suggesting allergy (see above). Recovery is usual. It is also caused by antidiabetic drugs (chlorpropamide, tolbutamide, glibenclamide), carbimazole, erythromycin and gold.

Type C (Continued use)

- *Chronic active hepatitis* may develop with prolonged use of methyldopa, isoniazid, dantrolene and nitrofurantoin.
- *Hepatic fibrosis* or *cirrhosis* may be caused by prolonged excess of alcohol, and therapeutic use of *methotrexate*, e.g. for psoriasis; in the latter case the risk is lessened by giving a large dose weekly rather than a smaller dose daily and by monitoring progress by liver biopsy after every 1.5–2 g of methotrexate. Chronic exposure to amiodarone may lead to cirrhosis.

Type D (Delayed effects)

Benign liver tumours may develop when *synthetic androgens*, e.g. anabolic steroids usually in high dose, and oral contraceptives are used for more than 5 years; there is also increased risk of hepatocellular *carcinoma*, although the absolute risk of either complication is very low. Malignant liver tumours associated with the contraceptive pill are highly vascular and may cause recurrent or acute abdominal pain if they rupture and bleed.

SUMMARY

Drugs may cause any of the common, and some of the uncommon, forms of liver disease.
Always think of the possibility of drug-induced injury when:

- Plasma transaminases of hepatic origin are raised
- Jaundice is unexplained
- Acute hepatitis, chronic active hepatitis or cirrhosis are diagnosed
- Primary hepatic tumour is present
- There is liver disease of obscure cause.

PHARMACOKINETIC AND PHARMACODYNAMIC CHANGES

Pharmacokinetic changes occur in liver disease because:

- Drug metabolising capacity is reduced where liver cells are either sick or, if functioning normally, are reduced in number
- Liver cells that metabolise drugs are bypassed when portal-systemic shunts develop in cirrhosis
- Liver disease may cause hypoproteinaemia leading to reduced drug-binding capacity, allowing more unbound and pharmacologically active drug to circulate.

The following discussion refers to stable liver disease such as cirrhosis or chronic active hepatitis; there is less information about altered pharmacokinetics in acute liver disease, e.g. viral hepatitis or toxic liver necrosis. The pattern of change that is induced by disease depends on the manner in which a drug is handled by the healthy liver and there are two general classes:

1. Drugs that are rapidly metabolised and highly extracted in a single pass through the liver.

Such drugs are said to undergo *presystemic* elimination after oral administration, i.e. to exhibit the hepatic first-pass effect (see Index). Poor liver cell function means that less drug is extracted from the blood as it passes through the liver and portal-systemic shunts allow a proportion of blood to bypass the liver altogether. Therefore the predominant change in the kinetics of drugs that are given orally is *increased systemic availability*, i.e. the amount that reaches the systemic circulation is larger than normal and its effect is correspondingly greater. Accordingly the initial doses of a drug should be smaller than usual, at least until some assessment of its effect has been obtained. The normally low systemic availability of, e.g. labetalol, propranolol, pentazocine, pethidine and chlormethiazole is much increased in cirrhotic patients. When liver function is severely impaired the $t^{1}/_{2}$ of drugs in this class may also be lengthened.

2. Drugs that are slowly metabolised and are poorly extracted in a single pass through the liver.

These drugs do not exhibit significant first-pass extraction after oral administration. The major change caused by liver disease is *prolongation of $t^{1}/_{2}$*. Consequently the interval between doses of such drugs may need to be lengthened and the time to reach steady-state concentration in the plasma ($5 \times t^{1}/_{2}$) is increased; the $t^{1}/_{2}$ of diazepam, lorazepam, phenobarbitone, theophylline and clindamycin is materially increased in patients with chronic liver disease.

Pharmacodynamic changes occur because:

- Cellular responses to drugs may alter. CNS sensitivity to opioids, sedatives and antiepilepsy drugs is increased; effect of oral anticoagulant is increased because synthesis of clotting factors is impaired.
- Fluid and electrolyte balance are altered. Sodium retention may be more readily induced by NSAIDs or corticosteroids; ascites and oedema may be more resistant to diuretics.

These issues are now discussed, as they affect the use of drugs.

PRESCRIBING IN LIVER DISEASE

It is especially important that drugs should be prescribed for patients with liver disease only if there is real need. Patients at greatest risk are those with ascites, jaundice or evidence of encephalopathy. The following examples provide a general guide.

Central nervous system. The brain receives concentrations of toxic substances (ammonia, amines) to which it is normally not exposed, as a result of failure of liver cells to metabolise naturally occurring substances and also of shunting of blood from the portal to the systemic circulation. CNS function becomes impaired (hepatic encephalopathy) and response to drugs is *qualitatively* abnormal.

Opioids should be avoided as coma may occur, but if an opioid is essential, pethidine is probably less dangerous than morphine. Lorazepam and oxazepam are preferred as anxiolytics and temazepam as an hypnotic. In patients with acute alcoholic liver disease who are withdrawing from alcohol, use of chlormethiazole should be particularly closely monitored. Antiepilepsy drugs should be monitored with particular care; phenobarbitone may induce coma. A tricyclic may be used when antidepressant therapy is deemed necessary but MAO inhibitors are hazardous.

Cardiovascular system. Beta-adrenoceptor blockers that are metabolised, e.g. propranolol, labetalol, should be given in reduced initial oral dose, as should calcium channel antagonists, e.g. nicardipine, nifedipine, verapamil. Hypokalaemia may precipitate coma so plasma electrolytes should be monitored carefully during diuretic therapy and a potassium-sparing drug should be included in the regimen.

Gastrointestinal system. Antacids that contain much sodium may cause fluid retention and those that contain aluminium and calcium may constipate, which predisposes to encephalopathy as there is greater opportunity for absorption of toxic substances from the gut.

Infection. Many antimicrobials are eliminated by the kidney, so ordinary doses of these are safe. Avoid, or use in reduced dose, those drugs that have known risk of hepatotoxicity, e.g. isoniazid, erythromycin, rifampicin, tetracyclines. Ketoconazole is contraindicated unless there is no alternative. The sodium content of some penicillins may be hazardously high.

Endocrine system. Avoid C–17α-substituted androgens and anabolic steroids for they are hepatotoxic (see above). Avoid combined oral contraceptives especially in cholestatic liver disease. Metformin is normally inactivated by the liver and should be avoided as it may cause lactic acidosis; chlorpropamide and tolbutamide are more likely to induce hypoglycaemia.

Respiratory system. Reduce the dose of theophylline.

ASPECTS OF THERAPY

Ascites. Standard therapy consists of dietary sodium restriction and diuretic; a weight loss of 0.5 kg/d is optimal as this is the rate at which ascites equilibrates with the vascular compartment. Abrupt diuresis, e.g. with large doses of a loop diuretic, may precipitate electrolyte imbalance, renal dysfunction and hepatic encephalopathy. In patients who fail to respond or who develop adverse effects of diuretic therapy, up to 4–6 litres of ascitic fluid may be removed per day by paracentesis, with simultaneous i.v. infusion of albumin (6–8 g per litre of ascitic fluid) to prevent hypovolaemia.

Portal hypertension and variceal bleeding. Bleeding from rupture of varices is serious, the mortality from an initial event being up to 50%, and 30% for subsequent bleeds.

- If endoscopic expertise is available, bleeding from oesophageal varices can be stopped by injection of a sclerosing substance or by band ligation.
- If endoscopic expertise is not immediately available, vasopressin or terlipressin (which has a weaker action), given by i.v. infusion or injection may cause bleeding to stop until injection sclerotherapy is undertaken. The vasopressin constricts splanchnic vessels, thus reducing flow to and pressure in the liver and the collateral (oesophageal) channels. Coronary vasoconstriction may be induced also and cause angina. Somatostatin or its synthetic analogue, octreotide, may also be used; they appear to cause fewer adverse effects but their efficacy has not been fully established. The major limitation of vasopressin and terlipressin is their failure to control massive or major haemorrhage; in such cases balloon tamponade should be used.
- Prophylactic therapy. β-blockade with propranolol reduces variceal bleeding especially in patients with mild (compensated) cirrhosis. It acts by reducing cardiac output, causing a fall in hepatic blood flow and with it portal pressure (but do not use when there is renal impairment). Other more complex mechanisms may be involved.

Viral hepatitis. Hepatitis A virus causes an acute, normally self-limiting, infection with a variable degree of hepatic damage. Chronic hepatitis caused by hepatitis B, C or D may lead to cirrhosis, hepatocellular failure or hepatocellular carcinoma. Collectively, hepatitis is probably the commonest of serious viral diseases in general, and constitutes a major health problem.

- Active immunity against hepatitis A is provided by *hepatitis A vaccine* which is formed from the inactivated virus. It should be used by frequent travellers to moderate to high risk areas and those who intend to stay for more than 3 months. The vaccine should be given at least 2 weeks before entering the risk area and a booster dose is needed 6–12 months after the initial dose. *Hepatitis B vaccine*, formed from the inactivated virus surface antigen and given i.m. takes up to 6 months to provide protection which lasts 3–5 years. It is provided for those deemed to be at special risk, e.g. people receiving frequent blood transfusions, health care personnel.
- Passive immunity is conferred immediately by *human normal immunoglobulin* which is prepared from pooled plasma and contains antibody to hepatitis A. It is used to prevent and control outbreaks of the disease, and for travellers to endemic areas. Specific *hepatitis B immunoglobulin* is available for those accidentally infected.
- **Therapy for chronic active hepatitis.** *Interferon alfa* is effective but the responses vary among the forms of hepatitis. In hepatitis B, interferon alfa 5 million units/d for 16 weeks by s.c. or i.m. injection clears the hepatitis B antigen and B virus DNA from the plasma in 30–40% of cases; serum aminotransaminases return to normal, liver histology improves and recurrence is unusual in those who respond. In 50% of hepatitis C cases, aminotransferases are normal and C virus RNA decreases after interferon alfa 3 million units × 3/week for 6 months but only 20–25% of cases show a sustained response. The cumulative incidence of hepatocellular carcinoma is reduced. About half of the cases of hepatitis D respond with normal serum aminotransferase concentrations and histological improvement after interferon alfa 9 million units × 3/week for 48 weeks, but the majority relapse. Further clinical trials will define the effects of this therapy on the outcome,

e.g. cirrhosis, carcinoma, in the various forms of hepatitis. Other antivirus drugs may also provide benefit: lamivudine (see HIV, p. 233) clears hepatitis B virus DNA from plasma.

Bile salts and gallstones

Human bile has a capacity for maintaining more cholesterol in solution than, say, an equivalent volume of water. The explanation is that bile contains bile acids (mainly cholic, deoxycholic and chenodeoxycholic) and phospholipids (mainly lecithin) which together form molecular aggregates called *mixed micelles* that are capable of keeping cholesterol dissolved within them. It follows that bile can become saturated and cholesterol can precipitate (forming gallstones) if:

- the concentration of bile acids is too low, or
- the concentration of cholesterol in the bile is too high.
- Reversing these two factors is the basis of medical treatment for cholesterol gallstone.

Chenodeoxycholic acid (CDCA) comprises about 40% of the naturally occurring bile acids, and when it is taken as a medicine to treat gallstones the proportion rises to 70%. It is effective for gallstone dissolution but causes diarrhoea in about 40% of patients and elevates plasma aspartate transaminase concentrations. Chenodeoxycholic acid should not be given to patients at risk of pregnancy or to patients with chronic liver disease or inflammatory bowel disease.

Ursodeoxycholic acid (UDCA) is a bile acid which occurs in small amounts in the human (but in large amounts in the bile of the bear family, *Ursidae*). It is effective at dissolving gallstones possibly by reducing cholesterol absorption from the gut, inhibiting cholesterol synthesis by the liver and, to a lesser extent, expanding the bile acid pool. The result is that bile contains less cholesterol and more bile acid, the endogenous bile acids being partially replaced by UDCA. Unlike CDCA, UDCA rarely causes diarrhoea and does not elevate transaminases; it is therefore usually preferred.

UDCA is hydrophilic and appears to provide benefit in primary biliary cirrhosis, possibly by substituting for the accumulating endogenous bile acids which are hydrophobic and cause damage to hepatocytes.

Use of CDCA and UDCA should be confined to patients who are not suitable for surgical treatment, who have mild symptoms, a functioning gallbladder, i.e. a normal oral cholecystogram, and small or medium sized radiolucent stones, for even a thin covering of calcium salts usually prevents dissolution. Only about 30% of patients are suitable for treatment. Bile salt therapy should continue for up to 24 months depending on the size of the stones and longterm prophylaxis may be needed after dissolution, monitored by gallbladder ultrasonography, as 30–50% stones recur in 3–5 years.

CONDITIONS CAUSED BY BILE ACIDS

Excess bile acids in the colon cause diarrhoea, e.g. after resection of the ileum, their normal site of reabsorption. In biliary obstruction pruritus is due to accumulation of bile acids. Both conditions may be helped by cholestyramine.

Cholestyramine is an anion-exchange resin that is used principally to treat hyperlipidaemias. Taken orally, it binds bile acids in the bowel, preventing their absorption, and is thus effective for diarrhoea due to bile acids in the colon; excess effect may cause steatorrhoea. Provided biliary obstruction is partial, i.e. that there is some escape of bile acids into the intestine where they can be bound, cholestyramine will reduce the accumulation of bile acids and help pruritus. It binds drugs in the gut including digoxin, thyroxine, warfarin, tetracycline.

Pancreas

DIGESTIVE ENZYMES

In pancreatic exocrine insufficiency, the aim of therapy is to prevent weight loss and diarrhoea and to maintain adequate growth in children. The problem of getting enough enzyme to the duodenum concurrently with food is not as simple as it might appear. Gastric emptying varies with the composition of meals, e.g. high fat, calories or protein cause delay, and the pancreatic enzymes taken by mouth

are destroyed by gastric juice. On the other hand, only one-tenth of the normal pancreatic output is sufficient to prevent excess fat (steatorrhoea) or excess nitrogen (azotorrhoea) loss, and it is not essential to eliminate these totally.

Preparations are of animal origin and of variable potency. Pancreatin as Cotazym and Nutrizym, appear to be satisfactory. A reasonable course is to start the patient on the recommended dose of a reliable formulation and to vary this according to the individual's needs, and the size and composition of meals. Some extract may be taken before, during and after food to limit destruction by gastric acid; antacids, cimetidine or ranitidine, taken 30–45 min before pancreatin, may improve its efficacy. Enteric-coated formulations (pancreatin granules, tablets) are available. High-potency pancreatic enzymes should not be used in patients with cystic fibrosis as they may cause ileocaecal and large bowel strictures.

Acute pancreatitis

Many drugs have been tested for specific effect, and none has shown convincing benefit. The main requirements of therapy are:

- To provide adequate analgesia. Opioids are generally satisfactory; their potential disadvantage of contracting the sphincter of Oddi (and retarding the flow of pancreatic secretion) appears to be outweighed by their analgesic efficacy; buprenorphine has less of this effect and may therefore be preferred.
- To correct hypovolaemia due to the exudation of large amounts of fluid around the inflamed pancreas. Plasma may be required, or blood if the haematocrit falls; in addition large volumes of electrolyte solution may be needed to maintain urine flow.

Drugs and the pancreas

The strongest association with acute pancreatitis is alcohol drinking. High plasma calcium, including that caused by hypervitaminosis D and parenteral nutrition also increase the risk. Corticosteroids, didanosine, azathoipurine, diuretics, including thiazides and frusemide, sodium valproate, mesalazine and paracetamol, in overdose, have also been causally related.

GUIDE TO FURTHER READING

Caraceni P, Van Thiel D H 1995 Acute liver failure. Lancet 345: 163

Di Bisceglie A M 1994 Interferon therapy for viral hepatitis. New England Journal of Medicine 330: 137

Hoofnagle J W, Lau D 1996 Chronic viral hepatitis — benefits of current therapies. New England Journal of Medicine 334: 1470

Johnston D E, Kaplan M M 1993 Pathogenesis and treatment of gallstones. New England Journal of Medicine 328: 412

Lau J Y N, Wright T L 1993 Molecular biology and pathogenesis of hepatitis B. Lancet 342: 1335

Lee W M 1995 Drug-induced hepatotoxicity. New England Journal of Medicine 333: 1118

Lim A G, Northfield T C 1994 Ursodeoxycholic acid and primary biliary cirrhosis. British Medical Journal 309: 491

Meyer K-H et al 1995 Autoimmune hepatitis. New England Journal of Medicine 333: 1004

Runyon B A 1994 Care of patients with ascites. New England Journal of Medicine 330: 337

Sherlock S 1986 The spectrum of hepatotoxicity to drugs. Lancet 2: 440

Shulkes A, Wilson J S 1994 Somatostatin in gastroenterology. British Medical Journal 308: 1381

Steer M L et al 1995 Chronic pancreatitis. New England Journal of Medicine 332: 1482

Steinberg W, Tenner S 1994 Acute pancreatitis. New England Journal of Medicine 330: 1198

Terrault N, Wright T L 1995 Interferon and hepatitis C. New England Journal of Medicine 332: 1509

Williams S G J, Westaby D 1994 Management of variceal haemorrhage. British Medical Journal 308: 1213

ENDOCRINE SYSTEM, METABOLIC CONDITIONS

35

Adrenal corticosteroids, antagonists, corticotrophin

In 1855, Dr Thomas Addison, assisted in his observations by three colleagues, published his famous monograph 'On the constitutional and local effects of disease of the suprarenal capsules' (Addison's disease). It was not until the 1920s that the vital importance of the adrenal cortex was appreciated and the distinction between the hormones secreted by the cortex and medulla.

By 1936, numerous steroids were being crystallised from cortical extracts, but not enough could be obtained to provide supplies for clinical trial.

In 1948 *cortisone* was made from bile acids in quantity sufficient for clinical trial, and the dramatic demonstration of its power to induce remission of rheumatoid arthritis was published in the following year. In 1950 it was realised that cortisone is biologically inert and that the active natural hormone is hydrocortisone (cortisol). Since then an embarrassingly large number of synthetic steroids has been made and offered to the clinician. They are made by a complicated process from natural substances (chiefly plant sterols), the constitutions of which approach most nearly to that of the steroids themselves. A principal aim in research is to produce steroids with more selective action than hydrocortisone, which induces a greater variety of effects than desired in any patient who is not suffering from adrenal insufficiency.

About the same time as cortisone was introduced, *corticotrophin* became available for clinical use.

Adrenal steroids and their synthetic analogues

Hormones normally produced by the adrenal cortex include hydrocortisone (cortisol), corticosterone, aldosterone and some androgens and oestrogens, but not cortisone. Cortisone is a prodrug, i.e. it is biologically inert and must be converted (largely in the liver) to hydrocortisone for biological activity; its use is obsolete for this reason.

Numerous analogues have been made in which the major actions have been separated.

When the adrenal cortex fails (Addison's disease) adrenocortical steroids are available for *replacement therapy*, but their chief use in medicine is for their *anti-inflammatory* and *immunosuppressive effects* (*pharmacotherapy*). These are only obtained when the drugs are given in doses far above those needed for physiological replacement. Various metabolic effects, which are of the greatest importance to the normal functioning of the body, then become adverse or side-effects. Much successful effort has gone into separating *glucocorticoid* from *mineralocorticoid* effects[1] and some steroids, e.g. dexamethasone, have virtually no mineralocorticoid activity. But it has not yet proved possible to separate the glucocorticoid effects from each other, so that if a steroid is used for its anti-inflammatory action the risks of osteoporosis, diabetes, etc., remain.

In the account that follows, the effects of hydrocortisone will be described and then other steroids in so far as they differ. In the context of this chapter 'adrenal steroid' means a substance with hydrocortisone-like activity. Androgens are described in Chapter 38.

MECHANISM OF ACTION

Adrenocortical steroids, being lipid soluble, enter inside their target cells, and combine with the glucocorticoid receptor in the cytoplasm. The unoccupied receptor is normally bound to the so-called heat shock protein HSP90. After occupation by a glucocorticoid steroid, the HSP90 is induced to change conformation and dissociate from the occupied glucocorticoid receptor. This translocates to the nucleus. The reason for the multiple actions of adrenocortical steroids is the presence of glucocorticoid response elements (GRE) in the promoter

---

[1] The mere introduction of a double bond transforms hydrocortisone to prednisolone, a big biological change: see Table 35.1 for relative potencies 1.0:1.0 to 4:0.8.

region of several genes; some of these are switched off by binding of the receptor to their GRE, whereas others are activated. A key protein in this complex process is the ubiquitous (intracellular) transcription factor, NF-κB; this is stimulated by a variety of inflammatory mediators to turn on production of *cytokines* (the term for several families of small proteins which are the key to the regulation of cell-to-cell interactions). Glucocorticoids induce transcription of a protein, IκB, which traps activated NF-κB in inactive cytoplasmic complexes. The lipocortins are another family of proteins which are activated by steroids; their actions are largely to inhibit pathways that normally lead to production of prostaglandins, leukotrienes and platelet activating factor. These mediators would normally contribute to increased vascular permeability and subsequent changes including oedema, leucocyte migration, fibrin deposition.

ACTIONS OF HYDROCORTISONE

Naturally there is a distinction between replacement therapy (physiological effects) and the higher doses of pharmacotherapy.

On inorganic metabolism (mineralocorticoid effects): increased retention of sodium by the renal tubule, and increased potassium excretion in the urine.

On organic metabolism (glucocorticoid effects):

- *Carbohydrate metabolism*: gluconeogenesis is increased and peripheral glucose utilisation (transport across cell membranes) may be decreased (insulin antagonism) so that hyperglycaemia and sometimes glycosuria result. Latent diabetes becomes overt, and this effect has been used as a test for the prediabetic state.

- *Protein metabolism*: *anabolism* (conversion of amino acids to protein) is decreased but catabolism continues unabated or even faster, so that there is a negative nitrogen balance with muscle wasting. Osteoporosis (reduction of bone protein matrix) occurs, growth slows in children, the skin atrophies and this, with increased capillary fragility, causes bruising and striae. Healing of peptic ulcers or of wounds is delayed, as is fibrosis.

- *Fat deposition*: this is increased on shoulders, face and abdomen.
- *Inflammatory response* is depressed, regardless of its cause, so that as well as being of great benefit in 'useless' or excessive inflammation, corticosteroids can be a source of danger in infections by limiting useful protective inflammation. Neutrophil and macrophage function is depressed, including the release of chemical mediators and the effects of these on capillaries.
- *Allergic responses* are suppressed. The antigen–antibody interaction is unaffected, but its injurious inflammatory consequences do not follow.
- *Antibody production* is reduced by heavy doses.
- *Lymphoid tissue* is reduced (including leukaemic lymphocytes).
- *Renal excretion of urate* is increased.
- *Blood eosinophils* are reduced in number.
- *Euphoria or psychotic states* may occur, perhaps due to CNS electrolyte changes.
- *Anti-vitamin D action*, see calciferol.
- *Reduction of hypercalcaemia* chiefly where this is due to excessive absorption of Ca from the gut (sarcoidosis, vitamin D intoxication).
- *Urinary calcium excretion* is increased and renal stones may form.
- *Growth reduction* where new cells are being *added* (growth in children), but not where they are *replacing* cells as in adult tissues.

- *Suppression of hypothalamic/pituitary/adrenocortical feedback system* (with delayed recovery) occurs with chronic use, so that abrupt withdrawal leaves the patient in a state of adrenocortical insufficiency.

Normal daily secretion of hydrocortisone is 10–30 mg. The exogenous daily dose that completely suppresses the cortex is hydrocortisone 40–80 mg, or prednisolone 10–20 mg, or its equivalent of other agents. Recovery of function is quick after a few days' use; but when used over months recovery takes months. A steroid-suppressed adrenal continues to secrete aldosterone.

INDIVIDUAL ADRENAL STEROIDS

The relative potencies[2] for glucocorticoid and mineralocorticoid (Na^+-retaining) effects which are shown in Table 35.1 are central to the choice of agent in relation to clinical indication.

[2] *Potency* rather than *efficacy*: see page 81. If a large enough dose of a glucocorticoid, e.g. prednisolone, were administered, the Na^+-retention would be almost as great as that caused by a mineralocorticoid. This is why, in practice, *different* (more selective) glucocorticoids, not higher doses of prednisolone, need to be used when maximal stimulation of glucocorticoid receptors is desired (e.g. in the treatment of acute transplant rejections).

Table 35.1 Relative potencies of adrenal steroids

Compound (tablet strength, mg)		Approximate relative potency		
		Anti-inflammatory (glucocorticoid) effect	Sodium-retaining (mineralocorticoid) effect	Equivalent[1] dosage (for anti-inflammatory effect, mg)[2]
Cortisone	(25)	0.8	1.0	25
Hydrocortisone	(20)	1.0	1.0	20
Prednisolone	(5)	4	0.8	5
Methylprednisolone	(4)	5	minimal	4
Triamcinolone	(4)	5	none	4
Dexamethasone	(0.5)	30	minimal	0.75
Betamethasone	(0.5)	30	negligible	0.75
Fludrocortisone	(0.1)	15	150	irrelevant
Aldosterone	none	none	500[3]	irrelevant

[1] Note that these equivalents are in approximate inverse accord with the tablet strengths.
[2] The doses in the final column are in the lower range of those that may cause suppression of the hypothalamic/pituitary/adrenocortical axis when given daily continuously. Much higher doses, e.g. 40 mg prednisolone, can be given on alternate days or daily for up to 5 days without causing clinically significant suppression.
[3] Injected.

All drugs in Table 35.1 except aldosterone are active when swallowed, being protected from hepatic first-pass metabolism by high binding to plasma proteins. Some details of preparations and equivalent doses are given in the table. Injectable and topical forms are available (creams, suppositories, eye drops).

The selectivity of hydrocortisone for the glucocorticoid receptor is not due to a different binding affinity of hydrocortisone to the two receptors but to the protection of the mineralocorticoid receptor by locally high concentrations of the enzyme 11β-steroid dehydrogenase, which converts cortisol (hydrocortisone) to the inactive cortisone. This enzyme is inhibited by one of the components of liquorice, and can occasionally harbour a genetic defect. Therefore both acquired (in liquorice addicts) and inherited syndromes of 'pseudohyperaldosteronism' can occasionally occur.

Hydrocortisone (cortisol) is the principal naturally occurring steroid; it is taken orally; a soluble salt can be given i.v. for rapid effect in emergency (whether due to deficiency, allergy or inflammatory disease). A suspension (Hydrocortisone Acetate Inj.) can be given intra-articularly.

Parenteral preparation for systemic effect: the soluble Hydrocortisone Sodium Succinate Inj. is used for quick (1–2 h) effect; for continuous effect about 8-hourly administration is appropriate. Prednisolone Acetate Inj. i.m. is an alternative, once or twice a week.

Oral tablet strengths, see Table 35.1.

Prednisolone is predominantly anti-inflammatory (glucocorticoid), biologically active and has little sodium-retaining activity; it is the standard choice for anti-inflammatory pharmacotherapy, orally or i.m.

Prednisone is a prodrug, i.e. it is biologically inert and converted into prednisolone in the liver. Since there is 20% less on conversion there seems no point in using it.

Methylprednisolone is similar to prednisolone; it is used i.v. for megadose pulse therapy (see below).

Fluorinated corticosteroids: triamcinolone has virtually no sodium-retaining (mineralocorticoid) effect but has the disadvantage that muscle wasting may occasionally be severe and anorexia and mental depression may be more common at high doses.

Dexamethasone and **betamethasone** are similar, powerful, predominantly anti-inflammatory steroids. They are longer acting than prednisolone and are used for therapeutic adrenocortical suppression.

Fludrocortisone has a very great sodium-retaining effect in relation to its anti-inflammatory action, and only at high doses need the nonelectrolyte effects be considered. It is used to replace aldosterone where the adrenal cortex is destroyed (Addison's disease). Fludrocortisone is also the drug of choice in most patients with autonomic neuropathy, in whom volume expansion is easier to achieve than a sustained increase in vasoconstrictor tone. Much higher doses of fludrocortisone (0.5–1 mg) are required when the cause of hypotension is a salt-losing syndrome of renal origin, e.g. following an episode of interstitial nephritis.

Aldosterone ($t^{1}/2$ 20 min), the principal natural salt-retaining hormone, has been used i.m. in acute adrenal insufficiency. After oral administration it is rapidly inactivated in the first pass through the liver and it has no place in routine therapeutics, as fludrocortisone is as effective and is active orally.

Spironolactone (see p. 489) is a competitive aldosterone antagonist which also blocks the mineralocorticoid effect of other steroids; it is used in treatment of *primary hyperaldosteronism* and as a diuretic, principally when severe peripheral oedema is due to *secondary hyperaldosteronism* (e.g. cirrhosis, congestive cardiac failure).

Beclomethasone and **budesonide** are used by inhalation for asthma (see p. 512). About 90% of an inhalation dose is swallowed and these steroids are inactivated by hepatic first-pass metabolism; the rest, absorbed from mouth and lungs, gives very low systemic plasma concentration. The risk of suppression of the hypothalamic/pituitary/adrenal axis is thus minimal (but it can happen). This property of extensive hepatic first-pass metabolism with low systemic availability is also an advantage in the topical treatment of inflammatory bowel disease with minimal risk of systemic adverse effects.

PHARMACOKINETICS OF CORTICOSTEROIDS

Absorption of the synthetic steroids given *orally* is rapid. The $t^{1/2}$ of most in plasma is 1–3 h but the maximum biological effect occurs after 2–8 h. They are usually given 2 or 3 times a day. They are metabolised principally in the liver and some are excreted unchanged by the kidney. The $t^{1/2}$ is prolonged in hepatic and renal disease and is shortened by hepatic enzyme induction to an extent that can be clinically important. For hepatic first-pass metabolism, see immediately above.

Topical application (skin, lung, joints) allows absorption which can be enough to cause systemic effects.

In the blood, adrenal steroids are carried in the free (biologically active) form (5%) and also bound (95% in the case of hydrocortisone) to *transcortin* (a globulin with high affinity, but low binding capacity) and, when this is saturated, to albumin (80% in the case of hydrocortisone). The concentration of the transcortin is increased by oestrogens, e.g. pregnancy, oral contraception, other oestrogen therapy, so that if plasma hydrocortisone concentration is measured the total will be found raised, but the amount of free hydrocortisone may be normal, being controlled by the normal feedback mechanism. Patients may be wrongly suspected of Cushing's syndrome if the fact that they are taking oestrogen is unrecognised and only the total concentration is measured (as is usual).

In patients with very low serum albumin, steroid doses should be lower than usual owing to the reduced binding capacity. In addition, low albumin concentration may be caused by *liver disease*, which also potentiates steroids by delaying metabolism ($t^{1/2}$ of prednisolone may be doubled).

DOSAGE SCHEDULES

Various spaced-out dosage schedules have been used in the hope of reducing hypothalamic/pituitary/adrenal suppression by allowing the plasma steroid concentration to fall enough between doses to provide time for pituitary recovery, e.g. prednisolone 40 mg on alternate days does not cause appreciable pituitary suppression. But none has been successful in both wholly avoiding suppression and at the same time controlling symptoms.

- Where a *single daily dose* is practicable it should be given in the early morning.
- *Alternate day schedules* are worth trying, especially where immunosuppression is the objective (organ transplants) rather than anti-inflammatory effect (rheumatoid arthritis); asthmatics taking a systemic steroid may or may not be manageable on such intermittent dosage.
- *Short courses* (a few days) may be practicable for some without significant suppression.
- Another variant is to give *enormous doses* (grams, not mg), orally or i.v., e.g. methylprednisolone 1.0 g i.v. on 3 successive days, at intervals of weeks or months (megadose pulses). The technique is used particularly in collagen diseases. Definitive evaluation of efficacy and side-effects is awaited.

Choice of adrenal steroid: summary

- **For oral replacement therapy** in adrenocortical insufficiency, *hydrocortisone* should be used to supply mineralocorticoid and some glucocorticoid activity. In Addison's disease a small dose of a hormone with only mineralocorticoid effect (*fludrocortisone*) is normally needed in addition. Prednisolone on its own is not effective replacement therapy.
- **For anti-inflammatory and anti-allergic (immunosuppressive) effect,** *prednisolone, triamcinolone* or *dexamethasone*. It is not possible to rank these in firm order of merit. One or other may suit an individual patient best, especially as regards incidence of side-effects such as muscle wasting. *By inhalation*: beclomethasone or budesonide.
- **For hypothalamic/pituitary/adrenocortical suppression**, e.g. in adrenal hyperplasia, prednisolone or dexamethasone.

ADVERSE EFFECTS OF SYSTEMIC ADRENAL STEROID PHARMACOTHERAPY

These consist largely of *too intense production* of the

physiological or pharmacological actions listed under actions of hydrocortisone. Some occur only with systemic use and for this reason local therapy, e.g. inhalation, intra-articular injection, is preferred where practicable.

Unwanted effects virtually do not occur with 1 or 2 doses though some occur with a few days' use, e.g. spread of infection. They follow prolonged administration and are sufficiently frequent and dangerous to warrant serious consideration by the physician whether 'the disease which he is attempting to suppress is more dangerous to the patient than the Cushing's syndrome which he might induce'.[3] The undesired effects recounted below should never be experienced in replacement therapy, but are sometimes unavoidable when the steroid is used as pharmacotherapy. Naturally, the nature of unwanted effects depends on the choice of steroid. Fludrocortisone in ordinary doses does not cause osteoporosis and prednisolone does not normally cause oedema.

In general, serious unwanted effects are unlikely if the daily dose is below the equivalent of hydrocortisone 50 mg or prednisolone 10 mg.

The principal evil effects of chronic corticosteroid administration are:

Iatrogenic Cushing's syndrome: moon face, characteristic deposition of fat on the body, oedema, hypertension, striae, bruising, acne, hirsutism, muscle wasting and *osteoporosis* of the spine (with fractures of vertebrae, ribs, femora and feet). Addition of a small dose of anabolic steroid in the hope of preventing osteoporosis and muscle wasting has been tried, but is usually ineffective. Oestrogens, as used for postmenopausal hormone replacement therapy, are more successful in women. Alternative steps are to supplement dietary calcium and add small doses of vitamin D to reduce progress of osteoporosis (which is largely irreversible).

Avascular necrosis of bone (femoral heads) is another serious complication (at higher doses); it appears to be due to restriction of blood flow through bone capillaries. Pain and restriction of

movement may occur months in advance of radiographic changes. **Diabetes mellitus** may appear. **Growth** in children is impaired.

Depression and psychosis can occur during the first few days of high dose administration, sometimes with suicide, especially in those with a history of mental disorder; *insomnia* is common.

Peptic ulceration. Patients taking continuous oral therapy probably have an excess incidence of peptic ulcer and haemorrhage of about 1–2%. It is plainly unreasonable to seek to protect all such patients by routinely giving prophylactic antiulcer therapy, i.e. to treat 98 patients unnecessarily in order to help two. But such therapy (histamine H_2-receptor blocker, sucralfate) may be used when ulcer is particularly likely, e.g. a patient with rheumatoid arthritis taking an NSAID, or when ulcer develops whilst taking the steroid. In patients with a history of peptic ulcer disease physicians will exercise their critical judgement.

Ulcer may occur with treatment as brief as 30 days.

Other effects include: posterior subcapsular lens cataract (risk if dose exceeds 10 mg prednisolone/day or equivalent for above a year), glaucoma (with prolonged use of eye drops), raised intracranial pressure and convulsions, blood hypercoagulability, menstrual disorders and fever. Delayed tissue healing following surgery is seldom important, but it can disagreeably complicate deep radiotherapy. Major skin damage can result from minor injury of any kind.

Suppression of the inflammatory response to infection and immunosuppression causes some patients to present with atypical symptoms and signs and quickly to deteriorate. The incidence of infection is increased with high dose therapy, and any infection can be more severe when it occurs. Previously dormant tuberculosis may become active insidiously. Intra-articular injections demand the strictest asepsis. *Live vaccines* become dangerous.

The incidence of unwanted effects of one kind or another depends on drug used, dosage and duration of therapy but can be as high as 50% of cases.

Hypothalamic/pituitary/adrenal (HPA) suppres-

---

[3] Liddle G W 1961 Clinical Pharmacology and Therapeutics 2: 615.

sion is dependent on the corticosteroid used, its dose, duration and the time of administration. A single morning dose of less than 20 mg of prednisolone may not be followed by suppression, whereas a dose of 5 mg given late in the evening is likely to suppress the essential early morning activation of the HPA axis (circadian rhythm). Substantial suppression of the HPA axis can occur within a week (but see Withdrawal of steroid therapy, below).

ADRENAL STEROIDS AND PREGNANCY

Adrenal steroids are teratogenic in animals. Although a relationship between steroid pharmacotherapy and cleft palate and other fetal abnormalities has been suspected in man, there is no doubt that many women taking a steroid throughout have both conceived and borne normal babies. Adrenal insufficiency due to hypothalamic/pituitary suppression in the newborn only occurs with high doses to the mother. Dosage during pregnancy should be kept as low as practicable and fluorinated steroids are best avoided as they are more teratogenic in animals (dexa- and betamethasone, triamcinolone and various topical steroids, e.g. fluocinolone). Hypoadrenal women who become pregnant may require an increase in hydrocortisone replacement therapy by about 10 mg per day to compensate for the increased binding by plasma proteins that occurs in pregnancy.

Labour should be managed as described for major surgery (below).

PRECAUTIONS DURING CHRONIC ADRENAL STEROID THERAPY

The most important precaution during replacement and pharmacotherapy is to see the patient regularly with an awareness of the possibilities of adverse effects including fluid retention (weight gain), hypertension, glycosuria, hypokalaemia (potassium supplement may be necessary) and back pain (osteoporosis); and of the serious hazard of patient noncompliance.

Mild withdrawal symptoms (iatrogenic cortical insufficiency) include conjunctivitis, rhinitis, weight loss, arthralgia and itchy skin nodules.

Patients must always

- carry a card giving details of therapy and simple instructions
- be impressed with the importance of compliance
- know what to do if they develop an intercurrent illness or other severe stress: double their next dose and to tell their doctor. If a patient omits a dose then it should be made up as soon as possible so that the total daily intake is maintained, because every patient should be taking the minimum dose necessary to control the disease.

Treatment of intercurrent illness

The normal adrenal cortex responds to severe *stress* by secreting more than 300 mg cortisol/day. Intercurrent illness is stress and treatment is urgent, particularly of *infections*; the dose of corticosteroid should be doubled during the illness and gradually reduced as the patient improves. Effective chemotherapy of bacterial infections is specially important.

Viral infections contracted during steroid therapy can be overwhelming because the immune response of the body may be largely suppressed. This is particularly relevant to immunosuppressed patients exposed to varicella/herpes zoster virus, which may cause fulminant illness; they may need passive protection with varicella/zoster immunoglobulin, VZIG, as soon as practicable. Continuous use of 20 mg prednisolone/day (or equivalent) is immunosuppressive. But a corticosteroid may sometimes be useful in therapy after the disease has begun (thyroiditis, encephalitis) and there has been time for the immune response to occur. It then acts by suppressing unwanted effects of immune responses and excessive inflammatory reaction.

Vomiting may require parenteral administration.

In the event of the misfortune of *surgery* being added to that of adrenal steroid therapy the patient should receive hydrocortisone 100–200 mg i.m. with premedication. If there is any sign suggestive that the patient may collapse, e.g. hypotension, during the operation, i.v. hydrocortisone (50–100 mg) should be infused at once. Otherwise, if there are no complications, the dose is repeated 6-hourly for 24–72 h and then reduced by half every 24 h until normal dose level is reached.

Minor operations, e.g. dental extraction, may be covered by hydrocortisone 100 mg orally 2–4 h before operation and the same dose afterwards.

In all these situations an i.v. infusion should be available for immediate use in case the above is not enough. These precautions should be used in patients who have received substantial treatment with corticosteroid within the past year, because their hypothalamic/pituitary/adrenal system, though sufficient for ordinary life, may fail to respond adequately to severe stress. If steroid therapy has been very prolonged, these precautions should be taken for as long as 2 years after stopping it. This will mean that some unnecessary treatment is given, but collapse due to acute adrenal insufficiency can be fatal and the ill-effects of short-lived increased dosage of steroid are less grave, being confined to possible increased incidence and severity of infection.

DOSAGE AND ROUTES OF ADMINISTRATION

Dosage depends very much on the purpose for which the steroid is being used and on individual response. It is impossible to suggest a single schedule that will suit every case.

Systemic commencing doses

- *For a serious disease* such as systemic lupus, dermatomyositis: prednisolone up to 60 mg/d orally in divided doses.
- If *life-threatening*, up to 70 mg, or its equivalent of another steroid. The dose is then increased if necessary until the disease is controlled or adverse effects occur; as much as prednisolone 300 mg/d can be needed. Cyclophosphamide or azathioprine (see p. 262) are valuable adjuncts to the use of prednisolone in inflammatory diseases. They may enhance the initial control of the disease and have a steroid-sparing effect on the maintenance dose of prednisolone required.
- *Alternatively* megadose pulses (methylprednisolone 1.0 g i.v. daily for 3 days); followed by oral maintenance.
- *For less dangerous disease*, such as rheumatoid arthritis: prednisolone 7.5–10.0 mg daily, adjusted later according to the response.
- In some special cases, including *replacement* of

adrenal insufficiency, dosage is mentioned in the account of the treatment of the disease.

- *For continuous therapy* the minimum amount to produce the desired effect must be used. Sometimes imperfect control must be accepted by the patient because full control, e.g. of rheumatoid arthritis, though obtainable, involves use of doses that must lead to longterm toxicity, e.g. osteoporosis, if continued for years. The decision to embark on such therapy is a serious matter for the patient.

Topical applications (creams, intranasal, inhalations, enemas) are used in attempts, often successful, to obtain local, whilst avoiding systemic, effects; suspensions of solutions are also injected into joints, soft tissues and subconjunctivally. However, all these can, with heavy dose, be sufficiently absorbed to suppress the hypothalamus and cause other unwanted effects. Individual preparations are mentioned in the text where appropriate.

The relatively high selectivity of *inhaled beclomethasone* in asthma is due to a combination of route of administration, high potency and rapid conversion to inactive metabolites by the liver of any drug that is absorbed (see Asthma, skin); but yet hypothalamic/pituitary suppression and systemic toxicity occasionally occur.

Contraindications to the use of adrenal steroids for suppressing inflammation are all relative, depending on the advantage to be expected. They should only be used for serious reasons in patients with: diabetes, a history of mental disorder or peptic ulcer, epilepsy, tuberculosis, hypertension or heart failure. The presence of any infection demands that effective chemotherapy be begun before the steroid, but there are exceptions (some viral infections, see above). Topical corticosteroid applied to an inflamed eye (with the very best of intention) can be *disastrous* if the inflammation is due to herpes virus.

Steroids containing fluorine (see above) intensify diabetes more than others and so should be avoided in that disease.

Longterm use of adrenal steroids in children presents essentially the same problems as in adults except that growth is retarded approximately in proportion to the dose. This is unlikely to be important unless therapy exceeds 6 months; there is a spurt of growth after withdrawal. Intermittent dosage schedules (alternate day) may reduce the risk (rarely, corticotrophin may be preferred, see p. 612).

Some other problems loom larger in children than in adults. Common childhood viral infections may be more severe, and if a nonimmune child taking an adrenal steroid is exposed to one, it is wise to try to prevent the disease with the appropriate specific immunoglobulin (if available).

Live virus vaccination is unsafe in immunosuppressed subjects, e.g. systemic prednisolone >2 mg/kg per day for >1 week in the preceding 3 months, as it may cause the disease, but active immunisation with killed vaccines or toxoids will give normal response unless the dose of steroid is high, when the response may be suppressed.

Raised intracranial pressure may occur more readily in children than in adults.

Fixed-dose combinations of adrenal steroids with other drugs in one tablet should *never* be used as they abrogate the principles for the use of such formulations (p. 106).

Indications for use of adrenal steroids

- Replacement of hormone deficiency
- Inflammation suppression
- Immunosuppression
- Suppression of excess hormone secretion

Nabarro[4] summarised *the place of adrenal steroids in therapeutics*, and his account of 1960 remains valid:

> The use of physiological amounts of hydrocortisone has greatly improved the replacement therapy available for patients with Addison's disease or hypopituitarism. Larger or pharmacological amounts of steroids have been used in the treatment of diseases unrelated to the adrenal gland. Adrenocortical steroids inhibit the inflammatory reaction, but in many instances the inflammatory reaction is part of the body's defence mechanism and is to be encouraged rather than inhibited. It has, however, become apparent that there are diseases which are really due to the body's reaction being quite disproportionate to the

noxious stimulus. The manifestations of the disease are, in fact, those of an exaggerated or inappropriate inflammatory response, and if steroid therapy can inhibit this inappropriate response the manifestations of the patient's disease will be suppressed. The underlying condition is not cured, though it may ultimately burn itself out.

The anti-inflammatory action of steroids is used for this purpose in allergic conditions and diseases like rheumatoid arthritis, rheumatic carditis, disseminated lupus erythematosus, and polyarteritis nodosa. Large doses of steroid will also inhibit antibody production and help in the management of auto-immune conditions like some of the haemolytic anaemias and thrombocytopenic purpuras. Steroid therapy may also be used to suppress the patient's adrenal glands; the doses required, however, are nearer the physiological levels. This may be needed in cases of adrenal dysfunction where abnormal androgenic steroids are being made, or in cases of disseminated breast cancer to inhibit adrenal secretion of oestrogens, the so-called medical adrenalectomy.

When large doses of steroids are given for their pharmacological action, the result will be to produce an iatrogenic Cushing's syndrome. There is a tendency to forget that Cushing's syndrome is a serious illness with a grave prognosis — so serious, in fact, that one has no hesitation in advising hypophysectomy or total adrenalectomy for its treatment. Admittedly, treatment with high doses of steroid may in some situations be life-saving, or produce a temporary remission in an incurable disease. There has been a tendency to overlook the dangers of treatment with adrenocortical steroids and to use them in cases where the treatment may prove more dangerous or disabling than the original disease.

USES OF ADRENOCORTICAL STEROIDS

REPLACEMENT THERAPY

Acute adrenocortical insufficiency
(Addisonian crisis)

This is an emergency and hydrocortisone sodium

---

[4] Nabarro J D N 1960 British Medical Journal 2: 553.

succinate 100 mg should be given i.v. immediately it is *suspected*, or the patient may die.

- An i.v. infusion of sodium chloride solution (0.9%) is set up immediately and a second 100 mg of hydrocortisone is added to the first litre, which may be given over 2 h (several litres of fluid may be needed in the first 24 h).
- The patient should then receive hydrocortisone 50–100 mg i.v. or i.m. 6–8 hourly for 24 h; then 12-hourly, initiating oral use when appropriate; then a total of 50–75 mg a day orally in 2 or 3 doses.

Other treatment to restore electrolyte balance will depend on the circumstances. The cause of the crisis should be sought and treated; it is often an infection. When the dose of hydrocortisone falls below 60 mg a day, supplementary mineralocorticoid (fludrocortisone) may be needed (see below).

The hyperkalaemia of Addison's disease will respond to the above regimen and must not be treated with insulin because of the risk of severe hypoglycaemia.

Chronic primary adrenocortical insufficiency
(Addison's disease)

Hydrocortisone orally is used (20–40 mg total daily) in the lowest dose that maintains well-being and body weight, with two-thirds of the total dose in the morning and one-third in the evening to mimic the natural *diurnal rhythm* of secretion.[5] Plainly corticotrophin is useless.

Some patients do well on hydrocortisone alone, with or without added salt, but most patients require a small amount of mineralocorticoid as well (fludrocortisone, 0.1–0.2 mg once a day, orally). If

the dose of fludrocortisone should exceed 0.5 mg a day, an unlikely event, then its glucocorticoid effect must be taken into account.

The dosage of the hormones is determined in the individual by following general clinical progress and particularly by observing: weight, blood pressure, appearance of oedema, serum sodium and potassium concentrations and haematocrit. The dose of fludrocortisone can be titrated against the plasma renin activity (routinely assayed in a number of chemical pathology laboratories by the radioimmunoassay of the amount of angiotensin I produced during a timed incubation of a plasma sample). Renin is secreted (by the juxtoglomerular apparatus of the kidney) in response to incomplete reversal of the sodium depletion in patients receiving inadequate replacement therapy. If any complicating disease arises, such as infection, a need for surgery or other stress, the hydrocortisone dosage should immediately be doubled, see above.

If there is vomiting, the replacement hormone must be given parenterally without delay.

There are no contraindications to replacement therapy. The risk lies in withholding rather than in giving it.

Some patients (particularly those with hypopituitarism), when first treated, cannot tolerate full doses of hydrocortisone because they become euphoric or otherwise mentally upset; 10 mg a day may be all they can take. The dose can usually soon be increased if it is done slowly. If diabetes is present the full dose is used and the diabetes controlled with insulin.

Chronic secondary adrenocortical insufficiency

This occurs in *hypopituitarism*. In theory the best treatment is corticotrophin, but the disadvantages of frequent injection are such that hydrocortisone is preferred. Usually less hydrocortisone is needed than in primary insufficiency. Special sodium-retaining hormone is seldom required, for the pituitary has little control over aldosterone production which responds principally to plasma K concentration and to the renin–angiotensin system. Thyroxine is given in appropriate dosage and sometimes sex hormones. The general conduct of therapy does not differ significantly from that in primary adrenal insufficiency.

---

[5] But this can be associated with an unphysiologically low plasma concentration of hydrocortisone in the late afternoon (with loss of well-being). Such patients may be best managed on 3 equal doses per day. *Air travellers* on long flights across longitude east to west (> 12 h, i.e. longer day): take an extra dose near the end of the flight. For west to east flights (> 8 h, i.e. shorter day): the normal evening dose may be taken sooner and the usual dose taken on the 'new' morning. *Night workers* may adjust their dosage to their work pattern (Drug and Therapeutics Bulletin 1990 28: 71).

Iatrogenic adrenocortical insufficiency: abrupt withdrawal

(See also Withdrawal of corticosteroid pharmacotherapy, below) This occurs in patients who have recently received prolonged pharmacotherapy with a corticosteroid which inhibits hypothalamic production of the corticotrophin releasing hormone and so results in *secondary* adrenal failure. It is treated by reinstituting therapy or as for acute insufficiency, as appropriate. To avoid an acute crisis on stopping, steroid therapy **must** be withdrawn gradually to allow the hypothalamus, the pituitary and the adrenal to regain normal function. Also, when patients taking steroids have an infection or surgical operation (major stress) they should be treated as for primary insufficiency.

After the use of large doses of hormone to suppress inflammation or allergy, sudden withdrawal may not only lead to an adrenal insufficiency crisis but to relapse of the disease, which has only been suppressed, not cured. Such relapse can be extremely severe, sometimes life-threatening.

PHARMACOTHERAPY

Suppression of adrenocortical function

In adrenogenital syndrome and adrenal virilism, an attempt may be made to suppress excess adrenal androgen secretion by inhibiting pituitary corticotrophin production by means of prednisolone or dexamethasone. Suppression of androgen production is effective if there is adrenal hyperplasia, but not if an adrenal tumour is present. Hairiness, which women especially dislike in themselves, is often unaffected even though good suppression is achieved, and menstruation recommences.

Use in inflammation and for immunosuppression

Adrenal steroids have been used in virtually every hitherto untreatable or obscure disease, e.g. immune complex diseases, nephrotic syndrome, sarcoidosis, with very variable results. Only a brief survey can be given here.

Drugs with primarily *glucocorticoid effects*, e.g. prednisolone, are chosen, so that dosage is not limited by the mineralocorticoid effects that are inevitable with hydrocortisone. But it remains essential to use only the *minimum dose* that will achieve the desired effect. Sometimes therapeutic effect must be partly sacrificed to avoid adverse effects, for it has not yet proved possible to separate the glucocorticoid effects from each other; indeed it is not known if it is possible to eliminate catabolic effects and at the same time retain anti-inflammatory action. In any case, in some conditions, e.g. nephrotic syndrome, the clinician cannot specify exactly what action they want the drug developer to provide.

Further uses

The decision to give a corticosteroid commonly depends on knowledge of the likelihood and amount of benefit (bearing in mind that very prolonged high dose inevitably brings serious complications such as osteoporosis), on the severity of the disease and on whether the patient has failed to respond usefully to other treatment. It often requires expertise that can only be imparted by those with wide experience of the disease concerned.

Adrenal steroids are used in all or nearly all cases of:

- *Exfoliative dermatitis* and pemphigus, if severe
- *Collagen diseases,* if severe, e.g. lupus erythematosus (systemic), polyarteritis nodosa, polymyalgia rheumatica and cranial giant cell arteritis (urgent therapy to save sight), dermatomyositis
- *Status asthmaticus*
- *Acute lymphatic leukaemia* (see Ch. 31)
- *Acquired haemolytic anaemia*
- *Severe allergic reactions* of all kinds, e.g. serum sickness, angioneurotic oedema, trichiniasis. Alone they will not control acute manifestations of anaphylactic shock as they do not act quickly enough
- *Organ transplant rejection*
- *Acute spinal cord injury:* early, brief, and high dose (to reduce the oedema/inflammation)
- *Active chronic hepatitis:* a corticosteroid improves well-being, liver function and histology and patient survival in the short term, but there is considerable uncertainty about the classes of

patient that will benefit long term. Prednisone should not be used because it is a prodrug and the liver may fail to transform it into the active prednisolone.

Adrenal steroids are used in some cases of:

- *Rheumatic fever*
- *Rheumatoid arthritis*
- *Ankylosing spondylitis*
- *Ulcerative colitis and proctitis*
- *Regional ileitis*
- *Bronchial asthma and hay-fever* (allergic rhinitis): also some bronchitics with marked airways obstruction.
- *Sarcoidosis*. If there is hypercalcaemia or threat to a major organ, e.g. eye, steroid administration is urgent. Pulmonary fibrosis may be delayed and central nervous system manifestations may improve.
- *Acute mountain/altitude sickness*, to reduce cerebral oedema.
- Prevention of *adverse reaction to radiocontrast media* in patients who have had a previous severe reaction.
- *Blood diseases due to circulating antibodies*, e.g. thrombocytopenic purpura (there may also be a decrease in capillary fragility with lessening of purpura even though thrombocytes remain few); agranulocytosis.
- *Eye diseases*. Allergic diseases and nongranulomatous inflammation of the uveal tract. But bacterial and virus infections may be made worse and use of steroids to suppress inflammation of infection is generally undesirable, is best left to ophthalmologists and must be accompanied by effective chemotherapy; this is of the greatest importance in herpes virus infection. Corneal integrity should be checked before use (by instilling a drop of fluorescein). Prolonged use of corticosteroid eye drops causes glaucoma in 1 in 20 of the population (a genetic trait). Application is generally as hydrocortisone, prednisolone or fluorometholone drops, or subconjunctival injection.
- *Nephrotic syndrome*. Patients with *minimal change disease* respond well to daily or alternate day therapy. With 60 mg/d total of prednisolone 90% of those who will lose their proteinuria will have done so within 4–6 weeks, the dose is tapered off over 3–4 months. Longer courses only induce adverse effects. Relapses are common (50%) and it is then necessary to find a minimum dose of steroid that will keep the patient well. If a steroid is for any reason undesirable, cyclophosphamide or chlorambucil may be substituted. *Membranous nephropathy* may respond to high dose corticosteroid with or without chlorambucil. The prognosis of other forms of glomerulonephritis is not improved by drugs, indeed for some patients the disease may even be made worse.
- *A variety of skin diseases*, such as eczema. Severe cases may be treated by occlusive dressings if a systemic effect is not wanted, though absorption can be substantial (see Ch. 16).
- *Acute gout* resistant to other drugs (see p. 263).
- *Hypercalcaemia* of sarcoidosis and of vitamin D intoxication responds to prednisolone 30 mg daily (or its equivalent of other steroid) for 10 days. Hypercalcaemia of myeloma and some other malignancies responds more variably. Hyperparathyroid hypercalcaemia does not respond.
- *Raised intracranial pressure due to cerebral oedema*, e.g. in cerebral tumour or encephalitis, probably an anti-inflammatory effect which reduces vascular permeability and acts in 12–24 h: give dexamethasone 10 mg i.m. or i.v. (or equivalent) initially and then 4 mg 6-hourly by the appropriate route, reducing dose after 2–4 days and withdrawing over 5–7 days; but much higher doses may be used in palliation of inoperable cerebral tumour.
- *Preterm labour*: (to mother) to enhance fetal lung maturation.
- *Mendelsohn's syndrome* (aspiration of gastric acid).
- *Myasthenia gravis*: see page 405.
- *Miscellaneous diseases*. In these other lines of treatment may be tried first, where they exist: steatorrhoea, severe nasal allergy (topical application), 'aphthous' mouth ulcers (suck a 2.5 mg hydrocortisone tablet (Corlan) 4 times daily), Bell's palsy, acute polyneuritis, toxic and virus encephalitis, post-irradiation fibrosis, Hunner's ulcer of the bladder, myotonia.
- *Cancer*, see Chapter 31.

Use in diagnosis: dexamethasone suppression test. Dexamethasone acts on the hypothalamus (like hydrocortisone), to reduce output of corticotrophin releasing hormone (CRH), but it does not interfere with measurement of corticosteroids in blood or urine. Normal suppression of cortisol production after administering dexamethasone indicates that the hypothalamic/pituitary/adrenal axis is intact. Failure of suppression implies pathological hypersecretion of ACTH by the pituitary or of cortisol by the adrenal. Dexamethasone is used because its action is prolonged (24 h). There is a number of ways of carrying out the test.

WITHDRAWAL OF PHARMACOTHERAPY

The longer the duration of therapy the slower must be the withdrawal. For use of less than 1 week (e.g. in severe asthma), although there is some hypothalamic suppression, withdrawal can be safely accomplished in a few steps. After use for 2 weeks, if rapid withdrawal is desired, a 50% reduction in dose may be made each day; but if the patient has been treated for a longer period, reduction in dose is accompanied by the dual risk of a flare up of the disease and of iatrogenic hypoadrenalism; then withdrawal should be done very slowly, e.g. 2.5–5 mg prednisolone or equivalent at intervals of 3–7 days.

An alternative scheme is to try halving the dose weekly until 25 mg prednisolone or equivalent is reached, after which it may be reduced by about 1 mg every third to seventh day. Paediatric tablets (1 mg) can be useful during withdrawal.

But these schemes may yet be found too fast (occurrence of fatigue, 'dish-rag' syndrome, or relapse of disease) and the rate may need to be even as slow as 1 mg prednisolone or equivalent per month, particularly as the dose approaches the level of physiological requirement (equivalent of 5–7 mg prednisolone daily).

The long tetracosactrin test or measurements of plasma corticotrophin concentration may be used to assess recovery of adrenal responsiveness, but a positive result should not be taken to indicate full recovery of the patient's ability to respond to stressful situations; the latter is best shown by an adequate response to insulin-induced hypoglycaemia (which tests the hypothalamic/pituitary capacity to respond).

Corticotrophin should not be used to hasten recovery of the atrophied cortex since its effects cause further suppression of the hypothalamic/pituitary axis, on the recovery of which the patient's future depends. Complete recovery of normal hypothalamic/pituitary/adrenal function sufficient to cope with severe intercurrent illnesses or surgery is generally complete in 2 months but may take as long as 2 years.

There have been many *reports of collapse*, even coma, occurring within a few hours of omission of steroid therapy, e.g. due to patients' ignorance of the risk to which their physicians are exposing them or failing to have their tablets with them and other trivial causes; but it is not invariable. Patients *must* be instructed on the hazards of omitting therapy and, during intercurrent disease, i.m. preparations should be freely used. Anaesthesia and surgery in adrenocortical insufficiency is discussed on page 609.

Inhibition of synthesis of adrenal and other steroid hormones

These agents have use in diagnosis of adrenal disease and in controlling excessive production of corticosteroids, e.g. by corticotrophin producing tumours of the pituitary (Cushing's syndrome) or by *adrenocortical adenoma or carcinoma* where the cause cannot be removed. They must be used with special care since they can precipitate acute adrenal insufficiency. Some members inhibit other steroid synthesis.

Metyrapone (Metopirone) inhibits the enzyme, steroid 11β-hydroxylase, that converts 11-deoxy precursors into hydrocortisone, corticosterone and aldosterone. It affects synthesis of aldosterone less than that of glucocorticoids.

Trilostane (Modrenal) blocks the synthetic path earlier (3β-hydroxysteroid dehydrogenase) and thus also inhibits aldosterone synthesis.

Formestane (Lentaron) is a specific inhibitor of the aromatase which converts androgens to oestrogens. A depot injection of 250 mg i.m. is given twice a month in the treatment of some patients with carcinoma of the breast who relapse on tamoxifen.

Aminoglutethimide (Orimeten) blocks even earlier, preventing the conversion of cholesterol to pregnenolone. It therefore blocks synthesis of all steroids, hydrocortisone, aldosterone and sex hormones (including the conversion of androgens to oestrogens); it has a use in breast cancer.

Ketoconazole (Nizoral) is an effective antifungal agent by virtue of its capacity to block sterol/steroid synthesis (ergosterol in the case of fungi). In man it inhibits steroid synthesis in gonads and adrenal cortex and it has been used in Cushing's syndrome and prostatic cancer.

COMPETITIVE ANTAGONISM OF ADRENAL STEROIDS

Spironolactone (Aldactone) and *potassium canrenoate* (see Index) antagonise the sodium-retaining effect of aldosterone and other mineralocorticoids. They are used to treat primary and secondary hyperaldosteronism (p. 602). *Mifepristone* (p. 652) weakly antagonises glucocorticosteroids.

Adrenocorticotrophic hormone (ACTH) (corticotrophin)

Natural corticotrophin is a 39-amino-acid polypeptide secreted by the anterior pituitary gland; it is obtained from animal pituitaries.

The physiological activity resides in the first 24 amino acids (which are common to many species) and most immunological activity resides in the remaining 15 amino acids.

The pituitary output of corticotrophin responds rapidly to physiological requirements by the familiar negative-feedback homeostatic mechanism. Since the $t^{1/2}$ of corticotrophin is 10 min and the adrenal cortex responds rapidly (within 2 min) it is plain that adjustments of steroid output can be quickly made.

Synthetic corticotrophins have the advantage that they are shorter amino acid chains (devoid of amino acids 25–39) and so are less likely to cause serious allergy, though this can happen. In addition they are not contaminated by animal proteins which are potent allergens.

Tetracosactrin consists of the biologically active first 24 amino acids of natural corticotrophin (from man or animals) and so it has similar properties, e.g. $t^{1/2}$ 10 min.

ACTIONS

Corticotrophin stimulates the synthesis of corticosteroids (of which the most important is *hydrocortisone*) and to a lesser extent of *androgens*, by the cells of the adrenal cortex. It has only a minor (transient) effect on aldosterone production, which can proceed independently; in the absence of corticotrophin the cells of the inner cortex atrophy.

The release of natural corticotrophin by the pituitary gland is controlled by the hypothalamus via *corticotrophin releasing hormone* (CRH or corticoliberin), production of which is influenced by environmental stresses as well as by the level of circulating hydrocortisone. High plasma concentration of any steroid with glucocorticoid effect prevents release of corticotrophin releasing hormone and so of corticotrophin, lack of which in turn results in adrenocortical hypofunction. This is the reason why catastrophe may follow sudden withdrawal of steroid therapy in the chronically treated patient who has an atrophied cortex.

The effects of corticotrophin are those of the *steroids* (*hydrocortisone, androgens*) liberated by its action on the adrenal cortex. Prolonged heavy dosage causes the clinical picture of Cushing's syndrome.

Uses. Corticotrophin is used principally in diagnosis and rarely in treatment. It is inactive if taken orally and has to be injected like other peptide hormones.

Diagnostic use: as a test of the capacity of the adrenal cortex to produce cortisol; the plasma cortisol (hydrocortisone) concentration is measured before and after an i.m. injection of tetracosactrin (Synacthen); a normal response is a rise of more than 200 nmol/1 in the plasma concentration of hydrocortisone. Variants of the test in cases of difficulty involve use of the depot (sustained-release) formulation i.m. For example, 1 mg of the depot is injected daily for 3 days at 9.00 am, with a short tetracosactrin test performed on day 3.

Therapeutic use is seldom appropriate because the peptide hormone has to be injected; selective glucocorticoid action (without mineralocorticoid effect) cannot be obtained, and clinical results are irregular. However, because androgens are secreted, corticotrophin is less liable to suppress growth in children, e.g. in severe chronic rheumatic disease it does not retard growth in children and adolescents and may occasionally be preferred for longterm therapy for this reason, despite the disadvantage of daily i.m. injection.

Corticotrophin is not useful during withdrawal of a steroid after prolonged therapy (it does not restore suppressed hypothalamic/pituitary function), but it can be used if these patients have an infection or other severe accidental stress during the succeeding 1–2 years when pituitary responsiveness may still be inadequate; though hydrocortisone is ordinarily preferred.

SUMMARY

- The zona fasciculata and zona glomerulosa of the adrenal cortex each make a steroid with a major role in physiology and pharmacology.
- The former secretes hydrocortisone (cortisol), the latter secretes aldosterone.
- Physiology levels of cortisol are essential for supporting the circulation and glucose production. Physiological levels of aldosterone are essential to prevent excessive Na^+ loss.
- For systemic pharmacological uses, prednisolone or other synthetic adrenocorticosteriod are used because they are more selective glucocorticoids (i.e. less Na^+-retaining activity).
- For local administration (skin, lung), more potent, fluorinated steroids may be required.
- Glucocorticoids inhibit the transcriptional activation of many of the inflammatory cytokines, giving them a versatile role in the treatment of many types of inflammation.
- Fludrocortisone is a valuable treatment for many Na^+-losing states, and for most causes of autonomic neuropathy.

Preparations

Tetracosactrin Injection is a powder dissolved in water immediately before injection i.v., i.m. or s.c.

Tetracosactrin Zinc Injection (Synacthen Depot) in which the hormone is adsorbed on to zinc phosphate from which it is slowly released. This is the form used in therapy, for it can be given i.m. twice a week and the doses then spaced according to response.

Corticotrophin preparations from animals (mixed with carboxymethylcellulose or gelatin for prolonged effect) remain available, but pure synthetic preparations are always preferable to inevitably impure biological preparations.

GUIDE TO FURTHER READING

Baylink D J 1983 Glucocorticoid-induced osteoporosis. New England Journal of Medicine 309: 306

Bone R C et al 1987 A controlled clinical trial of high-dose methylprednisolone in the treatment of severe sepsis and septic shock. New England Journal of Medicine 317: 653

Byyny R 1976 Withdrawal from glucocorticoid therapy. New England Journal of Medicine 295: 30

Downie W W et al 1977 Steroid cards: patient compliance. British Medical Journal 2: 428

Editorial 1983 Prednisolone pulses in collagen disease: grammes or milligrammes? Lancet 1: 280

English J et al 1983 Diurnal variation in prednisolone kinetics. Clinical Pharmacology and Therapeutics 33: 381

Freidy J F 1988 Reactions to contrast media and steroid pretreatment. British Medical Journal 296: 809

Hench P S et al 1949 The effect of a hormone of the adrenal cortex (17-hydroxy-11-dehydrocorticosterone: Compound E) and of pituitary adrenocorticotrophic hormone on rheumatoid arthritis. Proceedings of the Staff Meetings of the Mayo Clinic 24: 181, 277 (acute rheumatism). The classic studies of the first clinical use of an adrenocortical steroid in inflammatory disease. See also page 298 for an account by E C Kendall of the biochemical and pharmaceutical background to the clinical studies. Kendall writes of his collaboration with Hench, 'he can now say "17-hydroxy-11-dehydrocorticosterone" and in turn I can say "the arthritis of lupus erythematosus". In sophisticated circles, however, I prefer to say, "the arthritis of L.E."'.

Lavin M J et al 1986 Use of steroid eye drops in general practice. British Medical Journal 292: 1448

Marx J 1995 How the glucocorticoids suppress immunity. Science 270: 232

Newrick P G et al 1990 Self-management of adrenal insufficiency by rectal hydrocortisone. Lancet 335: 212

Newton R W et al 1978 Adrenocortical suppression in workers manufacturing synthetic glucocorticoids. British Medical Journal 1: 73

Orth D N 1995 Cushing's syndrome. New England Journal of Medicine 332: 791–803.

Swinburne C R et al 1988 Evidence of prednisolone induced mood change ('steroid euphoria') in patients with chronic obstructive airways disease. British Journal of Clinical Pharmacology 26: 709

Wolthers O D et al 1991 Growth of asthmatic children during treatment with budesonide: a double blind trial. British Medical Journal 303: 163

36

Diabetes mellitus, insulin, oral antidiabetes agents

SYNOPSIS

Diabetes mellitus affects 1–2% of many populations. Its successful management requires close collaboration between the patient and the doctor.

- Diabetes mellitus and insulin
- Insulins in current use (including choice, formulations, adverse effects, hypoglycaemia, insulin resistance)
- Oral antidiabetes drugs
- Treatment of diabetes mellitus
- Diabetic ketoacidosis
- Surgery in diabetic patients

Diabetes mellitus and insulin

HISTORY

Insulin (as pancreatic islet cell extract) was first administered to a 14-year-old insulin-deficient patient on 11 January 1922 in Toronto, Canada. An adult sufferer from diabetes who developed the disease in 1920 and who, because of insulin, lived until 1968, has told[1] how

Many doctors, after they have developed a disease, take up the speciality in it ... But that was not so with me. I was studying for surgery when diabetes took me up. The great book of Joslin said that by starving you might live four years with luck. [He went to Italy and, whilst his health was declining there, he received a letter from a biochemist friend which said] there was something called 'insulin' appearing with a good name in Canada, what about going there and getting it. I said 'No thank you; I've tried too many quackeries for diabetes; I'll wait and see'. Then I got peripheral neuritis ... So when [the friend] cabled me and said, 'I've got insulin – it works – come back quick', I responded, arrived at King's College Hospital, London, and went to the laboratory as soon as it opened ... It was all experimental for [neither of us] knew a thing about it ... So we decided to have 20 units a nice round figure. I had a nice breakfast. I had bacon and eggs and toast made on the Bunsen. I hadn't eaten bread for months and months ... by 3 o'clock in the afternoon my urine was quite sugar free. That hadn't happened for many months. So we gave a cheer for Banting and Best.[2]

But at 4 pm I had a terrible shaky feeling and a terrible sweat and hunger pain. That was my first experience of hypoglycaemia. We remembered that Banting and Best had described an overdose of insulin in dogs. So I had some sugar and a biscuit and soon got quite well, thank you.

[1] Abbreviated from Lawrence R D 1961 King's College Hospital Gazette 40: 220. Transcript from a recorded after dinner talk to students' Historical Society.

[2] F G Banting and C H Best of Toronto, Canada (see also Journal of Laboratory and Clinical Medicine (1922) 7: 251).

Diabetes mellitus is classified broadly as:

Type I (insulin dependent diabetes mellitus, IDDM) which typically occurs in younger people who cannot secrete insulin

Type II (non-insulin dependent diabetes mellitus, NIDDM), which typically occurs in older, often obese people who retain capacity to secrete insulin but who are resistant to its action.

These terms and abbreviations are used in this chapter.

Sources of insulin

Insulin is synthesised and stored (bound to zinc) in granules in the β-islet cells of the pancreas. Daily secretion amounts to 30–40 units, which is about 25% of total pancreatic insulin content. The principal factor that evokes insulin secretion is a high blood glucose concentration.

Insulin is a polypeptide with 2 peptide chains (A chain, 21 amino acids and B chain, 30) linked by 2 disulphide bridges. The basic structure having metabolic activity is common to all mammalian species but there are minor species differences, which result in the development of antibodies in all patients treated with animal insulins, as well as to unavoidable impurities in the preparations, minimal though these now are.

- **Bovine** insulin differs from human insulin by 3 amino acids and is *more antigenic* to man than is
- **Porcine** insulin, which differs from human by only 1 amino acid
- **Human** insulin (1980) is made either by enzyme modification of porcine insulin, or by using recombinant DNA to synthesise the proinsulin, precursor molecule for insulin. This is done by artificially introducing the DNA into either *Escherichia coli* or yeast. These 3 forms of insulin have the same amino acid sequence, but are separately designated as insulin *emp* (Enzyme Modified Porcine), *prb* (Proinsulin Recombinant in Bacteria) and *pyr* (Precursor insulin Yeast Recombinant). Although one of the incentives for introducing human insulin was avoidance of insulin antibody production, the allergies to older insulins were largely caused by impurities in the preparations, and are avoided equally well by using the highly purified,

monocomponent porcine and bovine insulins. Other preparations have been withdrawn. There is no systematic difference in activity between human and animal insulin, but any change in preparation prescribed to a patient should be monitored with care (see below).

Insulin receptors

Insulin is bound to a receptor (tyrosine kinase) on the surface of the target cell (mostly liver, muscle, fat) and the insulin/receptor complex enters the cell. Receptors vary in number inversely with the insulin concentration to which they are exposed, i.e. with high insulin concentration the number of receptors declines (*down-regulation*) and responsiveness to insulin also declines (insulin resistance); with low insulin concentration the number of receptors increases (*up-regulation*) and responsiveness to insulin increases. Obese Type II (NIDDM) tends to secrete excessive amounts of insulin and to have insulin resistance. In some patients the increased insulin secretion may be an attempt to overcome the insulin resistance; in others, the hypersecretion may be partly stimulated by overeating. These patients may recover insulin responsiveness as a result of dieting so that the insulin secretion diminishes, cellular receptors increase and insulin sensitivity is restored.

Actions of insulin

The effects of stimulation of the insulin receptors include activation of glucokinase and glucose phosphatase. Insulin also increases glucose transport as well as its utilisation, especially by muscle and adipose tissue. Its effects include:

- *Reduction in blood glucose* due to increased glucose uptake in the peripheral tissues (which convert it into glycogen or fat), and *reduction of hepatic output* of glucose (diminished breakdown of glycogen and diminished gluconeogenesis). When the blood–glucose concentration falls below the renal threshold (10 mmol/l or 180 mg/100 ml) glycosuria ceases, as does the osmotic diuresis of water and electrolytes. Polyuria with dehydration and excessive thirst are thus alleviated. If the blood glucose falls much below normal levels appetite is stimulated.

- *Other metabolic effects*. In addition to enabling glucose to pass across cell membranes, the transit of amino acids and potassium into the cell is enhanced. Insulin regulates carbohydrate utilisation and energy production. It *enhances* protein synthesis. It *inhibits* breakdown of fats (lipolysis). An insulin-deficient diabetic (Type 1) becomes dehydrated due to osmotic diuresis, and is *ketotic* because fats break down faster than the ketoacid metabolites can be metabolised.

Uses

Diabetes mellitus is the main indication. Insulin promotes the passage of potassium simultaneously with glucose into cells, and this effect is utilised in *hyperkalaemia* (see p. 490).

Insulin hypoglycaemia can also be used as a test of *anterior pituitary function* (growth hormone and corticotrophin are released).

Pharmacokinetics

- Insulin *naturally secreted* by the pancreas enters the portal vein and passes straight to the liver which takes up half of it. The rest enters the systemic circulation where its concentration is only about 15% (in fasting subjects) of that entering the liver.
- When insulin is *injected* s.c. it enters the systemic circulation and both liver and other peripheral organs receive the same concentration.

This difference may have clinical importance and this is why some continuous infusion pumps (see below) deliver insulin intraperitoneally rather than subcutaneously.

In conventional use, insulin is injected (s.c., i.m. or i.v.) as it is digested if swallowed. It is absorbed into the blood[3] and is inactivated in the liver and kidney; about 10% appears in the urine. The $t^{1/2}$ is about 5 min.

---

[3]Peak-plasma insulin (s.c.) concentration 60–90 min. Absorption is slower if there is peripheral vascular disease or smoking, and faster if the patient takes a hot bath or uses an ultraviolet light sunbed (which has induced a hypoglycaemic fit) or exercises. The effects are due to changes in peripheral blood flow.

In addition to needles and syringes, alternative techniques for insulin administration have been developed, some availing themselves of the kinetics of insulin: insulin pens (supplied preloaded or with replaceable cartridges), external infusions and implantable pumps. These latter are convenient for an accurately controlled continuously functioning biofeedback system, but pose difficulties for routine replacement in insulin deficiency. Therefore *sustained-release* (depot) *formulations* are used to provide an approach reasonably near to natural function and compatible with the convenience of daily living. An even closer approach is provided by the development of (at present inevitably expensive) miniaturised infusion pumps which can be used by *reliable* patients.

DIFFERENCES BETWEEN HUMAN AND ANIMAL INSULINS

Human insulin is absorbed from subcutaneous tissue slightly more rapidly than animal insulins and it has a slightly shorter duration of action.

Human insulin is less immunogenic than bovine, but not porcine, insulin. When changing from beef to human insulin patients taking <100 units of beef insulin are likely to require 10% less human insulin, and if taking >100 units beef insulin, 25% less human insulin. With pork insulin, dose reduction is not usually necessary.

There has been concern that patients taking human insulin may experience more frequent and more severe *hypoglycaemic attacks*, especially when transferring from animal insulins. Such occurrences are likely to be due to management problems rather than to pharmacological differences.

However there is some evidence of a lessened awareness of hypoglycaemia with human insulin, i.e. the counter-regulatory physiological responses to animal and human insulin may differ. It is claimed that with human insulin patients experience less *adrenergic* symptoms (sweating, tremor, palpitations), which are such a useful warning, although the *neurological* (neuroglycopenic) symptoms (dizziness, headache, inability to concentrate) are unchanged. It now seems likely that the reduced awareness is a paradoxical response to improved glycaemic control. Thus patients with a normal level of glycosylated haemoglobin (HbA1$_c$)

show no reduction in glucose uptake in the brain during episodes of hypoglycaemia that trigger a symptomatic and neuroendocrine response in patients with elevated levels of $HbA1_c$ (see Boyle et al 1995, in Guide to Further Reading).

PREPARATIONS OF INSULIN (Fig. 36.1)

There are three major factors:

- Strength (concentration)
- Source (human, porcine, bovine)
- Formulation
  — *short-acting* solution of insulin for use s.c., i.m. or i.v.
  — *intermediate and longer acting* (sustained release) preparations in which the insulin has been physically modified by combination with protamine or zinc to give an amorphous or crystalline suspension; this is given s.c. and slowly dissociates to release insulin in its soluble form (given i.m., which is not advised, the time course of release would be different).

Dosage is measured in international units now standardised by chemical assay.

Diabetes mellitus may be managed from a choice of four types of insulin (animal or human) preparations, having:

1. Short duration of action (and rapid onset): Soluble Insulin (neutral insulin). The most recent addition to this class of insulin, *insulin lispro (Humalog)*, is a modified human insulin in which the reversing of two amino acids has resulted in a very rapid onset of action, within 15 minutes of injection.

2. Intermediate duration of action (and slower onset): Isophane Insulin, a suspension with protamine; Insulin Zinc Suspensions, amorphous or a mixture of amorphous and crystalline

3. Longer duration of action: Insulin Zinc Suspension, crystalline, or Protamine Zinc Insulin (insulin in suspension with both zinc and protamine).

4. A mixture of soluble and isophane insulins, officially called biphasic insulins. Other mixtures are available, but infrequently used.

Insulin nomenclature

This is potentially confusing! The confusion has arisen from the fact that the insulin molecule itself is a naturally occurring molecule (differing slightly among species), which has been formulated in many different ways — partly to cater for differing patient requirements, and partly reflecting the different processes used to manufacture insulin preparations by different companies.

Fortunately, there has been considerable rationalisation of the preparations, helped by some rationalisation of the manufacturing companies. But it may be helpful to point out, and explain, some remaining ambiguities.

- *Soluble* and *neutral* insulin are the same; the British National Formulary favours the former term, but *neutral* is the INN (internationally approved) name, dating back to when there were acid and neutral pH formulations of soluble insulin. Human, porcine and beef are available.
- *Isophane* insulin is the only approved name for suspensions of insulin with protamine. Human, porcine and beef are available.
- *Biphasic* insulins are, with one exception, proprietary mixtures of *soluble* (neutral) insulin and *isophane* insulin, which provide soluble (neutral) insulin at concentrations between 10% and 50% of the total insulin concentration. Human, porcine and beef are available, but most preparations in this group are of human insulin. These preparations remove the need for patients to mix soluble and isophane insulins, without losing the flexible administration of the right amount of soluble (neutral) insulin to cover the meal following the dose.
- *Mixed* insulin zinc suspension is, confusingly, the approved name for proprietary mixtures of crystalline and amorphous zinc suspension. Mixed insulins are **not**, therefore, the same as biphasic insulins. While the different proprietary formulations in this group do have differing time courses of action (see Fig 36.1) depending on their (unstated) proportions of amorphous and crystalline suspension, it is **not** expected that doctors or patients would vary the formulation prescribed.

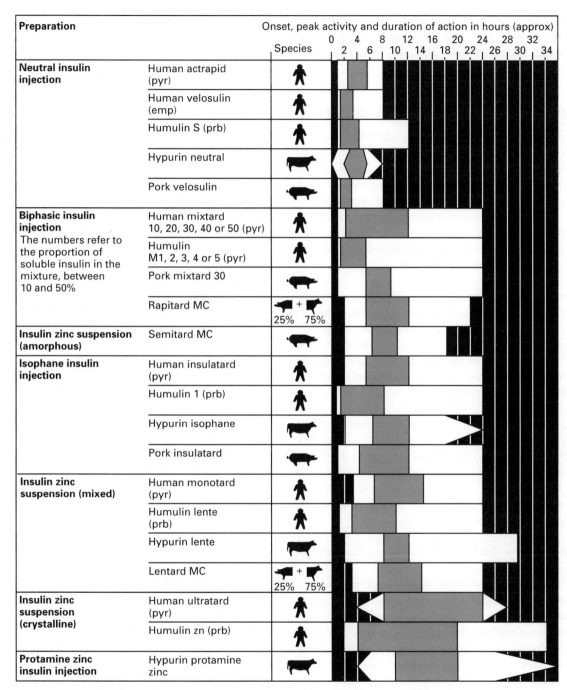

(prb) – produced from prc insulin synthesised by bacteria using recombinant DNA technology;
(pyr) – produced from a precursor synthesised by yeast using recombinant DNA technology;
(emp) – produced by enzymatic modification of porcine insulin.

Fig 36.1 Insulin chart. Reproduced with permission of MIMS, Haymarket Medical Publications, London. This chart is subject to change as companies develop their products.

The important thing is for the doctor to get to know well a range that will serve most patients. (For insulin regimens and injection techniques, see p. 627.)

NOTES FOR PRESCRIBING INSULIN

There is no need to change a stabilised diabetic from animal to human insulin. Unexplained requirement of above 100 units/d is usually due to noncompliance and less often to antibodies since the withdrawal of the older insulin preparations.

Allergy still occurs: to additives (protamine), to the preservative, e.g. phenol, cresol, or to insulin itself. It may take the form of local reactions (inflammatory or fat atrophy) or of insulin resistance.

Antibodies to insulin, provided they are moderate in amount, may be actually advantageous. They act as a carrier or store, binding insulin after injection and releasing it slowly as the free insulin in the plasma declines. In this way they smooth and prolong insulin action. But too high concentrations cause insulin resistance.

Compatibility. Soluble insulin may be mixed in the syringe with insulin zinc suspensions (amorphous, crystalline) and with isophane and mixed (biphasic) insulin, and used at once: but there are insulins in which *protamine* is used as a carrier, and spare protamine will bind some of the short-acting neutral insulin, thus blunting its effects.

Intravenous insulin. Only Soluble (neutral) Insulin Inj. should be used.

The standard strength of insulin preparations is 100 units per ml in a large and growing number of countries. Even very low doses can be accurately measured with modern special syringes. Solutions of 40 units and 80 units remain available in many countries.

Insulins in current use

CHOICE OF PREPARATION

That insulin preparations should be both precise and of uniform strength all over the world is vital to the health and safety of millions of diabetics. Advances in technology now allow biological standardisation in animal insulin to be replaced by physicochemical methods (high performance liquid chromatography: HPLC).

Soluble Insulin Inj. (neutral, regular insulin) is an aqueous solution of insulin. It is simple to use, being given s.c. 2–3 times a day, 30 min before meals. There is little risk of serious hypoglycaemic reaction if it is used sensibly. If it is known that a meal must be delayed, then the insulin injection can be postponed. The dose can easily be adjusted according to self-performed blood or urine glucose measurements.[4] For these reasons it is often used initially to balance diabetics needing insulin and always for the treatment of diabetic ketosis. The biggest disadvantages of soluble insulin for longterm use are the need for frequent injections, and the occurrence of high blood glucose before breakfast.

Soluble insulin is neutral, adjusted to pH 7.0. Acid formulations of soluble insulin are no longer available.

Intravenous soluble (neutral) **insulin** is used in diabetic ketoacidosis. It may be given intermittently (i.v. or i.m.) but continuous infusion is preferred. If the insulin is *infused by drip* in physiological saline (40 units/l) as much as 60–80% can be lost due to binding to the fluid container and tubing. It is necessary to take this into account in dosing. Polygeline (Haemaccel) may be added to bind the insulin in competition with the apparatus and so carry it into the body.

Use of a slow-infusion pump with a more concentrated solution (insulin 1.0 unit/ml) is preferred. Insulin loss is much less and control of dosage is

---

[4]An adverse effect of easy self-monitoring is that a minority of obsessional patients, told of the desirability of blood glucose concentrations being kept in the normal range to prevent diabetic complications, become obsessed with monitoring, and experience great anxiety when they find what are, in fact, normal fluctuations. They then anxiously change their insulin doses daily and as a result induce frequent hypoglycaemia, e.g. one patient had 33 episodes in 44 days, many with loss of consciousness (Beer S F et al 1989 British Medical Journal 298: 362).

more accurate when more concentrated solutions are infused by pump; at 1000 units/litre (1 unit/ml), such as is convenient for infusion by pump, losses are not of practical importance. (For i.v. doses see diabetic ketoacidosis, below.) Long-acting (sustained-release) preparations must not be given i.v.

The *time course* of soluble insulin given i.v. is shorter than when given s.c. (as in Table 36.1). The $t^{1/2}$ of insulin given i.v. is ~5 minutes; hence the use of continuous infusion when insulin is given by this route.

Insulin Zinc Suspensions and isophane insulin (see Fig 36.1) are sustained-release formulations in which rate of release is controlled by modifying particle size. Neutral pH, soluble insulin can be mixed with them without altering the time course of effect of either and these formulations can be a great convenience.

Duration of action. Patients live by a 24-hour cycle and plainly insulins having a duration of action exceeding 24 hours can cause problems, especially early morning hypoglycaemia.

DOSE OF INSULIN

The total daily output of endogenous insulin from pancreatic islet cells is 30–40 units (determined by the needs of completely pancreatectomised patients), and most insulin-deficient diabetics will need 30–50 unit/day (0.5–0.8 units/kg) of insulin (two-thirds in the morning and one-third in the evening).

Initial treatment for a Type I (IDDM) patient, who has not been in ketoacidosis, will usually be outside hospital with two injections of intermediate-acting insulin, or a mixed insulin. Other permutations, including soluble insulin before each meal, and an intermediate-acting insulin at bedtime, are possible. The following is a guide to initial daily dose requirements:

- 0.3 units/kg (16–20 units daily)
- increasing to 0.5 units/kg.

The dose is adjusted according to the usual monitoring of blood[5] and/or urine glucose. Daily (total) dose increments should be 4 units.

If it is decided to give the patient only one injection per day, then 10–14 units of an intermediate-acting isophane suspension may be given. Dose increments (4 units) may be given on alternate days.

Soluble insulin (neutral) may be added, or mixed (biphasic) insulins may be used, according to the patient's response. Excessive dose of insulin leads to overeating and obesity; it also leads to hypoglycaemia (especially nocturnal), that may be followed by rebound morning hyperglycaemia that is mistakenly treated by increased insulin, thus establishing a vicious cycle (Somogyi effect).

Muscular activity increases carbohydrate utilisation, so that hypoglycaemia is likely if a well-stabilised patient changes suddenly from an inactive hospital existence to a vigorous life outside. If this is likely to happen the diet may be increased by 250–500 calories[6] or the dose of insulin reduced by up to one-third and then readjusted according to need. This is less marked in patients on oral agents.

See also Choice of regimen and Ketoacidosis (below).

ADVERSE EFFECTS OF INSULIN

Adverse effects are mainly those of overdose.[7] Because the brain relies on glucose as its source of energy, an adequate blood–glucose concentration is just as essential as an adequate supply of oxygen, and hypoglycaemia may lead to coma, convulsions and even death (in 4% of diabetics under 50 years of age).

It is usually easier to differentiate **hypoglycaemia** from severe diabetic ketosis than from other causes of coma, which are as likely in a diabetic as in anyone else. If there is doubt as to the aetiology in a comatose patient it is reasonable to give glucose i.v., but only after taking blood for a glucose estimation. If hypoglycaemia of short duration is responsible, then a rapid improvement is usual; in any case

---

[5]The normal (fasting) blood glucose range is 3.9–5.8 mmol/l (70–105 mg/100 ml).

[6]1.0 calorie = 4.2 joules.

[7]Suicidal overdose (in diabetics) is well recorded. Surgical excision of the skin and subcutaneous tissue at the injection site of an enormous dose of long-acting insulin has been used.

a dose of glucose generally (but not always, see below) does no harm. Hypoglycaemia may manifest itself as disturbed sleep and morning headache. For details of treatment see below.

Other adverse reactions to insulin are **lipodystrophy** (atrophy or hypertrophy) at the injection sites (rare with purified pork and human insulin), after they have been used repeatedly. These are unsightly, but otherwise harmless. The site should not be used further, for absorption can be erratic, but the patient may be tempted to continue if local anaesthesia has developed, as it sometimes does. Lipoatrophy is probably allergic and lipohypertrophy is due to a local metabolic action of insulin. Local allergy also is manifested as itching or painful red lumps.

Generalised allergic reactions are very rare, but may occur to any insulin (including human) and to any constituent of the formulation. Change of brand of insulin, especially to highly purified preparations (or to one with a different mode of manufacture) may rectify allergic problems. But zinc occurs in all insulins (though very little in soluble insulin) and can be the allergen.

TREATMENT OF A HYPOGLYCAEMIC ATTACK

Prevention depends very largely upon patient education, but it is an unavoidable aspect of intensive glycaemic control. Patients should never miss meals, must know the early symptoms of an attack, and always carry glucose with them.[8] Treatment is to give sugar, either by mouth if the patient can still swallow or glucose (dextrose) i.v. (20–50 ml of 50% solution, i.e. 10–25 g; this concentration is thrombotic so do not withdraw the needle and compress the vein immediately after completion of injection); 20% glucose is less thrombotic, if available. The response is usually dramatic. The patient should be given a meal to avoid relapse. But if the patient does not respond within 30 min, it may be because of cerebral oedema, which recovers slowly and may require treatment with i.v. dexamethasone and perhaps mannitol. If the patient has been severely

hypoglycaemic for hours or if very large amounts of insulin or sulphonylurea have been taken, then large amounts of 20% glucose may have to be given by i.v. infusion for several days. Very severe attacks sometimes damage the central nervous system permanently. (See also Glucagon, below.)

After recovery from a severe attack and elucidation of the cause, the patient's treatment regimen should be carefully reviewed with appropriate educational input.

Some advocate (see above) giving i.v. glucose to comatose diabetics on the basis that it will revive them if they are hypoglycaemic and do no harm if they are hyperglycaemic. The latter assumption is unsound since a minority of comatose insulin-dependent diabetics have hyperkalaemia and added glucose can cause a brisk and potentially hazardous rise in serum potassium (mechanism uncertain), in contrast to nondiabetics in whom glucose causes a fall in serum potassium.

Hypoglycaemia due to other causes, e.g. alcohol, is treated similarly.

INSULIN RESISTANCE AND HORMONES THAT INCREASE BLOOD GLUCOSE

Insulin resistance may be due to a decline in *number* and/or *affinity* of receptors (see above) or to defects in *postreceptor mechanisms*.

A diabetic requiring more than 200 units/day is rare and regarded as insulin resistant (occasional patients have needed as much as 5000 units/day). Insulin resistance has become much less frequent with the wide availability of purified, mono-component and human insulins. If the requirement is acquired and genuine, it is due to *antibodies* binding insulin in a biologically inactive complex (though it can dissociate as with protein binding of drugs). De novo insulin resistance occurs in a small number of genetic syndromes, e.g. in combination with the skin condition, acanthosis nigricans.

Where animal insulins are still in use, change to a highly purified pork or human insulin may be successful in reducing resistance. Responsiveness to insulin may sometimes be restored by immunosuppression, e.g. an adrenocortical steroid (prednisolone 20–40 mg/d) over weeks (or a few months), to suppress antibody production.

---

[8]In the early stages of insulin treatment, it can be very useful training to allow a patient to experience hypoglycaemia once by delaying a meal.

Obviously, if this is successful, insulin dosage will have to be reduced in accordance with the unpredictable reduction in antibodies. Patients need to be carefully monitored to avoid severe hypoglycaemia. *Ketoacidosis* also reduces the effect of insulin.

Glucagon ($t^{1}/_{2}$ 4 min) is a polypeptide hormone (29 amino acids) from the α-islet cells of the pancreas. It is released in response to hypoglycaemia and is a physiological regulator of insulin effect. It releases liver glycogen as glucose. It has been used to treat insulin hypoglycaemia, but in about 45 min from onset of *coma* the hepatic glycogen will anyway be exhausted and glucagon will be useless. Its chief advantage would seem to be that, as it can be given s.c. or i.m. (1.0 mg), it can be used in severe hypoglycaemic attack by somebody, e.g. a member of the patient's family, who is unable to give an i.v. injection of glucose. If a comatose patient does not recover sufficiently in 20 min to allow oral therapy, i.v. glucose is essential. Glucagon is ineffective in substantial hepatic insufficiency.

Glucagon has a positive cardiac inotropic effect by stimulating adenylyl cyclase; it appears to have value in acute overdose of β-adrenoceptor blockers (see Index).

Adrenaline raises the blood sugar by mobilising liver and muscle glycogen; it does not antagonise the peripheral actions of insulin. Glycosuria and diabetic symptoms may occur in patients with phaeochromocytoma.

Adrenal steroids, either endogenous or exogenous, antagonise the actions of insulin, although this effect is only slight with the primarily mineralocorticoid group; the glucocorticoid hormones increase gluconeogenesis and reduce glucose uptake and utilisation by the tissues. Patients with Cushing's syndrome thus develop diabetes very readily and may be resistant to insulin. Patients with Addison's disease, hypothyroidism and hypopituitarism are abnormally sensitive to insulin action.

Oral contraceptives can impair carbohydrate tolerance.

Growth hormone antagonises the actions of insulin

in the tissues. Acromegalic patients may develop insulin-resistant diabetes.

Thyroid hormone increases the requirements for insulin.

Oral antidiabetes drugs

Oral antidiabetes drugs are of two kinds: sulphonamide derivatives (*sulphonylureas*) and guanidine derivatives (*biguanides*). They are used by 30% of all diabetics. Unlike insulin they are not essential for life.

Following the observation in 1918 that guanidine had hypoglycaemic effect, guanides were tried in diabetes in 1926, but were abandoned a few years later for fear of hepatic toxicity.

In 1930 it was noted that sulphonamides could cause hypoglycaemia, and in 1942 severe hypoglycaemia was found in patients with typhoid fever during a therapeutic trial of sulphonamide. In the 1950s a similar observation was made during a chemotherapeutic trial in urinary infections. This was followed up and effective drugs soon resulted. The first sulphonylureas were introduced into clinical practice in 1954.

Mode of action

Sulphonylureas activate receptors on the β cells of the pancreatic islets to release stored insulin in response to glucose. They do not increase insulin formation. Sulphonylureas appear to enhance insulin action on liver, muscle and adipose tissue by increasing insulin receptor number and by enhancing the postreceptor complex enzyme reactions mediated by insulin. The principal result is decreased hepatic glucose output and increased glucose uptake in muscle. They are ineffective in totally insulin-deficient patients and for successful therapy probably require about 30% of normal β-cell function to be present. They cause hypoglycaemia in normal subjects as well as in diabetics.

Gain in weight is liable to occur. Because of the mode of action, *secondary failure* (after months or a few years) occurs due to declining β-cell function and to increasing insulin resistance.

Biguanides. These agents have been in use since 1957, and metformin has remained a major agent in the management of NIDDM. The cellular mode of action is uncertain but the most important effect seems to be to reduce the production of glucose in the liver, mainly by inhibiting gluconeogenesis but also glycogenolysis. Other effects include enhancement of peripheral insulin sensitivity increasing glucose uptake in peripheral tissues; they do not act in the absence of insulin. They do not (used alone) cause hypoglycaemia in normal subjects nor in diabetics, but they can cause lactic acidosis. Secondary failure is not a problem.

Both groups of drugs are effective only in the presence of insulin.

Drugs of the two groups may be used either alone or in combination.

INDIVIDUAL DRUGS

Absorption from the alimentary tract is good for all the oral agents. It is advisable to take drugs ~30 min before a meal. If a patient fails to respond to one drug response to another of the same group may yet occur.

Sulphonylureas (see also Table 36.1)

Tolbutamide ($t^{1/2}$ 8 h) is rapidly metabolised by oxidation in the liver so that patients with hepatic disease should be treated with special caution, as always. It is the preferred sulphonylurea in the presence of impaired renal function. Adverse effects are unlikely to occur in more than 3% of patients. They usually consist of mild gastrointestinal upsets, which may be mitigated by taking the drug after food or by antacids, and of rashes. Alcohol intolerance (inhibition of metabolism) and alcohol-enhanced hypoglycaemia occur occasionally with all sulphonylureas. Other ill-effects are rare, but include blood disorders. The question of increased cardiovascular mortality with longterm use has been raised; it will not be resolved without further large and longterm studies.

Sulphonamides, as expected, potentiate sulpho-

Table 36.1 Principal oral antidiabetes drugs

Drug $t^{1/2}$ h	Total daily dose	Remarks
Sulphonylureas		
Tolbutamide (Rastinon) ($t^{1/2}$ 8)	0.5–2 g in 2–3 daily doses	Safe. Frequent administration
Chlorpropamide (Diabinese) ($t^{1/2}$ 36)	100–500 mg in 1 dose at breakfast	Less safe than tolbutamide. May succeed where tolbutamide fails. Taken only once daily. Avoid in elderly and patients with renal failure
Glibenclamide (Daonil) ($t^{1/2}$ 10)	2.5–15 mg in 1 dose at breakfast	Its $t^{1/2}$ allows once or twice daily dosing
Gliclazide (Diamicron) ($t^{1/2}$ 10)	40–320 mg daily, as single dose	
Glipizide (Glibenese) ($t^{1/2}$ 2.5)	2.5–15 mg daily as single dose; in divided doses up to 40 mg daily	
Biguanide		
Metformin (Glucophage) ($t^{1/2}$ 5)	1.5–2.0 g in 2–3 doses with meals	Preferred treatment for obese patients. Capable of controlling some patients when used alone. Also used as supplement for a sulphonylurea or insulin

Other sulphonylureas include gliquidone, glibornuride, tolazamide, glimepride.

nylureas by direct action and by plasma protein displacement.

Chlorpropamide is partly metabolised and largely excreted unchanged by the kidney. It is dangerous in patients with poor renal function because of its long $t^{1/2}$ (36 h) which is even longer in the elderly for whom the drug is unsuitable. Adverse effects are about twice as frequent as with tolbutamide: gastrointestinal upsets, rashes, vertigo, muscle weakness, headache, unpleasant taste, alcohol intolerance, jaundice and blood disorders; but the latter are rare and seldom serious (see Diabetes insipidus).

Glibenclamide ($t^{1/2}$ 10 h) is shorter-acting than chlorpropamide but is yet suitable for use in single daily dose; its action is terminated by metabolism.

Biguanide (diguanide) (see also Table 36.1)

Metformin ($t\frac{1}{2}$ 5 h) is taken with meals. Minor adverse gut reactions are common, including diarrhoea, and a metallic taste in the mouth. These symptoms are usually transient or subside after reduction of dose. Metformin is not metabolised and is excreted by the kidney and should not be used in the presence of renal impairment. Heavy prolonged use can cause vitamin B_{12} deficiency due to malabsorption. Its chief *use* is in the obese patient with NIDDM either alone or in combination with a sulphonylurea. Metformin has an anorexic effect which helps to reduce weight in the obese.

With a biguanide ketonuria may occur in the presence of normal blood sugar. This is not generally severe and may be treated by reducing the dose. More serious but rare is lactic acidosis, which has been reported with the older biguanide, phenformin, with an incidence of 0.25 to 1 case per 1000 patient years. The estimated incidence of metformin related lactic acidosis is 0.03 cases per 1000 patient years. When this condition does occur, it is usually against the background of a serious underlying medical condition such as renal impairment, liver failure or cardiogenic or septic shock. (Phenformin has now been abandoned in most countries.) Lactic acidosis is treated with large (i.v.) doses of sodium bicarbonate.

PRECAUTIONS WITH ORAL AGENTS

Hypoglycaemia is the most uncommon adverse effect with sulphonylureas, but is less common than with insulin therapy. However, it can be severe, prolonged for days, and may be fatal in 10% of cases, especially in the elderly and in patients with heart failure. Erroneous alternate diagnoses such as stroke may be made.

Renal and hepatic disease. A biguanide should not be used in patients with either; the risk of lactic acidosis is too great.

Sulphonylureas are potentiated in these diseases and a drug with a short $t\frac{1}{2}$ (not chlorpropamide) should be used in low doses.

Age and cardiac disease add to the hazard of oral agents.

Other adverse effects are rare but include skin rashes, gastrointestinal upset, minor derangement of haematological and hepatic indices (commoner with chlorpropamide).

OTHER ORAL AGENTS

Acarbose (Glucobay) is an α-glucosidase inhibitor. The reduced digestion of complex carbohydrates slows their absorption from the gut, and in high doses the drug may cause actual malabsorption. Acarbose reduces the glycaemic excursion after meals, and may improve overall glycaemic control. The usual dose is 150–300 mg daily. Adverse effects include abdominal bloating and diarrhoea. The drug may be combined with a sulphonylurea.

DIETARY FIBRE AND DIABETES

The addition of gel-forming (soluble) but unabsorbable fibre (*guar gum*, a hydrocolloidal polysaccharide of galactose and mannose from seeds of the 'cluster bean') to the diet of diabetics reduces carbohydrate absorption and flattens the postprandial blood glucose curve. Reduced need for insulin and oral agents has been reported, but adequate amounts (taken with lots of water) are unpleasant (flatulence) and patient compliance is therefore poor.

Treatment of diabetes mellitus

Both doctor and patient are faced with a lifetime of collaboration. Compliance is not a one-sided process, and the patients need all the consideration and support they can get. They should learn about their disease and its management, including home monitoring of blood glucose.

Good control of diabetes always involves diet and most patients need insulin or oral antidiabetes drugs in addition.

The aims of treatment are:

● to alleviate symptomatic hyperglycaemia and improve quality of life, while avoiding hypoglycaemia

- to avoid ketosis and infections
- to keep the fasting blood glucose <6 mmol/l
        the 2-hour postprandial concentration
        <9 mmol/l
        the glycosylated haemoglobin HbA1$_c$ as
        close to normal as possible
- by this regimen to avoid or delay the longterm complications and reduce mortality.

Each patient must be assessed individually; only an outline of the general principles involved can be given here.

Diet. Patients should be allowed to follow their own preferences as far as is practicable. Some carbohydrate restriction is necessary, but the amount varies from patient to patient according to their total energy requirements and whether weight increase or reduction is desired. The way in which carbohydrate is distributed through the day should correspond with the type of drug treatment, and especially the type of insulin in the IDDM.

In IDDM, patients are initially underweight, whereas the reverse is true of NIDDM. While carbohydrate intake needs to be controlled in both types, overall energy intake is restricted initially only in the obese NIDDM. *Other general factors which influence the diet*, in both IDDM and NIDDM, are

- High incidence of ischaemic heart disease, requiring some restriction of saturated fat intake (depending on measured levels of blood lipids)
- Need to reduce protein intake in patients with nephropathy.

Weight. Older overweight diabetics (70% of NIDDM) form a group whose blood often contains much insulin but who are resistant to its action; they seldom develop ketosis. In these patients, hypocaloric diet is vital, as weight loss dramatically improves glycaemic control. Glycosuria may cease when their weight is reduced. It is also likely that effective dieting is the most effective defence against macrovascular disease, both through influence on the glycaemia and through improved control of lipids and blood pressure. Biguanide treatment particularly helps weight reduction. Weight loss is associated with an increase in numbers of insulin receptors and so an increase in responsiveness to insulin. Patients should receive

dietary advice on a high complex carbohydrate diet (~55% of total calories) with low fat (<30% of calories) and emphasis on reduction in saturated fat in favour of mono- and polyunsaturates. Calories should be restricted and patients encouraged to achieve an ideal body weight. Diet should contain ~40 g of fibre/24 h.

Young patients with IDDM are often underweight and need insulin to restore normal weight. The blood of these young diabetics contains negligible insulin (they are sensitive to its action), and they readily become ketotic.

SELECTION OF THERAPY FOR DIABETES

Patients are treated with:

- Diet alone
- Diet plus oral agent
- Diet plus insulin
- For ketoacidosis: soluble insulin urgently.

Diabetics under 30 years: almost all need insulin; the exception is the rare single-gene disorder of Maturity Onset Diabetes of the Young (MODY) due to mutations in the glucokinase gene.

Diabetics over 30 years: approximately one-third need insulin, one-third oral agents and one-third diet only.

Type I (IDDM): human insulin is preferred for new patients (for regimen see below).

Type II (NIDDM): oral antidiabetics should only be used initially when there is no significant ketonuria.

NIDDM: treatment. In NIDDM, careful trial is the only sure way of deciding who can be maintained on oral therapy rather than on insulin. When diet alone has failed to control NIDDM it is necessary to add an oral agent; the choice should fall first on

- a sulphonylurea for the non-obese
- metformin for the obese patient.

A biguanide is also used as a supplement to a sulphonylurea when this is insufficient to give control.

Of the principal sulphonylureas, *tolbutamide* is the safest (short t$^{1/2}$), especially in the elderly, but has to given up to 4 times a day. *Chlorpropamide* is prone to accumulate, but can succeed where tolbutamide fails and need only be given once a day. They thus have their advantages and disadvantages and the choice in any patient is a matter of judgement and of trial. *Glibenclamide* is popular largely because its kinetics are intermediate.

To start a sulphonylurea: an example regimen would be glibenclamide 5 mg orally (or 2.5 mg in the aged) before breakfast. The dose is adjusted, according to response, at 2–4 weekly intervals by increments of 2.5 or 5 mg, to a maximum of 15 mg. If control is incomplete, metformin may be added.

To start metformin: the usual regimen is metformin 500 mg twice daily after the main meal, increasing at 2–4 weekly intervals to a maximum of 3 g daily.

Failure of oral agents. If the postprandial blood sugar does not fall below 10 mmol/l (180 mg/100 ml) on diet and maximal sulphonylurea treatment (primary failure), then insulin is needed, for not only is this state unsatisfactory but, on the same treatment, control may worsen over succeeding weeks (for Secondary failure, see p. 623).

Insulin treatment in NIDDM. Insulin treatment is needed in many patients with NIDDM to achieve adequate glycaemic control. Definitive evidence that this will reduce complications is still awaited, but there is certain improvement in quality of life with few patients requesting to stop insulin once they have started. Initial treatment with a single injection of long-acting insulin (see Fig 36.1) last thing at night, or intermediate-acting insulin twice daily, may control hyperglycaemia. Fluctuations in blood glucose levels may be controlled with twice daily mixed insulin or by multiple injections.

Withdrawal of oral agents, gradually, may be attempted after the patient has been controlled and stable for 3–6 months. About 30% of patients will be found not to need that drug any longer.

Monitoring of patients taking oral agents should be as close as of those on insulin and probably closer. The patient must be disabused of any notion that substitution of tablets to swallow for the tiresome routine of self-injection carries any implication that the condition is less serious, or that diet can be relaxed.

IDDM: treatment. The range of insulin formulations available allows flexible adjustment of the regimen to the patient's way of life. There is no reason to coerce patients into a regimen favoured by the physician. There is no single regimen that suits all patients.

One of the following regimens can suit most patients (see Fig 36.1):

- Three doses of soluble insulin (before the main meals) plus an intermediate-acting insulin at bedtime
- A biphasic or intermediate-acting insulin (see Fig 36.1) twice a day before morning and evening meals
- A single morning dose of a biphasic or intermediate-acting insulin before breakfast may suffice for some patients.

Injection technique has pharmacokinetic consequences according to whether the insulin is delivered into the subcutaneous tissue or muscle. Patients have been traditionally taught to pinch up a skin fold and inject obliquely, thus ensuring true subcutaneous injection. But, with the introduction of short needles and pen-shaped injectors, patients are often encouraged to inject perpendicularly to the skin, it being assumed that this will provide subcutaneous delivery. But the thickness of subcutaneous tissue is very variable between individuals and between different parts of the body and this technique may lead to superficial (and intermittent) i.m. injection, which may be unrecognised as i.m. injection is not necessarily more painful. The absorption of insulin is as much as 50% more rapid from shallow i.m. injection. Clearly factors such as heat or exercise which alter skin or muscle blood flow can markedly alter the rate of insulin absorption.

Patients should standardise their technique to ensure injection is s.c. Inadvertent i.m. injection of an overnight dose of an extended duration insulin can lead to inadequate early morning control of blood glucose. Sites of injection should be rotated to minimise the now rare local complications (lipodystrophy). Absorption is faster from arm and abdomen than it is from the thigh and buttock.

Diabetic complications. A well-controlled diabetic is less liable to ketosis, infections, neuropathy and cataract. It is now certain that good control of glycaemia at least mitigates the serious microvascular retinal and renal complication. Overzealous control of glycaemia can result in increase in hypoglycaemia attacks.

SOME FACTORS AFFECTING CONTROL OF DIABETES

Intercurrent illnesses, cause fluctuations in the patient's metabolic needs. If these are severe, e.g. myocardial infarction, it is prudent to substitute insulin for oral agents. An appropriate starting dose is biphasic (mixtard) insulin 10–15 units twice daily. Infections cause an increase in insulin need (about 20%), which may drop briskly on recovery. In patients with poor glycaemic control, it is preferable to use an insulin infusion and sliding scale, as described below for diabetic ketosis.

Surgery, see later.

Menstruation and oral contraception: insulin needs may rise slightly.

In pregnancy close control of diabetes is of the first importance to avoid fetal loss at all stages, and in the *first trimester* to reduce fetal malformations. Insulin requirements increase steadily after the third month. Ideally, women of childbearing age should be advised to conceive during a period of stable, euglycaemic control.

During labour soluble insulin should be given by continuous infusion at about 1–2 unit/h with i.v. infusion of 5% glucose 1.0 l in 8 h). Substantially less, e.g. 25%, insulin is likely to be needed immediately after delivery, when timing and dose of insulin injections should be carefully reconsidered lest hypoglycaemia occurs. Insulin need remains lower during the first 6 weeks of lactation.

Blood glucose estimations are necessary during pregnancy, for glycosuria is not then a reliable guide. The renal threshold for glucose (also of lactose) falls, so that glycosuria and lactosuria may occur in the presence of a normal blood glucose.

Maternal hyperglycaemia leads to fetal hyperglycaemia with consequent fetal islet cell hyperplasia, high birthweight babies, and postnatal hypoglycaemia.

Premature labour: use of β_2-adrenoceptor agonists and of dexamethasone (to prevent respiratory distress syndrome in the prematurely newborn) causes hyperglycaemia and increased insulin (and potassium) need.

Oral antidiabetes agents and pregnancy: the continued use of these during pregnancy is associated with fetal loss and insulin should be substituted. Young women on oral hypoglycaemic agents planning a pregnancy should be changed to insulin and continue on it throughout pregnancy.

INTERACTIONS WITH NONDIABETES DRUGS

The subject is ill-documented, but whenever a diabetic under treatment takes other drugs it is prudent to be on the watch for disturbance of control.

Adrenocorticosteroids antagonise insulin.

β-adrenoceptor blocking drugs impair the sympathetic mediated (β_2-receptor) release of glucose from the liver in response to hypoglycaemia and also reduce the adrenergic-mediated symptoms of hypoglycaemia (except sweating). Insulin hypoglycaemia is thus both more profound and less noticeable. A diabetic needing a β-adrenoceptor blocker should be given a β_1-cardioselective member, e.g. atenolol. *Thiazides* at a higher dose than generally now used in hypertension can precipitate diabetes, and it is wise to avoid high doses especially in established diabetes.

The action of sulphonylureas is intensified by heavy *sulphonamide* dosage and some sulphonamides increase free tolbutamide concentrations, probably by competing for plasma protein binding sites.

Monoamine oxidase inhibitors potentiate oral agents and perhaps also insulin. They can also reduce appetite and so upset control.

Interaction may occur with *alcohol* (hypoglycaemia with any antidiabetes drug, flushing with chlorpropamide). *Combined contraceptive pill* reduces hypoglycaemic effect.

Hepatic enzyme inducers may enhance the metabolism of sulphonylureas that are metabolised in the liver (tolbutamide). *Cimetidine*, an inhibitor of drug metabolising enzymes, increases metformin plasma concentration.

These examples suffice to show that the possibility of interactions of practical clinical importance is a real one.

DRUG-INDUCED DIABETES

After the introduction of *thiazide diuretics*, it was soon found that their prolonged use increased hyperglycaemia in diabetics and, later, that they impaired glucose tolerance in some nondiabetics.

Research for better antihypertensive thiazides resulted in the discovery of a nondiuretic derivative with antihypertensive effect, *diazoxide*; but it proved unsatisfactory for longterm use as it often caused diabetes, though it is effective short term (see p. 432). It is useful in treating hypoglycaemia due to islet-cell tumour (insulinoma).

An antibiotic (*streptozotocin*) is selectively toxic to malignant β-islet cell tumours. It has been used to treat functioning metastases. After a short course remission may occur in 3 weeks and last a year or longer.

Adrenocortical steroids and *oral contraceptives* are also diabetogenic.

Diuretics for diabetics. In general a nonthiazide should be chosen (see Ch. 27). Frusemide and bumetanide are less prone to precipitate diabetes.

Potassium-conserving diuretics should be avoided in patients with reduced renal function, because of the risk of hyperkalaemia.

Diabetic ketoacidosis

The condition is discussed in detail in medical texts and only the more pharmacological aspects will be dealt with here. Nevertheless, it should be emphasised that the patients are always severely dehydrated and that fluid replacement is the first priority.

In severe ketoacidosis the patient urgently needs insulin to stop ketogenesis. The objective is to supply, as continuously as possible, a moderate amount of insulin.

Soluble insulin, preferably from the same species the patient has been using (never a sustained-release form), should be given by continuous i.v. infusion (rather than by intermittent bolus injection) ideally by a pump (which allows independent control of insulin and electrolyte administration more readily than an i.v. drip) in a concentration of 0.1 unit/ml in isotonic sodium chloride, at a dose of 0.1 unit/kg/h, i.e. 7 units/h in a 70 kg adult. The dose is raised or lowered using a sliding scale of blood glucose concentrations (Table 36.2). If an i.v. drip is used instead of a pump the concentration should be lower (40 units/l); stringent precautions against septicaemia are necessary in these patients. It has been shown that continuous infusion i.m. (not s.c.) can be equally effective, provided the patient is not in shock and provided there is not an important degree of peripheral vascular disease.

Intermittent doses i.v. or i.m. may be used when circumstances require. If the i.m. route is used, a priming dose of 10–20 units should be given at the outset and then 10 units hourly.

Progress. When the blood glucose has fallen to 10 mmol/l the infusion rate may be reduced to,

Table 36.2 Sliding scale of insulin doses according to blood glucose concentrations in ketoacidosis (see text)

Blood glucose (mmol/l)	Infusion rate (ml/h = units/hour for 50 ml syringe containing 50 units of insulin)
> 16	8.0 + check pump and connections
12–16	4.0
8–12	2.0 + change from saline to glucose infusion if blood glucose <10 mmol/l
5–8	1.5
3–5	1.0
< 3	0.3 (+ increase glucose infusion)

say, 0.02 unit/kg per hour until the patient can eat and drink and s.c. insulin is restarted. Similar progression is used if the insulin is given i.m., e.g. lower doses 2-hourly. Doses are always tailored to the clinical situation, which requires *close* monitoring.

Less severe cases of ketosis can be treated with half the above doses (3 units/h) at the outset.

It has been shown that the rate of fall of blood glucose/hour is proportional to the rate of infusion of insulin over the range of 1–10 units/h. A reasonable rate of fall during treatment is 4–5.5 mmol/l (75–100 mg/100 ml) per hour.

Intravenous fluid and electrolytes.[9] Patients are often more deficient in water than in saline and although initial replacement is by *isotonic* (0.9%) *sodium chloride* solution, occurrence of hypernatraemia is an indication for half isotonic (0.45%) solution. A patient with diabetic ketoacidosis may have a fluid deficit of above 5 litres and may be given:

- 1 litre in the first hour,
- followed by 2 litres in 4 hours,
- then 4 litres in the next 24, watching the patient for signs of fluid overload.

Fluid replacement causes a fall in blood glucose by dilution.

Glucose should only be given when its concentration in blood falls below the renal threshold, in practice starting when the blood glucose falls to 10 mmol/l. If it is used at concentrations above the renal threshold it merely increases the diabetic osmotic diuresis, causing further dehydration and potassium and magnesium loss (but see Hypoglycaemia, above). When the blood glucose level falls to 10 mmol/l, the fluid replacement should be changed from saline to 5% glucose, at the same rate as detailed above.

Potassium. Even if plasma potassium is normal or high, patients have a substantial total body deficit,

and the plasma potassium will fall briskly with i.v. saline (dilution) and insulin which draws potassium into cells within minutes. KCl should be added to the second and subsequent litres of fluid according to plasma K^+ (only if passing urine):

- <3.5 mmol/l add 40 mmol/l of fluid
- 3.5–5.0 mmol/l add 20 mmol/l of fluid
- >5.0 mmol/l none.

Bicarbonate (isotonic) should be used only if plasma pH is <7.0 and peripheral circulation is good; insulin corrects acidosis.

Success in treatment of diabetic ketoacidosis and its complications (hypokalaemia, aspiration of stomach contents, infection, shock, thromboembolism, cerebral oedema) attends on *close, constant, informed supervision.*

Mild diabetic ketosis. If the patient is fully conscious and there has been no nausea or vomiting for at least 12 h, intravenous therapy is unnecessary. It is reasonable to give *small* doses of insulin s.c. 3–6-hourly and fluids by mouth.

Hyperosmolar diabetic coma occurs chiefly in non-insulin-dependent diabetics who fail to compensate for their continuing, osmotic glucose diuresis. It is characterised by severe dehydration, a very high blood sugar (>33 mmol/l: 600 mg/100 ml) and lack of ketosis and acidosis. Treatment is with isotonic or hypotonic saline with less potassium than in severe ketoacidosis and insulin according to blood glucose levels. Insulin requirements may be less than in ketoacidosis, where the acidosis causes resistance to the actions of insulin. Patients are more liable to thrombosis and heparin is used.

Surgery in diabetes patients

Principles of management

- Surgery constitutes a major stress
- Insulin needs increase with surgery
- Avoid ketosis
- Avoid hypoglycaemia

---

[9] In this situation glucose solution does not provide water replacement since the normal capacity to metabolise glucose is fully taken up.

- High blood glucose concentration matters little over short periods.

The programme for control should be agreed between anaesthetist and physician whenever *diabetics* must undergo *general anaesthesia* or modify their *diets*. There are many different techniques that can give satisfactory results.

TYPE I DIABETES (IDDM)

Elective major surgery

- Admit to hospital the day before surgery
- Arrange operation for morning
- Evening before surgery: give patient's usual insulin
- Day of operation: omit morning s.c. dose; set up i.v. infusion (glucose 10% + insulin 16 units/litre + KCl 10 mmol/litre) and infuse at 100 ml/h (or as appropriate for fluid requirements)
- Modify regimen during and after surgery according to monitoring; insulin doses should be adjusted according to similar scale as in Table 36.2
- Stop i.v. infusion one hour after first postsurgical s.c. insulin
- Insulin requirements may be as high as 20 units/h in cases of serious infection, corticosteroid use, obesity, liver disease.

Minor surgery

For example, simple dental extractions (for multiple extractions or when there is infection the patient should be admitted to hospital). A suitable postoperative diet of appropriate calorie and carbohydrate content must be arranged. Plan the operation for between 12 noon and 5 pm (17.00h). Omit the usual dose of long-acting insulin on the morning of the operation and substitute soluble insulin, one-quarter of the usual total daily dose, before a light breakfast 6 h preceding the operation. Arrange a light evening meal after the operation and soluble insulin, 10–30 units s.c., according to the blood tests. Return to the normal routine the next day.

Emergency surgery

When a surgical emergency is complicated by dia-

SUMMARY

- Diabetes mellitus is the most important chronic illness because of its high incidence and frequency of major complications. It is of **two kinds**: insulin dependent diabetes mellitus (IDDM) and non-insulin dependent diabetes (NIDDM).
- Insulin dependent diabetes (IDDM) is almost always present in young or thin patients with diabetes. Insulin may also be required when glycaemic control is not achieved by oral drugs in older patients.
- Insulin is given s.c. to stable patients, usually as a biphasic mixture of soluble, short-acting human insulin, and a longer acting suspension of insulin with protamine or zinc.
- In the treatment of comatose patients, in the perioperative patient, and at other times of changing insulin requirement, insulin is best given by i.v. infusion of the soluble form.
- Stable patients can also treat themselves by continuous s.c. infusion of soluble insulin.
- Diet plays a major role in the treatment of non-insulin dependent diabetes (NIDDM) with obesity.
- There is now a clear difference in the choice of first-line drug, if a drug is required, in NIDDM. A sulphonylurea is used for the non-obese, and metformin (a biguanide) for the obese.
- Aggressive treatment of IDDM, and probably NIDDM, successfully reduces the microvascular complications. Close attention to associated risk factors, especially hyperlipidaemia and hypertension, is important in reducing risk of macrovascular disease.

betic ketosis, an attempt should be made to control the ketosis before the operation. Management during the operation will be similar to that for major surgery except that more insulin will be needed.

In other cases small doses of soluble insulin are given 2–4-hourly (where pumps are not available), keeping the blood glucose between 8.5 and 10 mmol/l (150 and 300 mg/100 ml).

TYPE II DIABETES (NIDDM)

Elective and emergency surgery, and minor surgery if NIDDM is poorly controlled: use the same regimen as for IDDM.

Minor surgery: If NIDDM is well controlled, omit oral hypoglycaemic agent on the morning of surgery. If the surgery is more than trivial, monitor blood glucose carefully, and use soluble insulin s.c.

or by infusion if blood glucose rises. If vomiting is likely, use insulin.

Miscellaneous

Most patients with both IDDM and NIDDM succumb to either the macrovascular or microvascular complications — especially ischaemic heart disease and diabetic nephropathy, respectively. Indeed diabetes is the major indication for dialysis and transplantation. As discussed in other chapters, the treatment of hypertension and hyperlipidaemia is particularly important in patients with diabetes. A number of large outcome studies are currently investigating whether either antihypertensive drugs (especially the ACE inhibitors) or lipid-lowering drugs (especially the statins) should be used in all patients with diabetic nephropathy, regardless of baseline blood pressure or serum lipid profile.

GUIDE TO FURTHER READING

Bogardus C et al 1990 Where all the glucose doesn't go in non-insulin dependent diabetes mellitus. New England Journal of Medicine 322: 262

Boyle P J et al 1995 Brain glucose uptake and unawareness of hypoglycemia in patients with insulin-dependent diabetes mellitus. New England Journal of Medicine 333: 1726–1731

Clark C M Jr, Lee D A 1995 Prevention and treatment of the complications of diabetes mellitus. New England Journal of Medicine 332: 1210–1217

De Fronzo L, Goodman A M et al 1995 Efficacy of metformin in patients with non-insulin-dependent diabetes mellitus. New England Journal of Medicine 333: 541–549

Diabetes Control and Complications Trial Research Group 1993 The effect of intensive treatment of diabetes on the development and progression of long-term complications in insulin-dependent diabetes mellitus. New England Journal of Medicine 329: 977–986

Garner P 1995 Type I diabetes mellitus and pregnancy. Lancet 346: 157–161

Gerich J E 1989 Oral hypoglycaemic agents. New England Journal of Medicine 521: 1231

MacPherson J N et al 1990 Insulin. British Medical Journal 300: 731

Nathan D M 1993 Long-term complications of diabetes mellitus. New England Journal of Medicine 328: 1676–1685

Patrick A W et al 1991 Human insulin and awareness of acute hypoglycaemic symptoms in insulin-dependent diabetes. Lancet 338: 528

Stevens A B et al 1989 Motor vehicle driving amongst diabetics taking insulin and non-diabetics. British Medical Journal 299: 591

Stumvoll M et al 1995 Metabolic effects of metformin in non-insulin-dependent diabetes mellitus. New England Journal of Medicine 333: 550–554

Williams G 1994 Management of non-insulin-dependent diabetes mellitus. Lancet 343: 95–100

Thyroid hormones, antithyroid drugs

SYNOPSIS

- Thyroid hormones (thyroxine T_4, liothyronine T_3)
- Use of thyroid hormone: treatment of hypothyroidism
- Antithyroid drugs and hyperthyroidism: thionamides, drugs that block sympathetic autonomic activity, iodide and radioiodine ^{131}I, preparation of patients for surgery, thyroid storm, exophthalmos
- Drugs that cause unwanted hypothyroidism

Thyroid hormones

L-thyroxine (T_4 or tetraiodo-L-thyronine) and **liothyronine** (T_3 or triiodo-L-thyronine) are the natural hormones of the thyroid gland. T_4 is a less active precursor of T_3, which is the major mediator of physiological effect.

For convenience, the term *thyroid hormone* is used to comprise T_4 plus T_3. Both forms are available for oral use as therapy.

Calcitonin: see page 673.

PHYSIOLOGY AND PHARMACOKINETICS

Thyroid hormone is formed from dietary iodine by iodination of tyrosine to mono- and diiodotyrosine; 2 molecules of diiodotyrosine combine to form tetraiodotyrosine, T_4 or *thyroxine*.

Thyroid hormone is stored in the gland as thyroglobulin from which enzymatic hydrolysis releases T_4 and a little T_3 into the circulation. About 80% of the released T_4 is deiodinated in the peripheral tissues to the biologically active T_3 (30–35%) and biologically inactive *reverse* T_3 (45–50%); thus most circulating T_3 is derived from T_4. Further deiodination, largely in the liver, leads to loss of activity.

In the blood both T_4 and T_3 are extensively (99.9%) bound to plasma proteins (thyroxine-binding globulin, TBG, and thyroxine-binding prealbumin, TBPA). The concentration of TBG is *raised* by oestrogens (including doses used in oral contraceptives), clofibrate, and prolonged use of neuroleptics, and in pregnancy. The concentration of TBG is *lowered* by adrenocortical and androgen (including anabolic steroid) therapy and by urinary protein loss in nephrotic syndrome. Phenytoin and salicylates compete with thyroid hormone for TBG binding sites. Effects such as these obviously can interfere with the assessment of the clinical significance of measurements of total thyroid hormone concentration. But measurement of free thyroid hormone by ingenious techniques (free thyroxine index) largely avoids these complicating factors.

T_4 and T_3 are well absorbed from the gut except in severe hypothyroidism, when initial parenteral therapy is used.

T4 (thyroxine): a single dose reaches its maximum effect in about 10 days (its binding to plasma proteins is strong as well as extensive) and passes off in 2–3 weeks ($t^1\!/_2$ 7 d in euthyroid subjects; 14 d in hypothyroid; 3 d in hyperthyroid).

T3 (liothyronine) is about 5 times as biologically potent as T_4; a single dose reaches its maximum effect in about 24 h (its binding to plasma proteins is weak) and passes off in one week ($t^1\!/_2$ 2 d in euthyroid subjects: see T_4 above).

PHARMACODYNAMICS

Thyroid hormone passes into the cells of target organs, combines with specific nuclear receptors there and induces characteristic metabolic changes:

- *Protein synthesis* during growth
- Increased *metabolic rate* with raised oxygen consumption
- Increased *sensitivity to catecholamines* with proliferation of β-adrenoceptors (particularly important in the cardiovascular system).

Thyroid hormone for hypothyroidism

The main indication for thyroid hormone is treatment of *deficiency* (cretinism, hypothyroidism, myxoedema) from any cause. The adult requirement of hormone is remarkably constant, and dosage does not have to be altered once the optimum is found. Children naturally need more as they grow.

Early treatment of neonatal hypothyroidism (cretinism) (1:5000 births) is important if permanent mental defect is to be avoided. It must be life-long.

Hypothyroidism due to panhypopituitarism requires replacement with adrenocortical as well as with thyroid hormones. Use of thyroxine alone can cause acute adrenal insufficiency.

Small doses of thyroxine in normal subjects merely depress pituitary thyroid stimulating hormone (TSH) production and consequently reduce the output of thyroid hormone by an equivalent amount.

When thyroid enlargement is associated with *excess* TSH (puberty goitre, endemic iodine deficiency, Hashimoto's autoimmune thyroiditis), thyroxine administration can be effective in suppressing TSH secretion (by the usual feedback mechanism) with reduction in size of goitre.

Thyroxine should not be used to treat simple obesity (see Obesity).

A curious by-way of human nature that can cause diagnostic difficulty is secret thyroxine 'addiction'.[1] It is associated with overt psychiatric disease and/or emotional immaturity, and aggressive dependence on mothers or mother substitutes. The condition is uncommon, and afflicts women particularly.

Treatment of hypothyroidism

Thyroxine Tabs contain pure L-thyroxine sodium and should be used (preparations of dried animal glands are obsolete because they are unreliable and moulds grow on them).

The initial oral dose may be 50–100 micrograms daily; but in the old and patients with heart disease or hypertension, this should be achieved gradually (to minimise cardiovascular risk due to a too sudden increase in metabolic demand), starting with 25 micrograms daily for the first 2–4 weeks, and then increasing by 25–50 micrograms every fortnight until symptoms are relieved, usually at 100–200 micrograms as a single daily dose. This is usually sufficient to reduce plasma TSH to normal concentrations which is the *best indicator* of adequate treatment. Patients who appear to need more are probably not taking their tablets consistently. The maximum effect of a dose is not reached for about 10 days and passes off over about 2–3 weeks. Absorption is more complete and less variable if thyroxine is taken well apart from food.

Tablets containing supposedly physiological mixtures of thyroxine and liothyronine offer no advantage.

Hypothyroid patients tend to be *intolerant of drugs* owing to delayed metabolism.

---

[1] Harvey R F 1973 British Medical Journal 2: 35.

Liothyronine Tabs. Liothyronine is the most rapidly effective thyroid hormone, a single dose giving maximum effect within 24 h and passing off over 24–48 h. Its main uses are in hypothyroid coma and psychosis, both rare conditions. It is not used in routine treatment of hypothyroidism because its rapid onset of effect can induce heart failure but, in the above conditions, particularly in coma where death is inevitable in the absence of treatment, the risk may be justified.

Hypothyroid coma follows prolonged total hormone deficiency and constitutes an emergency. An untreated patient dies of hypothyroidism and a too vigorously treated patient dies from cardiovascular collapse due to a precipitate rise in metabolism. Thus the physician must steer between the Scylla[2] of undertreatment and the Charybdis[3] of overtreatment, both fatal. This may be done by giving thyroxine (T_4) i.v., if available. The biologically weaker T_4 is gradually converted into the highly active T_3. A single dose of 500 micrograms of thyroxine raises the plasma T_4 to about half the normal concentration and suffices for a week, after which routine oral maintenance dose may be used. Oral T_4 is too slow in the emergency.

Alternatively (or sometimes, judiciously, in addition in low dose) the quick-acting T_3 may be given by stomach tube, 5–10 micrograms 8–12-hourly (or i.v.). Maximum dose in the first 24 h should probably not exceed 50 micrograms since 100 micrograms is the full replacement dose. The dose may be raised after 3 days and the patient transferred to thyroxine after recovery.

Hydrocortisone i.v. is also needed, as prolonged hypothyroidism is associated with hypoadrenalism, and hydrocortisone is needed to cope with the increasing metabolism.

Adverse effects of thyroid hormone parallel the increase in metabolic rate. The symptoms and signs are those of hyperthyroidism, minus exophthalmos. Angina pectoris or heart failure are liable to be provoked by too vigorous therapy or in patients having serious ischaemic heart disease who may even be unable to tolerate optimal therapy. Should they occur thyroxine must be discontinued for at least a week and begun again at lower dosage. Only slight overdose is needed to precipitate atrial fibrillation in patients over 60 years.

In pregnancy a hypothyroid patient should be carefully assessed; a small increase in dose of thyroxine may be required; breast feeding is not contraindicated though the baby's thyroid status should be watched.

Antithyroid drugs and hyperthyroidism

Drugs used for the treatment of hyperthyroidism include:

- **Thionamides** which block the synthesis of thyroid hormone

- **Iodine:** radioiodine which destroys the cells making thyroid hormone; iodide, an *excess* of which reduces the production of thyroid hormone *temporarily* by an unknown mechanism (it is also necessary for the formation of hormone, and both excess and deficiency can cause goitre).

THIONAMIDES (THIOUREA DERIVATIVES)

Mode of action

The major action of thionamides is to *reduce the formation of thyroid* hormone by inhibiting the organification (incorporation into organic form) of iodine (iodotyrosines), and by inhibiting the cou-

---

[2] In classical mythology *Scylla* was a rival in love to Circe who, using her pharmacological expertise, changed Scylla into a monster having 12 feet, 6 heads and 3 rows of teeth. Terrified by this, Scylla threw herself into the sea and was transformed into rocks.

[3] *Charybdis* stole the oxen of Hercules, was struck by thunder, and became a whirlpool.

Ships passing between Sicily and Italy were liable to fall victim to one or other of these hazards. The Latin words *Incidit in Scyllam, qui vult vitare Charybdim* have become a proverb to show that, 'in our eagerness to avoid one evil, we often fall into a greater' (Lemprière).

pling of iodotyrosines to form T_4 and T_3. Maximum effect is delayed until existing hormone stores are exhausted (weeks, see below). With high dosage the reduction in hormone synthesis may be sufficient to induce the pituitary to produce more TSH, which in turn causes thyroid enlargement (hyperplasia and increase in vascularity).

Carbimazole and methimazole (the chief metabolite of carbimazole) ($t^1/2$ 5 h) and propylthiouracil ($t^1/2$ 2 h) are commonly used, but $t^1/2$ matters little since the drugs accumulate in the thyroid and act there for 30–40 h; thus a single daily dose suffices.

Propylthiouracil differs from other members of the group in that it also inhibits peripheral conversion of T_4 to T_3 (but this is not quick enough immediately to arrest a thyroid storm, see below).

Doses

- Carbimazole, initial, orally, 30–60 mg total/day until euthyroid:

  maintenance 5–15 mg total/day.
- Propylthiouracil, orally, 300–450 mg total/day until euthyroid:

  maintenance 50–150 mg total/day. Higher doses are sometimes needed (even 3 times the above).

Use

It is probable that no patient is wholly refractory to these drugs. Failure to respond is likely to be due to the patient not taking the tablets or to wrong diagnosis.

The drugs are used in hyperthyroidism as

- principal therapy,
- adjuvant to radioiodine to control the disease until the radiation achieves its effect,[4]
- to prepare patients for surgery.

Clinical improvement is noticeable in about a

---

[4] Use of a thionamide during the week before and after radioiodine therapy may impair the response to radiation (Velkeniers B et al 1988 Lancet 1: 1127) (see Mode of action of thionamides, above).

week, and the patient should be euthyroid in 8–12 weeks. The dose is then progressively reduced and adjusted monthly according to the clinical picture. The best guides to therapy are the patients' feelings, their weight and pulse rate, though measurements of the latter can be misleadingly high in a well-controlled patient if they are only taken in a clinic. Where biochemical tests for thyroid function (preferably plasma concentrations of free T_4 and TSH) are not readily accessible, the *ankle reflex time* (long in *hypo-* and short in *hyper-*thyroidism) is a useful guide to therapy (rather than to diagnosis) in both hyper- and hypothyroidism. Simple machines to record this are available.

Symptoms and signs are, of course, less valuable as guides if the patient is also taking a β-adrenoceptor blocker, and reliance is then put on tests, but β-blockers also prolong the ankle reflex time.

With optimal treatment the gland decreases in size, but *overtreatment* leading to low hormone concentrations in the blood activates the pituitary feedback system, inducing TSH secretion and goitre.

All three drugs give similar results.

Adverse reactions

These drugs are all liable to cause allergic effects including rashes, lymphadenopathy and, most serious of all, leucopenia sometimes proceeding to agranulocytosis (1:10 000) or aplastic anaemia (which may be due to idiosyncrasy rather than to allergy). Blood disorders are most common in the first 2 months of treatment. Repeated leucocyte counts are often advocated but agranulocytosis may be so acute that the counts give no warning; a leucocyte count should be done if the patient develops an infection (usually a sore throat, but infected haemorrhoids have heralded agranulocytosis). Patients should be warned to report this, and any suggestion of anaemia should be investigated. Cross allergy between the drugs occurs sometimes, but must be *assumed* for agranulocytosis.

Pregnancy. If a pregnant woman has hyperthyroidism (2/1000 pregnancies) she should be treated with the *smallest possible* amount of these drugs because they cross the placenta; with over-treatment fetal goitre occurs. Surgery in the second trimester may be preferred to continued drug therapy.

So little of propylthiouracil passes into breast milk that it may safely be used during breast feeding.

Goitre (fetal) may occur due to increased TSH secretion by the pituitary in response to decreased thyroxine production.

Control of antithyroid drug therapy

The aim of drug therapy is to control the hyperthyroidism until a natural remission takes place. Unfortunately, though usual, remission is not invariable and there is no way of predicting which patients will not remit and who should therefore be offered radiation or surgery at the outset.

Clinically, it is not possible to decide reliably when remission has occurred, although disappearance of bruit and reduction in gland size suggest it. Treatment should not be stopped whilst a bruit persists.

If there has never been a bruit, treatment may be stopped after the patient has been judged euthyroid for 4–6 months on the minimum dose of the drug. Lid retraction is the only eye sign that improves. But the duration of therapy that minimises the relapse rate is controversial, and 12–18 months' total therapy before withdrawal as a routine is commonly advised. Plasma concentrations of T_3 and T_4 (at withdrawal and 4 weeks later) can be used to determine if remission has occurred, along with clinical monitoring.

Relapse occurs in a few months or years in as many as 50–70% of cases, and this is the major disadvantage of thionamides; a second course of treatment may be successful. The use of *thyroxine concurrently with an antithyroid drug* ('block and replace regimen') is popular because carbimazole can be continued at a high dose for 12 months without such frequent supervision for titration of thyroid function. There is also some evidence that this high dose may have an immunosuppressive effect, and reduce the risk of relapse.

DRUGS THAT BLOCK SYMPATHETIC AUTONOMIC ACTIVITY

There is increased tissue sensitivity to catecholamines in hyperthyroidism with an increase in either the number of β-adrenoceptors or the second messenger response (i.e. intracellular cyclic AMP synthesis) to their stimulation. Therefore some of the unpleasant symptoms are adrenergic, and indeed phaeochromocytoma (p. 455) can enter into the differential diagnosis of hyperthyroidism.

Quick relief can be obtained with a β-adrenoceptor blocking drug (judge dose by heart rate) though these do not block all the metabolic effects of the hormone, e.g. on the myocardium, and the basal metabolic rate is unchanged. For this reason they should not be used as sole therapy; they do not alter the course of the disease, nor biochemical tests of thyroid function. Any effect on thyroid hormonal action on peripheral tissues is clinically unimportant. It is desirable to choose a drug that is nonselective for $β_1$ and $β_2$ receptors, and lacks partial agonist effect (intrinsic sympathomimetic activity).

β-adrenoceptor blockade is specially useful during the long wait (months) for the effect of radioiodine, though it may be used for any patient who feels uncomfortable.

Eye signs are due partly to excess adrenergic activity and may respond to eye drops of a β-adrenoceptor blocker (timolol) or of an adrenergic neuron blocker (guanethidine, but this can cause conjunctival fibrosis in prolonged use).

A hyperthyroid patient with urgent intercurrent disease, e.g. need for surgery, should at once be treated with a β-adrenoceptor blocker.

In hyperthyroid heart failure patients may occasionally be judged to need their adrenergic drive (β-adrenoceptor stimulation) to the heart to be intact. But it is more likely that the heart failure is secondary to hyperthyroid-induced tachydysrhythmia and that β-adrenoceptor blockade will be beneficial.

IODINE (IODIDE AND RADIOACTIVE IODINE)

Iodide is well absorbed from the intestine, is distributed like chloride in the body and is rapidly excreted by the kidney. It is selectively taken up and concentrated (about $\times 25$) by the thyroid gland, but more in hyperthyroidism and less in hypothyroidism. A *deficiency of iodide* reduces the amount of thyroid hormone produced, which stimulates the pituitary to secrete TSH. The result is hyperplasia and increased vascularity of the gland, with eventual goitre formation.

Effects

Iodide effects are complex and related to dose and to thyroid status of the subject.

In hyperthyroid subjects a moderate excess of iodide may enhance hormone production by providing 'fuel' for hormone synthesis. But a substantial excess inhibits hormone release and promotes storage of hormone and involution of the gland, making it firmer and less vascular so that surgery is easier. The effect is transient and its mechanism uncertain.

In euthyroid subjects with normal glands an excess of iodide from any source can cause goitre (with or without hyperthyroidism), e.g. use of iodide-containing cough medicines, iodine-containing radiocontrast media, amiodarone, seaweed eaters.

A euthyroid subject with an autonomous adenoma (hot nodule) becomes hyperthyroid if given iodide.

Uses

Iodide (large dose) is used for *thyroid crisis* (storm) and in *preparation for thyroidectomy* because it rapidly benefits the patient by reducing hormone release and renders surgery easier and safer (above).

Potassium iodide in doses of 60 mg orally 8-hourly (longer intervals allow some escape from the iodide effect) produces some effect in 1–2 days, maximal after 10–14 days, after which the benefit declines as the thyroid adapts. A traditional formulation is aqueous iodine oral solution (Lugol's Iodine) (5% iodine + 10% potassium iodide in water: 130 mg; iodine/ml: doses 0.1–0.3 ml 8-hourly). The iodine is rapidly converted into iodide in the liver.

Such therapy maximises iodide stores in the thyroid, which delays response to thionamides.

Prophylactic iodide (1 part in 100 000 parts) may be added to the salt, water or bread where goitre is endemic.

In economically deprived communities a method of prophylaxis is to inject iodised oil i.m. every 3–5 years; given early enough to women, this prevents endemic cretinism; but occasional hyperthyroidism occurs (see Autonomous adenoma, above).

As an antiseptic for use on the skin, povidone-iodine (a complex of iodine with a sustained-release carrier, povidone or polyvinyl-pyrrolidone) is used. It can be applied repeatedly and used as a surgical scrub.

Bronchial secretion. Iodide is concentrated in bronchial and salivary secretions. It acts as an expectorant (see Cough).

Organic compounds containing iodine are used as contrast media in radiology. It is essential to ask patients specifically whether they are allergic to iodine before they are used. An i.v. test dose ought to be given half an hour before the full i.v. dose if there is history of any allergy. Despite this, severe anaphylaxis, even deaths, occur every year in busy X-ray departments, and iodine containing contrast media are being superseded by so-called nonionic preparations.[5]

Adverse reactions

Patients vary enormously in their tolerance of iodine; some are intolerant or allergic to it both orally and when put on the skin.

Symptoms of iodism include: a metallic taste, excessive salivation with painful salivary glands, running eyes and nose, sore mouth and throat, a productive cough, diarrhoea, and various rashes that may mimic chicken-pox. Elimination can be enhanced by inducing a saline diuresis.

Goitre can occur (see above) with prolonged use of iodide-containing expectorant by bronchitics and asthmatics. Such therapy should therefore be intermittent, if it is used at all.

---

[5] The newer preparations approximately triple the cost of diagnostic investigations requiring contrast media. With a fatality rate of ~1/50 000 in patients receiving the older agents, hospitals are faced with an interesting cost-benefit equation.

Topical application of iodine-containing antiseptics to neonates has caused hypothyroidism. Iodide intake above that in a normal diet will depress thyroid uptake of *administered radioiodine*, because the two forms will compete.

In the case of diet, medication and water soluble radio-diagnostic agents, interference will cease 2–4 weeks after stopping the source, but with agents used for cholecystography it may last for 6 months or more (tissue binding).

RADIOIODINE (^{131}I)

^{131}I is treated by the body just like the ordinary non-radioactive isotope, so that when swallowed it is concentrated in the thyroid gland. It emits mainly β radiation (90%), which penetrates only 0.5 mm of tissue and thus allows therapeutic effect on the thyroid without damage to the surrounding structures, particularly the parathyroids. However, it also emits some γ rays, which are more penetrating and can be detected with a Geiger counter. ^{131}I has a physical (radioactive) t$\frac{1}{2}$ of 8 days.

^{131}I is increasingly used as treatment of choice in hyperthyroidism at all ages, and in combination with surgery in some cases of thyroid carcinoma, especially those in which metastases are sufficiently differentiated to take up iodide selectively.

In hyperthyroidism the beneficial effects of a single dose may be felt in one month but its action is not maximal for 3 months; β-adrenoceptor blockade and, in severe cases, antithyroid drug (but see footnote 4) will be needed to render the patient comfortable whilst waiting. Very rarely the radiation damage to the thyroid causes a release of hormone and a thyroid storm. Repeated doses are sometimes needed.

In the event of **inadvertent overdose,** large doses of sodium or potassium iodide should be given to compete with the radioiodine for thyroid uptake and to hasten excretion by increasing iodide turnover (increased fluid intake and a diuretic are adjuvants).

Radioiodine offers the **advantages** that treatment is simple and in no way unpleasant (the patient just drinks it) and it carries no immediate mortality. However, it is slow in acting and it is difficult to judge the dose that will render the patient euthyroid.

In the first year after treatment 6–15% or even more (depending on the dose) of patients will become **hypothyroid**. After this 2–3% of patients become hypothyroid annually, perhaps because the capacity of thyroid cells to divide is permanently abolished so that cell renewal ceases. Patients must therefore be followed up *indefinitely* after radioiodine treatment, for most are likely to need *treatment for hypothyroidism* eventually.

Because such follow-up over years may fail and because the onset of hypothyroidism may be insidious and not easily recognised, some physicians prefer deliberately to render patients hypothyroid with the first dose and to educate them on the use of replacement therapy which is safe and effective.

Risks

Experience has eliminated the fear that radioiodine causes carcinoma of the thyroid, and it is now used in patients of all ages. But *pregnant women* should not be treated with radioiodine (^{131}I) because it crosses the placenta.

There is a theoretical risk of germ cell mutagenic effect and patients should not reproduce for a few (say, 6) months after treatment.[6] Larger doses of radioiodine are used for *thyroid carcinoma* than for hyperthyroidism, and there is an increased incidence of late leukaemia in these patients. The treatment of thyroid carcinoma is highly specialised. It is not always required after resection of a papillary carcinoma, but is routinely used after resection of follicular cell carcinomas.

Tests

Radioiodine uptake can be used to test *thyroid function*. It has been largely superseded, except for the identification of solitary nodules, and in the differential diagnosis of Graves' disease from the less common thyroiditides (e.g. de Quervain's thyroidi-

---

[6] Even today it can be embarrassing to offer such advice to an excited hyperthyroid unmarried woman or man. Yet to fail to do so could have grave consequences for a child. It is rumoured that some physicians have prescribed an oral contraceptive without telling the patient what it is; a procedure that is understandable if not ethically justifiable.

tis). In the latter, excessive thyroxine release caused by follicular cell damage can cause clinical and biochemical features of hyperthyroidism, but ^{131}I uptake is reduced.

CHOICE OF TREATMENT OF HYPERTHYROIDISM

There are three possible lines of treatment, each with its special advantages and disadvantages:

- Antithyroid drug
- Radioiodine
- Surgery, after preparation as below.

Antithyroid drugs are generally preferred provided the goitre is small and diffuse. A nodular goitre is generally large enough to be a source of complaint, relapses when drug therapy is withdrawn (nodules are autonomous), and is best treated surgically. These drugs do not decrease thyroid size; it may even increase (see above). They may be used in pregnancy.

Radioiodine is now commonly used for patients of all ages; but not in pregnancy. It affects both diffuse and nodular goitre. The goitre becomes smaller. Hyperthyroidism due to a single hyperfunctioning adenoma ('hot nodule') is also suitable for this treatment, and higher doses may be used since the function of the rest of the gland is already suppressed by the familiar negative feedback regulatory process.

Surgery is indicated if obstruction of neck veins or trachea exists or is thought to be likely in the future, if the thyroid is nodular or there are grounds for fearing malignancy.

PREPARATION FOR SURGERY

Preparation of hyperthyroid patients for surgery can be satisfactorily achieved by making them euthyroid with one of the above drugs plus a β-adrenoceptor blocker for comfort (see below) and safety,[7] and *adding* iodide for 7–10 days before oper-

---

[7] No patient should be operated on with a resting pulse of 90/min or above, and no dose of β-adrenoceptor blocker, including the important postoperative dose, should be omitted. Toft A D et al 1978 New England Journal of Medicine 298: 643.

ation (not sooner) to reduce the surgically inconvenient vascularity of the gland. This procedure takes about 5 weeks.

An alternative is to prepare the patient with a β-adrenoceptor blocker (propranolol 6-hourly) for 4 days (adjust dose to eliminate tachycardia) and to continue thus through the operation and for 7–10 days after.

The important differences with this second technique are that the gland is smaller and less friable, although the patient's *tissues* are still hyperthyroid, and it is essential, in order to avoid a hyperthyroid crisis or storm, that the adrenoceptor blocker be continued as above without the omission of even a single 6-hourly dose of propranolol; but erratic plasma concentrations can be a cause of failure.

Thyroid crisis or **storm** is rare with modern methods of preparing hyperthyroid patients for surgery. It is probably due to liberation of large amounts of hormone into the circulation. Treatment is urgently required to save life. Propranolol should be given immediately (i.v. *slowly*, 1 mg/min to max of 10 mg, in severe cases, preceded by atropine 1–2 mg i.v. to prevent excessive bradycardia); iodide to inhibit further hormone release from the gland (say 600 mg–1.0 g iodide orally or i.v. in the first 24 h) (see Iodide), and hydrocortisone i.v. Mental disturbance may be treated by chlorpromazine; hyperthermia by cooling and aspirin; heart failure in the ordinary way.

Exophthalmos of hyperthyroidism

The cause may be related to an immunoglobulin that attacks the external ocular muscles and retrobulbar tissue. Antithyroid drugs do not help. TSH secretion is not responsible (it is high in primary thyroid gland failure in which exophthalmos rarely occurs). The patient should be rendered euthyroid. High systemic doses of prednisolone or less with another immunosuppressive (cyclosporin) may help, but in urgent cases surgery is necessary, i.e. orbital decompression. Artificial tears (hypromellose) are useful when natural tears and blinking are inadequate to maintain corneal lubrication.

SUMMARY

- Autoimmune disease of the thyroid can cause over- or underproduction of thyroxine.
- Hypothyroidism is readily treated by oral administration of L-thyroxine 50–200 micrograms daily. This needs to be continued indefinitely.
- The preferred treatment of hyperthyroidism due to Graves' disease is a single dose of [131]I. Alternatives are a minimum of 6 months' treatment with carbimazole or propylthiouracil, either alone or as a prelude to a partial thyroidectomy. These drugs do not have a place in the 5–10% of patients in whom thyrotoxicosis is due to a toxic adenoma or to subacute thyroiditis.
- The natural history of Graves' disease is of alternating remission and relapse. Progression to hypothyroidism can occur, especially after ^{131}I treatment. Such patients should have longterm follow-up, and are likely to require thyroxine replacement therapy.
- Most forms of thyroid eye disease are resistant to treatment. Urgent surgical decompression can be required for exophthalmos.

Drugs that cause unwanted hypothyroidism

In addition to drugs used for their antithyroid effects, the following substances can cause hypothyroidism: PAS (for tuberculosis), phenylbutazone (antirheumatic), iodide (see above), cobalt salts (for anaemia), sulphonylureas (for diabetes), resorcinol (for leg ulcers), lithium (for mania/depression), amiodarone (cardiac antidysrhyth-mic). Effects are generally reversible on withdrawal.

Miscellaneous

Treatment of thyroiditis (Hashimoto's thyroiditis, subacute thyroiditis of de Quervain). Where hyperthyroidism is a feature, treatment is by a β-adrenoceptor blocking drug. Antithyroid drugs should not be used. Where there is hypothyroidism, the treatment is thyroxine replacement.

Calcitonin: see Chapter 39.

GUIDE TO FURTHER READING

Franklyn J A et al 1990 Thyroxine replacement treatment and osteoporosis. British Medical Journal 300: 693

Franklyn J A 1994 The management of hyperthyroidism. New England Journal of Medicine 330: 1731–1738

Mandel S J et al 1990 Increased need for thyroxine during pregnancy in women with primary hypothyroidism. New England Journal of Medicine 323: 91

Mazzaferri E L 1993 Management of a solitary thyroid nodule. New England Journal of Medicine 328: 553–559

Surks M I, Sievert R 1995 Drug therapy: drugs and thyroid function. New England Journal of Medicine 333: 1688–1694

Toft A D 1994 Thyroxine therapy. New England Journal of Medicine 331: 174–180

Hypothalamic, pituitary and sex hormones

Hormones, analogues and antagonists

Once the structure of natural hormones, local or systemic (including hormone-releasing hormones),

is defined it becomes possible to synthesise not only the hormones themselves[1] but also *analogues* and *antagonists*. Thus, increasingly, substances become available differing in selectivity and duration of action, and active by various routes of administration.

These hormones, analogues (agonists) and antagonists can be used:

- to analyse the functional integrity of endocrine control systems
- as replacement in hormone deficiency states
- to modify malfunction of endocrine systems
- to alter normal function where this is inconvenient, e.g. contraception.

The scope of the specialist endocrinologist continues to increase in amount and in complexity and only an outline is appropriate here.

Hypothalamic and pituitary hormones

Hypothalamus: hormone-releasing hormones, hormone-releasing inhibiting hormones, gonadorelin.

Anterior pituitary: growth hormone, gonadotroph-

---

[1] Hormones can be synthesised directly in the chemical laboratory or by inserting mammalian genes into microbes, e.g. *Escherichia coli*, recombinant DNA technology.

ic hormones, corticotrophin, thyrotrophin, pro-lactin.

Posterior pituitary: vasopressin, oxytocin.

Hypothalamus and anterior pituitary

Some agents have restricted commercial availability. The $t^1/2$ of the polypeptide and glycoprotein hormones listed below is 5–30 min; they are digested if swallowed.

Corticotrophin releasing hormone (CRH), corti-coliberin, is a hypothalamic polypeptide that has diagnostic use; it is not generally available.

Corticotrophin, adrenocorticotrophic hormone (ACTH), see page 612.

Thyroid stimulating hormone (TSH), thy-rotrophin, a glycoprotein of the anterior pituitary, controls the release of thyroid hormone from the gland, and also the uptake of iodide by the thyroid gland. TSH secretion is inhibited (via the hypothalamus and TRH, see below) by a high level of thyroid hormone in the blood and stimulated by a low concentration, i.e. there is a negative feedback mechanism of control.

A stimulation test using TSH is no longer useful now that TSH blood concentration and free T_4 and T_3 can be measured.

Antithyroid drugs, by reducing thyroid hormone production, cause increased formation of TSH which is the cause of the thyroid enlargement that sometimes occurs during antithyroid drug therapy.

Thyrotrophin-releasing hormone (TRH) protire-lin, is a tripeptide formed in the hypothalamus and controlled by free plasma T_4, T_3 concentration. It has been synthesised and can be used in diagnosis to test the capacity of the pituitary to release thyroid-stimulating hormone (TSH), e.g. to determine whether hypothyroidism is due to primary thyroid gland failure or is secondary to pituitary disease or to a hypothalamic lesion.

Sermorelin is an analogue of the hypothalamic growth hormone releasing hormone (somatorelin); it is used in a diagnostic test for growth hormone secretion from the pituitary, or of somatostatin secretion from certain tumours.

Somatostatin, growth hormone release inhibiting hormone, occurs in other parts of the brain as well as in the hypothalamus, and also in some peripheral tissues, e.g. pancreas, stomach. In addition to the action implied by its name, it inhibits secretion of thyrotrophin, insulin, gastrin and serotonin.

Octreotide is a synthetic analogue of somatostatin having a longer action ($t^1/2$ 1.5 h). Uses include acromegaly, carcinoid (serotonin secreting) tumours and other rare tumours of the alimentary tract.

Somatropin, growth hormone (Genotropin, Humatrope), is a biosynthetic form (191 amino acids) of growth hormone prepared by recombinant DNA technology, as is somatrem. Naturally occurring human growth hormone obtained from dead people is no longer used because of the risk of transmitting Creutzfeldt-Jacob disease, the lethal prion infection. Growth hormone acts on many organs to produce a peptide (somatomedin) which causes muscle, bone and other tissues to increase growth, i.e. protein synthesis, and the size and number of cells.

It is used in childhood pituitary insufficiency (the bone epiphyses must be open) to prevent dwarfism and provide normal growth. Use simply to avoid low height for social reasons is controversial, and at ~£15 000 ($20 000) p.a. is certainly hard to justify.

About 50% of the elderly have growth hormone secretion below the norm for people in their twenties. The bodily changes of age are not simply due to growth hormone deficiency. Administration of growth hormone to the elderly for 6 months induces modest increase in lean body mass, in skin fold thickness, in vertebral bone density, and reduction in adipose tissue; also a small increase in isometric strength. In excess (as in acromegaly) growth hormone causes diabetes, hypertension and arthritis. There is a need for large, prolonged and detailed clinical studies before growth hormone can be considered for use to improve the quality of life of otherwise healthy elderly people.

Possibilities of *abuse* have also arisen, e.g. creation of 'super' sports people. Less dubious, but not yet a licensed indication, is the potential for accelerated wound healing reported in children with large cutaneous burns.[2]

Acromegaly. Excess growth hormone secretion is reduced by octreotide and by bromocriptine (see Index).

Gonadorelin: gonadotrophin releasing hormone (GnRH) releases luteinising hormone (LH) and follicle-stimulating hormone (FSH). Its full abbreviation is thus LH-FSH-RH, but it is commonly represented as LH-RH for brevity, or GnRH. It has use in assessment of pituitary function. Intermittent pulsatile administration evokes secretion of gonadotrophins (LH and FSH) and is used to treat infertility. But *continuous* use evokes tachyphylaxis due to down-regulation of its receptors, i.e. gonadotrophin release and therefore gonadal secretions are reduced. Longer-acting analogues, e.g. buserelin, goserelin, nafarelin, deslorelin and leuprorelin are used to suppress androgen secretion in prostatic carcinoma. Other uses may include endometriosis, precocious puberty and contraception. All these drugs need to be administered by a parenteral route, by i.m. injection or intranasally. Their use should generally be in the hands of a specialist endocrinologist, oncologist or gynaecologist.

Follicle-stimulating hormone (FSH) stimulates development of ova and of spermatozoa. It is prepared from the urine of postmenopausal women; menotrophin (Pergonal) also contains a small amount of LH, and urofollitrophin (Metrodin) is FSH alone. They are used in female and male hypopituitary infertility.

Chorionic gonadotrophin (human chorionic gonadotrophin: HCG) is secreted by the placenta and is obtained from the urine of pregnant women. Its predominant action is that of luteinising hormone (LH) (interstitial cell stimulating hormone) which induces progesterone production by the corpus luteum and, in the male, gonadal testosterone production. It is used in hypopituitary anovular and other infertility in both sexes (for LH effect is not confined to women despite its name). It is also used for cryptorchidism in prepubertal boys (about 6 years; if it fails to induce testicular descent, there is time for surgery before puberty to provide maximal possibility of a full functional testis). It may also precipitate puberty in men where this is delayed.

Prolactin is secreted in both women and men and, despite its name, it influences numerous biological functions (as many as 80), though not all of physiological importance. Prolactin secretion is controlled by an inhibitory dopaminergic path. Thus, dopamine *agonists*, e.g. bromocriptine, reduce prolactin secretion and dopamine *antagonists* increase secretion. This explains the use of bromocriptine to suppress hyperprolactinaemia, e.g. pituitary tumours, and occasionally to suppress lactation; also the occurrence of hyperprolactinaemia (causing galactorrhoea) during therapy with neuroleptic dopamine antagonist drugs, and with metoclopramide and methyldopa.

HYPOPITUITARISM

In hypopituitarism there is a deficiency of all the hormones secreted by the anterior lobe of the pituitary. The posterior lobe hormones (see below) may also be deficient in a few cases, e.g. when a tumour has destroyed the pituitary. Patients suffering from hypopituitarism may present in coma, in which case treatment is as for a severe acute adrenal insufficiency. Maintenance therapy is required, using adrenocortical and thyroid hormones. Sex hormones are not usually required, although androgens will help to establish a positive nitrogen balance in wasted patients.

Infertility: see page 653.

Posterior pituitary hormones and analogues

Vasopressin: antidiuretic hormone (ADH)

Vasopressin is a nonapeptide ($t^{1/2}$ 20 min) with two separate G-protein coupled target receptors responsible for its two roles. The V_1 receptor on vascular

[2] Gilpin D A et al 1994 Annals of Surgery 220: 19.

smooth muscle cells is coupled to Ca^{++}-ion entry. This receptor is not usually stimulated by physiological concentrations of the hormone. The V_2 receptor is coupled to adenylyl cyclase, and regulates opening of the water channel, aquaporin, in cells of the renal collecting duct.

Secretion of the antidiuretic hormone is stimulated by any increase in the osmotic pressure of the blood supplying the hypothalamus and by a variety of drugs, notably *nicotine*. Secretion is inhibited by a fall in blood osmotic pressure and by *alcohol*.

In large nonphysiological doses (pharmacotherapy) vasopressin causes *contraction of all smooth muscle*, raising the blood pressure and causing intestinal colic. The smooth-muscle stimulant effect provides an example of tachyphylaxis (frequently repeated doses give progressively less effect). It is not only inefficient when used to raise the blood pressure, but is also dangerous, since it causes constriction of the coronary arteries and sudden death has occurred following its use.

For replacement therapy of *pituitary diabetes insipidus* the longer acting desmopressin is preferred.

Desmopressin

Desmopressin (des-amino-D-arginine vasopressin) (DDAVP) has two major advantages: the vasoconstrictor effect has been reduced to near insignificance and the duration of action with nasal instillation, spray on or s.c. injection, is 8–20 h ($t^{1/2}$ 75 min) so that, using it 2–3 times a day, patients are not inconvenienced by frequent recurrence of polyuria during their waking hours and can also expect to spend the night continuously in bed. Duration of action of the alternative, *lypressin*, is 3–4 h. The dose for children is about half that for adults. The bioavailability of intranasal DDAVP is 10%. It is also the only peptide for which an oral formulation is currently available, albeit with a bioavailability of only 1%. The tablets of DDAVP are prescribed at 0.1–1.2 mg three times daily.

Nephrogenic diabetes insipidus, as is to be expected, does not respond to antidiuretic hormone.

Nocturnal enuresis: see page 335.

In *bleeding oesophageal varices* in hepatic cirrhosis, use is sometimes made of the vasoconstrictor effect of vasopressin (as terlipressin, a vasopressin prodrug): see page 592.

In *haemophilia* desmopressin can enhance blood concentration of factor VIII. Felypressin is used as a vasoconstriction with local anaesthetics.

DIABETES INSIPIDUS: VASOPRESSIN DEFICIENCY

Diabetes insipidus (DI) can be due to either pituitary or renal causes. The pituitary may be damaged by trauma, tumours, haemorrhage or infarction (Sheehan's syndrome is pituitary failure following the shock of postpartum haemorrhage). Nephrogenic DI has a larger number of causes including drugs (lithium), and several diseases affecting the renal medulla. The DNA sequencing of the V_2 receptor and aquaporins has also allowed identification of mutations in these which cause congenital DI.

Desmopressin replacement therapy is the first choice. *Thiazide diuretics* (and chlorthalidone) also have paradoxical antidiuretic effect in diabetes insipidus. That this is not due to Na depletion is suggested by the fact that the nondiuretic thiazide, diazoxide (see Index), also has this effect. It is probable that changes in the proximal renal tubule result in increased reabsorption and in delivery of less Na and water to the distal tubule, but the mechanism remains incompletely elucidated. Some cases of the *nephrogenic* form, which is not helped by antidiuretic hormone, may be benefited.

Drugs, e.g. lithium and demeclocycline, may cause nephrogenic diabetes insipidus.

Chlorpropamide. A patient with diabetes *insipidus*, wrongly believing himself to suffer from diabetes mellitus, 'at his own discretion' took chlorpropamide.[3] His physician was surprised at the apparent therapeutic effect and tried the drug on other patients, confirming it.

Chlorpropamide (but not other sulphonylureas) and *carbamazepine* are effective in *partial* pituitary diabetes insipidus, i.e. some natural hormone production remains, because they act on the kidney potentiating the effect of vasopressin on the renal

---

[3] Arduino F et al 1966 Journal of Clinical Endocrinology 26: 1325.

tubule. Hypoglycaemia may occur with chlorpropamide.

Evidently all these drugs may cause difficulty due to their other actions that are not desired, and none is drug of first choice for this disease.

SYNDROME OF INAPPROPRIATE ANTIDIURETIC HORMONE SECRETION (SIADH)

A variety of tumours, e.g. oat-cell lung cancer, can make vasopressin, and of course they are not subject to normal homeostatic mechanisms. Dilutional hyponatraemia may occur, and fludrocortisone may be needed along with fluid restriction (soon becomes intolerable) and infusion of hypertonic saline (in acute cases only). Demeclocycline, which inhibits the renal action of vasopressin, can be useful. Chemotherapy to the causative tumour is likely to be the most effective treatment.

Oxytocin: see page 665.

Sex (gonadal) hormones and antagonists: steroid hormones

Steroid hormone receptors (for gonadal steroids and adrenocortical steroids) are complex proteins inside the target cell. The steroid penetrates, is bound and translocates into the cell nucleus, which is the principal site of action and where RNA/protein synthesis occurs. Compounds that occupy the receptor without causing translocation into the nucleus or the replenishment of receptors act as antagonists, e.g. spironolactone to aldosterone, cyproterone to androgens, clomiphene to oestrogens.

Selectivity. Many synthetic analogues, although classed as, e.g. androgen, anabolic steroid, progestogen, are *nonselective* and bind to several types of receptor as agonist, partial agonist, antagonist. The result is that their effects are complex, as will be seen in the following account.

PHARMACOKINETICS

Steroid sex hormones are well absorbed through the skin (factory workers need protective clothing) and the gut. Most are subject to extensive hepatic metabolic inactivation (some so much that oral administration is ineffective or requires very large doses if a useful amount is to pass through the liver and reach the systemic circulation). There is some enterohepatic recirculation, especially of oestrogen, and this may be interrupted by severe diarrhoea to cause loss of efficacy. There are some nonsteroid analogues that are more slowly metabolised. Sustained-release (depot) preparations are used. The hormones are carried in the blood extensively bound to sex-hormone-binding globulin. In general the plasma $t^{1/2}$ relates to the duration of cellular action. Duration of action is implied in the recommended dosage schedules.

Androgens

Testosterone is the natural androgen secreted by the interstitial cells of the testis; it is necessary for normal spermatogenesis, for the development of the male secondary sex characteristics, and for the growth, at puberty, of the sexual apparatus. It is converted by hydroxylation to the active dihydrotestosterone.

Protein *anabolism* is increased by androgens, i.e., androgens increase the proportion of protein laid down as tissue, especially muscle (and, combined with training, increase strength). Growth of bone is promoted, but the rate of closure of the epiphyses is also hastened, causing short stature in cases of precocious puberty or of androgen overdose in the course of treating hypogonadal children.

INDICATIONS FOR ANDROGEN THERAPY

The prime indication is *testicular failure* which may be primary or secondary (due to lack of pituitary gonadotrophins). In either case replacement with androgens is often necessary. Unfortunately, sterility is not remedied, although loss of libido and of secondary sex characteristics can be greatly improved. Impotence is helped if it is hypogonadal, but not if it has a psychological cause (which is often the case).

For *male contraception* androgens are under trial; they inhibit pituitary gonadotrophin production and have a direct testicular action.

If androgen is given to a boy with delayed puberty, a growth spurt and sexual development will occur. Such treatment is not usually indicated until the age of 16 years since up to that age natural delay in pituitary secretion may be responsible and normal development may yet occur.

In *hepatic cirrhosis* degradation of oestrogens in the liver may be impaired, leading to raised blood concentrations of oestrogen with feminisation; androgens may help such patients. They may also stop the itching of *biliary obstruction*. Relatively small amounts of androgens can be used to increase the *formation of new tissue*, e.g. in osteoporosis in androgen deficient men (see below). Androgens may also help in some cases of *anaemia* due to bone marrow failure. Androgens are now little used in *metastatic breast cancer* because of their virilising effects.

PREPARATIONS AND CHOICE OF ANDROGENS

- *Testosterone* given orally is subject to extensive hepatic first-pass metabolism and is therefore most successful as an implant, but this is superseded by testosterone esters, e.g. enanthate, which may be given orally or as depot injections; these esters do not injure the liver (see below). Skin patches are available.
- *Mesterolone* provides oral therapy; its molecular structure is such that its hypothalamic feedback inhibition of pituitary gonadotrophin secretion is less and it does not cause liver injury (see below).
- See also: anabolic steroids, danazol.

ADVERSE EFFECTS

Adverse effects are mainly those to be expected of a male sex hormone (including hypothalamic-pituitary suppression of gonadotrophin production); increased libido may lead to undesirable

sexual activity, especially in mentally unstable patients, and virilisation is obviously undesired by most women. Androgens have a weak *salt and water retaining activity*, which is not often clinically important. Liver injury (cholestatic) can occur, particularly with 17α-alkyl derivatives (ethylestrenol, stanozolol, danazol, oxymetholone); it is reversible; these agents should be avoided in hepatic disease.

Effects on *blood lipids* are complex and variable, and the balance may be to disadvantage.

In patients with malignant disease of bone androgen administration may be followed by hypercalcemia. The less virilising androgens are used to promote anabolism and are discussed below.

Antiandrogens (androgen antagonists)

Plainly oestrogens and progestogens are physiological antagonists to androgens. But compounds which compete selectively for androgen receptors have been made.

Cyproterone

Cyproterone is a derivative of progesterone; its combination of structural similarities and differences results in the following:

- Competition with testosterone for receptors in target peripheral organs (but not causing feminisation as do oestrogens); it reduces spermatogenesis even to the level of azoospermia (reverses over about 4 months after the drug is stopped); abnormal sperm occurs during treatment.
- Competition with testosterone in the central nervous system, reducing sexual drive and thoughts, and causing impotence.
- Some agonist progestogenic activity on hypothalamic receptors, inhibiting gonadotrophin secretion, which also inhibits testicular androgen production.

Uses. Cyproterone is used for reducing male hypersexuality and in prostatic cancer and severe female hirsutism. A formulation of cyproterone plus ethinyloestradiol (Dianette) is offered for this latter purpose as well as for severe acne in women; this preparation acts as an oral contraceptive but should not be used primarily for this purpose. Plainly, longterm use of the drug poses both medical and ethical problems.[4] It is even advised that for management of male hypersexuality formally witnessed written consent be obtained.

Cyproterone causes hepatomas in rats.

Cyproterone is plainly unsuitable for male contraception (see actions above).

Flutamide and bicalutamide (Casodex) are non-steroidal antiandrogens available for use in conjunction with the gonadorelins (e.g. goserelin) in the treatment of prostatic carcinoma. Finasteride (p. 498), which inhibits conversion of testosterone to dihydrotestosterone, has localised antiandrogen activity in tissues where dihydrotestosterone is the principal androgen: this makes it a useful drug in the treatment of *benign prostatic hypertrophy*.

Spironolactone (p. 489) also has antiandrogen activity and may help hirsutism in women.

Androgen secretion may be diminished by continued use of a gonadorelin (LH-RH) analogue (see p. 644).

Ketoconazole (antifungal) interferes with androgen and corticosteroid synthesis and may be used in prostatic carcinoma.

Anabolic steroids

(See also above)

Androgens are effective protein anabolic agents, but their clinical use for this purpose is limited by the amount of virilisation that women will tolerate.

Attempts made to separate anabolic from androgenic action have been only partially successful and *all anabolic steroids also have androgenic effects*. They have little use in male osteoporosis. They can also prevent the calcium and nitrogen loss in the urine that occurs in patients bedridden for a long time and they have therefore been recommended in the treatment of some severe fractures.

The use of anabolic steroids in conditions of *general wasting* is justifiable in extreme debilitating disease, such as severe ulcerative colitis, after major surgery; in the later stages of malignant disease they may make the patient feel and look less wretched. Their general use as tonics is scandalous as is their use in sport (see Index).[5] They may be tried in *aplastic anaemia*.

The *itching of biliary obstruction* may be relieved and these drugs are perhaps preferable to testosterone for the purpose. There remains, however, a risk of increasing the degree of jaundice (see p. 590).

Anabolic steroids do not usefully counter the unwanted catabolic effects of adrenocortical hormones.

Hereditary angioedema (lack of inhibition of the complement C1 esterase) may be prevented by androgens (stanozolol and danazol are used).

None of these agents is free from virilising properties in high doses; acne and greasy skin may be the early manifestation of virilisation (see also, Adverse effects of androgens, p. 647; and Drugs and sport).

Oestrogens have only modest anabolic effect.

Administration should generally be intermittent in courses of 3–12 weeks with similar intervals, to reduce the occurrence of unwanted effects, especially liver injury.

There is little to choose between the principal available drugs, nandrolone (Durabolin) (i.m. once a week) and stanozolol (Stromba) (orally), except that the latter is contraindicated in liver disease.

---

[4] Individual problems can be quite trying and revealing. A 26-year-old woman with severe facial hirsutism was prescribed cyproterone from days 5 to 15 of each menstrual cycle. After 4 months, she reported to her doctor that her male Rottweiler would not leave her alone and repeatedly tried to mount her during these 10 days of each month. The patient managed to keep her Rottweiler and lose her hair by having the dog castrated (Cotterill J A 1992 Lancet 340: 986).

[5] While the misuse of anabolic steroids in sport is well known (infamous), a recent report has drawn attention to the increasing practice among some teenagers of using the drugs to improve their appearance and handsomeness, giving themselves the 'macho' look which they think girls like. (Nilsson S 1995 Androgenic anabolic steroid use among male adolescents in Falkenberg. European Journal of Clinical Pharmacology 48: 9–11).

Oestrogens and antioestrogens

Oestrone and oestradiol are both natural oestrogens secreted by the ovary. Oestrogens are responsible for the normal development of the female genital tract, of the breast and of the female secondary sex characteristics. The pubertal growth spurt is less marked in females than in males, probably because oestrogens have less protein anabolic action than do androgens, although they are as effective in promoting closure of epiphyses. Blood oestrogen concentrations must be above a critical level for the maintenance of both proliferative and (together with progesterone) secretory phases of the uterine endometrium. If the oestrogen level falls too low then the endometrium can no longer be maintained and uterine bleeding follows. Thus uterine bleeding may be stopped temporarily by giving large doses of oestrogens, or started by abrupt withdrawal (oestrogen-withdrawal bleeding). Bleeding may occur despite a high blood oestrogen concentration if large doses are given for a long time, due to infarctions in the greatly hypertrophied endometrium. Oestrogens are necessary for the maintenance of normal pregnancy and for the accompanying breast hyperplasia. The vagina is more sensitive to oestrogens than is the endometrium.

PHARMACOKINETICS: see page 646.

PREPARATIONS OF OESTROGENS

Innumerable oestrogen preparations are available, but the following selection should cover all needs. The dose varies greatly according to whether replacement of physiological deficiencies is being carried out (*replacement therapy*) or whether *pharmacotherapy* is being used.

- *Ethinyloestradiol* (t$\frac{1}{2}$ 13 h) is a synthetic agent of first choice for pharmacological (mainly contraceptive) uses; it is effective by mouth.
- *Oestradiol* and *oestriol* are orally active mixed natural oestrogens.
- *Conjugated oestrogens* (Premarin) are orally active mixed natural oestrogens obtained from the urine of pregnant mares.[6]

- *Estropipate* (piperazine oestrone sulphate) is an orally active synthetic conjugate.
- *Stilboestrol* (diethylstilbestrol) is the first synthetic oestrogen: its use is confined to androgen dependent cancers (breast, prostate).

CHOICE OF OESTROGEN

Ethinyloestradiol is a satisfactory first choice for pharmacotherapy, but the weaker endogenous oestrogen, oestradiol, is preferable for physiological replacement. However, individual patients may be intolerant of any one agent, when it is worth trying the others. It remains uncertain whether all oestrogens have exactly similar hormonal and nonhormonal effects, including adverse effects.

Transdermal formulations are available. They can be effective and convenient for women who dislike taking oral therapy.

INDICATIONS FOR OESTROGEN THERAPY

Replacement therapy in hypo-ovarian conditions. Ethinyloestradiol (up to 50 micrograms orally daily for 21 days) followed by a progestogen (norethisterone or medroxyprogesterone 5 mg orally) for 7–10 days per monthly cycle is generally acceptable.

Unless the cause of the hypo-ovarian state is primary ovarian failure, treatment should be stopped after every third cycle to see if spontaneous menstruation will occur.

For menopausal symptoms (flushes, dry vagina) severe enough to demand treatment combined oestrogen-progestogen formulations are used for one year or more. The oestrogen may be cyclical or continuous and the progestogen cyclical. Most women will experience intermittent withdrawal bleeding.

Special calendar packs of various regimens are available under a range of proprietary names, e.g. Menophase, Prempak. Oestrogens used include

---

[6] The mares are bred on 480 farms in the prairie provinces of Canada. The 80 000 foals that are produced each year have a less medicinal future than their mothers' urine: they are weaned at 120 days and sold for meat.

oestradiol and conjugated oestrogens; ethinyl-oestradiol should be used only at a low dose (10 µg/d) for a month to treat vaginal atrophy, and even here local application of an oestrogen cream is preferable. Either oestriol or conjugated oestrogens are available in this way; Ortho-Gynest, Ovestin, and Premarin contain oestriol 0.01%, oestriol 0.1% and conjugated oestrogens respectively. Progestogens are used mainly by mouth and include dihydrogesterone, medroxyprogesterone, norgestrel and norethisterone. Individual progestogens can be given orally in combination with an oestrogen given by subcutaneous depot injection or by transdermal patch. One patch (Estracombi) provides both hormones, but obviously the doses cannot be separately titrated to provide the minimum necessary to prevent both flushing and (if undesired) withdrawal bleeding.

A popular alternative to oestrogen therapy is the drug, tibolone (Livial), which is a synthetic steroid with weak oestrogenic, progestogenic and androgenic properties. It is administered as a daily oral dose of 2.5 mg. The main adverse effect is vaginal bleeding, which needs investigation if persistent. Vasomotor menopausal symptoms may occasionally be helped by *low doses* of clonidine (Dixarit). Neither of these drugs should be used for prevention of postmenopausal osteoporosis.

The oestrogen-progestogen formulations do not provide adequate contraception and nonhormonal methods should be used until it is quite certain that the menopause is fully accomplished (45–55 years).

But increasingly hormone therapy is prolonged, as follows:

Postmenopausal hormone replacement therapy (HRT) has been practised for many years (in the 1970s more than 30% of postmenopausal women in some rich countries were taking prescribed oestrogen) for its benefits on general well being including a hoped-for reduction in facial wrinkles, to prevent osteoporosis (certainly) and to prevent cardiovascular disease (possibly). However, all the longterm evidence of benefit from HRT accrued during trials of unopposed oestrogens, and it is not yet certain whether the addition of progestogens may nullify the benefits as well as the risks. The recent concerns about an increased risk of venous thrombosis with the third generation contraceptives emphasises the

dangers of extrapolating from trials of older therapies.

'Unopposed' oestrogen therapy, if prolonged for years, is associated with an increased incidence of endometrial carcinoma. This may obtain whether administration is continuous or cyclical. Addition of a progestogen ('opposed' oestrogen therapy) reduces the risk; but it is unnecessary in the absence of a uterus. The risk of breast cancer is also increased, by about 50% in older women, after prolonged use (> 5 years). Women should conduct careful self-examination. This risk will need to be weighed against the benefits, if proven, in reducing risks of osteoporosis and ischaemic heart disease. The evidence for the former at present derives from studies of bone density, where HRT prevents the postmenopausal loss, but has not yet been shown to reduce fracture incidence. Data for ischaemic heart disease for women receiving combined HRT formulations will not be available till the next decade, and rest meanwhile on surrogate measurements. These include falls in low density lipoprotein (LDL) and fibrinogen levels in plasma, and rises in high density lipoprotein (HDL).

Duration of therapy may be 10 years on present knowledge, perhaps longer. Currently used oestrogen-progestogen formulations, e.g. Menophase, Cyclo-Progynova, do not provide reliable contraception. Women requiring surgery should be treated as those using the combined contraceptive pill.

PHARMACOTHERAPY

Contraception: see below.

Menstrual disorders: see below.

Vaginitis. Senile vaginitis usually responds to daily use of an oestrogen pessary or cream (which can also be used in small girls with vaginitis). Absorption can occur sufficiently to cause systemic effects in both the subject and her male sexual partner.

Inhibition of lactation. Oestrogen, alone and in combination with a progestogen or androgen, has been used for 50 years. But it causes thromboembolism as well as stimulating the endometrium at a time when it should be undergoing involution. Such use is obsolete (see Bromocriptine, p. 663.)

Androgen-dependent carcinoma. High doses of oestrogens are used in prostatic carcinoma, which is an androgen-dependent neoplasm. Feminisation is inevitable and the gynaecomastia is often painful. Prevention of thrombosis is sought by concurrent use of aspirin for its antiplatelet effect.

To reduce sexual urge in men whose activities are qualitatively or quantitatively unacceptable to the community and/or to themselves is an occasional indication for oestrogens: 1 mg of stilboestrol daily should be enough (see also Antiandrogen (cyproterone) and benperidol).

Epistaxis: as a last resort in recurrent cases, e.g. telangiectasia.

Atrophic rhinitis may benefit, as also may **acne**.

ADVERSE EFFECTS

Adverse effects consist largely of overdose causing excess of the physiological actions. Withdrawal uterine bleeding is common but seldom prolonged; and bleeding occurs with prolonged high dose. In men, reduced libido, impotence and gynaecomastia (which may be painful) occur. In both sexes *oedema* due to salt and water retention, and *thromboembolism* occur. Natural oestrogens may cause less thromboembolism than do synthetic oestrogens (due to increased clotting factors and increased platelet adhesiveness).

● *Oral administration* is liable to cause nausea, vomiting and diarrhoea.
● Longterm unopposed oestrogen replacement therapy in postmenopausal women is associated with increased incidence of *gallbladder disease* and *endometrial carcinoma*.
● Stilboestrol (obsolete except in prostatic cancer) has been incriminated as a *transplacental carcinogen*, i.e. administered to the mother in the first 18 weeks of pregnancy (in an attempt to prevent miscarriage) it has caused vaginal adenocarcinoma in the offspring (peak age 18 years).
● *Blood lipids*: the effect of oestrogens is on bal-

ance favourable, but the addition of a progestogen (unless gestodene or desogestrel) reverses the balance.
● Oestrogens added to *cosmetics* (skin and hair creams) can cause precocious puberty in children and postmenopausal bleeding; and gynaecomastia in adults. Cosmetics are not subject to the same official controls as are medicines.

Contraindications to oestrogen therapy include women who may have an oestrogen-dependent neoplasm, e.g. breast cancer, who may be pregnant, or have a disposition to thromboembolism. Hypertension, liver disease or gallstones, migraine, diabetes, uterine fibroids or endometriosis may all be made worse by oestrogen. These are not necessarily absolute contraindications, and HRT should not for instance be denied to a polysymptomatic woman with mild hypertension. If necessary, it may be permissible to treat both the hypertension and the postmenopausal symptoms with separate drugs.

Antioestrogens

Obviously the virilising effects of androgens and progestogens antagonise physiologically many of the effects of oestrogens. But selective competitive agents blocking the oestrogen receptor are more likely to be clinically useful.

Clomiphene is structurally related to stilboestrol; it is a weak oestrogen agonist having less activity than natural oestrogens, so that its occupation of receptors results in antagonism, i.e. it is a partial agonist. Such partial agonists are sometimes referred to as 'impeded' oestrogens. Clomiphene blocks hypothalamic oestrogen receptors so that the negative feedback of natural oestrogens is prevented and the pituitary responds by increased secretion of gonadotrophins, which may induce ovulation. Clomiphene is used to treat anovulatory infertility. Multiple ovulation with multiple pregnancy may occur and this is its *principal adverse effect*. There have also been reports of an increased incidence of ovarian carcinoma following multiple exposure, and the number of consecutive cycles for which clomiphene may be used to stimulate ovulation should be limited to six.[7]

Cyclofenil acts similarly to clomiphene.

Tamoxifen is a nonsteroid competitive oestrogen antagonist on target organs; it is used for anovulatory infertility and for treatment of oestrogen-dependent *breast cancer*; it is under trial for the primary prevention of breast cancer in high risk groups.

Progesterone and progestogens

Progesterone (t$\frac{1}{2}$ 5 min) is produced by the corpus luteum and converts the uterine epithelium from the proliferative to the secretory phase. It is thus necessary for successful implantation of the ovum, and is essential throughout pregnancy in the last two-thirds of which it is secreted in large amounts by the placenta. It acts particularly on tissues that are sensitised by oestrogens. Some synthetic progestogens are less selective, having varying oestrogenic and androgenic activity, and these may inhibit ovulation, though not very reliably.

Progestogens are of two principal kinds:

- *Progesterone and its derivatives*: dydrogesterone, hydroxyprogesterone, medroxyprogesterone (t$\frac{1}{2}$ 28 h), etc.
- *Testosterone derivatives*: norethisterone and its prodrug ethynodiol (t$\frac{1}{2}$ 10 h), levonorgestrel, desogestrel, gestodene, gestronol, norgestimate.

All can virilise directly or via metabolites (except progesterone and dydrogesterone) and fetal virilisation to the point of sexual ambiguity has occurred with vigorous use during pregnancy (see also Contraception, p. 653).

Megestrol is used only in cancer; it causes tumours in the breasts of beagle dogs.

---

[7] Rossing M et al 1994 New England Journal of Medicine 331: 771–776.

PHARMACOKINETICS

USES

The clinical uses of progestational agents are ill-defined, apart from contraception (see below), the menopause and postmenopausal hormone replacement therapy (see above).

Other possible uses include

- *menstrual disorders*, e.g. menorrhagia, endometriosis, dysmenorrhoea and premenstrual syndrome (doubtful efficacy)
- *breast and endometrial cancer*.

PREPARATIONS

Available progestogens (some used only in combined formulations) include:

- *oral*: norethisterone, dydrogesterone, gestodene, desogestrel, levonorgestrel, megestrol, medroxyprogesterone
- *suppositories or pessaries*: progesterone
- *injectable*: progesterone, hydroxyprogesterone, medroxyprogesterone.

Adverse effects of prolonged use include virilisation (see above), raised blood pressure and adverse trend in blood lipids. Gestodene, desogestrel and norgestimate may have less affinity for androgen receptors and therefore less unfavourable effect on blood lipids; however the first two of these may have a higher risk of thrombosis.

Antiprogestogens

Menstruation (in its luteal phase) is dependent on progesterone, and uterine bleeding follows antagonism of progesterone. Pregnancy is dependent on progesterone (for implantation, endometrial stimulation, suppression of uterine contractions and placenta formation), and abortion follows progesterone antagonism in early pregnancy.

Mifepristone is a pure competitive antagonist at progesterone and glucocorticoid receptors. Clinical trials of oral use in hospital outpatients have shown it to be safe and effective in terminating pregnancy (used up to 3 weeks from the first missed period). Efficacy is enhanced if its use is followed by administration of a prostaglandin (gemeprost) (vaginally) to produce uterine contractions (the success rate is raised from 85% to above 95%). Adverse effects of the combined treatment include nausea and vomiting, dizziness, asthenia, abdominal pain; uterine bleeding may be heavy. Mifepristone also offers the opportunity for mid-trimester terminations. These are likely to become increasingly frequent as the number of inherited syndromes amenable to antenatal diagnosis at this stage increases.

Other progesterone derivatives

Danazol (Danol) is a derivative of the progestogen, ethisterone. It has partial agonist androgen activity and is described as an 'impeded' androgen; it has little progestogen activity. It is a relatively selective inhibitor of pituitary gonadotrophin secretion (LH, FSH) affecting the surge in the mid-menstrual cycle more than basal secretion. This reduces ovarian function, which leads to atrophic changes in endometrium, both uterine and elsewhere (ectopic), i.e. endometriosis. In males it reduces spermatogenesis. Androgenic unwanted effects occur in women (acne, hirsutism and, rarely, enlargement of the clitoris).

It is chiefly used for: *endometriosis, fibrocystic mastitis, gynaecomastia*, precocious puberty, menorrhagia and hereditary angioedema (p. 648).

Gestrinone is similar.

Fertility regulation

Infertility

The treatment of infertility in either sex is a highly specialised business, requiring a detailed understanding of reproductive physiology and analysis of the cause.

Depending on the cause, the following agents, already described, are used:

For women: to procure ovulation

- Hypothalamic hormone: gonadorelin (p. 644)
- Anterior pituitary hormones: follicle stimulating hormone (p. 644); chorionic gonadotrophin (p. 644)
- Antioestrogens: clomiphene, etc. (p. 651)
- Bromocriptine for hyperprolactinaemia (p. 665).

For men: to enhance spermatogenesis: the same agents as for ovulation are used; androgens are not useful unless there is hypogonadism.

Contraception by drugs and hormones

The requirements of a successful hormonal contraceptive are stringent, for it will be used by millions of healthy people who wish to separate sexual relations from physical reproduction. It must therefore be

- *extremely safe* as well as *highly effective*
- its action must be *quick in onset* and *quickly and completely reversible*, even after years of continuous use
- It must not affect libido.

The fact that alternative methods are less reliable implies that their use will lead to more unwanted pregnancies with their attendant inconvenience, morbidity and mortality, and this must be taken into account in deciding what risks of hormonal contraception are acceptable.

POSSIBLE MODES AND SITES OF ACTION

1. *Direct inhibition of spermatogenesis*: this presents many problems including the lag in onset of effect due to storage of mature spermatozoa until they are ejaculated or die of old age.

2. *Indirect inhibition of spermatogenesis* by suppression of hypothalamic/pituitary activity, which controls it, e.g. by progestogen-androgen combinations; see gonadorelin.

3. *Immunological techniques* (vaccines), to induce antibodies to pituitary gonadotrophins, sperm, or other components of the reproductive process in either sex: these are being developed.

4. *Inhibition of ovulation* presents a different and easier biological problem. There is no need to suppress continuous formation of the gametes, as in the male, but only to prevent their release from the ovary approximately 13 times a year.

Either the pituitary gonadotrophin may be inhibited or the ovary may be made unresponsive to it.

5. *Prevention of fertilisation*: the female genital tract may be made inhospitable to spermatozoa, e.g. by altering cervical mucus or fallopian tube function.

6. *Antizygotic drugs*: compounds effective in the rat have been developed.

7. *Inhibition of implantation*: implantation does not occur unless the endometrium is in the right state, and this depends on a delicate balance between oestrogen and progesterone. This balance can readily be disturbed.

Mice fail to become pregnant if, after mating, they are exposed to the smell of alien malts (via a chemical communicator or pheromone). This approach does not yet seem to have been explored in humans and 'it would be rash indeed to suppose that a contraceptive perfume is on the way'.[8]

8. *Use of spermicides in the vagina.*

Hormonal and chemical contraception in women

- Oestrogen and progestogen (combined and phased administration)
- Progestogen alone

COMBINED CONTRACEPTIVES (THE 'PILL')

Combined oestrogen-progestogen oral contraceptives have been extensively used since 1956. The principal mechanism is inhibition of ovulation (4, above) by action on the hypothalamus inhibiting the release of hormone-releasing hormones and so the pituitary. In addition the endometrium is altered, so that implantation is less likely (7, above) and cervical mucus becomes more viscous and impedes the passage of the spermatozoa (5, above).

Oestrogens alone can inhibit ovulation but, used alone, they are not completely reliable; they cause thromboembolism and endometrial cancer.

Progestogens used alone inhibit ovulation in up to 40% of cycles, render cervical mucus less easily penetrable by sperm and induce a premature secretory change in the endometrium so that implantation does not occur. There is liable to be break-through bleeding and some are a cause of raised blood pressure and an adverse trend in blood lipids and arterial disease.

An appropriate dose of oestrogen + progestogen gives complete reliability with good menstrual cycle control. The following account applies to these combined preparations.

The combination is conveniently started on the first day of the cycle (first day of menstruation) and continued for 21 days (this is immediately effective, inhibiting the first ovulation). Withdrawal bleeding usually begins 21 days after discontinuation. After an interval of 7 days,[9] regardless of menstruation, a new 21-day course is begun, and so on, i.e. active tablets are taken daily for 3 weeks out of 4. But packaging of numbered tablets (21 active: 7 dummy) so that the woman takes one every day without interruption may be best for easy compliance. If the course is not started on the first day of menstruation, but on the fifth day (to give a full month between the menses at the outset), an alternative method of contraception should be used until the 14th pill,[10] has been taken, since the first ovulation may not have been suppressed in women who have short menstrual cycles.

The pill should be taken at the same time every day and preferably not just before intercourse (for pharmacokinetic reasons).

The monthly bleeds that occur 1–2 days after the cessation of active hormone administration are hormone withdrawal bleeds not natural menstruation. They are not an essential feature of oral contraception (3-monthly bleed regimens, phased pills, are

---

[8] Parkes A S 1965 Practitioner 194: 455.

[9] A 7-day interval may be too long, i.e. follicles may develop. A safer regimen is 22 days' hormone administration with a 6-day interval.

[10] The word *pill* has gained currency in both professional and popular usage to mean 'oral contraceptive', losing its original precise technical pharmaceutical meaning.

available), but women are accustomed to monthly bleeds and they provide monthly reassurance of the absence of pregnancy.

Numerous field trials have shown that progestogen-oestrogen mixtures, if taken precisely as directed, are the most reliable reversible contraceptives known. (The only close competitors are depot progestogens and progestogen-releasing intrauterine devices.)

Important aspects

Subsequent fertility. After stopping the pill, fertility that is normal for the age the woman has now reached is restored in 99.9% of subjects, although conception may be delayed for a few months longer in younger and as much as a year in older users than if other methods had been used. Permanent damage to fertility is very rare.

Effect on an existing pregnancy. Although progestogens can masculinise the female fetus, the doses for contraception are so low that risk of harming an undiagnosed pregnancy is extremely low, probably less than 1 in 1000 (the background incidence of birth defects is 1–2%).

Carcinoma of the *breast and cervix* may be unaffected or very slightly increased; *hepatoma* (very rare) is increased. The risk to life seems to be less than that of moderate smoking (10 cigarettes/day). Carcinoma of the *ovary* and *endometrium* are substantially reduced. Total incidence of cancer is unaltered.

Effect on menstruation (it is not true menstruation, see above) is generally to regularise it, and often to diminish blood loss, but amenorrhoea can occur. In some women 'breakthrough' intermenstrual bleeding occurs, especially at the outset, but this seldom persists for more than a few cycles. *Premenstrual tension* and *dysmenorrhoea* are much reduced.

Libido is greatly subject to psychosocial influences, and removal of fear of pregnancy may permit enthusiasm for the first time. It is likely that direct pharmacological effect (reduction) is rare. There is evidence that the normal increase in female-initiated sexual activity at ovulation time is suppressed.[11]

Cardiovascular complications. Incidence of venous thromboembolism is increased in pill users. It is directly related to the amount of oestrogen in the preparation. The small increase in hypertension, cerebrovascular accident and acute myocardial infarction is principally confined to smokers.

Increased arterial disease also appears to be associated with the type of progestogen in the combined pill. The third generation pills containing gestodene or desogestrel appear to carry a higher risk of venous thrombosis, but may have a lower risk of arterial thrombosis because their lower androgen activity leads to slightly higher HDL levels than older pills.[12] It is possible that the higher incidence of venous thrombosis has been an artefact since there have been no prospective comparisons and there is always a tendency for newer agents to be given to patients who have had problems (such as previous thrombosis) on older agents. The progestogen-only pill does not affect coagulation.

Major surgery (in patients taking oestrogen-progestogen contraceptives and postmenopausal hormone replacement therapy). Because of the added risk of venous thromboembolism (surgery causes a fall in antithrombin III) it has been advised that these oral contraceptives should be withdrawn, if practicable, 4 weeks before all lower limb operations or any major elective surgery (and started again at the first menstruation to occur more than 2 weeks after surgery). But increases in clotting factors may persist for many weeks and there is also the risk of pregnancy to be considered (plainly, alternative contraception should be used). An alternative for emergencies is to use low-dose heparin (though this may not reverse all the oestrogen effects on coagulation) and other means (mechanical stimulation of venous return) to prevent post-

---

[11] Adams D B et al 1978 New England Journal of Medicine 299: 1145.

[12] Spitzer W O et al 1996 Third generation oral contraceptives and risk of venous thromboembolic disorders: an international case-control study. British Medical Journal 312: 83–88.

operative thrombosis. A similar problem arises with *prolonged immobilisation* from other causes.

Hepatic function may be impaired as may drug-metabolising capacity ($t^{1/2}$ antipyrine, a general indicator of drug-metabolising capacity, may increase by 30%). Gallbladder disease is more common, and highly vascular hepatocellular adenomas occur (rare).

Cervical erosion incidence is doubled (it is a harmless condition). **Crohn's disease** may be more frequent.

Decreased glucose tolerance occurs, perhaps due to a peripheral effect reducing the action of insulin.

Plasma lipoproteins may be adversely affected; least where the progestogen is desogestrel or low-dose norethisterone.

Plasma proteins. Oestrogens cause an increase in proteins, particularly globulins that bind hydrocortisone, thyroxine and iron. As a result, the *total* plasma concentration of the bound substances is increased, though the concentration of *free* and active substance remains normal. This can be misleading in diagnostic tests, e.g. of thyroid function. This effect on plasma proteins passes off about 6 weeks after cessation of the oestrogen.

Other adverse effects

Often more prominent at the outset and largely due to oestrogen, these include: nausea and, rarely, vomiting; breast discomfort, fluid retention, headache (increase in migraine), lethargy, abdominal discomfort, vaginal discharge or dryness. Depression may occur (and some patients have low blood concentration of pyridoxine); it may be benefited by pyridoxine (try 25 mg orally/day and stop after 4 weeks if there is no benefit). Most depression in pill users is not pill caused.

Benefits additional to contraception

Side-effects are commonly assumed always to be unpleasant aspects of drug action, but they can sometimes also be pleasant.

The oestrogen-progestogen pill is associated with *reduced* risk of functional ovarian cysts and cancer, of endometrial cancer and of benign breast disease; there is a reduced risk of uterine fibroids and they bleed less; there is perhaps less risk of autoimmune thyroid disease; menses are regular and blood loss is not excessive; menses are accompanied by less premenstrual tension and dysmenorrhoea; and there may even be less ear wax.

Contraindications

- Carcinoma of the breast or of the genital tract, past or present, is regarded as an absolute contraindication, as is a history of thromboembolic disease.
- In patients with a history of liver disease, they should only be used if liver function tests are normal.
- Diabetes may become more difficult to control or may be precipitated.
- Lactation may be reduced by combinations but not by progestogens alone.
- Migraine may be precipitated.
- Hypertension will be worsened.

Smoking (15 cigarettes/day) greatly enhances ($\times$ 3) the risks of circulatory disease, and constitutes a contraindication for women over 35 years. Other risk factors for circulatory disease are hyperlipidaemia, hypertension, obesity and age.

Duration of use does not enhance risks of itself. The increase in risk with increased duration of use is due to increasing age. The approaching menopause presents an obvious problem. Because cyclic bleeding will continue to occur under the influence of the drugs even after the natural menopause, the only way of deciding whether contraception can be permanently abandoned is by abandoning it (and using another technique) for 3 months annually to see if natural menstruation is resumed; or stop the combined pill for one month and measure LH/FSH concentration in the blood, which indicates the state of pituitary function.

Ex-users. There may be persistence of cardiovascular risk for a few years after stopping in those with cardiovascular risk factors.

Conclusions

- Pregnancy carries risk.
- *Serious* adverse effects of the combined pill are rare and 'several times a rare event is still a rare event'.[13]
- Precise figures on risk with current low-dose formulations are not available. The major studies, involving, e.g. 23 000 women, used higher dose formulations and cannot be repeatedly replicated (cost, logistics) to keep up with developments.
- Overall mortality amongst users (having low risk factors) is either unaffected or only slightly increased.

Formulations of oestrogen-progestogen combination

Oestrogen: ethinyloestradiol or mestranol
Progestogen: levonorgestrel, norethisterone, ethynodiol, gestodene, or desogestrel

The most important variable is the dose of oestrogen, which is usually between 20 and 50 micrograms. The incidence of thromboembolism has been found higher with high-dose oestrogen preparations, e.g. 100 micrograms, but it is not known if there is any difference between doses below 50 micrograms.

It is now appreciated that the earlier preparations had much more oestrogen than was necessary for efficacy. It seems probable that 20 micrograms is about the limit below which serious loss of efficacy can be expected. Indeed in hepatic enzyme-induced patients, e.g. using antiepileptics, some antirheumatics, it is advisable to use a preparation containing 50 micrograms of oestrogen or more to avoid loss of efficacy due to increased oestrogen metabolism (elimination of breakthrough bleeding is a guide to adequacy of dose).

As discussed above, the type of progestogen in the pill has also been reported to affect risk of venous, but not arterial thrombosis, possibly because they interfere with breakdown of the oestrogen.

Common problems

> **Missed pill.** Inadvertent omission of a dose is less serious on the higher dose preparations, e.g. if one active tablet is omitted the woman remains protected for 24 h if she has been taking a 50 micrograms oestrogen preparation, but for only 12 h if using a 30 micrograms oestrogen preparation.
>
> - If an omitted dose is remembered *within 12 hours* it should be taken at once and the next dose at the usual time, and all should be well (unless it is the *first or last* active pill in the packet, in which case follow the advice in the next paragraph).
> - *If more than 12 hours* has elapsed the same procedure should be followed but an alternative barrier method of contraception should be used for 7[14] days (or abstinence).
>
> Plainly a regimen in which a pill is taken every day (dummy pills) may confuse the subject who will then need advice.

Intercurrent gut upset. Obviously a patient may *vomit* the dose; if vomiting occurs <3 h after a pill, behave as under *missed pill* (above). The hormones are rapidly absorbed and only severe diarrhoea would interfere significantly with efficacy.[15] But if there is doubt, it would be prudent to use a barrier method during and for 14 days after the episode.

Changing of preparation. If a woman is uncomfortable on one preparation she should be changed to another containing a different dose of oestrogen and/or progestogen. The new preparation should start *the day after* she has finished a cycle on the previous preparation. If this is done no extra risk of pregnancy occurs.

Breakthrough bleeding (bleeding on days of active pill taking) can mean a higher dose of oestrogen or progestogen is required.

---

[13] Guillebaud J 1989 The pill. Oxford University Press. A general reference for all practical aspects of use.

[14] If these 7 unprotected days run beyond the beginning of the routine intended pill-free days, the next cycle (packet) should follow without a gap, thus postponing the menses by a month (Family Planning Assoc.).

[15] Orme M et al 1991 Unintended pregnancies and contraceptive use. British Medical Journal 302: 79.

Choice of oestrogen-progestogen combination

There is a wide choice of formulations:

- *Low oestrogen* (20–35 micrograms) plus *low progestogen*, e.g. Marvelon, Minulet, Femodene
- *Low oestrogen plus high progestogen*, e.g. Ovran 30, Eugynon 30
- *High oestrogen* (50 micrograms) plus *low or high progestogen*, e.g. Ovran, Norinyl-1.

In general users should employ the lowest total hormone dose that suits them (good cycle control and minimal side-effects) and should make a start with the first preparation given above.

POSTCOITAL ('morning after pill')[16] AND EMERGENCY CONTRACEPTION

Overall probability of pregnancy following unprotected intercourse is 1:25–1:50 (higher in mid-cycle, lower at end cycle); it may be prevented before implantation by disrupting the normal hormonal arrangements; mode of action is probably by delaying or preventing ovulation or by preventing implantation of the fertilised ovum, though there may also be a postimplantation action.

Postcoital contraception may be successful up to *72 hours* after the exposure. A usual technique is to take 2 tablets of an oestrogen-progestogen combined formulation (containing 50 micrograms of oestrogen and 250 micrograms of levonorgestrel) (Schering PC4) at the earliest opportunity, followed by a further 2 tablets exactly 12 hours later. Vomiting may occur and must be taken into account as a cause of failure (if tablets are vomited, repeat the dose with an antiemetic). The failure rate is hard to estimate (controlled trials are not practicable, but studies on rape and volunteer cases have been made) and may be about 1:200 (but higher in mid-cycle); ectopic pregnancy may perhaps be promoted. If pregnancy is present the procedure will not cause abortion. It is not known if injury to a pregnancy may occur; if so, the risk is probably less than 1:1000; some people will consider abortion. The procedure should not be used more than once in a cycle; nor where absolute contraindications for oestrogen exist.

---

[16] A popular term that misleads women (see text below).

PHASED-FORMULATION CONTRACEPTIVES

Phased pills employ low doses and variable ratios between oestrogen and progestogen, in 2 (*biphasic*) or 3 (*triphasic*) periods within the menstrual cycle. The dose of progestogen is low at the beginning and higher at the end, the oestrogen remaining either constant or rising slightly in mid-cycle. The objective is to achieve effective contraception with minimal distortion of natural hormonal rhythms.

The advantages claimed for these techniques are diminished adverse metabolic changes, e.g. blood lipids, and a particularly reliable monthly bleeding pattern without loss of contraceptive efficacy. But against these (potential) advantages, there is even less latitude of safety if a dose is forgotten. Preparations include BiNovum, TriNovum, Logynon.

PROGESTOGEN-ONLY CONTRACEPTION

Progestogen-only contraception ('mini-pill'): the oral formulation is taken every day throughout the 28-day cycle; a 3-month depot i.m. injection is an alternative.

Subcutaneous implantations that release hormone for several years are in use; they can be removed surgically, e.g. Norplant, if adverse effects develop or pregnancy is desired.

Oral progestogen-only contraception is less effective but safer (no effect on blood coagulation) than combined formulations. Intramuscular progestogen is equal in efficacy to the combined pill. It works by inhibiting ovulation, though much less effectively than the combined pill, but principally by rendering the cervical mucus inhospitable (thick and scanty) to spermatozoa maximally 5 hours after a daily dose (so time the oral dose appropriately where sexual practice is regular).

Progestogen-only contraception is particularly appropriate to women having an absolute contraindication for oestrogen, e.g. history of thromboembolism, smokers (who refuse to give it up), and for diabetics. Hypertension is not an absolute contraindication to the more effective combined pill since only a proportion of women have oestrogen dependent hypertension (and often such women are normotensive until exposed to increased levels of oestrogen). It is used by *lactating women* as it interferes with the milk less than the combined pill.

A missed oral dose allows even less latitude than the combined pill. If a dose is more than 3 *hours* late it should be taken at once and a barrier method used for 2 days (this short safety interval can be a great nuisance). Behave similarly in the presence of vomiting and severe diarrhoea.

A significant limitation to the use of the progestogen-only pill is erratic uterine bleeding which many women understandably dislike. There may be no bleeding for months or there may be frequent and irregular bleeding. Ectopic pregnancy may be more frequent due to a fertilised ovum being held up in a functionally depressed fallopian tube. Other adverse effects are generally less than the combined pill (blood coagulation is unaffected); data on breast cancer are conflicting but are largely reassuring.

The progestogens used (alone) orally include norgestrel, levonorgestrel, ethynodiol, norethisterone (e.g. Noriday, Micronor, Femulen); medroxyprogesterone (Depo-Provera) (t$\frac{1}{2}$ 28 h) is a sustained-release (aqueous suspension) i.m. injection given 3-monthly.

The use of i.m. *medroxyprogesterone* has been much criticised ('ban the jab') on ethical and social grounds, e.g. consent, and there are real ethical issues, especially with mentally retarded women. But it is important that criticism be properly directed (which it has not been) at the way the drug is used, not at the (safe) drug itself. Much has also been made of 'menstrual chaos' by the critics, but the tolerance of bleeding irregularities will be a matter of personality and counselling, and some patients will prefer the infrequent (and private) injection according to their own social situation. It is essential that a drug, useful to some, be not banned because some prescribers have used it wrongly or too casually, reprehensible though that may be.

DRUG INTERACTIONS WITH STEROID CONTRACEPTIVES

Particularly now that the lowest effective doses are in use there is little latitude between success and failure if the absorption, distribution and metabolism are disturbed. Any additional drug-taking must be looked at critically lest it reduces efficacy.

The classic example of interference with the combined pill is the increase of breakthrough bleeding and pregnancy in young women being treated with rifampicin for tuberculosis (1971). Rifampicin is a potent inducer of hepatic drug-metabolising enzymes. Enhanced metabolism of the steroids caused failure. Antiepileptics (phenytoin and carbamazepine but not sodium valproate) create a similar risk.

All drugs that induce metabolising enzymes (see p. 101) whether prescribed or self-administered (alcohol, tobacco smoking) constitute a risk to contraceptive efficacy and prescribing should be specifically reviewed for this effect. Pregnancies have occurred in women taking a contraceptive who commence an antiepileptic drug and doctors have been sued (for negligence) successfully in a court of law.

HYPOTHALAMIC/PITUITARY HORMONE APPROACH TO CONTRACEPTION (See gonadorelin)

OTHER METHODS OF CONTRACEPTION

Intrauterine devices that are also sustained-release formulations of a progestogen or copper to enhance their efficacy by local action on the endometrium have been developed.

Vaginal preparations, to immobilise or kill (spermicide) spermatozoa, are used to add safety to various mechanical contraceptives. They are very unreliable and should be used alone only in an emergency. Substances used include nonoxinols (surfactants that alter the permeability of the sperm lipoprotein membrane) as pessary, gel or foam.

Oil-based lubricants cause condom failure; many 'lubricants', e.g. hand or baby creams, wash off readily, but are oil-based.

RISKS OF CONTRACEPTION IN RELATION TO BENEFIT

Whether a drug should be prescribed involves an assessment of benefit to the patient versus risk to the patient. Even when there is a defined disease the decision can be difficult. It is even more so when the subject is healthy, as is the case with most contraception, and perception of benefit will vary widely between individuals.

It has been pointed out that a woman having regular sexual intercourse faces a finite chance of death from pregnancy, childbirth or from measures to avoid or interrupt pregnancy.

But as well as the risks of unwanted pregnancy, the risk of oral contraceptives (see above) should be viewed in the context of the risks of everyday life, which are substantial.

The death rate from taking oral contraceptives is probably about the same magnitude as deaths from cricket and football (in Britain) and much less than those from swimming (750 men, 250 women per annum in Britain). A car driver may expect, on average, to be admitted to hospital once in 20 years due to a road accident. A woman would have to use oral contraceptives for 2000 years for a similar chance due to a thrombotic episode. It has been calculated that a death in a family that has acquired an outboard motor boat is 10 times more likely than death where the mother is taking an oral contraceptive.[17]

Any danger oral contraceptives may have for the individual must also be seen in relation to their benefits, not only to the individual, but to the community, e.g. fewer self-induced and criminal abortions, fewer unwanted children, slowing down of the speed of increase of world population with less hunger and misery.

The debate will continue, and so will technical advances which will require to be tested on willing subjects (see Ethics of research, Ch. 4).

That research in this field has major ethical implications is illustrated by the now notorious San Antonio study[18] as follows.

In order to distinguish between genuine pharmacodynamic side-effects of an oral contraceptive and the symptoms of everyday life, women seeking contraception were entered into a randomised, placebo controlled, double blind, crossover study; they were not told of the placebo but were advised to use a spermicidal vaginal cream. Of the 76 subjects 11 became pregnant, 10 whilst taking placebo.

With the development of research ethics review committees, such studies, it is to be hoped, are now impossible. Indeed, such a study has never been ethically acceptable.

MALE CONTRACEPTION (systemic)

Suppression of spermatogenesis may be achieved by interfering with:

- extra-gonadal endocrine control, i.e. the hypothalamic/pituitary/gonadal axis
- direct action on gonadal spermatogenesis
- vaccines to produce antibodies to sperm.

Approaches include androgen or combinations of androgen with danazol, or progestogen, or oestrogen, also gonadorelin. Gossypol, a phenol from the cotton plant, has been under evaluation in China since about 1974[19] but it appears to have unacceptable adverse effects, e.g. hypokalaemia. In one study of injected testosterone enanthate, men became azoospermic in 120 days.

Natural regulators of mitosis (chalones) are tissue specific, and their identification should allow synthesis of analogues that might provide the necessary specificity and reversibility to deserve trial as male contraceptives. Whether a risk of genetic damage is inherent in drugs acting on spermatogenesis is unknown. The obvious biological problems of male contraception, delay in onset of effect, need for continuous effect as opposed to the elimination of a single regular event (ovulation) plus the ready availability of female contraception, plus the fact that men do not get pregnant, reduce the commercial incentives to seek and to use contraceptives for men.

Development of new contraceptives

Extension of the range of contraceptives (hormonal or nonhormonal) to include new mechanisms of action, and especially to include men, has been the

---

[17] Potts D M 1970 British Medical Bulletin 26: No 1, 27.

[18] Quoted from Levine R J 1986 Ethics and regulation of clinical research. Urban and Schwarzenburg: recommended reading.

[19] Attention was drawn to gossypol by the high prevalence of male infertility in rural areas where food was cooked in cotton-seed oil.

subject of social and political demand. This is partly because current contraceptives are still imperfect, not only with regard to safety, efficacy and convenience, but also with regard to cultural, socioeconomic and moral aspects. The first combined oestrogen-progestogen pill was developed over 5 years. Development of a new agent that is not just a variant of existing agents is now likely to require 15–20 years and the cost will be enormous. Regulatory requirements will be rigorous and extensive (see Chs 3, 5).

For the female contraceptive, regulatory bodies generally require that the preparation be used in at least 20 000 cycles with a quarter of the data derived from longterm use. New drugs or methods will be subject to close scrutiny as to whether they truly prevent conception or induce early abortion, a distinction that raises moral issues.

For a male systemic contraceptive the regulatory requirements remain undefined, but they will be strict.

Claims that pharmaceutical developers should compensate sufferers of adverse reactions also may deter all but the boldest and richest companies from making the necessary investment in research unless society, i.e. governments, accept at least some of the liability for injury where there is no fault on the part of the developer.

SUMMARY

- Many of the pituitary hormones and their hypothalamic releasing factors are used in diagnosis or therapy.
- Vasopressin (antidiuretic hormone) is used both for its vasoconstrictor effect (in the treatment of oesophageal varices) and for its antidiuretic action.
- The main therapeutic use of pituitary hormones is of growth hormone (anterior pituitary) and those from the posterior pituitary: oxytocin and vasopressin.
- The main hypothalamus-pituitary-target organ axis for therapeutic intervention is that controlling reproductive hormones, especially in women.
- Suppression of oestrogen and/or androgen production is used in the treatment of tumours stimulated by these: breast and prostate.
- Therapy in women is used to suppress ovulation (contraceptives), to stimulate ovulation (fertility treatment) or to mimic ovarian endocrine function (postmenopausal hormone replacement therapy, HRT).

Menstrual disorders

Only a note on the simpler uses of hormones is appropriate here.

Amenorrhoea, primary or secondary, requires specialist endocrinological diagnosis. Where the cause is failure of hormone production, cyclical replacement therapy is indicated.

Severe dysfunctional uterine bleeding (often due to oestrogen excess) can be controlled

- *during bleeding,* generally within 48 hours, by a *progestogen* (norethisterone) 5 mg/d for 10 days (a withdrawal bleed follows in 2–4 d)
- to prevent an *anticipated* excessive bleed: give 10 mg/d from 19th-26th days of the cycle (for 2–3 cycles). There will be withdrawal bleeding. This may be followed, if appropriate, by cycle control with an oestrogen-progestogen combination (particularly one with high progestogen content) (an oral contraceptive will serve).

Danazol continuously can also be effective. Other agents that may help resistant cases of dysfunctional uterine bleeding include antifibrinolytic agent (tranexamic acid), indomethacin or mefenamic acid (to inhibit prostaglandin synthesis given just before and during menstruation) and ethamsylate (by inhibiting prostaglandin synthesis and capillary fragility); but none of these is treatment of first choice. These treatments may be effective in the presence of an intrauterine contraceptive device; but not in the presence of fibroids.

Less severe cases, moderately heavy periods, are likely to respond to prostaglandin synthase inhibition, e.g. mefenamic acid 500 mg when the blood loss becomes heavy followed by 250 mg × 3/d for 3 days if necessary. Aspirin and paracetamol are ineffective. (see ethamsylate).

THE TIMING OF MENSTRUATION

Sometimes there are pressing reasons to prevent menstruation at the normal time, but obviously this cannot be done at the last moment.

Menstruation can be postponed by giving oral norethisterone 5 mg × 3/d, starting 3 days before the expected onset; bleeding occurs 2–3 d after withdrawal. Users of the combined oral contraceptive pill (having a 7-day break) can simply continue with active pills where they would normally stop for 7 days.

Although there is no evidence that harm follows such manoeuvres, it is obviously imprudent to practise them frequently.

Note. These uses of progestogen should not be undertaken if there is any possibility of pregnancy.

Endometriosis. It has been observed that endometriosis is benefited by pregnancy and so a 'pseudopregnancy treatment' has been practised, by giving an oestrogen-progestogen oral contraceptive for about 9 months; marked improvement and even cure may result. But danazol, taken continuously, or norethisterone can be effective; as can analogues of gonadorelin, e.g. goserelin; adverse reactions are troublesome.

Dysmenorrhoea is due to uterine contractions resulting from excess prostaglandins in the uterus during ovulatory cycles. It can be treated by suppressing ovulation (using the combined pill or norethisterone); also by using inhibitors of prostaglandin synthesis, e.g. aspirin, indomethacin, naproxen. The analgesic prostaglandin synthase inhibitor (NSAID) may need to be given for several days before menstruation or only at the time of the pain.

Premenstrual tension syndrome may be due to an imbalance of natural oestrogen and progesterone secretion, but knowledge of the syndrome remains imprecise. Psychosocial factors can be important. Placebo effects are strong. Drugs are not necessarily the preferred treatment.

There is evidence for and against:

- *Restriction of salt and fluid plus a thiazide diuretic* in the second half of the menstrual cycle where symptoms suggest fluid retention
- *Pyridoxine* (vitamin B$_6$, a coenzyme): try 100 mg/d orally (not more) for 3 months and abandon if there is no benefit. It may help depression and irritability particularly

- *Oestrogen-progestogen* oral contraceptive combination
- *Bromocriptine*, especially where there is breast pain
- *Prostaglandin synthase inhibition*. e.g. mefenamic acid.

Cyclical breast pain or mastalgia, when severe, may respond to continuous use of gamolenic acid (Efamast) (orally); it is an essential unsaturated fatty acid for cell membranes (patients have low concentrations); it may act by reducing cellular uptake of prolactin and ovarian hormones. Danazol and bromocriptine also help.

Myometrium

He gently prevails on his patient to try
The magic effects of the ergot of rye.
(attributed to Alfred, Lord Tennyson, 1809–1892)

Ergot and derivatives

Ergot is a fungus which preys on grasses, especially rye, bread made from which has caused epidemics of painful peripheral gangrene and abortion due to its smooth muscle stimulant actions. For medicinal production the plant is artificially infected.

Ergotism is now very rare but an epidemic was reported in England in 1928[20] and in France in 1951[21] although the genuineness of both these has been questioned.

The uterine effects of ergot have been known for at least 400 years and active alkaloids (ergotamine, ergotoxine, etc) were isolated at the beginning of the 20th century. But the identification of what is clinically the most important (ergometrine, ergonovine) had to wait until 1932 when a clinical

[20] Robertson J et al 1928 British Medical Journal 1: 302.

[21] Gabbai et al 1951 British Medical Journal 2: 650, editorial, ibid., 596.

obstetrician[22] was asked to investigate why extracts of ergot seemed to be active on the uterus when pharmacologists said they ought not to be.

Fortunately, the study was published in a journal that has a correspondence column so that the subsequent clash of opinion between clinician and pharmacologist could take place in public.

ASPECTS OF THE CURIOUSLY COMPLEX PHARMACOLOGY OF ERGOT

Ergot alkaloids[23] are related to lysergic acid and are based on ergoline which bears structural resemblance to the biogenic amines, noradrenaline (norepinephrine), dopamine and serotonin (5-HT). Therefore it is no surprise that ergot derivatives can act as agonists, antagonists or both simultaneously (partial agonists) at these amine receptors. Indeed, it is combinations of these actions on the specific receptors that largely account for the multifarious actions of *ergot derivatives*; none is completely receptor specific:

- Co-dergocrine (Hydergine) is the most active α-adrenoceptor antagonist.
- Ergotamine is the most active α-adrenoceptor agonist.
- Methysergide is the most active serotonin (5-HT) antagonist.
- Bromocriptine, lysuride, pergolide and cabergoline are the most active dopamine receptor agonists.
- (Methyl) ergometrine is the most active uterine α-adrenoceptor agonist. (But selectivity alters with changing drug concentrations and specificity may only be attained at carefully adjusted concentrations.)
- Lysergide (LSD) is the most active hallucinogen (mechanism uncertain). But all supply of and research on LSD was stopped by the pharmaceutical firm that invented it following the surge of hallucinogen abuse in the early 1960s.

Metabolism: ergot alkaloids are metabolised in the liver.

BROMOCRIPTINE

Bromocriptine ($t^{1/2}$ 6 h) provides an example of the exploitation of the extraordinarily wide spectrum of activities of ergot derivatives. Ergotoxine (a mixture) has oxytocic and cardiovascular effects. It also prevents, by a *dopamine receptor agonist* action on the anterior pituitary, the release of prolactin. Bromocriptine was the product of a research programme aimed at eliminating the oxytocic and cardiovascular effects whilst retaining the prolactin release-inhibiting effect. The result has been a useful dopamine receptor agonist which *suppresses lactation and prolactinomas, benefits cyclic mastalgia*, and suppresses types of *hypogonadism* associated with hyperprolactinaemia (which reduces gonadotrophin secretion); it also has some efficacy in parkinsonism (unrelated to prolactin) (see p. 360). It increases growth hormone release in healthy people and suppresses it in acromegaly (see also Index).

Cabergoline and *quinagolide* are newer alternatives which are more selective than bromocriptine at the dopamine (D_2) receptor and have longer $t^{1/2}$ permitting once daily dosing (see Parkinsonism).

Suppression of lactation

Inhibition of lactation is sometimes necessary, e.g. dead child, sick mother.

> One alternative which is not considered often enough is ... A tight binder, sympathy, and occasional sedatives (which) will carry many women through the initial discomfort of engorged breasts. Without the stimulus of suckling, the high prolactin concentrations at delivery fall to normal within a week and lactation soon peters out. Fluid restriction is unnecessary.[24]

The procedure is safe and cheap.

Pituitary secretion of prolactin is normally under inhibitory tone from the hypothalamus via prolactin release-inhibiting factor (PIF), which may be dopamine.

---

[22] Moir C 1932 British Medical Journal 1: 1119, 1189; 2: 75.

[23] Berde B, Schild H O (eds) 1978 Ergot alkaloids and related compounds. Springer, Berlin.

[24] Editorial 1977 British Medical Journal 1: 189.

Dopamine receptor agonists activate or mimic hypothalamic prolactin-inhibiting factor, the plasma prolactin concentration fails and lactation stops. Drugs are no longer recommended for the routine suppression of lactation. Exceptionally, *bromocriptine* or *cabergoline* may be used. A single dose of the latter prevents puerperal lactation; treatment is given for 2 days to suppress established lactation.

Oestrogens are effective but can cause thrombosis.

ERGOTAMINE (see Migraine)

Ergotamine causes vasoconstriction (arteries and veins), which may be sufficient to cause hypertension, by an α-adrenoceptor agonist action and also by sensitising to endogenously released noradrenaline. The degree of vasoconstriction is determined by the pre-existing vascular tone. The $t^{1}/_{2}$ of ergotamine is 2 h, but tissue storage allows prolonged action, so that if it is being given several times a day for migraine there is short-term accumulation that can be dangerous, causing peripheral gangrene, for which sodium nitroprusside i.v. may be used.

ERGOMETRINE (ergonovine)

Ergometrine ($t^{1}/_{2}$ 2 h) is now the only ergot alkaloid used for stimulating uterine activity (α-adrenoceptor and dopamine receptor agonist), as ergotamine is slow in acting even after i.v. injection, whereas ergometrine acts almost immediately when injected i.v. Serious circulatory side-effects are also less frequent (see below). The uterus is stimulated at all times, but is much more sensitive in late pregnancy.

Ergometrine and oxytocin (see below) differ in their actions on the uterus. In moderate doses oxytocin produces slow generalised contractions with full relaxation in between; ergometrine produces faster contractions superimposed on a tonic contraction. High doses of both substances produce sustained tonic contraction. It will be seen, therefore, that oxytocin is more suited to induction of labour and ergometrine to the prevention and treatment of postpartum haemorrhage, the incidence of which is reduced by its routine prophylactic use (generally i.m.).

Dosage

Ergometrine may be given:

- *Orally:* 0.5–1 mg, when action begins in about 8 min and lasts about 1 hour.
- *i.v.:* 100–500 micrograms; onset of action about 1 min; used as treatment of established postpartum haemorrhage.
- *i.m.:* 200–500 micrograms; action begins in about 6 min; the onset is speeded by mixing the injection with hyaluronidase (1500 units), which enhances tissue permeation and so speeds absorption.

This combination is appropriate for use by birth attendants who are not permitted to give an i.v. injection.

Oxytocin i.m. is an alternative for quick (but brief) action. Plainly speed of onset can be vital if the woman is bleeding profusely. *Oxytocin mixed with ergometrine* (Syntometrine: ergometrine 500 micrograms plus oxytocin 5 units, i.m.) has the advantages of quick (2 min) onset of action and prolonged effect.

When given during labour the timing of the injection is the subject of disagreement. It is commonly given when the anterior shoulder of the child is delivered, but some give it earlier at the crowning of the head (never before this) or later when the placenta has separated or has been delivered. Ergometrine tablets may be given orally (0.5 mg/ × 3/d) for 3 days in the early puerperium or in incomplete abortion.

Hypertension, lasting hours or even days after ergometrine, occurs occasionally. It seems that in some patients ergometrine is capable of inducing vascular effects of a magnitude similar to those of ergotamine. It is most likely to occur in toxaemic patients[25] and in cases where sympathomimetic vasoconstrictors have been used, e.g. with a local anaesthetic. It can be severe and complaints of headache post partum should be taken seriously. The blood pressure can be reduced by chlorpromazine (10–15 mg) i.v. or i.m. and then larger doses orally, or by any other α-adrenoceptor blocking drug. Ergometrine can also cause hypotension.

---

[25] Synthetic oxytocin (Syntocinon) is preferable in such patients.

Methysergide: see Migraine and above.

Co-dergocrine (Hydergine) is a mixture of hydrogenated alkaloids. There is weak evidence of modest beneficial effect in mild dementia in the elderly.

Adverse effects

Adverse effects of ergot derivatives are mostly predictable from the various receptor actions mentioned above.

CNS: vomiting due to dopaminergic effect on the chemoreceptor trigger zone; hypotension, especially postural, due to depression of the vasomotor centre, which is enhanced by peripheral α-adrenoceptor block (hydrogenated alkaloids).

Overdose causes: confusion, depression, convulsions and a variety of neurological syndromes, probably vascular in origin.

Peripheral vessels: constriction even to gangrene (ergotamine) occurs and this alkaloid is dangerous in patients with peripheral vascular or ischaemic cardiac disease.

Blood pressure may rise or fall according to the varying central and peripheral adrenoceptor agonist and antagonist effects.

Oxytocin

Oxytocin is a peptide hormone of the posterior pituitary gland. It stimulates the contractions of the pregnant uterus, which becomes much more sensitive to it at term. However, patients with posterior pituitary disease (diabetes insipidus) can go into labour normally.

Oxytocin is reflexly released from the pituitary following suckling (and manual stimulation) and causes almost immediate contraction of the myoepithelium of the breast; it can be used to enhance milk ejection (nasal spray). The only other clinically important effect is on the blood pressure, which may fall if an overdose is given.

Synthetic oxytocin (Syntocinon) is pure and is not contaminated with vasopressin as is the natural product, which is obsolete.

OXYTOCIN IN MANAGEMENT OF LABOUR

Oxytocin is used i.v. in the *induction of labour* and sometimes for uterine inertia, haemorrhage or during abortion. It produces, almost immediately, rhythmic contractions with relaxation between, i.e. it mimics normal uterine activity. The association of oxytocin with neonatal jaundice appears to be due to increased erythrocyte fragility causing haemolysis.

The decision to use oxytocin requires special skill. It has a $t^{1/2}$ of 6 min and is given by i.v. infusion at 1–3 milliunits per min; it *must* be closely supervised; the dose is adjusted by results; overdose can cause uterine tetany and even rupture. The dose may be increased every 10 min until contractions commence and then at intervals of at least 20 min. The utmost care is required.

Oxytocin is structurally close to vasopressin and it is no surprise that it also has antidiuretic activity. Serious water intoxication can occur with prolonged i.v. infusions, especially where accompanied by large volumes of fluid.

Oxytocin has been supplanted by ergometrine as prime treatment of postpartum haemorrhage except when, as occasionally happens, there is no response to ergometrine. There are advantages in a mixture of oxytocin and ergometrine (Syntometrine, see above).

Uterine relaxants

β_2-adrenoceptor agonists relax the uterus and are given by i.v. infusion by obstetricians to inhibit *premature labour*, e.g. isoxsuprine, terbutaline, ritodrine, salbutamol; their use is complicated by the expected cardiovascular effects, including tachycardia, hypotension. Less easy to explain, but more devastating on occasion to the patient, is severe left ventricular failure. Possibly the combination of fluid overload (due to the vehicle) and increased oxygen demand by the heart are factors, and the risk is higher in the presence of multiple pregnancy, pre-existing cardiac disease or maternal infection. It is important to administer the β_2-agonist using a syringe pump with 5% dextrose (**not saline**) as diluent, and to monitor the patient closely for signs of fluid overload.

Prostaglandins

(For a general account of prostaglandins see p. 250.)

Prostaglandins that soften the uterine cervix (by an action on collagen) and have a powerful oxytocic effect include:

Dinoprost (prostaglandin $F_2\alpha$, $PGF_2\alpha$) (Prostin F2 alpha) and **dinoprostone** (prostaglandin E_2; PGE_2) (Prostin E2). They are used to induce labour and to terminate pregnancy, including missed or partial abortion and in the treatment of hydatidiform mole; they are given by intra- or extra-amniotic injection, by vaginal tablet, or intracervical gel, by i.v. infusion or by mouth. Their safe and effective use (including choice of route) requires special skill.

Adverse effects include vomiting, diarrhoea, headache, pyrexia and local tissue reaction.

Gemeprost (prostaglandin E_1 analogue) (Cervagem) is used intravaginally to soften the cervix before operative procedures in the first trimester of pregnancy and for abortion, alone and in combination with an antiprogestogen (mifepristone, p. 652).

Carboprost (prostaglandin $F_2\alpha$ analogue) is used for postpartum haemorrhage (resistant to ergometrine and oxytocin) for its oxytocin action. It is highly effective. Adverse effects include hypertension, asthma and pulmonary oedema.

Use of drugs and morality

Increasingly, drug use is a cause of moral and social, as well as of technical, problems and this is particularly so in the field of reproduction (contraception and abortion).

Some doctors regard these uses as impermissible under any circumstances, some as permissible under certain circumstances; others see no moral issue. In any case it is desirable that all doctors should be technically informed if they are likely to meet patients who may be taking or seeking such treatment. Since pharmacological considerations are not fundamental to moral decisions, these contentious issues will not be discussed here.

GUIDE TO FURTHER READING

Bagatell C J, Bremner W J 1996 Androgens in men—uses and abuses. New England Journal of Medicine 334: 707

Belchetz P E 1994 Hormonal treatment of postmenopausal women. New England Journal of Medicine 330: 1062–1071

Collaborative Group on Hormone Factors in Breast Cancer 1996 Breast cancer and hormonal contraceptives: collaborative reanalysis of individual data on 53 297 women with breast cancer and 100 239 women without breast cancer from 54 epidemiological studies. Lancet 347: 1703, 1713

Conn P M et al 1991 Gonadotrophin-releasing hormone and its analogues. New England Journal of Medicine 324: 93

Donaldson M D C 1996 Jury still out for normal short stature and Turner's syndrome. Lancet 348: 3

Healy D L et al 1994 Female infertility: causes and treatment. Lancet 343: 1539–1544

Jacobs H S, Loeffler F E 1992 Postmenopausal hormone replacement therapy. British Medical Journal 305: 1403–1408

Magos A L 1990 Management of menorrhagia. British Medical Journal 300: 1537

McPherson K 1995 Breast cancer and hormonal supplements in postmenopausal women. British Medical Journal 311: 699–700

McPherson K 1996 Third generation oral contraception and venous thromboembolism. British Medical Journal 312: 68–69

Mishell D R 1989 Contraception. New England Journal of Medicine 320: 777

Posthuma W F et al 1994 Cardioprotective effect of hormone replacement therapy in postmenopausal women: is the evidence biased? British Medical Journal 308: 1268–1269

Seeley T 1992 Oestrogen replacement therapy after hysterectomy. British Medical Journal 305: 811–812

Silvestre L et al 1990 Voluntary interruption of pregnancy with mifepristone and a prostaglandin analogue. New England Journal of Medicine 322: 6451; editorial p. 691

Vance M 1990 Growth hormone for the elderly? New England Journal of Medicine 323: 52

Vessey M P et al 1989 Mortality among oral contraceptive users: 20 year follow-up of women in a cohort study. British Medical Journal 299: 1487

39

Vitamins, calcium, bone

SYNOPSIS

The principally *pharmacological* aspects of vitamins are described here. The *nutritional* aspects, physiological function, sources, daily requirements and deficiency syndromes (primary and secondary) are to be found in any textbook of medicine.

- Vitamin A: retinol
- Vitamin B: complex
- Vitamin C: ascorbic acid
- Vitamin D, calcium, parathyroid hormone, calcitonin, biphosphonates, bone
- Treatment of calcium and bone disorders
- Vitamin E: tocopherol

Vitamins are substances that are essential for normal metabolism and must be chiefly supplied in the diet.

Humans cannot synthesise any vitamins in the body except some vitamin D in the skin and nicotinamide from tryptophan. Lack of a particular vitamin may lead to a specific deficiency syndrome. This may be *primary* (inadequate diet), or *secondary*, due to failure of absorption (intestinal abnormality or chronic diarrhoea), or to increased metabolic need (growth, pregnancy, lactation, hyperthyroidism).

Vitamin deficiencies are commonly multiple, and complex clinical pictures occur. There are numerous single and multivitamin preparations to provide prophylaxis and therapy.

It has often been suggested, but never proved, that subclinical vitamin deficiencies are a cause of much chronic ill-health and liability to infections. This idea has led to enormous consumption of vitamin preparations, which, for most consumers, probably have no more than placebo value. Fortunately most of the vitamins are comparatively nontoxic, but *prolonged* administration of *vitamins A and D* can have *serious* ill-effects.

Vitamins fall into two groups:

- **water-soluble vitamins:** the B group and C
- **fat-soluble vitamins:** A, D, E and K

Vitamin A: retinol

Vitamin A is a generic term embracing substances having the biological actions of retinol and related substances (which are called *retinoids*). The principal functions of retinol are to:

- sustain normal epithelia
- form retinal photochemicals
- enhance immune functions
- protect against infections and probably some cancers.

Deficiency of retinol leads to metaplasia and hyperkeratosis throughout the body. This metaplasia is reminiscent of the early stage of transformation of normal tissue to cancer.

Retinol and derivatives are used in doses above

those needed for nutrition, i.e. pharmacotherapy, in dyskeratotic skin diseases (psoriasis, acne) and are being explored, with some success, in the prevention of cancers and infections.

Tretinoin is retinoic acid. It is used in acne by topical application, see page 280.

Isotretinoin is a retinoic acid isomer ($t^{1/2}$ 20 h). It is used orally in acne (see p. 280). It is effective in preventing second primary tumours in patients who have been treated for squamous cell carcinoma of the head and neck.

Acitretin is a retinoic acid derivative ($t^{1/2}$ 48 h). It is used orally for *psoriasis*, see p. 280.

Retinol itself is used in prevention and treatment of deficiency ($t^{1/2}$ 7–14 d).

Adverse effects

Toxic effects occur with prolonged high intake (in children 25 000–500 000 IU daily). A diagnostic sign of *chronic poisoning* is the presence of painful tender swellings on the long bones. Anorexia, skin lesions, hair loss, hepatosplenomegaly, papilloedema, bleeding and general malaise also occur. Vitamin A is very cumulative (it is stored in liver and fat) and effects take weeks to wear off. Most cases of vitamin A poisoning have been due to mothers administering large amounts of fish-liver oils to their children in the belief that it was good for them.

Chronic overdose also causes an increased liability of biological membranes and of the outer layer of the skin to peel. An extreme example of this is the case of the hungry Antarctic explorer who in 1913 ate the liver of his husky sledge dogs. His feet felt sore and

the sight of my feet gave me quite a shock, for the thickened skin of the soles had separated in each case as a complete layer . . . I did what appeared to be the best thing under the circumstances: smeared the new skin with lanolin . . . and with bandages bound the skin soles back in place.[1]

Vitamin A and its derivatives are *teratogenic* at above physiological doses, i.e. with pharmacotherapy (for precautions, see use in acne and psoriasis, p. 280). Misguided pregnant health enthusiasts may take enough self-prescribed supplements to hazard a fetus. The Teratology Society advises that supplements should not exceed 8000 IU (2400 micrograms) per day.

Acute overdose: travellers have been made ill by eating the livers of Arctic carnivores:

Eskimos never eat polar-bear liver, knowing it to be toxic, and husky dogs, with instinctive wisdom, also avoid it. Those who pooh-pooh the Eskimos' fears or the husky dogs' instincts and are tempted to enjoy a man's portion of polar-bear liver — appetites get sharp near the North Pole — will consume anything up to 10 000 000 IU of vitamin A (normal daily requirement is 5000 IU). This is too much of a good thing, and the diner will probably soon find himself drowsy then overcome by headache and vomiting, and finally losing the outer layer of his skin.[2]

Vitamin B complex

A number of widely differing substances are now, for convenience, classed the 'vitamin B complex'. Those used for pharmacotherapy include the following:

Thiamine (B_1) is used orally for nutritional purposes, but is given i.v. in serious emergencies, e.g. Wernicke–Korsakoff syndrome, when it can cause anaphylactic shock; the injection should be given over 10 min (or i.m.).

Cobalamins (B_{12}): see Chapter 30.

Folic acid: see Chapter 30.

Pyridoxine (B_6) is a coenzyme (including decar-

[1] Shearman J C 1978 Vitamin A and Sir Douglas Mawson. British Medical Journal 1: 283.

[2] Editorial 1962 British Medical Journal 1: 855.

boxylases) for transamination and is concerned with many metabolic processes. Normal adult requirements are about 2 mg/d. Apart from its use to correct nutritional vitamin B_6 deficiency, pyridoxine is given to treat certain pyridoxine-dependent inborn errors of metabolism, namely homocystinuria, hereditary sideroblastic anaemia and primary hyperoxaluria. Deficiency may be induced by drugs such as isoniazid, hydralazine and penicillamine; pyridoxine 10–50 mg/day prevents the development of peripheral neuritis without interfering with therapeutic action.

Pyridoxine is also used for a variety of conditions including premenstrual tension (100–400 mg/d), vomiting in pregnancy and radiation sickness.

Pyridoxine, even in small doses, can block the therapeutic effect of levodopa in parkinsonism, by enhancing its decarboxylation to dopamine, which does not enter the brain. It does not interfere with the combined levodopa/decarboxylase preparations because of the presence of the decarboxylase inhibitor. Heavy overdose of pyridoxine causes peripheral neuropathy.

Niacin (nicotinic acid, nicotinamide) (B_7) is an essential part of co-dehydrogenases I and II, and so it is present in every living cell.

Adverse effects do not occur with standard doses of nicotinamide. *Nicotinic acid*, which is converted into nicotinamide, causes peripheral vasodilatation accompanied by an unpleasant flushing and itching, and the patient may faint.

Nicotinic acid is used in some hyperlipidaemias, see page 481.

Vitamin C: ascorbic acid

Deficiency of ascorbic acid leads to *scurvy*,[3] which is characterised by petechial haemorrhages, haematomas, bleeding gums (if teeth are present) and anaemia. It has a memorable place in the history of therapeutic measurement.

Scurvy had been a scourge for thousands of years, particularly amongst sailors on long voyages. In 1753, Dr James Lind performed a simple controlled therapeutic trial on 12 sailors with advanced scurvy. They were all on the same basic diet and were living in the same quarters on board ship at sea. He divided them into pairs and dosed each pair separately on cider, sulphuric acid, sea-water, vinegar, a concoction of garlic, mustard, balsam and myrrh, and two oranges and a lemon. The pair receiving the oranges and lemon recovered and were back on duty within a week; of the others, only the pair taking cider was slightly improved. The efficacy of oranges and lemons in the prevention and cure of scurvy was repeatedly confirmed. Eventually the British Navy provided a regular daily allowance of lemon juice, unfortunately later replaced by the cheaper lime[4] juice which contained insufficient ascorbic acid to prevent scurvy completely.

Function

Ascorbic acid is required for the synthesis of collagen. It is also a powerful reducing agent (antioxidant) and plays a part in intracellular oxidation-reduction systems, and in mopping up oxidants (free radicals) produced endogenously or in the environment, e.g. cigarette smoke (see Vitamin E).

Indications for ascorbic acid

- The prevention and cure of scurvy
- Urinary acidification (rarely appropriate)
- Methaemoglobinaemia, for its properties as reducing agent (see below)
- Coryza: it is possible that large daily doses (1 g or more/d), of ascorbic acid (daily nutritional requirement 60 mg) may reduce the incidence and severity of coryza. Reliable trials in this disease are difficult and the results are inconclusive. To justify use of such doses in populations, benefit must be shown to be clinically, as well as statistically, significant;

---

[3] Only man (and other primates), guinea-pigs, the Indian fruit bat and the red-vented bulbul (a bird) get scurvy; other animals are able to synthesise ascorbic acid for themselves.

[4] Hence the term 'limey' for British sailors; generally used pejoratively, but obsolete except in Australia.

and harm insignificant. This has not been achieved.

Adverse effects

High doses may cause sleep disturbances, headaches and gut upsets. Ascorbic acid is partly eliminated in the urine unchanged and partly metabolised to oxalate. Doses above 4 g/d, which have been taken over long periods in the hope of preventing coryza, increase urinary oxalate concentration sufficiently to form oxalate stones. Intravenous ascorbic acid may precipitate a haemolytic attack in subjects with glucose-6-phosphate dehydrogenase deficiency.

METHAEMOGLOBINAEMIA

A reducing substance is needed to convert the methaemoglobin (ferric iron) back to oxyhaemoglobin (ferrous iron) whenever enough has formed seriously to impair the oxygen-carrying capacity of the blood. Ascorbic acid is nontoxic (it acts by direct reduction) but is less effective than *methylene blue*. Both can be given orally, i.v. or i.m. Excessive doses of methylene blue can cause methaemoglobinaemia (by stimulating NADPH-dependent enzymes).

Methaemoglobinaemia may be *drug-induced* by: sulphonamides, nitrites, nitrates (may occur in drinking water), primaquine, -caine local anaesthetics, dapsone, nitrofurantoin, nitroprusside, vitamin K analogues, chlorates, aniline and nitrobenzene. In the rare instance of there being urgency, methylene blue 1 mg/kg slowly i.v. benefits within 30 min. (Ascorbic acid competes directly with the chemical cause but is inadequate in severe cases, which are the only ones that need treatment.)

In the *congenital form*, oral methylene blue with or without ascorbic acid gives benefit in days to weeks.

Methylene blue turns the urine blue and high concentrations can irritate the urinary tract, so that fluid intake should be high when big doses are used.

Sulphaemoglobinaemia cannot be treated by drugs. It can be caused by sulphonamides, nitrites or nitrates.

Vitamin D, calcium, parathyroid hormone, calcitonin, biphosphonates, bone

The agents are closely interrelated and will be discussed together.

VITAMIN D

Vitamin D comprises a number of structurally related sterol compounds having similar biological properties in that they prevent or cure the vitamin D deficiency diseases, rickets and osteomalacia.

- **D$_2$ or ergocalciferol** (calciferol) made by ultraviolet irradiation of ergosterol
- **D$_3$ or cholecalciferol** made by ultraviolet irradiation of 7-dehydrocholesterol; it is the form that occurs in natural foods and is formed in the skin.

The above, D$_2$, D$_3$, are 25-hydroxylated into more active forms in the *liver*, which are then 1α-hydroxylated in the *kidney* (under the control of parathormone) into the most active form, 1α-25-dihydroxycholecalciferol; this, the most active natural form of vitamin D, is available as **calcitriol**. In renal disease this final rate-limited renal α-hydroxylation is inadequate, and administration of the less biologically active precursors is therefore liable to lack efficacy.

Subsequently there was introduced a 1α-hydroxylated form (1α-hydroxycholecalciferol) **alfacalcidol** (One-Alpha), that only requires hepatic hydroxylation to become the highly active 1α-25-dihydroxycholecalciferol (calcitriol). Alfacalcidol (and of course calcitriol) is therefore effective in the presence of renal failure since the defective renal hydroxylation stage has been bypassed. Its extraordinary potency and efficacy is indicated by the adult dose, often only 1–2 micrograms/d.

In addition there is a structural variant of vitamins D$_2$ and D$_3$, **dihydrotachysterol** (ATIO, Tachyrol), which is also biologically activated by hepatic 25-hydroxylation.

Advantages of alfacalcidol and dihydrotachysterol include a faster onset (below) and shorter duration of clinical effect (days) than vitamins D_2 and D_3 (weeks). But these factors are not relevant to the ordinary management of vitamin D deficiency.

Actions are complex. Vitamin D promotes the active transport (absorption) of calcium and therefore of phosphate from the gut, to control, with parathormone, the mineralisation of bone and to promote the renal tubular reabsorption of calcium and phosphate. The plasma calcium concentration rises. After a dose of D_2 or D_3 there is a lag of about 21 h before the intestinal effect begins and this is probably due to the time needed for its metabolic conversion to the more active forms. But after the biologically active calcitriol the lag is only 2 h.

A large single dose of vitamin D has biological effects for as long as 6 months (because of metabolism and storage, knowledge of the plasma $t^1/_2$ is of no practical importance). Thus the agent is cumulative and overdose by a mother anxious that her child shall have strong bones can cause serious toxicity.

Epileptic patients taking drugs that are enzyme inducers may develop osteomalacia (adults) or rickets (children). This may be due to enzyme induction increasing vitamin D metabolism and causing deficiency, or there may be inhibition of one of the hydroxylations that increase biological activity or an effect on calcium metabolism.

Indications for vitamin D are the prevention and cure of rickets of all kinds and osteomalacia, and the symptomatic treatment of some cases of hypoparathyroidism; also psoriasis.

In osteomalacia secondary to steatorrhoea or renal disease there is defective absorption of calcium from the gut and large amounts of vitamin D are often needed to enhance absorption.

Use of vitamin D as pharmacotherapy should in general be accompanied by monitoring of plasma calcium.

Dosage (1.0 microgram = 40 units). The therapeutic dose for primary, diet-deficiency rickets is 3000–4000 units per day, but much more may be needed daily in malabsorption syndromes, e.g.

40 000 units, or renal osteodystrophy, 200 000 units, and dosage must then be carefully controlled by measuring plasma calcium concentrations; a rise in total calcium above 2.75 mmol/l (11 mg/100 ml) is dangerous.

Prophylactic dose in diet-deficient people is about 1000 units/day for a few months, then adequate diet. Where there is doubt that an adequate diet will be maintained, calcium and ergocalciferol tabs (each containing ergocalciferol 10 micrograms) one daily, will suffice.

The maximum antirachitic effect of vitamin D is delayed for 1–2 months and the plasma calcium concentration reflects the dosage given days or weeks before. Frequent changes of dose are thus pointless and confuse the picture.

Preparations are many and the choice is not critical, though the elderly with nutritional osteomalacia due to malabsorption are often best managed by calciferol inj. i.m., 6–12 monthly (eliminating problems or patient compliance and gut malabsorption) with biochemical monitoring.

It is important to recognise that, because of the need for very big doses in certain vitamin D-resistant cases, there is an *unusually wide* scope of dosage in *single tablets* available. These range from Calcium and Ergocalciferol Tabs containing 10 micrograms (400 units) of ergocalciferol to tablets confusingly named Calciferol Tabs BP and containing enormous doses, i.e. 10 000 units (250 micrograms) and 50 000 units (1250 micrograms) of ergocalciferol. When these are prescribed the dose should be specified (and the terms 'strong' or 'high strength' should not be used). The large doses are for use only in exceptional circumstances, e.g. hypoparathyroidism or metabolic rickets; their inadvertent administration to children can lead to disaster.

Alfacalcidol is an alternative to calciferol that may be used for some forms of metabolic rickets; it acts more quickly, i.e. in days rather than in weeks (see above). *Calcipotriol* is an analogue used for psoriasis (p. 280).

Symptoms of overdose are due mainly to excessive rise in plasma calcium. General effects include: malaise, drowsiness, nausea, abdominal pain, thirst, constipation and loss of appetite. Other longterm effects include ectopic calcification almost anywhere in the body, renal damage and an increased calcium output in the urine; renal calculi may be formed. It is dangerous to exceed 10 000 units daily of vitamin D in an adult for more than about 12 weeks.

Much vitamin D toxicity is due to well-meaning, but needless, administration by parents. The US Food and Drug Administration warns that intake of fortified diet supplements should not exceed 400 units a day.

Patients with *sarcoidosis* are intolerant of vitamin D possibly even to the tiny amount present in a normal diet, and to that synthesised in their skin by sunlight. The intolerance may be due to overproduction of calcitriol (see above) by macrophages activated by interferon; the overproduction is reversed by corticosteroid.

Adrenal steroids antagonise vitamin D by an uncertain mechanism and are used in the treatment of hypercalcaemic sarcoidosis and of severe hypervitaminosis D.

Treatment of calcium and bone disorders

TETANY

In acute hypocalcaemia requiring systemic therapy *calcium gluconate* is given slowly i.v.; dihydrotachysterol is also used to increase calcium absorption; it acts quicker than vitamin D_2 or D_3. Dietary calcium is increased by giving calcium gluconate (an effervescent tablet is available) or lactate, and this plus vitamin D (in high dose) may be needed longterm for chronic cases, e.g. of hypoparathyroidism. *Aluminium hydroxide* binds phosphate in the gut causing hypophosphataemia, which stimulates renal formation of the most active vitamin D metabolite and so enhances calcium absorption.

Calcium gluconate inj. is administered i.v. as a 10% solution, 10–20 ml being given at the rate of about 2 ml per min and followed by a continuous i.v. infusion containing 40 ml (9 mmol) per day with monitoring of plasma calcium. It must not be given i.m. as it is painful and causes necrosis. *Calcium glubion-*

ate (Calcium Sandoz) can be given by deep i.m. injection in adults.

Adverse effects of intravenous calcium may be very dangerous. An early sign is a tingling feeling in the mouth and of warmth spreading over the body. Serious effects are those on the heart, which mimic and synergise with digitalis; fatal cardiac arrest may occur in digitalised animals and it would seem advisable to avoid i.v. calcium in any patient on a digitalis glycoside (except in severe symptomatic hypocalcaemia); indeed, reduction of ionised calcium by a chelating agent has been successful in treating digitalis dysrhythmia. The effect of calcium on the heart is antagonised by potassium and similarly the toxic effects of a high serum potassium in acute renal failure may be to some extent counteracted with calcium.

HYPERCALCAEMIA

Treatment of severe acute hypercalcaemia causing symptoms is needed whether or not the cause can be removed; generally a plasma concentration of 3.0 mmol/l (12 mg/100 ml) needs urgent treatment if there is also clinical evidence of toxicity (individual tolerance varies greatly).

Temporary measures

After taking account of the patient's cardiac and renal function, the following measures may be employed selectively:

● First, correct *dehydration* with physiological saline solution and even *force fluid* to enhance renal calcium elimination; consider adding a high-efficacy *loop diuretic* (frusemide) for further effect (not a thiazide which increases renal reabsorption of calcium). Rehydration may require 6–8 l given over 2 days with careful attention to fluid and electrolyte balance, including potassium.

● *Biphosphonates* (p. 674). Pamidronate is preferred; it is active in a wide variety of hypercalcaemic disorders. Fall in serum calcium begins in 1–2 d, reaches a nadir in 5–6 d and lasts 20–30 d. Etidronate is given i.v. in hypercalcaemia of malignant disease. It acts in 1–2 d and a dose lasts

3–4 weeks; it may also provide benefit for neoplastic metastatic disease in bone. Clodronate is an alternative (oral or i.v.).

● Hypercalcaemia due to cancer or hyperparathyroidism may be reduced by a single dose of *plicamycin* (p. 674); maximum effect is in 4 days.

● An *adrenocortical steroid*, e.g. prednisolone 20–40 mg/d orally, reduces intestinal absorption of calcium and may inhibit osteolytic cancer but it takes several days to work and has no effect in hyperparathyroidism. It is most effective in vitamin D intoxication and sarcoid.

● *Calcitonin.* When the hypercalcaemia is at least partly due to mobilisation from bone, calcitonin can be used to inhibit bone resorption, and it may enhance urinary excretion of calcium. The effect develops in a few hours, and responsiveness may be lost over a few days (but may sometimes be restored by an adrenal steroid).

● *Trisodium edetate* (therapeutically equivalent to disodium edetate) i.v. can be used; it chelates calcium and the inert complex is excreted by glomerular filtration; it is rapidly effective.

● *Dialysis* is quick and effective and is likely to be needed in severe cases or with renal failure.

● *Phosphate* i.v. is quickly effective but lowers calcium by precipitating calcium phosphate in bone and soft tissues; it should be used only when other methods have failed.

The above measures are temporary only, to give time to tackle the cause.

Longterm use

To bind dietary calcium in the gut sodium *cellulose phosphate* (Calcisorb) is an oral ion exchange substance with a particular affinity for calcium. Bound calcium is eliminated in the faeces. It is used particularly for patients who overabsorb dietary calcium and who develop hypercalciuria and renal stones.

Inorganic phosphate, e.g. sodium acid phosphate (Phosphate Sandoz) taken orally also binds calcium in the gut.

HYPERCALCIURIA

In renal stone formers, in addition to general measures (low calcium diet, high fluid intake), urinary calcium may be diminished by a thiazide diuretic (with or without citrate to bind calcium) and oral phosphate (see above). See also Nephrolithiasis (p. 497).

PARATHYROID HORMONE

Parathyroid hormone acts chiefly on bone and kidney, regulating calcium and phosphate passage; its effects on the gut are indirect due to alteration of renal synthesis of 1α-25-dihydroxycholecalciferol (see Vitamin D). It increases the rate of bone remodelling (mineral and collagen) and osteocyte activity with, at high doses, an overall balance in favour of resorption (osteoclast activity) with a rise in plasmal calcium concentration (and fall in phosphate); but, at low doses, the balance favours bone formation (osteoblast activity). Parathyroid hormone increases the gut absorption of calcium (probably via its effect on vitamin D metabolism).

Natural (animal) and synthetic forms (of the first and active 34 amino acids of the 84 amino acid peptide hormone) are available. Endocrinologists use them for diagnosis in parathyroid disorder. The possibility of use of low doses for osteoporosis has been raised.

CALCITONIN

Calcitonin is a peptide hormone produced by the C cells of the thyroid gland (in mammals). It acts on bone (inhibiting osteoclasis) to reduce the rate of bone turnover, and on the kidney to reduce reabsorption of calcium and phosphorus. It is obtained from natural sources (pork, salmon, eel), or synthesised. The $t^{1/2}$ varies according to source; $t^{1/2}$ human is 10 min. Antibodies develop particularly to pork calcitonin and neutralise its effect; synthetic salmon calcitonin (*salcatonin*) is therefore preferred for prolonged use; loss of effect may also be due to downregulation of receptors. Calcitonin is used (s.c., i.m. or intranasally) to control hypercalcaemia (rapid effect), Paget's disease (relief of pain, and to relieve compression of nerves, e.g. auditory cranial), metastatic bone cancer pain, and postmenopausal osteoporosis.

Adverse effects include allergy, nausea, flushing and tingling of the face and hands.

BIPHOSPHONATES (diphosphonates)

The biphosphonates (*alendronic acid, disodium etidronate, disodium pamidronate, sodium clodronate*) become adsorbed onto bone crystals (hydroxyapatite) conferring resistance to hydrolysis and prolongation of t$\frac{1}{2}$ in the skeleton. Also, when the complex is phagocytosed by an osteoclast that cell is inhibited and cannot resorb more bone. Their actions are more complex than this, however, and biphosphonates find use in treatment of Paget's disease, osteoporosis and hypercalcaemia due to cancer (pamidronate or clodronate). They may be given orally or i.v. and are eliminated unchanged by the kidney.

Adverse effects include pyrexia, diarrhoea, increased bone pain (as well as relief), fractures (high dose, prolonged use only) due to demineralisation of bone. Alendronic acid may cause oesophageal irritation.

PLICAMYCIN (mithramycin)

Plicamycin is a cytotoxic antibiotic (made by a Streptomyces), now used only in *Paget's disease* and *acute hypercalcaemia* due to malignant disease; it is relatively selective for osteoclasts and a single dose may give benefit for days. Its use should not exceed a few days because it depresses bone marrow.

OSTEOPOROSIS

One in 4 women in their 60s and one in 2 in their 70s in the UK experiences an osteoporotic fracture.

Osteoporosis is an abnormal decrease in amount of bone, but what there is, is of normal quality.

Postmenopausal osteoporosis is due to gonadal deficiency; it can be prevented.

Oestrogen arrests the process by reducing bone resorption.

Progestogen arrests the process by increasing bone formation, but therapeutic benefit is less than with oestrogen. A combination of the two may achieve some overall reversal of the osteoporotic process over the first 2 years of therapy, though the bones are unlikely to become fully normal. Unopposed oestrogen has been widely used and it is effective, but it carries a risk of endometrial cancer, which is diminished by added progestogen; therefore combinations of oestrogen and progestogen are used (see Postmenopausal hormone replacement therapy, p. 650). Such combinations are the mainstay of treatment for postmenopausal osteoporosis; they inhibit the rapid bone loss that occurs immediately after the menopause and should be continued for 5 years, perhaps even as long as 10 years. Prolonged oestrogen use reduces sensitivity of bone to natural resorbing agents and this results in compensatory stimulation of parathyroid hormone secretion. If the oestrogen is suddenly stopped there is a period (as long as 3 years) of enhanced bone loss due to the excess of parathyroid hormone.

Calcium dietary supplementation (Ca gluconate, carbonate, hydroxyapatite, citrate, maleate) reduces bone loss where intake may be inadequate, i.e. below 800 mg/d. Calcium is a weak inhibitor of bone resorption; it is not a substitute for hormones; they should be used together.

Calcitonin (see above) inhibits bone resorption.

The above treatments *arrest* progress of the disease, increasing bone mass a little or not at all.

Fluoride and biphosphonates may reverse osteoporosis.

Sodium fluoride increases bone mass by stimulating osteoblasts, but there is doubt about the quality of bone formed, e.g. there may be increased fragility. Its use remains controversial.

Biphosphonate, e.g. disodium etidronate (Didronel) (see above), used cyclically with a calcium supplement has been shown to decrease the incidence of vertebral fractures.

Parathyroid hormone (see above).

Secondary osteoporosis, e.g. due to intestinal malabsorption, corticosteroid therapy, hypoparathyroidism or alcoholism, may benefit from the above treatments.

Corticosteroids used longterm cause osteoporosis but the mechanism remains uncertain; treatment is as above.

OSTEOMALACIA

Osteomalacia is due to *primary* or *secondary* vitamin D deficiency. In secondary cases, e.g. malabsorption or renal disease, high doses of vitamin D are sometimes needed. Longterm therapy with some *antiepilepsy drugs* may cause osteomalacia (see Vitamin D).

PAGET'S DISEASE OF BONE

This disease is characterised by bone resorption and formation (bone turnover) increased as much as 50 times normal, the results of which are large, vascular, deformed, painful bones. *Biphosphonates* (e.g. disodium etidronate) are effective and have become the treatment of choice. They inhibit crystal formation, growth and dissolution, such as must occur in bone mineralisation and demineralisation (bone turnover), and are relatively nontoxic. The response is dose-related and remission after a course may last up to two years. Some therapeutic success has been found with *calcitonin* (which inhibits bone resorption) and with *cytotoxic agents* that inhibit osteoclasis, e.g. plicamycin, cactinomycin (dactinomycin).

Vitamin E: tocopherol

The functions of vitamin E may be to take up (scavenge) the free radicals generated by normal metabolic process and by substances in the environment, e.g. hydrocarbons, and so to prevent them attacking polyunsaturated fats in cell membranes with resultant cellular injury. A deficiency syndrome is now recognised, including peripheral neuropathy with spinocerebellar degeneration; and a haemolytic anaemia in premature infants.

Alpha tocopheryl acetate (Ephynal) pharmacotherapy may benefit the neuromuscular complications of congenital cholestasis and abetalipoproteinaemia. Studies in a wide variety of diseases, particularly cardiovascular, are proceeding.

Vitamin K: see page 519.

GUIDE TO FURTHER READING

Anderson D 1992 Osteoporosis in men. British Medical Journal 305: 489

Bates C J 1995 Vitamin A. Lancet 345: 31

Bilezikian J P 1992 Management of acute hypercalcaemia. New England Journal of Medicine 326: 1196

Compston J E 1994 The therapeutic use of biphosphonates. British Medical Journal 309: 711

Cooper C, Eastell R 1993 Bone gain and loss in premenopausal women. British Medical Journal 306: 1357

Dempster D W, Lindsay R 1993 Pathogenesis of osteoporosis. Lancet 341: 797

Editorial 1962 Arctic offal. British Medical Journal 1: 855

Fraser D R 1995 Vitamin D. Lancet 345: 104

Greenberg E R, Sporn M B 1996 Antioxidant vitamins, cancer and cardiovascular disease. New England Journal of Medicine 334: 1189

Lindsay R, Nieves J 1994 Milk and bones. British Medical Journal 308: 930

Manolagas S C et al 1995 Bone marrow, cytokines, and bone remodeling. New England Journal of Medicine 332: 305

Meydani M 1995 Vitamin E. Lancet 345: 170

Riggs B L, Melton L J 1993 The prevention and treatment of osteoporosis. New England Journal of Medicine 327: 620

Slemenda C W 1994 Cigarettes and the skeleton. New England Journal of Medicine 330: 430

Spector T D, Sambrook P N 1993 Steroid osteoporosis. British Medical Journal 307: 519

Index

Proprietary names (an incomplete list, inevitably) are in *italic type* followed by the non-proprietary name. Regarding the adoption of recommended International Non-proprietary Names, see Chapter 6.